ANSEL'S Pharmaceutical Dosage Forms and Drug Delivery Systems

ANSEL'S Pharmaceutical Dosage Forms and Drug Delivery Systems TWELFTH EDITION 2023

LOYD V. ALLEN, Jr, PhD, R.Ph

Professor Emeritus
Department of Medicinal Chemistry and Pharmaceutics
College of Pharmacy
University of Oklahoma
University of Oklahoma Health Sciences Center
Oklahoma City, Oklahoma

Editor-in-Chief
International Journal of Pharmaceutical Compounding

Editor-in-Chief
Remington—The Science and Practice of Pharmacy, 22nd *Edition*

And

TIMOTHY B. McPHERSON, PhD

Professor of Pharmaceutical Sciences
School of Pharmacy
Southern Illinois University Edwardsville
Edwardsville, Illinois

Philadelphia • Baltimore • New York • London
Buenos Aires • Hong Kong • Sydney • Tokyo

Not authorised for sale in United States, Canada, Australia, New Zealand, Puerto Rico, and U.S. Virgin Islands.

Acquisitions Editor: Matt Hauber
Development Editor: Tom Conville
Editorial Coordinator: Oliver Raj
Marketing Manager: Phyllis Hitner
Production Project Manager: Bridgett Dougherty
Design Coordinator: Stephen Druding
Manufacturing Coordinator: Margie Orzech
Prepress Vendor: SPi Global

Twelfth Edition

Library of Congress Cataloging-in-Publication Data
Names: Allen, Loyd V., Jr. author. | McPherson, Timothy B., author.
Title: Ansel's pharmaceutical dosage forms and drug delivery systems / Loyd V. Allen Jr. and Timothy B. McPherson.
Other titles: Pharmaceutical dosage forms and drug delivery systems
Description: Twelfth edition. | Philadelphia : Wolters Kluwer, 2023. | Includes bibliographical references and index. | Summary: "The purpose of this text is to introduce pharmacy students to the principles, practices, and technologies applied in the preparation of pharmaceutical dosage forms and drug delivery systems. An integrated presentation is used in this textbook to demonstrate the interrelationships between pharmaceutical and biopharmaceutical principles, product design, formulation, manufacture, compounding, and the clinical application of the various dosage forms in patient care. Regulations and standards governing the manufacturing and compounding of pharmaceuticals are also presented"—Provided by publisher.
Identifiers: LCCN 2021031414 (print) | LCCN 2021031415 (ebook) | ISBN 9781975171773 | ISBN 9781975171780 (epub)
Subjects: MESH: Dosage Forms | Drug Delivery Systems | Pharmaceutical Preparations—administration & dosage
Classification: LCC RS200 (print) | LCC RS200 (ebook) | NLM QV 786 | DDC 615/.1—dc23
LC record available at https://lccn.loc.gov/2021031414
LC ebook record available at https://lccn.loc.gov/2021031415

PREFACE

The purpose of this text is to introduce pharmacy students to the principles, practices, and technologies applied in the preparation of pharmaceutical dosage forms and drug delivery systems. An integrated presentation is used in this textbook to demonstrate the interrelationships between pharmaceutical and biopharmaceutical principles, product design, formulation, manufacture, compounding, and the clinical application of the various dosage forms in patient care. Regulations and standards governing the manufacturing and compounding of pharmaceuticals are also presented.

As has been the hallmark of this textbook since its first edition over 50 years ago, each chapter is written at a level consistent with the requirements of students being introduced to this area of study. Because this textbook often is used early in the professional curriculum, it contains important introductory topics, such as the historical development of drugs and pharmacy, the role of the pharmacist in contemporary practice, standards of the United States Pharmacopeia–National Formulary, systems and techniques of pharmaceutical measurement, pharmaceutical and biopharmaceutical principles applicable to drug product development, current good manufacturing practice and current good compounding practice standards, and the regulatory process by which manufactured pharmaceuticals are approved for marketing by the federal Food and Drug Administration.

The detailed presentation of each dosage form includes physical, physicochemical, and clinical discussions. The activities at the end of each chapter are designed to provide opportunities for creative thought and application of the content.

CONTINUING FEATURES IN THIS EDITION

The 12th edition presents an update and rewrite of sections of the previous edition and many updated and new colored figures and images. The eight divisions have been retained, containing 21 chapters, based upon traditional pharmaceutical pedagogy. This allows the systematic presentation of dosage forms according to their physical form and characteristics. The "Physical Pharmacy Capsules" introduced in the sixth edition continues to emphasize important underlying pharmaceutical and scientific principles.

Other features that we have retained from the 11th edition include the following:

1. Enhanced considerations of dosage form design and formulation.
2. Two case studies (one pharmaceutical and one clinical) in each of the dosage form chapters (see "Explanation of the SOAP Format for Case Studies" later in the preface).
3. An update of the current good compounding practices.
4. Expanded clinical considerations in the use of the dosage forms.
5. Two glossaries in the appendices, one listing the dosage forms and one listing pharmaceutical terms.
6. Chapter objectives that inform students what they will master in each chapter.
7. Chapter-at-a-Glance so the reader can easily see what is covered in the chapter.
8. An "Applying the Principles and Concepts" section at the end of each chapter that provides faculty and students with group and individual activities for the application of the material in each chapter.
9. In-depth information related to both nonsterile and sterile manufactured and compounded dosage forms. This is important because the contemporary practice of pharmacy requires the knowledge of both to effectively work with prescribers, patients, and other pharmacists.
10. Example manufactured and compounding formulas.
11. Ancillaries as described in the following section.
12. Appendix on active ingredient considerations in dosing.
13. The new chapter, "Clinical Pharmaceutics," has been modified and expanded as well as incorporation of this subject matter throughout other chapters in the book.

WHAT IS NEW IN THIS EDITION?

New features of this edition include the following:

- Updated content in each chapter.
- Over 90% of photos and figures are now in color.
- Expanded Patient Counseling information on the dosage forms.

ADDITIONAL RESOURCES

Ansel's Pharmaceutical Dosage Forms and Drug Delivery Systems, 12th edition, includes additional resources for both instructors and students that are available on the book's companion Web site at thePoint.lww.com/Allen12e.

Instructors

Approved adopting instructors will be given access to the following additional resources:

- Expanded PowerPoint slides
- Lecture support and handout material

Students

Students who have purchased *Ansel's Pharmaceutical Dosage Forms and Drug Delivery Systems*, 12th edition, have access to the following additional resources:

- An expanded quiz bank with NAPLEX-patterned questions

In addition, purchasers of the text can access the searchable full text online by going to the *Ansel's Pharmaceutical Dosage Forms and Drug Delivery Systems*, 12th edition, Web site at thePoint.lww.com/Allen12e. See the inside front cover of this text for more details, including the passcode you will need to gain access to the Web site.

EXPLANATION OF THE SOAP FORMAT FOR CASE STUDIES[1]

A common format for clinical case studies is referred to by the mnemonic SOAP, which stands for *S*ubjective information, *O*bjective information, *A*ssessment, and *P*lan.

---

[1]Adapted from O'Sullivan TA, Wittkowsky AK. Clinical drug monitoring. In: Stein S, ed. Boh's Pharmacy Practice Manual: A Guide to the Clinical Experience. 3rd Ed. Baltimore, MD: Lippincott Williams & Wilkins, 2010:483, with permission.

The first paragraph begins with "**S:**" and contains subjective information, which is obtained from the patient interview. Examples of subjective information include patient-provided information about disease symptoms, over-the-counter medications, drug allergy descriptions, and compliance.

The second paragraph begins with "**O:**" and contains objective information obtained by physically examining the patient, reviewing laboratory data, checking prescription records for doses and refill patterns, locating medication costs from a printed or online formulary, and so on. Some information can be either subjective or objective, depending on how it is obtained. The most important thing to remember when composing the subjective and objective portions of notes is that *only information pertaining directly to the assessment should be included.*

The third paragraph begins with "**A:**" and contains the pharmacist's assessment of the patient's medical and pharmacologic problem or problems. If the subjective and objective paragraphs are written well, the problem should be obvious to the reader. Other types of information included in the assessment paragraph are the therapeutic goals and a brief discussion of the therapeutic alternatives.

The fourth paragraph begins with either "**P:**" or "**R:**" and details either a plan (P) or a recommendation (R), whichever is more appropriate for the situation. The plan should include individualized instructions (drug by generic name, dose, route, frequency, and, when applicable, duration of therapy). The exact dose and frequency should be identified.

Also, the monitoring plan must be detailed, including specifically what should be measured (e.g., laboratory test, symptom), who should measure it (patient, caregiver, pharmacist), when and how frequently the measurement should be performed, and at what point changing therapy should be considered. A backup plan for use in the event of therapeutic failure should also be noted here. Finally, instructions for the proper use of prescribed medication or medications should be included to enhance the therapeutic outcome.

ACKNOWLEDGMENTS

We acknowledge with grateful appreciation the contributions and foresight of Howard C. Ansel, PhD, the originator of this textbook, whose guidance and hard work over the years have significantly contributed to the education of tens of thousands of pharmacists worldwide.

It is with distinct pleasure that Dr. Timothy B. McPherson, Professor of Pharmaceutical Sciences at the School of Pharmacy, Southern Illinois University Edwardsville, joins as coauthor on this 12th edition of the book.

We also acknowledge with appreciation those who have generously provided scientific, technical, and clinical information and updated the figures and photos for our use. Also, we gratefully acknowledge the many individuals who contributed to the development of this book through their critiques, reviews, suggestions, and contributions on the individual chapters as listed in previous editions. Finally, Dr. McPherson is acknowledged for his work on the online questions and lecture presentations.

We especially thank the staff at Wolters Kluwer who have contributed so expertly to the planning, preparation, and production of this 12th edition, particularly Matt Hauber, acquisitions editor; Oliver Raj, editorial coordinator; and Tom Conville, development editor.

Loyd V. Allen, Jr, PhD, R.Ph
Timothy B. McPherson, PhD

CONTENTS

LIST OF PHYSICAL PHARMACY CAPSULES

SECTION ONE

Introduction to Drugs, Drug Dosage Forms, and Drug Delivery Systems

1   Introduction to Drugs and Pharmacy
2   New Drug Development and Approval Process
3   Current Good Manufacturing Practices and Current Good Compounding Practices

Introduction to Drugs and Pharmacy

CHAPTER AT A GLANCE The Heritage of Pharmacy • Drug Standards • Drug Regulation and Control • The Federal Food, Drug, and Cosmetic Act of 1938 • The Pharmacist's Contemporary Role • Code of Ethics for Pharmacists of the American Pharmacists Association • Code of Ethics of the American Association of Pharmaceutical Scientists

OBJECTIVES

After reading this chapter, the student will be able to:

Describe the development and purpose of the *United States Pharmacopeia* (USP) and the *National Formulary* (NF)

Describe the composition of a typical drug monograph

Compare and contrast significant drug regulation and control federal laws and their impact on pharmacy

Explain the concept of pharmaceutical care

Summarize the Code of Ethics for Pharmacists of the American Pharmacists Association

Summarize the Code of Ethics of the American Association of Pharmaceutical Scientists (AAPS)

▋ INTRODUCTION

A drug is defined as an agent intended for use in the diagnosis, mitigation, treatment, cure, or prevention of disease in humans or in other animals (Food, Drug, and Cosmetic Act, 1938). One of the most astounding qualities of drugs is the diversity of their actions and effects on the body. This quality enables their selective use in the treatment of a range of common and rare conditions involving virtually every body organ, tissue, and cell.

Some drugs selectively stimulate the cardiac muscle, the central nervous system, or the gastrointestinal tract, whereas other drugs have the opposite effect. Mydriatic drugs dilate the pupil of the eye, and miotics constrict or diminish pupillary size. Drugs can render blood more coagulable or less coagulable; they can increase the hemoglobin content of the erythrocytes, reduce serum cholesterol, or expand blood volume.

Drugs termed emetics induce vomiting, whereas antiemetic drugs prevent vomiting. Diuretic drugs increase the flow of urine; expectorant drugs increase respiratory tract fluid; and cathartics or laxatives evacuate the bowel. Other drugs decrease the flow of urine, diminish body secretions, or induce constipation.

Drugs may be used to reduce pain, fever, thyroid activity, rhinitis, insomnia, gastric acidity, motion sickness, blood pressure, and mental depression. Other drugs can elevate mood, blood pressure, or activity of the endocrine glands. Drugs can combat infectious disease, destroy intestinal worms, or act as antidotes against the poisoning effects of other drugs. Drugs can assist in smoking cessation or alcohol withdrawal or can modify obsessive–compulsive disorders.

Drugs are used to treat common infections, AIDS, benign prostatic hyperplasia, cancer, cardiovascular disease, asthma, glaucoma, Alzheimer disease, and male impotence. They can protect against the rejection of transplanted tissues and organs and reduce the incidence of measles and mumps. Antineoplastic drugs provide one means of attacking the cancerous process; radioactive pharmaceuticals provide another. Drugs may be used to diagnose diabetes, liver malfunction, tuberculosis, or pregnancy. They can replenish a body deficient in antibodies, vitamins, hormones, electrolytes, protein, enzymes, or blood. Drugs can prevent pregnancy, assist fertility, and sustain life itself.

Certainly, the vast array of effective medicinal agents available today is one of our greatest scientific accomplishments. It is difficult to conceive our civilization devoid of these remarkable and beneficial agents. Through their use, many of the diseases that have plagued humans throughout history, such as smallpox and poliomyelitis, are now virtually extinct. Illnesses such as diabetes, hypertension, and mental depression are effectively controlled with modern drugs. Today's surgical procedures would be virtually impossible without the benefit of anesthetics, analgesics, antibiotics, blood transfusions, and intravenous fluids.

New drugs may be derived from plant or animal sources, as by-products of microbial growth, or through chemical synthesis, molecular modification, or biotechnology. Computer libraries and data banks of chemical compounds and sophisticated methods of screening for potential biologic activity assist drug discovery.

The process of drug discovery and development is complex. It entails the collective contributions of many scientific specialists, including organic, physical, and analytical chemists; biochemists; molecular biologists; bacteriologists; physiologists; pharmacologists; toxicologists; hematologists; immunologists; endocrinologists; pathologists; biostatisticians; pharmaceutical scientists; clinical pharmacists; physicians; and many others.

After a potential new drug substance is discovered and undergoes definitive chemical and physical characterization, a great deal of biologic information must be gathered. The basic pharmacology, or the nature and mechanism of action of the drug on the biologic system, must be determined including toxicologic features. The drug's site and rate of absorption, its pattern of distribution and concentration within the body, its duration of action, and the method and rate of its elimination or excretion must be studied. Information on the drug's metabolic degradation and the activity of any of its metabolites must be obtained. A comprehensive study of the short-term and long-term effects of the drug on various body cells, tissues, and organs must be made. Highly specific information, such as the effect of the drug on the fetus of a pregnant animal or its ability to pass to a nursing baby through the breast milk of its mother, may be obtained. Many a promising new drug has been abandoned because of its potential to cause excessive or hazardous adverse effects.

The most effective routes of administration (e.g., oral, rectal, parenteral, topical, transdermal) must be determined, and guidelines for the dosages recommended for persons of varying ages (e.g., neonates, children, adults, the elderly), weights, and states of illness have to be established. It has been said that the only difference between a drug and a poison is the dose. To facilitate administration of the drug by the selected routes, appropriate dosage forms, such as tablets, capsules, injections, suppositories, ointments, aerosols, and others, are formulated and prepared. Each dosage unit is designed to contain a specified quantity of medication for ease and accuracy of dosage administration. These dosage forms are highly sophisticated delivery systems. Their design, development, production, and use are the product of application of the pharmaceutical sciences—the blending of the basic, applied, and clinical sciences with pharmaceutical technology.

Each particular pharmaceutical product is a formulation unique unto itself. In addition to the active therapeutic ingredients, a pharmaceutical formulation contains a number of nontherapeutic or pharmaceutical ingredients. It is through their use that a formulation achieves its unique composition and characteristic physical appearance. Pharmaceutical ingredients include such materials as fillers, thickeners, solvents, suspending agents, tablet coatings and disintegrants, penetration enhancers, stabilizing agents, antimicrobial preservatives, flavors, colorants, and sweeteners.

To ensure the stability of a drug in a formulation and the continued effectiveness of the drug product throughout its usual shelf life, the principles of chemistry, physical pharmacy, pharmaceutics, microbiology, and pharmaceutical technology must be applied. The formulation must be such that all components are physically and chemically compatible, including the active therapeutic agents, the pharmaceutical ingredients, and the packaging materials. The formulation must be preserved against decomposition due to chemical degradation and protected from microbial contamination and the destructive influences of excessive heat, light, and moisture. The therapeutic ingredients must be released from the dosage form in the proper quantity and in such a manner that the onset and duration of the drug's action are that which are desired. The pharmaceutical product must lend itself to efficient administration and must possess attractive features of flavor, odor, color, and texture that enhance acceptance by the patient. Finally, the product must be effectively packaged and clearly and completely labeled according to legal regulations.

Once prepared, the pharmaceutical product must be properly administered if the patient is to receive maximum benefit. The medication must be taken in sufficient quantity, at specified intervals, and for an indicated duration to achieve the desired therapeutic outcomes. The effectiveness of the medication in achieving the prescriber's objectives should be reevaluated at regular intervals and necessary adjustments made in the dosage, regimen, schedule, or form or, indeed, in the choice of the drug administered. Patients' expressions of disappointment in the rate of progress or complaints of side effects to the prescribed drug should be evaluated and decisions made as to the continuance, adjustment, or major change in drug therapy. Before initially taking a medication, a patient should be advised of any expected side effects and of foods, beverages, and/or other drugs that may interfere with the effectiveness of the medication.

Through professional interaction and communication with other health professionals, the pharmacist can contribute greatly to patient care. An intimate knowledge of drug actions, pharmacotherapeutics, formulation and dosage form design, available pharmaceutical products, and drug information sources makes the pharmacist a vital member of the health care team. The pharmacist is entrusted with the legal responsibility for the procurement, storage, control, and distribution of effective pharmaceutical products and for the compounding and filling of prescription orders. Drawing on extensive training and knowledge, the pharmacist serves the patient as an advisor on drugs and encourages their safe and proper use through patient counseling. The pharmacist delivers pharmaceutical services in a variety of community and institutional health care environments and effectively uses medication records, patient monitoring, and assessment techniques in safeguarding the public health.

To appreciate the progress that has been made in drug discovery and development and to provide background for the study of modern drugs and pharmaceutical dosage forms, it is important to examine pharmacy's heritage.

THE HERITAGE OF PHARMACY

Drugs, in the form of vegetation and minerals, have existed as long as humans. Human disease and the instinct to survive have led to their discovery through the ages. The use of drugs, crude though they may have been, undoubtedly began long before recorded history, for, the instinct of primitive man to relieve the pain of a wound by bathing it in cool water or by soothing it with a fresh leaf or protecting it with mud is within the realm of belief. From experience, early humans would learn that certain therapy was more effective than others, and from these beginnings came the practice of drug therapy.

Among many early races, disease was believed to be caused by the entrance of demons or evil spirits into the body. The treatment naturally involved ridding the body of the supernatural intruders. From the earliest records, the primary methods of removing spirits were through the use of spiritual incantations, the application of noisome materials, and the administration of specific herbs or plant materials.

The First Apothecary

Before the days of the priestcraft, the wise man or woman of the tribe, whose knowledge of the healing qualities of plants had been gathered through experience or handed down by word of mouth, was called upon to attend to the sick or wounded and prepare the remedy. It was in the preparation of the medicinal materials that the art of the apothecary originated.

The art of the apothecary has always been associated with the mysterious, and its practitioners were believed to have connection with the world of spirits and thus performed as intermediaries between the seen and the unseen. The belief that a drug had magical associations

meant that its action, for good or for evil, did not depend upon its natural qualities alone. The compassion of a God, the observance of ceremonies, the absence of evil spirits, and the healing intent of the dispenser were individually and collectively needed to make the drug therapeutically effective. Because of this, the tribal apothecary was one to be feared, respected, trusted, sometimes mistrusted, worshipped, and revered, for it was through his or her potions that spiritual contact was made, and upon that contact the cures or failures depended.

Throughout history, the knowledge of drugs and their application to disease has always meant power. In the Homeric epics, the term *pharmakon* (Gr.), from which our word pharmacy was derived, connotes a charm or a drug that can be used for good or for evil. Many of the tribal apothecary's failures were doubtless due to impotent or inappropriate medicines, underdosage, overdosage, and even poisoning. Successes may be attributed to experience, mere coincidence of appropriate drug selection, natural healing, inconsequential effect of the drug, or placebo effects, that is, successful treatment because of psychological rather than therapeutic effects. Even today, placebo therapy with inert or inconsequential chemicals is used successfully to treat individual patients and is a routine practice in the clinical evaluation of new drugs, in which subjects' responses to the effects of the actual drug and the placebo are compared and evaluated.

As time passed, the art of the apothecary combined with priestly functions, and among the early civilizations, the priest–physician became the healer of the body as well as of the soul. Pharmacy and medicine are indistinguishable in their early history because their practice was the combined function of the tribal religious leaders.

The apothecary is listed in the Bible as one of the earliest trades or professions. It is evident that people experienced pain, disease, and suffering and that they used medicines of various types for healing, many obtained from the apothecary:

> "And thou shalt make it an oil of holy ointment, an ointment compound after the art of the apothecary: it shall be an holy anointing oil." (Exodus 30:25)

> "Dead flies cause the ointment of the apothecary to send forth a stinking savour; so doth a little folly him that is in reputation for wisdom and honour." (Ecclesiastes 10:1)

> "And by the river upon the bank thereof, on this side and on that side, shall grow all trees for meat, whose leaf shall not fade, neither shall the fruit thereof be consumed; it shall bring forth new fruit according to his months, because their waters they issued out of the sanctuary; and the fruit thereof shall be for meat, and the leaf thereof for medicine." (Ezekiel 47:12)

In many cases, the medicines used were either topical ointments or products such as wines and plant extracts that were taken internally. The apothecary was noted for the mixing of perfumes, ointments, and some medicines.

Early Drugs

Because of the patience and intellect of the archaeologist, the types and specific drugs used in the early history of drug therapy are not as indefinable as one might suspect. Numerous ancient tablets, scrolls, and other relics as early as 3000 BC have been uncovered and deciphered by archaeologic scholars to the gratitude of historians of both medicine and pharmacy (Fig. 1.1).

Perhaps the most famous of these surviving artifacts is the Ebers papyrus, a continuous scroll some 60 feet long and a foot wide dating to the 16th century BC. This document, which is now preserved at the University of Leipzig, is named for the noted German Egyptologist Georg Ebers, who discovered it in the tomb of a mummy and partly translated it during the last half of the 19th century. Since that time, many scholars have participated in the translation of the document's challenging hieroglyphics, and although they are not unanimous in their interpretations, there is little doubt that by 1550 BC, the Egyptians were using some drugs and dosage forms that are still used today.

The text of the Ebers papyrus is dominated by drug formulas, with more than 800 formulas or prescriptions being described and more than 700 drugs mentioned. The drugs are chiefly botanical, although mineral and animal drugs are also noted. Such botanical substances as acacia, castor bean (from which we express castor oil), and fennel are mentioned along with apparent references to such minerals as iron oxide, sodium carbonate, sodium chloride, and sulfur. Animal excrements were also used in drug therapy.

The vehicles of the day were beer, wine, milk, and honey. Many of the pharmaceutical formulas employed two dozen or more medicinal agents, a type of preparation later called polypharmacy. The Egyptians commonly used mortars and pestles, hand mills, sieves, and balances in their compounding of suppositories, gargles, pills, inhalations, troches, lotions, ointments, plasters, and enemas.

Introduction of the Scientific Viewpoint

Throughout history, many individuals have contributed to the advancement of the health sciences. Notable among those whose genius and creativeness had a revolutionary influence on the development of pharmacy and medicine were Hippocrates (ca. 460 to 377 BC), Dioscorides (first century AD), Galen (ca. 130 to 200 AD), and Paracelsus (1493 to 1541 AD).

Hippocrates, a Greek physician, is credited with the introduction of scientific pharmacy and medicine. He rationalized medicine, systematized medical knowledge, and put the practice of medicine on a high ethical plane. His thinking on the ethics and science of medicine dominated the medical writings of his and successive generations, and his concepts and precepts are embodied in the renowned Hippocratic oath of ethical behavior for the healing professions. His works included the descriptions of hundreds of drugs, and it was during this period that the term *pharmakon* came to mean a purifying remedy for good only, transcending the previous connotation of a charm or drug for good or for evil purposes. Because of his pioneering work in medical science and his inspirational teachings and advanced philosophies that have become a part of modern medicine, Hippocrates is honored by being called the Father of Medicine.

Dioscorides, a Greek physician and botanist, was the first to deal with botany as an applied science of pharmacy. His work, *De Materia Medica*, is considered a milestone in the development of pharmaceutical botany and in the study of naturally occurring medicinal materials. This area of study is today known as natural products chemistry and/or pharmacognosy, a term formed from two Greek words, *pharmakon*, drug, and *gnosis*, knowledge. Some of the drugs Dioscorides described, including opium, ergot, and hyoscyamus, continue to have use in medicine. His descriptions of the art of identifying and collecting natural drug products, the methods of their proper storage, and the means of detecting adulterants or contaminants were the standards of the period, established the need for additional work, and set guidelines for future investigators.

Claudius Galen, a Greek pharmacist–physician who attained Roman citizenship, aimed to create a perfect system of physiology, pathology, and treatment. Galen

FIGURE 1.1. Sumerian clay tablet from the third millennium BC on which are believed to be the world's oldest written prescriptions. Among them are a preparation of the seed of carpenter plant, gum resin of markhazi, and thyme, all pulverized and dissolved in beer, and a combination of powdered roots of "Moon plant" and white pear tree, also dissolved in beer. (Courtesy of the Penn Museum, object no. B14221.)

formulated doctrines that were followed for 1,500 years. He was one of the most prolific authors of his or any other era, having been credited with 500 treatises on medicine and some 250 others on philosophy, law, and grammar. His medical writings include descriptions of numerous drugs of natural origin with a profusion of drug formulas and methods of compounding. He originated so many preparations of vegetable drugs by mixing or melting the individual ingredients that the field of pharmaceutical preparations was once commonly referred to as "Galenic pharmacy." Perhaps the most famous of his formulas is one for a cold cream, called Galen's Cerate, which has similarities to some in use today, including theatrical cold cream and others that are slight modifications of his formula.

Pharmacy remained a function of medicine until the increasing variety of drugs and the growing complexity of compounding demanded specialists who could devote full attention to the art. Pharmacy was officially separated from medicine for the first time in 1240 AD, when a decree of Emperor Frederick II of Germany regulated the practice of pharmacy within the part of his kingdom called the Two Sicilies. His edict separating the two professions acknowledged that pharmacy required special knowledge, skill, initiative, and responsibility if adequate care to the medical needs of the people was to be guaranteed. Pharmacists were obligated by oath to prepare reliable drugs of uniform quality according to their art. Any exploitation of the patient through business relations between the pharmacist and the physician was strictly forbidden. Between that time and the evolution of chemistry as an exact science, pharmacy and chemistry became united as pharmacy and medicine had been.

Perhaps no person in history exercised such a revolutionary influence on pharmacy and medicine as did Aureolus Theophrastus Bombastus von Hohenheim (1493 to 1541), a Swiss physician and chemist who called himself Paracelsus. He influenced the transformation of pharmacy from a profession based primarily on botanical science to one based on chemical science. Some of his chemical observations were astounding for his time and for their anticipation of later discoveries. He believed it was possible to prepare a specific medicinal agent to combat each specific disease and introduced a host of chemical substances to internal therapy.

Early Research

As the knowledge of the basic sciences increased, so did their application to pharmacy. The opportunity was presented for the investigation of medicinal materials on a firm scientific basis, and the challenge was accepted by numerous pharmacists who conducted their research in the back rooms and basements of their pharmacies. Noteworthy among them was the Swede Karl Wilhelm Scheele (1742 to 1786), perhaps the most famous of all pharmacists because of his scientific genius and dramatic discoveries. Among his discoveries were the chemicals lactic acid, citric acid, oxalic acid, tartaric acid, and arsenic acid. He

identified glycerin, invented new methods of preparing calomel and benzoic acid, and discovered oxygen a year before Priestley.

The isolation of morphine from opium by the German pharmacist Friedrich Sertürner (1783 to 1841) in 1805 prompted a series of isolations of other active materials from medicinal plants by a score of French pharmacists. Joseph Caventou (1795 to 1877) and Joseph Pelletier (1788 to 1842) combined their talents and isolated quinine and cinchonine from cinchona and strychnine and brucine from nux vomica. Pelletier together with Pierre Robiquet (1780 to 1840) isolated caffeine, and Robiquet independently separated codeine from opium. Methodically, one chemical after another was isolated from plant drugs and identified as an agent responsible for the plants' medicinal activity. Today, we are still engaged in this fascinating activity as we probe nature for more useful and more specific therapeutic agents. Contemporary examples of drugs isolated from a natural source include paclitaxel (Taxol), an agent with antitumor activity derived from the Pacific yew tree (*Taxus baccata*) and employed in the treatment of metastatic carcinoma of the ovary; vincaleukoblastine, another antineoplastic drug, from *Vinca rosea*; and digoxin, a cardiac glycoside, from *Digitalis lanata*.

Throughout Europe during the late 18th century and the beginning of the 19th century, pharmacists like Pelletier and Sertürner were held in great esteem because of their intellect and technical abilities. They applied the art and the science of pharmacy to the preparation of drug products with the highest standards of purity, uniformity, and efficacy possible at that time. The extraction and isolation of active constituents from crude (unprocessed) botanical drugs led to the development of dosage forms of uniform strength containing singly effective therapeutic agents of natural origin. Many pharmacists of the period began to manufacture quality pharmaceutical products on a small but steadily increasing scale to meet the growing needs of their communities. Some of today's largest pharmaceutical research and manufacturing companies developed from these progressive prescription laboratories of two centuries ago.

Although many of the drugs indigenous to America and first used by the American Indians were adopted by the settlers, most drugs needed in this country before the 19th century were imported from Europe, either as the raw materials or as finished products. With the Revolutionary War, however, it became more difficult to import drugs, and the American pharmacist was stimulated to acquire the scientific and technologic expertise of his European contemporary. From this period until the Civil War, pharmaceutical manufacture was in its infancy in this country. A few of the pharmaceutical firms established during the early 1800s are still in operation. In 1821, the Philadelphia College of Pharmacy was established as the nation's first school of pharmacy. In 1820, the *United States Pharmacopeia* (USP) was created to aid in establishing standards for drugs in the United States.

DRUG STANDARDS

As the scientific basis for drugs and drug products developed, so did the need for uniform standards to ensure quality. This need led to the development and publication of monographs and reference books containing such standards to be used by those involved in the production of drugs and pharmaceutical products. Organized sets of monographs or books of these standards are called pharmacopeias or formularies.

The *United States Pharmacopeia* and the *National Formulary*

The term pharmacopeia comes from the Greek *pharmakon*, meaning drug, and *poiein*, meaning make, and the combination indicates any recipe or formula or other standards required to make or prepare a drug. The term was first used in 1580 in connection with a local book of drug standards in Bergamo, Italy. From that time on, countless city, state, and national pharmacopeias were published by various European pharmaceutical societies. As time passed, the value of a uniform set of national drug standards became apparent. In Great Britain, for example, three city pharmacopeias—the London, the Edinburgh, and the Dublin—were official until 1864, when they were replaced by the *British Pharmacopoeia* (BP).

In the United States, drug standards were first provided on a national basis in 1820, when the first USP was published. However, the need for drug standards was recognized in this country long before the first USP was published. For convenience and because of their familiarity with them, colonial physicians and apothecaries used the pharmacopeias and other references of their various homelands. The first American pharmacopeia was the so-called *Lititz Pharmacopeia*, published in 1778 at Lititz, Pennsylvania, for use by the Military Hospital of the United States Army. It was a 32-page booklet containing information on 84 internal and 16 external drugs and preparations.

During the last decade of the 18th century, several attempts were made by various local medical societies to collate drug information, set appropriate standards, and prepare an extensive American pharmacopeia of the drugs in use at that time. In 1808, the Massachusetts Medical Society published a 272-page pharmacopeia containing information or monographs on 536 drugs and pharmaceutical preparations. Included were monographs on many drugs indigenous to America, which were not described in the European pharmacopeias of the day.

On January 6, 1817, Lyman Spalding, a physician from New York City, submitted a plan to the Medical Society of the County of New York for the creation of a national pharmacopeia. Spalding's efforts were later to result in his being recognized as the Father of the *United States Pharmacopeia*. He proposed dividing the United States as then known into four geographic districts—northern, middle, southern, and western. The plan provided for a convention

FIGURE 1.2. The first United States Pharmacopeial Convention, held on January 1, 1820, in Washington, DC. (Reprinted with permission from the United States Pharmacopeial Convention.)

in each of these districts, to be composed of delegates from all medical societies and medical schools within them. Where there was as yet no incorporated medical society or medical school, voluntary associations of physicians and surgeons were invited to assist in the undertaking. Each district's convention was to draft a pharmacopeia and appoint delegates to a general convention to be held later in Washington, DC. At the general convention, the four district pharmacopeias were to be compiled into a single national pharmacopeia.

Draft pharmacopeias were submitted to the convention by only the northern and middle districts. These were reviewed, consolidated, and adopted by the first United States Pharmacopeial Convention assembled in Washington, DC, on January 1, 1820 (Fig. 1.2). The first USP was published on December 15, 1820, in English and Latin, then the international language of medicine, to render the book more intelligible to physicians and pharmacists of any nationality. Within its 272 pages were listed 217 drugs considered worthy of recognition; many of them were taken from the *Massachusetts Pharmacopeia*, which is considered by some to be the precursor to the USP. The objective of the first USP was stated in its preface and remains important. It reads in part:

> It is the object of a Pharmacopeia to select from among substances, which possess medicinal power, those, the utility of which is most fully established and best understood; and to form from them preparations and compositions, in which their powers may be exerted to the greatest advantage. It should likewise distinguish those articles by convenient and definite names, such as may prevent trouble or uncertainty in the intercourse of physicians and apothecaries (1).

Before adjourning, the convention adopted a constitution and bylaws, with provisions for subsequent meetings of the convention leading to a revised USP every 10 years. As many new drugs entered use, the need for more frequent issuance of standards became increasingly apparent. In 1900, the Pharmacopeial Convention granted authority to issue supplements to the USP whenever necessary to maintain satisfactory standards. At the 1940 meeting of the convention, it was decided to revise the USP every 5 years while maintaining the use of periodic supplements.

The first United States Pharmacopeial Convention was composed exclusively of physicians. In 1830 and again in 1840, prominent pharmacists were invited to assist in the revision, and in recognition of their contributions, pharmacists were awarded full membership in the convention of 1850 and have participated regularly ever since. By 1870, the USP was so nearly in the hands of pharmacists that vigorous efforts were required to revive interest in it among physicians. The present constitution and bylaws of the United States Pharmacopeial Convention provide for accredited delegates representing educational institutions, professional and scientific organizations, divisions of governmental bodies, non–U.S. international organizations and pharmacopeial bodies, persons who possess special scientific competence or knowledge of emerging technologies, and public members (2). Of the eight elected members of the board of trustees, at least two must be representatives of the medical sciences, two others must be representatives of the pharmaceutical sciences, one must be a public member, and three shall serve without restriction concerning their affiliation.

After the appearance of the first USP, the art and science of both pharmacy and medicine changed remarkably. Before 1820, drugs to treat disease had been the same for centuries. The USP of 1820 reflected the fact that the apothecary of that day was competent at collecting and identifying botanical drugs and preparing from them the mixtures and preparations required by the physician. The individual pharmacist seemed fulfilled as he applied his total art to the creation of elegant pharmaceutical preparations from crude botanical materials. It was a time that would never be seen again because of the impending upsurge in technologic capabilities and the steady development of the basic sciences, particularly synthetic organic chemistry.

The second half of the 19th century brought great and far-reaching changes. The industrial revolution was in full swing in the United States. The steam engine, which used water power to turn mills that powdered crude botanical drugs, was replaced by the gas, diesel, or electric motor. New machinery was substituted for the old whenever possible, and often, machinery from other industries was adapted to the special needs of pharmaceutical manufacturing. Mixers from the baking industry, centrifugal machines from the laundry industry, and sugarcoating pans from the candy industry were a few examples of improvisations. Production increased rapidly, but the new industry had to wait for the scientific revolution before it could claim newer and better drugs for mankind. A symbiosis between science and the advancing technology was needed.

By 1880, the industrial manufacture of chemicals and pharmaceutical products had become well established in this country, and the pharmacist was relying heavily on commercial sources for drug supply. Synthetic organic chemistry began to have its influence on drug therapy. The isolation of some active constituents of plant drugs led to the knowledge of their chemical structure. From this arose methods of synthetically duplicating the same structures, as well as manipulating molecular structure to produce organic chemicals yet undiscovered in nature. In 1872, the synthesis of salicylic acid from phenol inaugurated the synthesis of a group of analgesic compounds including acetylsalicylic acid (aspirin), which was introduced into medicine in 1899. Among other chemicals synthesized for the first time were sleep-producing derivatives of barbituric acid called barbiturates. This new source of drugs—synthetic organic chemistry—welcomed the turn into the 20th century.

Until this time, drugs created through the genius of the synthetic organic chemist relieved a host of maladies, but none had been found to be curative—none, that is, until 1910, when arsphenamine, a specific agent against syphilis, was introduced to medical science. This was the start of an era of chemotherapy, an era in which the diseases of humans became curable through the use of specific chemical agents. The concepts, discoveries, and inspirational work that led mankind to this glorious period are credited to Paul Ehrlich, the German bacteriologist who together with a Japanese colleague, Sahachiro Hata, discovered arsphenamine. Today, many of our drugs originate in the flask of the synthetic organic chemist.

The advancement of science, both basic and applied, led to drugs of a more complex nature and to more of them. The standards advanced by the USP were more than ever needed to protect the public by ensuring the purity and uniformity of drugs.

When the American Pharmaceutical Association (APhA) was organized in 1852, the only authoritative and recognized book of drug standards available was the third revision of the USP. To serve as a therapeutic guide to the medical profession, its scope, then as now, was restricted to drugs of established therapeutic merit. Because of strict selectivity, many drugs and formulas that were accepted and used by the medical profession were not granted admission to early revisions of the USP. As a type of protest, and in keeping with the original objectives of the APhA to standardize drugs and formulas, certain pharmacists, with the sanction of their national organization, prepared a formulary containing many of the popular drugs and formulas denied admission to the USP. The first edition was published in 1888 under the title *National Formulary of Unofficial Preparations* (3). The designation "unofficial preparations" reflected the protest mood of the authors, because the USP had earlier adopted the term "official" as applying to the drugs for which it provided standards. The title was changed to *National Formulary* (NF) on June 30,

1906, when President Theodore Roosevelt signed into law the first federal Pure Food and Drug Act, designating both the USP and NF as establishing legal standards for medicinal and pharmaceutical substances. Thus, the two publications became official compendia. Among other things, the law required that whenever the designation USP or NF was used or implied on drug labeling, the products must conform to the physical and chemical standards set forth in the compendium monograph.

The early editions of the NF served mainly as a convenience to practicing pharmacists by providing uniform names of drugs and preparations and working directions for the small-scale manufacture of popular pharmaceutical preparations prescribed by physicians. Before 1940, the NF, like the USP, was revised every 10 years. After that date, new editions appeared every 5 years, with supplements issued periodically as necessary. In 1975, the United States Pharmacopeial Convention, Inc., purchased the NF, unifying the official compendia and providing the mechanism for a single national compendium.

Today, the United States Pharmacopeia–National Formulary (USP/NF) is continuously revised. Revisions are available annually in hard copy and as online editions, including twice-yearly supplements and update notices on the USP Web site. Monographs for drug substances, dietary supplements, dosage forms, and compounded preparations are contained in the USP sections of the combined compendium, whereas monographs for pharmaceutical excipients are contained in the NF section.

The standards advanced by the USP and the NF are put to active use by all members of the health care industry who share the responsibility and enjoy the public's trust for ensuring the availability of quality drugs and pharmaceutical products and preparations. The term "products" is now generally used to refer to manufactured drugs and "preparations" to compounded drugs. The USP/NF is used by pharmacists, physicians, dentists, veterinarians, nurses, producers, and suppliers of bulk chemicals for use in drug production; large and small manufacturers of pharmaceutical products; drug procurement officers of various private and public health agencies and institutions; drug regulatory and enforcement agencies; and others.

The USP/NF consists of drug substance monographs, drug product monographs, compounding monographs, excipient monographs, dietary substance monographs, general chapters, and supportive information. The General Chapters are divided into those that are enforceable (numbered <1,000 of which there are ~200) and those that are informational (numbered >1,000 of which there are ~180). As the USP has no enforcement powers, it is dependent upon the FDA and the State Boards of Pharmacy for acceptance and enforcement of its standards. It should be noted that these are "standards" and not regulations or laws. Not all State Boards of Pharmacy have adopted the chapters specifically related to compounding and to the handling of hazardous drugs but have developed their own individual state standards for enforcement.

USP General Chapters

A few of the General Chapters of special interest to pharmacist practitioners include the following.

USP Chapter <795> Pharmaceutical Compounding—Nonsterile Preparations

Pharmaceutical compounding is an integral part of pharmacy practice and is essential to providing quality health care. This chapter provides pharmacists with guidance on applying good compounding practices for the preparation of nonsterile compounded formulations for dispensing and/or administration to humans or animals. There are 14 sections in this chapter related to categorization of compounding, compounder responsibilities, compounding processes, facilities, equipment, components, stability and beyond-use dating, packaging, documentation, quality control, patient counseling, personnel training, and compounding for animal patients.

USP Chapter <797> Pharmaceutical Compounding–Sterile Preparations

The objective of this chapter is to provide guidance (both environmental and practice) to prevent harm, including death, to patients that could result from nonsterility, excessive bacterial endotoxins, variations in intended strength, unintended chemical and physical contaminants, and ingredients of inappropriate quality. This chapter discusses responsibilities and training/evaluation of all personnel as well as facility and equipment requirements, quality control, risk levels, verification, standard operating procedures, finished preparation release checks and tests, storage and beyond-use dating, and many other topics.

USP Chapter <800> Hazardous Drugs—Handling in Health Care Settings

The purpose of USP Chapter <800> is to promote patient safety, worker safety, and environmental protection and can apply to all health care personnel who handle hazardous drug preparations and all entities that store, prepare, transport, or administer hazardous drugs (e.g., pharmacies, hospitals and other health care institutions, patient treatment clinics, physicians' practice facilities, or veterinarians' office). The chapter is divided into 18 sections covering general topics such as (*a*) Informational and Definitions, (*b*) Responsibilities, (*c*) Protection, (*d*) Communications and Training, (*e*) Processing Concerns, (*f*) Cleaning and Spill Control, and (*g*) Documentation and Surveillance. Hazardous drugs are based upon the NIOSH List of Antineoplastic and Other Hazardous Drugs in Healthcare Settings. This chapter has a great impact on compounding pharmacies and some impact on dispensing pharmacies.

USP <1160> Pharmaceutical Calculations in Pharmacy Practice

The purpose of this chapter is to provide general information to assist pharmacists and support personnel in performing required calculations for the compounding and dispensing of medications. It is not intended to be an all-inclusive chapter as additional support is provided in other official chapters and in pharmaceutical textbooks. This chapter is divided into 18 sections and an appendix covering most of the calculations a pharmacists will require for practice. It is very useful as a reference and for both teaching and review purposes.

USP <1163> Quality Assurance in Pharmaceutical Compounding

The safety and quality of compounded preparations depend upon correct ingredients and calculations, accurate and precise measurements, appropriate formulation, quality facilities and equipment, documented procedures, and well-founded pharmaceutical judgment. This chapter discusses training, standard operating procedures, documentation, verification, analytical/chemical testing, physical testing, microbiological testing, cleaning/disinfecting/safety, packaging, outsourcing, responsibilities, etc. The chapter concludes by summarizing that a quality assurance program is necessary to ensure the quality of compounded preparations. Pharmacists must determine the types and extent of testing for their quality assurance program and decide whether to perform testing in-house or outsource it to contract laboratories.

USP and NF Monographs

The USP and NF adopt standards for drug substances, pharmaceutical ingredients, and dosage forms reflecting the best in the current practices of medicine and pharmacy and provide suitable tests and assay procedures for demonstrating compliance with these standards. In fulfilling this function, the compendia become legal documents, every statement of which must be of a high degree of clarity and specificity.

In the United States, a drug with a name recognized in the USP/NF must comply with compendial identity standards or be deemed adulterated, misbranded, or both. To avoid being deemed adulterated, such drugs also must comply with compendial standards for strength, quality, or purity, unless labeled to show all respects in which the drug differs. In addition, to avoid being deemed misbranded, drugs recognized in the USP/NF also must comply with compendial standards for packaging and labeling.

Many pharmaceutical products on the market, especially combinations of therapeutic ingredients, are not described in formulation or dosage form monographs in the official compendia. However, the individual components in these products are described in monographs in the compendia, in supplements to the compendia, or in drug applications for marketing approved by the U.S. Food and Drug Administration (FDA).

An example of a typical monograph for a drug substance appearing in the USP is shown in Figure 1.3. This monograph demonstrates the type of information that appears for organic medicinal agents.

The initial part of the monograph consists of the official title (generic or nonproprietary name) of the drug substance. This is followed by its graphic or structural formula, empirical formula, molecular weight, established chemical names, and the drug's Chemical Abstracts Service (CAS) registry number. The CAS registry number identifies each compound uniquely in the CAS computer information retrieval system. Appearing next in the monograph is a statement of chemical purity, a cautionary statement that reflects the toxic nature of the agent, packaging and storage recommendations, and chemical and physical tests, and the prescribed method of assay to substantiate the identification and purity of the chemical.

In each monograph, the standards set forth are specific to the individual therapeutic agent, pharmaceutical material, or dosage form product/preparation to ensure purity, potency, and quality.

Other Pharmacopeias

In addition to the USP and the NF, other references to drug standards, such as the *Homeopathic Pharmacopeia of the United States* (HPUS) and the *Pharmacopoeia Internationalis*, or *International Pharmacopoeia* (IP), provide additional guidelines for drug quality required by certain practitioners and agencies. HPUS is used by pharmacists and homeopathists as well as by law enforcement agencies that must ensure the quality of homeopathic drugs. The term homeopathy was coined by Samuel Hahnemann (1755 to 1843) from the Greek *homoios*, meaning similar, and *pathos*, meaning disease. In essence, the basis of homeopathy is the law of similars, or that like cures like: that is, a drug that produces symptoms of the illness in healthy persons will also be capable of treating those same symptoms and curing the disease. Embodied in the homeopathic approach are (*a*) the testing of a drug on healthy persons to find the drug's effects so that it may be employed against the same symptoms manifesting a disease in an ill person; (*b*) the use of only minute doses of drugs in therapy, employed in dilutions expressed as "1×" (a 1:10 dilution), "2×" (a 1:100 dilution), and so on; (*c*) the administration of not more than one drug at a time; and (*d*) the treatment of the entire symptom complex of the patient, not just one symptom (4–6). The HPUS is essential for pharmacists who prepare drugs to be used in the practice of homeopathy.

The IP is published by the World Health Organization (WHO) of the United Nations with the cooperation of member countries. It is intended as a recommendation to national pharmacopeial revision committees to modify their pharmacopeias according to international standards. It has no legal authority, only the respect and recognition accorded it by the participating countries in their effort to provide acceptable drug standards on an international basis. The first volume of the IP was published in 1951. It has been revised periodically since that time.

Over the years, a number of countries have published their own pharmacopeias, including the United Kingdom,

$C_{16}H_{19}N_3O_5S \cdot 3H_2O$ 419.45

4-Thia-1-azabicyclo [3.2.0] heptane-2-carboxylic acid, 6-[[amino (4-hydroxyphenyl) acetyl]amino]-3, 3-dimethyl-7-oxo-,trihydrate [2S-[2α,5α,6β(S*)]]-; (2S,5R,6R)-6-[(R)-(−)-2-Amino-2-(p-hydroxyphenyl) acetamido]-3,3-dimethyl-7-oxo-4-thia-1-azabicyclo [3.2.0] heptane-2-carboxylic acid trihydrate [61336-70-7]. Anhydrous   365.41   [26787-78-0].

Definition—Amoxicillin contains NLT 900 µg and NMT 1,050 µg of $C_{16}H_{19}N_3O_5S$ per milligram, calculated on the anhydrous basis.

Identification—*Infrared absorption* (197K)

Assay
- **Procedure**
  Diluent: 6.8 g/L of monobasic potassium phosphate in water. Adjust with a 45% (w/w) solution of potassium hydroxide to a pH of 5.0 ± 0.1.
  Mobile phase: Acetonitrile and *Diluent* (1:24)
  Standard solution: 1.2 mg/mL of USP Amoxicillin RS in *Diluent*. (Note—Use this solution within 6 hours.)
  Sample solution: 1.2 mg/mL of Amoxicillin in *Diluent*. (Note—Use this solution within 6 hours.)
  Chromatographic system (see *Chromatography* [621], *System Suitability*)
  Mode: LC
  Detector: UV 230 nm
  Column: 4-mm × 25-cm; packing L1
  Flow rate: 1.5 mL/min
  Injection size: 10 µL
  System suitability
  Sample: Standard solution
  Suitability requirements
  Tailing factor: NMT 2.5
  Relative standard deviation: NMT 2.0%

  Analysis
  Samples: Standard solution and Sample solution
  Calculate the quantity, in µg/mg, of $C_{16}H_{19}N_3O_5S$ in the portion of Amoxicillin taken:

  $$Result = (r_U/r_S) \times (C_S/C_U) \times P$$

  r_U = peak response from the *Sample solution*
  r_S = peak response from the *Standard solution*
  C_S = concentration of USP Amoxicillin RS in the *Standard solution* (mg/mL)
  C_U = concentration of *Sample solution* (mg/mL)
  P = potency of amoxicillin in USP Amoxicillin RS (µg/mg)

  Acceptance criteria: 900 to 1050 µg of $C_{16}H_{19}N_3O_5S$ per milligram on the anhydrous basis

FIGURE 1.3. Amoxicillin.

Impurities

Organic Impurities

- **Procedure**
  Solution A: 2.72 g/L of monobasic potassium phosphate. Adjust with 1 N potassium hydroxide or 20% phosphoric acid to a pH of 5.0 ± 0.1.
  Solution B: Methanol
  Mobile phase: See the gradient table below.

TIME (MIN)	SOLUTION A (%)	SOLUTION B (%)
0	97	3
10	97	3
22	75	25
26	97	3

  Standard solution: 12.5 µg/mL of USP Amoxicillin RS in *Solution A*
  System suitability solution: 12.5 µg/mL each of USP Amoxicillin Related Compound A RS and USP Amoxicillin Related Compound D RS in *Solution A*
  Sample solution: 1.25 mg/mL of Amoxicillin in *Solution A*. (Note—Store this solution at 4 degrees and use within 4 hours)
  Chromatographic system (see *Chromatography* [621], *System Suitability*)
  Mode: LC
  Detector: UV 210 nm
  Column: 4.6-mm × 10-cm; 5-µm packing L1
  Column temperature: 40 degrees
  Flow rate: 1.5 mL/min
  Injection size: 10 µL
  Autosampler temperature: 4 degrees
  System suitability
  Samples: Standard solution and System suitability solution

Suitability requirements
(Note—Identify peaks by the relative retention times in *Impurity Table 1*.)
Resolution: NLT 1.5 between Amoxicillin related compound A and the second peak for Amoxicillin related compound D, *System suitability solution*
Relative standard deviation: NMT 10%, *Standard solution*

Analysis
Samples: Standard solution and Sample solution
Calculate the percentage of each impurity in the portion of *Amoxicillin* taken:

$$Result = (r_U/r_S) \times (C_S/C_U) \times F \times 100$$

r_U = peak response of each impurity from the *Sample solution*
r_S = peak response of amoxicillin from the *Standard solution*
C_S = concentration of USP Amoxicillin RS in the *Standard solution* (µg/mL)
C_U = nominal concentration of Amoxicillin in the *Sample solution* (mg/mL)
F = unit conversion factor (0.001 mg/µg)

(Continued)

Impurity Table 1

NAME	RELATIVE RETENTION TIME	ACCEPTANCE CRITERIA, NMT (%)
Amoxicillin related compound I[a] (D-hydroxyphenylglycine)	0.32	1.0
Amoxicillin related compound D[b,c] (amoxicillin open ring)	0.53	1.0
	0.68	1.0
Amoxicillin related compound A[d] (6-aminopenicillanic acid)	0.78	0.5
Amoxicillin related compound B[e,f] (L-amoxicillin)	0.87	—
Amoxicillin	1.0	—
Amoxicillin related compound G[g] (D-hydroxyphenylglycylamoxicillin)	2.9	1.0
Amoxicillin related compound E[h,i] (amoxicillin penilloic derivative)	4.5	1.0
Amoxicillin related compound M[j] (N-(penicillan-6-yl) open ring amoxicillinamide)	6.0	1.0
Amoxicillin related compound F[e,k] (phenylpyrazinediol)	6.3	—
Amoxicillin related compound C[l] (amoxicillin rearrangement product)	6.4	1.0
Amoxicillin related compound E[h,i] (amoxicillin penilloic derivative)	6.7	1.0
Amoxicillin related compound J[m] (amoxicillin open ring dimer)	8.8	1.0
Amoxicillin related compound L[n] (N-(penicillan-6-yl) amoxicillinamide)	9.0	1.0
Any unspecified individual impurity	—	1.0

[a](R)-2-Amino-2-(4-hydroxyphenyl)acetic acid.
[b]The chromatographic system resolves two penicilloic acids from each other.
[c](4S)-2-{[(R)-2-Amino-2-(4-hydroxyphenyl)acetamido](carboxy)methyl}-5,5-dimethylthiazolidine-4-carboxylic acid.
[d](2S,5R,6R)-6-Amino-3,3-dimethyl-7-oxo-4-thia-1-azabicyclo[3.2.0]heptane-2-carboxylic acid.
[e]These compounds are listed for information only and are not to be reported.
[f](2S,5R,6R)-6-[(S)-2-Amino-2-(4-hydroxyphenyl)acetamido]-3,3-dimethyl-7-oxo-4-thia-1-azabicyclo[3.2.0]heptane-2-carboxylic acid.
[g](2S,5R,6R)-6-{(R)-2-[(R)-2-Amino-2-(4-hydroxyphenyl)acetamido]-2-(4-hydroxyphenyl)acetamido}-3,3-dimethyl-7-oxo-4-thia-1-azabicyclo[3.2.0]heptane-2-carboxylic acid.
[h]The chromatographic system resolves two penilloic acids from each other.
[i](4S)-2-{[(R)-2-Amino-2-(4-hydroxyphenyl)acetamido]methyl}-5,5-dimethylthiazolidine-4-carboxylic acid.
[j](2S,5R,6R)-6-(2-[(R)-2-Amino-2-(4-hydroxyphenyl)acetamido]-2-((4S)-4-carboxy-5,5-dimethylthiazolidin-2-yl)acetamido)-3,3-dimethyl-7-oxo-4-thia-1-azabicyclo[3.2.0]heptane-2-carboxylic acid.
[k]3-(4-Hydroxyphenyl)pyrazin-2-ol.
[l](4S)-2-[5-(4-Hydroxyphenyl)-3,6-dioxopiperazin-2-yl]-5,5-dimethylthiazolidine-4-carboxylic acid.
[m](2S,5R,6R)-6-((2R)-2-{2-[(R)-2-Amino-2-(4-hydroxyphenyl)acetamido]-2-[(4S)-4-carboxy-5,5-dimethylthiazolidin-2-yl]acetamido}-2-(4-hydroxyphenyl)acetamido)-3,3-dimethyl-7-oxo-4-thia-1-azabicyclo[3.2.0]heptane-2-carboxylic acid.
[n](2S,5R,6R)-6-{(2S,5R,6R)-6-[(R)-2-Amino-2-(4-hydroxyphenyl)acetamido]-3,3-dimethyl-7-oxo-4-thia-1-azabicyclo[3.2.0]heptane-2-carboxamido}-3,3-dimethyl-7-oxo-4-thia-1-azabicyclo[3.2.0]heptane-2-carboxylic acid.

Acceptance criteria
(Note—The reporting limit is 0.03% of the amoxicillin peak from the *Standard solution.*)
Individual impurities: See *Impurity Table 1.*
Total impurities: NMT 5.0%

Specific Tests
- *Crystallinity (695):* Meets the requirements
- *Dimethylaniline (223):* Meets the requirement
- pH *(791):* 3.5–6.0
  Sample solution: 2 mg/mL
- *Water determination, Method I (921):* 11.5% to 14.5%
- *Sterility tests (71):* Where the label states that Amoxicillin is sterile, it meets the requirements when tested as directed in *Test for Sterility of the Product to Be Examined, Direct Inoculation of the Culture Medium,* except to use fluid thioglycollate medium containing polysorbate 80 solution (5 mg/mL) and an amount of sterile penicillinase sufficient to inactivate the amoxicillin in each tube, to use soybean–casein digest medium containing polysorbate 80 solution (5 mg/mL) and an amount of sterile penicillinase sufficient to inactivate the amoxicillin in each tube, and to shake the tubes once daily.
- *Bacterial endotoxins test (85):* Where the label states that Amoxicillin is sterile or Amoxicillin must be subjected to further processing during the preparation

of injectable dosage forms, it contains NMT 0.25 USP Endotoxin Unit/mg of amoxicillin.

Additional Requirements
- *Packaging and storage:* Preserve in tight containers, and store at controlled room temperature.
- *Labeling:* Where it is intended for use in preparing injectable dosage forms, the label states that it is intended for veterinary use only and that it is sterile or must be subjected to further processing during the preparation of injectable dosage forms. Label all other Amoxicillin to indicate that it is to be used in the manufacture of nonparenteral drugs only.
- USP *reference standards (11)*
  USP Amoxicillin RS
  USP Amoxicillin Related Compound A RS
  (2S,5R,6R)-6-Amino-3,3-dimethyl-7-oxo-4-thia-1-azabicyclo[3.2.0]heptane-2-carboxylic acid; 6-aminopenicillanic acid.
  $C_8H_{12}N_2O_3S$ 216.26
  USP Amoxicillin Related Compound D RS
  (4S)-2-{[(R)-2-Amino-2-(4-hydroxyphenyl)acetamido](carboxy)methyl}-5,5-dimethylthiazolidine-4-carboxylic acid; amoxicillin open ring.
  $C_{16}H_{21}N_3O_6S$ 383.42
  USP Endotoxin RS

FIGURE 1.3. *(Continued)*

France, Italy, Japan, India, Mexico, Norway, and the People's Republic of China. These pharmacopeias and the *European Pharmacopoeia* (EP or Ph Eur) are used within their legal jurisdictions and by multinational pharmaceutical companies that develop and market products internationally. Countries not having a national pharmacopeia frequently adopt one of another country for use in setting and regulating drug standards. Selection of the pharmacopeia is usually based on geographic proximity, a common heritage or language, or a similarity of drugs and pharmaceutical products used. For example, Canada, which does not have its own national pharmacopeia, has traditionally used USP/NF standards. The Mexican pharmacopeia (*Farmacopea de los Estados Unidos Mexicanos*) and the Brazilian Pharmacopoeia (*Farmacopeia Brasileira*) are the only other actively maintained pharmacopeias in this hemisphere. The Brazilian Pharmacopoeia is part of the MERCOSUR Pharmacopoeia, comprising Argentina, Brazil, Paraguay, and Uruguay (7).

Standards Set Forth in FDA-Approved New Drug Applications

In the United States, in addition to the official compendia, some initial drug and drug product standards and assay methods are established as set forth in new drug applications approved by the FDA (see Chapter 2). The manufacturer must rigidly adhere to these initial standards to maintain product quality and continued FDA approval for marketing. Ultimately, these or subsequently developed standards are adopted as new monographs by the USP/NF.

International Organization for Standardization

The International Organization for Standardization (ISO) is an international consortium of representative bodies constituted to develop and promote uniform or harmonized international standards. Representing the United States in the consortium is the American National Standards Institute.

Among the various ISO standards used in the pharmaceutical industry are those in the series ISO 9000 to ISO 9004. Included here are standards pertaining to development, production, quality assurance (QA), quality control (QC), detection of defective products, quality management (QM), and other issues, such as product safety and liability. Industry compliance with the standards is voluntary. However, many firms find it advantageous to their business to comply with ISO standards and to be identified within their industry as having an internationally recognized QM system. Some companies choose to become ISO certified through a rigorous evaluation and accreditation process (8).

DRUG REGULATION AND CONTROL

The first federal law in the United States designed to regulate drug products manufactured domestically was the Food and Drug Act of 1906. The law required drugs marketed interstate to comply with their claimed standards for strength, purity, and quality. Manufacturers' claims of therapeutic benefit were not regulated until 1912, when the passage of the Sherley Amendment specifically prohibited false claims of therapeutic effects, declaring such products misbranded.

THE FEDERAL FOOD, DRUG, AND COSMETIC ACT OF 1938

The need for additional drug standards was tragically demonstrated in 1938. The then-new wonder drug sulfanilamide, which was not soluble in most common pharmaceutical solvents of the day, was prepared and distributed by an otherwise reputable manufacturer as an elixir using as the solvent diethylene glycol, a highly toxic agent used in antifreeze solutions. Before the product could be removed from the market, more than 100 persons died of diethylene glycol poisoning. The necessity for proper product formulation and thorough pharmacologic and toxicologic testing of the therapeutic agent, pharmaceutical ingredients, and the completed product was painfully recognized. Congress responded with the passage of the Federal Food, Drug, and Cosmetic Act of 1938 and the creation of the FDA to administer and enforce it.

The 1938 Act prohibits the distribution and use of any new drug or drug product without the prior filing of a New Drug Application (NDA) and approval of the FDA. It became the responsibility of the FDA to either grant or deny permission to manufacture and distribute a new product after reviewing the applicant's filed data on the product's ingredients, methods of assay and quality standards, formulation and manufacturing processes, preclinical (animal, tissue, or cell culture) studies including pharmacology and toxicology, and clinical trials on human subjects.

Although the Act of 1938 required manufactured pharmaceutical products to be safe for human use, it did not require them to be efficacious. Subsequent legislation, as described later in this chapter, requires that a drug approved for marketing in the United States be both safe and effective for the condition for which it is intended. Many drugs that had been on the market prior to this Act were allowed to remain on the market if their formula was unchanged, and they were "grandfathered" in by the Act: examples include selected dosage forms of acetaminophen, codeine phosphate, codeine sulfate, hydrocodone, levothyroxine, morphine, nitroglycerin, oxycodone, pilocarpine hydrochloride, potassium chloride, potassium iodide, sodium fluoride, and others.

Durham-Humphrey Amendment of 1951

The Durham-Humphrey Amendment of the Federal Food Drug and Cosmetic Act established a legal distinction between prescription and over-the-counter (OTC) or nonprescription drugs. Until that time, all drugs could be purchased over the counter by consumers.

Medications deemed safe enough by the FDA for self-treatment are made available to consumers for direct purchase, whereas medications requiring professional diagnosis for their safe and effective use must be dispensed only upon a valid prescription or institutional medication order. Prescription drugs must bear the symbol "R$_x$ Only" or the legend "Caution: Federal Law Prohibits Dispensing Without Prescription." New drug substances are limited to prescription-only dispensing. However, their legal status may be changed to OTC, albeit usually at lower recommended dosage, should they later be considered useful and safe enough for the lay person's discretionary use. Examples of such drugs include cimetidine, ibuprofen, ketoprofen, loratadine, omeprazole, and ranitidine.

According to the Durham-Humphrey Amendment, prescriptions for legend drugs may not be refilled (dispensed again after the initial filling of the prescription) without the express consent of the prescriber. The refill status of prescriptions for certain legend drugs known to be subject to public abuse was further regulated with the passage of the Drug Abuse Control Amendments of 1965 and then by the Comprehensive Drug Abuse Prevention and Control Act of 1970.

Kefauver-Harris Amendments of 1962

A tragedy in 1960 led to the passage of the Kefauver-Harris Amendments to the Federal Food Drug and Cosmetic Act of 1938. A new synthetic drug, thalidomide, recommended as a sedative and tranquilizer, was being sold OTC in Europe. It was a drug of special interest because of its apparent lack of toxicity even at extreme dosage levels. It was hoped that it would replace the barbiturates as a sedative and therefore prevent the frequent deaths caused from accidental and intentional barbiturate overdosage. A pharmaceutical company was awaiting FDA approval for marketing in the United States when reports of a toxic effect of the drug's use in Europe began to appear. Thalidomide given to women during pregnancy produced birth defects, most notably phocomelia, an arrested development of the limbs of the affected newborn. Thousands of children were affected to various extents (9). Some were born without arms or legs and others, with partially formed limbs. The more fortunate were born with only disfigurations of the nose, eyes, and ears. The most severely afflicted died of malformation of the heart or gastrointestinal tract. This drug catastrophe spurred the Congress to strengthen the existing laws regarding new drugs. Without dissent, on October 10, 1962, the Kefauver-Harris Drug Amendments to the Food, Drug, and Cosmetic Act of 1938 were passed by both houses of Congress. The purpose of the enactment was to ensure a greater degree of safety for approved drugs, and manufacturers were now required to prove a drug both safe and effective before it would be granted FDA approval for marketing.

Under the Food, Drug, and Cosmetic Act as amended, the sponsor of a new drug is required to file an investigational new drug application (IND) with the FDA before the drug may be clinically tested on human subjects. Only after carefully designed and structured human clinical trials, in which the drug is evaluated for safety and effectiveness, may the drug's sponsor file an NDA seeking approval for marketing. The FDA was given authority to issue good manufacturing practice (GMP) guidelines governing how drugs were to be manufactured, access to facilities for inspection, and jurisdiction over prescription drug advertising. The requirements for these and other submissions to the FDA are presented in Chapter 2.

Interestingly, WHO now considers thalidomide to be the standard treatment for the fever and painful skin lesions associated with erythema nodosum leprosum (ENL) in patients with leprosy, and the FDA has approved its use for this purpose. Further, research into potential uses for thalidomide has determined that it is effective in the treatment of multiple myeloma, a blood and bone marrow cancer, and shows promise in certain inflammatory diseases, and in Kaposi sarcoma, a cancer of the blood vessel walls mostly found in people with HIV (10).

Comprehensive Drug Abuse Prevention and Control Act of 1970

The Comprehensive Drug Abuse Prevention and Control Act of 1970 (now referred to as the Controlled Substances Act [CSA]) served to consolidate and codify control authority over drugs of abuse into a single statute. Under its provisions, the Drug Abuse Control Amendments of 1965, the Harrison Narcotic Act of 1914, and other related laws governing stimulants, depressants, narcotics, and hallucinogens were repealed and replaced by regulatory framework now administered by the Drug Enforcement Administration (DEA) in the Department of Justice.

The Comprehensive Drug Abuse Prevention and Control Act of 1970 established five "schedules" for the classification and control of drug substances that are subject to abuse. These schedules provide for decreasing levels of control, from schedule I to schedule V. The drugs in the five schedules may be described as follows:

- Schedule I: Drugs with no accepted medical use, or other substances with a high potential for abuse. In this category are agents including heroin, lysergic acid diethylamide (LSD), mescaline, peyote, methaqualone, marijuana, and similar items. Any nonmedical substance that is being abused can be placed in this category.
- Schedule II: Drugs with accepted medical uses and a high potential for abuse that if abused may lead to severe psychological or physical dependence. In this category are morphine, cocaine, methamphetamine, amobarbital, and other such drugs.
- Schedule III: Drugs with accepted medical uses and a potential for abuse less than those listed in schedules I

and II that if abused may lead to moderate psychological or physical dependence. In this category are specified quantities of codeine, hydrocodone, and similar agents.

- Schedule IV: Drugs with accepted medical uses and low potential for abuse relative to those in schedule III that if abused may lead to limited physical dependence or psychological dependence relative to drugs in schedule III. In this category are specified quantities of difenoxin, diazepam, oxazepam, and similar agents.
- Schedule V: Drugs with accepted medical uses and low potential for abuse relative to those in schedule IV that if abused may lead to limited physical dependence or psychological dependence relative to drugs in schedule IV. Included in this category are specified quantities of dihydrocodeine, diphenoxylate, and similar agents.

FDA Pregnancy and Lactation Labeling

The FDA has amended its regulations governing the content and format of the "Pregnancy," "Labor and delivery," and "Nursing mothers" subsections of the "Use in Specific Populations" section of the labeling for human prescription drug and biological products. The pregnancy categories A, B, C, D, and X are removed from all human prescription drug and biological product labeling.

The requirement now is that the labeling includes a summary of the risks of using a drug during pregnancy and lactation, a discussion of the data supporting that summary, and relevant information to help health care providers make prescribing decisions and counsel women about the use of drugs during pregnancy and lactation.

The "Labor and delivery" subsection has been removed because this information is included in the "Pregnancy" subsection. The labeling also includes relevant information about pregnancy testing, contraception, and infertility for health care providers prescribing for females and males of reproductive potential. It creates a consistent format for providing information about the risks and benefits of prescription drug and/or biological product use during pregnancy and lactation and by females and males of reproductive potential.

Medication Exposures During Pregnancy and Lactation

Every woman in the general population has a 3% to 5% risk of having a child with a birth defect or mental retardation. Birth defects are the leading cause of infant mortality in the United States. Two important factors to consider when assessing the teratogenic potential of a medication are the stage of pregnancy at which the exposure occurred and the amount of medication taken. It is critical to evaluate each exposure on a case-by-case basis in order to give an accurate risk assessment. Some of the known, possible, and unlikely human teratogens are listed in Table 1.1. In a pregnant or breast-feeding patient who is currently taking, or considering taking, a medication, the patient needs to be counseled about potential adverse effects the medication could have on her fetus or infant (11). This counseling needs to be documented.

Black Box Warnings

A *black box warning* in prescription drug labeling is used to call attention to one of the following situations: (*a*) there is an adverse reaction so serious in proportion to the potential benefit that it be considered in assessing the risks and benefits of using the drug, (*b*) the risk of a serious adverse reaction can be prevented or reduced in severity by careful use of the drug (e.g., patient selection, special monitoring, certain concomitant therapy), or (*c*) the FDA has approved the drug *with restrictions* to prescribing/distribution to ensure its safe use (12).

Drug Listing Act of 1972

The Drug Listing Act was enacted to provide the FDA with the legislative authority to compile a list of marketed drugs to assist in the enforcement of federal laws requiring that drugs be safe and effective and not adulterated or misbranded. Under the regulations of the act, each firm that manufactures or repackages drugs for ultimate sale or distribution to patients or consumers must register with the FDA and submit appropriate information for listing. All foreign drug manufacturing and distributing firms whose products are imported into the United States are also included in this regulation. Exempt from the registration and listing requirements are hospitals, clinics, and the various health practitioners who compound pharmaceutical preparations for use in their respective institutions and practices. Also exempt are research and teaching institutions in which drug products are prepared for purposes other than sale. Each registrant is assigned a permanent registration number, following the format of the National Drug Code (NDC) numbering system. Under this system, the first four numbers, the labeler code of the 10-character code, identify the manufacturer or distributor. The last six numbers identify the drug formulation and the trade package size and type. The segment that identifies the drug formulation is the product code, and the segment that identifies the trade package size and type is the package code. The manufacturer or distributor determines the ratio of use of the last six digits for the two codes, as a 3:3 digit product code to package code configuration (e.g., 542 to 112) or a 4:2 digit configuration (e.g., 5421 to 12). Only one such type of configuration may be selected for use by a manufacturer or distributor, who then assigns a code number to each product to be included in the drug listing. A final code number is presented as the example: NDC 0081-5421-12.

The NDC numbers appear on all manufacturers' drug labeling. In some instances, manufacturers imprint the NDC number, or a part of the NDC number, directly on the dosage units, such as capsules and tablets, for rapid and positive identification when the number is matched in the NDC Directory or against a decoding list provided by the manufacturer. Once a number is assigned to a drug

TABLE 1.1. Some Known Teratogens

Radiation

Atomic weapons

Radioiodine

Therapeutic radiation

Infections

Cytomegalovirus

Herpes simplex virus I and II

Parvovirus B-19 (erythema infectiosum)

Rubella virus

Syphilis

Toxoplasmosis

Varicella virus

Venezuelan equine encephalitis virus

Maternal and Metabolic Imbalance

Alcoholism

Amniocentesis, early (before day 70 postconception)

Chorionic villus sampling (before day 60 postconception)

Cretinism, endemic

Diabetes

Folic acid deficiency

Hyperthermia

Myasthenia gravis

Phenylketonuria

Rheumatic disease

Sjögren syndrome

Virilizing tumors

Drugs and Environmental Chemicals

ACE inhibitors (benazepril, captopril, enalapril, fosinopril, lisinopril, moexipril, quinapril, ramipril, trandolapril)

Aminopterin

Androgenic hormones

Busulfan

Chlorobiphenyls

Cigarette smoking

Cocaine

Coumarin anticoagulants

Cyclophosphamide

Diethylstilbestrol

Etretinate

Fluconazole (high doses)

Iodides

Isotretinoin (Accutane)

Lithium

Mercury, organic

Methimazole

Methotrexate (methylaminopterin)

Methylene blue (via intra-amniotic injection)

Misoprostol

Penicillamine

Phenytoin

Tetracyclines

Thalidomide

Toluene (abuse)

Trimethadione

Valproic acid

Possible Teratogens

Binge drinking

Carbamazepine

Colchicine

Disulfiram

Ergotamine

Glucocorticoids

Lead

Primidone

Quinine (suicidal doses)

Streptomycin

Vitamin A (high doses)

Zidovudine (AZT)

Zinc deficiency

Unlikely Teratogens

Agent Orange

Anesthetics

Aspartame

Aspirin (but aspirin in the second half of pregnancy may increase cerebral hemorrhage during delivery)

Bendectin (antinauseant)

Electromagnetic waves

Hydroxyprogesterone

LSD

Marijuana

Medroxyprogesterone

Metronidazole

Oral contraceptives

Progesterone

Rubella vaccine

Spermicides

Video display terminals

Ultrasound

product, it is a permanent assignment. Even when a drug manufacturer discontinues the manufacture and distribution of a product, the number may not be used again. If a drug product is substantially changed, as through an alteration in the active ingredients, dosage form, or product name, the registrant assigns a new NDC number and advises the FDA accordingly.

The product information is now received by the FDA electronically from each registrant, processed and stored in computer files, and made available in Web-based format. A search of the Drug Code Directory may be done online by proprietary name, application number, active ingredient, NDC number, or labeler name.

Orphan Drug Act of 1983

Drugs intended for the treatment of "rare diseases and conditions" may be designated *orphan* drugs to help promote research on rare diseases. "Rare" diseases are defined as diseases affecting fewer than 200,000 people or diseases that affect more than 200,000 people but where circumstances are such that a company is unlikely to recover its research and development costs. The law provides tax credits and designated years of marketing exclusivity as incentives.

Drug Price Competition and Patent Term Restoration Act of 1984

Changes to speed FDA approval of generic drugs and the extension of patent life for innovative new drugs were the major components of the Drug Price Competition and Patent Restoration Act of 1984.

Under the provisions of the legislation, applications for generic copies of an originally approved new drug can be filed through an abbreviated new drug application (ANDA), and the extensive animal and human studies of an NDA are not required. This reduces considerably the time and expense of bringing a generic version of the drug to market. The FDA evaluates the chemistry, manufacturing, control (CMC) standards, and the drug's bioavailability in determining that the generic version is equivalent to the originally approved drug. In 2014, the unbranded generics dispensed in the United States were about 82% and the branded generics 5.6% (13).

For holders of patented drugs, the legislation provides an extension of patent life equal to the time required for FDA review of the NDA plus half the time spent in the testing phase, up to a maximum of 5 years and not to exceed the usual 20-year patent term. This extends the effective patent life and exclusive marketing period for innovative new drug products, thereby encouraging pioneering research and development.

Prescription Drug Marketing Act of 1987 and Prescription Drug Amendments of 1992

The Prescription Drug Marketing Act of 1987 established new safeguards on the integrity of the nation's supply of prescription drugs. The act is intended to reduce the risks of adulterated, misbranded, repackaged, or mislabeled drugs entering the legitimate marketplace through "secondary sources." The primary sections of the Act are summarized as follows:

1. Reimportation: Prohibits the reimportation of drug products manufactured in the United States except by the manufacturer of the product.
2. Sales restrictions: Prohibits selling, trading, purchasing, or the offer to sell, trade, or purchase a drug sample. It also prohibits resale by health care institutions of pharmaceuticals purchased explicitly for the use of the institution. Charitable institutions that receive drugs at reduced prices or no cost cannot resell the drugs.
3. Distribution of samples: Samples may be distributed only to (*a*) practitioners licensed to prescribe such drugs and, (*b*) at the written request of the practitioner, to pharmacies of hospitals or other health care institutions.
4. Wholesale distributors: Manufacturers are required to maintain a list of their authorized distributors.

Prescription Drug User Fee Act of 1992

The Prescription Drug User Fee Act, first passed in 1992 and subsequently renewed, allows the FDA to accept *user fees* from drug and biologic companies in return for committing to review new drug and biologic applications within certain time frames. The Act is credited with a more rapid application review process and the speedier approval of new drug products. The third enactment, passed as part of the "Public Health Security and Bioterrorism Preparedness and Response Act of 2002," included designated resources for postmarketing studies to monitor the continuing safety and efficacy of new drug products.

Dietary Supplement Health and Education Act of 1994 and the Dietary Supplement and Nonprescription Drug Consumer Protection Act of 2006

In passing the Dietary Supplement Health and Education Act (DSHEA) of 1994, Congress recognized the growing interest in the use of various herbs and dietary supplements and addressed the need to regulate the labeling claims made for these products. These products, which include vitamins, minerals, amino acids, and botanicals, legally are not considered drugs if they have not been submitted for review on NDAs and thus have not been evaluated for safety and efficacy by the FDA. However, as with drugs, their safe use is a concern to the FDA.

The act forbids manufacturers or distributors of these products to make any advertising or labeling claims that indicate that the use of the product can prevent or cure a specific disease. In fact, a disclaimer must appear on the product: "This product is not intended to diagnose, treat, cure, or prevent any disease." However, the law does permit claims of benefit as they may properly relate to a nutrient deficiency disease or, based on scientific evidence, how an ingredient may affect the body's "structure or function" (e.g., increase circulation or lower cholesterol) or how use of the product can affect a person's general well-being. But before any promotional or labeling claims may be made, they first must be submitted to the FDA as being truthful and not misleading (14).

The use of herbs and nutritional supplements is part of today's milieu of "alternative" therapies and as such is receiving increased attention on the part of the scientific community and the FDA. Many of these agents, including ginseng, *Ginkgo*, saw palmetto, St. John's wort, and *Echinacea*, are used worldwide and have been the subject of literature reports and research conducted in Europe and Asia. In 1997, a report of the U.S. Presidential Commission on Dietary Supplement Labels called for more research in this country on the health benefits of dietary supplements. In response, academic and National Institutes of Health (NIH) studies are assessing the therapeutic usefulness of some of these agents and to determine their safety. The USP/NF has adopted standards for many of these products using marker ingredients that must be present within specified ranges if the product is labeled USP/NF. The USP also has a voluntary Dietary Supplement Verification program in place. Participants who meet USP's criteria can place a logo on the label of their product signifying their compliance with USP standards (Fig. 1.4).

The "Dietary Supplement and Nonprescription Drug Consumer Protection Act of 2006" enabled the FDA to implement a policy of GMPs for dietary supplements similar to those in place for pharmaceutical products. This requires that dietary supplements are manufactured according to quality standards, that all ingredients listed are in the declared amounts, that they are properly packaged and accurately labeled, and that complete manufacturing and QC records are maintained along with a system for the identification and reporting of serious adverse events.

FIGURE 1.4. USP Verified Mark on dietary supplement label assures consumers receive expected value. (Reprinted with permission from *United States Pharmacopeia*.)

The FDA and the Food and Drug Administration Modernization Act of 1997 and the Food and Drug Administration Amendments Act of 2007

As noted previously, the FDA was established in 1938 to administer and enforce the Federal Food Drug and Cosmetic Act. Starting with this initial authority, today, the FDA is responsible for enforcing many additional pieces of legislation.

The mission of the FDA is to protect the public health against risks associated with the production, distribution, and sale of food and food additives, human drugs and biologicals, radiologic and medical devices, animal drugs and feeds, and cosmetics. In carrying out the intent of legislation, it is mandated to enforce the FDA

- Sets policies, establishes standards, issues guidelines, and promulgates and enforces rules and regulations governing the affected industries and their products
- Monitors for regulatory compliance through reporting requirements, product sampling and testing, and establishment inspections
- Establishes product labeling requirements, disseminates product use and safety information, issues product warnings, and directs product recalls
- Acts as the government's gatekeeper in making safe and effective new drugs, clinical laboratory tests, and medical devices available through a carefully conducted application and review process

The FDA, an agency of the Department of Health and Human Services, is organized into appropriate units to support its various responsibilities and functions. A complete and detailed FDA organizational chart may be found on the agency's Web site: http://www.fda.gov/AboutFDA/CentersOffices/OrganizationCharts/default.htm.

A listing of some primary offices include

- Office of the Commissioner
- Office of Policy and Planning
- Office of the Chief Scientist
- National Center for Toxicological Research
- Office of Women's Health
- Office of Minority Health
- Office of Foods
- Center for Veterinary Medicine
- Center for Food Safety and Applied Nutrition
- Office of Medical Products and Tobacco
- Center for Devices and Radiological Health
- Center for Biologics Evaluation and Research (CBER)
- Center for Drug Evaluation and Research (CDER)
- Office of Global Regulatory Operations and Policy
- Office of Regulatory Affairs

Each of these offices and centers has a highly organized substructure and personnel to address agency policy, regulations, and operational responsibilities.

The CDER and the CBER are responsible for the drug and biologicals approval process as described in Chapter 2.

The FDA Modernization Act of 1997 was enacted to streamline FDA policies and to codify many of the agency's newer regulations (15). The bill expanded patient access to investigational treatments for AIDS, cancer, Alzheimer disease, and other serious or life-threatening illnesses. It also provided for faster new drug approvals by using drug sponsors' fees to hire additional internal reviewers, by the authorized use of external reviewers, and by changes in the requirements demonstrating a drug's clinical effectiveness. It also provided incentives for investigations of drugs for children.

The legislation included provisions to track clinical trial data in a joint program with the NIH, established a system to follow and review studies of the safety and efficacy of marketed drug products, established a program for the dissemination of information on off-label uses of marketed drugs and encouraged applications for additional therapeutic indications, and fostered the expansion of the FDA's information management system and the agency's progress toward paperless systems for human drug applications.

To codify, enable, and enforce legislative authority, the FDA develops relevant guidelines and regulations. These are first published in the *Federal Register* (FR) for public comment, and when finalized, in the *Code of Federal Regulations* (CFR).

The Biologics Price Competition and Innovation Act (BPCI) of 2009

The Biologics Price Competition and Innovation Act (BPCI) of 2009, also called the biosimilar statute, established a shortened or accelerated approval pathway for biologic drugs that have demonstrated to be highly similar (biosimilar) to or interchangeable with FDA-licensed biological products. The Act provides 12 years of data exclusivity and prohibits the FDA from allowing another manufacturer of a very highly similar biologic to rely on the agency's prior findings of safety, purity, and potency from the innovator product. Also, the statute further prohibits any product from being granted more than one period of data exclusivity unless a manufacturer modifies an approved product to produce a change in safety, purity, or potency. In this case, the modified product would be considered a new product and would be entitled to new data exclusivity of 12 years. The BPCI became part of the Patient Protection and Affordable Care Act that was signed into law on March 23, 2010. On March 6, 2015, Zarxio (a biosimilar version of filgrastim [Neupogen] by Amgen manufactured by Sandoz) obtained the first approval of the FDA.

H.R. 3204 Drug Quality and Security Act (DQSA) of 2013

The DQSA incorporates and brings up to date the court decisions regarding the Food and Drug Modernization Act of 1997. It resulted from the New England Compounding Center (NECC) tragedy where there were 64 deaths and hundreds sickened in 14,000 patients. The outbreak of fungal meningitis occurred in 2012 and was traced to fungal contamination in three lots of compounded methylprednisolone suspension for epidural steroid injections.

The law amends the Federal Food, Drug, and Cosmetic Act (FFDCA) with respect to the regulation of compounding drugs; it exempts compounded drugs from new drug requirements, labeling requirements, and track and trace requirements if the drug is compounded by or under the direct supervision of a licensed pharmacist in a registered outsourcing facility and meets applicable requirements. It establishes requirements for 503a traditional compounding pharmacies and for 503b outsourcing facilities.

Globalization and the FDA

The responsibility of the Federal Food and Drug Administration to protect the public health by assuring the safety and efficacy of the drugs and other products it regulates has become increasingly complex in recent years by the rapidly expanding globalization of the marketplace. Data indicate that 80% of the active pharmaceutical ingredients used in the manufacture of pharmaceutical products and 40% of the finished dosage forms used in the United States are imported (16). FDA-regulated products originate in over 150 countries, are produced in approximately 300,000 foreign facilities, and are distributed by 130,000 importers (16).

In addressing this challenge, the FDA has established foreign operational offices in receptive supplier countries around the world and has increased inspections of foreign supplier facilities. In addition, the FDA is working to develop internationally accepted quality and safety standards through coalitions with foreign counterpart agencies, and together, they are generating global data information systems and mechanisms to identify and quickly address potential risks irrespective of geographic location (16).

It should be noted that the activities of the USP are also worldwide in scope nowadays, with physical operations in key international manufacturing and distribution sites.

Drug Product Recall

If the FDA or a manufacturer finds that a marketed product presents a threat or a potential threat to consumer safety, that product may be recalled or sought for return to the manufacturer from its depth of distribution. The pharmaceutical manufacturer is legally bound to report serious unlabeled adverse reactions to the FDA through the FDA MedWatch Program (800-FDA-1088 or www.FDA.gov). A practitioner also has a responsibility to report a problem with any drug product or medical device using the MedWatch program. Reported problems may include product defects, product adulteration, container leakage, improper labeling, unexpected adverse reactions, and others.

A drug product recall may be initiated by the FDA or by the manufacturer, the latter being termed a voluntary recall.

A numerical classification, as follows, indicates the degree of hazard associated with the product being recalled:

- Class I: There is a reasonable probability that the use of or exposure to a violative product will cause serious adverse health consequences or death.
- Class II: The use of or exposure to a violative product may cause temporary or medically reversible adverse health consequences or the probability of serious adverse health consequences is remote.
- Class III: The use of or exposure to a violative product is not likely to cause adverse health consequences.

The depth of recall, or the level of market removal or correction (e.g., wholesaler, retailer, consumer), depends on the nature of the product, the urgency of the situation, and depth to which the product has been distributed. The lot numbers of packaging control numbers on the containers or labels of the products help in identifying the product to be recalled.

Drug Products Removed or Withdrawn

The following drug products were withdrawn or removed from the market because such drug products or components of such drug products were found to be unsafe or not effective. Thus, the products as listed may not be compounded under the provisions of section 503A(a) of the Federal Food, Drug, and Cosmetic Act. It is important to note that not all dosage forms of the drugs listed have been removed or cannot be compounded because in some situations, it is select dosage forms. The Web site to obtain the current list is http://www.accessdata.fda.gov/scripts/cdrh/cfdocs/cfcfr/cfrsearch.cfm?fr=216.24

THE PHARMACIST'S CONTEMPORARY ROLE

Pharmacy graduates holding the Bachelor of Science (BS) in Pharmacy degree or the Doctor of Pharmacy (PharmD) degree practice in a variety of settings, applying the basic pharmaceutical sciences, the clinical sciences, and professional training and experience. This includes practice in community pharmacies, patient care institutions, managed care, home health care, military and government service, academic settings, professional associations, and the pharmaceutical research and manufacturing industry, as well as in other positions requiring the pharmacist's expertise. The former BS degree was 5 years in length with an additional year of internship required by state boards of pharmacy for licensure for a total of 6 years. The PharmD degree includes the internship experiences within the curriculum during the final year of the program and is still a total of 6 years education/training.

Historically, the abbreviation RPh (registered pharmacist) has been used as the professional designation of a pharmacist licensed by a state board of pharmacy to practice in that state. Doctors of Pharmacy use the PharmD after their name in place of RPh. To minimize any confusion from patients, some states instituted the title DPh (Doctor of Pharmacy)

to designate licensed pharmacists. This designation is used by pharmacists who have earned a BS in Pharmacy. Under this format, all pharmacists in the states where this has been implemented can be called doctors as are those who have earned the PharmD degree; one is a professional degree designation and the other a licensure designation.

Most pharmacists practice within an ambulatory care or community pharmacy setting. In either setting, the pharmacist plays an active role in the patient's use of prescription and nonprescription medication, diagnostic agents, durable medical equipment and devices, and other health care products. The pharmacist develops and maintains individual patient medication profiles, compounds drug preparations, dispenses drug products, issues patient information leaflets (PILs), counsels patients on their health status, and provides information on the use of drug and nondrug measures. As members of the health care team, pharmacists serve as an expert source of drug information and participate in the selection, monitoring, and assessment of drug therapy.

A substantial number of pharmacists practice in institutional settings, such as hospitals, clinics, extended care facilities, and health maintenance organizations (HMOs). In these settings, pharmacists manage drug distribution and control systems and provide a variety of clinical services, including drug utilization reviews (DURs), drug use evaluations, therapeutic drug monitoring, intravenous admixture programs, pharmacokinetic consulting services, investigational drug supplies, and poison control and drug information.

For most of its history as a profession, pharmacy was relatively undifferentiated. The emergence of some practice differentiation occurred in the late 1960s and early 1970s with the professional literature describing hospital pharmacists who had developed unique roles that were distinctive from the traditional dispensing roles of the pharmacist. The "clinical pharmacists" are associated with physicians in therapeutic decision-making, and it was suggested that their level of knowledge and practice skills required special preparation. Further, hospital pharmacists were encouraged to organize their departments to recognize and utilize these emerging "specialties" and proposed that the medical model of service organization might be applicable to pharmacy. Shortly thereafter, the Study Commission on Pharmacy (*syn* the Millis commission) was commissioned by the American Association of Colleges of Pharmacy (AACP). Its 1975 report acknowledged that differentiation in pharmacy practice was occurring and that this differentiation was, in general, expected and desirable. While not specifying specialty practice areas, the commission suggested that a structure be established to oversee all pharmacist credentialing. Actually, there has only been limited success in changing the pharmacists' role to be all clinically based.

The Board of Pharmaceutical Specialties (BPS) was officially established on January 5, 1976, when the American Pharmacists Association (APhA) membership approved the BPS bylaws under the aegis of the APhA structure. The initial mission of BPS was based on responsibilities outlined in its bylaws. The BPS recognizes appropriate specialties in pharmacy practice using specific criteria developed for this purpose. The BPS establishes standards for certification and recertification of pharmacists in designated areas of specialty practice. This is achieved primarily by individual specialty councils, within the BPS structure, that make recommendations to the full Board. The BPS administers the process of examination and evaluation of individuals who seek certification and recertification as specialists, and it serves as an information clearinghouse and coordinating agency for organizations and pharmacists with regard to the specialty practice of pharmacy. Currently, there are eight specialty areas as follows: ambulatory care, critical care, nuclear, nutrition support, oncology, pediatric, pharmacotherapy, and psychiatric pharmacy.

In recent years, managed health care programs have grown extraordinarily and managed health care organizations have enrolled a large and growing base of patients and thus have assumed major responsibilities in the delivery of health care, including the delivery of pharmaceutical services. A few new positions have been created for pharmacists within the managed care industry, including positions for pharmacy benefit managers, disease management specialists, drug formulary managers, therapeutic outcomes researchers, DUR specialists, and others (17). In these functions, managed care pharmacists apply administrative, epidemiological, clinical, financial, research, information technology, and communication skills in their practice.

A number of pharmacy graduates, particularly those having an interest in institutional practice, participate in postgraduate residency and/or fellowship programs to enhance their practice and/or research skills. A pharmacy residency is an organized, directed postgraduate training program in a defined area of practice. The chief purpose is to train pharmacists in professional practice and management skills. Residency programs are conducted primarily in institutional practice settings. A fellowship to develop skill in research is a directed, highly individualized postgraduate program designed to prepare the participant to become an independent researcher. Both pharmacy residencies and fellowships last 12 months or longer and require the close direction of a qualified preceptor.

Pharmacists working for pharmaceutical research, development, and manufacturing firms can participate in a range of activities, including drug discovery, drug analysis and QC, product development and production, clinical studies and drug evaluation, labeling and drug literature, marketing and sales, regulatory affairs, and management. The pharmacist's knowledge of the basic chemical, biological, and pharmaceutical sciences, along with technical knowledge of product formulation, dosage form design, and clinical use meshes well with the requirements of the pharmaceutical industry. Pharmacists with advanced degrees (Master of Science [MS] or Doctor of Philosophy [PhD]) in the basic or pharmaceutical sciences or in health care administration are highly sought in the pharmaceutical industry.

In government service, pharmacists perform professional and administrative functions in the development and implementation of pharmaceutical care delivery programs and in the design and enforcement of regulations involving drug distribution and drug quality standards. Career opportunities for pharmacists in government service at the federal level include positions in the military service, in the U.S. Public Health Service, and in such civil service agencies as the FDA, Veterans Administration, Department of Health and Human Services, DEA, NIH, the Indian Health Service, and others. At the state and local levels, many pharmacists find rewarding careers in health departments, family and children's services, drug investigation and regulatory control, clinics and other health care institutions, and state boards of pharmacy.

Schools of pharmacy enlist pharmacists, some with and some without advanced degrees (MS, PhD), to serve as preceptors within the practice setting, to teach specific courses and/or laboratories within the academic institution, to participate in extramural research, and to contribute to the service and continuing education mission of the school. Some pharmacists work full-time in the academic setting, whereas many others provide part-time professional instruction in community or hospital pharmacies, teaching hospitals and clinics, drug information centers, nursing homes and extended care facilities, health departments, home health care, managed care, and other areas in which pharmaceutical services are delivered.

A number of pharmacists serve their profession in volunteer or professional positions with local, state, and national pharmaceutical associations. For example, the APhA, the American Society of Health-Systems Pharmacists (ASHP), American College of Apothecaries (ACA), International Academy of Pharmaceutical Compounding, The International Academy of Pharmaceutical Compounding has been re-named to The Alliance for Pharmacy Compounding (APC) American College of Clinical Pharmacy (ACCP), the American Society of Managed Care Pharmacy (AMCP), and the AACP are national organizations with pharmacists in key leadership positions. Pharmacists are also active in international pharmacy organizations including International Pharmaceutical Federation (FIP) and the International Society of Pharmaceutical Compounding (ISPhC).

Pharmacists exercise a vital service health education role in their communities through participation in drug and health education community forums, by conducting "brown bag" sessions, by speaking on drug issues in schools, by conducting in-service education programs in patient care settings, and by providing input on drug and health issues to state and federal legislators and community leaders and officials.

The Mission of Pharmacy

In 1991, the House of Delegates of the APhA adopted the following mission statement for pharmacy practice (18):

> To serve society as the profession responsible for the appropriate use of medications, devices, and services to achieve optimal therapeutic outcomes.

And, in 2011, APhA's Board of Trustees adopted the following vision statement for the profession of pharmacy (18):

> Pharmacists are essential for optimizing medication use and improving patient health.

Definition of Pharmaceutical Care

Today, one role of the pharmacist in contemporary practice is the delivery of pharmaceutical care, which was first proposed in 1975 by Mikeal and others as "the care that a given patient requires and receives which assures rational drug usage" (19). Since then, the term has been redefined by many authors, including Strand and others who in 1992 stated (20):

> Pharmaceutical care is that component of pharmacy practice which entails the direct interaction of the pharmacist with the patient for the purpose of caring for that patient's drug-related needs.

The ASHP, a national organization that represents pharmacists who practice in hospitals, HMOs, long-term care facilities, home care agencies, and other components of health care systems, advanced the following statement on pharmaceutical care in 1993 (21):

> The mission of the pharmacist is to provide pharmaceutical care. Pharmaceutical care is the direct, responsible provision of medication-related care for the purpose of achieving definite outcomes that improve a patient's quality of life.

The APhA in 1996 issued its Principles of Practice for Pharmaceutical Care, including the following general statement (22):

> Pharmaceutical care is a patient-centered, outcomes-oriented pharmacy practice that requires the pharmacist to work in concert with the patient and the patient's other health care providers to promote health, to prevent disease, and to assess, monitor, initiate, and modify medication use to assure that drug therapy regimens are safe and effective.
>
> The goal of pharmaceutical care is to optimize the patient's health-related quality of life and achieve positive clinical outcomes, within realistic economic expenditures.

Implicit in all of these statements is the requirement of pharmacists to participate fully in all aspects of medication distribution (manufactured and compounded drugs) and their appropriate clinical use to achieve optimal therapeutic outcomes. The contemporary pharmacy literature contains research papers and articles in support of the concept and practice of pharmaceutical care, including clinical skill development (23), pharmaceutical care databases (24), information technology (25), literature retrieval (26), therapeutic drug monitoring and outcomes assessment (27–30), DUR (31), pharmacotherapy and medication therapy management (MTM) (32,33), drug treatment protocols (34), adverse drug reaction monitoring (35), pharmacokinetic services (36), and strategies to implement pharmaceutical care (37).

In 1997, the AACP's Janus Commission issued a report, *Approaching the Millennium*, which stated that to provide pharmaceutical care, the successful pharmacy graduate must be (38)

- A problem solver, capable of adapting to changes in health care
- Able to achieve health outcomes through effective medication use that are valued by the health care system
- Able to collaborate with and be a resource to physicians, nurses, and other health care team members
- A committed lifelong learner

Pharmacy Practice Standards

The scope and standards of pharmacy practice are established in each state through laws and regulations promulgated by the state's board of pharmacy. Together with applicable federal laws, they constitute the basis for the legal practice of pharmacy.

Over the years, various professional associations in pharmacy have developed documents termed standards of practice. One such document is the *Practice Standards of the ASHP*. In 1991, the APhA, the AACP, and the National Association of Boards of Pharmacy studied the scope of pharmacy practice to revalidate the Standards of Practice for the Profession of Pharmacy, which were published in 1979 and updated in 1986 as Competency Statements for Pharmacy Practice (39). They can be summarized as follows:

- General management and administration of the pharmacy: Selects and supervises pharmacists and non-professionals for pharmacy staff, establishes a pricing structure for pharmaceutical services and products, administers budgets and negotiates with vendors, develops and maintains a purchasing and inventory system for all drugs and pharmaceutical supplies, and initiates a formulary system. In general, establishes and administers pharmacy management, personnel, and fiscal policy.
- Processing the prescription: Verifies the prescription for legality and physical and chemical compatibility, checks the patient's record before dispensing prescription, measures quantities needed to dispense the prescription, performs final check of the finished prescription, and dispenses the prescription.
- Patient care functions: Clarifies the patient's understanding of dosage, integrates drug with patient information, advises the patient of potential drug-related conditions, refers the patient to other health care resources, monitors and evaluates therapeutic response of the patient, and reviews and/or seeks additional drug-related information.
- Education of health care professionals and patients: Organizes, maintains, and provides drug information to other health care professionals, organizes and/or participates in in-pharmacy education programs for other pharmacists, makes recommendations regarding drug therapy to the physician or patient, and develops and maintains system for drug distributions and QC.

In 1998, a consortium of 10 pharmacy organizations undertook a pharmacy practice activity classification project to develop uniform language in describing practice activities in such areas as pharmacotherapy, monitoring and therapeutic outcomes, dispensing medications, health promotion and disease prevention, and health systems management (40). The developed classification is intended to provide the common language to be used and understood within and outside of the profession in describing the practice activities of pharmacists.

The Omnibus Budget Reconciliation Act of 1990

The Omnibus Budget Reconciliation Act of 1990 (OBRA 90), which became effective on January 1, 1993, established a requirement for each state to develop and mandate DUR programs to improve the quality of pharmaceutical care provided to patients covered by the federal medical assistance (Medicaid) program (41). The statute was designed to ensure that prescriptions are appropriate, medically necessary, and not likely to result in adverse medical effects. The statute required that each state's plan provide for a review of drug therapy before each prescription is dispensed and delivered to an eligible patient.

The regulations required patient medication monitoring for therapeutic appropriateness, therapeutic duplication, overuse, underuse, drug–disease contraindications, drug–drug interactions with other prescribed and OTC medications, drug–allergy interactions, correct drug dosage, duration of treatment, and clinical abuse or misuse. They also required that pharmacists offer therapeutic counseling to each recipient of a prescription or the recipient's caregiver regarding the drug, dosage and duration of use, route of administration, side effects, contraindications, techniques for self-monitoring drug therapy, proper storage, refill information, and action to be taken in the event of a missed dose. Pharmacists are to maintain patient medication profiles and therapeutic counseling records. However, it should be mentioned that no reimbursement was defined in these new responsibilities.

In designing the DUR programs, state boards of pharmacy commonly included the federal requirements in the state's pharmacy practice regulations, thereby applying them to each recipient of a prescription, not only to patients receiving benefits under the Medicaid program. Many states used the model regulations for the practice of pharmaceutical care developed by the National Association of Boards of Pharmacy.

Patient Protection and Affordable Care Act of 2010

The Patient Protection and Affordable Care Act (PPACA) was enacted to decrease the number of medically uninsured while improving the quality and reducing the overall costs of health care in the United States. Among its many provisions are expanded prescription drug coverage for Medicare and Medicaid patients, programs for innovative methods of health care delivery, and a pathway for the approval of *biosimilars* (generic biological products) (42).

▌CODE OF ETHICS FOR PHARMACISTS OF THE AMERICAN PHARMACISTS ASSOCIATION

By definition, a profession is founded on an art, built on specialized intellectual training, and has as its primary objective the performing of a service. The principles on which the professional practice of pharmacy is based are embodied in the Code of Ethics of the APhA.

The APhA Code of Ethics has been revised over the years to reflect dynamic changes in the profession. The current version is as follows (43):

Code of Ethics for Pharmacists

PREAMBLE
Pharmacists are health professionals who assist individuals in making the best use of medications. This Code, prepared and supported by pharmacists, is intended to state publicly the principles that form the fundamental basis of the roles and responsibilities of pharmacists. These principles, based on moral obligations and virtues, are established to guide pharmacists in relationships with patients, health professionals, and society.

I.   **A pharmacist respects the covenantal relationship between the patient and pharmacist**.
    Considering the patient–pharmacist relationship as a covenant means that a pharmacist has moral obligations in response to the gift of trust received from society. In return for this gift, a pharmacist promises to help individuals achieve optimum benefit from their medications, to be committed to their welfare, and to maintain their trust.

II. **A pharmacist promotes the good of every patient in a caring, compassionate, and confidential manner**.
    A pharmacist places concern for the well-being of the patient at the center of professional practice. In doing so, a pharmacist considers needs stated by the patient as well as those defined by health science. A pharmacist is dedicated to protecting the dignity of the patient. With a caring attitude and a compassionate spirit, a pharmacist focuses on serving the patient in a private and confidential manner.

III. **A pharmacist respects the autonomy and dignity of each patient**.
    A pharmacist promotes the right of self-determination and recognizes individual self-worth by encouraging patients to participate in decisions about their health. A pharmacist communicates with patients in terms that are understandable. In all cases, a pharmacist respects personal and cultural differences among patients.

IV. **A pharmacist acts with honesty and integrity in professional relationships**.
    A pharmacist has a duty to tell the truth and to act with conviction of conscience. A pharmacist avoids discriminatory practices, behavior or work

conditions that impair professional judgment, and actions that compromise dedication to the best interests of patients.

V. **A pharmacist maintains professional competence**. A pharmacist has a duty to maintain knowledge and abilities as new medications, devices, and technologies become available and as health information advances.

VI. **A pharmacist respects the values and abilities of colleagues and other health professionals**.
When appropriate, a pharmacist asks for the consultation of colleagues or other health professionals or refers the patient. A pharmacist acknowledges that colleagues and other health professionals may differ in the beliefs and values they apply to the care of the patient.

VII. **A pharmacist serves individual, community, and societal needs**.
The primary obligation of a pharmacist is to individual patients. However, the obligations of a pharmacist may at times extend beyond the individual to the community and society. In these situations, the pharmacist recognizes the responsibilities that accompany these obligations and acts accordingly.

VIII. **A pharmacist seeks justice in the distribution of health resources**.
When health resources are allocated, a pharmacist is fair and equitable, balancing the needs of patients and society.

▌CODE OF ETHICS OF THE AMERICAN ASSOCIATION OF PHARMACEUTICAL SCIENTISTS

Like pharmacy practitioners, pharmaceutical scientists recognize their special obligation to society and to the public welfare. Members of the American Association of Pharmaceutical Scientists (AAPS) have adopted the following code of ethics (44).

In their scientific pursuits, they:

- Conduct their work in a manner that adheres to the highest principles of scientific research so as to merit the confidence and trust of peers and the public in particular regarding the rights of human subjects and concern for the proper use of animals involved and provision for suitable safeguards against environmental damage.
- Avoid scientific misconduct and expose it when encountered. AAPS uses the current federal definition of scientific misconduct, 65 FR 76260–76264: Fabrication, falsification, and plagiarism in proposing, performing, or reviewing research or reporting research results.
- Recognize latitude for differences of scientific opinion in the interpretation of scientific data and that such differences of opinion do not constitute unethical conduct.
- Disclose sources of external financial support for, or significant financial interests in the content of, research reports/publications and avoid the manipulation of the release of such information for illegal financial gain.
- Report results accurately, stating explicitly any known or suspected bias, opposing efforts to improperly modify data or conclusions, and offering professional advice only on those subjects concerning, which they regard themselves competent through scientific education, training, or experience.
- Respect the known ownership rights of others in scientific research and seek prior authorization from the owner before disclosure or use of such information including the contents of manuscripts submitted for prepublication review.
- Support in their research and among their employers the participation and employment of all qualified persons regardless of race, gender, creed, or national origin.

APPLYING THE PRINCIPLES AND CONCEPTS

GROUP ACTIVITIES

1. Develop a comparison chart of the drug regulations and control laws described in this chapter. Include when the law was initiated, why the law was created, what the law entails, and how the law affects everyday pharmacy practice.
2. Research and present a pharmacy practice area you are not familiar with and would desire to learn more about. Possibilities include ambulatory care, nuclear pharmacy, managed care, etc.
3. With a partner, role-play a provider–patient dialogue example of pharmaceutical care. Be sure the example encompasses all aspects of the definition.

4. After reviewing the APhA Code of Ethics, do you believe the principles are complete and inclusive? Are there any new aspects in the practice of pharmacy that may need to be incorporated in the future version of the Code of Ethics? Discuss, present, and defend your conclusions.

INDIVIDUAL ACTIVITIES

1. Describe the evolution of the USP and the NF since its inception up to the current date.
2. After reviewing the Competency Statements for Pharmacy Practice, evaluate how well the college/school of pharmacy you attend will prepare you to practice the profession of pharmacy.

REFERENCES

1. Mission and preface. USPNF: History. In: United States Pharmacopeia. Current Edition. Rockville, MD: United States Pharmacopeial Convention, Inc.

2. Constitution and Bylaws. USP-NF. Current Edition. Rockville, MD: United States Pharmacopeial Convention, Inc. Available at: http://www.usp.org/sites/default/files/usp_pdf/EN/aboutUSP/governance/article5.pdf

3. History of the National Formulary. In: National Formulary. 18th Ed. Rockville, MD: United States Pharmacopeial Convention, Inc., 1995:2196–2200.

4. Chavez ML. Homeopathy. Hosp Pharm 1998;33:41–49.

5. Der Marderosian AH. Understanding homeopathy. J Am Pharm Assoc 1996;36:317–321.

6. Pray WS. The challenge to professionalism presented by homeopathy. Am J Pharm Educ 1996;60:198–204.

7. International Meeting of World Pharmacopeias. World Health Organization, 2012. Available at: http://www.who.int/medicines/areas/quality_safety/quality_assurance/resources/Brazil_Pharmacopoeia.pdf. (Accessed July 20, 2020)

8. International Organization for Standardization. Available at: http://www.iso.org/iso/home/about.htm. (Accessed July 20, 2020)

9. FDA. The thalidomide tragedy—25 years ago. FDA Consum 1987;21:14–17.

10. Thalidomide: Research advances in cancer and other conditions. Mayo Clinic. Available at: http://www.mayoclinic.com/health/thalidomide/HQ01507. (Accessed July 20, 2020)

11. Summary of Proposed Rule on Pregnancy and Lactation Labeling U.S. Food and Drug Administration. Available at: http://www.fda.gov/Drugs/DevelopmentApprovalProcess/DevelopmentResources/Labeling/ucm093310.htm. (Accessed July 20, 2020)

12. Guidance for Industry, Warnings and Precautions, and Boxed Warning Sections of Labeling for Human Prescription Drugs and Biological Products. Food and Drug Administration. Available at: http://www.fda.gov/Drugs/GuidanceComplianceRegulatoryInformation/Guidelines/default.htm. (Accessed July 20, 2020)

13. http://www.statista.com/statistics/205042/proportion-of-brand-to-generic-prescriptions-dispensed/

14. Bonnell L. Packaging nutritional supplements. Pharm Med Packag News 1997;5:42–50.

15. Berger MS, Berger BA. FDA Overview Available at: http://www.emedicinehealth.com/fda_overview/article_em.htm. (Accessed July 20, 2020)

16. Autor DM. Globalization and the FDA. Presented at the 36th Good International Manufacturing Practices Conference. The University of Georgia, Athens, GA. March 12, 2012.

17. Vogenberg FR. Managed health care: A review. Hosp Pharm 1997;32:975–982.

18. Vision and mission for the pharmacy profession. Available at: http://www.pharmacist.com/vision-and-mission-pharmacy-profession. (Accessed July 20, 2020)

19. Mikeal RL, Brown TP, Lazarus HL, et al. Quality of pharmaceutical care in hospitals. Am J Hosp Pharm 1975;32:567–574.

20. Strand LM, Cipolle RJ, Morley PC. Pharmaceutical Care: An Introduction. Current Concepts. Kalamazoo, MI: Upjohn, 1992.

21. American Society of Health-System Pharmacists. ASHP guidelines on a standardized method of pharmaceutical care. Am J Health Syst Pharm 1996;53:1713–1716.

22. American Pharmacists Association. Principles of Practice for Pharmaceutical Care. Washington, DC: American Pharmacists Association. Available at: http://www.aphanet.org/pharmcare/prinprac.html. (Accessed July 20, 2020)

23. Barnette DJ, Murphy CM, Carter BL. Clinical skill development for community pharmacists. J Am Pharm Assoc 1996;NS36:573–579.

24. Rodriquez de Bittner M, Michocki R. Pharmaceutical care databases. J Am Pharm Assoc 1997;NS37:595–596.

25. West DS, Szeinbach S. Information technology and pharmaceutical care. J Am Pharm Assoc 1997;NS37:497–501.

26. Grant KL, Herrier RN, Armstrong EP. Teaching a systematic search strategy improves literature retrieval skills of pharmacy students. Am J Pharm Educ 1996;60:281–286.

27. Madan PL. Therapeutic drug monitoring. US Pharm 1996;21:92–105.

28. McDonough RP. Interventions to improve patient pharmaceutical care outcomes. J Am Pharm Assoc 1996;NS36:453–459.

29. Fera T, Bluml BM, Ellis WM, et al. The Diabetes Ten City Challenge: Interim clinical and humanistic outcomes of a multisite community pharmacy diabetes care program. J Am Pharm Assoc 2008;48(2):181–190.

30. Isetts BJ, Schondelmeyer SW, Artz MB, et al. Clinical and economic outcomes of medication therapy management services: The Minnesota experience. J Am Pharm Assoc 2008;48(2):203–211.

31. Kubacka RT. A primer on drug utilization review. J Am Pharm Assoc 1996;NS36:257–261.

32. McGivney MS, Meyer SM, Duncan-Hewitt W, et al. Medication therapy management: Its relationship to patient counseling, disease management, and pharmaceutical care. J Am Pharm Assoc 2007;47(5):620–625.

33. Nkansah NT, Brewer JM, Connores R, et al. Clinical outcomes of patients with diabetes mellitus receiving medication management by pharmacists in an urban private physician practice. Am J Health Syst Pharm 2008;65(2):145–149.

34. American Pharmacists Association. APhA Guide to Drug Treatment Protocols. Washington, DC: American Pharmacists Association, 1997.

35. American Society of Health-System Pharmacists. ASHP Guidelines on Adverse Drug Reaction Monitoring and Reporting. Bethesda, MD: American Society of Health-System Pharmacists, 1995.

36. American Society of Health-System Pharmacists. ASHP Statement on the Pharmacist's Role in Clinical Pharmacokinetic Services. Bethesda, MD: American Society of Health-System Pharmacists, 1998.

37. Berdine HJ, O'Neil CK. Development and implementation of a pharmacist-managed university-based wellness center. J Am Pharm Assoc 2007;47(3):390–397.

38. American Association of Colleges of Pharmacy. Approaching the Millennium: The Report of the AACP Janus Commission. Alexandria, VA: American Association of Colleges of Pharmacy, 1997.

39. Pancorbo SA, Campagna KD, Davenport JK, et al. Task force report of competency statements for pharmacy practice. Am J Pharm Educ 1987;51:196–206.

40. Maine LL. Pharmacy practice classification. J Am Pharm Assoc 1998;38:139–148.

41. Health Care Financing Administration. Medicaid program: Drug use review program and electronic claims management system for outpatient drug claims. Washington, DC: Health Care Financing Administration, Department of Health and Human Services. Fed Regist 1992;57:49397–49412.

42. PUBLIC LAW 111-148—MAR. 23, 2010. Available at: http://www.gpo.gov/fdsys/pkg/PLAW-111publ148/pdf/PLAW-111publ148.pdf. (Accessed July 20, 2020)

43. Code of Ethics. American Pharmacists Association. Available at: http://www.pharmacist.com/code-ethics. (Accessed July 20, 2020)

44. Code of Ethics. American Association of Pharmaceutical Scientists. Available at: http://www.aaps.org/uploadedFiles/Content/About_AAPS/Policies_and_Governance/AAPSCodeofEthics.pdf. (Accessed July 20, 2020)

New Drug Development and Approval Process

CHAPTER AT A GLANCE Drug Discovery and Drug Design • Biologic Characterization • Early Formulation Studies • The Investigational New Drug Application • Clinical Study Registry • The New Drug Application • Supplemental, Abbreviated, and Other Applications • International Conference on Harmonization of Technical Requirements for Registration of Pharmaceuticals for Human Use

OBJECTIVES

After reading this chapter, the student will be able to:

Compare and contrast an Investigational New Drug (IND) Application with a New Drug Application (NDA)

Differentiate between Phase 1, Phase 2, Phase 3, and Phase 4 clinical trials

Give examples of the sources of new drugs

Differentiate between the various methods of drug discovery

Delineate the circumstances whereby an old drug could be classified as "new"

Define pharmacology, drug metabolism, and toxicology

Explain a treatment IND

Define an orphan drug

Define a package insert and the information contained therein

▮ INTRODUCTION

The federal Food, Drug, and Cosmetic Act, as regulated through Title 21 of the U.S. Code of Federal Regulations (CFR), requires a new drug to be approved by the Food and Drug Administration (FDA) before it may be legally introduced in the interstate commerce (1). The regulations apply to the drug products manufactured domestically and those imported into the United States.

To gain approval for marketing, a drug's sponsor (e.g., a pharmaceutical company) must demonstrate, through supporting scientific evidence, that the new drug or drug product is safe and effective for its proposed use. The sponsor must also demonstrate that the various processes and controls used in producing the drug substance and in manufacturing, packaging, and labeling are properly controlled and validated to ensure that the product meets the established standards of quality. The process and time course from drug discovery to approval for marketing can be lengthy and tedious but are well defined and understood in the pharmaceutical industry. A schematic representation of the process for new drug development is shown in Figure 2.1, and the usual time course is depicted in Figure 2.2. Although these representations demonstrate the course for *new chemical entities* (usually small-molecule drugs), similar developmental schemes are followed for *new biological entities*, as described later in this chapter. After the discovery (e.g., synthesis) of a proposed new drug, the agent is biologically characterized for pharmacologic and toxicologic effects and for potential therapeutic application. Preformulation studies are initiated to define the physical and chemical properties of the agent. Formulation studies follow to develop the initial features of the proposed pharmaceutical product or dosage form.

New Chemical Entity
sources:
- Organic synthesis
- Molecular modification
- Isolation from plants

Preclinical Studies
including:
- Chemistry
- Physical properties
- Biological
  - Pharmacology
  - ADME
  - Toxicology
- Preformulation

Investigational New Drug Application (IND)
- Submission
- FDA review

Clinical Trials
- Phase I
- Phase II
- Phase III

Preclinical Studies *(continued)*
plus:
- Long-term animal toxicity
- Product formulation
- Manufacturing and controls
- Package and label design

New Drug Application (NDA)
- Submission
- FDA review
- Preapproval plant inspection
- FDA action

Postmarketing
- Phase IV clinical studies
  - Clinical pharmacology/ Toxicology
  - Additional indications
- Adverse reaction reporting
- Product defect reporting
- Product line extension

FIGURE 2.1. The new drug development process of a new chemical entity from discovery through preclinical and clinical studies, FDA review of the NDA, and postmarketing activities. A variation of this process is followed for the discovery and development of new biological entities, as described later in this chapter.

To obtain the required evidence demonstrating the drug's safety and effectiveness for its proposed use, a carefully designed and progressive sequence of preclinical (e.g., cell culture, whole animal) and clinical (human) studies is undertaken.

Only when the preclinical studies demonstrate adequate safety and the new agent shows promise as a useful drug will the drug's sponsor file an *Investigational New Drug (IND) Application* with the FDA for initial testing in humans. If the drug demonstrates adequate safety in these initial human studies, termed Phase 1, progressive human trials through Phases 2 and 3 are undertaken to

assess safety and efficacy. As the clinical trials progress, laboratory work continues toward defining the agent's basic and clinical pharmacology and toxicology, product design and development, manufacturing scale-up and process controls, analytical methods development, proposed labeling and package design, and initial plans for marketing. At the completion of the carefully designed preclinical and clinical studies, the drug's sponsor may file a *New Drug Application (NDA)* seeking approval to market the new product. The FDA's approval of an NDA indicates that the body of scientific evidence submitted sufficiently demonstrates that the drug or the drug product

FIGURE 2.2. Time course for the development of a new drug. (Adapted from The Pharmaceutical Research and Manufacturers of America (PhRMA), 2012. Available at: http://www.phrma.org/research)

is safe and effective for the proposed clinical indications, that there is adequate assurance of its proper manufacture and control, and that the final labeling accurately presents the necessary information for its proper use. Some products, however, have been approved and later removed from the market for safety reasons, including alosetron HCl (Lotronex), aprotinin (Trasylol), astemizole (Hismanal), bromfenac sodium (Duract), butamben (Efocaine, Butoforme), cerivastatin (Baycol), cisapride (Propulsid), dexfenfluramine HCl (Redux), dipyrone (Metamizole), fenfluramine HCl (Pondimin), flosequinan (Manoplax), grepafloxacin HCl (Raxar), levamisole (Ergamisol), lorcaserin (Belviq), mibefradil (Posicor), natalizumab (Tysabri), oxyphenisatin (Phenisatin), pemoline (Cylert), pergolide (Permax), phenylpropanolamine (Propagest, Dexatrim), rofecoxib (Vioxx), terfenadine (Seldane), tegaserod (Zelnorm), ticrynafen (Tienilic acid), troglitazone (Rezulin), and valdecoxib (Bextra).

The content of a product's approved labeling, represented by the package insert, is a summary of the entire drug development process because it contains the essential chemistry, pharmacology, toxicology, indications and contraindications for use, adverse effects, formulation composition, dosage, and storage requirements, as ascertained during the research and development (R&D).

In addition to the general new drug approval process, special regulations apply for the approval of certain new drugs to treat serious or life-threatening illnesses, such

as AIDS and cancer. These may be placed on an accelerated or fast-track program for approval. Also, if there are no satisfactory approved drugs or treatment alternatives for a serious medical condition, special protocols may be issued permitting the use of an investigational drug to treat some patients prior to approval of the NDA. This type of protocol is termed a treatment IND. Treatment INDs often are sought for orphan drugs, which are targeted for small numbers of patients who have rare conditions or diseases for which there are no satisfactory alternative treatments.

An abbreviated new drug application (ANDA) is used to gain approval to market a generic equivalent of a product that is already approved and being marketed by the pioneer, or the original sponsor, of the drug. In these instances, the sponsor of the ANDA provides documentation on the chemistry, manufacturing, controls (CMCs), and bioavailability of the proposed product to demonstrate biologic equivalency to the original product (2). Clinical data on the drug's safety and efficacy are not required because clinical studies were provided by the pioneer sponsor.

Federal regulations are varied and specific for orphan drugs (3); for biologics, such as human blood products and vaccines, which require approval of a biologics licensing application (BLA) for distribution (4); for over-the-counter (OTC) drugs (5); and for animal drugs, which may require an investigational new animal drug application (INADA), a new animal drug application (NADA), or a supplemental new animal drug application (SNADA) (6). Medical devices, such as catheters and cardiac pacemakers, follow a separate approval process (7). These regulations and others governing foods and drugs are found in the CFR Title 21 and may be accessed at http://www.accessdata.fda.gov/scripts/cdrh/cfdocs/cfCFR/CFRSearch.cfm.

The following sections are intended to serve as an overview of the new drug development and approval process. More specific and detailed information may be obtained directly from the referenced sections of the CFR (1–7), from relevant entries in the Federal Register (8), and from other treatises on the topic (9–13).

DRUG DISCOVERY AND DRUG DESIGN

The discovery of new drugs and their development into commercial products take place across the broad scope of the pharmaceutical industry. The basic underpinning for this effort is the cumulative body of scientific and biomedical information generated worldwide in research institutes, academic centers, and industry. The combined efforts of chemists, biologists, molecular biologists, pharmacologists, toxicologists, statisticians, physicians, pharmacists and pharmaceutical scientists, engineers, and many others participate in drug discovery and development.

Some pharmaceutical firms focus their R&D activities on new prescription drugs for human use, whereas other firms concentrate on the development of OTC medications, generic drugs, biotechnology products, animal health care drugs, diagnostic products, and/or medical devices. Many of the large pharmaceutical companies develop and manufacture products of various types, with some firms having subsidiary companies for specialized functions and products.

The pharmaceutical industry in the United States grew rapidly during World War II and in the years immediately following. The upsurge in the domestic production of drugs and pharmaceutical products stemmed in part from the wartime hazards and consequent undependability of overseas shipping, the unavailability of drugs from previous sources, and the increased need for drugs of all kinds, but especially those with lifesaving capabilities. One such drug is penicillin, the antibiotic that became commercially available in 1944, 15 years after its discovery in England by Sir Alexander Fleming and 1 year before the end of the war. In every year since, scientific discoveries and technological advancements have enabled the development of new drugs and therapies that have enhanced the lives of countless millions worldwide. Today, the scientific exploration of *disease mechanisms* is leading to the discovery and development of agents that specifically impact these mechanisms, resulting in new therapeutic modalities. There is a dramatic advance in the development of *biologic drugs*, including monoclonal antibodies, therapeutic proteins, immunotherapies, and vaccines, which is transforming the treatment of many diseases. Presently, biologics is the fastest growing segment within the new prescription drug market and is expected to continue as such in the years ahead. Annually, approximately 40 new molecular entities receive FDA approval for marketing. In addition, many new dosage strengths and dosage forms of previously approved drugs, new generic products, and new biologics are approved each year.

Not all drugs are discovered, developed, and first approved in the United States. Many pharmaceutical companies do drug R&D in other countries, and many drugs are first marketed abroad. Many of the world's largest pharmaceutical companies are multinational firms with facilities for R&D, manufacturing, and distribution in countries around the world. Irrespective of the country of origin, a drug may be proposed by its sponsor for regulatory approval for marketing in the United States and/or in other countries. These approvals do not occur simultaneously, as they are subject to the laws, regulations, and requirements peculiar to each country's governing authority. However, the international effort to harmonize the regulations through the work of the International Conference on Harmonization (ICH) as described at the end of this chapter fosters multinational drug approvals.

Sources of New Drugs

New drugs may be discovered from a variety of natural sources (e.g., plants), synthesized in the laboratory, or created through processes of biotechnology. Historically, some drugs were found by accident, others by serendipity, but most through years of largely random but tireless pursuit by the synthetic organic chemist. Nowadays, new drugs are the chemical or engineered biologic material resulting from research that is more targeted: that is, directed specifically toward the identified physiologic/metabolic process or biomolecular target of a disease. Current methods of drug discovery are discussed later in this chapter.

Throughout history, plant materials have served as a reservoir of potential new drugs. Yet, only a small portion of the approximately 270,000 known plants thus far have been investigated for medicinal activity. Certain major contributions to modern drug therapy may be attributed to the successful conversion of botanic folklore remedies into modern wonder drugs. The chemical reserpine, a tranquilizer and a hypotensive agent, is an example of a medicinal chemical isolated by design from the folklore remedy *Rauwolfia serpentina*. Another plant drug, periwinkle, or *Vinca rosea*, was first scientifically investigated as a result of its reputation in folklore as an agent useful in the treatment of diabetes mellitus. Plant extracts from *V. rosea* yield two potent drugs that, when screened for pharmacologic activity, surprisingly exhibited antitumor capabilities. These two materials, vinblastine and vincristine, have been used successfully in the treatment of certain types of cancer, including acute leukemia, Hodgkin disease, lymphocytic lymphoma, and other malignancies. Another example, paclitaxel (Taxol), prepared from an extract of the Pacific yew tree, is used in the treatment of ovarian cancer.

After the isolation and structural identification of active plant constituents, organic chemists may recreate them by total synthesis in the laboratory or, more importantly, use the natural chemical as the starting material in the creation of slightly different chemical structures through molecular manipulation. The new structures, termed semisynthetic drugs, may have a slightly or vastly different pharmacologic activity from that of the starting substance, depending on the nature and extent of chemical alteration. Other plant constituents that in themselves may be inactive or rather unimportant therapeutically may be chemically modified to yield important drugs with profound pharmacologic activity. For example, the various species of *Dioscorea*, popularly known as Mexican yams, are rich in the chemical steroid structure from which cortisone and estrogens are semisynthetically produced.

Animals have served humans in their search for drugs in a number of ways. They not only have yielded to drug testing and biologic assay but also have provided drugs that are mannered from their tissues or through their biologic processes. Hormonal substances, such as thyroid extract, insulin, and pituitary hormone obtained from the endocrine glands of cattle, sheep, and swine, are lifesaving drugs used daily as replacement therapy in the human body. The urine of pregnant mares is a rich source of estrogens. Knowledge of the structural architecture of the individual hormonal substances has produced a variety of synthetic and semisynthetic compounds with hormone-like activity. The synthetic chemicals used as oral contraceptives are notable examples.

The use of animals in the production of various biologic products, including serums, antitoxins, and vaccines, has had lifesaving significance ever since the pioneering work of Edward Jenner on the smallpox vaccine in England in 1796. Today, the poliomyelitis vaccine is prepared in cultures of monkey renal tissue, the mumps and influenza vaccines in fluids of chick embryo, the rubella (German measles) vaccine in duck embryo, and the smallpox vaccine from the skin of bovine calves inoculated with vaccinia virus. New vaccines for diseases such as AIDS and cancer are being developed through the use of cell and tissue cultures.

Today, we are witnessing a new era in the development of pharmaceutical products as a result of the advent of genetic engineering, the submicroscopic manipulation of the double helix, and the spiral DNA chain of life. Through this process will come more abundant and vastly purer antibiotics, vaccines, and yet unknown chemical and biologic products to combat human diseases.

The two basic technologies that drive the genetic field of drug development are recombinant DNA and monoclonal antibody (mAb) production (14–16). Common to each technique is the ability to manipulate and produce proteins, the building blocks of living matter. Proteins are an almost infinite source of drugs. Made up of long chains of amino acids, their sequence and spatial configuration offer a staggering number of possibilities. Both recombinant rDNA and mAb production techniques influence cells' ability to produce proteins.

The more fundamental of the two techniques is recombinant DNA. It has the potential to produce almost any protein. Genetic material can be transplanted from higher species, such as humans, into a lowly bacterium. This so-called gene splicing can induce the lower organism to make proteins it would not otherwise have made. Such drug products as human insulin, human growth hormone, hepatitis B vaccine, epoetin alfa, and interferon are being produced in this manner. Human insulin was the first recombinant biopharmaceutical approved in the United States, in 1982.

Whereas recombinant DNA techniques involve the manipulation of proteins within the cells of lower animals, mAb production is conducted entirely within the cells of higher animals, including the patient. The technique exploits the ability of cells with the potential to produce a desired antibody and stimulates an unending stream of pure antibody production. These antibodies have the capacity to combat the specific target.

The development and use of monoclonal antibodies is having a profound impact in both diagnostic medicine and in the treatment of disease. Diagnostically, for example, monoclonal antibodies are used in home pregnancy testing products. In these tests, the mAb is highly sensitive to binding on one site on the human chorionic gonadotropin (HCG) molecule, a specific marker to pregnancy because in healthy women, HCG is synthesized exclusively by the placenta. The first FDA-approved therapeutic mAb was muromonab, a transplant rejection drug, approved in 1986. Since then, many additional mAbs have received FDA approval for marketing with hundreds of others undergoing clinical trials. Among those in current use are belimumab (lupus erythematosus), brentuximab (Hodgkin lymphoma), cetuximab (colorectal cancer), natalizumab (multiple sclerosis), ofatumumab (lymphocytic leukemia), ranibizumab (macular degeneration), and tocilizumab (rheumatoid arthritis).

Human gene therapy, used to prevent, treat, cure, diagnose, or mitigate human diseases caused by genetic disorders, is another promising new technology. The human body contains up to 100,000 genes. Genes that are aligned on a double strand of DNA in the nucleus of every cell control all of the body's functions. Base pairs of adenine and thymine (A and T, respectively) and cytosine and guanine (C and G, respectively) constitute the instructions on a gene. Only genes necessary for a specific cell's function are active or expressed. When a gene is expressed, a specific type of protein is produced. In genetic diseases, gene expression may be altered and/or gene sequences may be mismatched, partly missing, or repeated too many times, causing cellular malfunction and disease.

Gene therapy is a medical intervention based on the modification of the genetic material of living cells. Cells may be modified outside the body (ex vivo) for subsequent administration, or they may be modified within the body (in vivo) by gene therapy products given directly to the patient. In either case, gene therapy entails the transfer of new genetic material to the cells of a patient with a genetic disease. The genetic material, usually cloned DNA, may be transferred into the patient's cells physically, as through microinjection, through chemically mediated transfer procedures, or through disabled retroviral gene transfer systems that integrate genetic material directly into the host cell chromosomes (17–19).

The first human gene therapy used was to treat adenosine deaminase (ADA) deficiency, a condition that results in abnormal functioning of the immune system. Therapy consisted of the administration of genetically modified cells capable of producing ADA (18). Many emerging biopharmaceutical companies are exploring the application of gene therapy to treat sickle cell anemia, malignant melanoma, renal cell cancer, heart disease, familial hypercholesterolemia, cystic fibrosis, lung and colorectal cancer, and AIDS (20). The FDA has established guidelines for cellular and gene therapy (21).

A Goal Drug

In theory, a goal drug would produce the specifically desired effect, be administered by the most desired route (generally orally) at minimal dosage and dosing frequency, have optimal onset and duration of activity, and exhibit no side effects and, following its desired effect, would be eliminated from the body efficiently, completely, and without residual effect. It would also be easily produced at low cost, pharmaceutically elegant, and physically and chemically stable in various conditions of use and storage. Although not completely attainable in practice, these qualities and features are sought in drug and dosage form design.

Methods of Drug Discovery

Although some drugs may be the result of fortuitous discovery, most drugs are the result of carefully designed research programs of screening, molecular modification, and mechanism-based drug design (11–13,22–25).

Random or untargeted screening involves the testing of large numbers of synthetic organic compounds or substances of natural origin for biologic activity. Random screens may be used initially to detect an unknown activity of the test compound or substance or to identify the most promising compounds to be studied by more sophisticated nonrandom or targeted screens to determine a specific activity.

Although random and nonrandom screening programs can examine a host of new compounds for activity, sometimes promising compounds may be overlooked if the screening models are not sensitive enough to reflect accurately the specific disease against which the agent or its metabolites may be useful (25).

To detect and evaluate biologic activity, bioassays are used to differentiate the effect and potency (strength of effect) of the test agent from those of controls of known action and effect. The initial bioassays may be performed in vitro using cell cultures to test the new agent's effect against enzyme systems or tumor cells, whereas subsequent bioassays may be performed in vivo and may use more expensive and disease-specific animal models.

Newer methods, such as high-throughput screening, are capable of examining 15,000 chemical compounds a week using 10 to 20 biologic assays (23). To be effective, this requires a sizable and chemically diverse collection of compounds to examine, which many pharmaceutical and chemical companies have in chemical libraries. Frequently these libraries, which may contain hundreds of thousands of compounds, are purchased or licensed from academic or commercial sources. With the advent of techniques like combinatorial chemistry, it has become feasible to increase substantially the size and diversity of a chemical library (23).

Molecular modification is a chemical alteration of a known and previously characterized organic compound (frequently a lead compound; see "A Lead Compound") for the purpose of enhancing its usefulness as a drug. This could mean enhancing its specificity for a particular body target site, increasing its potency, improving its rate and extent of absorption, modifying to advantage its time course in the body, reducing its toxicity, or changing its physical or chemical properties (e.g., solubility) to provide desired features (23). The molecular modifications may be slight or substantial, involving changes in functional groups, ring structures, or configuration. Knowledge of chemical structure–pharmacologic activity relationships plays an important role in designing new drug molecules. Molecular modification produces new chemical entities and improved therapeutic agents. Figure 2.3 shows the molecular modifications that led to the discoveries of the first commercial beta-blocker, propranolol, and the first commercial histamine H2-receptor blocking agent, cimetidine.

Mechanism-based drug design is molecular modification to design a drug that interferes specifically with the known or suspected biochemical pathway or mechanism of a disease process. The intention is the interaction of the drug with specific cell receptors, enzyme systems, or the metabolic processes of pathogens or tumor cells, resulting in a blocking, disruption, or reversal of the disease process. For this, it is essential to understand the biochemical pathway of the disease process and the manner in which it is regulated. Molecular graphics, the use of computer graphics to represent and manipulate the structure of the drug molecule to fit the simulated molecular structure of the receptor site, is a useful complementary tool in drug molecule design.

An example of mechanism-based drug design is the compound enalaprilat, the active metabolite of enalapril (Vasotec), which inhibits the angiotensin-converting enzyme (ACE) that catalyzes the conversion of angiotensin I to the vasoconstrictor substance angiotensin II. Inhibition

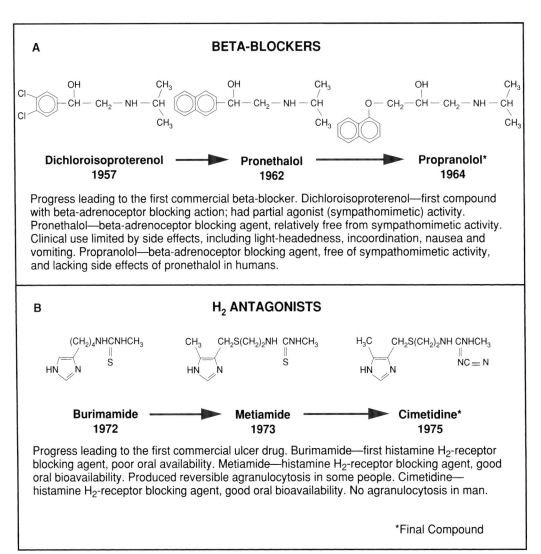

FIGURE 2.3. Molecular modifications leading to the development of the first commercial beta-blocker, propranolol, and the first commercial histamine H2-receptor blocking agent, cimetidine. (Reprinted from Maxwell RA. The state of the art of the science of drug discovery. Drug Dev Res 1984;4:375–389; through Pharmaceutical Research: Therapeutic and Economic Value of Incremental Improvements, 1990:12, with permission. Courtesy of National Pharmaceutical Council, Reston, VA. Reprinted with permission from John Wiley & Sons, Inc.)

of the enzyme results in decreased plasma angiotensin II, leading to decreased vasopressor effects and lower blood pressure. Another example is ranitidine (Zantac), an inhibitor of histamine at the histamine H2 receptors, including receptors on the gastric cells. This inhibits gastric acid secretion, making the drug effective in the treatment of gastric ulcers and other gastrointestinal conditions related to the production of gastric acid. A third example is sertraline (Zoloft), which inhibits the central nervous system's neuronal uptake of serotonin, making the drug useful in the treatment of depression.

A Lead Compound

A lead compound is a prototype chemical compound that has a fundamental desired biologic or pharmacologic

activity. Although active, the lead compound may not possess all of the features desired, such as potency, absorbability, solubility, low toxicity, and so forth. Thus, the medicinal chemist may seek to modify the lead compound's chemical structure to achieve the desired features while reducing the undesired ones. The chemical modifications produce analogs with additional or different functional chemical groups, altered ring structures, or different chemical configurations. The results are modified chemical compounds capable of having different interactions with the body's receptors, thereby eliciting different actions and intensities of action.

The synthesis of derivatives of the prototype chemical may ultimately lead to successive generations of new compounds of the same pharmacologic type. This may be exemplified by the development of new generations of cephalosporin antibiotics, additional H2 antagonists from the pioneer drug cimetidine, and the large series of anti-anxiety drugs derived from the benzodiazepine structure and the innovator drug chlordiazepoxide (Librium).

Most drugs exhibit activities secondary to their primary pharmacologic action. It is fairly common to take advantage of a secondary activity by using molecular modification to develop new compounds that amplify the secondary use of the drug or by gaining approval to market the drug for a secondary indication. For example, the drug finasteride (Proscar) was originally developed and approved to treat benign prostatic hyperplasia. Later, the same drug (as Propecia) was approved at a lower recommended dosage to treat male pattern baldness.

Prodrugs

Prodrug is a term used to describe a compound that requires metabolic biotransformation after administration to produce the desired pharmacologically active compound. The conversion of an inactive prodrug to an active compound occurs primarily through enzymatic biochemical cleavage. Depending on the specific prodrug–enzyme interaction, the biotransformation may occur anywhere along the course of drug transit or at the body site where the requisite enzymes are sufficiently present. An example of a prodrug is enalapril maleate (Vasotec), which, after oral administration, is bioactivated by hydrolysis to enalaprilat, an ACE inhibitor used in the treatment of hypertension. Prodrugs may be designed preferentially for solubility, absorption, biostability, and prolonged release (24).

Solubility

A prodrug may be designed to possess solubility advantages over the active drug, enabling the use of specifically desired dosage forms and routes of administration. For example, if an active drug is insufficiently soluble in water to prepare a desired intravenous injection, a water-soluble prodrug, for example, hydrocortisone sodium succinate, could be prepared through the addition of a functional group that later would be detached by the metabolic process to yield, once again, the active drug molecule.

Absorption

A drug may be made more water or lipid soluble, as desired, to facilitate absorption via the intended route of administration. For example, for patients requiring prolonged antipsychotic therapy, the addition of the decanoate ester to the haloperidol molecule makes the molecule less water soluble. Subsequently, when it is administered by a deep intramuscular injection, the molecule provides a sustained effect that lasts up to 4 weeks.

Biostability

If an active drug is prematurely destroyed by biochemical or enzymatic processes, the design of a prodrug may

protect the drug during its transport in the body. For example, valacyclovir is a prodrug of acyclovir. Normally, the bioavailability of acyclovir is 10% to 20% after oral administration. Valacyclovir is converted to acyclovir by liver esterases via the first-pass metabolism resulting in a 55% bioavailability. In addition, the use of a prodrug could result in site-specific action of greater potency. For example, dopamine in the treatment of Parkinson disease is unable to cross the blood–brain barrier. However, its prodrug, levodopa, is able to cross the blood–brain barrier and then is converted to dopamine.

Prolonged Release

Depending on a prodrug's rate of metabolic conversion to an active drug, it may provide prolonged drug release and extended therapeutic activity.

FDA's Definition of a New Drug

A new molecular entity (NME) is defined by the FDA as an active ingredient that has never before been marketed in the United States in any form (26). However, a drug need not be a new chemical entity to be considered new. A change in a previously approved drug product's formulation or method of manufacture constitutes newness under the law because such changes can alter the therapeutic efficacy and/or safety of a product.

A combination of two or more old drugs or a change in the usual proportions of drugs in an established combination product is considered new if the change introduces a question of safety or efficacy.

A proposed new use for an established drug, a new dosage schedule or regimen, a new route of administration, or a new dosage form makes a drug or a drug product's status new and triggers reconsideration for safety and efficacy.

Drug Nomenclature

When first synthesized or identified from a natural source, an organic compound is represented by an empirical formula, for example, $C_{16}H_{19}N_3O_5S \cdot 3H_2O$ for amoxicillin, which indicates the number and relationship of the atoms in the molecule. As knowledge of the relative locations of these atoms increases, the compound receives a systematic chemical name, such as 4-thia-1-azabicylco[3.2.0] heptane-2-carboxylic acid, 6-[amino(4-hydroxyphenyl) acetyl]amino-3,3-dimethyl-7-oxo, trihydrate 2S-[2[alpha], [5[alpha], 6[beta](S*)]]. To be adequate and fully specific, the name must reveal every part of the compound's molecular structure, so that it describes only that compound and no other. The systematic name is generally so formidable that it soon is replaced in scientific communication by a shortened name, which, although less descriptive chemically, is understood to refer only to that chemical compound. This shortened name is the chemical's nonproprietary (or generic) name (e.g., amoxicillin; see Fig. 1.3). A nonproprietary name of a drug serves numerous and varied purposes, its principal function being to identify the substance to which it applies by means of a designation that may be used by the professional and lay public free from the restrictions associated with registered trademarks.

Today, many companies give their new compounds code numbers before assigning a nonproprietary name. These code numbers take the form of an identifying prefix letter or letters that identify the drug's sponsor, followed by a number that further identifies the test compound (e.g., SQ 14,225, the investigational code number for the drug captopril, initially developed by Squibb). The code number frequently stays with a compound from its initial preclinical laboratory investigation through human clinical trials.

When the results of testing indicate that a compound shows sufficient promise of becoming a drug, the sponsor may formally propose a nonproprietary name to the U.S. Adopted Names (USAN) Council. The Council is trisponsored by the American Medical Association (AMA), the United States Pharmacopeial Convention (USP), and the American Pharmacists Association (APhA). In addition, the FDA cooperates with and is represented on the Council. Should the drug receive recognition in an official compendium, the nonproprietary name established during the drug's early usage is adopted. Nonproprietary names are issued only for single agents. An updated list of adopted names may be found on the Web site http://www.ama-assn.org/ama/pub/physician-resources/medical-science/united-states-adopted-names-council/adopted-names.page.

Guiding principles for the coining of a nonproprietary name are comprehensive (27). Among the stated principles are the following: (*a*) the name should be useful primarily to health care practitioners particularly in its safety for use in the routine processes of prescribing, dispensing, and administering drugs; (*b*) the name should be a single word, preferably with no more than four syllables, and should be free from conflict with other nonproprietary names and should be neither confusing nor misleading; and (*c*) distinctive terminology should be used for specific drugs or drug groups (e.g., beta-blockers).

The USP/NF titles for monograph articles (drug substance and drug products/preparations) are legally recognized under the Federal Food, Drug, and Cosmetic Act as the designations for use in labeling articles; this is also known as the nonproprietary or generic name. The USP is a cosponsor of the USAN program and the USP Council of Experts considers the adoption of the U.S. Adopted Name, if any, as the official title for any compound that attains compendial recognition. The USAN program started in 1961 and publishes the U.S. Adopted Names (USAN). The USP Dictionary of USAN and International Drug Names serves as a book of names useful for identifying and distinguishing all kinds of names for drug substances, whether public, proprietary, chemical, or code-designated names. This official or nonproprietary name serves to identify the substance to which it applies by means of a designation

that is used by the professional and lay public free from registered trademarks and other restrictions.

Salt Nomenclature

USP monographs for drug products and compounded preparations containing a salt of an acid or base use the name of the active moiety and the strength of the product or preparation is also expressed in terms of the active moiety. An active moiety is the molecule or ion, excluding those appended portions of the molecule that cause the drug to be a salt or other noncovalent derivative of the molecule. The active moiety is responsible for the physiological or pharmacological action of the drug substance without regard to the actual charged state of the molecule in vivo. This nomenclature is used by the USP in naming drug products and compounded preparations that are newly recognized in the USP. Products already on the market are not generally affected.

Nomenclature Forms

There are some general guidelines the USP uses for naming drug products and preparations.

- The general format is [DRUG][DOSAGE FORM].
- The [ROUTE OF ADMINISTRATION] is omitted when it is obvious.
- Some drugs require some step in preparation prior to administration. Their general format is [DRUG][DOSAGE FORM] for [ROUTE OF ADMINISTRATION][DOSAGE FORM]. An example would be "Aspirin Effervescent Tablets for Oral Solution."
- The term "for" is used for solid preparations that must be dissolved or suspended in a suitable liquid to obtain a dosage form suitable for administration. Their general format is [DRUG] for [ROUTE OF ADMINISTRATION][DOSAGE FORM]. An example would be "Amoxicillin for Oral Suspension."
- The term "Vaginal Inserts" is used rather than vaginal tablets, vaginal capsules, or vaginal suppositories to minimize the potential for incorrect administration.
- The term "Suppositories" is used for solid preparations intended for rectal administration.
- [DRUG] Injection is used for liquid preparations that are administered by injection.
- [DRUG] for Injection is used for dry solids requiring addition of a suitable vehicle.
- [DRUG] Injectable Emulsion is used for liquid preparations dissolved or dispersed in a suitable emulsion medium.
- [DRUG] Injectable Suspension is used for liquid preparations of solids suspended in a suitable liquid medium.
- [DRUG] for Injectable Suspension is used for dry solids that, upon the addition of suitable vehicles, yield suspensions suitable for injection.
- [DRUG] Extended-Release Injectable Suspension is used for liquid preparations of solids suspended in a

suitable liquid designed to make the drug available over an extended period of time.

- [DRUG] for Extended-Release Injectable Suspension is used for dry solids that, upon adding a suitable vehicle, produces preparations for releasing the injectable drug over an extended period of time.
- [DRUG] in [VEHICLE] is used for injections intended to be administered through an intravenous secondary line ("piggyback") formulated in vehicles other than Water for Injection. An example would be [DRUG] in Dextrose Injection.
- [DRUG] Compounded [DOSAGE FORM].
- [DRUG] Compounded [DOSAGE FORM], Veterinary.

▌BIOLOGIC CHARACTERIZATION

Prospective drug substances must undergo preclinical testing for biologic activity to assess their potential as useful therapeutic agents. These studies, which fall into the general areas of pharmacology, drug metabolism, and toxicology, involve many types of scientists, including general biologists, microbiologists, molecular biologists, biochemists, geneticists, pharmacologists, physiologists, pharmacokineticists, pathologists, toxicologists, statisticians, and others. Their work leads to the determination of whether a chemical agent possesses adequate features of safety and sufficient promise of usefulness to pursue as a prospective new drug.

To judge whether a drug is safe and effective, information must be gained on how it is absorbed, distributed throughout the body, stored, metabolized, and excreted and how it affects the action of the body's cells, tissues, and organs. Scientists have developed studies that may be conducted outside the living body by using cell and tissue culture and computer programs that simulate human and animal systems. Cell cultures are being used increasingly to screen for toxicity before progressing to whole-animal testing.

Pharmacology

Within its broad definition, pharmacology is the science concerned with drugs, their sources, appearance, chemistry, actions, and uses. The term in general can be expanded to include biochemical and physiologic effects, mechanisms of action, absorption, distribution, biotransformation, and excretion. From this basic field of study come such subareas as pharmacodynamics, the study of the biochemical and physiologic effects of drugs and their mechanisms of action; pharmacokinetics, which deals with the rates of absorption, distribution, metabolism or biotransformation, and excretion (ADME) of drugs; and clinical pharmacology, which applies pharmacologic principles to the study of the effects and actions of drugs in humans.

Today's emphasis in the development of new drugs is on identifying the cause and process of a disease and then designing molecules capable of interfering with that process. Although the precise cause of each disease is not yet known, what is known is that most diseases arise from a biochemical imbalance, an abnormal proliferation of cells, an endogenous deficiency, or an exogenous chemical toxin or invasive pathogen.

The biochemical processes in the body's cells involve intricate enzymatic reactions. An understanding of the role of a particular enzyme system in the body's healthy state and disease state can lead to the design of drugs that affect the enzyme system with positive results, as exemplified earlier in this chapter for the drug enalaprilat.

Different drug substances produce different effects on the biologic system because of the specific interactions between a drug's chemical structure and specific cells or cellular components of a particular tissue or organ, termed receptor sites (Fig. 2.4). The action of most drugs takes place at the molecular level, with the drug molecules interacting with the molecules of the cell structure or its contents. The selectivity and specificity of drugs for a certain body tissue—for example, drugs that act primarily on the nerves, heart, or kidney—are related to specific sites on or within the cells, receptive only to chemicals of a particular

FIGURE 2.4. Receptor site and substrate (drug). (Reprinted from Clark FH, ed. *How Modern Medicines Are Discovered.* Mount Kisco, NY: Futura, 1973, with permission. Courtesy of Futura Publishing.)

chemical structure and configuration. This is the basis for structure–activity relationships established for drugs and for families of drugs within therapeutic categories. Studies of the pharmacologic activities of a series of analogs with varied functional groups and side chains can reveal the most specific structure for a given drug–cell or drug–enzyme interaction.

Although receptors for many drugs have yet to be identified, they, like the active centers of enzymes, are considered to be carboxyl, amino, sulfhydryl, phosphate, and similar reactive groups oriented on or in the cell in a pattern complementary to that of the drugs with which they react. The binding of a drug to the receptor is thought to be accomplished mainly by ionic, covalent, and other relatively weak reversible bonds. Occasionally, firm covalent bonding is involved, and the drug effect is then slowly reversible.

There is a relationship between the quantity of drug molecules available for interaction and the capacity of the specific receptor site. For instance, after a dose of drug and its transit to the site of action, the cell's receptors may or may not become fully saturated with the interacting drug. When the receptors are saturated, the effects of the specific interaction are maximized. Any additional drug present (as in the circulation) and not participating in the interaction may serve as a reservoir to replace the drug molecules released from the complex. Two drugs in a biologic system may compete for the same binding sites, with the drug having the stronger bonding attraction for the site generally prevailing. Already bound molecules of the more weakly bound drug may be displaced from the binding site and left free in the circulation.

Certain cells within the body are capable of binding drugs without eliciting a drug effect. These cells act as carriers and may be important to a drug's transport to active sites or to sites of the drug's biotransformation and elimination.

The process of evaluating chemical compounds for biologic activity and the determination of their mechanisms of action are the responsibilities of the pharmacologist. In vitro cultures of cells and enzyme systems and in vivo animal models are used to define a chemical's pharmacologic profile.

To define a pharmacologic profile, pharmacologists progress stepwise through increasingly sophisticated levels of evaluation, based on the test compound's success in prior studies. Whole-animal studies are reserved for the test compounds that have demonstrated reasonable potential as a drug candidate.

Among the early studies are the determination of a compound's selectivity for various receptors and its activity against select enzyme systems. Studies of the compound's effects on cell function are then performed to detect evidence of efficacy and to determine whether the compound is an agonist or antagonist. These are followed by studies with isolated animal tissues to define further the compound's activity and selectivity. Then, whole-animal studies are used to evaluate the pharmacologic effects of the agent on specific organ systems. Finally, studies are undertaken using animal models of human disease for which the compound is considered a drug candidate.

Most animal testing is performed on small animals, usually rodents (mouse, rat) for a number of reasons including cost, availability, the small amount of drug required for a study, the ease of administration by various routes (oral, inhalation, and intravenous), and experience with drug testing in these species. However, in final pharmacologic and toxicologic studies, two or more animal species are used as required by the FDA, including a rodent and an animal from another nonrodent mammalian order, such as a dog. Drugs are studied at various dose levels to determine the effect, potency, and toxicity.

The primary objective of the animal studies is to obtain basic information on the drug's effects that may be used to predict safe and effective use in humans. This is a difficult task because of species variation and the fact that animals are not absolute predictors of human response. However, a number of animal models have been developed to mimic certain human diseases, and these are used effectively. For instance, there are animal models for type I diabetes and hypertension, using genetically diabetic and hypertensive animals, respectively, and for tumor growth, using tumor transplants in various species. Certain animal species have been determined to be the best for certain studies of organ systems, or as human disease models, including dogs and rats for hypertension, dogs and guinea pigs for respiratory effects, dogs for diuretic activity, rabbits for blood coagulation, and mice and rats for central nervous system studies (28). Unfortunately, useful animal models are not available for every human disease. As a drug candidate progresses in its preclinical pharmacologic evaluation, drug metabolism and toxicity tests are initiated.

Drug Metabolism

A series of animal studies of a proposed drug's ADME are undertaken to determine (*a*) the extent and rate of drug absorption from various routes of administration, including the one intended for human use; (*b*) the rate of distribution of the drug through the body and the site or sites and duration of the drug's residence; (*c*) the rate, primary and secondary sites, the mechanism of the drug's metabolism in the body, and the chemistry and pharmacology of any metabolites; and (*d*) the proportion of administered dose eliminated from the body and its rate and route of elimination. In these studies, a minimum of two animal species are employed (generally the same as used in the pharmacologic and toxicologic studies), a rodent and one other, usually a dog.

The biochemical transformation or metabolism of drug substances is the body's means of transforming nonpolar drug molecules into polar compounds, which are more readily eliminated. Specific and nonspecific enzymes participate in drug metabolism, primarily in the liver but also in the kidneys, lungs, and gastrointestinal tract. Drugs that enter the hepatic circulation after absorption from the gut, as after oral administration, are particularly exposed to rapid drug metabolism. This transit through the liver and exposure to the hepatic enzyme system is termed the first-pass effect. If the first-pass effect is to be avoided, other routes of administration (buccal, rectal) may be used that allow the drug to be absorbed into the systemic circulation through blood vessels other than hepatic.

Drug metabolism or biotransformation frequently results in the production of one or more metabolites of the administered drug, some of which may be pharmacologically active compounds, whereas others may not. As noted previously, drug metabolism may be essential to convert prodrugs to active compounds. For reasons of safety, it is important to determine whether a drug's metabolic products are toxic or nontoxic to the animal and later to the human. When metabolites are found, they are chemically and biologically characterized for activity and toxicity. Some new drugs have been discovered as metabolic by-products, or metabolites, of parent compounds.

ADME studies are performed through the timely collection and analysis of urine, blood, and fecal samples and through a careful examination of animal tissues and organs upon autopsy. In addition, special studies are undertaken to determine the presence, if any, of a test drug or its metabolites in the milk of lactating animals; the ability of the drug to cross the placental barrier and enter the fetal blood supply; and the long-term retention of drugs or metabolites in the body. In studying the formation and disposition of metabolites, a radioactive label is commonly incorporated into the administered compound and traced in the animal's waste products and tissues.

The relationship between ADME and drug product development is discussed in Chapter 5.

Toxicology

Toxicology deals with the adverse or undesired effects of drugs. Although the ability to predict the safe use of a new drug in humans based on preclinical animal studies is desirable, it is not entirely achievable. The direct extrapolation of preclinical animal safety data to humans is difficult because of species variation, different dose–response relationships, immunologic differences, subjective reactions that are not deducible in animals (such as headache), and other reasons. Although many adverse reactions in humans cannot be predicted in advance through animal studies, the greater the number of animal species tested that demonstrate a toxic effect, the greater the likelihood that the effect will also be seen in humans.

In drug development programs, preclinical drug safety evaluation or toxicity studies are undertaken to determine (*a*) the substance's potential for toxicity with short-term (acute effects) or long-term use (chronic effects); (*b*) the substance's potential for specific organ toxicity; (*c*)

the mode, site, and degree of toxicity; (*d*) dose–response relationships for low, high, and intermediate doses over a specified time; (*e*) gender, reproductive, or teratogenic toxicities; and (*f*) the substance's carcinogenic and genotoxic potential.

As a part of an application to initiate human studies (IND), the FDA requires an integrated summary of the toxicological effects of the drug in animals and in vitro. Depending on the nature of the drug, the application is required to include the results of acute, subacute, and chronic toxicity tests; tests of the drug's effects on reproduction and the developing fetus; and any special toxicity test related to the drug's particular mode of administration or conditions of use, for example, inhalation, dermal, or ocular toxicology (9,29,30).

Acute or Short-Term Toxicity Studies

These studies are designed to determine the toxic effects of a test compound when administered in a single dose and/or in multiple doses over a short period, usually a single day. Although various routes of administration may be used (such as lavage dosing via gastric tube), the studies should be conducted to represent the intended route for human use.

The test compound is administered at various dose levels, with toxic signs observed for onset, progression or reversal, severity, mortality, and rates of incidence. Doses are ranged to find the largest single dose of the test compound that will not produce a toxic effect, the dose level at which severe toxicity occurs, and intermediate toxicity levels. The animals are observed and compared with controls for eating and drinking habits, weight change, toxic effects, psychomotor changes, and any other signs of untoward effects, usually over a 30-day postdose period. Feces and urine specimens are collected and clinical laboratory tests are performed to detect changes in clinical chemistry and other changes that could indicate toxicity. When they occur, animal deaths are recorded, studied by histology and pathology, and statistically evaluated on the basis of dose–response, gender, age, and intraspecies and interspecies findings and against laboratory controls.

Subacute or Subchronic Studies

In designing an animal toxicology program, relationships to projected human clinical studies for safety must be considered. For example, animal toxicity studies of a minimum of 2 weeks of daily drug administration at three or more dosage levels to two animal species are required to support the initial administration of a single dose in human clinical testing (8). These studies are termed subacute or subchronic. The initial human dose is usually one-tenth of the highest nontoxic dose (in milligrams per kilogram of subject's weight) shown during the animal studies. For drugs intended to be given to humans for a week or more, animal studies of 90 to 180 days must demonstrate safety. These are termed chronic toxicity studies. And if the drug

FIGURE 2.5. A researcher examining research data. (Courtesy of ARL BioPharma, Inc. d/b/a Analytical Research Laboratories.)

is to be used for a chronic human illness, animal studies for 1 year or longer must be undertaken to support human use. Some animal toxicity studies last 2 years or longer and may be used to corroborate findings obtained during the course of the human clinical trials.

Included in the subchronic and chronic studies are comparative data of test and control animal species, strain, sex, age, dose levels and ranges, routes of administration, duration of treatment, observed effects, mortality, body weight changes, food and water consumption, physical examinations (e.g., electrocardiography, ophthalmic examination), hematology, clinical chemistry, organ weights, gross pathology, neoplastic pathology, histopathology, urinalysis, ADME data, and other factors. Figure 2.5 shows a toxicologist examining research data of body weight changes during preclinical rodent studies.

Carcinogenicity Studies

Carcinogenicity testing is usually a component of chronic testing and is undertaken when the compound has shown sufficient promise as a drug to enter human clinical trials. Carcinogenicity studies are usually carried out in a limited number of rat and mouse strains for which there is reasonable information on spontaneous tumor incidence.

Dose-ranging studies are done with female and male animals using high, intermediate, and low doses over a 90-day period. For carcinogenicity studies, the high dose should be only high enough (the maximum tolerated dose) to elicit signs of minimal toxicity without significantly altering the animal's normal life span by effects other than carcinogenicity (31).

Carcinogenicity studies are long term (18 to 24 months), with surviving animals killed and studied at defined weeks during the test period. Data on the causes of animal death (other than killing), tumor incidence, type and site, and necropsy findings are collected and evaluated. Any preneoplastic lesions and/or tissue-specific proliferative effects are important findings.

Reproduction Studies

Reproduction studies are undertaken to reveal any effect of an active ingredient on mammalian reproduction. Included in these studies are fertility and mating behavior; early embryonic, prenatal, and postnatal development; multigenerational effects; and teratology. The combination of studies allows exposure from conception to sexual maturity and allows immediate and latent effects to be detected through complete life cycles and through successive generations.

In these studies, the maternal parent, fetus, neonates, and weaning offspring are evaluated for anatomic abnormalities, growth, and development. The same species of animal used in other toxicity studies are used in reproductive studies, usually the rat. In embryotoxicity studies only, a second mammalian species traditionally has been required.

In reproductive studies, as is the case for other toxicity studies, the doses selected and the routes of administration used are critical. A high dose, based on previous acute and chronic toxicity and pharmacokinetic studies, is selected, with lower dosages chosen in descending sequence. Setting close dosage intervals is useful to reveal trends in dose-related toxicity. Although once-daily dosing is usual, the drug's pharmacokinetics may influence the frequency of dosing (32). The route or routes of administration used should be similar to those intended for human use. A single route of administration may be acceptable if it can be shown that a similar drug distribution (kinetic profile) results from different routes of administration.

Genotoxicity or Mutagenicity Studies

Genotoxicity studies are performed to determine whether the test compound can affect gene mutation or cause chromosome or DNA damage. Strains of *Salmonella typhimurium* are routinely used in assays to detect mutations (9,33).

▌ EARLY FORMULATION STUDIES

As a promising compound is characterized for biologic activity, it is also evaluated with regard to chemical and physical properties that have a bearing on its ultimate and successful formulation into a stable and effective pharmaceutical product. This is the area of responsibility of pharmaceutical scientists and formulation pharmacists. When sufficient information is gleaned on the compound's physical and chemical properties, initial formulations of the dosage form are developed for use in human clinical trials. During the course of the clinical trials, the proposed product is developed further, from initial formulation to final formulation and from pilot plant (or small-scale production) to scale-up, in preparation for large-scale manufacturing.

To provide sufficient quantities of the bulk chemical (drug) compound for the sequence of preclinical studies, clinical trials, and small-scale and large-scale dosage form production, the careful planning, scheduling, and implementation of the bulk chemical's production must be undertaken by chemical engineers. Quality control and validation must be built into each step of the process.

Full documentation of the CMCs is an essential part of all drug applications filed with the FDA (1,34).

Preformulation Studies

Each drug substance has intrinsic chemical and physical characteristics that must be considered before the development of a pharmaceutical formulation. Among these are the drug's solubility, partition coefficient, dissolution rate, physical form, and stability. These and other factors, discussed in detail in Chapter 4 and in the Physical Pharmacy Capsules throughout the text, are briefly noted here as an introduction to their importance in the preparation of dosage forms for drug evaluation in human clinical trials and in the development of a final product submitted to the FDA for marketing approval. The FDA's protocols seek to correlate in vitro drug product dissolution and in vivo bioavailability, because drug dissolution and gastrointestinal permeability are the fundamental parameters controlling the rate and extent of drug absorption (35).

Drug Solubility

A drug substance administered by any route must possess some aqueous solubility for systemic absorption and therapeutic response. Poorly soluble compounds (e.g., <10 mg/mL aqueous solubility) may exhibit incomplete, erratic, and/or slow absorption and thus produce a minimal response at desired dosage. Enhanced aqueous solubility may be achieved by preparing more soluble derivatives of the parent compound, such as salts or esters, by chemical complexation, or by reducing the drug's particle size.

Partition Coefficient

To produce a pharmacologic response, a drug molecule must first cross a biologic membrane of protein and lipid, which acts as a lipophilic barrier to many drugs. The ability of a drug molecule to penetrate this barrier is based in part on its preference for lipids (lipophilic) versus its preference for an aqueous phase (hydrophilic). A drug's partition coefficient is a measure of its distribution in a lipophilic-hydrophilic phase system and indicates its ability to penetrate biologic multiphase systems.

Dissolution Rate

The speed at which a drug substance dissolves in a medium is called its dissolution rate. Dissolution rate data, when considered along with data on a drug's solubility, dissolution constant, and partition coefficient, can provide an indication of the drug's absorption potential. For a chemical entity, its acid, base, or salt forms, as well as its physical form (e.g., particle size), may result in substantial differences in the dissolution rate.

Physical Form

The crystal or amorphous forms and/or the particle size of a powdered drug can affect the dissolution rate, and thus the rate and extent of absorption, for a number of drugs. For example, by reducing the particle size and increasing the powder fineness and therefore the surface area of a poorly soluble drug, its dissolution rate in the gut is enhanced (through greater exposure of the drug to gastrointestinal fluid) and its biologic absorption increased. Small and controlled particle size is also critical for drugs administered to the lung by inhalation. The smaller the particle, the deeper is the penetration into the alveoli. Thus, by selective control of the physical parameters of a drug, biologic response may be optimized.

Stability

The chemical and physical stability of a drug substance alone, and when combined with formulation components, is critical to preparing a successful pharmaceutical product. For a given drug, one type of crystal structure may provide greater stability than other structures and may therefore be preferred. For drugs susceptible to oxidative decomposition, the addition of antioxidant stabilizing agents to the formulation may be required to protect the potency. For drugs destroyed by hydrolysis, protection against moisture in formulation, processing, and packaging may be required to prevent decomposition. In every case, drug stability testing at various temperatures, conditions of relative humidity (RH)—as 40°C 75% RH/30°C 60% RH—durations, and environments of light, air, and packaging is essential in assessing drug and drug product stability. Such information is vital in developing label instructions for use and storage, assigning product expiration dating, and packaging and shipping.

Initial Product Formulation and Clinical Trial Materials

An initial product is formulated using the information gained during the preformulation studies and with the consideration of the dose or doses, dosage form, and route of administration desired for the clinical studies and for the proposed marketed product. Thus, depending upon the design of the clinical protocol and desired final product, formulation pharmacists are called upon to develop a specific dosage form (e.g., capsule, suppository, solution) of one or more dosage strengths for administration by the intended route of administration (e.g., oral, rectal, intravenous). Additional dosage forms for other than the initial route of administration may later be developed, depending on patients' requirements, therapeutic utility, and marketing assessments. This is especially important if the drug may be administered to children.

The initial formulations prepared for Phase 1 and Phase 2 of the clinical trials, although not as sophisticated and elegant as the final formulation, should be of high pharmaceutical quality; meet analytical specifications for composition, manufacturing, and control; and be sufficiently stable for the period of use.

Often during Phase 1 studies, for orally administered drugs, capsules are employed containing the active ingredient alone, without pharmaceutical excipients. Excipients are included in the formulation for Phase 2 trials. During human trials, studies of the drug's ADME are undertaken to obtain a profile of the drug's human pharmacokinetics and biologic availability from the formulation administered. Different formulations may be prepared and examined to develop the one having the desired characteristics. During Phase 2, the final dosage form is selected and developed for Phase 3 trials; this is the formulation that is submitted to the FDA for marketing approval.

Clinical supplies or clinical trial materials comprise all dosage formulations used in the clinical evaluation of a new drug. This includes the proposed new drug, placebos (inert substances), and drug products against which the new drug is to be compared (comparator drugs or drug products). They all must be prepared in indistinguishable dosage forms (look alike, taste alike, and so on) and packaged with coded labels to reduce possible bias when blinded studies are called for in the clinical protocol. Blinded studies are controlled studies in which at least one of the parties (e.g., patient, physician) does not know which product is being administered. At the conclusion of the clinical study, the codes for the products administered are broken and the clinical results statistically evaluated. Some studies are open label, in which case, all parties may know what products are administered.

Some pharmaceutical companies have special units for the preparation, analytical control, coding, packaging, labeling, shipping, and record maintenance of clinical supplies. Other companies integrate this activity within their existing drug product development and production operations. Still other companies employ contract firms specializing in this field to prepare and manage their clinical trial materials program.

In all clinical study programs, the package label of the investigational drug must bear the statement "Caution: new drug—limited by federal [or United States] law to investigational use." Once received by the investigator, the clinical supplies may be administered only to subjects in the study. Blister packaging is commonly used in clinical studies, with immediate labels containing the clinical study or protocol number; patient identification number; sponsor number; directions for use; code number to distinguish between investigational drug, placebo, and/or comparator product; and other relevant information. Records of the disposition of the drug must be maintained by patient number, dates, and quantities administered. When there is a department of pharmacy at the site of the clinical study (e.g., university teaching hospital), pharmacists frequently assist in the control and management of clinical supplies. When an investigation is terminated, suspended, discontinued, or complete, all unused clinical supplies must be returned to the sponsor and an accounting made of used and unused products.

All formulations, from those developed initially through the final marketed version, must be prepared under the conditions and procedures set out by the FDA in its Current Good Manufacturing Practice guidelines (36), as outlined in Chapter 3.

THE INVESTIGATIONAL NEW DRUG APPLICATION

Under the Food, Drug, and Cosmetic Act as amended, the sponsor of a new drug is required to file with the FDA an IND before the drug may be given to human subjects (1). This is to protect the rights and safety of the subjects and to ensure that the investigational plan is sound and is designed to achieve the stated objectives. The sponsor of an IND takes responsibility for and initiates a clinical investigation. The sponsor may be an individual (a sponsor–investigator), a pharmaceutical company, governmental agency, academic institution, or some other private or public organization. The sponsor may actually conduct the study or employ, designate, or contract other qualified persons to do so. Nowadays, many contract research organizations conduct all or designated portions of clinical studies or clinical drug trials for others through contractual arrangements.

After submission of the IND, the sponsor must delay the use of the drug in human subjects for not less than 30 days from the date the FDA acknowledges the receipt of the application. An IND automatically goes into effect following this period unless the FDA notifies the sponsor that as a result of its review of the submission, it is waiving the period and the sponsor may initiate the study early or the investigation is being placed on a clinical hold (37).

A *clinical hold* is an order issued by the FDA to delay the start of a clinical investigation or to suspend an ongoing study. During a clinical hold, the investigational drug may not be administered to human subjects (unless specifically permitted by the FDA for individual patients in an ongoing study). A clinical hold is issued when there is concern that human subjects will be exposed to unreasonable and significant risk of illness or injury, when there is a question of the qualifying credentials of the clinical investigators, or when the IND is considered incomplete, inaccurate, or misleading. If the concerns raised are addressed to the FDA's satisfaction, a clinical hold may be lifted and clinical investigations resumed; if not, an IND may be maintained in a clinical hold, declared inactive, withdrawn by the sponsor, or terminated by the FDA.

Content of the IND

The content of an IND is prescribed in the CFR and is submitted under a cover sheet (Form FDA-1571) (38).

Among the items required

- Name, address, and telephone number of the sponsor of the drug
- Date of submission
- Name(s) of the drug, including all available names (generic, trade name, chemical, code)
- IND number (if one has been previously assigned)
- Indications for the proposed drug's use
- Indication of whether the application is a new submission, a response to a clinical hold, or an amendment to a previously submitted IND application
- Name and title of the person responsible for monitoring the conduct and progress of the investigation
- Names and titles of the persons responsible for the review and evaluation of the information relevant to the safety of the drug
- Name and address of any contract research organization involved in the study
- Identification of the phase or phases of the clinical investigation to be conducted
- Introductory statement and general investigational plan: the name of the drug and all active ingredients, the drug's structural formula and pharmacologic class, the formulation of the dosage form and route of administration, and the broad objectives and planned duration of the study
- Description of the investigational plan: the rationale for the drug or research study, the indication or indications to be studied, the approach to evaluating the drug, the types of studies to be conducted, the estimated number of subjects to be given the drug, and any serious risks anticipated based on animal studies or other human experiences with the drug
- Brief summary of previous human experience with the drug (domestic or foreign), including the reasons if the drug has been withdrawn from any other investigation and/or marketing
- CMC information: a complete description of the drug substance, including its physical, chemical, and biologic characteristics; its method of preparation and analytical methods to ensure its identity, strength, quality, purity, and stability; a quantitative list of the active and inactive components of the dosage form to be administered; the methods, facilities, and controls employed in the manufacture, processing, packaging, and labeling

of the new drug to ensure appropriate qualitative and quantitative standards; and product stability during the clinical investigation
- Pharmacology and toxicology information: the drug's mechanism of action if known; information on the drug's absorption, distribution, metabolism, and excretion; and acute, subacute, chronic, and reproductive and developmental toxicity studies
- If the new drug is a combination of previously investigated components, a complete preclinical and clinical summary of these components when administered singly and any data or expectations relating to the effect when combined
- Clinical protocol for each planned study
- Commitment that an institutional review board (IRB) has approved the clinical study and will continue to review and monitor the investigation (discussed in the next section)
- Investigator brochure (discussed in the next section)
- Indication if any part of the study is to be conducted by a contract research organization and, if so, the name and address of that organization
- Commitment not to begin clinical investigations until the IND is in effect, the signature of the sponsor or authorized representative, and the date of the signed application

The Clinical Protocol

As a part of the IND application, a clinical protocol must be submitted to ensure the appropriate design and conduct of the investigation. Clinical protocols include the following:

- Statement of the purpose and objectives of the study
- Outline of the investigational plan and study design, including the kind of control group and methods to minimize bias on the part of the subjects, investigators, and analysts
- Estimate of the number of patients to be involved
- Basis for subject selection, with inclusion and exclusion criteria
- Description of the dosing plan, including dose levels, route of administration, and duration of patient exposure
- Description of the patient observations, measurements, and tests to be used
- Clinical procedures, laboratory tests, and monitoring to be used in minimizing patient risk
- Names, addresses, and credentials of the principal investigators and coinvestigators
- Locations and descriptions of the clinical research facilities to be used
- Approval of the authorized IRB

Once an IND is in effect, a sponsor must submit an amendment for approval of any proposed changes. This may involve changes of dosing levels, testing procedures, the addition of new investigators, additional sites for the study, and so on.

For many years, women and the elderly were included only rarely in clinical drug investigations. Women of childbearing age were excluded from early drug tests out of fear that the subject would become pregnant during the investigation with possible harm to the fetus. Exceptions were made only in cases of potentially lifesaving drugs. However, in recognition that the general exclusion of women from drug investigations results in inadequate data on any gender-based differences in a drug's effects, the FDA now calls for the inclusion of women in numbers adequate to allow detection of clinically significant differences in drug response.

The FDA Guideline for the Study and Evaluation of Gender Differences in the Clinical Evaluation of Drugs issued in 1993 states the agency's gender inclusion policy (39). Although the guideline does not require participation of women in any particular trial, it sets forth FDA's general expectations regarding the inclusion of both women and men in drug development, analysis of clinical data by gender, and assessment of potential pharmacokinetic differences between genders. In 1994, the National Institutes of Health (NIH) similarly issued its policy that women and minorities be included in all NIH-supported biomedical and behavioral research projects involving human subjects "unless there is a clear and compelling rationale and justification that their inclusion is inappropriate with respect to the health of the subjects or the purpose of the research" (40).

Pregnancy is a concern in drug investigations because drugs are readily transported from the maternal to the fetal circulation. Because of undeveloped drug detoxication and excretion mechanisms in the fetus, concentrations of drugs may actually reach a higher level in the fetus than in the maternal circulation, with toxic levels resulting. To reduce the risk of fetal exposure to investigational drugs in women of childbearing age, the FDA guideline calls for pregnancy testing, use of contraception, and full information disclosure of potential fetal risks to prospective study subjects. The FDA has made a special effort to ensure that women who have a life-threatening disease (e.g., AIDS-related) are not automatically excluded from investigational trials of drug products for that disease because of a perceived risk of reproductive or developmental toxicity from use of the investigational drug. There are other instances in which drug studies or drug use during pregnancy is justified, for example, agents intended to prevent Rh immunization and hemolytic disease of the newborn (41).

When a proposed drug is likely to have significant use in the elderly, elderly patients are required to be included in clinical studies to yield age-related data of a drug's effectiveness and any adverse effects. Older people handle a drug differently because of altered body functions such as diminished liver and kidney function, reduced circulation, and changes in drug ADME. Furthermore, the elderly have a greater incidence of chronic illness and multiple disease states than younger adults and, as a result, take multiple medications daily, increasing the potential for drug–drug interactions. This potential is studied and defined.

Recognition of the need to examine in children new drugs intended for the pediatric patient has a similar requirement to ensure a drug's safe and effective use in this population. Also, differentiation in a drug's activity in minority groups and their subpopulations is important in the full assessment of a drug's potential. It is well known that there are interethnic variations both in disease incidence and in biologic response to some medications, and these factors must be considered in the clinical evaluation of drug substances (42).

Each IND submission must have the prior approval of the IRB with jurisdiction over the site of the proposed clinical investigation. An IRB is a body of professional and public members that has the responsibility for reviewing and approving any study involving human subjects in the institution they serve. The purpose of the IRB is to protect the safety of human subjects by assessing a proposed clinical protocol, evaluating the benefits against risks, and ensuring that the plan includes all needed measures for subject protection. By law, the IRB shall be constituted to include persons competent to review clinical research proposals and be diverse in membership, with consideration of race, gender, cultural background, and sensitivity to issues affecting the subjects and the community (43). Any substantive change or amendment to an originally approved clinical protocol must be submitted, reviewed, and approved by the IRB and the FDA before implementation.

Each clinical investigator must receive from the sponsor an investigator's brochure, which contains all of the pertinent information developed during the preclinical studies, including summary information on the drug's chemistry, pharmacology, toxicology, and pharmacokinetics; formulation of the clinical trial materials; any known information related to the drug's safety and effectiveness; a description of possible risks and side effects that may be anticipated and special monitoring required; the clinical protocol and study design; criteria for patient inclusion and exclusion; laboratory and clinical tests to be performed; and drug control and record-keeping information.

Each study has defined criteria for subject inclusion or exclusion. These criteria may relate to age, sex (as qualified earlier), smoking, health status (e.g., liver and/or renal function), and other factors deemed necessary in a given phase of investigation. Each subject in a clinical investigation must participate willingly and with full knowledge of the benefits and risks associated with the investigation.

The sponsor of the study must certify that each person who will receive the investigational drug has given informed consent—that is, he or she has been informed of the following: participation in the study is voluntary; the purpose and nature of the study; the procedures involved; a description of any foreseeable risks or discomforts; the potential benefits for patients; disclosure of alternative procedures or courses of treatments, if any; the extent of confidentiality of records; conditions under which the subject's participation in the study may be terminated; consequences of a patient's decision to withdraw from the study; the approximate number of subjects to be enrolled; and whom to contact for answers to pertinent questions and/or in case of research-related illness or injury. These elements of informed consent, and additional protections that apply to prisoners in clinical investigations, must be in conformance with the CFR (44). Individuals who agree to be subjects in an investigation indicate their consent by signing the form or document containing this information.

Investigators selected by the sponsor to conduct a clinical investigation must be qualified as experts by training and experience to investigate a particular drug. Each investigator's qualifications are submitted to the FDA as a part of the IND application. To participate in an investigation, each investigator signs a form agreeing to comply with and to be responsible for ensuring that the study is conducted according to the IND's investigational plan and clinical protocol; protecting the rights, safety, and welfare of the human subjects; control of the investigational drug; written records of case histories and clinical observations; and the timely submission of progress reports, safety reports, and a final report. It is the responsibility of the sponsor to monitor the progress of all clinical investigations under its IND. If a sponsor discovers that an investigator is not in compliance with the investigational plan, it is the sponsor's responsibility to gain compliance or to terminate the investigator's participation in the study.

Any serious, unexpected, life-threatening, or fatal adverse experience that may be associated with the use of the drug during a clinical investigation must be reported promptly to the sponsor and subsequently to the FDA for investigation. Depending on the severity and assessment of the adverse experience, an alert notice may be sent to other investigators, a clinical hold may be placed on the study for further evaluation and assessment, or the IND may be withdrawn by the sponsor, placed on inactive status, or terminated by the FDA.

Pre-IND Meetings

On request, the FDA will advise a sponsor on scientific, technical, or formatting concerns relating to the preparation and submission of an IND. This may include advice on the adequacy of data to support an investigational plan, the design of a clinical trial, or whether the proposed investigation is likely to produce the data needed to meet the requirements of the next step, the filing of an NDA to gain approval for marketing.

FDA Review of an IND Application

The FDA's objectives in reviewing an IND are to protect the safety and rights of the human subjects and to help ensure that the study allows the evaluation of the drug's safety and effectiveness. These objectives are best met by the accuracy and completeness of the IND submission, the design and conduct of the investigational plan, and the expertise and diligence of the investigators.

When received by the FDA, the IND submission is stamped with the date of receipt, assigned an application number, and forwarded to either the Center for Drug Evaluation and Research (CDER) or the Center for Biologics Evaluation and Research (CBER) for review. Applications for chemical agents are sent to CDER and applications for biologics to CBER.

Within CDER, applications are forwarded to the appropriate office of drug evaluation and then to one of its divisions for review (45).

After assignment to one of the divisions, the content of the application is thoroughly reviewed to determine whether the preclinical data indicate that the drug is sufficiently safe for administration to human subjects and that the proposed clinical studies are designed to provide the desired data on drug safety and efficacy while not exposing the human subjects to unnecessary risks.

Although the discussion in this chapter is based principally on the evaluation and approval of new chemical entities and products, for biologic products, there is a similar but necessarily distinct procedure of application review and product licensing for biologics through CBER and its divisions (4).

FDA Drug Classification System

The FDA's CDER has established a drug classification system for the review of drug applications. Within 14 days of receipt of an original new drug or new biologic application, the agency determines whether the application will receive a *Priority (P) Review* or a *Standard (S) Review* (45). A priority review is considered if the proposed drug product provides a significant improvement compared to marketed products or provides safe and effective therapy where no satisfactory alternative therapy exists.

Phases of a Clinical Investigation

An IND may be submitted for one or more phases of a clinical investigation, namely, Phase 1, Phase 2, or Phase 3 (Fig. 2.2; Table 2.1). Although the phases are conducted sequentially, certain studies may overlap.

Phase 1 includes the initial introduction of an investigational drug into humans and is primarily for the purpose of assessing safety. The studies are closely monitored by clinicians expert in such investigations. The human subjects are usually healthy volunteers, although, in certain protocols, they may be patients. The total number of subjects included in Phase 1 studies varies with the drug but is usually in the range of 20 to 100. The initial dose of the drug is usually low, usually one-tenth of the highest no-effect dose observed during the animal studies. If the first dose is well tolerated, the investigation continues with the administration of progressively greater doses (to new subjects) until some evidence of the drug's effects is observed.

TABLE 2.1. Testing in Humans

Phase	Number of Patients	Length	Purpose	Percentage of Drugs Successfully Tested
Phase 1	20–100	Up to 1 year	Mainly safety	70%
Phase 2	100–500	Several months to 2 years	Some short-term safety but mainly effectiveness	33%
Phase 3	1,000–5,000	1–4 years	Safety, effectiveness, dosage	25%–30%

For example, of 100 drugs for which investigational new drug applications are submitted to the FDA, about 70% will clear Phase 1 and go on to Phase 2. About 33 of the original 100 drugs will clear Phase 2 and go on to Phase 3. About 25 to 30 of the original 100 drugs will clear Phase 3 and go on to Phase 4. Finally, on average, 20 of the original 100 drugs ultimately will be approved for marketing. www.centerwatch.com/clinical-trials/overview.aspx

Reproduced from © 2006, North Carolina Association for Biomedical Research (NCABR). Mapping Your Future: Careers in Biomanufacturing, 2014. Available at: http://www.ncabr.org/wp-content/uploads/2015/12/mapping-your-future.pdf.

Phase 1 studies are designed to determine the human pharmacology of the drug, structure–activity relationships, side effects associated with increasing doses, and, if possible, early evidence of effectiveness. Among the basic data collected are the rate of absorption; the concentration of drug in the blood over time; the rate and mechanism of drug metabolism and elimination; toxic effects, if any, in body tissues and major organs; and changes in physiologic processes from baseline. The subjects' ability to tolerate the drug and any unpleasant effects of the drug is observed and recorded. Phase 1 studies are often useful in selecting from among different chemical analogs of a lead compound. As noted previously, capsules without excipients are used for orally administered drugs in Phase 1 studies. If the studies demonstrate sufficient merit and if the order of drug toxicity is low, Phase 2 begins, studying up to several hundred patients.

Phase 2 trials are controlled clinical studies to evaluate the effectiveness of a drug in patients with the condition for which the drug is intended and to assess side effects and risks that may be revealed. Because this phase uses patients as subjects, side effects or toxicity symptoms that were not shown in the preclinical animal studies or in Phase 1 studies with healthy volunteers may be revealed for the first time. Only clinicians expert in the disease being treated are used as investigators during Phase 2 studies (Fig. 2.6). During this phase, additional data are collected on the drug's pharmacokinetics and studies undertaken to determine dose–response and dose ranging (often called Phase 2a studies). Each patient is monitored for the appearance of the drug's effects while the dose is carefully increased to determine the minimal effective dose. Then, the dose is extended beyond the minimally effective dose to the level at which a patient reveals extremely undesirable or intolerable toxic or adverse effects. The greater the range between the dose of the drug determined to be minimally effective and that which causes severe side effects, the greater is the drug's safety margin. These dose determination studies (often called Phase 2b studies) result in the specific doses and the dose range to be used in Phase 3 studies. During Phase 2 trials, the drug product is refined, with the final formulation developed for use during late Phase 2 and Phase 3 trials.

If the clinical results of Phase 2 trials indicate continued promise for the new drug and if the margin of safety appears to be good, end-of-Phase 2 meetings between the drug's sponsor and the FDA's review division are held to analyze the data from Phases 1 and 2. This resolves any questions and issues and to establish investigational plans for Phase 3 studies.

Phase 3 studies may include several hundred to several thousand patients in controlled and uncontrolled trials. The objective is to determine the usefulness of the drug in an expanded patient base. Many additional clinicians having patients with the condition for drug's intended use are recruited to participate in this trial. Several dosage strengths of the proposed drug may be evaluated during this phase, using formulations intended to be proposed in the NDA and for marketing. Sufficient information on the drug's effectiveness and safety is expected to be gathered during Phase 3 to evaluate the overall benefit–risk relationship of the drug and to file a complete NDA.

It is fairly common for certain Phase 3 studies to be continued after an NDA is filed but prior to approval. In these instances, the completed studies (Phase 3a studies) are considered sufficient for the NDA. The additional studies (Phase 3b studies) are used to gather supplemental

FIGURE 2.6. Equipment for monitoring the effects for cardiac function of a patient (Ex. As part of an investigational drug clinical evaluation). (Courtesy of Pulsar Imagens/Alamy Stock Photo.)

information that may support certain labeling requests, provide information on patients' quality of life issues, reveal product advantages over already marketed competing drugs, provide evidence in support of possible additional drug indications, or provide other clues for prospective postmarketing studies (Phase 4).

Clinical Study Controls and Designs

As indicated, Phase 2 and some Phase 3 studies are controlled, that is, the effects of the investigational drug are compared with another agent. The second agent may be a placebo (placebo control) or an active drug (positive control), a standard or comparator drug product. Both a placebo and an active drug may be used as controls in the same study. For studies that are blinded, the identities of the investigational drug and the control or controls are not revealed to certain participants to decrease bias. In single-blind studies, the patient is unaware of the agent administered. In double-blind studies, neither the patient nor the clinician is aware of the agent administered. In preparing dosage forms for blinded studies, all of the agents administered, investigational drug, placebo, and/or comparator drug must be indistinguishable to the blinded individuals. This requires the preparation of clinical trial materials of the same dosage form, having the same size, shape, color, flavor, texture, and so forth. Indistinguishable clinical trial materials are not necessary for open-label studies, in which all parties are aware of the identities of the agents administered.

In designing a clinical trial, many additional factors are considered, including the scheme of the study design and the duration of the treatment period. Before treatment, baseline data are obtained on each subject through physical examination and appropriate laboratory tests and procedures. Subjects are randomly assigned to different treatment groups to allow treatment comparisons. Some common parallel and crossover study designs are depicted in Figure 2.7 (46). These studies may be blinded or not, using placebo and/or active drug controls. The parallel designs are applicable to most clinical trials. Crossover designs are useful in comparing different treatments within individuals because following one treatment, a patient is crossed over to a different treatment. Between treatment periods, subjects may be given no drugs as a washout period to allow return to baseline.

Drug Dosage and Terminology

A major part of any clinical drug study is the determination of a drug's safe and effective dose. As noted earlier, dose and dose-ranging studies are conducted during Phase 2 and concluded during Phase 3 clinical trials.

The safe and effective dose of a drug depends on a number of factors, including characteristics of the drug substance, the dosage form and its route of administration, and a variety of patient factors including age, body weight, general health status, any pathologic conditions, and

SOME CLINICAL TRIAL PARALLEL STUDY DESIGNS

1. COMMON PARALLEL DESIGNS

2. TWO-PART PARALLEL DESIGN

3. INTRODUCTION OF PLACEBO DURING TREATMENT

Treatment Group I	Placebo	Treatment Group I
Treatment Group II	Placebo	Treatment Group II
Treatment Group III	Placebo	Treatment Group III

4. MULTIPLE DOSES WITHIN EACH TREATMENT GROUP

| Treatment Group I | Dose A | Dose B | Dose C | Dose D |
| Treatment Group II | Dose E | Dose F | Dose G | Dose H |

SOME CLINICAL TRIAL CROSSOVER STUDY DESIGNS

1. SINGLE CROSSOVER WITH NO INTERVENING BASELINE

2. SINGLE CROSSOVER WITH INTERVENING BASELINE

3. EXTRA PERIOD CROSSOVER

FIGURE 2.7. Some common clinical study designs. (Reprinted from Spilker B. Guide to Clinical Trials. New York, NY: Raven, 1991, with permission.)

concomitant drug therapy. All of these factors and others are integral to clinical drug trials.

For convenience of dosage administration, most products are formulated to contain a drug's usual dose within a single unit (e.g., capsule) or within a specified volume (e.g., 5 mL or a teaspoonful) of a liquid dosage form. To serve varying dosage requirements, manufacturers often formulate a drug into more than one dosage form and in more than a single strength.

The dose of a drug may be described as an amount that is enough but not too much; the idea is to achieve the drug's optimum therapeutic effect with safety but at the lowest possible dose. The effective dose of a drug may be different for different patients. The familiar bell curve presented in Figure 2.8 shows that in a normal distribution sample, a drug's dose will provide what might be called an average effect in most individuals. However, in a portion of the population, the drug will produce little effect, and in another portion, the drug will produce an effect greater than average. The amount of drug that will produce the desired effect in most adult patients is considered the drug's usual adult dose and the likely starting dose for a patient. From this initial dose, the physician may, if necessary, increase or decrease subsequent doses to meet the particular requirements of the patient. Certain drugs may produce more than one effect, depending on the dose. For example, a low dose of a barbiturate produces sedation, whereas a larger dose produces hypnotic effects. The usual dosage range indicates the quantitative range or amounts of the drug that may be prescribed safely within the framework of usual medical practice. Doses falling outside of the usual range may result in underdosage or overdosage or may reflect a patient's special requirements. For drugs administered to children, a usual pediatric dose may be determined, as discussed later in this section.

The schedule of dosage, or the dosage regimen, is determined during the clinical investigation and is based largely on a drug's inherent duration of action, its pharmacokinetic profile, and the characteristics of the dosage form (e.g., immediate release or modified release). Because of these factors, some drugs are recommended for once-a-day dosage and others more frequently.

For certain drugs, an initial, priming, or loading dose may be required to attain the desired concentration of the drug in the blood or tissues, after which the blood level may be maintained through subsequent administration of regularly scheduled maintenance doses.

Certain biologic products, such as tetanus immune globulin, may have two usual doses, a prophylactic dose,

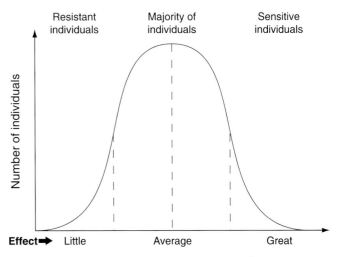

FIGURE 2.8. Drug effect in a population sample.

or the amount administered to protect the patient from contracting the illness, and the therapeutic dose, which is administered to a patient after exposure or contraction of the illness. The doses of vaccines and other biologic products often are expressed in units of activity rather than in specific quantitative amounts of the drug. This is because the unavailability of suitable chemical assay methods for the active biologic component necessitates the use of biologic assays to determine a product's potency.

To provide systemic effects, a drug must be absorbed from its route of administration at a suitable rate, be distributed in adequate concentration to the receptor sites, and remain there for a sufficient period. One measure of a drug's absorption characteristics is its blood serum concentration at various intervals after administration. Certain drugs have a correlation between blood serum concentration and the presentation of drug effects. For these drugs, an average blood serum concentration represents the minimum concentration that can be expected to produce the drug's desired effects in a patient. This concentration is the minimum effective concentration (MEC). As shown in Figure 2.9, the serum concentration of a hypothetical

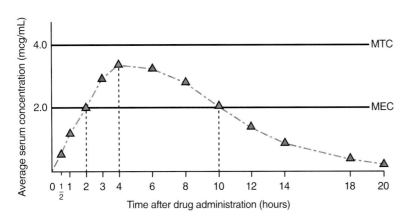

FIGURE 2.9. Example of a blood level curve for a hypothetical drug as a function of time following oral administration. MEC, minimum effective concentration; MTC, minimum toxic concentration.

drug reaches the MEC 2 hours after its administration, achieves a peak concentration in 4 hours, and decreases below the MEC in 10 hours. If it were desired to maintain the drug serum concentration above the MEC for a longer period, a second dose of the drug would be required at approximately 8 hours. The time–blood level curve presented in Figure 2.9 is hypothetical. In practice, the curve would vary, depending on the nature of the drug substance, its chemical and physical characteristics, the dosage form administered, and the individual patient factors. The second level of serum concentration of drug refers to the minimum toxic concentration (MTC). Drug serum concentrations above this level would be expected to produce dose-related toxic effects in the average individual. Ideally, the serum drug concentration in a well-dosed patient would be maintained between the MEC and the MTC (the therapeutic window for the drug) for the period that drug effects are desired. Table 2.2 presents examples of therapeutic, toxic, and considered lethal concentrations for some selected drug substances. The values in this table do not apply to infants and children. Further, the portrayed values should not be considered absolute but used as a guideline. Actual values of drugs can be influenced by a number of factors that are described later in this section. The median effective dose of a drug is the amount that will produce the desired intensity of effect in 50% of the individuals tested. The median toxic dose is the amount that will produce a defined toxic effect in 50% of the individuals tested. The relationship between the desired and undesired effects of a drug is commonly expressed as the therapeutic index and is defined as the ratio between a drug's median toxic dose and its median effective dose,

TD50/ED50. Thus, a drug with a therapeutic index of 15 would be expected to have a greater margin of safety in its use than a drug with a therapeutic index of 5. For certain drugs, the therapeutic index may be as low as 2, and extreme caution must be exercised in their administration. Table 2.3 demonstrates drugs and pharmacological classes of drugs that have narrow therapeutic indices and, therefore, should be monitored closely in patients receiving them. Some factors of patients considered in determining a drug's dose in clinical investigations and in medical practice include the following.

Age

The age of the patient may be a consideration in the determination of drug dosage. Age is particularly important in the treatment of neonatal, pediatric, and geriatric patients.

TABLE 2.3. Therapeutic Indices for Various Drug Substances

Less than 5	Between 5 and 10	Greater than 10
Amitriptyline	Barbiturates	Acetaminophen
Chlordiazepoxide	Diazepam	Bromide
Diphenhydramine	Digoxin	Chloral hydrate
Ethchlorvynol	Imipramine	Glutethimide
Lidocaine	Meperidine	Meprobamate
Methadone	Paraldehyde	Nortriptyline
Procainamide	Primidone	Pentazocine
Quinidine	Thioridazine	Propoxyphene

From Niazi S. Textbook of Biopharmaceutics and Clinical Pharmacokinetics. New York, NY: Appleton-Century-Crofts, 1979:254.

TABLE 2.2. Therapeutic and Toxic Blood Level Concentrations of Some Drug Substances

Drug Substance	Drug Substance Concentration, mg/L		
	Therapeutic	Toxic	Lethal
Acetaminophen	10–20	400	1,500
Amitriptyline	0.5–0.20	0.4	10–20
Barbiturates			
Short acting	1	7	10
Intermediate acting	1–5	10–30	30
Long acting	~10	40–60	80–150
Diazepam	0.5–2.5	5–20	50
Digoxin	0.0006–0.0013	0.002–0.009	—
Imipramine	0.05–0.16	0.7	2
Lidocaine	1.2–5.0	6	—
Lithium	4.2–8.3	13.9	13.9–34.7
Meperidine	0.6–0.65	5	30
Morphine	0.1	—	0.05–4
Phenytoin	5–22	50	100
Quinidine	3–6	10	30–50
Theophylline	20–100	—	—

Infants, especially newborns and those born prematurely, have immature hepatic and renal function, the means by which drugs are normally inactivated and eliminated from the body. A reduced capacity to detoxify and eliminate drugs can result in drug accumulation in the tissues to toxic levels. Often, drug blood levels are determined in these patients and are carefully monitored.

Before there was sufficient understanding of the capacity of the young to detoxify and eliminate drugs, infants and children were dosed by fractions of the adult dose determined by age-based or weight-based formulas. Age or weight alone is no longer considered to be a particularly valid criterion in the determination of pediatric dosage. Today, doses for many drugs are determined through pediatric clinical trials under special protocols and subject safeguards (47). Many pediatric doses are based on body weight or body surface area (BSA), as noted later in this section.

Elderly persons also present unique therapeutic and dosing problems that require special attention. Most physiologic functions begin to diminish in adults after the third decade of life. For example, cardiac output declines approximately 1% per year from age 20 to age 80. Glomerular filtration rate falls progressively until age 80, at which time it is only about half of what it was at age 20. Vital capacity, immune capacity, and liver microsomal enzyme function also decrease (48). The decline in renal and hepatic function in the elderly slows the drug clearance rate and increases the possibility of drug accumulation and toxicity. Elderly persons may also respond differently to drugs than do younger patients because of changes in drug receptor sensitivity or because of age-related alterations in target tissues or organs (49).

Furthermore, the chronic disorders in most geriatric patients require concomitant drug therapy, increasing the possibility of drug–drug interactions and adverse drug effects. In the clinical evaluation of a new drug, consideration is given to other drugs most likely to be taken concomitantly by the intended patient, with studies directed toward determining the potential drug–drug effects or interactions.

Among the references to assist the prescriber and pharmacist in neonatal, pediatric, and geriatric dosing are the following: *Pediatric and Neonatal Dosing* and *Geriatric Dosing* (50).

Pharmacogenetics

Pharmacogenetic research in the last two decades has uncovered significant differences among racial and ethnic groups in the metabolism, clinical effectiveness, and adverse effects of therapeutically important drugs. Clinical studies have been conducted on cardiovascular agents, for example, beta-blockers, diuretics, calcium channel blockers, ACE inhibitors, or psychotropic and central nervous system agents, for example, tricyclic antidepressants (51) and neuroleptics. Antihistamines, alcohol, and analgesics, for example, acetaminophen and codeine, have also demonstrated varying effects among different ethnic and racial populations. Common genetic polymorphisms, that is, multiple forms of enzymes governing drug metabolism, affect the clearance from the blood of many therapeutically important drugs used in large patient populations. These polymorphisms are the rule rather than the exception, and genetic diversity is a major source of interindividual, interethnic, and racial differences in drug response. These genetic polymorphisms may influence a drug's action by altering its pharmacokinetic profile and/or pharmacodynamic properties. The result could be an increase or a decrease in the intensity of the patient's response and duration of the drug activity. Thus, dosage adjustments may be necessary for individuals from minority populations.

Body Weight

The usual doses for drugs are considered generally suitable for 70-kg (150-lb) individuals. The ratio between the amount of drug administered and the size of the body influences drug concentration in body fluids. Therefore, drug dosage may require adjustment from the usual adult dose for abnormally lean or heavy patients. The doses for certain drugs are based on body weight and are expressed on a milligram (drug) per kilogram (body weight) basis (e.g., 1 mg/kg).

As noted earlier, body weight is considered more dependable than age as determinant of drug dosage for youngsters, and for many drugs, the dose is based on milligrams per kilogram. In some instances, a pediatric dose may be based on a combination of age and weight (e.g., 6 months to 2 years of age: 3 mg/kg/d).

Body Surface Area

Because of the correlation between a number of physiologic processes and BSA, some drug doses are based on this relationship (e.g., 1 mg/m^2 BSA). The BSA for a child or adult may be determined using a nomogram (Fig. 2.10). The BSA is determined at the intersect of a straight line drawn to connect an individual's height and weight. For example, an adult measuring 67 inches in height and weighing 132 lb would have a BSA of approximately 1.7 m^2.

Sex

Because biochemical and physiologic factors produce different responses to certain drugs and drug dosages in men and women, both sexes should be included in clinical drug trials. Pharmacokinetic differences between women and men may be particularly important for drugs having a narrow therapeutic index, in which the smaller average size of women may necessitate modified dosing. Drugs with narrow therapeutic indices carry the inherent risk that drug blood levels may increase to toxic levels or decrease to ineffective levels with minimal dosing changes. Other important studies on women include the effects of the menstrual cycle and menopausal status on a drug's

A Nomogram for Calculating the Body Surface Area of Children

B Nomogram for Calculating the Body Surface Area of Adults

FIGURE 2.10. Nomograms for calculating the BSA. **A:** For children. **B:** For adults. (From the formula of DuBois D, DuBois EF. A formula to estimate the approximate surface area if height and weight be known. Arch Intern Med 1916;17:863. S = W0.425 × H0.725 × 71.84, or log S = log W × 0.425 + log H × 0.725 + 1.8564, where S = body surface in square centimeters, W = weight in kilograms, H = height in centimeters.) (Reprinted from Novartis AG. Documenta Geigy Scientific Tables. 7th Ed. Basel: Ciba-Geigy, 1970:537–538, with permission.)

pharmacokinetics and the drug interaction potential of concomitant estrogen or oral contraceptive use (52).

Because virtually no clinical investigations have included pregnant women in their study protocols and thus drug effects are undetermined in these circumstances, great caution is advised for the use of most drugs during pregnancy and in women of childbearing age. Similar caution is applicable to drug use in nursing mothers because transfer from mother's milk to an infant is well documented for a variety of drugs (53,54).

Pathologic State

The effects of certain drugs may be modified by the pathologic condition of the patient. For example, if certain drugs are used in the presence of renal impairment, excessive systemic accumulation of the drug may occur, risking toxicity. In such conditions, lower than usual doses are indicated, and if therapy is prolonged, blood serum levels of the drug should be assessed and the patient monitored at regular intervals to ensure the maintenance of nontoxic levels of the drug. In these instances, pharmacokinetic dosing is an integral part of the clinical study protocol and of the approved product labeling.

Tolerance

The ability to endure the influence of a drug, particularly during continued use, is referred to as drug tolerance. It is usually developed to a specific drug and to its chemical congeners; in the latter instance, it is referred to as cross-tolerance. The result is that drug dosage must be increased over time to maintain a desired therapeutic response. Tolerance is common with the use of antihistamines and narcotic analgesics. After the development of tolerance, normal response may be regained by suspending the drug's administration for a while.

Concomitant Drug Therapy

The effects of a drug may be modified by the prior or concurrent administration of another drug. Such interference, a drug–drug interaction, may be due to a chemical or physical interaction between the drugs or to an alteration of the absorption, distribution, metabolism, or excretion patterns of one of the drugs. Certain clinical protocols include the evaluation of a new drug in the presence of other drugs most likely to be included in the target patient's therapeutic regimen.

Important drug–drug interactions that are identified during a drug's clinical trials are included in approved product labeling. Additional drug interactions that become known after the drug is marketed are added in labeling revisions. Drug–drug interactions may include "social" agents such as tobacco and alcohol, which affect the pharmacokinetics of a number of drugs and require an alteration in a drug's usual dose.

Time and Conditions of Administration

The time at which a drug is administered may influence the dosage. This is true especially for oral therapy in relation to meals. Absorption proceeds more rapidly if the stomach and the upper portions of the intestinal tract are empty of food. A dose of a drug that is effective when taken before a meal may be less effective if administered during or after eating. Drug–food interactions can affect a drug's usual absorption pattern. When such interactions are determined, appropriate guidance is provided in the product and professional literature.

Dosage Form and Route of Administration

The effective dose of a drug may vary with the dosage form and the route of administration. Drugs administered intravenously enter the bloodstream directly and completely. In contrast, drugs administered orally are rarely, if ever, fully absorbed into the bloodstream because of the various physical, chemical, and biologic barriers to their absorption. Thus, in many instances, a lower parenteral (injectable) dose of a drug is required than the oral dose to achieve the same blood levels or clinical effects. Varying rates and degrees of absorption can occur from drug administration in the rectum, in the gastrointestinal tract, under the tongue, via the skin, and to other sites. Therefore, for a given drug, different dosage forms and routes of administration are considered new by the FDA and must be evaluated individually through clinical studies to determine the effective doses.

Treatment IND

A treatment IND or a treatment protocol permits the use of an investigational drug in the treatment of patients who are not enrolled in the clinical study but who have a serious or immediately life-threatening disease for which there is no satisfactory alternative therapy. The objective is to make promising new drugs available to desperately ill patients as early as possible in the drug development process. By FDA definition, "immediately life-threatening" means "a stage of a disease in which there is a reasonable likelihood that death will occur within a matter of months or in which premature death is likely without early treatment" (1). This includes such conditions as advanced cases of AIDS, herpes simplex encephalitis, advanced metastatic refractory cancers, bacterial endocarditis, Alzheimer disease, advanced multiple sclerosis, advanced Parkinson disease, and others.

For products to be considered for a treatment IND, the drug must be under active investigation in a controlled clinical trial with sufficient evidence of its safety and efficacy demonstrated to support its use in the intended patients. Depending on the sponsor's clinical safety and efficacy data, a drug may be approved for treatment use during Phase 2 or Phase 3 of the clinical trials. In applying for a drug's treatment use, a sponsor must submit a treatment protocol in addition to the information normally included in an IND application. In making its decision, the FDA renders a risk–benefit judgment after considering the severity of the disease, any alternative therapy, and the potential benefits of the drug against the known and possible risks.

A "Group C" treatment IND was established by agreement between FDA and the National Cancer Institute (NCI). The Group C program is a means for the distribution of investigational agents to oncologists for the treatment of cancer under protocols outside the controlled clinical trial. Group C drugs are generally Phase 3 study drugs that have shown evidence of relative and reproducible efficacy in a specific tumor type. They can generally be administered by properly trained physicians without the need for specialized supportive care facilities. Group C drugs are distributed only by the NIH under NCI protocols. Although treatment is the primary objective and patients treated under Group C guidelines are not part of a clinical trial, safety and effectiveness data are collected. Because administration of Group C drugs is not done with research intent, FDA has generally granted a waiver from the IRB review requirements (55).

The need for an investigational drug may arise in an emergency situation that does not allow time for submission of an IND in the usual manner. In such cases, FDA may authorize an "emergency use IND" and shipment of the drug for a specified use. Such authorization is usually conditioned upon the sponsor filing an appropriate application as soon as practicable. Prospective IRB review and informed consent are required (55).

IND for an Orphan Drug

Under the Orphan Drug Act of 1983 as amended, an orphan disease is defined as a rare disease or condition that affects fewer than 200,000 people in the United States and for which there is no reasonable expectation that costs of R&D for the indication can be recovered by sales of the product in the United States. Examples of such illnesses are chronic lymphocytic leukemia, Gaucher disease, cystic fibrosis, and conditions related to AIDS.

The FDA Office of Orphan Products Development was established to identify and facilitate the development of orphan products, including drugs, biologics, and medical devices. To foster the necessary R&D, the FDA provides support grants to conduct clinical trials on safety and effectiveness. Applicants first request orphan status designation for the disease and file an IND or an investigational device exemption with their grant application. In most cases, grants are awarded for Phase 2 and Phase 3 clinical studies based on preliminary clinical research. Regular and treatment IND protocols may be included in orphan drug clinical trials. An incentive to orphan product development is a provision for a 7-year period of exclusive marketing rights after regulatory approval of a product.

Withdrawal or Termination of an IND

A sponsor may withdraw an IND at any time, ending all clinical investigations. All stock of clinical supplies must be returned to the sponsor or otherwise destroyed. If an IND is withdrawn for safety reasons, the FDA, IRB, and all investigators must be so advised.

If no subjects are entered in an IND for 2 years or more or if investigations remain on a clinical hold for 1 year or more, the FDA may place the IND on inactive status upon proper notification of the sponsor. An IND may also be placed on inactive status on the initiative of the sponsor.

The FDA may terminate an IND and end-related clinical investigations for reasons of safety, efficacy, or regulatory compliance.

CLINICAL STUDY REGISTRY

The National Library of Medicine (NLM) at the U.S. NIH at the Web site *ClinicalTrials.gov* provides a registry and database of clinical studies conducted around the world. This Web-based resource provides the general public, patients, their family members, health care professionals, and researchers with easy access to information on publicly and privately supported clinical studies on a wide range of diseases and conditions. The Web site facilitates basic and advanced searches and is continually updated by the sponsor or principal investigator of the clinical study.

THE NEW DRUG APPLICATION

If the three phases of clinical testing during the IND period demonstrate sufficient drug safety and therapeutic effectiveness, the sponsor may file an NDA with the FDA. This filing may be preceded by a pre-NDA meeting between the sponsor and the FDA to discuss the content and format of the NDA. The purpose of the NDA is to gain permission to market the drug product in the United States.

General Content of the NDA Submission

An NDA contains a complete presentation of all of the preclinical and clinical results that the sponsor has obtained during the investigation of the drug. It is a highly organized document that may contain several hundred volumes of information. In recent years, a computer-assisted NDA process has been implemented whereby the sponsor may interact by computer with the FDA reviewers to facilitate the application review.

The applicant submits three copies of the NDA: an archival copy, maintained by the FDA as the reference document; a review copy, used by the FDA review division; and a field copy, used by the FDA district office and field inspectors in an on-site preapproval inspection (1). The preapproval inspection is conducted in the facilities in which the approved product is to be produced. The inspectors assess the sponsor's capability to comply with all control and quality standards contained in the application, including the FDA's Current Good Manufacturing Practice standards (discussed in Chapter 3). Final approval of an NDA can be contingent upon this inspection.

In part, an application for a new chemical entity contains the following components:

- Application form (form FDA 356h) with the name, address, date, and signature of the applicant or the applicant's authorized representative
- Chemical, nonproprietary, code, and proprietary names of the drug, the dosage form, its strength, and route of administration
- Statement regarding the applicant's proposal to market the drug product as prescription only or as an OTC product
- Detailed summary of all aspects of the application, including the proposed text of the product's intended labeling, CMCs, nonclinical and clinical pharmacology and toxicology, human pharmacokinetics and bioavailability, statistical analysis, clinical trial data, benefit and risk considerations, and proposed additional or planned postmarketing studies
- Detailed technical sections on the CMCs for the drug substance, including its physical and chemical characteristics, methods of identification, assay, and controls, and the drug product, including its composition, specifications, methods of manufacture and equipment used, in-process controls, batch and master production records, container and closure systems, stability, and expiration dating
- Detailed technical sections for nonclinical pharmacology and toxicology in relation to the proposed therapeutic indication, including acute, subacute, and chronic toxicology, carcinogenicity, reproductive toxicology, and animal studies of absorption, distribution, metabolism, and excretion
- Detailed technical sections for human pharmacokinetics and bioavailability along with microbiology for antibiotic applications
- Detailed technical sections for clinical data for each controlled and uncontrolled study relating to the proposed indication, a copy of the study protocol, effectiveness and safety data including any updates on safety information, comparison of human and animal pharmacology and toxicology data, and support for the dosage and dose intervals and modifications for specific subgroups such as pediatric, geriatric, and renally impaired subjects
- Statement regarding compliance to IRB and informed consent requirements
- Statistical methods and analysis of the clinical data
- Samples of the drug substance, drug product proposed for marketing, reference standards, and finished market package, as requested
- Clinical case report forms for the archival copy of the application

The FDA accepts foreign clinical data if they are applicable to the U.S. population and domestic medical practice, if the studies were conducted by clinical investigators of recognized competence, and if the FDA considers the data to be valid without the need for an on-site inspection. The FDA has entered into bilateral agreements with some countries whereby inspections performed by the regulatory personnel of those countries are acceptable to the FDA.

Drug Product Labeling

The labeling of all drug products distributed in the United States must meet the specific labeling requirements set forth in the CFR and approved for each product by the FDA (56). Specific labeling requirements differ for prescription drugs, nonprescription drugs, and animal drugs. In each instance, however, the objective is the same—to ensure the appropriate and safe use of the approved product.

According to federal regulations, drug labeling includes not only the labels placed on an immediate container but also the information on the packaging, in package inserts, and in company literature, advertising, and promotional materials.

For prescription drugs, labeling is a summary of all of the preclinical and clinical studies conducted over the period from drug discovery through product development to FDA approval. The essential prescribing information for a human prescription drug is provided in the package insert, which by law contains a balanced presentation of the usefulness and the risks associated with the product to enable safe and effective use. The package insert is required to contain the following summary information in the order listed.

Highlights of Prescribing Information section, containing a summary of the critical or most frequently used drug information.
Full prescribing information section.
Boxed warning—if any.

1. Indications and usage, including the FDA-approved indications in the treatment, prevention, or diagnosis of a disease or condition, evidence of effectiveness demonstrated by results of controlled clinical trials, and special conditions to the drug's use for short-term or long-term use.
2. Dosage and Administration, stating the important administration instructions and recommended usual dose, the usual dosage range, the safe upper limit of dosage, duration of treatment, modification of dosage in special patient populations (children, elders, and patients with kidney and/or liver dysfunction), and special rates of administration (as with parenteral medications).
3. Dosage Forms and Strengths, listing the available forms of the product.
4. Contraindications, situations in which the drug should not be used because the risk of use clearly outweighs any possible beneficial effect. Contraindications may be associated with drug hypersensitivity, concomitant therapy, disease state, pregnancy, and/or factors of age or gender.

WARNING

An increased rate of mortality secondary to malignancy was observed in patients treated with 3 or more tubes of REGRANEX Gel in a post-marketing retrospective cohort study. REGRANEX Gel should only be used when the benefits can be expected to outweigh the risks. REGRANEX Gel should be used with caution in patients with known malignancy. (See **CONTRAINDICATIONS** and **WARNINGS**)

FIGURE 2.11. Example warning for REGRANEX® Gel 0.01% (becaplermin).

5. Warnings and Precautions, including descriptions of serious adverse reactions and potential safety hazards, limitations to use imposed by them, and steps to be taken if they occur. See Figure 2.11 for example.
6. Adverse reactions, including predictable and potential unpredictable undesired (side) effects, categorized by organ system or severity of reaction and frequency of occurrence, with specific reference to the experience of patients in clinical trials.
7. Drug Interactions, listing those drugs that are known to interact with the product and the nature of the interaction in patients.
8. Use in Specific Populations, including use in pregnancy, lactation, females and males of reproductive potential, pediatric, geriatric use, renal impairment, and hepatic impairment.
9. Drug Abuse and Dependence, if relevant, including legal schedule if a controlled substance, types of abuse and resultant adverse reactions, psychological and physical dependence potential, and treatment of withdrawal.
10. Overdosage, including signs, symptoms, and laboratory findings of acute overdosage, along with specifics or principles of treatment.
11. Description, including the proprietary and nonproprietary names, dosage form and route of administration, quantitative product composition, pharmacologic or therapeutic class of the drug, chemical name and structural formula of the drug compound, and important chemical and physical information (e.g., pH, sterility).
12. Clinical Pharmacology, including a summary of actions of the drug in humans, relevant in vitro and animal studies essential to the biochemical and/or physiologic basis for action, pharmacokinetic information on rate and degree of absorption, biotransformation, and metabolite formation, degree of drug binding to plasma proteins, rate or half-time of elimination, uptake by a particular organ or fetus, and any toxic effects.
13. Nonclinical Toxicology, including data on carcinogenesis, mutagenesis, and impairment of fertility, and animal toxicology and/or pharmacology.
14. Clinical Studies, with an overview of the clinical studies experience and more detailed descriptions of relevant individual clinical trials with the drug.
15. References, if any.
16. How Supplied/Storage and Handling, including information on available dosage forms, strengths, and means of dosage form identification, as color, coating, scoring, and National Drug Code.
17. Patient Counseling Information, which instructs medical professionals in the information to give patients for safe and effective use of the drug. A Medication Guide section is included for many products, which provides patient counseling information in layman's terms and is intended to be given as a handout to patients.

FDA Review and Action Letters

The completed NDA is carefully reviewed by the FDA, which decides whether to allow the sponsor to market the drug, to disallow marketing, or to require additional data before rendering a judgment. By regulation, the FDA must respond within 180 days of receipt of an application. This 180-day period is called the review clock and is often extended by agreement between the applicant and the FDA, as additional information, studies, or clarifications are sought.

The NDA is reviewed by the same FDA division that reviewed the sponsor's original IND. However, for the NDA review, the FDA also obtains the recommendation of an outside advisory review committee composed of persons of recognized competence and stature in the clinical area of the proposed drug's use. Although not binding, this committee's recommendation has influence in the FDA's decision to issue an action letter after the entire review of the application is completed. The FDA can respond to a sponsor of an NDA with one of the following types of letters:

1. Approval, meaning the drug has met agency standards for safety and efficacy and the drug can be marketed for sale in the United States.
2. Complete response, letting a company know that the review period for a drug is complete and that the application is not yet ready for approval. The letter will describe specific deficiencies and, when possible, will outline the recommended actions the applicant might take to get the application ready for approval.

After an NDA is approved and the product marketed, the FDA requires periodic safety and other reports, schedules plant inspections, and requires continued compliance with control and quality standards and current good manufacturing practices.

Phase 4 Studies and Postmarketing Surveillance

The receipt of marketing status for a new drug product does not necessarily end a sponsor's investigation of the drug. Continued clinical investigations, often called Phase 4 studies, may contribute to the understanding of the drug's mechanism or scope of action, may indicate possible new therapeutic uses for the drug, and/or may demonstrate the need for additional dosage strengths, dosage forms, or routes of administration. Postmarketing studies may also reveal additional side effects, serious and unexpected adverse effects, and/or drug interactions.

In applying for a new use, strength, dosage form, or route of administration for a previously approved drug, the sponsor must file a new IND, conduct all necessary additional nonclinical and clinical studies, and file a new NDA for FDA review.

Postmarketing Reporting of Adverse Drug Experience

A drug's sponsor is required to report to the FDA each adverse drug experience that is both serious (life threatening or fatal) and unexpected (not contained in the approved drug product labeling), regardless of the source of the information, within 15 working days of receipt of the information. These 15-day alert reports must then be investigated by the sponsor with a follow-up report submitted to the FDA, again within 15 working days. Other adverse events, not considered serious and unexpected, are reported quarterly for 3 years following the date of approval of the NDA and annually thereafter. Practicing pharmacists and other health care professionals participate in adverse drug experience reporting through the FDA's MedWatch program, using forms provided for this purpose at http://fda.gov/Safety/MedWatch/HowToReport/DownloadForms/default.htm (57). Two forms are available: Form FDA 3500 is for voluntary reporting by health care professionals, consumers, and patients; Form FDA 3500 A is for mandatory reporting by IND reporters, manufacturers, distributors, importers, and other specified parties.

Depending on the nature, causal relationship, and seriousness of an adverse drug reaction report, the FDA may require revised product labeling to reflect the new findings, ask the sponsor to issue special warning notices to health care professionals, undertake or require the sponsor to undertake a review of all available clinical data, restrict the marketing of the product during a review period, issue a product recall notice, or withdraw the product approval for marketing.

In the event of information on or a confirmed incident of a mislabeled, contaminated, or deteriorated product in distribution, the sponsor is required to file an NDA field alert report to the FDA district office by telephone or other rapid communication within 3 working days of receipt of the information. The FDA follows up with appropriate action.

Annual Reports

Each year, the sponsor of an approved drug must file with the FDA division responsible for the NDA review a report containing the following information:

- An annual summary of significant new information that might affect the safety, effectiveness, or labeling of the drug product
- Data on the quantity of dosage units of the drug product distributed domestically and abroad
- A sample of professional labeling, patient brochures, or package inserts and a summary of any changes since the previous report
- Reports of experiences, investigations, studies, or tests involving chemical or physical properties of the drug that may affect its safety or effectiveness
- A full description of any manufacturing and controls changes not requiring a Supplemental New Drug Application (SNDA)
- Copies of unpublished reports and summaries of published reports of new toxicologic findings in vitro and animal studies conducted or obtained by the sponsor
- Full or abstract reports on published clinical trials of the drug, including studies on safety and effectiveness; new uses; biopharmaceutical, pharmacokinetic, clinical pharmacologic, and epidemiologic reports; pharmacotherapeutic and lay press articles on the drug; and summaries of unpublished clinical trials or prepublication manuscripts, as available, conducted, or obtained by the sponsor
- A statement on the current status of any postmarketing studies performed by or on behalf of the sponsor
- Specimens of mailing pieces or other forms of promotion of the drug product

Failure to make required reports may lead to FDA withdrawal of approval for marketing.

◼ SUPPLEMENTAL, ABBREVIATED, AND OTHER APPLICATIONS

In addition to the IND and NDA, the following types of applications are filed with the FDA for the purposes described.

Supplemental New Drug Application

A sponsor of an approved NDA may make changes in that application through the filing of an SNDA. Depending on the changes proposed, some require FDA approval before implementing; others do not. Among the changes requiring prior approval are the following:

- A change in the method of synthesis of the drug substance
- Use of a different facility to manufacture the drug substance where the facility has not been approved through inspection for Current Good Manufacturing Practice standards within the previous 2 years
- Change in the formulation, analytical standards, method of manufacture, or in-process controls of the drug product

- Use of a different facility or contractor to manufacture, process, or package the drug product
- Change in the container and closure system for a drug product
- Extension of the expiration date for a drug product based on new stability data
- Any labeling change that does not add to or strengthen a previously approved label statement

Examples of changes that may be made without prior approval are minor editorial or other changes in the labeling that add to or strengthen an approved label section, any analytical changes made to comply with the USP/NF, an extension of the product's expiration date based on full shelf-life data obtained from a protocol in the approved application, and a change in the size (not the type of system) of the container for a solid dosage form.

Abbreviated New Drug Application

An ANDA is one in which nonclinical laboratory studies and clinical investigations may be omitted, except those pertaining to the drug's bioavailability. These applications are usually filed for duplicates (generic copies) of drug products previously approved under a full NDA and for which the FDA has determined that information on the exempted nonclinical and clinical studies is already available at the agency. ANDAs commonly are filed by competing companies following the expiration of patent term protection of the innovator drug or drug product. Bioavailability and product bioequivalency are discussed in Chapter 5.

The Patient Protection and Affordable Care Act of 2010 created an abbreviated licensure pathway for biological products that are demonstrated to be "biosimilar" to or "interchangeable" with an FDA-licensed biological product. Under the Act, a biological product may be deemed to be "biosimilar" if data show that, among other things, the product is "highly similar" to an already-approved biological product.

Biologics License Application

BLAs are submitted to the FDA's CBER for the manufacture of biologics such as blood products, vaccines, and toxins. The applications for biologics approvals follow the regulatory requirements as stated specifically for these products in the relevant parts of the CFR (4).

Animal Drug Applications

The Federal Food, Drug, and Cosmetic Act, as amended, contains specific regulations pertaining to the approval for the marketing and labeling of drugs intended for animal use (6).

Included are NADAs, supplemental applications to an approved drug (SNADA), abbreviated new animal drug applications (ANADAs) for generic equivalents, and CNADAs, which are applications for conditional approval of new animal drugs, which allow a drug sponsor to legally market a new animal drug intended for a minor use or a minor species after proving it is safe but before collecting all the necessary effectiveness data. The drug's sponsor can keep the product on the market for up to 5 years while collecting the effectiveness data required for an NADA application.

Medical Devices

The FDA has regulatory authority over the manufacture and licensing of all medical devices, from surgical gloves and catheters to cardiac pacemakers and cardiopulmonary bypass blood gas monitors (7). Included in the regulations are standards and procedures for manufacturer registration, investigational studies, good manufacturing practices, and premarket approval.

▌ INTERNATIONAL CONFERENCE ON HARMONIZATION OF TECHNICAL REQUIREMENTS FOR REGISTRATION OF PHARMACEUTICALS FOR HUMAN USE

In recognition of the international marketplace for pharmaceuticals and in an effort to achieve global efficiencies for both regulatory agencies and the pharmaceutical industry, the FDA, the counterpart agencies of the European Union and Japan, and geographic representatives of the pharmaceutical industry formed a tripartite organization in 1991 to discuss, identify, and address relevant regulatory issues. This organization, named the ICH of Technical Requirements for Registration of Pharmaceuticals for Human Use, has worked toward harmonizing, or bringing together, the regulatory requirements with the long-range goal of establishing a uniform set of standards for drug registration within these geographic areas.

▌ APPLYING THE PRINCIPLES AND CONCEPTS ▌

GROUP ACTIVITIES

1. Given a new FDA approval, research and present its progression from a new chemical entity to its NDA. Identify pertinent dates, preclinical trials, and clinical trials.
2. Within the last 2 years, identify a drug that was given a treatment IND, a drug approved for an SNDA, a drug that was approved for an ANDA, and

an example of a drug that was withdrawn from its IND.
3. Draw a timeline of the steps taken for a drug to gain approval after an IND is submitted to the FDA.
4. Create a table of patient factors considered in determining a drug's dose in clinical investigations and in medical practice, and provide three examples of drug dosages/regimens influenced by the specific factor.

INDIVIDUAL ACTIVITIES

1. Identify a drug that had previous FDA approval; however, it has recently been submitted as a new drug under the FDA definition.
2. Identify a drug that had postmarketing reporting that resulted in the drug being withdrawn from the market; identify a drug whose postmarketing surveillance reporting resulted in the addition of a black box warning.
3. Determine how much money a drug company typically spends before a drug is FDA approved. How much does a drug company allocate for marketing a new product? Explain how this accounts for the cost of new prescription medications.

REFERENCES

1. Code of Federal Regulations, Title 21, Parts 300–314.
2. Code of Federal Regulations, Title 21, Part 320.
3. Code of Federal Regulations, Title 21, Part 316.
4. Code of Federal Regulations, Title 21, Parts 600–680.
5. Code of Federal Regulations, Title 21, Parts 330.
6. Code of Federal Regulations, Title 21, Parts 510–555.
7. Code of Federal Regulations, Title 21, Parts 800–895.
8. Federal Register, U.S. Washington: Government Printing Office, Superintendent of Documents. Available at: http://www.gpo.gov/fdsys/browse/collection.action?collectionCode=FR. (Accessed July 20, 2020)
9. Mathieu M. New Drug Development: A Regulatory Overview. 8th Ed. Cambridge, MA: PAREXEL International, 2008.
10. Mathieu M. Biologics Development: A Regulatory Overview. 1348321086 false—1 5 5 4. Cambridge, MA: PAREXEL International, 2004.
11. Chorghade MS, ed. Drug Discovery and Development. Volume 1: Drug Discovery. Hoboken, NJ: Wiley-Interscience, 2006.
12. Kayser O, Warzecha H, eds. Pharmaceutical Biotechnology: Drug Discovery and Clinical Applications. 2nd Ed. Hoboken, NJ: Wiley, 2012.
13. Ng R. Drugs, from Discovery to Approval. 2nd Ed. Hoboken, NJ: Wiley-Blackwell, 2008.
14. Portfolio management solutions. JamesSamanenConsulting.com. Available at: http://www.portfoliomanagementsolutions.com/overall-outline/. (Accessed July 20, 2020)
15. Tami JA, Parr MD, Brown SA, et al. Monoclonal antibody technology. Am J Hosp Pharm 1986;43:2816–2826.
16. Brodsky FM. Monoclonal antibodies as magic bullets. Pharm Res 1988;5:1–9.
17. Parasrampuria DA, Hunt CA. Therapeutic delivery issues in gene therapy, part 2: Targeting approaches. Pharm Technol 1998;22:34–43.
18. Chew NJ. Cellular and gene therapies, part 1: Regulatory health. BioPharmacy 1995;8:22–23.
19. Smith TJ. Gene therapy: Opportunities for pharmacy in the 21st century. Am J Pharm Ed 1996;60:213–215.
20. Milestones in gene therapy. BioPharmacy 1997;10:17.
21. Cellular and Gene Therapy Guidance Documents. Rockville, MD: Food and Drug Administration. Available at: https://www.fda.gov/vaccines-blood-biologics/biologics-guidances/cellular-gene-therapy-guidances. (Accessed July 20, 2020)
22. Kauvar LM. Affinity fingerprinting: Implications for drug discovery. Pharm News 1996;3:12–15.
23. Harris AL. High throughput screening and molecular diversity. Pharm News 1995;2:26–30.
24. Silverman RB. Drug discovery, design, and development. In: Silverman RB, ed. The Organic Chemistry of Drug Design and Drug Action. New York, NY: Academic Press, 1992:4–51.
25. Perun TJ, Propst CL, eds. Computer-Aided Drug Design: Methods and Applications. New York, NY: Marcel Dekker, 1989.
26. FDA Glossary of Terms. Rockville, MD: Food and Drug Administration. Available at: http://www.fda.gov/Drugs/InformationOnDrugs/ucm079436.htm. (Accessed July 20, 2020)
27. United States Adopted Names. Chicago, IL: American Medical Association. Available at: USAN http://www.ama-assn.org/ama/pub/physician-resources/medical-science/united-states-adopted-names-council/adopted-names.page. (Accessed July 20, 2020)
28. Spilker B. Extrapolation of preclinical safety data to humans. Drug News Perspect 1991;4:214–216.
29. Code of Federal Regulations Title 21, 312.23. Rockville, MD: Food and Drug Administration. Available at: http://www.accessdata.fda.gov/scripts/cdrh/cfdocs/cfcfr/CFRSearch.cfm?fr=312.23. (Accessed July 20, 2020)
30. 60 Federal Register 11263–11268. International conference on harmonization; guideline on the assessment of systemic exposure in toxicity studies, 1995.
31. 60 Federal Register 11277–11281. International conference on harmonization; guidance on dose selection for carcinogenicity study of pharmaceuticals, 1995.
32. 58 Federal Register 21073–21080. International conference on harmonization; draft guideline on detection of toxicity to reproduction for medicinal products, 1993.
33. 59 Federal Register 48734–48737. International conference on harmonization, draft guideline on specific aspects of regulatory genotoxicity tests, 1994.
34. Guideline for the Format and Content of the Chemistry, Manufacturing, and Controls Section of an Application. Rockville, MD: Food and Drug Administration, 1987.
35. The Biopharmaceutics Classification System. Rockville, MD: Food and Drug Administration. Available at: http://www.fda.gov/downloads/Drugs/GuidanceComplianceRegulatoryInformation/Guidances/UCM070246.pdf. (Accessed July 20, 2020)
36. Code of Federal Regulations, Title 21, Parts 210–211.
37. Center for Drug Evaluation and Research. IND Process and Review Procedures. Manual of Policies and Procedures. Rockville, MD: Food and Drug Administration. Available at: http://www.fda.gov/downloads/AboutFDA/CentersOffices/OfficeofMedicalProductsandTobacco/CDER/ManualofPoliciesProcedures/UCM082022.pdf. (Accessed July 20, 2020)
38. Investigational New Drug Application (FDA Form 1571). Available at: http://www.fda.gov/downloads/AboutFDA/ReportsManualsForms/Forms/UCM083533.pdf. (Accessed July 20, 2020)
39. 58 Federal Register 39405–39416. Guideline for the study and evaluation of gender differences in the clinical evaluation of drugs, 1993.
40. 59 Federal Register 11145–11151. NIH guidelines on the inclusion of women and minorities as subjects in clinical research, 1994.
41. Wright DT, Chew NJ. Women as subjects in clinical research. Appl Clin Trials 1996;5:44–52.
42. Wick JY. Culture, ethnicity, and medications. J Am Pharm Assoc (Wash) 1996;NS36:555–563.
43. Code of Federal Regulations, Title 21, Part 56.
44. Code of Federal Regulations, Title 21, Part 50.
45. Manual of Policies & Procedures (CDER). Rockville, MD: Food and Drug Administration. Available at: http://www.fda.gov/AboutFDA/CentersOffices/OfficeofMedicalProductsandTobacco/CDER/ManualofPoliciesProcedures/default.htm#ode2. (Accessed July 20, 2020)
46. Spilker B. Guide to Clinical Trials. New York, NY: Raven, 1991.
47. Bush C. When your subject is a child. Appl Clin Trials 1997;6:54–56.
48. Cohen HJ. The elderly patient: A challenge to the art and science of medicine. Drug Ther 1983;13:41.
49. Futerman SS. The geriatric patient: Pharmacy care can make a difference. Apothecary 1982;94:34.

50. Taketomo CK, ed. Pediatric and Neonatal Dosage Handbook. 22nd Ed. Hudson OH: Lexi-Comp Inc., 2015.

51. Kim H, Lim SW, Kim S, et al. Monoamine transporter gene polymorphisms and antidepressant response in Koreans with late-life depression. JAMA 2006;296:1609–1618.

52. Food and Drug Administration. New labeling to provide information about contraceptives and STDs. FDA Med Bull 1993;23:2–4.

53. Logsdon BA. Drug use during lactation. J Am Pharm Assoc (Wash) 1997;NS37:407–418.

54. Drug safety in lactation. Available at: https://medsafe.govt.nz/Profs/PUarticles/lactation.htm. (Accessed July 20, 2020)

55. Treatment Use of Investigational Drugs—Information Sheet. Rockville, MD: Food and Drug Administration. Available at: https://www.fda.gov/regulatory-information/search-fda-guidance-documents/treatment-use-investigational-drugs. (Accessed July 20, 2020)

56. Code of Federal Regulations, Title 21. Part 201.

57. MedWatch. Rockville, MD: Food and Drug Administration.

CHAPTER

Current Good Manufacturing Practices and Current Good Compounding Practices

CHAPTER AT A GLANCE Standards for Current Good Manufacturing Practice • cGMP for Finished Pharmaceuticals • Additional cGMP Regulatory Requirements • Current Good Compounding Practices • Packaging, Labeling, and Storage of Pharmaceuticals

OBJECTIVES

After reading this chapter, the student will be able to:

- List common terms used in the Current Good Manufacturing Practice (cGMP) for finished pharmaceuticals
- Describe the organization and personnel required by cGMP
- Describe the intent and importance of written procedures within the various components of cGMP
- Describe the various types of tamper-evident packaging, and provide a product example of each type
- Differentiate between pharmaceutical manufacturing and extemporaneous compounding
- Describe the USP chapters related to pharmacy compounding

▐ STANDARDS FOR CURRENT GOOD MANUFACTURING PRACTICE

Current Good Manufacturing Practice (cGMP or GMP) regulations are established by the Food and Drug Administration (FDA) to ensure that minimum standards are met for drug product quality in the United States (1). The first GMP regulations were promulgated in 1963 under the provisions of the Kefauver-Harris Drug Amendments, and since then, they have been periodically revised and updated.

The cGMP regulations establish requirements for all aspects of pharmaceutical manufacture. They apply to domestic and to foreign suppliers and manufacturers whose bulk components and finished pharmaceutical products are imported, distributed, or sold in this country. To ensure compliance, the FDA inspects the facilities and production records of all firms covered by these regulations.

The Code of Federal Regulations (CFR) contains (*a*) requirements for the "Current Good Manufacturing Practice for Finished Pharmaceuticals" and (*b*) additional cGMP requirements for biologic products, (*c*) medicated articles, and (*d*) medical devices. Currency and compliance with

cGMP regulations are supported through notices in the Federal Register and through the FDA's Compliance Policy Guide and various other guidances issued by the FDA.

A topical outline of the cGMP regulations for finished pharmaceuticals is presented in Table 3.1 and summarized in the sections that follow.

▐ cGMP FOR FINISHED PHARMACEUTICALS

General Provisions: Scope and Definitions

The regulations in 21 CFR, part 211, contain the minimum GMP requirements for the preparation of finished pharmaceutical products for administration to humans or animals.

Common terms used in these regulations are defined as follows:

- Active ingredient or active pharmaceutical ingredient (API): Any component that is intended to furnish pharmacologic activity or other direct effect in the diagnosis,

TABLE 3.1. Topical Outline of Current Good Manufacturing Practice Regulations

A. General Provisions	Equipment identification
Scope	Sampling and testing of in-process materials and drug products
Definitions	Time limitations on production
B. Organization and Personnel	Control of microbiological contamination
Responsibilities of quality control unit	Reprocessing
Personnel qualifications	G. Packaging and Labeling Control
Personnel responsibilities	Materials examination and usage criteria
Consultants	Labeling issuance
C. Buildings and Facilities	Packaging and labeling operations
Design and construction features	Tamper-resistant packaging requirements for OTC human drug products
Lighting	Drug product inspection
Ventilation, air filtration, air heating, and cooling	Expiration dating
Plumbing	H. Holding and Distribution
Sewage and refuse	Warehousing procedures
Washing and toilet facilities	Distribution procedures
Sanitation	I. Laboratory Controls
Maintenance	General requirements
D. Equipment	Testing and release for distribution
Equipment design, size, and location	Stability testing
Equipment construction	Special testing requirements
Equipment cleaning and maintenance	Reserve samples
Automatic, mechanical, and electronic equipment	Laboratory animals
Filters	Penicillin contamination
E. Control of Components and Drug Product Containers and Closures	J. Records and Reports
General requirements	General requirements
Receipt and storage of untested components, drug product containers, and closures	Equipment cleaning and use log
Testing and approval or rejection of components, drug product containers, and closures	Component, drug product container, closure, and labeling records
Use of approved components, drug product containers, and closures	Master production and control records
Retesting of approved components, drug product containers, and closures	Batch production and control records
Rejected components, drug product containers, and closures	Production record review
Drug product containers and closures	Laboratory records
F. Production and Process Controls	Distribution records
Written procedures, deviations	Complaint files
Charge-in of components	K. Returned and Salvaged Drug Products
Calculation of yield	Returned drug products
	Drug product salvaging

Code of Federal Regulations 21, Part 211. Revised April 1, 2012. Available at: http://www.accessdata.fda.gov/scripts/cdrh/cfdocs/cfcfr/CFRSearch.cfm?CFRPart=211. (Accessed September 25, 2012)

cure, mitigation, treatment, or prevention of disease or to affect the structure or function of the body of man or other animals

- Batch: A specific quantity of a drug of uniform specified quality produced according to a single manufacturing order during the same cycle of manufacture

- Batchwise control: The use of validated in-process sampling and testing methods in such a way that results prove that the process has done what it purports to do for the specific batch concerned

- Certification: Documented testimony by qualified authorities that a system qualification, calibration, validation, or revalidation has been performed appropriately and that the results are acceptable

- Compliance: Determination through inspection of the extent to which a manufacturer is acting in accordance with prescribed regulations, standards, and practices
- Component: Any ingredient used in the manufacture of a drug product, including those that may not be present in the finished product
- Drug product: A finished form that contains an active drug and inactive ingredients. The term may also include a form that does not contain an active ingredient, such as a placebo
- Inactive ingredient: Any component other than the active ingredients in a drug product
- Lot: A batch or any portion of a batch having uniform specified quality and a distinctive identifying lot number
- Lot number, control number, or batch number: Any distinctive combination of letters, numbers, or symbols from which the complete history of the manufacture, processing, packaging, holding, and distribution of a batch or lot of a drug product may be determined
- Master record: Record containing the formulation, specifications, manufacturing procedures, quality assurance requirements, and labeling of a finished product
- Quality assurance: Provision to all concerned the evidence needed to establish confidence that the activities relating to quality are being performed adequately
- Quality audit: A documented activity performed in accordance with established procedures on a planned and periodic basis to verify compliance with the procedures to ensure quality
- Quality control: The regulatory process through which industry measures actual quality performance, compares it with standards, and acts on the difference
- Quality control unit: An organizational element designated by a firm to be responsible for the duties relating to quality control
- Quarantine: An area that is marked, designated, or set aside for the holding of incoming components prior to acceptance testing and qualification for use
- Representative sample: A sample that accurately portrays the whole
- Reprocessing: The activity whereby the finished product or any of its components is recycled through all or part of the manufacturing process
- Strength: The concentration of the drug substance per unit dose or volume
- Verified: Signed by a second individual or recorded by automated equipment
- Validation: Documented evidence that a system (e.g., equipment, software, controls) does what it purports to do
- Process validation: Documented evidence that a process (e.g., sterilization) does what it purports to do
- Validation protocol: A prospective experimental plan to produce documented evidence that the system has been validated

Organization and Personnel

The organization and personnel section of the regulations deals with the responsibilities of the quality control unit, employees, and consultants. The regulations require that a quality control unit have the authority and responsibility for all functions that may affect product quality. This includes accepting or rejecting product components, product specifications, finished products, packaging, and labeling. Adequate laboratory facilities shall be provided, written procedures followed, and all records maintained.

All personnel engaged in the manufacture, processing, packing, or holding of a drug product, including those in supervisory positions, are required to have the education, training, and/or experience needed to fulfill the assigned responsibility. Appropriate programs of skill development, continuing education and training, and performance evaluations are essential for maintaining quality assurance. Any consultants advising on scientific and technical matters should possess requisite qualifications for the tasks.

Buildings and Facilities

As outlined in Table 3.1, the regulations in this section include the design, structural features, and functional aspects of buildings and facilities. Each building's structure, space, design, and placement of equipment must be such to enable thorough cleaning, inspection, and safe and effective use for the designated operations. Proper considerations must be given to such factors as water quality standards; security; materials used for floors, walls, and ceilings; lighting; segregated quarantine areas for raw materials and product components subject to quality control approval; holding areas for rejected components; storage areas for released components; weighing and measuring rooms; sterile areas for ophthalmic and parenteral products; flammable materials storage areas; finished products storage; control of heat, humidity, temperature, and ventilation; waste handling; employee facilities and safety procedures in compliance with the Occupational Safety and Health Administration regulations; and procedures and practices of personal sanitation.

All work in the manufacture, processing, packaging, or holding of a pharmaceutical product must be logged in, inspected by a supervisor, and signed off. Similarly, a log of building maintenance must be kept to document this component of the regulations.

Equipment

Each piece of equipment must be of appropriate design and size and suitably located to facilitate operations for its intended use, cleaning, and maintenance. The equipment's surfaces and parts must not interact with the processes or product's components so as to alter the purity, strength, or quality.

Standard operating procedures must be written and followed for the proper use, maintenance, and cleaning of each piece of equipment, and appropriate logs and records must be kept. Automated equipment and computers used in the processes must be routinely calibrated, maintained, and validated for accuracy.

Filters used in the manufacture or processing of injectable drug products shall not release fibers into such products. If fiber-releasing filters must be used, non–fiber-releasing filters also must be used to reduce any fiber content.

Control of Components, Containers, and Closures

Written procedures describing the receipt, identification, storage, handling, sampling, testing, and approval or rejection of all drug product components, product containers, and closures must be maintained and followed. Bulk pharmaceutical chemicals, containers, and closures must meet the exact physical and chemical specifications established with the supplier at the time of ordering.

When product components are received from a supplier, each lot must be logged in with the purchase order number, date of receipt, bill of lading, name and vital information of the supplier, supplier's stock or control number, and quantity received. The component is assigned a control number that identifies both the component and the intended product. Raw materials are quarantined until they are verified through representative sampling and careful qualitative and quantitative analysis. The quality control unit approves and releases for use in manufacture only those that meet the specifications. The assigned control number follows the component throughout production so it can be traced if necessary.

Rejected components, drug product containers, and closures are identified and controlled under a quarantine system to prevent their use in manufacturing and processing operations. As the majority of bulk chemicals (APIs) are synthesized overseas (primarily in China and India), it is important to confirm their identity and purity and conformance with U.S. Pharmacopeia (USP) and National Formulary (NF) standards prior to use in finished pharmaceuticals.

Production and Process Controls

Written procedures are required for production and process controls to ensure that the drug products have the correct identity, strength, quality, and purity. These procedures, which include the charge-in of all components, use of in-process controls, sample testing, and process and equipment validation, must be followed for quality assurance. Any deviation from the written procedures must be recorded and justified. In most instances, the operator records time and date of each key operation, and the supervisor signs off on it. When operations are controlled by automated equipment, such equipment must be validated regularly for precision.

All product ingredients, equipment, and drums or other containers of bulk finished product must be distinctively identified by labeling as to content and/or status.

In-process samples are taken from production batches periodically for product control. In-process controls are of two general types: (*a*) those performed by production personnel at the time of operation to ensure that the machinery is producing output within preestablished control limits (e.g., tablet size, hardness) and (*b*) those performed by the quality control laboratory personnel to ensure compliance with all product specifications (e.g., tablet content, dissolution) and batch-to-batch consistency. Product found out of standard sometimes may be reprocessed for subsequent use. However, in this, as in all instances, procedures must be performed according to established protocol, and all materials must be accounted for, all specifications met, and all records meticulously maintained.

Packaging and Labeling Control

Written procedures are required for the receipt, identification, storage, handling, sampling, and testing of drug product and issuance of labeling and packaging materials. Labeling for each variation in drug product—strength, dosage form, or quantity of contents—must be stored separately with suitable identification. Obsolete and outdated labels and other packaging materials must be destroyed. Access to the storage area must be limited to authorized personnel.

All materials for use in the packaging and labeling of product must be withheld until approved and released by the quality control unit. Control procedures must be followed and records maintained for the issuance and use of product labeling. Quantities issued, used, and returned must be reconciled and discrepancies investigated. Before labeling operations commence, the labeling facilities must be inspected to ensure that all drug products and labels have been removed from the previous operations. There must be dedicated labeling and packaging lines for *each different strength of each different drug product.* There must be use of appropriate electronic or electromechanical equipment to conduct a 100% examination for correct labeling during or after completion of finishing operations or use of visual inspection to conduct a 100% examination for correct labeling during or after completion of finishing operations for hand-applied labeling. Such examination shall be performed by one person and independently verified by a second person. All of these procedures are essential to avoid label mix-ups and the mislabeling of products. All records of inspections and controls must be documented in the batch production records.

Labels must meet the legal requirements for content as outlined in Chapter 2 and later in this chapter. Each label must contain expiration dating and the production batch or lot number to facilitate product identification.

Expiration Dating

To assure that a drug product meets applicable standards of identity, strength, quality, and purity at the time of use, it must bear an expiration date determined by appropriate stability testing. Exempt from this requirement are homeopathic drug products, allergenic extracts, and investigational drugs that meet the standards established during preclinical and clinical studies.

Tamper-Evident Packaging

On November 5, 1982, the FDA published initial regulations on tamper-resistant packaging in the *Federal Register*. These regulations were promulgated after criminal tampering with over-the-counter (OTC) drug products earlier in that year resulted in illness and deaths. In the primary incident, cyanide was surreptitiously placed in acetaminophen capsules in commercial packages.

Today, the cGMP regulations require tamper-evident packaging for OTC drug products to improve their security and to assure their safety and effectiveness. All OTC drug products offered for retail sale are required to have tamper-evident packaging except for some categories, such as dentifrices, dermatologicals, insulin, and throat lozenges. For other product categories, a manufacturer may file with the FDA a Request for Exemption from Tamper-Evident Rule. The petition is required to contain specific information on the drug product, the reasons the requirement is unnecessary or cannot be achieved, and alternative steps the petitioner has taken or may take to reduce the likelihood of malicious adulteration of the product. Generally exempt from these regulations are products not packaged for retail sale but rather distributed to hospitals, nursing homes, and health care clinics for institutional use.

A tamper-evident package is defined as "one having one or more indicators or barriers to entry which, if breached or missing, can reasonably be expected to provide visible evidence to consumers that tampering has occurred" (1). The indicators or barriers may involve the immediate drug product container and/or an outer container or carton. For two-piece hard gelatin capsule products, a minimum of two tamper-evident packaging features is required unless the capsules are sealed with tamper-resistant technology.

Even with these safeguards in effect, the possibility of drug product tampering requires the pharmacist and consumer to remain constantly vigilant for signs of product entry. Pharmaceutical manufacturers have the option of determining the type of tamper-resistant packaging to use. Table 3.2 presents some examples of tamper-evident packaging.

Holding and Distribution

Written procedures must be established and followed for the holding and distribution of product. Finished pharmaceuticals must be quarantined in storage until released by the quality control unit. Products must be stored and shipped under conditions that do not affect product quality. Ordinarily, the oldest approved stock is distributed first. The distribution control system must allow the distribution point of each lot of drug product to be readily determined to facilitate its recall if necessary.

Laboratory Controls

Laboratory controls are requirements for the establishment of and conformance to written specifications, standards, sampling plans, test procedures, and other such mechanisms. The specifications, which apply to each batch of drug product, include provisions for sample size, test intervals, sample storage, stability testing, and special testing requirements for certain dosage forms, including parenterals, ophthalmics, controlled-release products, and radioactive pharmaceuticals. Reserve samples must be retained for distributed products for specified periods depending on their category. Animals used in testing components, in-process materials, or drug products for compliance with established specifications shall be maintained and controlled in a manner that assures their suitability for their intended use. They shall be identified, and adequate records shall be maintained showing the history of their use.

Records and Reports

Production, control, and distribution records must be maintained for at least a year following the expiration date of a product batch. This includes equipment cleaning and maintenance logs; specifications and lot numbers of product components, including raw materials and product

TABLE 3.2. Examples of Tamper-Evident Packaging

Package Type	Tamper Protection
Film wrapper	Sealed around product and/or product container; film must be cut or torn to remove product
Blister/strip pack	Individually sealed dose units; removal requires tearing or breaking individual compartment
Bubble pack	Product and container sealed in plastic, usually mounted on display card; plastic must be cut or broken open to remove product
Shrink seal, band	Band or wrapper shrunk by heat or drying to conform to cap; must be torn to open package
Bottle seal	Paper or foil sealed to mouth of container under cap; must be torn or broken to reach product
Tape seal	Paper or foil sealed over carton flap or bottle cap; must be torn or broken to reach product
Breakable cap	Plastic or metal tearaway cap over container; must be broken to remove
Sealed tube	Seal over mouth of tube; must be punctured to reach product
Sealed carton	Carton flaps sealed; carton cannot be opened without damage
Aerosol container	Tamper-resistant by design

containers and closures; and label records. Complete master production and control records for each batch must be kept.

These master records must document that each step in the production, control, packaging, labeling, and distribution of the product was accomplished and approved by the quality control unit. Depending on the operation, the operator's and/or supervisor's full signatures, initials, or other written or electronic identification codes are required.

Records of written and oral complaints regarding a drug product (e.g., product failure, adverse drug experience) must also be maintained, along with information regarding the internal disposition of each complaint. All records must be made available at the time of inspection by FDA officials.

Returned and Salvaged Drug Products

Returned drug products (e.g., from wholesalers) must be identified by lot number and product quality determined through appropriate testing. Drug products that meet specifications may be salvaged or reprocessed. Those that do not, along with those that have been subjected to improper storage (e.g., extremes in temperature), shall not be returned to the marketplace. Records for all returned products must be maintained and must include the date and reasons for the return; quantity and lot number of product returned; procedures employed for holding, testing, and reprocessing the product; and the product's disposition.

Information Technology and Automation

Although not part of the cGMP requirements, the effective deployment of information technologies and automated systems can enhance pharmaceutical process development, production efficiencies, product quality, and regulatory compliance (2).

Computers are used extensively in plant operations such as production scheduling, in-process manufacturing, quality control, and packaging and labeling. The networking of computers in the production and quality control areas fully integrates laboratory information and manufacturing operations into sophisticated management systems. These integrated systems support cGMP compliance, process validation, resource management, and cost control. Figure 3.1 presents an example of computer use in the pharmaceutical industry for the management of plant operations. Robotic devices increasingly are being employed to replace manual operations in production lines, analytical sampling, and packaging. Figure 3.2 presents an example of robot use in the laboratory. Laboratory robotics provides automation in areas such as sample preparation and handling, wet chemistry procedures, laboratory process control, and instrumental analysis (3). Pharmaceutical applications of robotics include automated product handling in production lines and in procedures such as sampling and analysis, tablet content uniformity, and dissolution testing.

FIGURE 3.1. Example of computer use in the pharmaceutical industry. (Courtesy of Fishman64/Shutterstock.)

ADDITIONAL cGMP REGULATORY REQUIREMENTS

Active Pharmaceutical Ingredients and Pharmaceutical Excipients

The manufacture of APIs comes under the *aegis* of cGMP regulations and requirements. The FDA publication *Guide to the Inspection of Bulk Pharmaceutical Chemicals* (4) identifies the inspection program for manufacture of chemical components of pharmaceutical products to assure that all required standards for quality are met. Because the quality of any finished pharmaceutical product depends on the quality of the various components, including the active ingredients, compliance with cGMPs is a critical part of the FDA's preapproval inspection program for new drug applications (NDAs) and abbreviated new drug applications (ANDAs).

The broad cGMP areas described previously for finished pharmaceuticals apply but are directed toward the process-specific aspects of bulk pharmaceutical chemicals. The application of the regulations is focused on all

FIGURE 3.2. Robotics in laboratory use. (Courtesy of Cylonphoto/Shutterstock.)

of the defining elements of chemical purity and quality, including the following (5):

- Specifications and analytical methods for all reactive and nonreactive components used in synthesis
- Critical chemical reaction steps
- Handling of chemical intermediates
- Effect of scale-up of chemical batches on the yield
- Quality of the water systems
- Solvent handling and recovery systems
- Analytical methods to detect impurities or chemical residues and the limits set
- Stability studies of the bulk pharmaceutical chemical

Pharmaceutical excipients, as they, too, are components of finished pharmaceutical products, must be produced in accordance with cGMP standards as certified on the application by each sponsor of an NDA or ANDA (6,7).

Clinical Trial Materials

Clinical trial materials (CTMs) must be produced in conformance with cGMP regulations. This applies to both the production of the APIs and investigational drug products.

The API used in a clinical investigation is subject to all of the requirements for the production of bulk pharmaceutical chemicals. However, the batch size is different from the commercial scale used in the production of an FDA-approved product. In some cases, technology transfer in the production of an API from one production site or laboratory to another may require validation to ensure purity and quality standards.

The CTMs used in clinical investigations must be produced in compliance with the cGMP regulatory requirements and standardized as to identity, purity, strength, and quality (8). However, during preclinical testing and the early phases of clinical evaluation, a product's formulation and many of the production processes and analytical controls are still under development. Thus, during this period, the regulatory requirements are applied with flexibility. As the clinical trials progress from Phase 1 to Phase 2, the processes are being characterized and refined, and during Phase 3, they are expected to meet all regulatory requirements. It is during Phase 3 that process optimization is demonstrated to the FDA by the production of at least one-tenth of a commercial-size batch (e.g., 100,000 capsules) of the proposed product. Prior to that, adequate supplies of dosing units from a few hundred to a few thousand may be prepared by hand or in pilot plant–scale operations as is necessary for the clinical trials (8).

In addition to the active drug product, matching placebo and/or comparator products must be prepared. Specific labeling, coding, packaging design, assembly, and distribution protocols are in effect for CTMs to accommodate the clinical trial design and the requirements for investigational drugs as discussed in Chapter 2.

Biologics

As noted previously, cGMP standards are defined for biologic products in the *Code of Federal Regulations* (1). Although the basic regulations for finished pharmaceuticals apply to biologic products as well, the nature of blood, bacterial, and viral products requires specific additional mandates, which are detailed in the regulations.

Medical Devices

Medical devices follow a path for FDA approval that resembles that for pharmaceuticals. For instance, clinical investigations of devices are conducted on approval of an investigational device exemption and approved for marketing when shown to be safe and effective through a premarket approval application, similar to an investigational new drug and NDA, respectively. Medical devices also are subject to the reporting of adverse events, to recall, and to termination of approval.

The regulations for "good manufacturing practice for medical devices" are similar in organizational structure to those for finished pharmaceuticals. Literally, thousands of medical devices are regulated by the provisions of the *Code of Federal Regulations* (1). Each device has a specific design with individual performance features and utility. For many devices, specific standards are stated in the regulations. Devices covered by cGMP regulations include intraocular lenses, hearing aids, intrauterine devices, cardiac pacemakers, clinical chemistry analyzers, catheters, cardiopulmonary bypass heart–lung machine console, dental x-ray equipment, surgical gloves, condoms, prosthetic hip joints, traction equipment, computed tomography equipment, and powered wheelchairs.

Noncompliance with cGMP Regulations

Noncompliance with cGMP regulations can lead to a number of regulatory actions by the FDA. Noncompliance determined during a premarket approval inspection of facilities as part of an NDA or ANDA application likely would result in a delay of approval of an otherwise approvable application. Noncompliance with cGMP regulations during a regularly scheduled FDA inspection can lead to various actions, depending on the severity of the offenses. In most instances, time for corrective action is given, with the firm required to institute and document corrective measures and undergo another inspection. In a worst-case scenario, the FDA is empowered to remove violative products from the market, withdraw product approvals, and restrict further applications. All FDA actions are subject to appeal.

cGMP Requirements for Manufacturing in Pharmacies

The FDA's cGMP regulations apply to community or institutional pharmacies engaged in the manufacture, repackaging, or relabeling of drugs and drug products in a supplier function and beyond the usual conduct of professional dispensing. Pharmacies that engage in such activities must register with the FDA as a 503b compounder as a manufacturer or distributor and be subject to FDA inspection at regular intervals.

Professional, legislative, and regulatory attention has been directed toward differentiating between pharmaceutical manufacturing and compounding as practiced by community pharmacists (9). Pharmaceutical manufacturing is large-scale production of drugs or drug products for distribution and sale, whereas compounding is professional preparation of prescriptions for specific patients as a part of the traditional practice of pharmacy. This was affirmed by provision in the Food and Drug Administration Modernization Act of 1997.

CURRENT GOOD COMPOUNDING PRACTICES

In recent years, pharmacists have increased the practice of compounding patient-specific medications. A number of reasons have been presented for the increase in preparing patient-specific medications, including the following:

1. Many patients need drug dosages or strengths that are not commercially available.
2. Many patients need dosage forms, such as suppositories, oral liquids, or topicals, that are not commercially available.
3. Many patients are allergic to excipients in commercially available products.
4. Children's medications must be prepared as liquids, flavored to enhance compliance, and prepared in alternative dosage forms, such as lozenges, gumdrops, popsicles, and lollipops.
5. Some medications are not very stable and require preparation and dispensing every few days; they are not suitable to be manufactured products.
6. Many physicians desire to deliver products in innovative ways, and pharmacists can work with them to solve medication problems.
7. Most products are not available for veterinary patients and must be compounded.
8. Home health care and the treatment of an increasing number of patients at home have resulted in many community pharmacies and home health care pharmacies preparing sterile products for home use.
9. Hospice care has resulted in new approaches to pain management that employ higher drug concentrations and innovative combinations of drugs that are not commercially available.
10. Many drugs are reported in the literature but are not yet manufactured, so pharmacists can compound them for their physicians' and patients' use.

As the extent of compounding increased, many standard-setting agencies and regulatory bodies wanted to ensure quality compounded products; consequently, there was a lot of activity during the mid-1990s to establish guidelines for pharmaceutical compounding.

U.S. Pharmacopeia–National Formulary

In 1990, the U.S. Pharmacopeial Convention initiated a number of activities related to contemporary pharmaceutical compounding. Guidance chapters related to pharmacy compounding were developed and published starting in 1996 (10). In addition, the first of the compounded preparation monographs became official in 1998, and they provide a tested, uniform formulation with valid beyond-use dating.

The USP-NF presently contains the following general guidance chapters related to pharmaceutical compounding:

<795> Pharmaceutical Compounding—Nonsterile Preparations
<797> Pharmaceutical Compounding—Sterile Preparations
<800> Hazardous Drugs—Handling in Healthcare Settings
<1160> Pharmaceutical Calculations in Prescription Compounding
<1163> Quality Assurance in Pharmaceutical Compounding
<1176> Prescription Balances and Volumetric Apparatus

In addition, the following are related chapters:

<71> Sterility Tests
<85> Bacterial Endotoxins Test
<1151> Pharmaceutical Dosage Forms

This present discussion will highlight chapters <795>, <797>, and <800>.

Chapter <795> Pharmacy Compounding—Nonsterile Preparations contains the following sections: (1) Introduction; (2) Definitions; (3) Categories of Compounding; (4) Responsibilities of the Compounder; (5) Compounding Process; (6) Compounding Facilities; (7) Compounding Equipment; (8) Component Selection, Handling, and Storage; (9) Stability Criteria and Beyond-Use Dating; (10) Packaging and Drug Preparation Containers; (11) Compounding Documentation; (12) Quality Control; (13) Patient Counseling; (14) Training; and (15) Compounding for Animal Patients. The purpose of this chapter is to include information to enhance the compounder's ability to extemporaneously compound preparations that are of acceptable strength, quality, and purity.

Chapter <797> Pharmacy Compounding—Sterile Preparations contains the following sections: (1) Definitions; (2) Responsibility of Compounding Personnel; (3) CSP Microbial Contamination Risk Levels; (4) Personnel Training and Evaluation in Aseptic Manipulation Skills; (5) Immediate-Use CSPs; (6) Single-Dose and Multiple-Dose Containers; (7) Hazardous Drugs as CSPs; (8) Radiopharmaceuticals as CSPs; (9) Allergen Extracts as CSPs; (10) Verification of Compounding Accuracy and Sterility; (11) Environmental Quality and Control; (12) Suggested

Standard Operating Procedures; (13) Elements of Quality Control; (14) Verification of Automated Compounding Devices for Parenteral Nutrition Compounding; (15) Finished Preparation Release Checks and Tests; (16) Storage and Beyond-Use Dating; (17) Maintaining Sterility, Purity, and Stability of Dispensed and Distributed CSPs; (18) Patient or Caregiver Training; (19) Patient Monitoring and Adverse Events Reporting; (20) Quality Assurance Program; (21) Abbreviations and Acronyms; and four appendices. The overall objective of the chapter is to describe conditions and practices to prevent harm, including death, to patients that could possibly result from microbial contamination, excessive bacterial endotoxins, variability in the intended strength and composition, unintended chemical and physical contaminants, and ingredients of inappropriate quality in CSPs (10).

Chapter <800> Hazardous Drugs—Handling in Healthcare Settings describes practice and quality standards for handling hazardous drugs (HDs) to promote patient safety, worker safety, and environmental protection. It contains the following sections: (1) Introduction and Scope; (2) List of Hazardous Drugs; (3) Types of Exposure; (4) Responsibilities of Personnel Handling Hazardous Drugs; (5) Facilities and Engineering Controls; (6) Environmental Quality and Control; (7) Personal Protective Equipment; (8) Hazard Communication Program; (9) Personnel Training; (10) Receiving; (11) Labeling, Packaging, Transport, and Disposal; (12) Dispensing Final Dosage Forms; (13) Compounding; (14) Administering; (15) Deactivating, Decontaminating, Cleaning, and Disinfecting; (16) Spill Control; (17) Documentation and Standard Operating Procedures; and (18) Medical Surveillance, along with a glossary, appendices, and references.

National Association of Boards of Pharmacy

"The Good Compounding Practices Applicable to State-Licensed Pharmacies" (11), developed by the National Association of Boards of Pharmacy, discusses eight recommendations. The subparts include (A) General Provisions and Definitions; (B) Organization and Personnel; (C) Drug Compounding Facilities; (D) Equipment; (E) Control of Components and Drug Product Containers and Closures; (F) Drug Compounding Controls; (G) Continuous Quality Improvement Program; (H) Labeling Control of Excess Products; and (I) Records and Reports. Details are available and the Model Act may be downloaded at https://www.nabp.net/publications/model-act.

Some individual states have used this model and/or implemented their own version. All pharmacists and pharmacy students should become familiar with the individual state requirements in the state in which they practice.

It will be important as compounding pharmacy increases to ensure reasonable agreement between the national and state agencies so pharmacists will have a set of guidelines within which they can work to provide their patients the needed individualized medications.

PACKAGING, LABELING, AND STORAGE OF PHARMACEUTICALS

The proper packaging, labeling, and storage of pharmaceutical products are all essential for product stability and efficacious use. The purpose of packaging is to protect the product from the environment, to protect the environment from the product, and to provide an appropriate presentation of the product to the consumer. Packaging is important to maintain the physical and chemical stability of the product by being an effective barrier to light, moisture, oxygen, bacteria, volatiles, etc. It also must protect the product from damage and maintain the product integrity during transit from the manufacturer to the consumer or patient.

Containers

Standards for the packaging of pharmaceuticals by manufacturers are contained in the "Current Good Manufacturing Practice" section of the *Code of Federal Regulations* (1), in the USP–NF (10), and in the FDA's *Guideline for Submitting Documentation for Packaging for Human Drugs and Biologics* (12). When submitting an NDA, the manufacturer must include all relevant specifications for packaging the product. During the initial stages of clinical investigations, the packaging must be shown to provide adequate drug stability for the duration of the clinical trials. As the clinical trials advance to their final stage, information on the chemical and physical characteristics of the container, closure, and other component parts of the package system for the proposed product must be developed to ensure drug stability for its anticipated shelf life.

Different specifications are required for parenteral, nonparenteral, pressurized, and bulk containers and for those made of glass, plastic, and metal. In each instance, the package and closure system must be shown to be effective for the particular product for which it is intended. Depending on the intended use and type of container, among the qualities tested are the following:

- Physicochemical properties
- Light transmission for glass or plastic
- Drug compatibility
- Leaching and/or migration
- Vapor transmission for plastics
- Moisture barrier
- Toxicity for plastics
- Valve, actuator, metered dose, particle size, spray characteristics, and leaks for aerosols
- Sterility and permeation for parenteral containers
- Drug stability for all packaging

Compendial terms applying to types of containers and conditions of storage have defined meanings (10). According to the USP, a container is "that which holds the article and is or may be in direct contact with the article." The immediate container is "that which is in direct contact with the article at all times." The closure is part of the container. The container, including the closure, should be clean and dry before it is filled with the drug. The container must not interact physically or chemically with the drug so as to alter its strength, quality, or purity beyond the official requirements. An example would be the sorption of lipophilic drugs, such as diazepam, to low-density plastics resulting in a loss of drug that is available for administration. The problem can be avoided with the use of glass containers.

The USP classifies containers according to their ability to protect their contents from external conditions (10). The minimally acceptable container is termed a well-closed container. It "protects the contents from extraneous solids and from loss of the article under ordinary conditions of handling, shipment, storage, and distribution." A tight container "protects the contents from contamination by extraneous liquids, solids, or vapors; from loss of the article; and from efflorescence, deliquescence, or evaporation under the ordinary or customary conditions of handling, shipment, storage, and distribution and is capable of tight reclosure." A hermetic container "is impervious to air or any other gas under the ordinary or customary conditions of handling, shipment, storage, and distribution." Sterile hermetic containers generally hold preparations intended for injection or parenteral administration. A single-dose container is one that holds a quantity of drug intended as a single dose and, when opened, cannot be resealed with assurance that sterility has been maintained. These containers include fusion-sealed ampuls and prefilled syringes and cartridges. A multiple-dose container is a hermetic container that permits withdrawal of successive portions of the contents without changing the strength or endangering the quality or purity of the remaining portion. These containers are commonly called vials. Examples of single-dose and multiple-dose products are shown in Figure 3.3.

Dosage forms, such as tablets, capsules, and oral liquids, may be packaged in single-unit or multiple-unit containers. A single-unit container is designed to hold a quantity of drug intended for administration as a single dose promptly after the container is opened (Fig. 3.4). Multiple-unit containers contain more than a single unit or dose of the medication. A single-unit package is termed a unit-dose package. The single-unit packaging of drugs may be performed on a large scale by a manufacturer or distributor or on a smaller scale by the pharmacy dispensing the medication. In either instance, the single-unit package must be appropriately labeled with the product identity,

FIGURE 3.3. Injectable products packaged in multiple-dose (vial) and single-dose (ampul) containers.

FIGURE 3.4. Single-unit packaging, including patient cup and blister packaging of single capsule. (Reprinted from Lacher BE. Pharmaceutical Calculations for the Pharmacy Technician. Baltimore, MD: Lippincott Williams & Wilkins, 2008, with permission.)

quality and/or strength, name of manufacturer, lot number, and expiration date to ensure positive identification of the medication.

Although single-unit packaging has a particular usefulness in institutional settings, for example, hospitals and extended care facilities, it is not limited to them. Many

FIGURE 3.5. Strip packaging equipment capable of producing 50 packages per minute. Seals solid dosage units in a variety of wrapping materials and labels each package simultaneously. (Courtesy of Packaging Machinery Associates.)

outpatients find single-unit packages a convenient and sanitary means of maintaining and using their medication. Among the advantages cited for single-unit packaging and unit-dose dispensing are positive identification of each dosage unit and reduction of medication errors (many are bar coded), reduced contamination of the drug because of its protective wrapping, reduced dispensing time, greater ease of inventory control in the pharmacy or nursing station, and elimination of waste through better medication management with less discarded medication.

Many hospitals with unit-dose systems strip-package oral solids (Fig. 3.5). Such equipment seals solid dosage forms into four-sided pouches and imprints dose identification on each package at the same time. The equipment can be adjusted to produce individual single-cut packages or perforated strips or rolls of doses. The packaging materials may be combinations of paper, foil, plastic, or cellophane. Some drugs must be packaged in foil-to-foil wrappings to prevent the deteriorating effects of light or permeation of moisture. The packaging of solid dosage forms in clear plastic or aluminum blister wells is perhaps the most popular method of single-unit packaging (Fig. 3.6).

Oral liquids may be dispensed in single units in paper, plastic, or foil cups or prepackaged and dispensed in glass containers having threaded caps or crimped aluminum caps. A number of hospital pharmacies package oral liquids for children's use in disposable plastic oral syringes with rubber or plastic tips on the orifice for closure. In these instances, the nursing staff must be fully aware of the novel packaging and special labeling used to indicate that

they are not for injection. These oral syringes are designed so they will not accept a needle. Other dosage forms, such as suppositories, powders, ointments, creams, and ophthalmic solutions, are also commonly found in single-unit packages provided by their manufacturers. However, the relatively infrequent use of these dosage forms in a given hospital, extended care facility, or community pharmacy does not generally justify the expense of purchasing the specialized packaging machinery necessary for the small-scale repackaging of these forms.

Some pharmaceutical manufacturers use unit-of-use packaging, that is, the quantity of drug product prescribed is packaged in a container. For example, if certain antibiotic capsules are usually prescribed to be taken two times a day for 10 days, unit-of-use packaging would contain 20 capsules. Other products may be packaged to contain a month's supply.

Many pharmaceutical products require light-resistant containers. In most instances, a container made of a good quality of amber glass or a light-resistant opaque plastic will reduce light transmission sufficiently to protect a light-sensitive pharmaceutical. Agents termed ultraviolet absorbers may be added to plastic to decrease the transmission of short ultraviolet rays. The USP provides tests and standards for glass and plastic containers with respect to their ability to prevent the transmission of light (10). Containers intended to provide protection from light or those offered as light-resistant containers must meet the USP standards that define the acceptable limits of light transmission at any wavelength between 290 and 450 nm. A recent innovation in plastic packaging is the coextruded two-layer high-density polyethylene bottle, which has an inner layer of black polyethylene coextruded with an outer layer of white polyethylene. The container provides light resistance (exceeding amber glass) and moisture protection. It is increasingly being used in the packaging of tablets and capsules.

The glass used in packaging pharmaceuticals falls into four categories, depending on the chemical constitution of the glass and its ability to resist deterioration. Table 3.3 presents the chemical makeup of the various glasses; types I, II, and III are intended for parenteral products, and type NP is intended for other products. Each type is tested according to its resistance to water attack. The degree of attack is determined by the amount of alkali released from the glass in the specified test conditions. Obviously, leaching of alkali from the glass into a pharmaceutical solution or preparation could alter the pH and, thus, the stability of the product. Pharmaceutical manufacturers must use

FIGURE 3.6. Commercial blister packaging of pharmaceuticals.

TABLE 3.3. Constitution of Official Glass Types

Type	General Description
I	Highly resistant borosilicate glass
II	Treated soda lime glass
III	Soda lime glass
NP	General purpose soda lime glass

containers that do not adversely affect the composition or stability of their products. Type I is the most resistant glass of the four categories.

Today, most pharmaceutical products are packaged in plastic. The modern compact-type container used for oral contraceptives, which contains sufficient tablets for a monthly cycle of administration and permits the scheduled removal of one tablet at a time, is a prime example of contemporary plastic packaging (Fig. 3.6). Plastic bags for intravenous fluids, plastic ointment tubes, plastic film–protected suppositories, and plastic tablet and capsule vials are other examples of plastics used in pharmaceutical packaging.

The widespread use of plastic containers arose from a number of factors, including the following:

- Its advantage over glass in lightness of weight and resistance to impact, which reduces transportation costs and losses because of container damage
- The versatility in container design and consumer acceptance
- Consumer preference for plastic squeeze bottles in administration of ophthalmics, nasal sprays, and lotions
- The popularity of blister packaging and unit-dose dispensing, particularly in health care institutions

The term *plastic* does not apply to a single type of material but rather to a vast number of materials, each developed to have desired features. For example, the addition of methyl groups to every other carbon atom in the polymer chains of polyethylene will give polypropylene, a material that can be autoclaved, whereas polyethylene cannot. If a chlorine atom is added to every other carbon in the polyethylene polymer, polyvinyl chloride (PVC) is produced. This material is rigid and has good clarity, making it particularly useful in the blister packaging of tablets and capsules. However, it has a significant drawback for packaging medical devices (e.g., syringes): it is unsuitable for *gamma* sterilization, a method that is being used increasingly. The placement of other functional groups on the main chain of polyethylene or added to other types of polymers can give a variety of alterations to the final plastic material. Among the newer plastics are polyethylene terephthalate (PET), amorphous polyethylene terephthalate glycol (APET), and polyethylene terephthalate glycol (PETG). Both APET and PETG have excellent transparency and luster and can be sterilized with *gamma* radiation (13).

Among the problems encountered in the use of plastics in packaging are (*a*) permeability of the containers to atmospheric oxygen and to moisture vapor, (*b*) leaching of the constituents of the container to the internal contents, (*c*) absorption/adsorption of drugs into/to the container, (*d*) transmission of light through the container, and (*e*) alteration of the container upon storage. Agents frequently added to alter the properties of plastic include plasticizers, stabilizers, antioxidants, antistatic agents, antifungal agents, colorants, and others.

Permeability is considered a process of solution and diffusion, with the penetrant dissolving in the plastic on one side and diffusing through to the other side. Permeability should not be confused with porosity, in which minute holes or cracks in the plastic allow gas or moisture vapor to move through directly. The permeability of a plastic is a function of several factors, including the nature of the polymer itself; the amounts and types of plasticizers, fillers, lubricants, pigments, and other additives; pressure; and temperature. Generally, increases in temperature, pressure, and the use of additives tend to increase the permeability of the plastic. Glass containers are less permeable than plastic containers.

The movement of moisture vapor or gas, especially oxygen, through a pharmaceutical container can pose a threat to the stability of the product. In the presence of moisture, solid dosage forms may lose their color or physical integrity. A host of pharmaceutical adjuncts, especially those used in tablet formulations, as diluents, binders, and disintegrating agents, are affected by moisture. Most of these adjuncts are carbohydrates, starches, and natural or synthetic gums, and because of their hygroscopicity, they hold moisture and may even serve as nutrient media for the growth of microorganisms. Many of the tablet-disintegrating agents act by swelling, and if they are exposed to high moisture vapor during storage, they can cause tablet deterioration. Many medicinal agents, including aspirin and nitroglycerin, are adversely affected by moisture and require special protection. Sublingual nitroglycerin tablets must be dispensed in their original glass container.

Specially developed high-barrier packaging can provide added protection to pharmaceutical products against the effects of humidity. Such packaging meets the drug stability requirements adopted by the International Committee on Harmonization, which call for testing of packaged products for a minimum for 12 months at 25°C (77°F) at 60% relative humidity (14). Many capsule and other products are liable to deteriorate in humidity unless protected by high-barrier packaging. Desiccant protectants, such as silica gel in small packets, are commonly included in solid-form packaging as added protection against the effects of moisture vapor.

Drug substances that are subject to oxidative degradation may undergo a greater degree of degradation when packaged in plastic than in glass. In glass, the container's void space is confined and presents only a limited amount of oxygen to the drug contents, whereas a drug packaged in a gas-permeable plastic container may be constantly exposed to oxygen because of the replenished air supply entering through the container. Liquid pharmaceuticals packaged in permeable plastic may lose drug molecules or solvent to the container, altering the concentration of the drug in the product and affecting its potency. An example of solvent loss involves large volume parenterals that are packaged in 1-L plastic bags that are packaged with an "overwrap" that is removed to yield the container of fluid that is actually used. The inside bag may feel slightly damp because of the loss of fluid from the primary container that is entrapped between the primary container and the overwrap.

Leaching is a term used to describe the movement of components of a container into the contents. Compounds leached from plastic containers are generally the polymer additives, such as the plasticizers, stabilizers, or antioxidants. The leaching of these additives occurs predominantly when liquids or semisolids are packaged in plastic. Little leaching occurs when tablets or capsules are packaged in plastic.

Leaching may be influenced by temperature, excessive agitation of the filled container, and the solubilizing effect of liquid contents on one or more of the polymer additives. The leaching of polymer additives from plastic containers of fluids intended for intravenous administration is a special concern that requires careful selection of the plastic used. Leached material, whether dissolved in an intravenous fluid or in minute particles, poses a health hazard to the patient. Thus, studies of the leaching characteristics of each plastic considered for use are undertaken as a part of the drug development process. Soft-walled plastic containers of PVC are used to package intravenous solutions and blood for transfusion.

Sorption, a term used to indicate the binding of molecules to polymer materials, includes both adsorption and absorption. Sorption occurs through chemical or physical means because of the chemical structure of the solute molecules and the physical and chemical properties of the polymer. Generally, the unionized species of a solute has a greater tendency to be bound than the ionized species. Because the degree of ionization of a solute may be affected by the pH of a solution, the pH may influence the sorption tendency of a particular solute. Furthermore, the pH of a solution may affect the chemical nature of a plastic container so as to increase or decrease the active bonding sites available to the solute molecules. Plastic materials with polar groups are particularly prone to sorption. Because sorption depends on the penetration or diffusion of a solute into the plastic, the pharmaceutical vehicle or solvent used can also play a role by altering the integrity of the plastic.

Sorption may occur with active pharmacologic agents or with pharmaceutical excipients. Thus, each ingredient must be examined in the proposed plastic packaging to determine its tendency. Sorption may be initiated by the adsorption of a solute to the inner surface of a plastic container. After saturation of the surface, the solute may diffuse into the container and be bound within the plastic. The sorption of an active pharmacologic agent from a pharmaceutical solution would reduce its effective concentration and render the product's potency unreliable. The sorption of pharmaceutical excipients such as colorants, preservatives, or stabilizers would likewise alter the quality of the product. Methylparaben may be sorbed to some types of plastics, resulting in a decrease in the available concentration of the preservative; this may be reflected in a lowering of its preservative effectiveness.

Deformations, softening, hardening, and other physical changes in plastic containers can be caused by the action of the container's contents or external factors, including changes in temperature and the physical stress placed upon the container in handling and shipping.

It is always good practice to dispense medication to patients in the same type and quality of container as that used by the manufacturer. In some instances, the original container may be used to dispense the medication.

Child-Resistant and Adult-Senior Use Packaging

The U.S. Consumer Product Safety Commission (CPSC) was created in 1972 through the Consumer Product Safety Act to protect "against unreasonable risks of injuries associated with consumer products." Today, the CPSC regulates the sale and manufacture of more than 15,000 different consumer products, including the packaging of legend and OTC medications. At present, all legend drugs intended for oral use must be dispensed by the pharmacist to the patient in a container having a child-resistant closure unless the prescriber or the patient specifically requests otherwise or unless the product is specifically exempt from the requirement.

The CPSC may propose exemption of certain drugs and drug products from the regulations based on toxicologic data or on practical considerations. For instance, certain cardiac drugs, such as sublingual tablets of nitroglycerin, are exempt from the regulations because of the importance of a patient's immediate access to the medication. Exemptions are also permitted in the case of OTC products for one package size or specially marked package to be available to consumers for whom safety closures are unnecessary or too difficult to manipulate. These consumers include childless persons, arthritic patients, and the debilitated. These packages must be labeled "This package for households without young children" or "Package not child resistant."

A child-resistant container is defined as one that is significantly difficult for children under 5 years of age to open or to obtain a harmful amount of its contents within a reasonable time and that is not difficult for "normal adults" to use properly (15,16). The CPSC evaluates the effectiveness of such containers using children aged 42 to 51 months. The four basic designs commonly used are align the arrows, press down and turn, squeeze and turn, and latch top. A child-resistant prescription container is shown in Figure 3.7.

In recognition that many adults, particularly the elderly and those with arthritis or weakened hand strength, have

FIGURE 3.7. Child-resistant safety closure on a prescription container. (Courtesy of Owens-Brockway Prescription Products.)

difficulty opening child-resistant packages, the regulations were amended to require that child-resistant containers be readily opened by senior adults.

Drugs that are used or dispensed in patient care institutions, including hospitals, nursing homes, and extended care facilities, need not be dispensed with safety closures unless they are intended for patients who are leaving the institution.

Compliance Packaging

Many patients are not compliant with the prescribed schedule for taking their medications. The many factors associated with noncompliance include misunderstanding the dosing schedule, confusion because the patient is taking multiple medications, forgetfulness, and a feeling of well-being leading to premature discontinuance of medication.

To assist patients in taking their medications on schedule, manufacturers and pharmacists have devised numerous educational techniques, reminder aids, compliance packages, and devices. The oral contraceptive compact was among the earliest packages developed to assist adherence to a prescribed dosing schedule. Many subsequent packaging innovations, as the methylprednisolone "dose pack," provide scheduled doses. For prescriptions dispensed in traditional containers (e.g., capsule vials), pharmacists often provide calendar medication schedules or commercial pillboxes with daily or weekly compartments. These medication compliance techniques and devices are particularly useful for patients taking multiple medications.

Labeling

All drug products distributed in the United States must meet the labeling requirements in the *Code of Federal Regulations* (1,17,18). Different labeling requirements apply to investigational drugs, manufacturer's prescription drugs, controlled substances, dispensed prescription medication, OTC products, products for animals, medical devices, and other specific categories and specific products. In every instance, federal labeling requirements may be strengthened by state law.

According to federal regulations, manufacturers' drug product labeling includes not only the labels on the immediate container and packaging but also inserts; company literature; advertising and promotional material, including brochures, booklets, mailing pieces, file cards, bulletins, price lists, catalogs, sound recordings, film strips, motion picture films, slides, exhibits, displays, literature reprints, and computer-accessed information; and other materials related to the product.

Important information for a prescription-only drug is provided to health professionals through the manufacturer's product package insert. As discussed in Chapter 2, the package insert must provide full disclosure, that is, a full and balanced presentation of the drug product to enable the prescriber to use the drug with sufficient knowledge of important benefit to risk factors.

Manufacturer's Label

Included in the information usually appearing on the manufacturer's or distributor's immediate label affixed to the container of legend drugs is the following:

1. The established or nonproprietary name of the drug or drugs and the proprietary name of the product if one is used
2. The name of the manufacturer, packer, or distributor of the product
3. A quantitative statement of the amount of each drug per unit of weight, volume, or dosage unit, whichever is most appropriate
4. The pharmaceutical type of dosage form constituting the product
5. The net amount of drug product contained in the package, in units of weight, volume, or number of dosage units, as appropriate
6. The logo "Rx only" or the federal legend "Caution—Federal law prohibits dispensing without prescription" or a similar statement
7. A label reference to refer to the accompanying package insert or other product literature for dosage and other information
8. Special storage instructions when applicable
9. The National Drug Code identification number for the product and a bar code
10. An identifying lot or control number
11. An expiration date
12. For controlled drug substances, the DEA symbol "C" together with the schedule assigned (e.g., III). The statement "Warning—May be habit forming" may also appear

Prescription Label

When dispensing a prescription, by federal law, the pharmacist must include the following information on the label of the dispensed medication:

- The name and address of the pharmacy
- The serial number of the prescription
- The date of the prescription or the date of its filling or refilling (state law often determines which date is to be used)
- The name of the prescriber
- The name of the patient
- Directions for use, including any precautions, as indicated on the prescription

In addition, state laws may require additional information:

- The address of the patient
- The initials or name of the dispensing pharmacist
- The telephone number of the pharmacy
- The drug name, strength, and manufacturer's lot or control number
- The expiration date of the drug
- The name of the manufacturer or distributor

- In an effort to decrease medication errors, there is thought to include the "indication" on the prescription label to help the pharmacist assure the prescribed drug is appropriate

Over-the-Counter Labeling

The FDA now requires a standardized format for the manufacturers' labeling of more than 100,000 OTC products (19,20). In addition to the name of the product, the name and address of the manufacturer or distributor, the quantity of net contents, the bar code and other product-identifying items, the expiration date, and the other drug-specific required information, the following "drug facts" (Fig. 3.8) must appear in this listed order (20):

- The product's active ingredients, including the amount in each dosage unit.
- The purpose of the product.
- The uses (indications) for the product.
- Specific warnings, including when the product should not be used under any circumstances and when it is appropriate to consult with a doctor or pharmacist. This section also describes side effects that could occur and substances or activities to avoid.

- Dosage instructions—when, how, and how often to take the product.
- The product's inactive ingredients and important information to help consumers avoid ingredients that may cause an allergic reaction.

The format and design of the label are intended to be easily read and understood, particularly by seniors who purchase over 30% of the OTC pharmaceutical products sold in the United States.

Dietary Supplement Labeling

Dietary supplements are defined, in part, as products intended to supplement the diet that bear or contain one or more of the following dietary ingredients (21):

- A vitamin
- A mineral
- An herb or other botanical
- An amino acid
- A dietary substance for use by man to supplement the diet by increasing the total dietary intake
- A concentrate, metabolite, constituent, extract, or a combination of any ingredient mentioned above

FIGURE 3.8. Example drug facts label.

The manufacturers of dietary supplements must follow the FDA's cGMP guidelines for dietary supplements, including labeling requirements (21). Labels must include, on the principal display panel or on the "supplement facts" panel (Fig. 3.9), a statement of identity (name of the dietary supplement), the net quantity of contents statement (amount of the dietary supplement), the nutrition values, the ingredient list, and the name and place of business of the manufacturer, packer, or distributor.

Under the Dietary Supplement Health Education Act (1994), supplement manufacturers are permitted to make certain label claims. However, the claims must be accurate and truthful. This act disallows "disease claims" that infer or imply that the product can be used to prevent, treat, cure, mitigate, or diagnose a disease. Thus, "structure/function" claims are allowed on the label. An example would be a claim that a product helps "improve mood" rather than treat depression. Statements can also be made relative to classical dietary nutrient deficiency disease and state of the prevalence of the disease in the United States.

In those instances when a manufacturer makes a permissible claim, the label must also bear the disclaimer, "This statement has not been evaluated by the FDA. This product is not intended to diagnose, treat, cure, or prevent any disease." For herbal products, the label must also state the part of the plant used to make the product, for example, root, stem, or leaf. A standardized format provides the patient with certain minimum information about the product prior to its use. See Figure 3.9 for an example.

In 2009, the U.S. Pharmacopeial Convention initiated publication of the USP Dietary Supplements Compendium (DSC), a collection of standards designed to assist dietary supplement manufacturers in providing quality products to consumers. The DSC contains quality specifications for the identity, strength, purity, and performance characteristics (e.g., dissolution, disintegration) of dietary supplements included in the monographs. It also includes general and regulatory information and guidance to help manufacturers comply with FDA's cGMPs. Since its first publication, the DSC has been expanded and continually updated (10).

The USP also offers *verification services* for dietary supplement finished products and the ingredients used to make them. Products and ingredients that meet all USP verification requirements—including a GMP audit, product and ingredient testing, and manufacturing documentation review—are awarded use of a distinctive "USP Verified Mark" or logo, which may be displayed on product labeling. Participation is voluntary.

Storage

To ensure the stability of a pharmaceutical preparation for the period of its intended shelf life, the product must be stored in proper conditions. The labeling of each product includes the desired conditions of storage. The terms generally employed in such labeling have meanings defined by the USP (10):

Freezer: A place in which the temperature is controlled between −25°C and −10°C (−13°F and 14°F). In some cases, a drug or drug product may have a recommended storage condition below −20°C.

Cold: Any temperature not exceeding 8°C (46°F). A refrigerator is a cold place in which the temperature is maintained thermostatically between 2°C and 8°C (36°F and 46°F). A freezer is a cold place in which the temperature is maintained thermostatically between −25°C and −10°C (−13°F and 14°F).

Cool: Any temperature between 8°C and 15°C (46°F and 59°F). An article for which storage in a cool place is directed may alternatively be stored in a refrigerator unless otherwise specified in the individual monograph.

Room temperature: The temperature prevailing in a working area; also called "ambient temperature." A controlled room temperature encompasses the usual working environment of 20°C to 25°C (68°F to 77°F) but also allows for temperature variations between 15°C and 30°C (59°F and 86°F) that may be found in pharmacies, hospitals, and drug warehouses. The Mean Kinetic Temperature (MKT) should not exceed 25°C. MKT is a weighted average value that represents the overall effect of temperature variations over a period of time on the stability of a drug product.

Warm: Any temperature between 30°C and 40°C (86°F and 104°F).

Excessive heat: Above 40°C (104°F).

Protection from freezing: Where in addition to the risk of breakage of the container, freezing subjects a product to loss of strength or potency or to destructive alteration of the dosage form, the container label bears an appropriate instruction to protect the product from freezing.

Protect from light: Packaging should be in a light-resistant container or package.

Transportation

The stability protection of a pharmaceutical product during transportation is an important consideration. Temperature and humidity variations may occur during shipment from a manufacturer to a wholesaler or to a pharmacy and from a pharmacy to a patient, during mail order shipment of prescriptions and their time in the mailbox, and in emergency care vehicles. Transportation to and within geographic areas of extreme temperatures and humidity requires special consideration.

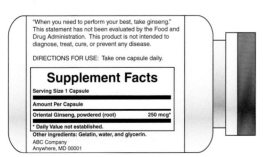

FIGURE 3.9. Example dietary supplement label.

APPLYING THE PRINCIPLES AND CONCEPTS

GROUP ACTIVITIES

1. Make a listing of issues that prevent pharmacies from compounding more than they do currently.
2. Compare and contrast pharmaceutical manufacturing and extemporaneous compounding. Give examples of each.
3. Develop a chart summarizing the eight recommendations of "The Good Compounding Practices Applicable to State-Licensed Pharmacies."
4. Provide examples of drugs that have been demonstrated to interact with their container and describe the type of interaction.

5. Compare and contrast a label from a prescription drug product with that of a nonprescription product label and a dietary supplement label.

INDIVIDUAL ACTIVITIES

1. Given a specific dosage form, determine why the container used to hold the drug is important.
2. What are the problems encountered in the use of plastics in packaging drugs?
3. Given an OTC drug, identify and list all FDA-required labeling information.
4. Create a product prescription label. Include all information required by federal law and respective state laws.

REFERENCES

1. Available at: http://www.accessdata.fda.gov/scripts/cdrh/cfdocs/cfCFR/CFRSearch.cfm
2. A Strategic View of Information Technology in the Pharmaceutical Industry. Philadelphia, PA: Deloitte & Touche, 1994. Available at: http://www.pharmait.co.uk/. (Accessed July 21, 2020)
3. Laboratory Robotics Handbook. Hopkinton, MA: Zymark, 1988. Available at: http://www.labautopedia.com/mw/index.php/The_Zymark_Story. (Accessed July 21, 2020)
4. Guide to Inspection of Bulk Pharmaceutical Chemicals. Rockville, MD: Food and Drug Administration, 1991.
5. Moore RE. FDA's guideline for bulk pharmaceutical chemicals: A consultant's interpretation. Pharm Technol 1992;16:88–100.
6. Guidance for Industry: Nonclinical Studies for the safety Evaluation of Pharmaceutical Excipients. Rockville, MD: Food and Drug Administration, 2005. Available at: http://www.scribd.com/doc/80945199/FDA-Guidance-on-Excipients. (Accessed July 21, 2020)
7. Mercill A. A good manufacturing practices guide for bulk pharmaceutical excipients. Pharm Technol 1995;19:34–40.
8. Bernstein DF. Investigational clinical trial material supply operations in new product development. Appl Clin Trials 1993;2:59–69.
9. Compliance Policy Guidance for FDA Staff and Industry: Pharmacy Compounding. Rockville, MD: Food and Drug Administration, 2002.
10. United States Pharmacopeial Convention, Inc USP/NF. Current Edition. Rockville, MD: US Pharmacopeial Convention, Inc.
11. Model State Pharmacy Act and Model Rules of the National Association of Boards of Pharmacy. Mount Prospect, IL: National Association of Boards of Pharmacy, 2008.
12. Guideline for Submitting Documentation for Packaging Drug Products. Rockville MD: Food and Drug Administration, 1999. (Accessed July 21, 2020)
13. Hacker D. Extruder sees future of medical market: Rigid PET. Pharm Med Pack News 1994;2:22.
14. Wagner J. Pending ICH guidelines and sophisticated drugs add up to the need for higher moisture protection. Pharm Med Pack News 1996;4:20–24.
15. 60 Federal Register 38671–38674.
16. 60 Federal Register 37709–37744.
17. Code of Federal Regulations, Title 21, Parts 111, 201, 210–211. Available at: http://www.accessdata.fda.gov/scripts/cdrh/cfdocs/cfCFR/CFRSearch.cfm. (Accessed July 21, 2020)
18. Code of Federal Regulations, Title 21, Part 1302. Available at: http://www.accessdata.fda.gov/scripts/cdrh/cfdocs/cfCFR/CFRSearch.cfm. (Accessed July 21, 2020)
19. Code of Federal Regulations, Title 21, Section 201, 2012. Available at: http://www.accessdata.fda.gov/scripts/cdrh/cfdocs/cfcfr/CFRSearch.cfm?FR=201.66. (Accessed July 21, 2020)
20. OTC Facts Label. Rockville, MD: Food and Drug Administration, 2002. Available at: http://www.fda.gov/Drugs/ResourcesForYou/Consumers/ucm143551.htm. (Accessed July 21, 2020)
21. General Dietary Supplement Labeling. Rockville, MD: Food and Drug Administration, 2005. Available at: http://www.fda.gov/Food/GuidanceComplianceRegulatoryInformation/GuidanceDocuments/DietarySupplements/DietarySupplementlabelingguide/ucm070519.htm. (Accessed July 21, 2020)

SECTION TWO

Drug Dosage Form and Drug Delivery System Design

Dosage Form Design: Pharmaceutical and Formulation Considerations

CHAPTER AT A GLANCE The Need for Dosage Forms • General Considerations in Dosage Form Design • Chemicals, Bonds, and Properties for Preformulation • Pharmaceutical Ingredients and Excipients

OBJECTIVES

After reading this chapter, the student will be able to:

List reasons for the incorporation of drugs into various dosage forms

Compare and contrast the advantages/disadvantages of various drug dosage forms

Describe the information needed in preformulation studies to characterize a drug substance for possible inclusion into a dosage form

Describe the mechanisms of drug degradation and provide examples of each

Describe the five types of drug instability of concern to the practicing pharmacist

Describe the purpose and general protocol for accelerated stability studies

Summarize approaches employed to stabilize drugs in pharmaceutical dosage forms

Calculate rate reactions for various liquid dosage forms

Categorize various pharmaceutical ingredients and excipients

INTRODUCTION

Drug substances are seldom administered alone; rather they are given as part of a formulation in combination with one or more nonmedicinal agents that serve varied and specialized pharmaceutical functions. Selective use of these nonmedicinal agents, referred to as pharmaceutical ingredients or excipients, produces dosage forms of various types. The pharmaceutical ingredients solubilize, suspend, thicken, dilute, emulsify, stabilize, preserve, color, flavor, and fashion medicinal agents into efficacious and appealing dosage forms. Each type of dosage form is unique in its physical and pharmaceutical characteristics. These varied preparations provide the manufacturing and compounding pharmacist with the challenges of formulation and the physician with the choice of drug and delivery system to prescribe. The general area of study concerned with the formulation, manufacture, stability, and effectiveness of pharmaceutical dosage forms is termed pharmaceutics.

The proper design and formulation of a dosage form require consideration of the physical, chemical, and biologic characteristics of all of the drug substances and pharmaceutical ingredients to be used in fabricating the product. The drug and pharmaceutical materials must be compatible with one another to produce a drug product that is stable, efficacious, attractive, easy to administer, and safe. The product should be manufactured with appropriate measures of quality control and packaged in containers that keep the product stable. The product should be labeled to promote correct use and be stored under conditions that contribute to maximum shelf life.

Methods for the preparation of specific types of dosage forms and drug delivery systems are described in subsequent chapters. This chapter presents some general considerations regarding physical pharmacy, drug product formulation, and pharmaceutical ingredients.

THE NEED FOR DOSAGE FORMS

The potent nature and low dosage of most of the drugs in use today preclude any expectation that the general public

TABLE 4.1. Examples of Low-Dosage Drugs Manufactured into Capsule or Tablet Dosage Forms[a]

Drug Content Per Capsule or Tablet	Indication or Category
Donepezil hydrochloride 5 mg	Dementia
Lisinopril 5 mg	Antihypertensive
Trandolapril 2 mg	Antihypertensive
Rivastigmine tartrate 1.5 mg	Dementia
Colchicine 0.6 mg	Gout
Rasagiline mesylate 0.5 mg	Parkinson disease
Nitroglycerine 0.3 mg	Angina pectoris
Everolimus 0.25 mg	Organ rejection (transplant)
Digoxin 0.125 mg (125 μg)	Heart failure; atrial fibrillation
Fentanyl 0.100 mg (100 μg)	Pain (severe)
Levothyroxine sodium 0.025 mg (25 μg)	Hypothyroidism
Lubiprostone 0.008 mg (8 μg)	Irritable bowel syndrome
Paricalcitol 0.002 mg (2 μg)	Hyperparathyroidism

[a]Examples are of the lowest strength capsule or tablet commercially available for each listed drug.

could safely obtain the appropriate dose of a drug from the bulk material. Most drug substances are administered in milligram quantities, much too small to be weighed on anything but a sensitive prescription or electronic analytical balance. For instance, how could the lay person accurately obtain from a bulk supply the 325 mg of aspirin found in the common tablet? Not possible. Yet compared with many other drugs, the dose of aspirin is formidable (Table 4.1). For example, the dose of ethinyl estradiol, 0.05 mg, is 1/6,500 the amount of aspirin in an aspirin tablet. To put it another way, 6,500 ethinyl estradiol tablets, each containing 0.05 mg of drug, could be made from an amount of ethinyl estradiol equal to the amount of aspirin in just one standard tablet. When the dose of the drug is minute, as with ethinyl estradiol, solid dosage forms such as tablets and capsules must be prepared with fillers or diluents so that the dosage unit is large enough to pick up with the fingertips. Table 4.1 presents some examples of drugs with low dosage that are formulated and manufactured into capsules and tablets for oral administration.

Besides providing the mechanism for the safe and convenient delivery of accurate dosage, dosage forms are needed for additional reasons:

- To protect the drug substance from the destructive influences of atmospheric oxygen or humidity (coated tablets, sealed ampuls)
- To protect the drug substance from the destructive influence of gastric acid after oral administration (enteric-coated tablets)
- To conceal the bitter, salty, or offensive taste or odor of a drug substance (capsules, coated tablets, flavored syrups)

- To provide liquid preparations of drug substances, either as dispersions (suspensions) or as clear preparations (solutions)
- To provide rate-controlled drug action (various controlled-release tablets, capsules, and suspensions)
- To provide optimal drug action from topical administration sites (ointments, creams, transdermal patches, and ophthalmic, ear, and nasal preparations)
- To provide for insertion of a drug into one of the body's orifices (rectal or vaginal suppositories)
- To provide for placement of drugs directly in the bloodstream or body tissues (injections)
- To provide for optimal drug action through inhalation therapy (inhalants and inhalation aerosols)

GENERAL CONSIDERATIONS IN DOSAGE FORM DESIGN

Before formulating a drug substance into a dosage form, the desired product type must be determined insofar as possible to establish the framework for product development. Then, various initial formulations of the product are developed and examined for desired features (e.g., drug release profile, bioavailability, clinical effectiveness) and for pilot plant studies and production scale-up. The formulation that best meets the goals for the product is selected to be its *master formula*. Each batch of product subsequently prepared must meet the specifications established in the master formula.

There are many different forms into which a medicinal agent may be placed for the convenient and efficacious treatment of disease. Most commonly, a manufacturer prepares a drug substance in several dosage forms and strengths for the efficacious and convenient treatment of disease (Fig. 4.1). Before a medicinal agent is formulated into one or more dosage forms, among the factors

FIGURE 4.1. Various forms of a drug substance marketed by a pharmaceutical company to meet the special requirements of the patient.

considered are the physical and chemical properties of the drug substance (discussed later in this chapter) and various therapeutic considerations.

If the medication is intended for systemic use and oral administration is desired, tablets and/or capsules are usually prepared because they are easily handled by the patient and are most convenient in the self-administration of medication. If a drug substance has application in an emergency in which the patient may be comatose or unable to take oral medication, an injectable form of the medication may also be prepared. Many other examples of therapeutic situations affecting dosage form design could be cited, including motion sickness, nausea, and vomiting, for which tablets and skin patches are used for prevention and suppositories and injections for treatment.

The age of the intended patient also plays a role in dosage form design. For infants and children younger than 5 years of age, pharmaceutical liquids rather than solid forms are preferred for oral administration. These liquids, which are flavored aqueous solutions, syrups, or suspensions, are usually administered directly into the infant's or child's mouth by drop, spoon, or oral dispenser (Fig. 4.2) or incorporated into the child's food. The palatability of some commercial products may not be acceptable to some patients, so different flavoring additives may be indicated to enhance compliance; an example would be the FLAVORx or similar commercial flavoring system. A single liquid pediatric preparation may be used for infants and children of all ages, with the dose of the drug varied by the volume administered. When a young patient has a productive cough or is vomiting, gagging, or simply rebellious, there may be some question as to how much of the medicine administered is actually swallowed and how much is expectorated. In such instances, injections may be required. Infant-size rectal suppositories may also be employed, although drug absorption from the rectum is often erratic.

During childhood and even adulthood, a person may have difficulty in swallowing solid dosage forms, especially uncoated tablets. For this reason, some medications are formulated as chewable tablets. Many of these tablets are comparable in texture to an after-dinner mint and break down into a pleasant-tasting creamy material. Newly available tablets dissolve in the mouth in about 10 to 15 seconds; this allows the patient to take a tablet but actually swallow a liquid. Capsules have been found by many to be more easily swallowed than whole tablets. If a capsule is moistened in the mouth before it is swallowed, it becomes slippery and readily slides down the throat with water. Also, a teaspoonful of gelatin dessert, liquid candy, or syrup placed in the mouth and partially swallowed before placing the solid dosage form in the mouth aids in swallowing them. Also, if a person has difficulty in swallowing a capsule, the contents may be emptied into a spoon; mixed with jam, honey, or other similar food to mask the taste of the medication; and swallowed. There is also a device called the Pill Glide that can be used to help swallow solid dosage forms. Medications intended for the elderly are commonly formulated into oral liquids or may be extemporaneously prepared into an oral liquid by the pharmacist. In many patient care facilities, as nursing homes, tablet-crushing devices are utilized by the nursing staff preparatory to mixing with food (as applesauce) for administration. However, certain tablets and capsules that are designed for controlled release should not be crushed or chewed, because that would interfere with their integrity and intended performance.

Many patients, particularly the elderly, take multiple medications daily. The more distinctive the size, shape, and color of solid dosage forms, the easier is proper identification of the medications. Errors in taking medications among the elderly occur frequently because of their multiple drug therapy and impaired eyesight. Dosage forms that allow reduced frequency of administration without sacrifice of efficiency are particularly advantageous.

In dealing with the problem of formulating a drug substance into a proper dosage form, research pharmacists employ knowledge gained through experience with other chemically similar drugs and through the proper use of the physical, chemical, biologic, and pharmaceutical sciences. The early stages of any new formulation include studies to collect basic information on the physical and chemical characteristics of the drug substance. These basic studies are the *preformulation* work needed before actual product formulation begins.

FIGURE 4.2. Oral dosage devices to assist in measuring doses for children.

CHEMICALS, BONDS, AND PROPERTIES FOR PREFORMULATION

Pharmaceutics includes the scientific and technological aspects of the design, compounding, and manufacture of dosage forms. Considerations in the design of dosage forms include the (a) physicochemical properties of the drug itself; (b) biopharmaceutical considerations; and (c) therapeutic considerations of the disease state to be treated. In order to understand the physicochemical properties of the drug, it is beneficial to understand the basic chemistry of the molecules, bonds, and their contribution to the physicochemical properties and uses of the drug.

Forces and Bonds

Atoms possess forces properly maintaining the electrons, protons, and neutrons in relative positions. If we consider the hydrogen atom, it is about 99.9999999999996% empty space, and in general, atoms are about 99.999999999999% empty space. The nucleus of protons and neutrons balance the encircling electrons, which form a type of "shell" around the atom giving it certain characteristics, including negative or positive charges. The shells are not always full of electrons and can share or join with other atoms forming molecules. The composition and arrangement of the atoms in molecules provide for properties of the molecules. Molecules can exist as gases, liquids, and/or solids because there are intermolecular forces that help hold them together (cohesion) and push them apart (repulsion). For molecules to interact, these forces must be balanced in an energy-favored arrangement. Knowing about these forces is important not only for studying them as gases, liquids, and solids but also for their properties, interfacial phenomena, flocculation in suspensions, stabilization of emulsions, compaction of powders in capsules, dispersion of powders or liquid droplets in aerosols, and the compression of granules to form tablets. There are numerous forces working simultaneously depending upon the system being studied, as follows:

- *van der Waals*: van der Waals forces involve nonionic interactions between molecules but involve charge–charge interactions. These can include permanent dipole, Keesom forces (dipole–dipole), Debye forces (dipole–induced dipole), and London forces (induced dipole–induced dipole). These relatively weak bonds are involved with condensation of gases, solubility of some drugs, formation of some metal complexes and molecular addition compounds, and certain biologic processes and drug actions.
- *Ion–dipole and ion-induced dipole*: In addition to the van der Waals forces, polar or nonpolar molecules and ions exhibit other types of attractions such as ion–dipole and ion-induced dipole forces. This may be involved in the formation of the iodine solutions involving the iodide complex ($I_2 + K^+I^- = K^+I_3^-$), which is important in the formation of the commonly used iodine solutions.
- *Ion–ion*: The strongest bonding interaction that can persist over the longest distance is the ionic, electrovalent bond between two counter ions. Also, there are weaker ion–ion interactions like those in some salt formations that exist and influence pharmaceutical systems. These ion–ion interactions are usually looked at as attractive forces. These forces are important in physical property characteristics of drugs including salt form selection, solid crystalline habit, solubility, dissolution, pH and pK determination, and solution stability.
- *Hydrogen*: Interactions between molecules containing a hydrogen atom can form an electrostatic type of union called a hydrogen bond or a hydrogen bridge. This exists in ice as well as in liquid water and accounts for many of the unusual properties of water such as its high dielectric constant, low vapor pressure, and high boiling point. Hydrogen bonds also are involved with alcohols, carboxylic acids, aldehydes, esters, and polypeptides.

Another type of bond is the covalent bond, which includes chemical bonds that involve the sharing of electron pairs between atoms. These electron pairs are known as shared pairs or bonding pairs, and the stable balance of attractive and repulsive forces between atoms, when they share electrons, is known as covalent bonding.

Regarding bond strengths, van der Waals forces and other interactions generally involve bond energies of 1 to 10 kcal/mol, hydrogen bonds about 2 to 8 kcal/mol, chemical covalent bonds about 50 to 100 kcal/mol, and over 100 kcal/mol for the ionic bonds.

States of Matter

The three primary states of matter involve gases, liquids, and solids, the actual state dependent upon intermolecular, interatomic, or ionic forces. In solids, the atoms can only move about fixed positions. With energy added, in the form of heat, the atoms can acquire sufficient energy to break the lattice bonds and move into a liquid form (this can occur at what is defined as a melting point). As additional energy/heat is applied, the molecules acquire sufficient energy to break out from the liquid state and into the gaseous state. Note that some solids with high vapor pressures (iodine, camphor, dry ice, etc.) can pass directly from the solid to the gaseous state bypassing the liquid state (sublimation).

Gaseous State: Characteristics of the gaseous state include rapid movement and collisions with each other and the walls of the container; hence, they exert a "pressure" or force per unit area. They tend to escape into the atmosphere unless restricted by a container. Another characteristic is that they occupy a "volume." The usefulness of these characteristics is discussed further in the chapter on disperse systems.

Liquid State: Liquids are in between gases and solids; they contain more energy than when a solid but less energy than when in the gaseous state. Liquids are more dense than gases and occupy certain volume and flow unless restricted by a container. Transitions from a gas to a liquid and from a liquid to a solid depend not only upon temperature but on pressure. Liquids are easier to work with than gases. An aerosol propellant container contains the propellant in both the liquid and gaseous phase, maintained under pressure. Generally, liquids have characteristics that are useful, including density, vapor pressure, etc., and are valuable for their solvent properties.

Liquids have a vapor pressure immediately above the surface of the liquid. If heat is applied to a liquid to the point that the vapor pressure of the liquid is the same as the external or atmospheric pressure, this is known as the boiling point. At this point, the incoming heat is used to change the liquid to vapor and the temperature will not rise until the liquid is completely vaporized. Moving in the opposite direction, when heat is removed, the energy loss in the liquid results in immobilization of the atoms to form a solid at its freezing point. This temperature is important especially in stability situations where one is trying to extend the beyond-use date of the expiration date of a drug. Freezing point is also important in lyophilization procedures.

Solid State: Solids are arranged in fixed geometric lattices or patterns. Examples include ice, sodium chloride, prednisone, etc., and occur as crystals. Crystalline solids exhibit definite shapes and an orderly arrangement of units. There are six crystalline systems, based on symmetry, including cubic (sodium chloride), tetragonal (urea), hexagonal (iodoform), rhombic (iodine), monoclinic (sucrose), and triclinic (boric acid). Solids are practically incompressible and are similar to liquids in this respect. Heating a solid will result in reaching a point at which it passes sharply from solid to liquid, and this is known as its melting point. The melting point is defined as the temperature at which the pure liquid and solid exist in equilibrium.

Some crystalline materials may exist in more than one crystalline form and are called polymorphic. Polymorphs can have different solubilities, melting points, x-ray crystal and diffraction patterns, and stabilities although they are the identical chemical composition. Most long-chain organic compounds exhibit polymorphism. One of the most common polymorphic materials is cocoa butter (theobroma oil) commonly used in suppositories. Others examples include chloramphenicol, cortisone acetate (at least five different forms), tamoxifen citrate, carbamazepine, estrogens, etc.

Another characteristic of solids is that some exist as solvates where residual solvents can be trapped in the crystalline lattice. The USP standards for these substances place limits on the amount of solvent(s) that can be present.

Amorphous solids are sometimes called supercooled liquids because the molecules are arranged in a random manner that is similar to the liquid state, but they are solid. Examples include synthetic plastics, pitch, and especially "glass." These do not have definite melting points, and whether a drug is amorphous or crystalline has been demonstrated to affect its therapeutic effectiveness. If used to prepare a solution, there may be a difference in the rate of dissolution, but once dissolved, the molecules are the same and act identically.

To obtain information on the characteristics related to many of these substances, various analytical methods are used, as shown in Physical Pharmacy Capsule 4.18. These methods provide valuable information on various aspects of molecules, drugs, and dosage forms. Many of the properties and analytical methods are related to their bonding structure/composition, intramolecular and intermolecular forces, etc., and these can be studied based on physical testing and chemical and other testing methods to characterize the molecules and substances. Spectroscopic methods are based on the interaction of the substance with electromagnetic radiation. Conductometric methods are based upon hydrogen ion concentrations and ionization; chromatographic methods are based upon separation of components/analytes under various conditions.

Preformulation Studies

Before the formulation of a drug substance into a dosage form, it is essential that it be chemically and physically characterized. The following *preformulation studies* (1) and others provide the type of information needed to define the nature of the drug substance. This information provides the framework for the drug's combination with pharmaceutical ingredients in the fabrication of a dosage form.

Preformulation is the process of optimizing a drug through the determination and/or definition of those physical and chemical properties considered important in the formulation of a stable, effective, and safe dosage form. Also considered are the possible interactions with the various components intended for use in the final drug product. It involves parameters as dissolution, polymorphic forms and crystal size and shape, pH profile of stability, and drug–excipient interactions, which may have a profound effect on a drug's physiological availability and physical and chemical stability.

Because the stability of a drug candidate will be related to the degree of crystallinity, it is important to identify all the possible crystalline forms of the compound that may be encountered. If a compound can exist in more than one crystalline state, it is important to identify the most stable polymorph. Different crystalline polymorphs will generally exhibit different melting points, with the highest melting form being regarded as the most stable.

Particle size distributions of drugs and excipients will exert profound effects on mixing phenomena and on possible segregation in mixed materials. In the absence of electrostatic effects, it is easiest to produce homogenous powders if the individual components are of about the same particle size. Adsorbed air is problematic. Particle size reduction to less than 10 μm may be inadvisable for some drug substances.

Physical Description

It is important to understand the physical description of a drug substance prior to dosage form development. Most drug substances in use today are solid materials, pure chemical compounds of either crystalline or amorphous constitution. The purity of the chemical substance is essential for its identification and for evaluation of its chemical, physical, and biologic properties. Chemical properties include structure, form, and reactivity. Physical properties include such characteristics as its physical description, particle size, crystalline structure, melting point, and solubility. Biologic properties relate to its ability to get to a site of action and elicit a biologic response. Some of this information can be obtained from Certificates of Analysis and from Safety Data Sheets (SDSs).

A Certificate of Analysis (COA) is important in evaluating whether or not a drug substance or excipient meets the physical and chemical requirements of compendial monographs, if the substance is official. If the ingredient is not an official substance, reasonable standards can be applied for acceptance as use in manufacturing or compounding. Bulk drug substances must be accompanied by a lot-specific, valid COA.

A COA is an authenticated document issued by an appropriate authority that certifies the quality and purity of not only pharmaceutical substances but also animal and plant products. COAs accompanying materials are generally designed to be as clear and concise as possible, while complying with the appropriate International Organization for Standardization (ISO) guide requirements.

For official ingredients, a *monograph* in the *USP/NF* provides the article's name, definition, specifications, and other requirements related to packaging, storage, and labeling. The specification consists of tests, procedures, and acceptance criteria that help ensure the identity, strength, quality, and purity of the article.

A SDS [formerly Material Safety Data Sheet (MSDS)] is a written document that outlines information and procedures for handling and working with chemicals. The SDS is an important component of compounding or manufacturing records. It is intended to provide workers and emergency personnel with procedures for handling or working with a specific substance in a safe manner. A SDS includes information such as physical data (melting point, boiling point, flash point, etc.), toxicity, health effects, first aid, reactivity, storage, disposal, protective equipment, and spill-handling procedures. SDS formats can vary from source to source within a country depending on national requirements. The sheet identifies the manufacturer of the material (name, address, phone and fax numbers) and usually includes (*a*) chemical identity; (*b*) hazardous ingredients; (*c*) physical and chemical properties; (*d*) fire and explosion data; (*e*) reactivity data; (*f*) health hazards data; (*g*) exposure limits data; (*h*) precautions for safe storage and handling; (*i*) need for protective gear; and (*j*) spill control, cleanup, and disposal procedures. SDSs are generally not lot specific.

SDSs should be maintained for any drug substance or bulk chemical located in the pharmacy. These data sheets are not required for commercially available finished preparations; the ingredient information on the commercial product label or package insert is sufficient. The ingredient information consists mainly of physicochemical, toxicity, and handling information. Precautions, information about potential hazards, and shipping instructions are also included. This information should be reviewed for the protection of a pharmacist as well as for that of a patient.

Drugs can be used therapeutically as solids, liquids, and gases. Liquid drugs are used to a much lesser extent than are solid drugs, and gases even less frequently.

Liquid drugs pose an interesting problem in the design of dosage forms and delivery systems. Many liquids are volatile and must be physically sealed from the atmosphere to prevent evaporation loss. Amyl nitrite, for example, is a clear yellowish liquid that is volatile even at low temperatures and is also highly flammable. It is kept for medicinal purposes in small sealed glass cylinders wrapped with gauze or another suitable material. When amyl nitrite is administered, the glass is broken between the fingertips, and the liquid wets the gauze covering, producing vapors that are inhaled by the patient requiring vasodilation. Propylhexedrine is another volatile liquid that must be contained in a closed system. This drug is used as a nasal inhalant for its vasoconstrictor action. A cylindrical roll of fibrous material is impregnated with propylhexedrine, and the saturated cylinder is placed in a suitable, usually plastic, sealed nasal inhaler. The inhaler's cap must be securely tightened each time it is used. Even then, the inhaler maintains its effectiveness for only a limited time because of the volatility of the drug.

Another problem associated with liquid drugs is that those intended for oral administration cannot always be formulated into tablet form, the most popular form of oral medication, without chemical modification or formulation alternatives. An exception to this is the liquid drug nitroglycerin, which is formulated into sublingual tablets that disintegrate within seconds after placement under the tongue. However, because the drug is volatile, it has a tendency to escape from the tablets during storage, and it is critical that the tablets be stored in a tightly sealed glass container. For the most part, when a liquid drug is to be administered orally and a solid dosage form is desired, one of two approaches is used. First, the liquid substance may be sealed in a soft gelatin capsule. Vitamins A, D, and E and ergoloid mesylates are liquids commercially available in capsule form. Second, the liquid drug may be developed into a solid ester or salt form that will be suitable for tablets or drug capsules. For instance, scopolamine hydrobromide is a solid salt of the liquid drug scopolamine and is easily pressed into tablets. Another approach to formulate liquids into solids is by mixing the drug with a solid or melted semisolid material, such as a high molecular weight polyethylene glycol. The melted mixture is poured into hard gelatin capsules to harden, and the capsules are sealed.

For certain liquid drugs, especially those taken orally in large doses or applied topically, their liquid nature may have some advantage in therapy. For example, 15-mL doses of mineral oil may be administered conveniently as such. Also, the liquid nature of undecylenic acid certainly does not hinder but rather enhances its use topically in the treatment of fungus infections of the skin. However, for the most part, pharmacists prefer solid materials in formulation work because they can easily form them into tablets and capsules.

Formulation and stability difficulties arise less frequently with solid dosage forms than with liquid preparations, and for this reason, many new drugs first reach the market as tablets or dry-filled capsules. Later, when the pharmaceutical problems are resolved, a liquid form of the same drug may be marketed. This procedure is doubly advantageous, because for the most part, physicians and patients alike prefer small, generally tasteless, accurately dosed tablets or capsules to the analogous liquid forms. Therefore, marketing a drug in solid form first is more practical for the manufacturer and suits most patients. It is estimated that tablets and capsules constitute the dosage form dispensed 70% of the time by community pharmacists, with tablets dispensed twice as frequently as capsules.

Microscopic Examination

Microscopic examination of the raw drug substance is an important step in preformulation work. It gives an indication of particle size and size range of the raw material along with the crystal structure. Photomicrographs of the initial and subsequent batch lots of the drug substance can provide important information in case of problems in formulation processing attributable to changes in particle or crystal characteristics of the drug. During some processing procedures, the solid drug powders must flow freely and not become entangled. Spherical and oval powders flow more easily than do needle-shaped powders and make processing easier.

Heat of Vaporization

The use of vapor pressure is important in the operation of implantable pumps delivering medications as well as in aerosol dosage forms. Another application is the use of nasal inhalants (propylhexedrine with menthol and lavender oil—Benzedrex) for treating nasal congestion. In this latter dosage form, the quantity of drug required for effectiveness and a reasonable estimate of time of usefulness can be determined. Also, in the case of spills in inaccessible places, the time to evaporation of a substance can also be calculated. Some volatile drugs can even migrate

within a tablet dosage form so the distribution may not be uniform any longer. This may have an impact in tablets that are scored for dosing where the drug in one portion may be higher or lower than in the other portion.

Exposure of personnel to hazardous drugs because of handling, spilling, or aerosolizing of drugs that may vaporize (oncology agents) is another application as the increase in mobility of the hazardous drug molecules may be related to temperature of the environment. Some drugs, such as carmustine, experience greater vapor pressures with increased temperature as compared to cyclophosphamide, etoposide, cisplatin, and 5-fluorouracil, as illustrated in Physical Pharmacy Capsule 4.1, Heat of Vaporization.

Melting Point Depression

A characteristic of a pure substance is a defined melting point or melting range. If not pure, the substance will exhibit a change in melting point. This phenomenon is commonly used to determine the purity of a drug substance and, in some cases, the compatibility of various substances before inclusion in the same dosage form. This characteristic is further described in Physical Pharmacy Capsule 4.2, Melting Point Depression.

The Phase Rule

Phase diagrams are often constructed to provide a visual picture of the existence and extent of the presence of solid and liquid phases in binary, ternary, and other mixtures. Phase diagrams are normally two-component (binary) representations, as shown in Physical Pharmacy Capsule 4.3, The Phase Rule, but can also be three-component representations, as shown in Physical Pharmacy Capsule 4.4, Triangular Phase Diagram.

Particle Size

Certain physical and chemical properties of drug substances, including dissolution rate, bioavailability, content uniformity, taste, texture, color, and stability, are affected by the particle size distribution. In addition, flow characteristics and sedimentation rates, among other properties, are important factors related to particle size. It is essential to establish as early as possible how the particle size of the drug substance may affect formulation and efficacy. Of special interest is the effect of particle size on absorption. Particle size significantly influences the oral absorption profiles of certain drugs, including griseofulvin, nitrofurantoin, spironolactone, and procaine penicillin. Also, satisfactory content uniformity in solid dosage forms depends to a large degree on particle size and the equal distribution of the active ingredient throughout the formulation. Sieve analysis is the simplest method for determining particle sizes but does not provide much

PHYSICAL PHARMACY CAPSULE 4.1 Heat of Vaporization

The amount of heat absorbed when 1 g of a liquid vaporizes is known as the heat of vaporization of that liquid and is measured in calories. The heat of vaporization of water at 100°C is 540 cal/g or about 9.720 cal/mol. This is the same quantity of heat energy that is released when 1 g of steam condenses to water at 100°C. This energy exchange is important in processes like steam sterilization as it is this energy transfer that results in death of microorganisms.

The movement of molecules varies with temperature. In liquids, this results in a tendency of the molecules to escape the liquid environment into a gaseous environment and possibly loss of the liquid. In the case of solids that sublime, the movement of the molecules is from the solid state to the vapor state. As an example, if one looks at an older bottle containing aspirin, there may be crystals of aspirin on the inside walls of the container. With ibuprofen, the walls of the container may become cloudy as the ibuprofen sublimes.

The use of vapor pressure is important in the operation of implantable pumps delivering medications as well as in aerosol dosage forms. Exposure of personnel to hazardous drugs because of handling, spilling, or aerosolizing of drugs that may vaporize (oncology agents) is another application as the increase in mobility of the hazardous drug molecules may be related to temperature of the environment. Some drugs, such as carmustine, experience greater vapor pressures with increased temperature as compared to cyclophosphamide, etoposide, cisplatin, and 5-fluorouracil, as illustrated in the table below. Particle size affects vapor pressure; the smaller the particle size, the greater the vapor pressure. This demonstrates the importance of personnel protection with working with micronized hazardous powders. The time to evaporation of a substance can also be calculated.

The variation of vapor pressure with temperature is described by the form of the Clausius-Clapeyron equation, as follows:

$$\frac{d \ln P}{dT} = \frac{\Delta H_{vap}}{RT^2}$$

assuming that δH_{vap} is constant, integration of the equation gives:

$$\log P = \frac{-\Delta H_{vap}}{2.303\,RT} + constant$$

A plot of the log of the vapor pressure versus 1/T should be linear and the slope will be equal $-\Delta H_{vap}/2.303R$ from which the enthalpy of vaporization can be calculated. With data obtained from Kiffmeyer et al. (2002), the following table can be constructed:

Compound	Measured Vapor Pressure (Pa)	
	20°C	40°C
Carmustine	0.019	0.530
Cisplatin	0.0018	0.0031
Cyclophosphamide	0.0033	0.0090
Etoposide	0.0026	0.0038
Fluorouracil	0.0014	0.0039

Source: Kiffmeyer TK, Kube C, Opiolka S, et al. Vapour pressures, evaporation behaviour and airborne concentrations of hazardous drugs: Implications for occupational safety. Pharm J 2002;68:331–337. ∎

PHYSICAL PHARMACY CAPSULE **4.2** Melting Point Depression

The *melting point*, or *freezing point*, of a pure crystalline solid is defined as the temperature at which the pure liquid and solid exist in equilibrium. Drugs with a low melting point may soften during a processing step in which heat is generated, such as particle size reduction, compression, sintering, and so on. Also, the melting point or range of a drug can be used as an indicator of purity of chemical substances (a pure substance is ordinarily characterized by a very sharp melting peak). An altered peak or a peak at a different temperature may indicate an adulterated or impure drug. This is explained as follows.

The *latent heat of fusion* is the quantity of heat absorbed when 1 g of a solid melts; the molar heat of fusion (ΔH_f) is the quantity of heat absorbed when 1 mole of a solid melts. High–melting point substances have high heat of fusion, and low–melting point substances have low heat of fusion. These characteristics are related to the types of bonding in the specific substance. For example, ionic materials have high heats of fusion (NaCl melts at 801°C with a heat of fusion of 124 cal/g), and those with weaker van der Waals forces have low heats of fusion (paraffin melts at 52°C with a heat of fusion of 35.1 cal/g). Ice, with weaker hydrogen bonding, has a melting point of 0°C and a heat of fusion of 80 cal/g.

The addition of a second component to a pure compound (A), resulting in a mixture, will result in a melting point that is lower than that of the pure compound. The degree to which the melting point is lowered is proportional to the mole fraction (N_A) of the second component that is added. This can be expressed thus:

$$\Delta T = \frac{2.303\,RTT_0}{\Delta H_f} \log N_A$$

where

ΔH_f is the molar heat of fusion,
T is the absolute equilibrium temperature,
T_0 is the melting point of pure A, and
R is the gas constant.

Two noteworthy things contribute to the extent of lowering of the melting point:

1. Evident from this relationship is the inverse proportion between the melting point and the heat of fusion. When a second ingredient is added to a compound with a low molar heat of fusion, a large lowering of the melting point is observed; substances with a high molar heat of fusion will show little change in melting point with the addition of a second component.
2. The extent of lowering of the melting point is also related to the melting point itself. Compounds with low melting points are affected to a greater extent than compounds with high melting points upon the addition of a second component (i.e., low–melting point compounds will result in a greater lowering of the melting point than those with high melting points). ■

PHYSICAL PHARMACY CAPSULE **4.3** The Phase Rule

A phase diagram, or temperature–composition diagram, represents the melting point as a function of composition of two- or three-component systems. The figure is an example of such a representation for a two-component mixture.

This phase diagram depicts a two-component mixture in which the components are completely miscible in the molten state and no solid solution or addition compound is formed in the solid state. As is evident, starting from the extremes of either pure component A or pure component B, as the second component is added, the melting point of the pure component decreases.

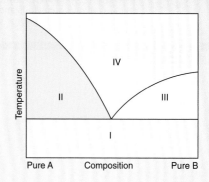

(continued)

There is a point on this phase diagram at which a minimum melting point occurs (i.e., the eutectic point). As is evident, four regions, or phases, in this diagram, represent the following:

   I. Solid A + solid B
  II. Solid A + melt
  III. Solid B + melt
  IV. Melt

Each phase is a homogenous part of the system, physically separated by distinct boundaries.

A description of the conditions under which these phases can exist is called the *Phase Rule*, which can be presented thus:

$$F = C - P + X$$

where

    F is the number of degrees of freedom,
    C is the number of components,
    P is the number of phases, and
    X is a variable dependent upon selected considerations of the phase diagram (1, 2, or 3).

C describes the minimum number of chemical components to be specified to define the phases. F is the number of independent variables that must be specified to define the complete system (e.g., temperature, pressure, concentration).

■ EXAMPLE 1

In a mixture of menthol and thymol, a phase diagram similar to that illustrated can be obtained. To describe the number of degrees of freedom in the part of the graph moving from the curved line starting at pure A, progressing downward to the eutectic point, and then following an increasing melting point to pure B, it is evident from this presentation that either temperature or composition will describe this system because it is assumed in this instance that pressure is constant. Therefore, the number of degrees of freedom to describe this portion of the phase diagram is given thus:

$$F = 2 - 2 + 1 = 1$$

In other words, along this line, either temperature or composition will describe the system.

■ EXAMPLE 2

When in the area of a single phase of the diagram, such as the melt (IV), the system can be described thus:

$$F = 2 - 1 + 1 = 2$$

In this portion of the phase diagram, two factors, temperature and composition, can be varied without a change in the number of phases in the system.

■ EXAMPLE 3

At the eutectic point,

$$F = 2 - 3 + 1 = 0$$

and any change in the concentration or temperature may cause disappearance of one of the two solid phases or the liquid phase.

Phase diagrams are valuable for interpreting interactions between two or more components, relating not only to melting point depression and possible liquefaction at room temperature but also to the formation of solid solutions, coprecipitates, and other solid-state interactions. ■

PHYSICAL PHARMACY CAPSULE **4.4** Triangular (Three-Component) Phase Diagram

Athree-component phase diagram has four degrees of freedom: F = 3 − 1 + 2 = 4. In this case, temperature and pressure are two of the conditions and the concentrations of two of the three components make up the rest. Only two concentrations are required because the third will be the difference between 100% and the sum of the other two components.

These systems are used for determining miscibility/solubility, coacervation regions, gel-forming regions for multicomponent mixtures, etc. To read a three-phase diagram, each of the three corners of the triangle represent 100% by weight of one of the components (A, B, C) and 0% by weight of the other two (A, B, C). The lines joining the corner points forming the triangle each represent two component mixtures of the three possible combinations (AB, BC, and CA). If two of the components are known, the third is known by difference. Any combination of the three components is described by a single point on the diagram. Combining different proportions of the three components and observing for an end point (solubility, gel formation, haziness, etc.), the phase differences can be visualized, as follows:

The following is a stack of four separate pseudoternary phase diagrams for a quaternary system composed of Brij 96, glycerin, mineral oil, and water. The Brij 96:glycerin ratio is noted on the diagram and is considered one of the three components. The shaded regions represent gel systems, whereas the clear regions represent fluid systems.

In addition to observing the phase changes in a single plane, the use of stacked ternary phase diagrams enables one to visualize the change using different ratios of one of the components (in this case, the Brij 96:glycerin ratios). Constructions like this enable a pharmaceutical scientist to select the best ratios and combinations of components for a formulation. ∎

information on particle shape. Particle size is discussed further in Chapter 6. Figure 4.3 shows a particle size analyzer.

Polymorphism

An important factor in formulation is the crystal or amorphous form of the drug substance. The specific conditions used for precipitation or recrystallization of a substance following the drug synthesis process determine the type of solid formed. Polymorphic forms are different crystal packing systems a compound may take and they usually exhibit different physicochemical properties, including melting point and solubility. Polymorphic forms in drugs are relatively common. It has been estimated that at least one-third of all organic compounds exhibit polymorphism. In addition to polymorphic forms, compounds may occur in noncrystalline or amorphous forms. Methods used to prepare amorphous solids do not allow the drug molecules sufficient time to form orderly arrays, and consequently, they solidify in a disordered state. Methods to form amorphous solids include rapid precipitation from solvent, rapid cooling of a melt of the drug, spray drying

and freeze-drying. Amorphous materials exhibit the lowest melting point and highest solubility for a drug. The energy required for a molecule of drug to escape from a crystal is much greater than is required to escape from an amorphous powder. Therefore, the amorphous form of a compound is always more soluble than a corresponding crystal form.

Evaluation of crystal structure, polymorphism, and solvate form is an important preformulation activity. Changes in crystal characteristics can influence bioavailability and chemical and physical stability and can have important implications in dosage form process functions. For example, it can be a significant factor relating to tablet formation because of flow and compaction behaviors, among others. Various techniques are used to determine crystal properties. The most widely used methods are hot stage microscopy, thermal analysis, infrared spectroscopy, and x-ray diffraction.

Solubility

An important physicochemical property of a drug substance is solubility, especially aqueous system solubility. A drug

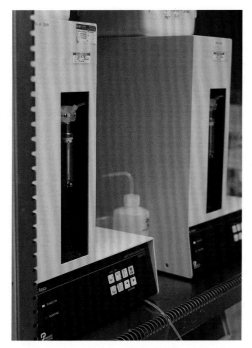

FIGURE 4.3. HIAC particle counter/analyzer. (Courtesy of ARL BioPharma, Inc. d/b/a Analytical Research Laboratories.)

must possess some aqueous solubility for therapeutic efficacy. For a drug to enter the systemic circulation and exert a therapeutic effect, it must first be in solution. Relatively insoluble compounds often exhibit incomplete or erratic absorption. If the solubility of the drug substance is less than desirable, consideration must be given to improve its solubility. The methods to accomplish this depend on the chemical nature of the drug and the type of dosage form under consideration. Chemical modification of the drug into salt or ester forms is frequently used to increase solubility.

A drug's solubility is usually determined by the equilibrium solubility method, by which an excess of the drug is placed in a solvent and shaken at a constant temperature over a long period until equilibrium is obtained. Chemical analysis of the drug content in solution is performed to determine degree of solubility.

Solubility and Particle Size

Although solubility is normally considered a physicochemical constant, small increases in solubility can be accomplished by particle size reduction as described in the Physical Pharmacy Capsule 4.5, Solubility and Particle Size.

PHYSICAL PHARMACY CAPSULE 4.5 Solubility and Particle Size

The particle size and surface area of a drug exposed to a medium can affect actual solubility within reason, for example, in the following relationship:

$$\log\frac{S}{S_0} = \frac{2\gamma V}{2.303\,RTr}$$

where

S is the solubility of the small particles,
S_0 is the solubility of the large particles,
γ is the surface tension,
V is the molar volume,
R is the gas constant,
T is the absolute temperature, and
r is the radius of the small particles.

The equation can be used to estimate the decrease in particle size required to increase solubility. For example, a desired increase in solubility of 5% would require an increase in the S/S_0 ratio to 1.05; that is, the left term in the equation would become log 1.05. If a powder has a surface tension of 125 dynes/cm, molar volume of 45 cm³, and temperature of 27°C, what is the particle size required to obtain the 5% increase in solubility?

$$\log 1.05 = \frac{(2)(125)(45)}{(2.303)(8.314\times10^7)(300)r}$$
$$r = 9.238\times10^{-6} \text{ cm or } 0.0238\,\mu$$

A number of factors are involved in actual solubility enhancement, and this is only an introduction to the general effects of particle size reduction. ■

Solubility and pH

Another technique to enhance solubility, if the drug is to be formulated into a liquid product, is adjustment of the pH of the solvent. However, for many drug substances, pH adjustment is not an effective means of improving solubility. Weak acidic or basic drugs may require extremes in pH that are outside accepted physiologic limits or that may cause stability problems with formulation ingredients. Adjustment of pH usually has little effect on the solubility of substances other than electrolytes. In many cases, it is desirable to use cosolvents or other techniques such as complexation, micronization, or solid dispersion to improve aqueous solubility. A review of pH is provided in Physical Pharmacy Capsule 4.6, Principles of pH. The effect of pH on solubility is illustrated in Physical Pharmacy Capsule 4.7, Solubility and pH.

In recent years, more and more physicochemical information on drugs is being made available to pharmacists in routinely used reference books. This type of information is important for pharmacists in different types of practice, especially those who compound and do pharmacokinetic monitoring.

Dissolution

Variations in the biologic activity of a drug substance may be brought about by the rate at which it becomes available to the organism. In many instances, dissolution rate, or the time it takes for the drug to dissolve in the fluids at the absorption site, is the rate-limiting step in absorption. This is true for drugs administered orally in solid forms, such as tablets, capsules, or suspensions, and for those administered intramuscularly. When the dissolution rate is the rate-limiting step, anything that affects it will also affect absorption. Consequently, dissolution rate can affect the onset, intensity, and duration of response and control the overall bioavailability of the drug from the dosage form, as discussed in the previous chapter.

The dissolution rate of drugs may be increased by decreasing the drug's particle size. It may also be increased by increasing its solubility in the diffusion layer, the small volume of solvent directly in contact with the solid particle. The most effective means of obtaining higher dissolution rates is to use a highly water-soluble salt of the parent substance. Although a soluble salt of a weak acid will precipitate as the free acid in the bulk phase of an acidic solution, such as gastric fluid, it will do so in the form of fine particles with a large surface area.

The dissolution rates of chemical compounds are determined by two methods: the constant surface method, which provides the intrinsic dissolution rate of the agent, and particulate dissolution, in which a suspension of the agent is added to a fixed amount of solvent without exact control of surface area.

The constant surface method uses a compressed disc of known area. This method eliminates surface area

PHYSICAL PHARMACY CAPSULE **4.6** Principles of pH

pH is a critical variable in pharmaceutics, and a basic understanding of its principles and measurement is important. Let's begin with a definition of the term pH. The p comes from the word power. The H, of course, is the symbol for hydrogen. Together, the term pH means the hydrogen ion exponent.

The pH of a substance is a measure of its acidity, just as a degree is a measure of temperature. A specific pH value tells the exact acidity. Rather than stating general ideas, such as cherry syrup is acidic or the water is hot, a specific pH value gives the same relative point of reference, thus providing more exact communication. "The cherry juice has a pH of 3.5" or "the water is at 80°C" provides an exact common language.

pH is defined in terms of the hydrogen ion activity:

$$pH = -\log_{10} a_{H^+} \quad \text{or} \quad 10^{-pH} = a_{H^+}$$

pH equals the negative logarithm of the hydrogen ion activity or the activity of the hydrogen ion is 10 raised to the exponent—pH. The latter expression renders the use of the p exponent more obvious. The activity is the effective concentration of the hydrogen ion in solution. The difference between effective and actual concentration decreases as one moves toward more dilute solutions, in which ionic interaction becomes progressively less important.

Normally, reference is made to the hydrogen ion when reference should be made to the hydronium ion (H_3O^+). It is a matter of convenience and brevity that only the hydrogen ion is mentioned, even though it is normally in its solvated form:

$$H^+ + H_2O = H_3O^+$$

(continued)

The complexing of the hydrogen ion by water affects activity and applies to other ions, which partially complex or establish an equilibrium with the hydrogen ion. In other words, equilibrium such as

$$H_2CO_3 = H^+ + HCO_3^-$$
$$HC_2H_3O_2 = H^+ + C_2H_3O_2^-$$

complexes the hydrogen ion so that it is not sensed by the pH measuring system. This is why an acid–base titration is performed if the total concentration of acid (H^+) is needed. These effects on hydrogen ion activity are obvious, but other more subtle effects are involved in the correlation of activity and concentration.

The activity of the hydrogen ion can be defined by its relation to concentration (C_{H^+}, molality) and the activity coefficient f_{H^+}:

$$aH^+ = f_H + C_{H^+}$$

If the activity coefficient is unity, activity is equal to concentration. This is nearly the case in dilute solutions, whose ionic strength is low. Because the objective of most pH measurements is to find a stable and reproducible reading that can be correlated with the results of some process, it is important to know what influences the activity coefficient and therefore the pH measurement.

The factors that affect the activity coefficient are the temperature (T), the ionic strength (μ), the dielectric constant (ε), the ion charge (Z_i), the size of the ion in angstroms (Å), and the density of the solvent (d). All of these factors are characteristics of the solution that relate the activity to the concentration by two main effects: the salt effect and the medium effect; the latter relates the influence that the solvent can have on the hydrogen ion activity. Thus, hydrogen activity is related to concentration through a salt effect and a solvent effect. Because of these influences, a sample pH value cannot be extrapolated to another temperature or dilution. If the pH value of a particular solution is known at 40°C, it is not automatically known at 25°C.

■ THE pH SCALE

In pure water, hydrogen and hydroxyl ion concentrations are equal at 10^{-7} M at 25°C. This is a neutral solution. Because most samples encountered have less than 1 M H^+ or OH^-, the extremes of pH 0 for acids and pH 14 for bases are established. Of course, with strong acids or bases, pH values below 0 and above 14 are possible but infrequently measured.

■ MEASUREMENT OF pH

The activity of the hydrogen ion in solution is measured with a glass electrode, a reference electrode, and a pH meter.

■ COMBINATION ELECTRODES

A combination electrode is a combination of the glass and reference electrodes into a single probe. The main advantage in using a combination electrode is with the measurement of small volume samples or samples in limited-access containers. ■

PHYSICAL PHARMACY CAPSULE **4.7** Solubility and pH

pH is one of the most important factors in the formulation process. Two areas of critical importance are the effects of pH on solubility and stability. The effect of pH on solubility is critical in the formulation of liquid dosage forms, from oral and topical solutions to intravenous solutions and admixtures.

The solubility of a weak acid or base is often pH dependent. The total quantity of a monoprotic weak acid (HA) in solution at a specific pH is the sum of the concentrations of both the free acid and salt (A^-) forms. If excess drug is present, the quantity of free acid in solution is maximized and constant because of its saturation solubility.

(continued)

PHYSICAL PHARMACY CAPSULE **4.7** Solubility and pH *(continued)*

As the pH of the solution increases, the quantity of drug in solution increases because the water-soluble ionizable salt is formed. The expression is

$$HA \overset{K_a}{\leftrightarrow} H^+ + A^-$$

where K_a is the dissociation constant.

There may be a certain pH level reached where the total solubility (S_T) of the drug solution is saturated with respect to both the salt and acid forms of the drug, that is, the pH_{max}. The solution can be saturated with respect to the salt at pH values higher than this but not with respect to the acid. Also, at pH values less than this, the solution can be saturated with respect to the acid but not to the salt. This is illustrated in the accompanying figure.

To calculate the total quantity of drug that can be maintained in solution at a selected pH, either of two equations can be used, depending on whether the product is to be in a pH region above or below the pH_{max}. The following equation is used when below the pH_{max}:

$$S_T = S_a \left[1 + \frac{K_a}{H^+} \right] \qquad \text{Equation 4.1}$$

The next equation is used when above the pH_{max}:

$$S_T = S_a' \left[1 + \frac{K_a}{H^+} \right] \qquad \text{Equation 4.2}$$

where

S_a is the saturation solubility of the free acid and
S_a' is the saturation solubility of the salt form.

■ EXAMPLE

A pharmacist prepares a 3% solution of an antibiotic as an ophthalmic solution and dispenses it to a patient. A few days later, the patient returns the eye drops to the pharmacist because the product contains a precipitate. The pharmacist, checking the pH of the solution and finding it to be 6, reasons that the problem may be pH related. The physicochemical information of interest on the antibiotic includes the following:

Molecular weight	285 (salt) 263 (free acid)
3% solution of the drug	0.1053-M solution
Acid form solubility (S_a)	3.1 mg/mL (0.0118 M)
K_a	5.86×10^{-6}

Using equation (Equation 4.1, the pharmacist calculates the quantity of the antibiotic in solution [dissolved] at a pH of 6) (*Note:* pH of 6.0 = [H⁺] of 1×10^{-6})

$$S_T = 0.0118 \left[1 + \left(5.86 \times 10^{-6} \right) / \left(1 \times 10^{-6} \right) \right] = 0.0809 \text{ molar}$$

From this, the pharmacist knows that at a pH of 6, a 0.0809-M solution can be prepared. However, the concentration that was to be prepared was a 0.1053-M solution; consequently, the drug will not be in solution at that pH. The pH may have been all right initially but shifted to a lower pH over time, resulting in precipitation of the drug. The question is at what pH (hydrogen ion concentration) the drug will remain in solution. This can be calculated using the same equation and information. The S_T value is 0.1053 M.

$$0.1053 = 0.0118 \left[1 + \frac{5.86 \times 10^{-6}}{H^+} \right]$$

$$\left[H^+ \right] = 7.333 \times 10^{-7}, \text{ or a pH of 6.135}$$

(continued)

The pharmacist prepares a solution of the antibiotic, adjusting the pH to above about 6.2, using a suitable buffer system, and dispenses the solution to the patient—with positive results.

An interesting phenomenon concerns the close relationship of pH to solubility. At a pH of 6, only a 0.0809-M solution could be prepared, but at a pH of 6.13, a 0.1053-M solution could be prepared. In other words, a difference of 0.13 pH units resulted in

$$\frac{0.1053 - 0.0809}{0.0809} = 30.1\%$$

more drugs going into solution at the higher pH than at the lower pH. In other words, a very small change in pH resulted in about 30% more drugs going into solution. According to the figure, the slope of the curve would be very steep for this example drug, and a small change in pH (x-axis) results in a large change in solubility (y-axis). From this, it can be reasoned that if one observes the pH–solubility profile of a drug, it is possible to predict the magnitude of the pH change on its solubility.

In recent years, more and more physicochemical information on drugs is being made available to pharmacists in routinely used reference books. This type of information is important for pharmacists in different types of practice, especially those involved in compounding and pharmacokinetic monitoring. ∎

and surface electrical charges as dissolution variables. The dissolution rate obtained by this method, the *intrinsic dissolution rate*, is characteristic of each solid compound and a given solvent in the fixed experimental conditions. The value is expressed as milligrams dissolved per minute per square centimeter. It has been suggested that this value is useful in predicting probable absorption problems because of dissolution rate. In particulate dissolution, a weighed amount of powdered sample is added to the dissolution medium in a constant agitation system. This method is frequently used to study the influence of particle size, surface area, and excipients upon the active agent. Occasionally, the surface properties of the drug produce an inverse relationship of particle size to dissolution. In these instances, surface charge and/or agglomeration result in the drug particles presenting a lower effective surface area to the solvent because of incomplete wetting, thus negating the expected benefits of particle size reduction. Fick laws describe the relationship of diffusion and dissolution of the active drug in the dosage form and when administered in the body, as shown in Physical Pharmacy Capsule 4.8, Fick Laws of Diffusion and the Noyes-Whitney Equation.

Early formulation studies should include the effects of pharmaceutical ingredients on the dissolution characteristics of the drug substance.

Membrane Permeability

Modern preformulation studies include an early assessment of passage of drug molecules across biologic membranes. To produce a biologic response, the drug molecule must first cross a biologic membrane. The biologic membrane acts as a lipid barrier to most drugs and permits the absorption of lipid-soluble substances by passive diffusion, whereas lipid-insoluble substances can diffuse across the barrier only with considerable difficulty if at all. The interrelationship of the dissociation constant, lipid solubility, and pH at the absorption site with the absorption characteristics of various drugs are the basis of the pH partition theory.

Data obtained from the basic physicochemical studies, specifically, pK_a, solubility, and dissolution rate, provide an indication of absorption. To enhance these data, a technique using the everted intestinal sac may be used to evaluate absorption characteristics of drug substances. In this method, a piece of the intestine is removed from an intact animal, is everted (turned inside out), and is filled with a solution of the drug substance, and the degree and rate of passage of the drug through the membrane sac are determined. This method allows evaluation of both passive and active transport. The importance of active transport in drug absorption, distribution, and elimination has been recognized in the past decade and screening for interaction with common transporters is now required for FDA approval of new chemical entities.

In the latter stages of preformulation testing or early formulation studies, animals and humans must be studied to assess the absorption efficiency and pharmacokinetic parameters and to establish possible in vitro and in vivo correlation for dissolution and bioavailability.

Partition Coefficient

The use of the partition coefficient is described in some detail in Physical Pharmacy Capsule 4.9, Partition Coefficient. Inherent in this procedure is the selection of appropriate extraction solvents, drug stability, use of salting-out additives, and environmental concerns. The octanol–water partition coefficient is commonly used in formulation

PHYSICAL PHARMACY CAPSULE **4.8** Fick Laws of Diffusion and the Noyes-Whitney Equation

All drugs must diffuse through various barriers when administered to the body. For example, some drugs must diffuse through the skin, gastric mucosa, or some other barrier to gain access to the interior of the body. Parenteral drugs must diffuse through muscle, connective tissue, and so on, to get to the site of action; even intravenous drugs must diffuse from the blood to the site of action. Drugs must also diffuse through various barriers for metabolism and excretion.

Considering all the diffusion processes that occur in the body (passive, active, and facilitated), it is not surprising that the laws governing diffusion are important to drug delivery systems. In fact, diffusion is important not only in the body but also in some quality control procedures used to determine batch-to-batch uniformity of products (dissolution test for tablets based on the Noyes-Whitney equation, which can be derived from Fick law).

When individual molecules move within a substance, diffusion is said to occur. This may occur as the result of a concentration gradient or by random molecular motion.

Probably the most widely used laws of diffusion are known as Fick first and second laws. Fick first law involving steady-state diffusion (where dc/dx does not change) is derived from the following expression for the quantity of material (M) flowing through a cross section of a barrier (S) in unit time (t) expressed as the flux (J):

$$J = dM / (Sdt)$$

Under a concentration gradient (dc/dx), Fick first law can be expressed thus:

$$J = D\left[(C_1 - C_2) / h \right] \text{ or } J = -D (dC / dx)$$

where

J is the flux of a component across a plane of unit area,
C_1 and C_2 are the concentrations in the donor and receptor compartments,
h is the membrane thickness, and
D is the diffusion coefficient (or diffusivity).

The sign is negative, denoting that the flux is in the direction of decreasing concentration. The units of J are grams per square centimeter; C, grams per cubic centimeter; M, grams or moles; S, square centimeters; x, centimeters; and D, square centimeters per second.

D is appropriately called a diffusion coefficient, not a diffusion constant, as it is subject to change. D may change in value with increased concentrations. Also, D can be affected by temperature, pressure, solvent properties, and the chemical nature of the drug itself. To study the rate of change of the drug in the system, one needs an expression that relates the change in concentration with time at a definite location in place of the mass of drug diffusing across a unit area of barrier in unit time; this expression is known as Fick second law. This law can be summarized as stating that the change in concentration in a particular place with time is proportional to the change in concentration gradient at that particular place in the system.

In summary, Fick first law relates to a steady-state flow, whereas Fick second law relates to a change in concentration of drug with time, at any distance, or an unsteady state of flow.

The diffusion coefficients ($D \times 10^{-6}$) of various compounds in water (25°C) and other media have been determined as follows: ethanol, 12.5 cm²/s; glycine, 10.6 cm²/s; sodium lauryl sulfate, 6.2 cm²/s; and glucose, 6.8 cm²/s.

The concentration of drug in the membrane can be calculated using the partition coefficient (K) and the concentration in the donor and receptor compartments.

$$K = (C_1 / C_d) = (C_2 / C_r)$$

where

C_1 and C_d are the concentrations in the donor compartment (g/cm³) and
C_2 and C_r are the concentrations in the receptor compartment (g/cm³).

K is the partition coefficient of the drug between the solution and the membrane. It can be estimated using the oil solubility of the drug versus the water solubility of the drug. Usually, the higher the partition coefficient, the more the drug will be soluble in a lipophilic substance. We can now write the expression:

$$dM / dt = \left[DSK (C_d - C_r) \right] / h$$

(continued)

or in sink conditions,

$$dM/dt = DSKC_d/h = PSC_d$$

The permeability coefficient (centimeters per second) can be obtained by rearranging to:

$$P = DK/h$$

■ EXAMPLE 1

A drug passing through a 1-mm-thick membrane has a diffusion coefficient of 4.23×10^{-7} cm^2/s and an oil–water partition coefficient of 2.03. The radius of the area exposed to the solution is 2 cm, and the concentration of the drug in the donor compartment is 0.5 mg/mL. Calculate the permeability and the diffusion rate of the drug.

$h = 1$ mm $= 0.1$ cm
$D = 4.23 \times 10^{-7}$ cm^2/s
$K = 2.03$
$r = 2$ cm, $S = \pi(2$ cm$)^2 = 12.57$ cm^2
$C_d = 0.5$ mg/mL
$P = [(4.23 \times 10^{-7}$ cm^2/s$)(2.03)]/0.1$ cm $= 8.59 \times 10^{-6}$ cm/s
$dM/dt = (8.59 \times 10^{-6}$ cm/s$)(12.57$ cm$^2)(0.5$ mg/mL$) = 5.40 \times 10^{-5}$ mg/s
$(5.40 \times 10^{-5}$ mg/s$)(3,600$ s/h$) = 0.19$ mg/h

In the dissolution of particles of drug, the dissolved molecules diffuse away from the individual particle body. An expression to describe this, derived from Fick equations, is known as the Noyes and Whitney expression, proposed in 1897. It can be written as follows:

$$dC/dt = (DS/Vh)(Cs - C)$$

where

C is the concentration of drug dissolved at time t,
D is the diffusion coefficient of the solute in solution,
S is the surface area of the exposed solid,
V is the volume of solution,
h is the thickness of the diffusion layer,
Cs is the saturation solubility of the drug, and
C is the concentration of solute in the bulk phase at a specific time, t.

It is common practice to use sink conditions in which C does not exceed about 20% of the solubility of the drug being investigated. Under these conditions, the expression simplifies to

$$dC/dt = (DSCs/Vh)$$

and incorporating the volume of solution (V), the thickness of the diffusion layer (h), and the diffusivity coefficient (D) into a coefficient k (to take into account the various factors in the system), the expression becomes

$$dC/dt = kSCs$$

As the factors are held constant, it becomes apparent that the dissolution rate of a drug can be proportional to the surface area exposed to the dissolution medium. A number of other expressions have been derived for specific application to various situations and conditions.

These relationships expressed as Fick first and second laws and the Noyes-Whitney equation have great importance and relevance in pharmaceutical systems.

■ EXAMPLE 2

The following information was obtained using the USP 32–NF 27 dissolution apparatus I. The drug is soluble at 1 g in 3 mL of water, so sink conditions were maintained; the surface area of the tablet exposed was 1.5 cm^2 (obtained by placing the tablet in a special holder exposing only one side to the dissolution medium); and the dosage form studied was a 16-mg sustained-release tablet; the release pattern should be zero order. What is the rate of release of drug?

(continued)

PHYSICAL PHARMACY CAPSULE **4.8** Fick Laws of Diffusion and the Noyes-Whitney Equation (continued)

Time (Hours)	Drug Concentration (mg/900 mL of Solution)	Graph of Release Profile
0.0	0.0	
0.5	1.0	
1.0	1.9	
2.0	4.1	
4.0	8.0	
6.0	11.8	
8.0	15.9	

In this problem, because the surface area (S) was maintained constant at 1.5 cm^2 and the solubility (Cs) of the drug is constant at 1 g in 3 mL of water, the plot of concentration versus time (t) yields a slope with a value of kSCs, or k$_2$, expressing the rate of release of the drug as

$$dC/dt = kSCs$$

$$\text{The slope of the line} = \Delta y / \Delta x = (y_2 - y_1)/(x_2 - x_1)$$
$$= (15.9\ mg - 0\ mg)/(8.0\ h - 0\ h)$$
$$= 15.9/8 = 1.99\ mg/h$$

Therefore, the rate of release of the sustained-release preparation is 1.99 or approximately 2 mg/h. From this, the quantity of drug released at any time (t) can be calculated. ■

development. Following the illustrations provided earlier, it is defined as

$$P = \frac{(\text{Concentration of drug in octanol})}{(\text{Concentration of drug in water})}$$

P depends on the drug concentration only if the drug molecules have a tendency to associate in solution. For an ionizable drug, the following equation is applicable:

$$P = \frac{(\text{Concentration of drug in octanol})}{[1-\alpha](\text{Concentration of drug in water})}$$

where α equals the degree of ionization.

pK$_a$/Dissociation Constants

Among the physicochemical characteristics of interest is the extent of dissociation or ionization of drug substances. This is important because the extent of ionization has an important effect on the formulation and pharmacokinetic parameters of the drug. The extent of dissociation or ionization in many cases is highly dependent on the pH of the medium containing the drug. In formulation, often the vehicle is adjusted to a certain pH to obtain a certain level of ionization of the drug for solubility and stability. In the pharmacokinetic area, the extent of ionization of a drug has a strong effect on its extent of absorption, distribution, and elimination. The dissociation constant, or pK$_a$, is usually determined by potentiometric titration. For the practicing pharmacist, it is important in predicting precipitation in admixtures and in calculating the solubility of drugs at certain pH values. Physical Pharmacy Capsule 4.10, pK$_a$/Dissociation Constants, presents a brief summary of dissociation and ionization concepts.

Hydrates and Solvates

Many active pharmaceutical agents exist as hydrates or solvates; some are hygroscopic, deliquescent, and/or efflorescent. Hygroscopic powders are those that will tend to absorb moisture from the air. Deliquescent powders are those that will absorb moisture from the air and even liquefy. Efflorescent powders are those that may give up their water of crystallization and may even become damp and pasty. When working with these powders, extra care must be taken. Generally, the USP description of a powder will state whether it has hygroscopic, deliquescent, or efflorescent properties.

One other factor is that if a hygroscopic or deliquescent powder is being weighed on a balance, the powder may

PHYSICAL PHARMACY CAPSULE **4.9** Partition Coefficient

The oil–water partition coefficient is a measure of a molecule's lipophilic character; that is, its preference for the hydrophilic or lipophilic phase. If a solute is added to a mixture of two immiscible liquids, it will distribute between the two phases and reach an equilibrium at a constant temperature. The distribution of the solute (unaggregated and undissociated) between the two immiscible layers can be described thus:

$$K = C_U / C_L$$

where

K is the distribution constant or partition constant,
C_U is the concentration of the drug in the upper phase, and
C_L is the concentration of the drug in the lower phase.

This information can be effectively used in

1. Extraction of crude drugs
2. Recovery of antibiotics from fermentation broth
3. Recovery of biotechnology-derived drugs from bacterial cultures
4. Extraction of drugs from biologic fluids for therapeutic drug monitoring
5. Absorption of drugs from dosage forms (ointments, suppositories, and transdermal patches)
6. Study of the distribution of flavoring oil between oil and water phases of emulsions
7. Other applications

This basic relationship can be used to calculate the quantity of drug extracted from or remaining behind in a given layer and to calculate the number of extractions required to remove a drug from a mixture.

The concentration of drug found in the upper layer (U) of the two immiscible layers is given thus:

$$U = Kr/(Kr + 1)$$

where

K is the distribution partition constant and
r is V_U/V_1 or the ratio of the volume of upper and lower phases.

The concentration of drug remaining in the lower layer (L) is given thus:

$$L = 1/(Kr + 1)$$

If the lower phase is successively extracted again with n equal volumes of the upper layer, each upper phase (U_n) contains the following fraction of the drug:

$$U_n = Kr/(Kr + 1)^n$$

where

U_n is the fraction contained in the nth extraction and
n is the nth successive volume.

The fraction of solute remaining in the lower layer (L_n) is given thus:

$$L_n = 1/(Kr + 1)^n$$

More efficient extractions are obtained using successive small volumes of the extraction solvent than single larger volumes. This can be calculated as follows when the same volume of extracting solvent is used in divided portions. For example, the fraction L_n remaining after the nth extraction:

$$L_n = \frac{1}{\left(\dfrac{Kr}{n} + 1\right)^n}$$

(continued)

PHYSICAL PHARMACY CAPSULE **4.9** Partition Coefficient *(continued)*

■ EXAMPLE 1

At 25°C and pH 6.8, the K for a second-generation cephalosporin is 0.7 between equal volumes of butanol and the fermentation broth. Calculate the U, L, and L_n (using the same volume divided into fourths).

$$U = 0.7 / (0.7 + 1) = 0.41, \text{ the fraction of drug extracted into the upper layer}$$
$$L = 1 / (0.7 + 1) = 0.59, \text{ the fraction of drug remaining in the lower layer}$$

The total of the fractions in the U and L = 0.41 + 0.59 = 1.

If the fermentation broth is extracted with four successive extractions accomplished by dividing the quantity of butanol used into fourths, the quantity of drug remaining after the fourth extraction is

$$L_{4th} = \frac{1}{\left(\dfrac{0.7 \times 1}{4} + 1\right)^4} = 0.525$$

From this, the quantity remaining after a single volume, single extraction is 0.59, but when the single volume is divided into fourths and four successive extractions are done, the quantity remaining is 0.525; therefore, more was extracted using divided portions of the extracting solvent. Inherent in this procedure is the selection of appropriate extraction solvents, drug stability, use of salting-out additives, and environmental concerns. ■

absorb moisture from the air and weigh heavier than it should. Therefore, weighings should be made quickly after opening the bulk chemical containers and then resealing them.

Solvates and hydrates must be packaged in "tight" containers to prevent the loss or gain of moisture. In fact, it is best to have all chemicals stored in "tight" containers and to keep them thoroughly closed at all times except for the short time when a weighing step is involved. Storage at the indicated temperatures is also important and to minimize any exposure to very high humidity levels. More on hydrates and solvates is presented in Physical Pharmacy Capsule 4.11, Hydrates and Solvates.

Organic Salt Considerations

Because many drugs are either weak acids or weak bases and have limited water solubility, they are often used as their "salts" to increase their aqueous solubility. For example, sodium salts are often made from weak acids (sodium salicylate is the salt of the weak acid, salicylic acid, and a strong base, sodium hydroxide). Also, a salt such as ephedrine hydrochloride can be prepared between a weak base, ephedrine, and a strong acid, hydrochloric acid. Third, the combination of a weak base, codeine, and a weak acid, phosphoric acid, can be used, as in codeine phosphate.

The purpose of the "salt" form is usually to enhance the solubility of the drug; but it may also enhance the stability and change other attributes of the drug that make it easier to handle and manipulate for producing dosage forms.

The "unionized" portion of the drug that will ultimately exert its effect in the body, as the remainder of the salt molecule may no longer follow the base, or unionized, form of the drug into the body.

When salts are placed in an aqueous environment, they will dissolve to some extent, based upon their solubility in the aqueous media and the pH of the media. There will be a portion of the drug that is dissolved, and some may remain undissolved. Of the dissolved portion, there will be a part that is "ionized" and the remainder will be "unionized," depending upon the pH of the media. Generally, it is the "unionized" portion of the drug in solution that will be absorbed for systemic effect. This is described by the "dissociation constant" or "pK_a" of the drug.

Because the bulk substance or active pharmaceutical ingredient (API) in a salt form is not 100% active drug, it is important to know whether or not the dose of the drug is based upon the drug salt or drug base form. Many drugs are "salts," and the dose may be based on the "total salt" form or just the "base" form of the drug.

Sources of information that can be used to determine the "form" of the drug (base, salt, or ester) include the wording of commercial products (package inserts) and the USP/NF. For example, Albuterol Sulfate Tablets USP are based on the "albuterol" content (present as the sulfate form). The USP states "Albuterol Tablets USP contain an amount of albuterol sulfate equivalent to not less than 90% and not more than 110% of the labeled amount of albuterol ($C_{13}H_{21}NO_3$)." In other words, sufficient albuterol sulfate is present to provide the labeled amount of the albuterol base.

PHYSICAL PHARMACY CAPSULE **4.10** pKₐ/Dissociation Constants

The dissociation of a weak acid in water is given by this expression:

$$HA \leftrightarrow H^+ + A^-$$

$$K_1[HA] \leftrightarrow K_2[H^+][A^-]$$

At equilibrium, the reaction rate constants K_1 and K_2 are equal. This can be rearranged, and the dissociation constant is defined as

$$K_a = \frac{K_1}{K_2} = \frac{[H^+][A^-]}{[HA]}$$

where K_a is the acid dissociation constant.

For the dissociation of a weak base that does not contain a hydroxyl group, the following relationship can be used:

$$BH^+ \leftrightarrow H^+ + B$$

The dissociation constant is described by

$$K_a = \frac{[H^+][B]}{[BH^+]}$$

The dissociation of a hydroxyl-containing weak base,

$$B + H_2O \leftrightarrow OH^- + BH^+$$

The dissociation constant is described by

$$K_b = \frac{[OH^-][BH^+]}{B}$$

The hydrogen ion concentrations can be calculated for the solution of a weak acid using

$$[H^+] = \sqrt{K_a C}$$

Similarly, the hydroxyl ion concentration for a solution of a weak base is approximated by

$$[OH^-] = \sqrt{K_b C}$$

Some practical applications of these equations are as follows.

■ EXAMPLE 1

The K_a of lactic acid is 1.387×10^{-4} at 25°C. What is the hydrogen ion concentration of a 0.02 M solution?

$$[H^+] = \sqrt{1.387 \times 10^{-4} \times 0.02} = 1.665 \times 10^{-3} \text{ G-ion/L}$$

■ EXAMPLE 2

The K_b of morphine is 7.4×10^{-7}. What is the hydroxyl ion concentration of a 0.02 M solution?

$$[OH^-] = \sqrt{7.4 \times 10^{-7} \times 0.02} = 1.216 \times 10^{-4} \text{ G-ion/L} \quad ■$$

PHYSICAL PHARMACY CAPSULE **4.11** Hydrates and Solvates

When a substance is a hydrate and water is present in the molecule, more of the chemical must be weighed to obtain the actual active drug. As a drug example that is available with different amounts of water, let us look at different forms of dexamethasone.

- Dexamethasone contains less than 0.5% of its weight in water.
- Dexamethasone acetate has one molecule of water of hydration and contains between 3.5% and 4.5% of water; the anhydrous form contains less than 0.4% water.
- Dexamethasone sodium phosphate contains a sum of water and alcohol that may be up to 16%.

Another example is lidocaine hydrochloride. Lidocaine hydrochloride occurs as a monohydrate and as the anhydrous form. The water content may be between 5% and 7%.

■ CALCULATIONS

How much adjustment should be made if using lidocaine hydrochloride monohydrate in place of lidocaine hydrochloride anhydrous for a compounded prescription?

Lidocaine HCl monohydrate $C_{14}H_{22}N_2O \cdot HCl \cdot H_2O$ MW 288.81
Lidocaine HCl anhydrous $C_{14}H_{22}N_2O \cdot HCl$ MW 270.80
A comparison of the molecular weights reveals a factor of 1.066 can be used for the adjustment:

$$(288.81) / (270.80) = 1.066$$

■ EXAMPLE

If a prescription for lidocaine hydrochloride 2% gel (100 g) is to be made, then 2 g of anhydrous lidocaine HCl could be used, OR:

2 g × 1.066 = 2.132 g of lidocaine HCl monohydrate.
Also, a direct comparison of the molecular weights and the physical quantity required can be used, as follows:

$$\frac{MW\ hydrate}{MW\ anhydrous} = \frac{weight\ of\ hydrated\ form}{weight\ of\ anhydrous\ form}$$

$$\frac{288.81}{270.80} = \frac{X}{2\ g}$$

$$X = 2.133\ g$$

Further, the USP monograph for lidocaine hydrochloride Jelly, USP states "It contains not less than 95% and not more than 105.09% of the labeled amount of lidocaine hydrochloride ($C_{14}H_{22}N_2O \cdot HCl$)." Note that this is the anhydrous form. It is important to also check the C of A for the lidocaine hydrochloride being used to determine the water content. Fortunately, most pure powders (anhydrous) generally only contain 0.2% to 0.5% moisture, which can be insignificant but need to be checked, nevertheless. ■

In another scenario, the dose of Diphenhydramine Hydrochloride Capsules USP is based on the total molecule, that is, diphenhydramine hydrochloride. The USP states "Diphenhydramine Hydrochloride Capsules USP contain not less than 90% and not more than 110% of the labeled amount of diphenhydramine hydrochloride ($C_{17}H_{21}NO \cdot HCl$)." As one can see, the weight of the "HCl" is considered in the dose of the drug.

The purpose of the "salt" form is usually to enhance the solubility of the drug; but it may also enhance the stability and change other attributes of the drug that make it easier to handle and manipulate for producing dosage forms. Also, it is the "unionized" portion of the drug that will ultimately exert its effect in the body, as the remainder of the salt molecule may no longer follow the base, or unionized, form of the drug into the body.

Why do we have some drugs that are dosed on the "base" form of the drug and some drugs that are dosed on the total weight of the "salt" form of the drug? In reviewing the USP revisions, it appears that this has always been an issue for many years with no apparent basis for which way the salts are dosed. However, both the official monographs and the U.S. Food and Drug Administration (FDA)-approved drug products appear to be inconsistent in how they determine how a drug is dosed. It is the responsibility of the pharmacist to know whether or not the base/acid of the salt form of the drug is to be used in the calculations for the amount of API to actually be used, if compounding.

The new "Monograph Naming Policy for Salt Drug Substances in Drug Products and Compounded Medications" (USP General Chapter <1121> Nomenclature) states the following:

"The titles of USP monographs for drug products and compounded preparations formulated with a salt of an acid or base use the name of the active moiety, as defined below. The strength of the product or preparation also is expressed in terms of the active moiety.

An active moiety is the molecule or ion, excluding those appended portions of the molecule that cause the drug to be an ester, salt (including a salt with hydrogen or coordination bonds), or other noncovalent derivative (such as a complex, chelate, or clathrate) of the molecule, responsible for the physiological or pharmacological action of the drug substance without regard to the actual charged state of the molecule in vivo.

For example, the active moiety of a hydrochloride salt of a base will be the free base and not the protonated form of the base. The active moiety of a metal salt of a weak acid will be the free acid.

This Policy is followed by USP in naming drug products and compounded preparations that are newly recognized in the USP. Revising existing monographs to conform to this Policy is not intended, except where the USP Council of Experts determines that, for reasons such as safety, a nomenclature change is warranted."

See example organic salt considerations in Physical Pharmacy Capsule 4.12, Organic Salts.

Organic Ester Considerations

Many drugs are available as the base form or as an "ester," and the dose may be based on the total ester form or just

PHYSICAL PHARMACY CAPSULE 4.12 Organic Salts

It is important to know whether or not a drug is "dosed" on the base or the salt form. Consider that the fentanyl dose is calculated on the "base" form but the "salt" is the form that is used in the dosage form. For example:
A prescription calls for 10 mL of fentanyl 50 µg/0.1 mL (as the citrate) topical gel. How much fentanyl citrate will be required?

1. 50 µg/0.1 mL = X µg/10 mL, X = 5 mg
2. Fentanyl MW = 336.47
   Fentanyl citrate MW = 528.59
3. 336.47/5 mg = 528.59/X, X = 7.85 mg
4. Each mg of fentanyl equals 528.59/336.47 = 1.57 mg fentanyl citrate

In a different example, Diphenhydramine Hydrochloride Capsules USP are based on the total molecule, that is, diphenhydramine hydrochloride. The USP states "Diphenhydramine Hydrochloride Capsules USP contain not less than 90% and not more than 110% of the labeled amount of diphenhydramine hydrochloride ($C_{17}H_{21}NO \cdot HCl$)." As one can see, the weight of the "HCl" is considered in the dose of the drug. For example:
A prescription calls for 30 capsules of diphenhydramine hydrochloride 35 mg each. How much diphenhydramine hydrochloride will be required?

1. Because the total salt molecule is part of the dose:
2. 30 × 35 mg = 1.05 g of diphenhydramine hydrochloride is required.

UXP XII (1942) lists about 20 tablet monographs that are all based on the "salt" form of the drug, for example, Morphine Sulfate Tablets USP contain not less than 93% and not more than 107% of the labeled amount of morphine sulfate [$(C_{17}H_{19}O_3N)_2 \cdot H_2SO_4 \cdot 5H_2O$]. The names of the monographed items in this time period were quite clear as the salt names were a part of the official name if it was to be used. For example, Barbital Tablets USP are based on the labeled amount of barbital ($C_8H_{12}N_2O_3$), but Barbital Sodium Tablets were based on the labeled amount of barbital sodium ($C_8H_{11}N_2O_3Na$).

USP XVI (1960) monograph for Amodiaquine Hydrochloride Tablets USP states "Amodiaquine Hydrochloride Tablets contain an amount of amodiaquine hydrochloride ($C_{20}H_{22}ClN_3O \cdot 2HCl \cdot 2H_2O$) equivalent to not less than 93% and not more than 107% of the labeled amount of amodiaquine base ($C_{20}H_{22}ClN_3O$)." It is evident in this monograph that the dose is calculated on the "base" form of the drug.

It is the responsibility of the formulator to determine whether or not the base/acid of the salt form of the drug is to be used in the calculations for the amount of API to actually be used. ■

the base form of the drug. If a number of factors are not considered, a final manufactured product or compounded preparation may not fall within the strength requirements, for example, 90% to 110% for compounded preparations or the USP monographs.

Some drugs are esters by virtue of their internal chemical structure (atropine, cocaine, many local anesthetics, etc.), and others are esters by the addition of a moiety that will form an ester for certain purposes. It is only the latter that are discussed here; those that are esters because of their basic molecular structure are not included.

An ester is a compound of the general formula R-C-O-R1 where R and R1 may be the same or different and may be either aliphatic or aromatic. The term "aliphatic" refers to an acyclic or cyclic, saturated or unsaturated carbon compounds excluding aromatic compounds; the term "aromatic" was originally used to describe compounds that "smelled" but were later found to contain either benzene or a fused benzene rings in the structure. The term has been generalized to include aromatic heterocyclic structures.

The dehydration reaction between a molecule of an alcohol and a molecule of an organic acid can form an ester. For example, ethanol reacts with acetic acid to form ethyl acetate, an ester:

$$C_2H_5OH + CH_3COOH \rightarrow CH_3CH_2$$
$$-O-CO-CH_3 + H_2O$$

Following salts, esters are the most important acid derivatives used in pharmacy. Esters can be prepared for a number of reasons, including solubility, stability, resistance to degradation after administration, use as prodrugs, etc.

Some drugs are very soluble but tend to degrade rapidly when in solution. One approach to increase their stability, and shelf life, is to prepare esters that are poorly soluble. This results in a "suspension" dosage form in place of a "solution" dosage form. A drug in a suspension dosage form degrades at a much slower rate than one in solution. After oral administration, the ester is cleaved and the active drug moiety released for absorption.

Some drugs may cause pain at the site of injection, especially if they precipitate and damage the surrounding tissue. This can be overcome by preparing a drug with increased solubility. Chloramphenicol has low water solubility, but the succinate ester is formed to increase the water solubility of the drug and facilitate parenteral administration. This succinate ester is inactive but is hydrolyzed to release the active chloramphenicol moiety.

Esters are an important means of preparing prodrugs because of the number of esterases present in various parts of the body that will cleave the ester linkage, releasing the active moiety. Carboxylic acid esters are common in pharmacy and are neutral liquids or solids, which can be hydrolyzed slowly by water and rapidly by acids or alkalis into their components. Some of the simple esters are soluble in water, but those with more than four carbon atoms are practically insoluble in water. See examples in Physical Pharmacy Capsule 4.13, Organic Esters.

Potency-Designated Active Pharmaceutical Ingredients

In the case of "potency-designated drugs," the bulk substance, or API, is not 100% active drug in all cases. It is important to know the assayed potency designation of the ingredient so that appropriate allowances can be made to obtain the correct amount. This may be on the label or on the COA.

Some APIs, including some antibiotics, endocrine products, biotechnology-derived products, biologics, etc., have potencies that are based on "activity" and are expressed in terms of "units of activity," "micrograms per milligram," or other standard terms of measurements. These are described for each API in the USP.

Regarding biologicals, the following is found in the General Notices of the USP:

"5.50.10 Units of Potency (Biological)"

For substances that cannot be completely characterized by chemical and physical means, it may be necessary to express quantities of activity in biological units of potency, each defined by an authoritative, designated reference standard.

Units of biological potency defined by the World Health Organization (WHO) for International Biological Standards and International Biological Reference Preparations are termed international units (IUs). Monographs refer to the units defined by USP Reference Standards as "USP units." For biological products, units of potency are defined by the corresponding U.S. Standard established by the FDA, whether or not IUs or USP units have been defined. There is no relationship between the units of potency of one drug with that of another different drug.

In the case of potency-designated drugs, there must be a "reference standard" for comparison. In actual usage, the potency specifications often include a range or "not less than __" and "not more than ___." In some cases, only a lower range is given, and in a few cases, there is no upper limit.

The determinations of potency are generally done on the "dried or anhydrous basis." In the case of hygroscopic APIs, one must exercise precautions to maintain the substance in a dried state in tight containers. In some cases, there is a designation of specified solvent-free conditions.

See examples in Physical Pharmacy Capsule 4.14, Potency-Designated Active Pharmaceutical Ingredients.

PHYSICAL PHARMACY CAPSULE **4.13** Organic Esters

Esters are quite interesting because one cannot simply look at the title and determine whether or not the drug is a salt or an ester. For example, "*acetate salts*" include calcium acetate, chlorhexidine acetate, desmopressin acetate, flecainide acetate, gonadorelin acetate, guanabenz acetate, leuprolide acetate, lysine acetate, mafenide acetate, and zinc acetate, and "*acetate esters*" include cortisone acetate, desoxycorticosterone acetate, dexamethasone acetate, fludrocortisones acetate, fluorometholone acetate, hydrocortisone acetate, isoflupredone acetate, medroxyprogesterone acetate, megestrol acetate, melengestrol acetate, methylprednisolone acetate, norethindrone acetate, paramethasone acetate, prednisolone acetate, trenbolone acetate, and betamethasone acetate.

Further, "*succinate salts*" include sumatriptan succinate, doxylamine succinate, loxapine succinate, and metoprolol succinate, and "*succinate esters*" include chloramphenicol sodium succinate, hydrocortisone sodium succinate, hypromellose acetate succinate, methylprednisolone sodium succinate, and prednisolone sodium succinate.

Let's look at cefuroxime axetil as an example of an ester that is dosed on the base form.

1. Cefuroxime axetil is $C_{20}H_{22}N_4O_{10}S$, with a molecular weight of 510.47. Cefuroxime axetil is described as a mixture of the diastereoisomers of cefuroxime axetil and contains the equivalent of not less than 745 μg and not more than 875 μg of cefuroxime ($C_{16}H_{16}N_4O_8S$) per mg, calculated on the anhydrous basis.
2. Cefuroxime Axetil Tablets USP contain the equivalent of not less than 90% and not more than 110% of the labeled amount of cefuroxime ($C_{16}H_{16}N_4O_8S$).
3. Ceftin Tablets (cefuroxime axetil tablets) provide the equivalent of 250 or 500 mg of cefuroxime as cefuroxime axetil.
4. Ceftin for Oral Suspension (cefuroxime axetil powder for oral suspension) provides the equivalent of 125 or 250 mg of cefuroxime as cefuroxime axetil per 5 mL of suspension.
5. After oral administration, cefuroxime axetil is absorbed from the gastrointestinal tract and rapidly hydrolyzed by nonspecific esterases in the intestinal mucosa and blood to cefuroxime; the axetil moiety is metabolized to acetaldehyde and acetic acid.
6. The molecular weight of cefuroxime axetil is 510.47. The molecular weight of cefuroxime is 424.39. Therefore, 1 mg of cefuroxime is contained in 510.47/424.39 = 1.2 mg of cefuroxime axetil. A 250 mg of cefuroxime tablet will contain 250 × 1.2 = 300 mg of cefuroxime axetil.
7. Therefore, if using a commercial product to prepare a dosage form, no conversion should be required. However, if using a bulk active ingredient, then the required amount of cefuroxime axetil that is equivalent to the desired dosage of cefuroxime must be calculated.

Dexamethasone-labeled strengths pose an interesting problem as they are not consistent in naming either the base or the ester form, for example:

"Dexamethasone" dosage form monographs are based on the labeled amount of "dexamethasone."
"Dexamethasone acetate" dosage form monograph is based on the labeled amount of "dexamethasone."
"Dexamethasone sodium phosphate" dosage form monographs are based upon the labeled amount of "dexamethasone phosphate," not "dexamethasone."

An example of a drug that occurs both as salt and ester forms is the drug erythromycin: erythromycin estolate is a salt; erythromycin ethylsuccinate is an ester; erythromycin gluceptate is a salt; erythromycin lactobionate is a salt; and erythromycin stearate is a salt. ∎

Complex Organic Molecules

Most complex molecules and biotechnology products are proteins; however, some may be smaller peptide-like molecules. Proteins are inherently unstable molecules and require special handling; also, their degradation profiles can be quite complex. Pharmacists involved in working with or handling biologically active proteins must be interested in their stabilization, formulation, and delivery to the site of action.

In working with complex molecules, one must be cognizant of both the active drug constituent and the total drug formulation in which it is contained. This is true when converting a commercial product into a compounded preparation. Protein drugs are very potent and are generally

PHYSICAL PHARMACY CAPSULE 4.14 Potency-Designated Active Pharmaceutical Ingredients

For those APIs, including some antibiotics, endocrine products, biotechnology-derived products, biologics, etc., that have potencies that are based on "activity" and are expressed in terms of "units of activity," "micrograms per milligram," or other standard terms of measurements, calculations must be made to ensure that the correct quantity of active drug is used.

In the case of dihydrostreptomycin, there are different potencies depending upon the use of the API. The potency may be not less than 450, 650, or 725 µg, depending upon its form or usage (route of administration).

In some cases, as in erythromycin ethylsuccinate and erythromycin stearate, the potency is based on the sum of the percentages of three different erythromycins that make up the API. Generally, the potency designation is determined on the "base" of the drug, but in few instances, the salt or ester form is used.

The potency of antibiotics is commonly expressed as "µg of activity per mg of substance." Obviously, there will be different equivalents for the base versus the salt forms of the drug. Tobramycin has not less than 900 µg of tobramycin per mg, and tobramycin sulfate has a potency of not less than 634 µg of tobramycin per mg, all on the anhydrous basis. As another example, ampicillin contains not less than 900 µg and not more than 1,050 µg of ampicillin per mg, and ampicillin sodium contains not less than 845 µg and not more than 988 µg of ampicillin per mg, both calculated on the anhydrous basis. So, one can tell that it is extremely important to check the labels accompanying each batch of each API for the necessary values to be used in calculations.

In some drugs, the actual dose may be expressed in units instead of mg. Examples of this include heparin and insulin. Other examples include enzymes (pancreatin, pancrelipase, papain) and antibiotics.

Each container must be labeled with the actual potency, and this information is to be used in calculations involving dosing prior to compounding activities. These calculations must be done and checked and documented, as different lots of the same API may have different potencies. An example of a calculation follows.

■ EXAMPLE

A formula calls for 500 mg of neomycin sulfate. The label on the API shows 650 µg of neomycin activity per mg of powder. How much of this powder is required to provide the 500 mg of neomycin sulfate?

$$\frac{650 \, \mu g}{1{,}000 \, \mu g} = \frac{500 \, mg}{X}$$

X = 769 mg of the powder is required to provide 500 mg of actual neomycin sulfate. ■

used in quite low concentrations. The bulk of many manufactured products and compounded preparations may be the excipients. These excipients include the vehicle, buffers, stabilizers, and others that are often incorporated in these products. A number of different stabilizers can be used from different chemical classes and include surfactants, amino acids, polyhydric alcohols, fatty acids, proteins, antioxidants, reducing agents, and metal ions. See Physical Pharmacy Capsule 4.15, Complex Organic Molecules, for further considerations.

Concentrates, Dilutions, and Triturations

Many drug substances and excipients are available as dilutions (triturations) and concentrates and do not consist of 100% drug or chemical, as shown in Table 4.2. Since the bulk substance, or API or excipient, is not 100% in all cases, then it is important to know the strength of the item so that appropriate allowances can be made to obtain the correct amount. Terminology used to describe the new sources of APIs is not well defined but the following definitions are available and commonly used.

Trituration: a dilution of a potent solid substance to a specific concentration by mixing it thoroughly with a suitable diluent.

Dilution: A diluted solution or mixture. A diluted substance.

Concentrates: A liquid preparation of increased strength and reduced volume, which is usually diluted prior to administration or use. Something concentrated. To make less dilute. Concentrates can also be nonliquid preparations.

Stock preparations: Concentrated products of API or excipient and are used as a convenience to compound preparations of lesser concentration.

Substances are available as dilutions (triturations) and concentrates for a number of reasons. First, the quantities required for dosing or compounding are so small they

PHYSICAL PHARMACY CAPSULE 4.15 Complex Organic Molecules

Most complex molecules and biotechnology products are proteins; however, some may be smaller peptide-like molecules. Proteins are inherently unstable molecules and require special handling; also, their degradation profiles can be quite complex. Pharmacists involved in compounding with biologically active proteins must be interested in their stabilization, formulation, and delivery to the site of action.

Protein drugs are potent and are generally used in low concentrations; consequently, the bulk of many manufactured products and compounded preparations may be the excipients, including the vehicle, buffers, stabilizers, and others that are often incorporated in these products.

■ FACTORS

pH: pH is one of the key important factors in formulating a stable preparation. The optimal pH range can be achieved through the selection of appropriate physiologic buffers, usually in buffer concentration ranges of 0.01 to 0.1 M. In general, an increase in the buffer concentration means an increase in pain on injection so is generally kept as low as reasonable.

Chelating agents: Chelating agents are incorporated to bind trace metals such as copper, iron, calcium, and manganese and minimize rates of degradation. Ethylenediaminetetraacetic acid (EDTA) is commonly used at a concentration of about 0.01% to 0.05%.

Antioxidants: Antioxidants are often used because oxidation is one of the major factors in protein degradation. Examples include ascorbic acid, sodium disulfide, monothioglycerol, and α-tocopherol and are frequently used at a concentration of about 0.05% to 0.1%.

Preservatives: Preservatives are used, especially if multiple dose vials are indicated. Examples include phenol (0.3% to 0.5%), chlorobutanol (0.3% to 0.5%), and benzyl alcohol (1% to 3%).

Others: Others may include the polyols, which are good stabilizers and are commonly used in concentrations from 1% to 10%, and tonicity-adjusting agents, which include sodium chloride and dextrose in concentrations necessary to achieve isotonicity of approximately 290 mOsm/L.

The use of filters in manipulating biotechnology products can result in "sorption" or the loss of some of the drug available to the patient. Sorption is "sticking" either by "absorption" into the filter or by "adsorption" onto the surface of the filter. Special filters have been prepared to minimize this problem. For example, muromonab-CD3 (Orthoclone OKT3) injection should be filtered with a low–protein-binding filter of 0.2 to 0.22 μm. Many biotechnology products should not be filtered at all. If a filtration device is part of the IV administration apparatus, large molecule drugs should generally be administered distal to the site of the filter. Filters that have been shown to minimize protein adsorption are those made from polyvinylidene difluoride, polycarbonate, polysulfone, and regenerated cellulose. As a precaution, low–protein-binding filters should be used.

Sorption of proteins to containers (glass or plastic) can result in drug loss. This loss can be minimized either by the use of albumin or by siliconization. Adding about 0.1% albumin to the product can decrease the sorption of proteins to containers. If glass containers are used, the albumin solution should be added and manipulated to coat the interior surface before adding the drug. If siliconization is used, one can prepare a silicon solution or emulsion and soak or rinse the glass vials in it. The drained vials should then be placed in an oven at about 250°C for 5 to 6 hours. This procedure will minimize protein adsorption to the glass; it can be used for both the preparation equipment and the packaging containers.

Specific issues relevant to large molecule drugs include the following:

- Effect of agitation and/or frothing on a preparation's stability.
- High molecular weight and potential for aggregation (i.e., a small change in structure can result in a change in activity).
- Assignment of potency to the reference standards (when traditional pharmaceuticals are about 98% pure, these materials may be only 0.1% to 1% active, with their activity assigned by potentially variable assays).
- Use of micropipets, which can require frequent calibration.
- Stability may be less than lyophilized preparations.
- Interaction of the product with the inner wall of the glass vial and with the elastomeric closure.
- Effectiveness of the preservative if a multidose product is mixed with other products.
- Immunogenic potential, because some are produced by a fermentation-type process and proteins can copurify with proteins.

Sorption is a problem with colony-stimulating factors and with aldesleukin (Proleukin) at low concentrations. To minimize "sticking" of the protein to the glass, the addition of about 0.1% albumin to the product to occupy the potential binding sites in the container is often helpful. Pharmacists must consider this problem before making any changes in packaging.

(continued)

PHYSICAL PHARMACY CAPSULE 4.15 Complex Organic Molecules (continued)

Agitation resulting in frothing can create difficulties in two ways. First, frothing can cause difficulties in using a syringe to withdraw the required amount of drug from a vial. To avoid this problem, the formulator should mix the product by rolling the vial in the hands or gently swirling it. Second, excessive agitation can cause changes in a protein's quaternary structure that often reduce or eliminate a drug's therapeutic activity. Some products, such as filgrastim (Neupogen) and sargramostim (Leukine), are reconstituted by directing a soft stream of diluent against the inside of the container wall. Others, such as recombinant tissue plasminogen activator (tPA; alteplase), are reconstituted by directing a stream of diluent directly into the product at the bottom of the vial.

Storage: The recommended storage temperature depends on the specific preparation and may include room temperature (15°C to 25°C), refrigerator temperature (2°C to 8°C), frozen (−20°C), or ultra frozen temperature (down to −80°C). Freezing does affect the activity of certain products; for instance, the activity of filgrastim decreases if it is frozen. Some products can retain potency at room temperature after reconstitution. Sargramostim retains potency for up to 30 days at 25°C. However, most manufacturers recommend refrigeration at 2°C to 8°C, regardless of the product's potency at room temperature.

The short shelf life of these products after reconstitution can be due to chemical, physical, or microbiological instability. The manufacturer's recommendations or those validated by the published literature should be followed for products after they are reconstituted and manipulated. One example is tPA, which has been used in treating intraocular fibrin formation after a vitrectomy and in managing subconjunctival hemorrhage after glaucoma filtration surgery. The prepared solution is stable in a pH range of 5 to 7.5 and is incompatible with bacteriostatic agents. To prepare a compounded preparation, the commercial product is reconstituted according to the manufacturer's directions, using sterile water for injection without preservatives to yield a concentration of 1 mg/mL. This solution is further diluted with 0.9% sodium chloride injection to yield a concentration of 25 µg/100 µL. Aliquots of 0.3 mL are withdrawn into 1-mL tuberculin syringes and capped. The syringes are stored in an ultra freezer at −70°C. This product has been shown, by both bioassay and clinical use, to retain its activity for at least 1 year. This type of specific product information is not included in the manufacturer's label information and is usually obtained from the literature or by asking the manufacturer directly.

Physical stability: This can involve degradation by aggregation, denaturation, and precipitation. *Aggregation* can be the result of covalent or noncovalent processes and can be either physical or chemical in nature. Aggregate formation can actually begin when primary particles are formed from protein molecules as a result of Brownian movement.

Denaturation can result from heat, cold, extreme pH values, organic solvents, hydrophilic surfaces, shear, agitation, mixing, filtering, shaking, freeze–thaw cycles, ionic strength, and other factors. Denaturation can be quite complex and can be either reversible or irreversible.

Precipitation can result from shaking, heating, filtration, pH, and chemical interactions. The first step in a precipitation process is generally aggregation. When the aggregates gain a sufficient size, they precipitate out of solution and are clearly evident. Precipitation can occur on membrane filters, in equipment, in tubing, and in contact with other equipment and supplies. ∎

cannot be accurately weighed so dilutions or triturations are prepared, assayed, and utilized. Second, some items, for example, nitroglycerin, are explosive and must be diluted in order to be safely handled. Third, many substances, such as acids and bases, are commercially available in percentage strengths that varies from one acid to another and depends on the solubility and stability of the solute in water and on the manufacturing process. The diluted acids are aqueous solutions usually 10% w/v but diluted acetic acid is 6% w/v. The concentrations of the official undiluted acids are expressed as percentages weight in weight (w/w) but the strengths of official diluted acids are expressed as percentages weight in volume (w/v). Therefore, it is necessary to consider the specific gravities of the concentrated acids when calculating the volume required to prepare a given quantity of

diluted acid. Table 4.2 lists a number of official and nonofficial solids and liquids available as dilutions or concentrates.

Solid Dilutions, Stable

Dilutions, also called triturations, were at one time official and consisted of diluting one part by weight of the drug with nine parts of finely powdered lactose; they were 10% mixtures of the drug. The purpose of these dilutions was for a means of conveniently obtaining small quantities of a drug for compounding purposes. Today, the strengths vary but the concept is the same.

Solid Dilutions, Unstable-Nitroglycerin

Diluted nitroglycerin contains the cautionary labeling: [Caution-Taking into consideration the concentration and

TABLE 4.2. Example Substances (Official and Nonofficial) Available as Concentrates/Dilutions/Triturations

Item	Percent Strength	Comment
Acetic Acid NF	36.0–37.0% w/w	
Acetic Acid, Diluted NF	5.7–6.3% w/v	
Alcohol, USP	94.9–96.0% v/v; 92.3–93.8% w/w	Sp Gr 0.812–0.816
Alcohol, Diluted NF	48.4–49.5% v/v	Sp Gr 0.935–0.937
Aluminum Sulfate USP	54.0–59.0%	
Amifostine USP	78.0–82.0%	
Aminophylline USP	84.0–87.4%	
Ammonia Solution, Strong NF	27–31% w/w	
Ammonium Lactate 70% Solution	70%	
Ammonium Lauryl Sulfate 28%	28%	
Benzalkonium Chloride Solution NF	Varies; 17% and 50% available. Check label.	
Benzoyl Peroxide USP	65.0–82.0%; Usually 70%	Note: Store in original container—Explosive
Beta Carotene Beadlets	10%	
Boron Citrate 5% Powder	5%	
Curcumin Powder 95%	95%	
Formaldehyde Solution USP	Nlt 34.5% w/w	
Glutaraldehyde 25% Aqueous Solution		
Glycolic Acid 70%		
Hydrochloric Acid NF	36.5–38.0% w/w	
Hydrochloric Acid, Diluted NF	9.5–10.5% w/v	
Hydrofluoric Acid 49%		
Hydrogen Peroxide Concentrate USP	29.0–32.0% w/w	Strong oxidant
Hydrogen Peroxide Topical Solution USP	2.5–3.5% w/v	
Hypophosphorous Acid NF	30.0–32.0%	
Isopropyl Rubbing Alcohol USP	68.0–72.0%	Sp Gr 0.872–0.883
Isosorbide Concentrate USP	70.0–80.0% w/w	
Isosorbide Dinitrate, Diluted USP	Varies-usually about 25% w/w	
Isosorbide Mononitrate, Diluted USP	See label	Explosive
Lactic Acid USP	88.0–92.0% w/w	
Lutein 5% Beadlets		
Maltitol Solution NF	Nlt 50.0%	
Misoprostol 1% HPMC Dispersion		
Nitroglycerin, Diluted USP	10% usually w/w	
Pamabrom USP	72.2–76.6%	
Phenol, Liquified USP	90% w/w	
Phytic Acid 50% in Water		
Phosphatidylserine 40%		
Phosphoric Acid NF	85.0–88.0% w/w	
Phosphoric Acid, Diluted NF	9.5–10.5% w/v	
Sodium Hypochlorite Solution USP	4.0–6.0% w/w	
Sodium Lactate Solution USP	NLT 50.0% w/w	
Sorbitol Solution	Nlt 64.0%	
Zinc Pyrithione 48% (min) Aqueous Dispersion		

amount of nitroglycerin ($C_3H_5N_3O_9$) in diluted nitroglycerin, exercise appropriate precautions when handling this material. Nitroglycerin is a powerful explosive and can be detonated by percussion or excessive heat. Do not isolate nitroglycerin ($C_3H_5N_3O_9$).] Isosorbide dinitrate and isosorbide mononitrate have similar warnings.

Undiluted nitroglycerin occurs as a white to pale yellow, thick, flammable, explosive liquid that is soluble in alcohol and slightly soluble in water. Diluted nitroglycerin with lactose is a white, odorless powder; when diluted with propylene glycol or alcohol, is a clear, colorless, or pale yellow liquid. Dilutions are safer to handle.

Liquid-Aqueous Concentrates

Many aqueous concentrates are available and are convenient to use; a notable example in compounding is benzalkonium chloride antiseptic/disinfectant solutions.

Benzalkonium chloride occurs as white or yellowish-white, thick gel or gelatinous pieces. It is very soluble in water and in alcohol. Benzalkonium chloride solution occurs as a clear liquid that is colorless or slightly yellow unless a color has been added. It is commonly available as 17% and 50% concentrates.

Methods of calculations using dilutions/triturations can include ratio and proportion, allegation alternate and allegation medial. One can consult pharmacy calculation texts for these procedures.

Acids and Bases

It is important to check the label of each lot of concentrated acid or base when utilizing for a prescription or procedure as they can sometimes vary. Dilutions can be prepared by allegation, ratio and proportion, or other calculation methods. As previously mentioned, these methods are detailed in pharmacy calculations textbooks.

Liquid-Oil Concentrates of Liquids

Vitamin A is available as the palmitate in oil (50% and 75%) and as the acetate (1,000,000, 2,500,000, and 2,800,000 IU/g). Vitamin A in liquid form occurs as a light-yellow to red oil that may solidify upon refrigeration. In solid form, it has the appearance of any diluent that has been added. In liquid form, it is soluble in absolute alcohol and in vegetable oils but insoluble in water and in glycerin. In solid form, it may be dispersible in water.

Vitamin E is available a 400 U/mL. Vitamin E occurs as the alpha tocopherols and alpha tocopheryl acetates as clear yellow, or greenish yellow, viscous oils. Alpha tocopherol acid succinate occurs as a white powder that is soluble in alcohol and in vegetable oils. Other forms of vitamin E are insoluble in water, soluble in alcohol, and miscible with vegetable oils.

Dilutions and concentrates are a way of life in pharmaceutical compounding and offer means of convenience, increased accuracy and quality, and safety for personnel. It is incumbent on compounding pharmacists to be aware of the strength of the drug substances used and whether or not they are available as aliquots, dilutions, and concentrates.

Drug and Drug Product Stability

One of the most important activities of preformulation work is evaluation of the physical and chemical stability of the pure drug substance. It is essential that these initial studies be conducted using drug samples of known purity. The presence of impurities can lead to erroneous conclusions in such evaluations. Stability studies conducted in the preformulation phase include solid-state stability of the drug alone, solution-phase stability, and stability in the presence of expected excipients. Initial investigation begins with knowledge of the drug's chemical structure, which allows the preformulation scientist to anticipate the possible degradation reactions. In practice, if a patient's response to a medication is not what is expected, the pharmacist may consider drug instability among the different possible causes of a lack of response, or an unexpected response.

Drug Stability: Mechanisms of Degradation

Chemical instability of medicinal agents may take many forms because the drugs in use today are of such diverse chemical constitution. Chemically, drug substances are alcohols, phenols, aldehydes, ketones, esters, ethers, acids, salts, alkaloids, glycosides, and others, each with reactive chemical groups having different susceptibilities to chemical instability. Chemically, the most frequently encountered destructive processes are hydrolysis and oxidation.

Hydrolysis is a solvolysis process in which (drug) molecules interact with water molecules to yield breakdown products. For example, aspirin, or acetylsalicylic acid, combines with a water molecule and hydrolyzes into one molecule of salicylic acid and one molecule of acetic acid.

Hydrolysis is probably the most important single cause of drug decomposition, mainly because a great number of medicinal agents are esters or contain such other groupings as substituted amides, lactones, and lactams, which are susceptible to the hydrolytic process (2).

Another destructive process is oxidation, which destroys many drug types, including aldehydes, alcohols, phenols, sugars, alkaloids, and unsaturated fats and oils. Chemically, oxidation is loss of electrons from an atom or a molecule. Each electron lost is accepted by some other atom or molecule, reducing the recipient. In inorganic chemistry, oxidation is accompanied by an increase in the positive valence of an element, for example, ferrous (+2) oxidizing to ferric (+3). In organic chemistry, oxidation is frequently considered synonymous with the loss of hydrogen (dehydrogenation) from a molecule. Oxidation frequently involves free chemical radicals, which are molecules or atoms containing one or more unpaired electrons, such as molecular (atmospheric) oxygen ($\bullet O\!-\!O\bullet$) and free hydroxyl ($\bullet OH$). These radicals tend to take electrons from other chemicals, thereby oxidizing the donor.

Many of the oxidative changes in pharmaceutical preparations have the character of autoxidations. Autoxidations occur spontaneously under the initial influence of atmospheric oxygen and proceed slowly at first and then more rapidly. The process has been described as a type of chain reaction commencing with the union of oxygen with the drug molecule and continuing with a free radical of this oxidized molecule participating in the destruction of other drug molecules and so forth.

In drug product formulation work, steps are taken to reduce or prevent deterioration due to hydrolysis, oxidation, and other processes. These techniques are discussed later.

Drug and Drug Product Stability: Kinetics and Shelf Life

Stability is the extent to which a product retains within specified limits and throughout its period of storage and use (i.e., its shelf life) the same properties and characteristics that it possessed at the time of its manufacture.

Five types of stability concern pharmacists:

1. *Chemical*: Each active ingredient retains its chemical integrity and labeled potency within the specified limits.
2. *Physical*: The original physical properties, including appearance, palatability, uniformity, dissolution, and suspendability, are retained.
3. *Microbiologic*: Sterility or resistance to microbial growth is retained according to the specified requirements. Antimicrobial agents retain effectiveness within specified limits.
4. *Therapeutic*: The therapeutic effect remains unchanged.
5. *Toxicologic*: No significant increase in toxicity occurs.

Chemical stability is important for selecting storage conditions (temperature, light, humidity), selecting the proper container for dispensing (glass vs. plastic, clear vs. amber or opaque, cap liners), and anticipating interactions when mixing drugs and dosage forms. Stability and expiration dating are based on reaction kinetics, that is, the study of the rate of chemical change and the way this rate is influenced by concentration of reactants, products, and other chemical species and by factors such as solvent, pressure, and temperature.

In considering chemical stability of a pharmaceutical, one must know the reaction order and reaction rate. The reaction order may be the overall order (the sum of the exponents of the concentration terms of the rate expression) or the order with respect to each reactant (the exponent of the individual concentration term in the rate expression).

In practice, one should be aware that many types of instability, especially chemical instability involving process such as hydrolysis, oxidation, photolytic reactions, and others, are not always visually apparent and require analytical instrumentation for detection.

Rate Reactions

The reaction rate is a description of the drug concentration with respect to time. Most commonly, zero-order and first-order reactions are encountered in pharmacy. These are presented in Physical Pharmacy Capsule 4.16, Rate Reactions, along with some appropriate examples.

Q_{10} Method of Shelf Life Estimation

The Q_{10} method of shelf life estimation lets the pharmacist estimate shelf life for a product that has been stored or is going to be stored under a different set of conditions than specified in the product labeling. It is explained in Physical Pharmacy Capsule 4.19, Q_{10}, Method of Shelf Life Estimation.

Enhancing Stability of Drug Products

Many pharmaceutical ingredients may be used to prepare the desired dosage form of a drug substance. Some of these agents may be used to achieve the desired physical and chemical characteristics of the product or to enhance its appearance, odor, and taste. Other substances may be used to increase the stability of the drug substance, particularly against hydrolysis and oxidation. In each instance, the added pharmaceutical ingredient must be compatible with and must not detract from the stability of the drug substance.

There are several approaches to the stabilization of pharmaceutical preparations containing drugs subject to hydrolysis. Perhaps the most obvious is the reduction or elimination of water from the pharmaceutical system. Even solid dosage forms containing water-labile drugs must be protected from humidity in the atmosphere. This may be accomplished by applying a waterproof protective coating over tablets or by keeping the drug in a tightly closed container. It is fairly common to detect hydrolyzed aspirin by noticing an odor of acetic acid upon opening a bottle of aspirin tablets. In liquid preparations, water can frequently be replaced or reduced in the formulation through the use of substitute liquids such as glycerin, propylene glycol, and alcohol. In certain injectable products, anhydrous vegetable oils may be used as the drug's solvent to reduce the chance of hydrolytic decomposition.

Decomposition by hydrolysis may be prevented in other liquid drugs by suspending them in a nonaqueous vehicle rather than dissolving them in an aqueous solvent. In still other instances, particularly for certain unstable antibiotic drugs, when an aqueous preparation is desired, the drug may be supplied to the pharmacist in a dry form for *reconstitution* by adding a specified volume of purified water just before dispensing. The dry powder is actually a mixture of the antibiotic, suspending agents, flavorants, and colorants; when reconstituted by the pharmacist, it remains stable for the period over which the preparation is normally consumed. Refrigeration is advisable for most

PHYSICAL PHARMACY CAPSULE **4.16** Rate Reactions

■ ZERO-ORDER RATE REACTIONS

If the loss of drug is independent of the concentration of the reactants and constant with respect to time (i.e., 1 mg/mL/h), the rate is called zero order. The mathematical expression is

$$\frac{-dC}{dt} = k_0$$

where k_0 is the zero-order rate constant (concentration [C]/time [t]).

The integrated and more useful form of the equation:

$$C = -k_0 t + C_0$$

where C_0 is the initial concentration of the drug.

The units for a zero rate constant k_0 are concentration per unit time, such as moles per liter second or milligrams per milliliter per minute.

It is meaningless to attempt to describe the time required for *all* material in a reaction to decompose, that is, infinity. Therefore, reaction rates are commonly described by k or by their half-life, $t_{1/2}$.

The half-life equation for a zero-order reaction:

$$t_{1/2} = (1/2)(C_0 / k_0)$$

If the C_0 changes, the $t_{1/2}$ changes. There is an inverse relationship between the $t_{1/2}$ and k.

■ EXAMPLE 1

A drug suspension (125 mg/mL) decays by zero-order kinetics with a reaction rate constant of 0.5 mg/mL/h. What is the concentration of intact drug remaining after 3 days (72 hours), and what is its $t_{1/2}$?

$$C = -(0.5 \text{ mg/mL/h})(72 \text{ h}) + 125 \text{ mg/mL}$$
$$C = 89 \text{ mg/mL after 3 d}$$
$$t_{1/2} = 1/2(125 \text{ mg/mL})/(0.5 \text{ mg/mL/h})$$
$$t_{1/2} = 125 \text{ h}$$

■ EXAMPLE 2

How long will it take for the suspension to reach 90% of its original concentration?

$$90\% \times 125 \text{ mg/mL} = 112.5 \text{ mg/mL}$$

$$t = \frac{C - C_0}{-k_0} - \frac{112.5 \text{ mg/mL} - 125 \text{ mg/mL}}{-0.5 \text{ mg/mL/h}} = 25 \text{ h}$$

Drug suspensions are examples of pharmaceuticals that ordinarily follow zero-order kinetics for degradation.

■ FIRST-ORDER RATE REACTIONS

If the loss of drug is directly proportional to the concentration remaining with respect to time, it is called a first-order reaction and has the units of reciprocal time, that is, $time^{-1}$. The mathematical expression is

$$\frac{-dC}{dt} = kC$$

where

C is the concentration of intact drug remaining,
t is time,
(dC/dt) is the rate at which the intact drug degrades, and
k is the specific reaction rate constant.

The integrated and more useful form of the equation:

$$\log C = \frac{-kt}{2.303} + \log C_0$$

where C_0 is the initial concentration of the drug.

(continued)

In natural log form, the equation is

$$\ln C = -kt + \ln C_0$$

The units of k for a first-order reaction are per unit of time, such as per second.

The half-life equation for a first-order reaction is

$$t_{1/2} = 0.693/k$$

and can be easily derived from the first-order equation by substituting values of C = 50% and C_0 = 100%, representing a decrease in concentration by 50%.

■ EXAMPLE 3

An ophthalmic solution of a mydriatic drug at 5 mg/mL exhibits first-order degradation with a rate of 0.0005/d. How much drug will remain after 120 days, and what is its half-life?

$$\ln C = -(0.0005/d)(120) + \ln (5 \text{ mg/mL})$$
$$\ln C = -0.06 + 1.609$$
$$\ln C = 1.549$$
$$C = 4.71 \text{ mg/mL}$$
$$t_{1/2} = 0.693/0.0005/d$$
$$t_{1/2} = 1{,}386 \, d$$

■ EXAMPLE 4

In Example 3, how long will it take for the drug to degrade to 90% of its original concentration?

$$90\% \text{ of } 5 \text{ mg/mL} = 4.5 \text{ mg/mL}$$
$$\ln 4.5 \text{ mg/mL} = -(0.0005/d)t + \ln (5 \text{ mg/mL})$$
$$t = \frac{\ln 4.5 \text{ mg/mL} - \ln 5 \text{ mg/mL}}{-0.0005/d}$$
$$t = 210 \, d$$

■ ENERGY OF ACTIVATION: ARRHENIUS EQUATION

Stability projections for shelf life (t_{90} or the time required for 10% of the drug to degrade with 90% of the intact drug remaining) are commonly based on the Arrhenius equation:

$$\log = \frac{k_2}{k_1} = \frac{Ea(T_2 - T_1)}{2.3 \, RT_1T_2}$$

which relates the reaction rate constants (k) to temperatures (T) with the gas constant (R) and the energy of activation (Ea).

The relationship of the reaction rate constants at two different temperatures provides the energy of activation for the degradation. By performing the reactions at elevated temperatures instead of allowing the process to proceed slowly at room temperature, the Ea can be calculated and a k value for room temperature determined with the Arrhenius equation.

■ EXAMPLE 5

The degradation of a new cancer drug follows first-order kinetics and has first-order degradation rate constants of 0.0001/h at 60°C and 0.0009/h at 80°C. What is its Ea?

$$\log = \frac{(0.0009)}{(0.0001)} = \frac{Ea(353 - 333)}{(2.3)(1.987)(353)(333)}$$
$$Ea = 25{,}651 \text{ kcal/mol}$$

■

preparations considered subject to hydrolysis. Together with temperature, pH is a major determinant of the stability of a drug prone to hydrolytic decomposition. Hydrolysis of most drugs depends on the relative concentrations of the hydroxyl and hydronium ions, and a pH at which each drug is optimally stable can be easily determined. For most hydrolyzable drugs, optimum stability is on the acid side, somewhere between pH 5 and 6. Therefore, through judicious use of buffering agents, the stability of otherwise unstable compounds can be increased. Buffers are used to maintain a certain pH, as described in Physical Pharmacy Capsule 4.17, Buffer Capacity.

Pharmaceutically, oxidation of a susceptible drug substance is most likely to occur when it is not kept dry in the presence of oxygen or when it is exposed to light or combined with other chemical agents without proper regard to their influence on oxidation. Oxidation of a chemical in a pharmaceutical preparation is usually accompanied by an alteration in the color of that preparation. It may also result in precipitation or a change in odor.

The oxidative process is diverted and the stability of the drug is preserved by agents called *antioxidants*, which react with one or more compounds in the drug to prevent progress of the chain reaction. In general, antioxidants act

PHYSICAL PHARMACY CAPSULE **4.17** Buffer Capacity

pH, buffers, and buffer capacity are especially important in drug product formulation, because they affect the drug's solubility, activity, absorption, and stability and the patient's comfort.

A buffer is a system, usually an aqueous solution, that can resist changes in pH upon addition of an acid or a base. Buffers are composed of a weak acid and its conjugate base or a weak base and its conjugate acid. Buffers are prepared by one of these processes:

1. Mixing a weak acid and its conjugate base or a weak base and its conjugate acid
2. Mixing a weak acid and a strong base to form the conjugate base or a weak base and a strong acid to form the conjugate acid

Using the Henderson-Hasselbalch equation:

$$pH = pK_a + \log(base/acid)$$

Remember that the acid is the proton donor and the base is the proton acceptor.

■ EXAMPLE 1

A buffer is prepared by mixing 100 mL of 0.2 M phosphoric acid with 200 mL of 0.08 M sodium phosphate monobasic. What is the pH of this buffer? (K_a of phosphoric acid = 7.5×10^{-3})

Moles acid = (0.2 mol/1,000 mL) (100 mL) = 0.02 mol; (0.02 mol)/(0.3 L) = 0.067 M

Moles base = (0.08 mol/1,000 mL) (200 mL) = 0.016 mol; (0.016 mol)/(0.3 L) = 0.053 M

$pK_a = \log 7.5 \times 10^{-3} = 2.125$

pH 2.125 + log (0.016 mol/0.02 mol) = 2.028

■ EXAMPLE 2

Determine the pH of the buffer prepared as shown:

Sodium acetate 50 g
Conc. HCl 10 mL
Water qs 2 L
Helpful numbers:
pK_a acetic acid = 4.76
MW sodium acetate = 82.08
MW acetic acid = 60.05
MW HCl = 36.45
Conc. HCl, 44% HCl w/v

(continued)

NaAc + HCl → NaCl + HAc + NaAc

(0.609 mol) (0.121 mol) (0.121 mol) (0.121 mol) (0.488 mol)

HCl: {(10 mL) [(44 g) / (100 mL)] (1 mol) / (36.45 g)} = 0.121 mol

NaAC: {(50 g) [(1 mol) / (82.08 g)]} = 0.609 mol (0.609 mol) − (0.121 mol) = 0.488 mol

pH = 4.76 + log (0.488 mol) / (0.121 mol) = 5.367

The ability of a buffer solution to resist changes in pH upon the addition of an acid or a base is called buffer capacity (b) and is defined thus:

$$\beta = \Delta B / \Delta pH$$

where

ΔB is molar concentration of acid or base added,
ΔpH is change in pH due to addition of acid or base, and
ΔpH can be determined experimentally or calculated using the Henderson-Hasselbalch equation.

■ EXAMPLE 3

If 0.2 mole of HCl is added to a 0.015-M solution of ammonium hydroxide and the pH falls from 9.5 to 8.9, what is the buffer capacity?

$$\Delta pH = 9.5 - 8.9 = 0.6$$
$$\Delta B = 0.2 \text{ mol/L} = 0.2 \text{ M}$$
$$\beta = 0.2 \text{ M} / 0.6 = 0.33 \text{ M}$$

■ EXAMPLE 4

If 0.002 mole of HCl is added to the buffer in Example 1, what is its buffer capacity? After adding 0.002 mole HCl:

$$H_3PO_4 : 0.02 \text{ mol} + 0.002 \text{ mol} = 0.022 \text{ mol}$$
$$NaH_2PO_4 : 0.016 \text{ mol} - 0.002 \text{ mL} = 0.014 \text{ mol}$$
$$pH = 2.125 + \log(0.014 \text{ mol} / 0.022 \text{ mol}) = 1.929$$
$$\Delta pH = 2.028 - 1.929 = 0.099$$
$$\Delta AB = 0.002 \text{ mol} / 0.3 \text{ L} = 0.0067 \text{ M}$$
$$\beta = 0.0067 \text{ M} / 0.099 = 0.067 \text{ M}$$

Another approach to calculating buffer capacity involves the use of Van Slyke equation:

$$\beta = 2.3C\{Ka\left[H^+\right] / (Ka[H^+])^2\}$$

where
C is the sum of the molar concentrations of the acid and base, and $[H^+]$ = 10^{-pH}.

■ EXAMPLE 5

What is the Van Slyke buffer capacity of the buffer prepared in Example 1?

$C = 0.0067 \text{ M} + 0.0053 \text{ M} = 0.12 \text{ M}$

$Ka = 7.5 + 10^{-3}$

$[H^+] = 10^{-2.028} = 9.38 \times 10^{-3} \text{ M}$

$\beta = 2.3(0.12 \text{ M})\{[(7.5 \times 10^{-3} \text{ M})(9.38 \times 10^{-3} \text{ M})] / [(7.5 \times 10^{-3} \text{ M}) / (9.38 \times 10^{-3} \text{ M})^2]\} = 0.68 \text{ M}$ ■

by providing electrons and easily available hydrogen atoms that are accepted more readily by the free radicals than are those of the drug being protected. Various antioxidants are employed in pharmacy. Among those, most frequently used in aqueous preparations are sodium sulfite (Na_2SO_3, at high pH values), sodium bisulfite ($NaHSO_3$, at intermediate pH values), sodium metabisulfite ($Na_2S_2O_5$, at low pH values), hypophosphorous acid (H_3PO_2), and ascorbic acid. In oleaginous (oily or unctuous) preparations, alpha-tocopherol, butyl hydroxy anisole, and ascorbyl palmitate find application.

In its labeling regulations for pharmaceutical products containing sulfites, the FDA requires a warning about possible allergic-type reactions, including possible life-threatening anaphylaxis symptoms and/or asthma episodes, in susceptible persons (3). Sulfites are used as preservatives in many injectable drugs, such as antibiotics and local anesthetics. Some inhalants and ophthalmic preparations also contain sulfites, but relatively few oral drugs contain these chemicals. The purpose of the regulation is to protect the estimated 0.2% of the population who are subject to allergic reactions to the chemicals. Many sulfite-sensitive persons have asthma or other allergic conditions. Previous to the regulations dealing with prescription medication, the FDA issued regulations for the use of sulfites in food. Asthmatics and other patients who may be sulfite sensitive should be reminded to read the labels of packaged foods and medications to check for the presence of these agents. Sulfite agents covered by the regulations are potassium bisulfite, potassium metabisulfite, sodium bisulfite, sodium metabisulfite, sodium sulfite, and sulfur dioxide. The FDA permits the use of sulfites in prescription products, with the proper labeling, because there are no generally suitable substitutes for sulfites to maintain potency in certain medications. Some but not all epinephrine injections contain sulfites.

The proper use of antioxidants permits their specific application only after appropriate biomedical and pharmaceutical studies. In certain instances, other pharmaceutical additives can inactivate a given antioxidant. In other cases, certain antioxidants can react chemically with the drugs they were intended to stabilize without a noticeable change in the appearance of the preparation.

Because oxygen may adversely affect their stability, certain pharmaceuticals require an oxygen-free atmosphere during preparation and storage. Oxygen may be present in pharmaceutical liquids in the airspace within the container or may be dissolved in the liquid vehicle. To avoid these exposures, oxygen-sensitive drugs may be prepared in the dry state and packaged in sealed containers with the air replaced by an inert gas such as nitrogen, as may liquid preparations. This is a common practice in commercial production of vials and ampuls of easily oxidizable preparations intended for parenteral use.

Trace metals originating in the drug, solvent, container, or stopper are a constant source of difficulty in preparing stable solutions of oxidizable drugs. The rate of formation of color in epinephrine solutions, for instance, is greatly increased by the presence of ferric, ferrous, cupric, and chromic ions. Great care must be taken to eliminate these trace metals from labile preparations by thorough purification of the source of the contaminant or by chemically complexing or binding the metal through the use of specialized agents that make it chemically unavailable for participation in the oxidative process. These chelating agents are exemplified by calcium disodium edetate and EDTA.

Light can also act as a catalyst to oxidation reactions, transferring its energy (photons) to drug molecules, making the latter more reactive through increased energy capability. As a precaution against acceleration of oxidation, sensitive preparations are packaged in light-resistant or opaque containers.

Because most drug degradations proceed more rapidly as temperature increases, it is also advisable to maintain oxidizable drugs in a cool place. Another factor that can affect the stability of an oxidizable drug in solution is the pH of the preparation. Each drug must be maintained in solution at the pH most favorable to its stability. This varies from preparation to preparation and must be determined on an individual basis for the drug in question.

Statements in the USP warn of the oxidative decomposition of susceptible drugs and preparations. In some instances, the specific agent to employ as a stabilizer is mentioned in the monograph, and in others, the term "suitable stabilizer" is used. An example in which a particular agent is designated for use is in the monograph for Potassium Iodide Oral Solution, USP. Potassium iodide in solution is prone to photocatalyzed oxidation and the release of free iodine, with a resultant yellow-to-brown discoloration of the solution. The use of light-resistant containers is essential to its stability. As a further precaution against decomposition if the solution is not to be used within a short time, the USP recommends the addition of 0.5 mg of sodium thiosulfate for each gram of potassium iodide. In the event that free iodine is released during storage, sodium thiosulfate converts it to colorless and soluble sodium iodide:

$$I_2 + 2Na_2S_2O_3 \rightarrow 2NaI + Na_2S_4O_6$$

In summary, for easily oxidizable drugs, the formulation pharmacist may stabilize the preparation by the selective exclusion from the system of oxygen, oxidizing agents, trace metals, light, heat, and other chemical catalysts to the oxidation process. Antioxidants, chelating agents, and buffering agents may be added to create and maintain a favorable pH.

In addition to oxidation and hydrolysis, destructive processes include polymerization, chemical decarboxylation, and deamination. However, these processes occur less frequently and are peculiar to only small groups of chemical substances.

Stability Testing

FDA's Current Good Manufacturing Practice regulations include sections on stability and stability testing of pharmaceutical components and finished pharmaceutical products (4). In addition, FDA and International Conference on Harmonization guidelines and guidances provide working recommendations to support the regulatory requirements. Among these are the following (5):

- "Stability Testing of New Drug Substances and Products"
- "Quality of Biotechnological Products: Stability Testing of Biotechnology/Biological Drug Products"
- "Photostability Testing of New Drug Substances and Products"
- "Stability Testing of New Dosage Forms"

Drug and drug product stability testing during every stage of development is critical to the quality of the product. Physical Pharmacy Capsule 4.18, Analytical Methods

and Standard Curves, provides a summary of the procedures required for the analysis of drug substances, and Table 4.3 lists a number of testing protocols that can be used for both stability testing and characterization. Drug stability is important during preclinical testing and in clinical (human) trials to obtain a true and accurate assessment of the product being evaluated. For a marketed drug product, assurance of stability is vital to its safety and effectiveness during the course of its shelf life and use.

The FDA-required demonstration of drug stability is necessarily different for each stage of drug development, such as for a 2-week preclinical study, an early phase I study, a limited phase II trial, or a pivotal phase III clinical study or for a new drug application. As a drug development program progresses, so do the requisite data to demonstrate and document the product's stability profile. Before approval for marketing, a product's stability must be assessed with regard to its formulation; the influence of its pharmaceutical ingredients; the influence of the

PHYSICAL PHARMACY CAPSULE **4.18** Analytical Methods and Standard Curves

Any study involving concentration of a drug requires an analytical method and the development of standard curves. There are numerous analytical methods used in pharmacy. It is important for pharmacists to have a basic understanding of pharmaceutical analysis to ensure that valid results are obtained when tests are being conducted. It is important to know (*a*) when to test; (*b*) what to test; (*c*) what method(s) to use; (*d*) how to interpret the results; (*e*) the limits of the test; and (*f*) the importance of analytical testing in the overall quality program in pharmacy.

The goal in analytical testing is to produce results as accurately, efficiently, and quickly as possible. Any analytical method used should have accuracy, speed, reproducibility, and specificity. No single analytical method is ideally suited for all drugs; each method has its own strengths and weaknesses, and there are a number of factors that determine the validity and reliability of results.

■ SELECTION OF AN ANALYTICAL METHOD

One general consideration in analytical method selection is the type of information that is needed: quantitative (potency, concentration), semiquantitative (where a "cutoff" level is involved, as in endotoxin levels), or qualitative (yes/no type of testing, including substance identification, sterility). Another consideration involves the physical and chemical characteristics of the analyte, including its solubility, partition coefficient, dissociation constant (pK_a), volatility, binding, and the quantity present.

One must consider the degree of quantitative measurement in the validation process, for example, accuracy, repeatability/reproducibility, and precision are required; generally, the greater the level that is required, the more sophisticated and expensive the analytical methods that must be used. This is also governed by the types of instrumentation that are on hand or available and the standards available for comparison.

■ FACTORS INVOLVED IN METHODS SELECTION

The ultimate analytical method selected depends upon a number of factors, including sample requirements, sample handling/preparation/purification requirements, type of data needed, and levels of specificity and accuracy required.

■ SAMPLING REQUIREMENTS

In any analytical method, there may be certain sample requirements that impact one's choice, such as the number of samples needed, the difficulty in obtaining a representative sample, the physical state of the sample (solid,

(continued)

PHYSICAL PHARMACY CAPSULE **4.18** Analytical Methods and Standard Curves (continued)

liquid, or gas), the type of container required for collection and storage of the sample (some analytes may sorb to the walls or cap liner of the sample containers), and leaching of the container material into the sample, if a liquid, may occur. All these may cause problems in analysis. In the event of sorption, siliconization of the sample vials may sometimes help.

The storage requirements for the sample after collection must be specified (type of container, material used, UV protection, latex contamination, etc.). The effects of air, such as oxidation of the sample ingredients, the presence of carbon dioxide, and the formation of insoluble carbonates, pH changes, free versus bound drug, etc., must be considered. The sample must be stored at the proper temperature (refrigerated, frozen, or controlled room) prior to shipment and during shipment. Procedures to follow if the sample is accidentally frozen or experiences a freeze–thaw cycle should be detailed.

In considering the chemical and physical stability of the sample, the effects of water must also be considered. If the sample must be maintained in a dry environment, including a desiccant, this should be detailed. The stability of the sample during storage, extraction, and preparation must be determined. The potential for enzymatic breakdown, or other adverse effects of pH, temperature, solvents, bacterial growth, etc., must be addressed. If volatile solvents are required, special handling must be implemented to prevent evaporation because if some of the solvent is allowed to evaporate, the resulting concentration may be falsely elevated.

The sample matrix effects must be determined. Any effects caused by sample viscosity (pipetting, aspiration), ionic strength (immunoassays, dialysis), buffers (ionized/unionized ratio can alter the extraction efficiency of an analyte prior to analysis), and vapor pressure, where drug can be lost, must be considered. If any sample pretreatment is required prior to shipment or working in-house, consider any inaccuracies that may occur from pipetting, which is one of the most common sources of analytical errors when working with small volumes.

There must be a consideration of any physical methods of separation and purification that might be used. Most analytical methods require some degree of sample pretreatment to prepare it for analysis. These may include crystallization from solution, distillation, sublimation, solvent extraction, solid-phase extraction, chromatography, and centrifugation; the proper choice of separation and purification depends upon the physical and chemical properties of the sample, including its solubility, volatility, binding, quantity present, etc. The effect of any substances in the formulation that may interfere or alter the results must be known beforehand.

■ DATA INTERPRETATION REQUIREMENTS

The collection of raw data from the analytical process must be done appropriately. One must ensure that appropriate and valid descriptive statistics are used to analyze the data and that the operating parameters of the analytical instruments are well established. Reference values, if available, should be provided with the analytical results. A description of the analytical controls used by the laboratory is important for documentation, as well as the source of reference standards used to establish standard curves.

■ ANALYTICAL METHODS

In pharmaceutical analysis, analytical methods can be generally divided into physical testing methods, methods that interact with electromagnetic radiation, conductometric techniques, immunoassay methods, separation techniques, and others.

Nonspecific methods generally include melting, freezing, and boiling points; density; refractive index; polarimetry; ultraviolet/visible spectroscopy; and pH. Methods that are somewhat more specific include infrared spectroscopic, mass spectroscopy, ion-selective electrodes, immunoassay methods, and chromatographic methods (high-performance liquid chromatography [HPLC] and gas chromatography [GC]), provided proper standards are used.

Methods that can be routinely used for testing incoming bulk materials, whether active or excipients, include melting, freezing, and boiling points; density; refractive index; UV/visible spectroscopy; infrared spectroscopy; polarimetry; pH; and the separation methods. Final products may generally require a method such as HPLC or GC. A classification of analytical methods follows along with suggested analytical methods that can be used for different dosage forms.

(continued)

■ CLASSIFICATION OF ANALYTICAL AND MICROBIOLOGICAL METHODS

Physical testing procedures

Melting point

Freezing point

Boiling point

Density

Refractive index

Optical rotation (polarimetry)

Thermal analysis

Color change

Precipitate formation

Viscosity change

Interaction of electromagnetic radiation

Ultraviolet/visible spectroscopy

Infrared spectroscopy

Fluorescence/phosphorescence spectroscopy

Raman spectroscopy

X-ray spectroscopy

Flame emission and atomic absorption spectroscopy

Polarimetry

Refractometry

Interferometry

Conductance methods

pH

Ion-selective electrodes

Polarography

Immunoassay

Radioimmunoassay

Enzyme-multiplied immunoassay technique

Enzyme-linked immunosorbent assay

Fluorescent immunoassay

Separation techniques

HPLC

GC

Thin-layer chromatography

Paper chromatography

Column chromatography

Gravimetric

Balance

Others

Osmolality

Microbiological methods

Sterility testing

Endotoxin testing

Preservative effectiveness testing

(continued)

PHYSICAL PHARMACY CAPSULE **4.18** Analytical Methods and Standard Curves *(continued)*

Suggested analytical methods for various dosage forms, depending upon the active drug:

Dosage Form	Wt	Vol	pH	Osm	RI	Sp Gr	MP	UV/vis	HPLC	GC	IR	Steril	Endo
Bulk substances	—	—	*	—	*	—	*	*	*	*	*	—	—
Powders	*	—	—	—	—	—	—	—	*	*	—	—	—
Capsules	*	—	—	—	—	—	—	—	*	*	—	—	—
Tablets	*	—	—	—	—	—	—	—	*	*	—	—	—
Lozenges	*	—	—	—	—	—	—	—	*	*	—	—	—
Suppositories	*	—	—	—	—	*	*	—	*	*	—	—	—
Sticks	*	—	—	—	—	*	*	—	*	*	—	—	—
Solutions	*	*	*	*	*	*	—	*	*	*	—	—	—
Suspensions	*	*	*	—	—	*	—	—	*	*	—	—	—
Emulsions	*	*	*	—	—	*	—	—	*	*	—	—	—
Semisolids	*	—	—	—	—	*	*	—	*	*	—	—	—
Gels	*	*	*	—	*	*	—	—	*	*	—	—	—
Ophthalmics, otics, and nasals	*	*	*	*	*	*	—	*	*	*	—	*(Ophthalmic only)	—
Inhalations	*	*	*	*	*	—	—	*	*	*	—	*	—
Injections	*	*	*	*	*	*	—	*	*	*	—	*	*

■ CONSTRUCTION OF A STANDARD CURVE

A standard curve is constructed by analyzing samples (standards) of known composition, generally in increasing concentrations. As each standard is analyzed, an instrumental response (absorbance, peak height, peak area, other numerical value) will be obtained. The standard concentrations are plotted as the "x" axis on a graph and the instrumental responses are plotted on the "y" axis. As an example,

The following table represents the results from an HPLC analytical method of methotrexate.

Concentration (µg/mL)	0	10	20	30
Response (peak height in units)	0	2,600	5,190	7,780

When plotted on a graph, one obtains the following:

The next step involves analyzing the unknown sample to obtain a response from the instrument. For example, if the unknown sample provided an instrumental response of 3,895, checking that value on the y-axis and moving toward the right on the graph until it intersects the plotted line and dropping down to the x-axis, we can read a value of 15 µg/mL of the methotrexate. As an option, the equation of the line can be calculated and the concentration determined by substituting the values of "y" and "b" with the slope of the line to obtain the drug concentration, as follows:

$$m = \Delta y / \Delta / x = (7{,}780 - 0) / (30 - 0) = 7{,}780 / 30 = 259.3$$

$y = mx + b$
$3{,}895 = 259.3x + 0$
$x = 15.02 \ \mu g/mL$ ■

container and closure; the manufacturing and processing conditions (e.g., heat); packaging components; conditions of storage; anticipated conditions of shipping, temperature, light, and humidity; and anticipated duration and conditions of pharmacy shelf life and patient use. Holding intermediate product components (such as drug granulations for tablets) for long periods before processing into finished pharmaceutical products can affect the stability of both the intermediate component and the finished product. Therefore, in-process stability testing, including retesting of intermediate components, is important.

Product containers, closures, and other packaging features must be considered in stability testing. For instance, tablets or capsules packaged in glass or plastic bottles require different stability test protocols from those for blister packs or strip packaging. Drugs particularly subject to hydrolysis or oxidative decomposition must be evaluated accordingly. And sterile products must meet sterility test standards to ensure protection against microbial contamination. All preservatives must be tested for effectiveness in the finished product.

As noted elsewhere in this section, drug products must meet stability standards for long-term storage at room temperature and relative humidity. Products are also subjected to accelerated stability studies as an indication of shelf life stability. Drug instability in pharmaceutical formulations may be detected in some instances by a change in the physical appearance, color, odor, taste, or texture of the formulation, whereas in other instances, chemical changes may not be self-evident and may be ascertained only through chemical analysis. Scientific data pertaining to the stability of a formulation can lead to prediction of the expected shelf life of the proposed product and when necessary to redesign of the drug (e.g., into more stable salt or ester form) and to reformulation of the dosage form. Obviously, the rate at which a drug product degrades is of prime importance. The study of the rate of chemical change and the way it is influenced by such factors as the concentration of the drug or reactant, the solvent, temperature and pressure, and other chemical agents in the formulation is reaction kinetics.

In general, a kinetic study begins by measuring the concentration of the drug at given intervals under a specific set of conditions, including temperature, pH, ionic strength, light intensity, and drug concentration. The measurement of the drug's concentration at the various times reveals the stability or instability of the drug under the specified conditions with the passage of time. From this starting point, each of the original conditions may be varied to determine the influence of such changes on the drug's stability. For example, the pH of the solution may be changed, whereas the temperature, light intensity, and original drug concentration are held constant.

The findings may be presented graphically, by plotting the drug concentration as a function of time. From the experimental data, the reaction rate may be determined and a rate constant and half-life calculated.

Accelerated Stability Studies

The purpose of stability testing is to provide evidence on how the quality of a drug substance or drug product varies with time under the influence of a variety of environmental factors, such as temperature, humidity, and, where appropriate, oxidation, light, and microbial exposure. Stability testing is also used to establish the shelf life for a drug product and recommended storage conditions (6,7).

Among the definitions applied in stability testing are as follows (7):

Accelerated testing: Studies designed to increase the rate of chemical degradation or physical change of a drug substance or drug product by using exaggerated storage conditions as part of long-term, intermediate, and accelerated studies. Data from these studies are used to assess degradation that might occur under normal (nonexaggerated) or slight deviations in storage conditions as during shipping and storage. Results allow the development of product labeling with regard to expiration dating and recommended conditions for storage.

Drug product: The dosage form in the final immediate packaging intended for marketing.

Drug substance: The unformulated drug substance that may subsequently be formulated with excipients to produce the dosage form.

Excipient: Anything other than the drug substance in the dosage form.

Expiration date: The date placed on the container label of a drug product designating the time prior to which a batch of the product is expected to remain within the approved shelf life specification, if stored under defined conditions, and after which it must not be used.

Shelf life (also referred to as expiration dating period): The time period during which a drug product is expected to remain within the approved shelf life specification, provided that it is stored under the conditions defined on the container label.

Stress testing (drug substance): Studies undertaken to elucidate the intrinsic stability of a drug substance. Such testing is part of the drug development process and is normally carried out under more severe conditions than those used for accelerated testing.

Stress testing (drug product): Studies undertaken to assess the effect of severe conditions on the drug product. Such studies include photostability testing as well as the specific testing of certain product types (e.g., metered-dose inhalers, creams, emulsions).

For the drug substance, the testing should evaluate its susceptibility to hydrolysis across a wide range of pH values when in solution or suspension. Photostability testing should be an integral part of stress testing. Data should be obtained from at least three pilot scale batches of the drug substance, manufactured by the method and procedures that mirror the process to be used for final full scale production batches. Stability studies also should be conducted on the drug substance packaged in the container

TABLE 4.3. Example Protocol for Drug and/or Drug Product Stability Studies[a]

Study Type	Storage Condition	Minimum Time Period
Long term	25°C ± 2°C @ 60% RH ± 5% RH	12 mo
Intermediate	30°C ± 2°C @ 65% RH[a] ± 5% RH	6 mo
Accelerated	40°C ± 2°C @ 75% RH[a] ± 5% RH	6 mo

[a]For chemical entities.
RH, relative humidity.
Adapted from Stability and Testing of New Drug Substances and Products. Available at http://www.fda.gov/downloads/RegulatoryInformation/Guidances/ucm128204.pdf. (Accessed September 28, 2012)

closure system that is the same or simulates the packaging proposed for the final product.

For the drug product, the design of the stability studies should be based on knowledge gained from those studies of the drug substance. Stability studies should be conducted on at least three batches of the manufactured dosage form, packaged in the container and closure system, including all secondary packaging (e.g., outer carton) proposed for marketing. The studies should include testing of those attributes of the product that are susceptible to change during storage, thereby affecting quality and efficacy. The testing should cover, as appropriate, the physical, chemical, biological, and microbiological attributes; preservative content (e.g., antioxidant, antimicrobial preservative); and functionality tests (e.g., metered-dose delivery system).

Table 4.3 presents an example protocol for long-term, intermediate, and accelerated stability studies for a chemical drug entity and dosage form product. Protocols vary for products intended to be maintained under conditions of refrigeration, for those to be frozen, for products known to be destined for geographic areas of temperature extremes, and for biotechnological/biological products, which have separate protocols for stability studies. Physical Pharmacy Capsule 4.19 presents the Q_{10} Method of Shelf Life Estimation.

Following FDA product approval and initial marketing, pharmaceutical manufacturers retain production samples of drug/drug product for 5 years or longer and continue studies for signs of degradation under various conditions of storage. Pharmacy practitioners should also observe signs of product instability (e.g., color change, distorted capsules, softened tablets, etc.) and report such findings.

Prescriptions requiring extemporaneous compounding by the pharmacist do not require the extended shelf life that commercially manufactured and distributed products do because they are intended to be used immediately on receipt by the patient and used only during the immediate course of the prescribed treatment. However, these compounded prescriptions must remain stable and efficacious during the course of use, and the compounding pharmacist must employ formulative components and techniques that will result in a stable product (7).

Today, there are a number of literature sources for the pharmacist to utilize in the compounding of high-quality and stable prescriptions. Several of these are listed among the references, including the USP chapters on the compounding of sterile and nonsterile preparations (8–12).

USP guidelines on stability of extemporaneous compounded formulations state that in the absence of stability information applicable to a specific drug and preparation, the following guidelines can be used: nonaqueous liquids and solid formulations in which the manufactured drug is the source of the active ingredient, not later than 25% of the time remaining until the product's expiration date or 6 months, whichever is earlier; nonaqueous liquids and solid formulations in which a USP or National Formulary (NF) substance is the source of active ingredient, a beyond-use date of 6 months; for water-containing formulations prepared from ingredients in solid form, a beyond-use date not later than 14 days in storage at cold temperatures; and for all other formulations, a beyond-use date of the intended duration of therapy or 30 days, whichever is earlier (8). Thus, if an oral aqueous liquid preparation is made from a tablet or capsule formulation, the pharmacist should make up only at most 14 days' supply, and it must be stored in a refrigerator. Furthermore, the pharmacist must dispense the medication in a container conducive to stability and use and must advise the patient of the proper method of use and conditions of storage of the medication.

Finally, when compounding on the basis of extrapolated or less than concrete information, the pharmacist is well advised to keep the formulation simple and not to shortcut but use the necessary pharmaceutical adjuvants to prepare the prescription.

PHARMACEUTICAL INGREDIENTS AND EXCIPIENTS

Definitions and Types

To produce a drug substance in a final dosage form requires pharmaceutical ingredients. For example, in the preparation of solutions, one or more *solvents* are used to dissolve the drug substance, *flavors* and *sweeteners* are used to make the product more palatable, *colorants* are added to enhance appeal, *preservatives* may be added to prevent microbial growth, and *stabilizers*, such as antioxidants and chelating agents, may be used to prevent decomposition, as previously discussed. In the preparation of tablets, *diluents* or *fillers* are commonly added to increase the bulk of the formulation, *binders* to cause adhesion of the powdered drug and pharmaceutical substances, *antiadherents* or *lubricants* to assist smooth tablet formation, *disintegrating agents* to promote tablet breakup after administration, and coatings to improve stability, control disintegration, or enhance appearance. Ointments, creams, and suppositories acquire their characteristic features from their pharmaceutical bases. Thus, for each dosage form, the pharmaceutical ingredients establish the primary features of the product and contribute

PHYSICAL PHARMACY CAPSULE **4.19** Q_{10} **Method of Shelf Life Estimation**

The Q_{10} approach, based on Ea, which is independent of reaction order, is described as

$$Q_{10} = e^{\{(Ea/R)[(1/T+10)-(1/T)]\}}$$

where

Ea is the energy of activation,
R is the gas constant, and
T is the absolute temperature.

In usable terms, Q_{10}, the ratio of two different reaction rate constants, is defined thus:

$$Q_{10} = \frac{K_{(T+10)}}{K_T}$$

The commonly used Q values of 2, 3, and 4 relate to the energies of activations of the reactions for temperatures around room temperature (25°C). For example, a Q value of 2 corresponds to an Ea (kcal/mol) of 12.2, a Q value of 3 corresponds to an Ea of 19.4, and a Q value of 4 corresponds to an Ea of 24.5. Reasonable estimates can often be made using the value of 3.

The equation for Q_{10} shelf life estimates is

$$t_{90}(T_2) = \frac{t_{90}(T_1)}{Q_{10}^{(\Delta T/10)}}$$

where

$t_{90}T_2$ is the estimated shelf life,
$t_{90}T_1$ is the given shelf life at a given temperature, and
ΔT is the difference in the temperatures T_1 and T_2.

As is evident from this relationship, an increase in ΔT will decrease the shelf life and a decrease in ΔT will increase the shelf life. This is the same as saying that storing at a warmer temperature will shorten the life of the drug and storing at a cooler temperature will increase the life of the drug.

■ EXAMPLE 1

An antibiotic solution has a shelf life of 48 hours in the refrigerator (5°C). What is its estimated shelf life at room temperature (25°C)?

Using a Q value of 3, we set up the relationship as follows:

$$t_{90}(T_2) = \frac{t_{90}(T_1)}{Q_{10}^{(\Delta T/10)}} = \frac{48}{3^{[(25-5)/10]}} = \frac{48}{3^2} = 5.33 \text{ hours}$$

■ EXAMPLE 2

An ophthalmic solution has a shelf life of 6 hours at room temperature (25°C). What is the estimated shelf life in a refrigerator at 5°C? (*Note*: Because the temperature is decreasing, ΔT will be negative.)

$$t_{90}(T_2) = \frac{6}{3^{[(5-25)/10]}} = \frac{6}{3^{-2}} = 6 \times 3^2 = 54 \text{ hours}$$

These are estimates, and actual energies of activation can often be obtained from the literature for more exact calculations. ■

to the physical form, texture, stability, taste, and overall appearance.

Table 4.4 presents the principal categories of pharmaceutical ingredients, listing some of the official and commercial agents in use. Additional discussion of many ingredients may be found in the chapters where they are most relevant; for example, pharmaceutical materials used in tablet and capsule formulations are discussed in

TABLE 4.4. Examples of Pharmaceutical Ingredients

Ingredient Type	Definition	Examples
Acidifying agent	Used in liquid preparations to provide acidic medium for product stability	Citric acid Acetic acid Fumaric acid Hydrochloric acid Nitric acid
Alkalinizing agent	Used in liquid preparations to provide alkaline medium for product stability	Ammonia solution Ammonium carbonate Diethanolamine Monoethanolamine Potassium hydroxide Sodium bicarbonate Sodium borate Sodium carbonate Sodium hydroxide Trolamine
Adsorbent	An agent capable of holding other molecules onto its surface by physical or chemical (chemisorption) means	Powdered cellulose Activated charcoal
Aerosol propellant	Agent responsible for developing the pressure within an aerosol container and expelling the product when the valve is opened	Carbon dioxide Dichlorodifluoromethane Dichlorotetrafluoroethane Trichloromonofluoromethane
Air displacement	Agent employed to displace air in a hermetically sealed container to enhance product stability	Nitrogen Carbon dioxide
Antifungal preservative	Used in liquid and semisolid preparations to prevent growth of fungi. Effectiveness of parabens is usually enhanced by use in combination	Butylparaben Ethylparaben Methylparaben Benzoic acid Propylparaben Sodium benzoate Sodium propionate
Antimicrobial preservative	Used in liquid and semisolid preparations to prevent growth of microorganisms	Benzalkonium chloride
Antioxidant	Used to prevent deterioration of preparations by oxidation	Ascorbic acid Ascorbyl palmitate Butylated hydroxyanisole Butylated hydroxytoluene Hypophosphorous acid Monothioglycerol Propyl gallate Sodium ascorbate Sodium bisulfite Sodium formaldehyde Sulfoxylate Sodium metabisulfite
Buffering agent	Used to resist change in pH upon dilution or addition of acid or alkali	Potassium metaphosphate Potassium phosphate, monobasic Sodium acetate Sodium citrate, anhydrous and dihydrate
Chelating agent	Substance that forms stable water-soluble complexes (chelates) with metals; used in some liquid pharmaceuticals as stabilizers to complex heavy metals that might promote instability. In such use, they are also called *sequestering* agents	Edetic acid Edetate disodium
Colorant	Used to impart color to liquid and solid (e.g., tablets and capsules) preparations	FD&C Red No. 3 FD&C Red No. 20 FD&C Yellow No. 6 FD&C Blue No. 2 D&C Green No. 5 D&C Orange No. 5 D&C Red No. 8 Caramel Ferric oxide, red

TABLE 4.4. Examples of Pharmaceutical Ingredients (*Continued*)

Ingredient Type	Definition	Examples
Clarifying agent	Used as a filtering aid for its adsorbent qualities	Bentonite
Emulsifying agent	Used to promote and maintain dispersion of finely subdivided particles of liquid in a vehicle in which it is immiscible. End product may be a liquid emulsion or semisolid emulsion (e.g., a cream)	Acacia Cetomacrogol Cetyl alcohol Glyceryl monostearate Sorbitan monooleate Polyoxyethylene 50 stearate
Encapsulating agent	Used to form thin shells to enclose a drug for ease of administration	Gelatin
Flavorant	Used to impart a pleasant flavor and often odor to a preparation. In addition to the natural flavorants listed, many synthetic ones are used	Anise oil Cinnamon oil Cocoa Menthol Orange oil Peppermint oil Vanillin
Humectant	Used to prevent drying of preparations, particularly ointments and creams	Glycerin Propylene glycol Sorbitol
Levigating agent	Liquid used as an intervening agent to reduce the particle size of a powder by grinding, usually in a mortar	Mineral oil Glycerin Propylene glycol
Ointment base	Semisolid vehicle for medicated ointments	Lanolin Hydrophilic ointment Polyethylene glycol ointment Petrolatum Hydrophilic petrolatum White ointment Yellow ointment Rose water ointment
Plasticizer	Component of film-coating solutions to make film more pliable, enhance spread of coat over tablets, beads, and granules	Diethyl phthalate Glycerin
Solvent	Used to dissolve another substance in preparation of a solution; may be aqueous or not (e.g., oleaginous). Cosolvents, such as water and alcohol (hydroalcoholic) and water and glycerin, may be used when needed. Sterile solvents are used in certain preparations (e.g., injections)	Alcohol Corn oil Cottonseed oil Glycerin Isopropyl alcohol Mineral oil Oleic acid Peanut oil Purified water Water for injection Sterile water for injection Sterile water for irrigation
Stiffening agent	Used to increase thickness or hardness of a preparation, usually an ointment	Cetyl alcohol Cetyl esters wax Microcrystalline wax Paraffin Stearyl alcohol White wax Yellow wax
Suppository base	Vehicle for suppositories	Cocoa butter Polyethylene glycols (mixtures) PEG 3350
Surfactant (surface active agent)	Substances that absorb to surfaces or interfaces to reduce surface or interfacial tension. May be used as wetting agents, detergents, or emulsifying agents	Benzalkonium chloride Nonoxynol 10 Octoxynol 9 Polysorbate 80 Sodium lauryl sulfate Sorbitan monopalmitate

(*Continued*)

TABLE 4.4. Examples of Pharmaceutical Ingredients (*Continued*)

Ingredient Type	Definition	Examples
Suspending agent	Viscosity-increasing agent used to reduce sedimentation rate of particles in a vehicle in which they are not soluble; suspension may be formulated for oral, parenteral, ophthalmic, topical, or other route.	Agar Bentonite Carbomer (e.g., Carbopol) Carboxymethylcellulose sodium Hydroxyethyl cellulose Hydroxypropyl cellulose Hydroxypropyl methylcellulose Kaolin Methylcellulose Tragacanth Veegum
Sweetening agent	Used to impart sweetness to a preparation	Aspartame Dextrose Glycerin Mannitol Saccharin sodium Sorbitol Sucrose
Tablet antiadherents	Prevent tablet ingredients from sticking to punches and dies during production	Magnesium stearate
Tablet binders	Substances used to cause adhesion of powder particles in tablet granulations	Acacia Alginic acid Carboxymethylcellulose sodium Compressible sugar (e.g., Nu-Tab) Ethylcellulose Gelatin Liquid glucose Methylcellulose Povidone Pregelatinized starch
Tablet and capsule diluent	Inert filler to create desired bulk, flow properties, and compression characteristics of tablets and capsules	Dibasic calcium phosphate Kaolin Lactose Mannitol Microcrystalline cellulose Powdered cellulose Precipitated calcium carbonate Sorbitol Starch
Tablet-coating agent	Used to coat a tablet to protect against decomposition by atmospheric oxygen or humidity, to provide a desired release pattern, to mask taste or odor, or for aesthetic purposes. Coating may be sugar, film, or thick covering around a tablet. Sugar-coated tablets generally start to break up in the stomach. Film forms a thin cover around a formed tablet or bead. Unless it is enteric, film dissolves in the stomach. Enteric coating passes through the stomach to break up in the intestines. Some water-insoluble coatings (e.g., ethylcellulose) are used to slow the release of drug in the gastrointestinal tract	
Sugar coating		Liquid glucose Sucrose
Film coating		Hydroxyethyl cellulose Hydroxypropyl cellulose Hydroxypropyl methylcellulose Methylcellulose (e.g., Methocel) Ethylcellulose (e.g., Ethocel)
Enteric coating		Cellulose acetate phthalate Shellac (35% in alcohol, pharmaceutical glaze)

TABLE 4.4. Examples of Pharmaceutical Ingredients (*Continued*)

Ingredient Type	Definition	Examples
Tablet direct-compression excipient	Used in direct-compression tablet formulations	Dibasic calcium phosphate (e.g., Ditab)
Tablet disintegrant	Used in solid forms to promote disruption of the mass into smaller particles more readily dispersed or dissolved	Alginic acid Polacrilin potassium (e.g., Amberlite) Sodium alginate Sodium starch glycolate Starch
Tablet glidant	Used in tablet and capsule formulations to improve flow properties of the powder mixture	Colloidal silica Cornstarch Talc
Tablet lubricant	Used in tablet formulations to reduce friction during tablet compression	Calcium stearate Magnesium stearate Mineral oil Stearic acid Zinc stearate
Tablet or capsule opaquant	Used to render a coating opaque. May be used alone or with a colorant	Titanium dioxide
Tablet polishing agent	Used to impart an attractive sheen to coated tablets	Carnauba wax White wax
Tonicity agent	Used to render solution similar in osmotic-dextrose characteristics to physiologic fluids, for example, in ophthalmic, parenteral, and irrigation fluids	Sodium chloride
Vehicle	Carrying agent used in formulating a variety of liquids for oral and parenteral administration Generally, oral liquids are aqueous (e.g., syrups) or hydroalcoholic (e.g., elixirs). Solutions for intravenous use are aqueous, whereas intramuscular injections may be aqueous or oleaginous	
Flavored, sweetened		Acacia syrup Aromatic syrup Aromatic elixir Cherry syrup Cocoa syrup Orange syrup Syrup
Oleaginous		Corn oil Mineral oil Peanut oil Sesame oil
Sterile		Bacteriostatic sodium chloride injection
Viscosity-increasing agent	Used to render preparations more resistant to flow. Used in suspensions to deter sedimentation, in ophthalmic solutions to enhance contact time (e.g., methylcellulose), to thicken topical creams, etc.	Alginic acid Bentonite Carbomer Carboxymethyl cellulose Sodium Methylcellulose Povidone Sodium alginate Tragacanth

Chapters 7 and 8, and those used in modified-release solid oral dosage forms and drug delivery systems in Chapter 9.

All drug products should be labeled to state the identity of all added substances (excipients). Such listing should be in alphabetical order by name and be distinguished from the identification statement of the active ingredient(s). The name of the inactive ingredient should be taken from the current edition of one of the following reference works (in the following order of precedence): (*a*) the USP or the NF, (*b*) USAN and the USP Dictionary of Drug Names, (*c*) CTFA Cosmetic Ingredient Dictionary, and (*d*) Food Chemicals Codex. If not listed in the above, then the reference works should be identified by the common or usual name or, if no common or usual name is available, by its chemical or other technical name. If an ingredient may or may not be present, it should be qualified by words such as "or" or "may also contain." If an ingredient is a trade secret, it may be omitted from the list if the list states "and other ingredients." If an ingredient is only present in a trace amount and has no functional or technical effect on the product, it does not need to be listed unless it has been shown to cause sensitivity reactions or allergic responses.

Handbook of Pharmaceutical Excipients

The *Handbook of Pharmaceutical Excipients* (10) presents monographs on more about 400 excipients used in dosage form preparation. Each monograph includes such information as nonproprietary, chemical, and commercial names; empirical and chemical formulas and molecular weight; pharmaceutical specifications and chemical and physical properties; incompatibilities and interactions with other excipients and drug substances; regulatory status; safety, stability, and handling information; and applications in pharmaceutical formulation or technology.

Appearance and Palatability

Although most drug substances in use today are unpalatable and unattractive in their natural state, their preparations present them to the patient as colorful, flavorful formulations attractive to the sight, smell, and taste. These qualities, which are the rule rather than the exception, have virtually eliminated the natural reluctance of many patients to take medications because of disagreeable odor or taste. In fact, the inherent attractiveness of today's pharmaceuticals has caused them to acquire the dubious distinction of being a source of accidental poisonings in the home, particularly among children who are lured by their organoleptic appeal.

There is some psychologic basis to drug therapy, and the odor, taste, and color of a pharmaceutical preparation can play a part. An appropriate drug has its most beneficial effect when it is accepted and taken properly by the patient. The proper combination of flavor, fragrance, and color in a pharmaceutical product contributes to its acceptance.

An "electronic tongue" is used to aid in providing a global "taste fingerprint" during formulation development. It provides information on bitterness levels and the stability of flavors in terms of taste (Fig. 4.4).

FIGURE 4.4. Electronic tongue to assist in formulation development. (Courtesy of Alpha MOS.)

Flavoring Pharmaceuticals

The flavoring of pharmaceuticals applies primarily to liquids intended for oral administration. The 10,000 taste buds on the tongue, roof of the mouth, cheeks, and throat have 60 to 100 receptor cells each (13). These receptor cells interact with molecules dissolved in the saliva and produce a positive or negative taste sensation. Medication in liquid form comes into immediate and direct contact with these taste buds. The addition of flavoring agents to liquid medication can mask the disagreeable taste. Drugs placed in capsules or prepared as coated tablets may be easily swallowed with no contact between the drug and the taste buds. Tablets containing drugs that are not especially distasteful may remain uncoated and unflavored. Swallowing them with water usually is sufficient to avoid undesirable taste sensations. However, chewable tablets, such as certain antacid and vitamin products, usually are sweetened and flavored to improve acceptance.

The flavor sensation of a food or pharmaceutical is actually a complex blend of taste and smell, with lesser influences of texture, temperature, and even sight. In flavor-formulating a pharmaceutical product, the pharmacist must give consideration to the color, odor, texture, and taste of the preparation. It would be incongruous, for example, to color a liquid pharmaceutical red and give it a banana taste and a mint odor. The color of a pharmaceutical must have a psychogenic balance with the taste, and the odor must also enhance that taste. Odor greatly affects the flavor of a preparation or foodstuff. If one's sense of smell is impaired, as during a head cold, the usual flavor sensation of food is similarly diminished.

The medicinal chemist and the formulation pharmacist are well acquainted with the taste characteristics of certain chemical types of drugs and strive to mask the unwanted taste through the appropriate use of flavoring agents. Although there are no rules for unerringly predicting the taste sensation of a drug based on its chemical constitution, experience permits the presentation of several observations. For instance, although we recognize and assume the salty taste of sodium chloride, the formulation pharmacist knows that not all salts are salty but that their taste is a function of both cation and anion. Whereas salty tastes are evoked by chlorides of sodium, potassium, and ammonium and by sodium bromide, bromides of potassium and ammonium elicit bitter and salty sensations, and potassium iodide and magnesium sulfate (Epsom salt) are predominantly bitter. In general, low molecular weight salts are salty, and high molecular weight salts are bitter.

With organic compounds, an increase in the number of hydroxyl groups (–OH) seems to increase the sweetness of the compound. Sucrose, which has eight hydroxyl groups, is sweeter than glycerin, another pharmaceutical sweetener, which has three hydroxyl groups. In general, the organic esters, alcohols, and aldehydes are pleasant to the taste, and because many of them are volatile, they also contribute to the odor and thus the flavor of preparations in which they are used. Many nitrogen-containing compounds, especially the plant alkaloids (e.g., quinine), are extremely bitter, but certain other nitrogen-containing compounds (e.g., aspartame) are extremely sweet. The medicinal chemist recognizes that even the most simple structural change in an organic compound can alter its taste. D-Glucose is sweet, but L-glucose has a slightly salty taste; saccharin is very sweet, but N-methyl-saccharin is tasteless (14).

Thus, prediction of the taste characteristics of a new drug is only speculative. However, it is soon learned, and the formulation pharmacist is then put to the task of increasing the drug's palatability in the environment of other formulative agents. The selection of an appropriate flavoring agent depends on several factors, primarily the taste of the drug substance itself. Certain flavoring materials are more effective than others in masking or disguising the particular bitter, salty, sour, or otherwise undesirable taste of medicinal agents. Although individuals' tastes and flavor preferences differ, cocoa-flavored vehicles are considered effective for masking the taste of bitter drugs. Fruit or citrus flavors are frequently used to combat sour or acid-tasting drugs, and cinnamon, orange, raspberry, and other flavors have been successfully used to make preparations of salty drugs more palatable.

The age of the intended patient should also be considered in the selection of the flavoring agent, because certain age groups seem to prefer certain flavors. Children prefer sweet candy-like preparations with fruity flavors, but adults seem to prefer less sweet preparations with a tart rather than a fruit flavor.

Flavors can consist of oil- or water-soluble liquids and dry powders; most are diluted in carriers. Oil-soluble carriers include soybean and other edible oils; water-soluble carriers include water, ethanol, propylene glycol, glycerin, and emulsifiers. Dry carriers include maltodextrins, corn syrup solids, modified starches, gum arabic, salt, sugars, and whey protein. Flavors can degrade as a result of exposure to light, temperature, headspace oxygen, water, enzymes, contaminants, and other product components, so they must be carefully selected and checked for stability.

Flavoring agents may be derived from natural sources (e.g., fruit components) or prepared artificially. They may be either water soluble or oil soluble. Their selected use in pharmaceutical products is based on desired flavor, their solubility characteristics, and their chemical and physical compatibility with the active therapeutic agent and other components of the formulation.

Flavoring agents in liquid pharmaceutical products are added to the solvent or vehicle component of the formulation in which it is most soluble or miscible. That is, water-soluble flavorings are added to the aqueous component of a formulation and oil-soluble flavorings are added to the nonaqueous components. In general, artificial flavors are used in liquid pharmaceutical at levels of 0.1% to 0.2%, whereas natural flavors are used within the 1% to 2% range.

Sweetening Pharmaceuticals

In addition to sucrose, other naturally occurring sweeteners, including stevia (*Stevia rebaudiana*) (Asteraceae), are also used. A number of artificial sweetening agents have been used in foods and pharmaceuticals over the years. Some of these, including aspartame, saccharin, and cyclamate, have faced challenges over their safety by the FDA and restrictions to their use and sale.

A review of the history of safety concerns over the use of artificial sweeteners, current scientific findings, and related FDA and legislative actions may be found at the Web site: http://www.cancer.gov/cancertopics/factsheet/Risk/artificial-sweeteners.

At the present time, the following artificial sweeteners are approved by the FDA with, in parenthesis, the number of times (×) each one is sweeter than table sugar:

- Acesulfame potassium (~200×)
- Aspartame (~180 to 200×)
- Sucralose (~600×)
- Saccharin (~300×)

Most large pharmaceutical manufacturers have special laboratories for taste-testing proposed formulations of their products. Panels of employees or interested community participants participate in evaluating the various formulations, and their assessments become the basis for the firm's flavoring decisions.

Coloring Pharmaceuticals

Coloring agents are used in pharmaceutical preparations for esthetics. A distinction should be made between agents that have inherent color and those that are employed as colorants. An example of a natural substance with inherent color that is employed as a colorant is red ferric oxide. It is mixed in small proportions with zinc oxide powder to give calamine its characteristic pink color, which is intended to match the skin tone upon application.

Most agents employed today to impart color to foods, drugs, cosmetics, and medical devices are synthetic. Synthetic coloring agents were first prepared in the middle of the 19th century from principles of coal tar. Coal tar (*pix carbonis*), a thick, black viscid liquid, is a by-product of the destructive distillation of coal. Its composition is extremely complex, and many of its constituents may be separated by fractional distillation. Among its products are anthracene, benzene, naphtha, creosote, phenol, and pitch. About 90% of the dyes used in the products FDA regulates are synthesized from a single colorless derivative of benzene called aniline. These aniline dyes are also known as synthetic organic dyes or as coal tar dyes, because aniline was originally obtained from bituminous coal. Aniline dyes today come mainly from petroleum.

Many coal tar dyes were originally used indiscriminately in foods and beverages to enhance their appeal without regard to their toxic potential. It was only after careful scrutiny that some dyes were found to be hazardous to health because of either their own chemical nature or the impurities they carried. As more dyestuffs became available, some expert guidance and regulation were needed to ensure the safety of the public. After passage of the Food and Drug Act in 1906, the

U.S. Department of Agriculture established regulations by which a few colorants were *permitted* or *certified* for use in certain products. Today, the FDA regulates the use of color additives in foods, drugs, and cosmetics through the provisions of the Federal Food, Drug, and Cosmetic Act of 1938, as amended in 1960 with the Color Additive Amendments. Lists of color additives *exempt* from certification and those *subject* to certification are codified into law and regulated by the FDA (15). Certified color additives are classified according to their approved use: (*a*) FD&C color additives, which may be used in foods, drugs, and cosmetics; (*b*) D&C color additives, some of which are approved for use in drugs, some in cosmetics, and some in medical devices; and (*c*) external D&C color additives, the use of which is restricted to external parts of the body, not including the lips or any other body surface covered by mucous membrane. Each certification category has a variety of basic colors and shades for coloring pharmaceuticals. A current list of certified color additives may be found at 21CFR74 (http://www.accessdata.fda.gov/scripts/cdrh/cfdocs/cfcfr/CFRSearch.cfm?CFRPart=74). One may select from a variety of FD&C, D&C, and external D&C reds, yellows, oranges, greens, blues, and violets. Each is identified by category, color, and number, as for example, "D&C Yellow No. 8" and "FD&C Red No. 4." By selective combinations of the colorants, one can create distinctive colors (Table 4.5).

As a part of the National Toxicology Program of the U.S. Department of Health and Human Services, various substances, including color additives, are studied for toxicity and carcinogenesis. For color additives, the study protocols usually call for a 2-year study in which groups of male and female mice and rats are fed diets containing various quantities of the colorant. The killed and surviving animals are examined for evidence of long-term toxicity and carcinogenesis. Five categories of evidence of carcinogenic activity are used in reporting observations: (*a*) "clear evidence" of carcinogenic activity; (*b*) "some evidence"; (*c*) "equivocal evidence," indicating uncertainty; (*d*) "no evidence," indicating no observable effect; and (*e*) "inadequate study," for studies that cannot be evaluated because of major flaws.

The certification status of the colorants is continually reviewed, and changes are made in the list of certified colors in accordance with toxicology findings. These changes may be (*a*) the withdrawal of certification, (*b*) the transfer of a colorant from one certification category to another, or (*c*) the addition of new colors to the list. Before gaining certification, a color additive must be demonstrated to be safe. By FDA definition, "*safe*" means that there is convincing evidence that establishes with reasonable certainty that no harm will result from the intended use of the color additive (16).

It should be borne in mind, however, that on an individual basis, some persons may demonstrate an allergic-type response to certain color additives and should avoid such agents accordingly.

Each certified color additive is subject to a host of chemical standards that must be met, including chemical identity, purity, and specifically stated levels of allowable impurities (17).

TABLE 4.5. Examples of Color Formulations

Shade or Color	FD&C Dye	% of Blend
Orange	Yellow No. 6	95
	or	
	Yellow No. 5	5
	Red No. 40	100
Cherry	Red No. 40	100
	or	
	Red No. 40	99
	Blue No. 1	1
Strawberry	Red No. 40	100
	or	
	Red No. 40	95
	Red No. 3	5
Lemon	Yellow No. 5	100
Lime	Yellow No. 5	95
	Blue No. 1	5
Grape	Red No. 40	80
	Blue No. 1	20
Raspberry	Red No. 3	75
	Yellow No. 6	20
	Blue No. 1	5
Butterscotch	Yellow No. 5	74
	Red No. 40	24
	Blue No. 1	2
Chocolate	Red No. 40	52
	Yellow No. 5	40
	Blue No. 1	8
Caramel	Yellow No. 5	64
	Red No. 3	21
	Yellow No. 6	9
	Blue No. 1	6
Cinnamon	Yellow No. 5	60
	Red No. 40	35
	Blue No. 1	5

In addition, they must be shown to not interfere with the therapeutic efficacy of a pharmaceutical product nor should they interfere with the performance of quality control assay procedures.

A colorant becomes an integral part of a pharmaceutical formulation, and its exact quantitative amount must be reproducible each time the formulation is prepared or else the preparation would have a different appearance from batch to batch. This requires a high degree of skill, for the amount of colorant generally added to liquid preparations ranges from 0.0005% to 0.001% depending upon the colorant and the depth of color desired. Because of their color potency, dyes generally are added to pharmaceutical preparations in the form of diluted solutions rather than as concentrated dry powders. This permits greater accuracy in measurement and more consistent color production (18).

In addition to liquid dyes in the coloring of pharmaceuticals, lake pigments may also be used. An FD&C lake is a pigment consisting of a substratum of alumina hydrate on which the dye is adsorbed or precipitated. Having aluminum hydroxide as the substrate, the lakes are insoluble in nearly all solvents.

Lakes in pharmaceuticals are commonly used in the form of fine dispersions or suspensions. The pigment particles may range in size from less than 1 μm up to 30 μm. The finer the particle, the less chance for color speckling in the finished product. Blends of various lake pigments may be used to achieve a variety of colors, and various vehicles, such as glycerin, propylene glycol, and sucrose-based syrup, may be employed to disperse the colorants.

Colored empty gelatin capsule shells may be used to hold a powdered drug mixture. Many commercial capsules are prepared with a capsule body of one color and a cap of a different color, resulting in a two-colored capsule. This makes certain commercial products more readily identifiable than solid-colored capsules. For powdered drugs dispensed as such or compressed into tablets, a generally larger proportion of dye is required (about 0.1%) to achieve the desired hue than with liquid preparations.

Both dyes and lakes are used to color sugar-coated tablets, film-coated tablets, direct-compression tablets, pharmaceutical suspensions, and other dosage forms (19). Traditionally, sugar-coated tablets have been colored with syrup solutions containing varying amounts of the water-soluble dyes, starting with very dilute solutions, working up to concentrated color syrup solutions. As many as 30 to 60 coats are common. With the lakes, fewer color coats are used. Appealing tablets have been made with as few as 8 to 12 coats using lakes dispersed in syrup. Water-soluble dyes in aqueous vehicles or lakes dispersed in organic solvents may be effectively sprayed on tablets to produce attractive film coatings. There is continued interest today in chewable tablets, because of the availability of many direct-compression materials such as dextrose, sucrose, mannitol, sorbitol, and spray-dried lactose. The direct-compression colored chewable tablets may be prepared with 1 lb of lake per 1,000 lb of tablet mix. For aqueous suspensions, FD&C water-soluble colors or lakes may be satisfactory. In other suspensions, FD&C lakes are necessary. The lakes, added to either the aqueous or the nonaqueous phase, generally at a level of 1 lb of color per 1,000 lb of suspension, require homogenization or mechanical blending to achieve uniform coloring.

For the most part, ointments, suppositories, and ophthalmic and parenteral products assume the color of their ingredients and do not contain color additives. Should a dye lose the certification status it held when a product was first formulated, manufactured, and marketed, the manufacturer must reformulate within a reasonable length of time, using only color additives certified at the new date of manufacture.

In addition to esthetics and the certification status of a dye, a formulation pharmacist must select the dyes to be used in a particular formula on the basis of their physical and chemical properties. Of prime importance is the solubility of a prospective dye in the vehicle to be used for a liquid formulation or in a solvent to be employed during a pharmaceutical process, as when the dye is sprayed on a batch of tablets. In general, most dyes are broadly grouped into those that are water soluble and those that are oil soluble; few if any dyes are both. Usually, a water-soluble dye is also adequately soluble in commonly used pharmaceutical liquids like glycerin, alcohol, and glycol ethers. Oil-soluble dyes may also be soluble to some extent in these solvents and in liquid petrolatum (mineral oil), fatty acids, fixed oils, and waxes. No great deal of solubility is required, because the concentration of dye in a given preparation is minimal.

Another important consideration when selecting a dye for use in a liquid pharmaceutical is the pH and pH stability of the preparation to be colored. Dyes can change color with a change in pH, and the dye must be selected so that no anticipated pH change will alter the color during the usual shelf life. The dye also must be chemically stable in the presence of the other formulative ingredients and must not interfere with the stability of the other agents. To maintain their original colors, FD&C dyes must be protected from oxidizing agents, reducing agents (especially metals, including iron, aluminum, zinc, and tin), strong acids and alkalis, and excessive heating. Dyes must also be reasonably photostable; that is, they must not change color when exposed to light of anticipated intensities and wavelengths under the usual conditions of shelf storage. As required, amber or opaque glass or plastic containers may be used to protect photolabile ingredients, including active therapeutic ingredients and colorants.

Preservatives

In addition to the stabilization of pharmaceutical preparations against chemical and physical degradation due to changed environmental conditions within a formulation, certain liquid and semisolid preparations must be preserved against microbial contamination.

Sterilization and Preservation

Although some types of pharmaceutical products, for example, ophthalmic and injectable preparations, are sterilized by physical methods (autoclaving for 20 minutes at 15 lb pressure and 121°C, dry heat at 180°C for 1 hour, or bacterial filtration) during manufacture, many of them also require an antimicrobial preservative to maintain their aseptic condition throughout storage and use. Other types of preparations that are not sterilized during their preparation but are particularly susceptible to microbial growth because of the nature of their ingredients are protected by the addition of an antimicrobial preservative. Preparations that provide excellent growth media for microbes are most aqueous preparations, especially syrups, emulsions, suspensions, and some semisolid preparations, particularly creams. Certain hydroalcoholic and most alcoholic preparations may not require the addition of a chemical preservative when the alcoholic content is sufficient to prevent microbial growth. Generally, 15% v/v alcohol will prevent microbial growth in acid media and 18% v/v in alkaline media. Most alcohol-containing pharmaceuticals, such as elixirs, spirits, and tinctures, are self-sterilizing and do not require additional preservation. The same applies to other individual pharmaceuticals that by virtue of their vehicle or other formulative agents may not permit the growth of microorganisms.

Preservative Selection

When experience or shelf storage experiments indicate that a preservative is required in a pharmaceutical preparation, its selection is based on many considerations, including some of the following:

- The preservative prevents the growth of the type of microorganisms considered the most likely contaminants of the preparation.
- The preservative is soluble enough in water to achieve adequate concentrations in the aqueous phase of a system with two or more phases.
- The proportion of preservative remaining undissociated at the pH of the preparation makes it capable of penetrating the microorganism and destroying its integrity.
- The required concentration of the preservative does not affect the safety or comfort of the patient when the pharmaceutical preparation is administered by the usual or intended route; that is, it is nonirritating, nonsensitizing, and nontoxic.
- The preservative has adequate stability and will not be reduced in concentration by chemical decomposition or volatilization during the desired shelf life of the preparation.
- The preservative is completely compatible with all other formulative ingredients and does not interfere with them nor do they interfere with the effectiveness of the preservative agent.
- The preservative does not adversely affect the preparation's container or closure.

General Preservative Considerations

Microorganisms include molds, yeasts, and bacteria, with bacteria generally favoring a slightly alkaline medium and the others an acid medium. Although few microorganisms can grow below pH 3 or above pH 9, most aqueous pharmaceutical preparations are within the favorable pH range and therefore must be protected against microbial growth. To be effective, a preservative agent must be dissolved in sufficient concentration in the aqueous phase of a preparation. Furthermore, only the undissociated fraction or molecular form of a preservative possesses preservative capability, because the ionized portion is incapable of penetrating the microorganism. Thus, the preservative selected must be largely undissociated at the pH of the formulation being prepared. Acidic preservatives like benzoic, boric, and sorbic acids are more undissociated and thus more effective as the medium is made more acid. Conversely, alkaline preservatives are less effective in acid or neutral media and more effective in alkaline media. Thus, it is meaningless to

suggest preservative effectiveness at specific concentrations unless the pH of the system is mentioned and the undissociated concentration of the agent is calculated or otherwise determined. Also, if formulative materials interfere with the solubility or availability of the preservative agent, its chemical concentration may be misleading, because it may not be a true measure of the effective concentration. It is essential for the research pharmacist to examine all formulative ingredients as one affects the other to ensure that each agent is free to do its job. In addition, the preservative must not interact with a container or closure.

The FDA recommends that in the pharmaceutical development process, the lowest effective concentration of an antimicrobial preservative should be used and that it should be demonstrated to be effective by an antimicrobial preservative effectiveness test. The concentration used should be validated in terms of efficacy and safety, with the effectiveness confirmed to last throughout the intended shelf life of the product (19).

Mode of Action

Preservatives interfere with microbial growth, multiplication, and metabolism through one or more of the following mechanisms:

- Modification of cell membrane permeability and leakage of cell constituents (partial lysis)
- Lysis and cytoplasmic leakage
- Irreversible coagulation of cytoplasmic constituents (e.g., protein precipitation)
- Inhibition of cellular metabolism, such as by interfering with enzyme systems or inhibition of cell wall synthesis
- Oxidation of cellular constituents
- Hydrolysis

Examples of the preservatives and their concentrations commonly employed in pharmaceutical preparations are benzoic acid (0.1% to 0.2%), sodium benzoate (0.1% to 0.2%), alcohol (15% to 20%), phenylmercuric nitrate and acetate (0.002% to 0.01%), phenol (0.1% to 0.5%), cresol (0.1% to 0.5%), chlorobutanol (0.5%), benzalkonium chloride (0.002% to 0.01%), and combinations of methylparaben and propylparaben (0.1% to 0.2%), the latter being especially good against fungus. The required proportion varies with the pH, dissociation, and other factors already indicated as well with the presence of other formulative ingredients with inherent preservative capabilities.

For each type of preparation to be preserved, the research pharmacist must consider the influence of the preservative on the comfort of the patient. For instance, a preservative in an ophthalmic preparation must have an extremely low degree of irritant qualities, which is characteristic of chlorobutanol, benzalkonium chloride, and phenylmercuric nitrate, frequently used in ophthalmic preparations. In all instances, the preserved preparation must be biologically tested to determine its safety and efficacy and shelf tested to determine its stability for the intended shelf life of the product.

CLINICAL CASE STUDY

SUBJECTIVE INFORMATION

HPI: Jen, an 8-year-old female, is 4'1" tall, weighs 27 kg, and has no known allergies.

She was brought to the clinic by her mother to seek advice on treating a "dry hacking" cough. Her mother states that Jen has had the cough for the past 4 weeks; it is a dry, hacking cough that does not produce any mucous. She experiences these coughs in 2- to 3-minute bouts once or twice daily, after coming in from recess or playing outside. At school, the nurse's office gives her water and a lozenge. After school and at bedtime, she also occasionally experiences the cough. Jen does not complain of stuffiness or increased nasal discharge. However, she has recently complained of a headache that was successfully treated with acetaminophen.

PMH: Over the past 2 months, Jen has had two episodes of sinusitis requiring antibiotic treatment. Her vaccinations are up to date and the rest of her history is negative.

MEDICATION RECORD

1/21 Augmentin 400/5 100 mL 1 tsp bid × 10 days.
4/14 Cefdinir 125/5 200 mL 7 mL bid × 10 days.

FH: The father (age 44) has diabetes mellitus type 2 treated with oral agents and high blood pressure. The mother (age 39) denies any health problems. Two other siblings are reported healthy.

OBJECTIVE INFORMATION

A physical exam reveals a well-nourished, well-developed female child who appears normal for her age. BP, 92/64; HR, 74 bpm; RR, 23 rpm; and temperature of 38°C.

ASSESSMENT

Patient is an 8-year-old female with a dry, hacking cough. She is not on any medications at this time. Cough seems to be aggravated after periods of exertion or exercise. The mother says she is concerned that some medicines might make Jen tired or drowsy while she is at school, so she would like one that is least likely to produce drowsiness/sedation.

Jen's mother also wants a product she can give to Jen before school (7:30 AM) that will last until the evening when she returns home. Also, she says that Jen does not like the taste of many medications and is concerned that Jen may not like what is recommended and refuse to take it. Also, she says that Jen prefers strawberry flavors.

PLAN

Three commonly used systemic antitussive medications include codeine, dextromethorphan, and diphenhydramine. Only dextromethorphan will not cause significant drowsiness as will codeine and diphenhydramine. One product that last up to 12 hours is Delsym. Dextromethorphan products do not necessarily taste very good. An option for improving the flavor of Delsym would be to add a commercial flavor. For example, FLAVORx flavorings could be used as follows: for Delsym, 120 mL, strawberry cream 24 drops or 0.7 mL, with vanilla 24 drops or 0.7 mL. ■

APPLYING THE PRINCIPLES AND CONCEPTS

GROUP ACTIVITIES

1. Develop a listing of examples where patients misunderstand the intent of the administration of a pharmaceutical dosage form.
2. Develop a listing of examples where patients misuse/abuse a pharmaceutical dosage form.
3. Explain the appropriate use of specific dosage forms for different patient types, for example, geriatric, pediatric, visually impaired, and hearing impaired. Identify and list the most common hurdles or obstacles for these patient populations with respect to medication compliance and discuss ways to overcome these barriers, that is, FLAVORx for liquids for children and Pill Glide for children transitioning to tablets.
4. Identify four ophthalmic products with differing preservative agents and provide a rationale for the selection of the specific preservative in the product.
5. Identify elixir dosage form products that contain minimal or no alcohol content. Explain the reasons for this misnomer.
6. Prepare a chart listing which flavors pair well with certain medications based upon their chemical structure and their palatability issues (bitter, salty, etc.). Different groups can select medications with different chemical structures.

INDIVIDUAL ACTIVITIES

1. Given a specific dosage form, list the signs of degradation a pharmacist might observe indicating product instability.
2. Given a concentration of drug in a liquid dosage form, determine its type of degradation rate and calculate its half-life and when its concentration will be 90% of the labeled amount.

3. Compare and contrast a zero-order rate of degradation and a first-order rate of degradation.
4. Make a listing of drugs that follow a zero-order rate of degradation in a liquid dosage form.
5. Make a listing of drugs that follow first-order rates of degradation in a liquid dosage form.

REFERENCES

1. Poole JW. Preformulation. FMC Corporation, 1982.
2. Brange J, Langkjaer L, Havelund S, et al. Chemical stability of insulin: Hydrolytic degradation during storage of pharmaceutical preparations. Pharm Res 1991;9:715–726.
3. 21CFR201.22. Drugs: Labeling. Available at: http://www.accessdata.fda.gov/scripts/cdrh/cfdocs/cfcfr/CFRSearch.cfm?fr=201. (Accessed July 22, 2020)
4. 21CFR211. Current Good Manufacturing Practice for Finished Pharmaceuticals. Available at: http://www.accessdata.fda.gov/scripts/cdrh/cfdocs/cfcfr/CFRSearch.cfm?CFRPart=211. (Accessed July 22, 2020)
5. Stability. International Conference on Harmonization. Available at: http://www.ich.org/about/organisation-of-ich/coopgroup/gcc.html. (Accessed July 22, 2020)
6. FDA & ICH Guidelines on Accelerated Shelf-life Testing. Available at: http://www.fdaregulatory.net/index.php/component/content/article/115-fda-a-ich-guidelines-on-accelerated-shelf-life-testing.html. (Accessed July 22, 2020)
7. Stability and Testing of New Drug Substances and Products. Available at: http://www.fda.gov/downloads/RegulatoryInformation/Guidances/ucm128204.pdf. (Accessed July 22, 2020)
8. General Chapter <795> Pharmaceutical Compounding-Nonsterile Preparations, and General Chapter <797> Pharmaceutical Compounding-Sterile Preparations. U.S. Pharmacopoeia—National Formulary. Current Ed. Rockville, MD: U.S. Pharmacopoeial Convention, Inc.
9. Trissel L, Ashworth LD, Ashworth J. Trissel's Stability of Compounded Formulations. 6th Ed. Washington, DC: American Pharmaceutical Association, 2018.
10. Sheskey PJ, Cook WG, Cable CG, eds. Handbook of Pharmaceutical Excipients. 8th Ed. London: Pharmaceutical Press, 2017.
11. Allen LV Jr, ed. Int J Pharm Compd. Edmond, OK. Available at: http://www.ijpc.com/
12. Allen LV Jr. The Art, Science, and Technology of Pharmaceutical Compounding. 5th Ed. Washington, DC: American Pharmacists Association, 2016.
13. Lewis R. When smell and taste go awry. FDA Consum 1991;25: 29–33.
14. Hornstein I, Teranishi R. The chemistry of flavor. Chem Eng News 1967;45:92–108.
15. 21CFR172 Food Additives. Available at: http://www.accessdata.fda.gov/scripts/cdrh/cfdocs/cfCFR/CFRSearch.cfm?CFRPart=172&showFR=1&subpartNode=21:3.0.1.1.3.9. (Accessed July 22, 2020)
16. 21CFR80 Color Additive Certification. Available at: http://www.gpo.gov/fdsys/pkg/CFR-2011-title21-vol1/pdf/CFR-2011-title21-vol1-part80.pdf. (Accessed July 22, 2020)
17. 21CFR 74. Listing of Color Additives Subject to Certification. Available at: http://www.gpo.gov/fdsys/pkg/CFR-2011-title21-vol1/pdf/CFR-2011-title21-vol1-part80.pdf. (Accessed July 22, 2020)
18. Colorants for drug tablets and capsules. Drug Cosmet Ind 1983;133(2):44–48, 107.
19. Guidance for Industry: Pharmaceutical Development. Rockville, MD: Food and Drug Administration, 2009. Available at: http://www.fda.gov/downloads/Drugs/GuidanceComplianceRegulatoryInformation/Guidances/UCM073507.pdf. (Accessed July 22, 2020)

Dosage Form Design: Biopharmaceutical and Pharmacokinetic Considerations

CHAPTER AT A GLANCE Principles of Drug Absorption • Dissolution and Drug Absorption • Bioavailability and Bioequivalence • Bioequivalence of Drug Products • Routes of Drug Administration • Fate of Drug After Absorption • Pharmacokinetic Principles

OBJECTIVES

After reading this chapter, the student will be able to:

1. Differentiate between *passive drug diffusion* and *active drug transport*
2. Discuss key data points in a blood plasma concentration–time curve following the oral administration of a drug
3. Differentiate between the terms *biopharmaceutics*, *bioavailability*, and *bioequivalence*
4. Discuss the importance of a drug's dissolution rate following the oral administration of a solid dosage form
5. Describe the sequence of events and the processes that occur to a drug during its course of bodily transit, from the time of its oral administration and absorption through its excretion
6. Perform various basic pharmacokinetic calculations
7. List the factors that a pharmacist must consider when determining a dosage regimen for a specific patient

INTRODUCTION

As discussed in Chapter 2, the biologic response to a drug is the result of an interaction between the drug substance and functionally important cell receptors or enzyme systems. The response is due to an alteration in the biologic processes that were present prior to the drug's administration. The magnitude of the response is related to the concentration of the drug achieved at the site of its action. This drug concentration depends on the dosage of the drug administered, the extent of its absorption and distribution to the site, and the rate and extent of its elimination from the body. The physical and chemical constitution of the drug substance—particularly its lipid solubility, degree of ionization, and molecular size—determines to a great extent its ability to carry out its biologic activity. The area of study embracing this relationship between the physical, chemical, and biologic sciences as they apply to drugs, dosage forms, and drug action has been given the descriptive term *biopharmaceutics*.

In general, for a drug to exert its biologic effect, it must be transported by the body fluids, traverse the required biologic membrane barriers, escape widespread distribution to unwanted areas, endure metabolic attack, penetrate in adequate concentration to the sites of action, and interact in a specific fashion, causing an alteration of cellular function. A simplified diagram of this complex series of events between a drug's administration and its elimination is presented in Figure 5.1.

The absorption, distribution, biotransformation (metabolism), and elimination of a drug from the body are dynamic processes that continue from the time a drug is taken until drug has been removed from the body entirely. The *rates* at which these processes occur affect the onset, intensity, and duration of the drug's activity within the body. The area of study that elucidates the time course of drug concentration in the blood and tissues is termed *pharmacokinetics*. It is the study of the kinetics of absorption, distribution, metabolism, and excretion (ADME) of drugs and their corresponding pharmacologic,

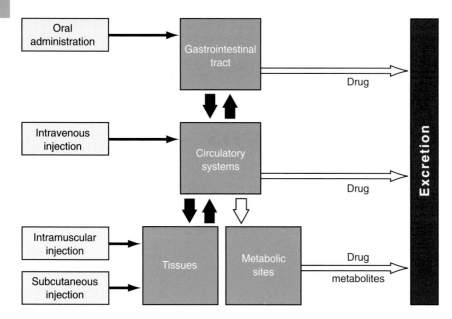

FIGURE 5.1. Events of absorption, metabolism, and excretion of drugs after their administration by various routes.

therapeutic, or toxic effects in animals and man. Furthermore, because one drug may alter the ADME of another drug, pharmacokinetics may be applied in the study of interactions between drugs.

Once a drug is administered and absorption begins, the drug does not remain in a single body location but rather is distributed throughout the body until its ultimate elimination. For instance, following the oral administration of a drug and its entry into the gastrointestinal tract, a portion of the drug is absorbed into the circulatory system, from which it is distributed to the various other body fluids, tissues, and organs. From these sites, the drug may return to the circulatory system and be excreted through the kidney as such or be metabolized by the liver or other cellular sites and be excreted as one or more metabolites. As demonstrated in Figure 5.1, drugs administered by intravenous injection are introduced directly into the circulatory system, avoiding absorption, which is required for systemic effects from all other routes of administration.

The various body locations to which a drug travels may be viewed as separate compartments, each containing some fraction of the administered dose of drug. The transfer of drug from the blood to other body locations is generally a rapid and reversible process; that is, the drug may diffuse back into the circulation. The drug in the blood therefore exists in equilibrium with the drug in the other compartments. However, in this equilibrium state, the concentration of the drug in the blood may be quite different (greater or lesser) than the concentration of the drug in the other compartments. This is due largely to the physicochemical properties of the drug and its resultant ability to leave the blood and traverse the biologic membranes. Certain drugs leave the circulatory system rapidly and completely, whereas other drugs do so slowly and with difficulty. A number of drugs become bound to blood proteins, particularly the albumins, and only a small fraction of the drug administered may actually be found outside of the circulatory system at a given time. The transfer of drug from one compartment to another is mathematically associated with a specific rate constant describing that particular transfer. Generally, the rate of transfer of a drug from one compartment to another is proportional to the concentration of the drug in the compartment from which it exits; the greater the concentration, the greater is the amount of drug transfer.

Metabolism is the major process by which foreign substances, including drugs, are eliminated from the body. During metabolism, a drug substance may be biotransformed into pharmacologically active or inactive metabolites, or both. Often, both the drug substance and its metabolite or metabolites are active and exert pharmacologic effects. For example, the anticonvulsant drug carbamazepine is metabolized in the liver to an active epoxide metabolite. In some instances, a pharmacologically inactive drug (termed a *prodrug*) may be administered for the known effects of its active metabolites. Dipivefrin, for example, is a prodrug of epinephrine formed by the esterification of epinephrine and pivalic acid. This enhances the lipophilic character of the drug, and as a consequence, its penetration into the anterior chamber of the eye is 17 times that of epinephrine. Within the eye, dipivefrin HCl is converted by enzymatic hydrolysis to epinephrine.

Usually, the metabolism of a drug to inactive products is an irreversible process that culminates in the excretion of the drug from the body, usually via the urine. The pharmacokineticist may calculate an elimination rate constant (K_{el}) for a drug to describe its rate of elimination from the body. The term *elimination* refers to both metabolism and excretion. For drugs that are administered intravenously and, therefore, are not absorbed, the task is much less complex than for drugs administered by other routes. Except with intravenous administration, absorption and elimination occur simultaneously but at different rates.

PRINCIPLES OF DRUG ABSORPTION

Before an administered drug can arrive at its site of action in effective concentrations, it must surmount a number of barriers. These barriers are chiefly a succession of biologic membranes such as those of the gastrointestinal epithelium, lungs, blood, and brain. Body membranes are generally classified as three main types: (*a*) those composed of several layers of cells, like the skin; (*b*) those composed of a single layer of cells, like the intestinal epithelium; and (*c*) those less than one cell thick, like the membrane of a single cell. In most instances, a drug substance must pass more than one of these membrane types before it reaches its site of action. For instance, a drug taken by mouth must first traverse the gastrointestinal membranes (stomach and intestines), gain entrance to the general circulation, pass to the organ or tissue with which it has affinity, gain entrance to that tissue, and then enter its individual cells.

Although the chemistry of body membranes differs one from another, the membranes may be viewed in general as a bimolecular lipid (fat-containing) layer attached on both sides to a protein layer. Drugs are thought to penetrate these biologic membranes in two general ways: (*a*) by passive diffusion and (*b*) through specialized transport mechanisms. Within each of these main categories, more clearly defined processes have been ascribed to drug transfer.

Passive Diffusion

The term *passive diffusion* is used to describe the passage of (drug) molecules through a membrane that does not actively participate in the process. Drugs absorbed according to this method are said to be *passively absorbed*. The absorption process is driven by the concentration gradient (i.e., the differences in concentration) across the membrane, with the passage of drug molecules occurring primarily from the side of high concentration. Most drugs pass through biologic membranes by diffusion; processes include transcellular diffusion, paracellular diffusion, utilization of transporter proteins, and via endocytosis.

Epithelial membranes utilize transcellular permeation or diffusion across the lipid bilayer for drug movement. The drug molecule encountering an epithelial membrane first goes through the apical cell membrane, through the aqueous intracellular compartment, and out through the cells basal membrane, possibly traversing two or more cell layers prior to encountering the connective tissue, capillaries, or lymph vessels. Since capillaries and lymph vessels distribute drug molecules to other sites in the body, the drug molecule must also penetrate the capillary and lymphatic system membranes as well. The permeability of capillary membranes varies from tissue to tissue but generally consists of a single layer of highly permeable endothelial cells that create a lesser barrier to drug diffusion.

Passive diffusion is described by *Fick first law* (Physical Pharmacy Capsule 4.8), which states that the rate of diffusion or transport across a membrane (dc/dt) is proportional to the difference in drug concentration on both sides of the membrane:

$$-\frac{dc}{dt} = P(C_1 - C_2)$$

where

C$_1$ and C$_2$ are the drug concentrations on each side of the membrane and
P is a permeability coefficient or constant.

The term C$_1$ is customarily used to represent the compartment with the greater concentration of drug, and thus the transport of drug proceeds from compartment 1 (e.g., absorption site) to compartment 2 (e.g., blood).

The concentration of drug at the site of absorption (C$_1$) is usually much greater than on the other side of the membrane because of the rapid dilution of the drug in the blood and its subsequent distribution to the tissues, so for practical purposes, the value of C$_1$ − C$_2$ may be taken simply as that of C$_1$ and the equation written in the standard form for a first-order rate equation:

$$-\frac{dc}{dt} = PC_1$$

The gastrointestinal absorption of most drugs from solution occurs in this manner in accordance with *first-order kinetics*, in which the rate depends on drug concentration; that is, doubling the dose doubles the transfer rate. The magnitude of the permeability constant depends on the diffusion coefficient of the drug, the thickness and area of the absorbing membrane, and the permeability of the membrane to the particular drug.

Because of the lipoid nature of the cell membrane, it is highly permeable to lipid-soluble substances. The rate of diffusion of a drug across the membrane depends not only on its concentration but also on the relative extent of its affinity for lipid and rejection of water (a high lipid partition coefficient). The greater its affinity for lipid and the more hydrophobic it is, the faster will be its rate of penetration into the lipid-rich membrane. Erythromycin base, for example, possesses a higher partition coefficient than do other erythromycin compounds, for example, estolate and gluceptate. Consequently, the base is the preferred agent for the topical treatment of acne where penetration into the skin is desired.

Because biologic cells are also permeated by water and lipid-insoluble substances, it is thought that the membrane also contains water-filled pores or channels that permit the passage of these types of substances. As water passes in bulk across a porous membrane, any dissolved solute with small enough molecules to traverse the pores passes in by *filtration*. Aqueous pores vary in size from membrane to membrane and thus in their individual permeability characteristics for certain drugs and other substances.

Most drugs today are weak organic acids or bases. Knowledge of their individual ionization or dissociation characteristics is important, because their absorption is governed to a large extent by their degrees of ionization as they are presented to the membrane barriers. Cell membranes are more permeable to the unionized forms of drugs than to their ionized forms, mainly because of the greater lipid solubility of the unionized forms and the highly charged nature of the cell membrane, which results in binding or repelling of the ionized drug and thereby decreases cell penetration. Also, ions become hydrated through association with water molecules, resulting in larger particles than the undissociated molecule and again decreased penetrating capability.

The degree of a drug's ionization depends both on the pH of the solution in which it is presented to the biologic membrane and on the pK_a, or dissociation constant, of the drug (whether an acid or base). The concept of pK_a is derived from the Henderson-Hasselbalch equation.

For an acid,

$$pH = pK_a + \log \frac{\text{ionized conc. (salt)}}{\text{unionized conc. (acid)}}$$

For a base,

$$pH = pK_a + \log \frac{\text{un ionized conc. (base)}}{\text{ionized conc. (acid)}}$$

Because the pH of body fluids varies (stomach, pH 1; lumen of the intestine, pH 6.6; blood plasma, pH 7.4), the absorption of a drug from various body fluids will differ and may dictate to some extent the type of dosage form and the route of administration preferred for a given drug.

Rearranging the equation for an acid yields

$$pK_a - pH =$$
$$\log \frac{\text{un ionized concentration (acid)}}{\text{ionized concentration (acid)}}$$

and one can theoretically determine the relative extent to which a drug remains unionized under various conditions of pH. This is particularly useful when applied to body fluids. For instance, if a weak acid having a pK_a of 4 is assumed to be in an environment of gastric juice with a pH of 1, the left side of the equation yields the number 3, which means that the ratio of unionized to ionized drug particles is about 1,000:1 and gastric absorption is excellent. At the pH of plasma, the reverse is true, and in the blood, the drug is largely in the ionized form. Table 5.1 presents the effect of pH on the ionization of weak electrolytes, and Table 5.2 offers some representative pK_a values of common drug substances.

The equation and Table 5.1 show that a drug substance is half ionized at a pH value equal to its pK_a. Thus, pK_a may be defined as the pH at which a drug is 50% ionized. For example, phenobarbital has a pK_a value of about 7.4, and in plasma (pH 7.4), it is present as ionized and unionized forms in equal amounts. However, a drug substance cannot reach the blood plasma unless it is placed there directly through intravenous injection or

TABLE 5.1. The Effect of pH on the Ionization of Weak Electrolytes pK_a–pH % Unionized

	If Weak Acid	If Weak Base
−3.0	0.10	99.90
−2.0	0.99	99.00
−1.0	9.09	90.90
−0.7	16.60	83.40
−0.5	24.00	76.00
−0.2	38.70	61.30
0.0	50.00	50.00
+0.2	61.30	38.70
+0.5	76.00	24.00
+0.7	83.40	16.60
+1.0	90.90	9.09
+2.0	99.00	0.99
+3.0	99.90	0.10

TABLE 5.2. pK_a Values for Some Acidic and Basic Drugs

	pK_a
Acids	
Acetylsalicylic acid	3.5
Barbital	7.9
Benzylpenicillin	2.8
Boric acid	9.2
Dicoumarol	5.7
Phenobarbital	7.4
Phenytoin	8.3
Sulfanilamide	10.4
Theophylline	9.0
Thiopental	7.6
Tolbutamide	5.5
Warfarin sodium	4.8
Bases	
Amphetamine	9.8
Apomorphine	7.0
Atropine	9.7
Caffeine	0.8
Chlordiazepoxide	4.6
Cocaine	8.5
Codeine	7.9
Guanethidine	11.8
Morphine	7.9
Procaine	9.0
Quinine	8.4
Reserpine	6.6

is favorably absorbed from a site along its route of entry, such as the gastrointestinal tract, and allowed to pass into the general circulation. As shown in Table 5.2, phenobarbital, a weak acid with a pK_a of 7.4, would be largely undissociated in the gastric environment of pH 1 and would likely be well absorbed. A drug may enter the circulation rapidly and at high concentrations if membrane penetration is easily accomplished or at a low rate and low level if the drug is not readily absorbed from its route of entry. The pH of the drug's current environment influences the rate and degree of its further distribution because under one condition of pH, it becomes more or less unionized and therefore more or less lipid penetrating than under another. If an unionized molecule is able to diffuse through the lipid barrier and remain unionized in the new environment, it may return to its former location or go on to a new one. However, if in the new environment it is greatly ionized because of the influence of the pH of the second fluid, it likely will be unable to cross the membrane with its former ability. Thus, a concentration gradient of a drug usually is reached at equilibrium on each side of a membrane because different degrees of ionization occur on each side. A summary of the concepts of dissociation and ionization is found in Physical Pharmacy Capsules 4.8 and 4.10.

It is often desirable for pharmaceutical scientists to make structural modifications in organic drugs and thereby favorably alter their lipid solubility, partition coefficients, and dissociation constants while maintaining the same basic pharmacologic activity. These efforts frequently result in increased absorption, better therapeutic response, and lower dosage.

Specialized Transport Mechanisms

In contrast to the passive transfer of drugs and other substances across a biologic membrane, certain substances, including some drugs and biologic metabolites, are conducted across a membrane through one of several postulated *specialized transport* mechanisms. This type of transfer seems to account for substances, many naturally occurring as amino acids and glucose, that are too lipid insoluble to dissolve in the boundary and too large to flow or filter through the pores. This type of transport is thought to involve membrane components that may be enzymes or some other type of agent capable of forming a complex with the drug (or other agent) at the surface membrane. The complex moves across the membrane, where the drug is released, with the carrier returning to the original surface. Figure 5.2 presents the simplified scheme of this process. Specialized transport may be differentiated from passive transfer in that the former process may become saturated as the amount of carrier for a given substance becomes completely bound with that substance, resulting in a delay in transport. Other features of specialized transport include the specificity by a carrier for a particular type of chemical structure, so that if two substances are transported by the same mechanism or carrier, one will compet-

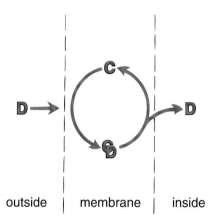

FIGURE 5.2. Active transport mechanism. D, drug molecule; C, the carrier in the membrane. (Adapted from O'Reilly WJ. Biological factors in dosage design I: Membranes and drug absorption. Aust J Pharm 1966;47(Supp 42):S51, with permission.)

itively inhibit the transport of the other. Furthermore, the transport mechanism is inhibited in general by substances that interfere with cell metabolism. The term *active transport* as a subclassification of specialized transport denotes a process with the additional feature of the solute or drug being moved across the membrane against a concentration gradient, that is, from a solution of lower concentration to one of a higher concentration or, if the solute is an ion, against an electrochemical potential gradient. In contrast to active transport, *facilitated diffusion* is a specialized transport mechanism having all of the described characteristics except that the solute is not transferred against a concentration gradient and may attain the same concentration inside the cell as on the outside.

Many body nutrients, such as sugars and amino acids, are transported across the membranes of the gastrointestinal tract by carrier processes. Certain vitamins, such as thiamine, niacin, riboflavin, and pyridoxine, and drug substances, such as methyldopa and 5-fluorouracil, require active transport mechanisms for their absorption.

Investigations of intestinal transport have often used in situ (at the site) or in vivo (in the body) animal models or ex vivo (outside the body) transport models; however, recently cell culture models of human small intestine absorptive cells have become available to investigate transport across intestinal epithelium (1). Both passive and transport-mediated studies have been conducted to investigate mechanisms and rates of transport.

DISSOLUTION AND DRUG ABSORPTION

For a drug to be absorbed, it must first be dissolved in the fluid at the absorption site. For instance, a drug administered orally in tablet or capsule form cannot be absorbed until the drug particles are dissolved by the fluids in the gastrointestinal tract. When the solubility of

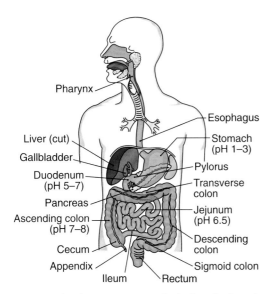

FIGURE 5.3. The digestive system, including the locations of drug absorption and their respective pH values. (Adapted from Cohen BJ, Wood DL. Memmler's the Human Body in Health and Disease. 11th Ed. Baltimore, MD: Lippincott Williams & Wilkins, 2009, with permission.)

a drug depends on either an acidic or basic medium, the drug dissolves in the stomach or intestines, respectively (Fig. 5.3). The process by which a drug particle dissolves is termed *dissolution*.

As a drug particle undergoes dissolution, the drug molecules on the surface are the first to enter into solution, creating a saturated layer of drug solution that envelops the surface of the solid drug particle. This layer of solution is the *diffusion layer*. From this diffusion layer, the drug molecules pass throughout the dissolving fluid and make contact with the biologic membranes and absorption ensues. As the molecules of drug continue to leave the diffusion layer, the layer is replenished with dissolved drug from the surface of the drug particle, and the process of absorption continues.

If the dissolution of a given drug particle is rapid or if the drug is administered as a solution and remains present in the body as such, the rate at which the drug becomes absorbed depends mainly on its ability to traverse the membrane barrier. However, if the rate of dissolution for a drug particle is slow because of the physicochemical characteristics of the drug substance or the dosage form, dissolution itself is a rate-limiting step in absorption. Slowly soluble drugs such as digoxin may not only be absorbed at a slow rate; they may be incompletely absorbed or in some cases largely unabsorbed following oral administration because of the natural limitation of time that they may remain within the stomach or the intestinal tract. Thus, poorly soluble drugs or poorly formulated drug products may be incompletely absorbed and pass unchanged out of the system via the feces.

Under normal circumstances, a drug may be expected to remain in the stomach for 2 to 4 hours (*gastric emptying time*) and in the small intestine for 4 to 10 hours, although there is substantial variation between people and even in the same person on different occasions. Various techniques have been used to determine gastric emptying time and the gastrointestinal passage of drug from various oral dosage forms, including tracking dosage forms labeled with gamma-emitting radionuclides through gamma scintigraphy (2,3). The gastric emptying time for a drug is most rapid with a fasting stomach, becoming slower as the food content is increased. Changes in gastric emptying time and/or in intestinal motility can affect drug transit time and thus the opportunity for drug dissolution and absorption.

These changes can be affected by drugs. Certain drugs with anticholinergic properties, for example, dicyclomine HCl and amitriptyline HCl, can slow gastric emptying. This can enhance the rate of absorption of drugs normally absorbed from the stomach and reduce the rate of absorption of drugs that are primarily absorbed from the small intestine. Alternatively, drugs that enhance gastric motility, for example, laxatives, may cause some drugs to move through the gastrointestinal system and past their absorptive site at such a rate as to reduce the amount of drug absorbed. This effect has been demonstrated with digoxin, whose absorption is significantly decreased by accelerating gastrointestinal motility.

Aging may also influence gastrointestinal absorption. In the elderly, gastric acidity, the number of absorptive cells, intestinal blood flow, the rate of gastric emptying, and intestinal motility are all decreased. However, drugs in which absorption depends on passive processes are not affected by these factors as much as are those that depend on active transport mechanisms, such as calcium, iron, thiamine, and sugars. A decrease in gastric emptying time is advantageous for drugs that are absorbed from the stomach but disadvantageous for those that are prone to acid degradation, such as penicillins and erythromycin, or inactivated by stomach enzymes, such as L-dopa.

The dissolution of a substance may be described by the modified Noyes-Whitney equation:

$$\frac{dc}{dt} = kS(C_s - C_t)$$

where

dc/dt is the rate of dissolution,
k is the dissolution rate constant,
S is the surface area of the dissolving solid,
C_s is the saturation concentration of drug in the diffusion layer (which may be approximated by the maximum solubility of the drug in the solvent, because the diffusion layer is considered saturated), and
C_t is the concentration of the drug in the dissolution medium at time t ($c_s - c_t$ is the concentration gradient).

The rate of dissolution is governed by the rate of diffusion of solute molecules through the diffusion layer into the body of the solution. The equation reveals that the dissolution rate of a drug may be increased by increasing the surface area (reducing the particle size) of the drug, by increasing the solubility of the drug in the diffusion layer, and by factors embodied in the dissolution rate constant, k, including the intensity of agitation of the solvent and the diffusion coefficient of the dissolving drug. For a given drug, the diffusion coefficient and usually the concentration of the drug in the diffusion layer will increase with increasing temperature. Also, increasing the rate of agitation of the dissolving medium will increase the rate of dissolution. A reduction in the viscosity of the solvent employed is another means to enhance the dissolution rate of a drug. Changes in the pH or the nature of the solvent that influence the solubility of the drug may be used to advantage in increasing dissolution rate. Effervescent, buffered aspirin tablet formulations use some of these principles to their advantage. The alkaline adjuvants in the tablet enhance the solubility of the aspirin within the diffusional layer, and the evolution of carbon dioxide agitates the solvent system, that is, gastric juices. Consequently, the rate of absorption of aspirin into the bloodstream is faster than from a conventional aspirin tablet formulation. If this dosage form is acceptable to the patient, it provides a quicker means for the patient to gain relief from a troublesome headache. Many manufacturers use

a particular amorphous, crystalline, salt, or ester form of a drug that will exhibit the solubility characteristics needed to achieve the desired dissolution characteristics. Some of these factors that affect drug dissolution briefly are discussed in the following paragraphs, whereas others will be discussed in succeeding chapters in which they are relevant.

The chemical and physical characteristics of a drug substance that can affect safety, efficacy, and stability must be carefully defined by appropriate standards in an application for U.S. Food and Drug Administration (FDA) approval and then sustained and controlled throughout product manufacture.

Surface Area

When a drug particle is broken up, the total surface area is increased. For drug substances that are poorly or slowly soluble, this generally results in an increase in the *rate* of dissolution. This is explained in Physical Pharmacy Capsule 5.1, Particle Size, Surface Area, and Dissolution Rate.

Increased therapeutic response to orally administered drugs due to smaller particle size has been reported for a

PHYSICAL PHARMACY CAPSULE **5.1** Particle Size, Surface Area, and Dissolution Rate

Particle size has an effect on dissolution rate and solubility. As shown in the Noyes-Whitney equation,

$$\frac{dC}{dT} = kS(C_s - C_t)$$

where

> dC/dT is the rate of dissolution (concentration with respect to time);
> k is the dissolution rate constant;
> S is the surface area of the particles;
> C_s is the concentration of the drug in the immediate proximity of the dissolving particle, that is, the solubility of the drug; and
> C_t is the concentration of the drug in the bulk fluid.

It is evident that C_s cannot be significantly changed, C_t is often under sink conditions (an amount of the drug is used that is <20% of its solubility), and k comprises many factors, such as agitation and temperature. This leaves the S, surface area, as a factor that can affect the rate of dissolution.

An increase in the surface area of a drug will, within reason, increase the dissolution rate. Circumstances in which it may decrease the rate include a decrease in the effective surface area, that is, a condition in which the dissolving fluid cannot wet the particles. Wetting is the first step in dissolution. This can be demonstrated by visualizing a tablet of diameter 0.75 inch by thickness 0.25 inch. The surface area of the tablet can be increased by drilling a series of 0.0625-inch holes in the tablet. However, even though the surface area has been increased, the dissolution fluid—water—because of surface tension and so on cannot necessarily penetrate the new holes and displace the air. Adsorbed air and other factors can decrease the effective surface area of a dosage form, including powders. This is the reason that particle size reduction does not always raise the dissolution rate. One can also visualize a powder that has been comminuted to a very fine state of subdivision; when it is placed in a beaker of water, the powder floats because of the entrapped and adsorbed air. The effective surface area is not the same as the actual surface area of the powder. ■

number of drugs, among them theophylline, a xanthine derivative used to treat bronchial asthma; griseofulvin, an antibiotic with antifungal activity; sulfisoxazole, an anti-infective sulfonamide; and nitrofurantoin, a urinary anti-infective drug. To increase surface area, pharmaceutical manufacturers frequently use *micronized* powders in their solid products. Although not officially defined, micronized powders generally consist of drug particles reduced in size to about 5 mm and smaller. A slight variation on this is accomplished by blending and melting poorly water-soluble powders with a water-soluble polymer, such as polyethylene glycol (PEG). A molecular dispersion of the drug in the carrier can be made by dissolving the drug powder in the molten carrier. Cooling the solution produces a solid dispersion that can be pulverized and formed into tablets or capsules. When this powder is placed in water, the water-soluble carrier rapidly dissolves, leaving the poorly soluble drug molecules enveloped in water, thus forming a solution.

The use of micronized drugs is not confined to oral preparations. For example, ophthalmic and topical ointments use micronized drugs for their preferred release characteristics and nonirritating quality after application.

Because of the different rates and degrees of absorption obtainable from drugs of various particle sizes, products of the same drug substance prepared by two or more reliable pharmaceutical manufacturers may result in different degrees of therapeutic response in the same individual. A classic example of this occurs with phenytoin sodium capsules, which have two distinct forms. The first is the rapid-release type, that is, Prompt Phenytoin Sodium Capsules, USP, and the second is the slow-dissolution type, that is, Extended Phenytoin Sodium Capsules, USP. The former has a dissolution rate of not less than 85% in 30 minutes and is recommended for use three to four times per day. The latter has a slower dissolution rate, for example, 15% to 35% in 30 minutes, which lends itself to use in patients who can be dosed less frequently. Because of such differences in formulation for a number of drugs and drug products, it is generally advisable for a person to continue taking the same brand of medication, provided it produces the desired therapeutic effect. Patients who are stabilized on one brand of drug should not be switched to another unless necessary. However, when a change is necessary, appropriate blood or plasma concentrations of the drug should be monitored until the patient is stabilized on the new product.

Occasionally, a rapid rate of drug absorption is not desired in a pharmaceutical preparation. Research pharmacists who wish to provide sustained rather than rapid action may employ agents of varying particle size to provide controlled dissolution and absorption. Summaries of the physicochemical principles of particle size reduction and the relation of particle size to surface area, dissolution, and solubility may be found in Physical Pharmacy Capsule 4.5.

Crystal or Amorphous Drug Form

Solid drug materials may occur as pure crystalline substances of definite identifiable shape or as amorphous particles without definite structure. The amorphous or crystalline character of a drug substance may be of considerable importance to its ease of formulation and handling, its chemical stability, and as has been recently demonstrated, even its biologic activity. Certain medicinal agents may be produced to exist in either a crystalline or an amorphous state. Because the amorphous form of a chemical is usually more soluble than is the crystalline form, different extents of drug absorption may result with consequent differences in the degree of pharmacologic activity obtained from each. Two antibiotic substances, novobiocin and chloramphenicol palmitate, are essentially inactive when administered in crystalline form, but when they are administered in the amorphous form, absorption from the gastrointestinal tract proceeds rapidly, with good therapeutic response. In other instances, crystalline forms of drugs may be used because of greater stability than the corresponding amorphous forms. For example, the crystalline forms of penicillin G as the potassium salt or sodium salt are considerably more stable than are the analogous amorphous forms. Thus, in formulation work on penicillin G, the crystalline forms are preferred and result in excellent therapeutic response.

The hormone insulin presents another striking example of the different degree of activity that may result from the use of different physical forms of the same medicinal agent. Insulin is the active principle of the pancreas and is vital to the body's metabolism of glucose.

It is indispensable in the treatment of patients with type 1 diabetes, who depend upon an external source of the hormone for survival.

Prior to the development of insulin by the biosynthetic process using recombinant DNA technology, insulin was obtained for therapeutic use through its extraction and purification from animal pancreas glands, primarily pork. Today, the vast majority of insulin currently used worldwide is biosynthetic recombinant "human" insulin and its analogs. Although the therapeutic use of insulin from animal origin is largely diminished, the discussion, which follows, remains important from the physical pharmacy standpoint.

Insulin is a protein that forms an extremely insoluble zinc–insulin complex when combined with zinc in the presence of acetate buffer. The complex may be crystalline or amorphous, depending upon the pH of the buffer solution. Each form of the complex has been utilized in the formulation of insulin products to take advantage of the different absorption and retention rates following injection. The amorphous form (or prompt insulin suspension) is rapidly absorbed following intramuscular or subcutaneous injection, whereas the larger crystalline form (extended insulin zinc suspension) is more slowly absorbed and has a longer retention time and duration of action. By combining the two types, 70% of the crystalline form and 30% of the amorphous form, an intermediate-acting insulin product is prepared.

Nowadays, different absorption and retention rates for insulin are achieved through analogs of human insulin developed though biotechnology.

Some crystalline medicinal chemicals are capable of forming different types of crystals, depending on the conditions (temperature, solvent, time) under which crystallization is induced. This property, whereby a single chemical substance may exist in more than one crystalline form, is polymorphism. Only one form of a pure drug substance is stable at a given temperature and pressure, with the other higher-energy forms, called metastable forms, converting in time to the stable crystalline form. It is therefore fairly common for a metastable form of a medicinal agent to change form even in a completed pharmaceutical preparation, although the time required for a complete change may exceed the normal shelf life of the product. However, from a pharmaceutical point of view, any change in the crystal structure of a medicinal agent may critically affect the stability and even the therapeutic efficacy of the product in which the conversion takes place.

The various polymorphic forms of the same chemical generally differ in many physical properties, including solubility and dissolution, which are of prime importance to the rate and extent of absorption. These differences are manifest so long as the drug is in the solid state. Once solution is effected, the different forms become indistinguishable one from another. Therefore, differences in drug action, pharmaceutically and therapeutically, can be expected from polymorphs contained in solid dosage forms as well as in liquid suspension. The use of metastable forms generally results in higher solubility and dissolution rates than does that of the respective stable crystal forms of the same drug. If all other factors remain constant, more rapid and complete drug absorption will likely result from the metastable forms than from the stable form of the same drug. On the other hand, the stable polymorph is more resistant to chemical degradation and, because of its lower solubility, is frequently preferred in pharmaceutical suspensions of insoluble drugs. If metastable forms are employed in the preparation of suspensions, their gradual conversion to the stable form may be accompanied by an alteration in the consistency of the suspension itself, which affects its stability. In all instances, the advantages of the metastable crystalline forms in terms of increased physiologic availability of the drug must be balanced against the increased product stability when stable polymorphs are employed. Sulfur and cortisone acetate exist in more than one crystalline form and are frequently prepared in pharmaceutical suspensions. In fact, cortisone acetate is reported to exist in at least five crystalline forms. It is possible for the commercial products of two manufacturers to differ in stability and therapeutic effect, depending on the crystalline form of the drug used in the formulation.

Salt Forms

The dissolution rate of a salt form of a drug is generally quite different from that of the parent compound. Sodium and potassium salts of weak organic acids and hydrochloride salts of weak organic bases dissolve much more readily than do the respective free acids or bases. The result is a more rapid saturation of the diffusion layer surrounding the dissolving particle and the consequent more rapid diffusion of the drug to the absorption sites.

Numerous examples could be cited to demonstrate the increased rate of drug dissolution due to the use of the salt form of the drug rather than the free acid or base, but the following will suffice: the addition of the ethylenediamine moiety to theophylline increases the water solubility of theophylline fivefold. The use of the ethylenediamine salt of theophylline has allowed the development of oral aqueous solutions of theophylline and diminished the need to use hydroalcoholic mixtures such as elixirs.

Other Factors

The *state of hydration* of a drug molecule can affect its solubility and pattern of absorption. Usually, the anhydrous form of an organic molecule is more readily soluble than is the hydrated form. This characteristic was demonstrated with the drug ampicillin, when the anhydrous form was found to have a greater rate of dissolution and accompanying greater rate of absorption than that for the trihydrate form of the drug (4).

A drug's solubility in the gastrointestinal tract can be affected not only by the pH of the environment but also by the normal components of the tract and any foodstuffs. A drug may interact with one of the other agents present to form a chemical complex that may result in reduced drug solubility and decreased drug absorption. The classic example of this complexation is the one between tetracycline analogs and certain cations, for example, calcium, magnesium, and aluminum, resulting in decreased absorption of the tetracycline derivative. Also, if the drug becomes *ad*sorbed onto insoluble material in the tract, its availability for absorption may be correspondingly reduced.

BIOAVAILABILITY AND BIOEQUIVALENCE

The term *bioavailability* describes the *rate* and *extent* to which an active drug ingredient or therapeutic moiety is absorbed from a drug product and becomes available at the site of action. The term *bioequivalence* refers to the *comparison* of bioavailabilities of different formulations, drug products, or batches of the same drug product.

The availability to the biologic system of a pharmaceutical product is integral to the goals of dosage form design and paramount to the effectiveness of the medication. The study of a drug's bioavailability depends on the drug's absorption or entry into the systemic circulation, and it is necessary to study the pharmacokinetic profile of the drug or its metabolite or metabolites over time in the appropriate biologic system, for example, blood, plasma, and urine. Graphically, bioavailability of a drug is portrayed by a concentration–time curve of the administered drug in an appropriate tissue system, for example, plasma (Fig. 5.4). Bioavailability data are used to determine (*a*) the amount or proportion of drug absorbed from a formulation or dosage form, (*b*) the rate at which the drug was absorbed, (*c*) the duration of the drug's presence in the biologic fluid or tissue correlated with the patient's response, and (*d*) the relationship between drug blood levels and clinical efficacy and toxicity.

During the product development stages of a proposed drug product, pharmaceutical manufacturers employ bioavailability studies to compare different formulations of the drug substance to ascertain which one allows the most desirable absorption pattern. Later bioavailability studies may be used to compare the availability of the drug substance in different production batches. They may also be used to compare the availability of the drug substance in different dosage forms (e.g., tablets, capsules, elixirs) or in the same dosage form produced by different (competing) manufacturers.

According to the FDA (5), the in vivo bioavailability of a drug product may be determined by measurements of the concentration of the active drug ingredient, its therapeutic moiety, or its metabolite(s) in the blood or urine or by pharmacological effects. For drug products that are not intended to be absorbed into the bloodstream, bioavailability may be assessed by measurements of the rate and extent to which the active drug moiety becomes available at the site of action. Two drug products may be considered *bioequivalent* if their rates and extents of absorption do not show a significant difference when administered at the same molar dose under similar experimental conditions, either single dose or multiple dose.

Single-Dose and Multiple-Dose Bioavailability Studies

Single-dose bioavailability studies compare the drug product to be tested against the appropriate reference material. Studies are conducted in normal adults generally in the fasting state. A single-dose study is usually crossover in design, unless a parallel design or other design is more appropriate for valid scientific reasons (refer to Fig. 2.7 for study designs). The sampling time for blood and/or urine is usually at least three times the half-life of the active drug ingredient or therapeutic moiety, its metabolite(s), or at least three times the half-life of the acute pharmacological effect. Measured are the peak concentration in the blood and the total area under the curve (discussed later in this chapter).

Multiple-dose bioavailability studies compare the test product and the reference material after repeated administration to determine steady-state levels of the active drug ingredient or therapeutic moiety in the body. Studies are conducted in human subjects in the fasting or nonfasting state, depending upon the conditions reflected in the proposed labeling of the test product.

A multiple-dose study may be required for a test product if (*a*) there is a difference in the rate of absorption but not in the extent of absorption; (*b*) there is excessive variability in bioavailability from subject to subject; (*c*) the concentration of the active drug ingredient or therapeutic moiety, or its metabolites, in the blood resulting from a single dose is too low for accurate determination by the analytical method; or (*d*) the drug product is an extended-release dosage form. A multiple-dose study is generally crossover in design unless scientific reasons dictate otherwise (e.g., if the study is designed to establish the pharmacokinetic profile of a new drug product, a new drug delivery system, or an extended-release dosage form). At least five times the half-life of the active drug ingredient, its therapeutic moiety, or its active metabolite(s) is measured in the blood or urine.

FIGURE 5.4. Serum concentration–time curve showing peak height concentration, time of peak concentration, and AUC. (Courtesy of D. J. Chodos and A. R. Disanto, Upjohn.)

FDA Bioavailability Submission Requirements

The FDA requires bioavailability data submissions in the following instances (5):

1. *New Drug Applications* (*NDAs*): A section of each NDA is required to describe the human pharmacokinetic data and human bioavailability data, or information supporting a waiver of the bioavailability data requirement (see waiver provisions following).
2. *Abbreviated New Drug Applications* (*ANDAs*): In vivo bioavailability data are required unless information is provided and accepted supporting a waiver of this requirement (see waiver provisions following).
3. *Supplemental Applications*: In vivo bioavailability data are required if there is a change in the following:
   a. Manufacturing process, product formulation, or dosage strength beyond the variations provided for in the approved NDA
   b. Labeling to provide for a new indication for use of the drug product and if clinical studies are required, to support the new indication
   c. Labeling to provide for a new or additional dosage regimen for a special patient population (e.g., infants) if clinical studies are required to support the new or additional dosage regimen

Conditions under which the FDA *may* waive the in vivo bioavailability requirement are as follows:

1. The drug product is a parenteral, ophthalmic, or otic solution and contains the same active agent in the same concentration and solvent as a product previously approved through a full NDA.
2. The drug product is administered by inhalation as a gas or vapor and contains the same active agent in the same dosage form as a product previously approved through a full NDA.
3. The drug product is an oral solution, elixir, syrup, tincture, or similar other solubilized form and contains the same active agent in the same concentration as a previously approved drug product through a full NDA and contains no inactive ingredient known to significantly affect absorption of the active drug ingredient.
4. The drug product is a topically applied preparation (e.g., ointment) intended for local therapeutic effect.
5. The drug product is an oral form that is not intended to be absorbed (e.g., antacid or radiopaque medium).
6. The drug product is a solid oral form that has been demonstrated to be identical or sufficiently similar to a drug product that has met the in vivo bioavailability requirement.

Most bioavailability and bioequivalence studies are applied to drugs prepared into solid dosage forms intended to be administered orally. This is due to the fact that the majority of new pharmaceutical products are first developed and marketed as tablets and capsules, and later, competing nonproprietary (generic) products are developed in the same forms. Consequently, much of the discussion, which follows, focuses on studies of orally administered dosage forms. However, this is not to imply that other dosage forms and routes of administration are free from bioavailability studies.

Blood, Serum, or Plasma Concentration–Time Curve

Following oral administration of a medication, if blood samples are drawn from the patient at specific time intervals and analyzed for drug content, the resulting data may be plotted on ordinary graph paper to yield the type of drug blood level curve presented in Figure 5.4. The vertical axis of this type of plot characteristically presents the concentration of drug in the blood (or serum or plasma), and the horizontal axis presents the time the samples were obtained following the administration of the drug. When the drug is first administered (time zero), the blood concentration of the drug should also be zero. As the drug passes into the stomach and/or intestine, it is released from the dosage form, eventually dissolves, and is absorbed. As the sampling and analysis continue, the blood samples reveal increasing concentrations of drug (positive slope of the curve) until the maximum (peak) concentration (C_{max}) is reached. Then, the blood level of the drug decreases (negative slope of the curve), and if no additional dose is given, it eventually falls to zero. The diminished blood level of drug after the peak height is reached indicates that the rate of elimination from the bloodstream is greater than the rate of absorption into the circulatory system. Absorption does not terminate after the peak blood level is reached; it may continue for some time. Similarly, the process of drug elimination is continuous. It begins as soon as the drug first appears in the bloodstream and continues until all of the drug has been eliminated. The positive or negative slope of the curve indicates which process is faster. When the drug leaves the blood, it may be found in various body tissues and cells for which it has an affinity until ultimately it is excreted as such or as drug metabolites in the urine or via some other route (Fig. 5.5). A urinalysis for the drug or its metabolites may be used to indicate the extent of absorption and/or the rate of elimination.

Parameters for Assessment and Comparison of Bioavailability

In discussing the important parameters to be considered in the comparative evaluation of the blood level curves following the oral administration of single doses of two formulations of the same drug entity, Chodos and DiSanto (6) list the following:

- The peak height concentration (C_{max})
- The time of the peak concentration (T_{max})
- The area under the blood (or serum or plasma) concentration–time curve (AUC)

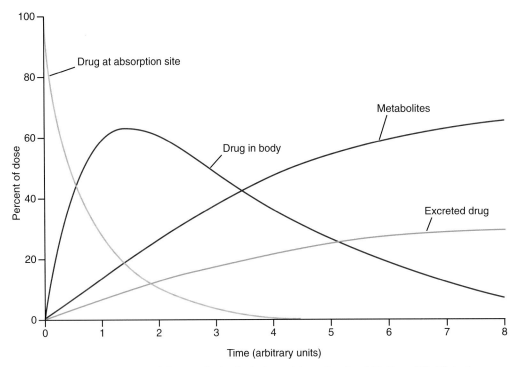

FIGURE 5.5. Time course of drug in the body. (Adapted from Rowland M, Tozer TN. Clinical Pharmacokinetics and Pharmacodynamics. 4th Ed. Baltimore, MD: Lippincott Williams & Wilkins, 2011, with permission.)

Using Figure 5.4 as an example, the height of the peak concentration is equivalent to 4.0 µg/mL of drug in the serum, the time of the peak concentration is 2 hours after administration, and the AUC from 0 to 12 hours is calculated as 21.5 µg/mL × hours. The meaning and use of these parameters are further explained as follows.

Peak Height

Peak height concentration is the C_{max} observed in the blood plasma or serum following a dose of the drug, indicating a slope of zero, meaning the rates of absorption and elimination are equal. For conventional dosage forms, such as tablets and capsules, the C_{max} will usually occur at only a single time, T_{max}. The amount of drug is usually expressed in terms of its concentration in relation to a specific volume of blood, serum, or plasma. For example, the concentration may be expressed as grams per 100 mL, micrograms per milliliter, or milligrams per 100 mL. Figure 5.6 depicts concentration–time curves showing different peak height concentrations for *equal* amounts of drug from two different formulations following oral administration. The horizontal line drawn across the figure indicates that the minimum effective concentration (MEC) for the drug substance is 4.0 µg/mL. This means that for the patient to exhibit an adequate response to the drug, this concentration in the blood must be achieved. Comparing the blood

FIGURE 5.6. Serum concentration–time curve showing different peak height concentrations for equal amounts of drug from two different formulations following oral administration. MEC, minimum effective concentration. (Courtesy of D. J. Chodos and A. R. Disanto, Upjohn, with permission from Elsevier.)

FIGURE 5.7. Serum concentration–time curve showing peak height concentrations, peak height times, times to reach MEC, and areas under the curves for equal amounts of drug from two different formulations following oral administration. MEC, minimum effective concentration; MTC, minimum toxic concentration. (Courtesy of D. I. Chodos and A. R. Disanto, Upjohn.)

levels of drug achieved after oral administration of equal doses of formulations A and B in Figure 5.6, formulation A will achieve the required blood levels of drug to produce the desired pharmacologic effect, whereas formulation B will not. On the other hand, if the MEC for the drug is 2.0 µg/mL and the minimum toxic concentration (MTC) is 4.0 µg/mL, as depicted in Figure 5.7, equal doses of the two formulations result in toxic effects produced by formulation A but only desired effects by formulation B. The objective in the individual dosing of a patient is to achieve the MEC but not the MTC.

The *size* of the dose influences the blood level concentration and C_{max} for that substance. Figure 5.8 depicts the influence of dose on the blood level–time curve for a hypothetical drug administered by the same route and in the same dosage form. In this example, it is assumed that all doses are completely absorbed and eliminated at the same rates. As the dose increases, the C_{max} is proportionately higher and the AUC proportionately greater. T_{max} is the same for each dose.

Time of Peak

The second important parameter in assessing the comparative bioavailability of two formulations is T_{max}. In Figure 5.6, T_{max} is 1 hour for formulation A and 4 hours for formulation B. This parameter reflects the *rate* of absorption from a formulation, which determines the time needed for the MEC to be reached and thus for initiation of the desired effect. The rate of absorption also influences the period over which the drug enters the bloodstream and therefore affects the duration that the drug is maintained in the blood. In Figure 5.7, formulation A allows the drug to reach the MEC within 30 minutes following administration and a peak concentration in 1 hour. Formulation B has a slower rate of release. Drug from this formulation reached the MEC 2 hours after administration and its peak concentration 4 hours after administration. Thus, formulation A permits the greater rate of drug absorption; it allows drug to reach both the MEC and its peak height sooner than does formulation B. On the other hand, formulation B provides more time for drug concentrations maintained above the MEC, 8 hours (2 to 10 hours following administration) compared to 5.5 hours (30 minutes to 6 hours following administration) for formulation A. Thus, if a rapid onset of action is desired, a formulation similar to A is preferred, but if a long duration rather than a rapid onset of action is desired, a formulation similar to B is preferred.

In summary, changes in the *rate* of drug absorption change the values of both C_{max} and T_{max}. Each product has its own characteristic rate of absorption. When the *rate* of absorption is decreased, the C_{max} is lowered and T_{max} occurs at a later time. If the doses of the drugs are the same and presumed completely absorbed, as in Figure 5.7, the AUC for each is essentially the same.

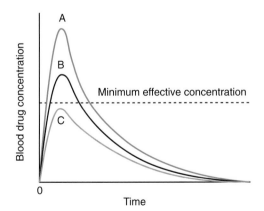

FIGURE 5.8. The influence of dose size on the blood drug concentration–time curves when three different doses of the same drug are administered and the rates of drug absorption and elimination are equal after the three doses. A, 100 mg; B, 80 mg; C, 50 mg. (Adapted from Ueda CT. Concepts in Clinical Pharmacology: Essentials of Bioavailability and Bioequivalence. Kalamazoo, MI: Upjohn, 1979, with permission.)

Area Under the Serum Concentration–Time Curve

The AUC of a concentration–time plot (Fig. 5.4) is considered representative of the total amount of drug absorbed into the circulation following the administration of a single dose of that drug. Equivalent doses of a drug, when fully absorbed, produce the same AUC. Thus, two curves dissimilar in terms of peak height and time of peak, like those in Figure 5.7, may be similar in terms of AUC and thus in the amount of drug absorbed. As indicated in Figure 5.7, the AUC for formulation A is 34.4 μg/mL × hours and for formulation B is 34.2 μg/mL × hours, essentially the same. If equivalent doses of drug in different formulations produce *different* AUC values, differences exist in the *extent* of absorption between the formulations. Figure 5.9 depicts concentration–time curves for three different formulations of equal amounts of drug with greatly different AUC. In this example, formulation A delivers a much greater amount of drug to the circulatory system than do the other two formulations. In general, the smaller the AUC, the lesser drug absorbed.

The fraction (F) (or bioavailability) of an orally administered drug may be calculated by comparison of the AUC after oral administration with that obtained after intravenous administration:

$$F = (AUC)_{oral} / (AUC)_{intravenous}$$

In practice, it is rare for a drug to be completely absorbed into the circulation following oral administration. As noted earlier, many drugs undergo a first-pass effect resulting in some degree of metabolic degradation before entering the general circulation. In addition, factors of product formulation, dissolution, chemical and physical interactions with the gastrointestinal contents, gastric emptying time, intestinal motility, and others limit the absorption of an administered dose of a drug. The oral dosage strengths of many commercial products are based on considerations of the proportion of the dose administered that is expected to be absorbed and available to its site of action to produce the desired drug blood level and/or therapeutic response.

The absolute bioavailability following oral dosing is generally compared to intravenous dosing. As examples, the reported mean oral bioavailability of ciprofloxacin hydrochloride tablets (Cipro) is 70%, levothyroxine sodium tablets (Synthroid) is 40% to 80%, fentanyl buccal tablets (Fentora) is 65%, lisinopril tablets (Prinivil) is 25%, and alendronate sodium tablets (Fosamax) is 0.64%. However, for most drugs, there is large intersubject variability, and the absorbed doses may vary from patient to patient.

BIOEQUIVALENCE OF DRUG PRODUCTS

A great deal of discussion and scientific investigation has been devoted recently to the problem of determining the equivalence between drug products of competing manufacturers.

The rate and extent to which a drug in a dosage form becomes available for biologic absorption or use depend in great measure on the materials in the formulation and on the method of manufacture. Thus, the same drug when formulated in *different* dosage forms may be found to possess different bioavailability characteristics and hence exhibit different clinical effectiveness. Furthermore, two seemingly identical or equivalent products of the same drug in the same dosage strength and in the *same* dosage form but differing in formulative materials or method of manufacture may vary widely in bioavailability and, thus, in clinical effectiveness.

Dissolution requirements for capsules and tablets are included in the USP and are integral to bioavailability. Experience has shown that where bioinequivalence has been found between two supposedly equivalent products, dissolution testing can help to define the product differences. According to the USP, significant bioavailability and bioinequivalence problems that may be revealed through dissolution testing are generally the result of one or more of the following factors: the drug's particle size, excessive amounts of a lubricant such as magnesium stearate in the

FIGURE 5.9. Serum concentration–time curve showing peak height concentrations, peak height times, and areas under the curves for equal amounts of drugs from three different formulations following oral administration. (Courtesy of D. I. Chodos and A. R. Disanto, Upjohn.)

formulation, coating materials, and inadequate amounts of tablet or capsule disintegrants.

The FDA uses the following terms to define the type or level of equivalency between drug products (5).

Pharmaceutical equivalents are drug products that contain identical amounts of the identical active drug ingredient, that is, the same salt or ester of the same therapeutic moiety, in identical dosage forms but not necessarily containing the same inactive ingredients and that meet the identical compendial or other applicable standard of identity, strength, quality, and purity, including potency and, where applicable, content uniformity, disintegration times, and/or dissolution rates.

Pharmaceutical alternatives are drug products that contain the identical therapeutic moiety or its precursor but not necessarily in the same amount or dosage form or as the same salt or ester. Each such drug product individually meets either the identical or its own compendial or other applicable standard of identity, strength, quality, and purity, including potency and, where applicable, content uniformity, disintegration times, and/or dissolution rates.

Bioequivalent drug products are pharmaceutical equivalents or pharmaceutical alternatives whose rate and extent of absorption do not show a significant difference when administered at the same molar dose of the therapeutic moiety under similar experimental conditions, either single dose or multiple dose. Some pharmaceutical equivalents or pharmaceutical alternatives may be equivalent in the extent of their absorption but not in their rate of absorption and yet may be considered bioequivalent because such differences in the rate of absorption are intentional and are reflected in the labeling, are not essential to the attainment of effective body drug concentrations on chronic use, or are considered medically insignificant for the particular drug product studied.

In addition, the term *therapeutic equivalents* has been used to indicate pharmaceutical equivalents that provide essentially the same therapeutic effect when administered to the same individuals in the same dosage regimens, that is, drugs that are both pharmaceutical equivalents and bioequivalent.

Differences in bioavailability have been demonstrated for a number of products involving the following and other drugs: tetracycline, chloramphenicol, digoxin, warfarin sodium, diazepam, and L-dopa. Not only has bio*in*equivalence been demonstrated to exist in products of different manufacturers; there have also been variations in the bioavailability of different batches of drug products from the same manufacturer. Variations in the bioavailability of certain drug products have resulted in some therapeutic failures in patients who took two inequivalent drug products in the course of their therapy.

The most common experimental plan to compare the bioavailability of two drug products is the simple *crossover design study*. In this method, each of the 12 to 24 individuals in the group of carefully matched subjects (usually healthy men aged 18 to 40 years and having similar height and weight) is administered both products under fasting conditions and essentially serves as his own control. To avoid bias of the test results, each test subject is randomly assigned one of the two products for the first phase of the study. Once the first assigned product is administered, samples of blood or plasma are drawn from the subjects at predetermined times and analyzed for the active drug moiety and its metabolites as a function of time. The same procedure is then repeated (*crossover*) with the second product after an appropriate interval, that is, a washout period to ensure that there is no residual drug from the first administered product that would artificially inflate the test results of the second product. Afterward, the patient population data are tabulated and the parameters used to assess and compare bioavailability; that is, C_{max}, T_{max}, and AUC are analyzed with statistical procedures. Statistical differences in bioavailability parameters may not always be clinically significant in therapeutic outcomes.

Inherent differences in individuals result in different patterns of drug absorption, metabolism, and excretion. These differences must be statistically analyzed to separate them from the factors of bioavailability related to the products themselves. The value in the crossover experiment is that each individual serves as his own control by taking each of the products. Thus, inherent differences between individuals are minimized.

Absolute bioequivalency between drug products rarely if ever occurs. Such absolute equivalency would yield serum concentration–time curves for the products that would be exactly superimposable. This simply is not expected of products that are made at different times, in different batches, or indeed by different manufacturers. However, some expectations of bioequivalency are expected of products considered to have equivalent merit for therapy.

In most studies of bioavailability, the originally marketed product (often called the prototype, pioneer, innovator, or brand-name drug product) is recognized as the established product of the drug and is used as the standard for the bioavailability comparative studies.

As is recalled from Chapter 2, an applicant seeking FDA approval for the marketing of a generic version of a previously approved drug product must file an Abbreviated New Drug Application (ANDA). The application is reviewed and acted upon by FDA's Center for Drug Evaluation and Research, Office of Generic Drugs. An approved generic product must be comparable to the innovator drug product in active ingredient, strength, dosage form, intended route of administration, therapeutic indication, and manufacturing and quality standards.

An ANDA application must contain data from in vitro studies, which demonstrate that the proposed product is "bioequivalent" to the approved comparator product. The applicant may request the FDA to *waive* the requirement for the submission of in vivo bioequivalence data based on an assessment that such bioequivalence may be considered self-evident as demonstrated by other data in the application or based on some of the following criteria (5):

- The drug product contains the same active drug ingredient, in the same concentration and dosage form as the comparator-approved product, and is intended to be administered by the same route.
- The drug product contains no inactive ingredient or other change in formulation from the approved drug product that may significantly affect the systemic absorption or therapeutic effectiveness of the active ingredient/product.
- The drug product is a parenteral, ophthalmic, nasal, oral, or otic solution; an inhalation; or a dermatologic preparation.
- The drug product is not a delayed-release or extended-release dosage form.
- The drug product meets an approved in vitro test comparable to the in vitro test of the approved drug, which has been correlated with in vivo data.
- The drug product is manufactured in accord with all Current Good Manufacturing Practice regulations.

The FDA may require in vivo studies if the agency determines that some differences between the proposed drug product and the previously approved drug product may affect the bioavailability, bioequivalence, or therapeutic equivalence of the proposed product.

The variables that can contribute to the differences between products are many (Table 5.3). For instance, in the manufacture of a tablet, different materials or amounts of such formulative components as fillers, disintegrating agents, binders, lubricants, colorants, flavorants, and coatings may be used. The particle size or crystalline form of a therapeutic or pharmaceutical component may vary between formulations. The tablet may vary in shape, size, and hardness, depending on the punches, dies, and compression forces used in the process. During packaging, shipping, and storage, the integrity of the tablets may be altered by physical impact, by changes in humidity and temperature, or through interactions with the components of the container. Each of these factors may affect the rates of tablet disintegration, drug dissolution, and consequently the rate and extent of drug absorption. Although the bioequivalency problems are perhaps greater among tablets than for other dosage forms because of the multiplicity of variables, the same types of problems exist for the other dosage forms and must be considered in assessing bioequivalency.

Sometimes even therapeutically equivalent drugs are not equally suitable for a particular patient. For example, a patient may be hypersensitive to an inert ingredient in one product (brand name or generic) that another product does not contain. Or a patient may become confused or upset if dispensed an alternative product that differs in color, flavor, shape, or packaging from that to which he or she is accustomed. Switching between products can gen-

TABLE 5.3. Some Factors That Influence Bioavailability of Oral Drugs

Drug Substance Physicochemical Properties

Particle size

Crystalline or amorphous form

Salt form

Hydration

Lipid or water solubility

pH and pK_a

Pharmaceutical Ingredients

Fillers

Binders

Coatings

Disintegrating agents

Lubricants

Suspending agents

Surface active agents

Flavoring agents

Coloring agents

Preservative agents

Stabilizing agents

Dosage Form Characteristics

Disintegration rate (tablets)

Dissolution time of drug in dosage form

Product age and storage conditions

Physiologic Factors and Patient Characteristics

Gastric emptying time

Intestinal transit time

Gastrointestinal abnormality or pathologic condition

Gastric contents

Other drugs

Food

Fluids

Gastrointestinal pH

Drug Metabolism (Gut and During First Passage Through Liver)

erate concern, and thus pharmacists need to be prudent in both initial selection and interchange of products.

ROUTES OF DRUG ADMINISTRATION

Drugs may be administered using a variety of dosage forms and routes of administration, as presented in Tables 5.4 and 5.5. One of the fundamental considerations in dosage form design is whether the drug is intended for local or systemic effects. *Local* effects are achieved by direct application of the drug to the desired site of action, such as the eye, nose, or skin. *Systemic* effects result from the entrance of the drug into the circulatory system and transport to

TABLE 5.4. Routes of Drug Administration

Term	Site
Oral	Mouth
Per oral (per os[a])	Gastrointestinal tract via mouth
Sublingual	Under the tongue
Parenteral	Other than the gastrointestinal tract (by injection)
Intravenous	Vein
Intra-arterial	Artery
Intracardiac	Heart
Intraspinal or intrathecal	Spine
Intraosseous	Bone
Intra-articular	Joint
Intrasynovial	Joint fluid area
Intracutaneous, intradermal	Skin
Subcutaneous	Beneath the skin
Intramuscular	Muscle
Epicutaneous (topical)	Skin surface
Transdermal	Skin surface
Conjunctival	Conjunctiva
Intraocular	Eye
Intranasal	Nose
Aural	Ear
Intrarespiratory	Lung
Rectal	Rectum
Vaginal	Vagina

[a]The abbreviation *PO* is commonly used on prescriptions to indicate oral administration.

TABLE 5.5. Route of Administration and Delivery System of Primary Dosage Forms

Oral	Tablets
	Capsules
	Solutions
	Syrups
	Elixirs
	Suspensions, emulsions
	Magmas
	Gels
	Powders
Sublingual	Tablets
	Troches, lozenges
	Drops (solutions, suspensions)
Parenteral	Solutions
	Suspensions, emulsions
	Infusion pumps
Epicutaneous, transdermal	Ointments, gels
	Creams
	Pastes
	Plasters
	Powders
	Aerosols
	Lotions (solutions, suspensions, emulsions)
	Transdermal patches, disks, solutions
Conjunctival	Contact lens inserts
	Ointments
Intraocular, intra-aural	Solutions
	Suspensions
Intranasal	Solutions, suspensions
	Sprays
	Inhalants
	Ointments
Intrarespiratory	Aerosols
Rectal	Solutions, suspensions
	Ointments
	Suppositories
	Gels
Vaginal	Solutions
	Ointments
	Emulsion foams
	Gels
	Tablets
	Inserts, suppositories, sponge
Urethral	Solutions
	Inserts

the cellular site of its action. For systemic effects, a drug may be placed directly in the bloodstream via intravenous injection or absorbed into the venous circulation following oral or other route of administration.

An individual drug substance may be formulated into multiple dosage forms that result in different drug absorption rates and times of onset, peak, and duration of action. Figure 5.10 and Table 5.6 demonstrate this for the drug nitroglycerin in various dosage forms. The sublingual, intravenous, and buccal forms present extremely rapid onsets of action, whereas the oral (swallowed), topical ointment, and topical patch present slower onsets of action but greater durations of action. The patch provides the longest duration of action, up to 14 hours following application of a single patch to the skin. The transdermal nitroglycerin patch allows a single daily dose, whereas the other forms require multiple dosing to maintain drug levels within the therapeutic window.

The difference in absorption between dosage forms is a function of the formulation and the route of administration. For example, a problem associated with the oral

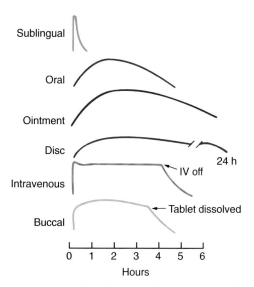

FIGURE 5.10. Blood level curves of nitroglycerin following administration of dosage forms by various routes. (Adapted from Abrams J. Proceedings of the First North American Conference on Nitroglycerin Therapy. Nitroglycerin and long-acting nitrates in clinical practice. Am J Med 1983;74(6):85–94, with permission from Elsevier.)

administration of a drug is that once absorbed through the lumen of the gastrointestinal tract into the portal vein, the drug may pass directly to the liver and undergo the *first-pass effect*. In essence, some or all of the drug may be metabolized by the liver. Consequently, its bioavailability is decreased. Thus, the bioavailable fraction is determined by the fraction of drug that is absorbed from the gastrointestinal tract and the fraction that escapes metabolism during its first pass through the liver. The bioavailable fraction (f) is the product of these two fractions as follows:

$$f = \text{fraction of drug absorbed} \times \text{fraction}$$
$$\text{escaping first-pass metabolism}$$

The bioavailability is lowest, then, for drugs that undergo a significant first-pass effect. For these drugs, a hepatic extraction ratio, or the fraction of drug metabolized, E, is calculated. The fraction of drug that enters the systemic circulation and is ultimately available to exert its effect then is equal to the quantity (1 − E). Table 5.7 lists some drugs according to their pharmacologic class that undergo a significant first-pass effect when administered by the oral route.

To compensate for this marked effect, the manufacturer may consider other routes of administration, for example, intravenous, intramuscular, or sublingual, that avoid the first-pass effect. Use of these routes must be accompanied by a corresponding adjustment in the dosage.

Another consideration centers on the metabolites themselves and whether they are pharmacologically active or inactive. If they are inactive, a larger oral dose is required to attain the desired therapeutic effect than with a lower dosage in a route with no first-pass effect. The classic example of drug that exhibits this effect is propranolol. However, if the metabolites are the active species, the oral dosage must be carefully tailored to the desired therapeutic effect. First-pass metabolism in this case will result in a quicker therapeutic response than that achieved by a route with no first-pass effect.

Also, the flow of blood through the liver can be decreased under certain conditions. Consequently, the bioavailability of drugs that undergo a first-pass effect can be expected to increase. For example, during cirrhosis, the blood flow to the kidney is dramatically decreased, and efficient hepatic extraction by enzymes responsible for a drug's metabolism also falls off. Consequently, in cirrhotic patients, the dosage of drug that undergoes a first-pass effect from oral administration will have to be reduced to avoid toxicity.

Oral Route

Drugs are most frequently taken by oral administration. Although a few drugs taken orally are intended to be dissolved in the mouth, nearly all drugs taken orally are swallowed. Of these, most are taken for the *systemic* drug effects that result after absorption from the various surfaces along the gastrointestinal tract. A few drugs, such as antacids, are swallowed for their local action in the gastrointestinal tract.

Compared with alternative routes, the oral route is considered the most natural, uncomplicated, convenient, and safe means of administering drugs. Disadvantages of the oral route include slow drug response (compared with parenterally administered drugs); chance of irregular

Nitroglycerin, Dosage Form	Usual Dose (mg)	Onset of Action (min)	Peak Action (min)	Duration
Sublingual	0.3–0.8	2–5	4–8	10–30 min
Buccal	1–3	2–5	4–10	30–300 min[a]
Oral	6.5–19.5	20–45	45–120	2–6 h[b]
Ointment (2%)	0.5–2 in.	15–60	30–120	3–8 h
Transdermal infusion system	20–160	30–60	60–180	12–14 h

TABLE 5.6. Dosage and Kinetics of Nitroglycerin in Various Dosage Forms

[a]Effect persists so long as tablet is intact.
[b]Some short-term dosing studies have demonstrated effects to 8 hours.
Reprinted from Abrams J. Proceedings of the First North American Conference on Nitroglycerin Therapy. Nitroglycerin and long-acting nitrates in clinical practice. Am J Med 1983;74(6):85, with permission from Elsevier.

TABLE 5.7. Some Drugs That Undergo Significant Liver Metabolism and Exhibit Low Bioavailability When Administered by First-Pass Routes

Drug Class	Examples
Analgesic	Aspirin, meperidine, pentazocine, propoxyphene
Antianginal	Nitroglycerin
Antiarrhythmic	Lidocaine
Beta-adrenergic blocker	Labetalol, metoprolol, propranolol
Calcium channel blocker	Verapamil
Sympathomimetic amine	Isoproterenol
Tricyclic antidepressant	Desipramine, imipramine, nortriptyline

absorption of drugs, depending upon such factors as constitutional makeup and the amount or type of food in the gastrointestinal tract; and the destruction of certain drugs by the acid reaction of the stomach or by gastrointestinal enzymes. Factors that can increase the rate of drug absorption include an empty stomach, low-viscosity fluids, higher pH liquids, isosmotic liquids, low calories, low fat, and larger volume liquids. Factors that can decrease the rate of drug absorption include food in the stomach, high-viscosity fluids, lower pH liquids, hyper- or hypotonic liquids, high caloric content, high-fat content, and small volume liquids.

Dosage Forms Applicable

Drugs are administered by the oral route in a variety of pharmaceutical forms. The most popular are tablets, capsules, suspensions, and various pharmaceutical solutions. Briefly, *tablets* are solid dosage forms prepared by compression or molding that contains medicinal substances with or without suitable diluents, disintegrants, coatings, colorants, and other pharmaceutical adjuncts. Diluents are

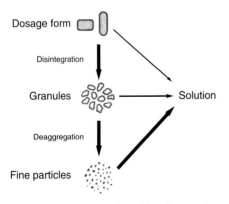

FIGURE 5.11. Disintegration of a tablet dosage form and direct availability of the contents in a capsule dosage form for dissolution and drug absorption after oral administration. (Adapted from Rowland M, Tozer TN. Clinical Pharmacokinetics and Pharmacodynamics. 4th Ed. Baltimore, MD: Lippincott Williams & Wilkins, 2011, with permission.)

fillers used to prepare tablets of the proper size and consistency. Disintegrants are used for the breakup or separation of the tablet's compressed ingredients. This ensures prompt exposure of drug particles to the dissolution process, enhancing drug absorption, as demonstrated in Figure 5.11. Tablet coatings are of several types and for several purposes. Some, called *enteric coatings*, are employed to permit safe passage of a tablet through the acid environment of the stomach, where certain drugs may be destroyed, to the more suitable juices of the intestines, where tablet dissolution safely takes place. Other coatings protect the drug substance from the destructive influences of moisture, light, and air during storage or to conceal a bad or bitter taste from the taste buds of a patient. Commercial tablets, because of their distinctive shapes, colors, and frequently employed monograms of company symbols and code numbers, facilitate identification by persons trained in their use and serve as an added protection to public health.

Capsules are solid dosage forms in which the drug substance and appropriate pharmaceutical adjuncts, such as fillers, are enclosed in either a hard or a soft shell, generally composed of a form of gelatin. Capsules vary in size, depending on the amount of drug to be administered, and have distinctive shapes and colors when produced commercially. Drug materials are released from capsules faster than from tablets. Capsules of gelatin, a protein, are rapidly hydrated and dissolved within the gastrointestinal tract, permitting the gastric juices to permeate and reach the contents. Because unsealed capsules have been subject to tampering by unscrupulous individuals, many capsules nowadays are sealed by fusion of the capsule shells where the two sections overlap. Also, capsule-shaped and coated tablets, called caplets, are increasingly used. These are easily swallowed, but their contents are sealed and protected from tampering like tablets.

Suspensions are preparations of finely divided drugs in a suitable fluid vehicle. Suspensions taken orally generally employ an aqueous vehicle, whereas those employed for other purposes may use a different vehicle. Suspensions of certain drugs to be used for intramuscular injection, for instance, may be maintained in a suitable oil. To be suspended, the drug particles must be insoluble in the vehicle. Nearly all suspensions must be shaken before use because they tend to settle. This ensures both uniformity of the preparation and, more importantly, the administration of the proper dosage. Suspensions are a useful means to administer large amounts of solid drugs that would be inconvenient to take in tablet or capsule form. In addition, suspensions have the advantage over solid dosage forms in that they are presented to the body in fine particle size, ready for dissolution immediately upon administration. However, not all oral suspensions are intended to be dissolved and absorbed by the body. For instance, some antidiarrheal preparations contain a kaolin mixture with pectin or attapulgite. The suspended kaolin or attapulgite acts in the intestinal tract by adsorbing excessive intestinal fluid on the large surface area of its particles.

Drugs administered in aqueous *solution* are absorbed much more rapidly than are those administered in solid form, because disintegration and dissolution are not required. Pharmaceutical solutions may differ in the type of solvent employed and therefore in their fluidity characteristics. Among the solutions frequently administered orally are *elixirs*, which are solutions in a sweetened hydroalcoholic vehicle and are more mobile than water; *syrups*, which generally use a sucrose solution as the sweet vehicle, resulting in a viscous preparation; and *solutions* themselves, which officially are preparations in which the drug substance is dissolved predominantly in an aqueous vehicle and do not for reasons of their method of preparation (e.g., injections, which must be sterilized) fall into another category of pharmaceutical preparations.

Absorption

Absorption of drugs after oral administration may occur at the various body sites between the mouth and rectum. In general, the higher up a drug is absorbed along the alimentary tract, the more rapid will be its action, a desirable feature in most instances. Because of the differences in chemical and physical nature among drug substances, a given drug may be better absorbed from one site than from another in the alimentary tract.

Sometimes the oral cavity is the absorption site. Physically, oral absorption of drugs is managed by allowing the drug substance to dissolve within the oral cavity with little or no swallowing until the taste of the drug has dissipated. This process is accommodated by providing the drug as extremely soluble and rapidly dissolving uncoated tablets. Drugs capable of being absorbed in the mouth present themselves to the absorbing surface in a much more concentrated form than when swallowed, because drugs become progressively more diluted with gastrointestinal secretions and contents as they pass along the alimentary tract.

The oral or *sublingual* (beneath the tongue) administration of drugs is regularly used for only a few drugs, with nitroglycerin and certain steroid sex hormones being the best examples. Nitroglycerin, a coronary vasodilator used in the prophylaxis and treatment of angina pectoris, is available in the form of tiny tablets that are allowed to dissolve under the tongue, producing therapeutic effects a few minutes after administration. The dose of nitroglycerin is so small (usually 400 mcg or 0.4 mg) that if it were swallowed, the resulting dilute gastrointestinal concentration might not result in reliable and sufficient drug absorption. Even more important, however, is the fact that nitroglycerin is rapidly destroyed by the liver through the *first-pass effect*. Many sex hormones have been shown to be absorbed materially better from sublingual administration than when swallowed. Although the sublingual route is probably an effective absorption route for many other drugs, it has not been extensively used, primarily because other routes have proven satisfactory and more convenient for the patient. Retaining drug substances in the mouth is unattractive because of the bitter taste of most drugs.

Drugs may be altered within the gastrointestinal tract to render them less available for absorption. This may result from the drug's interaction with or binding to some normal constituent of the gastrointestinal tract or a foodstuff or even another drug. For instance, the absorption of the tetracycline group of antibiotics is greatly interfered with by the simultaneous presence of calcium. Because of this, tetracycline drugs must not be taken with milk or other calcium-containing foods or drugs.

Sometimes the pharmacist intends to prepare a formulation that releases the drug slowly over an extended time. There are many methods by which slow release is accomplished, including the complexation of the drug with another material, the combination of which is only slowly released from the dosage form. An example of this is slow-release wax-matrix potassium chloride tablets. These are designed to release their contents gradually as they are shunted through the gastrointestinal tract. Because their contents are leached out gradually, there is little incidence of gastric irritation. The intermingling of food and drug generally results in delayed drug absorption. Because most drugs are absorbed more effectively from the intestines than from the stomach, when rapid absorption is intended, it is generally desirable to have the drug pass from the stomach into the intestines as rapidly as possible. Therefore, gastric emptying time is an important factor in drug action dependent on intestinal absorption. Gastric emptying time may be increased by a number of factors, including the presence of fatty foods (more effect than proteins, which in turn have more effect than carbohydrates) or lying on the back when bedridden (lying on the right side facilitates passage in many instances), or decreased, as by the presence of drugs (e.g., morphine) that have a quieting effect on the movements of the gastrointestinal tract. If a drug is administered in the form of a solution, it may be expected to pass into the intestines more rapidly than drugs administered in solid form. As a rule, large volumes of water taken with medication facilitate gastric emptying and passage into the intestines.

The pH of the gastrointestinal tract increases progressively along its length from about pH 1 in the stomach to approximately pH 8 at the far end of the intestines. pH has a definite bearing on the degree of ionization of most drugs, and this in turn affects lipid solubility, membrane permeability, and absorption. Because most drugs are absorbed by passive diffusion through the lipoid barrier, the lipid–water partition coefficient and the pK_a of the drugs are of prime importance to both the degree and the site of absorption within the gastrointestinal tract. As a general rule, weak acids are largely *unionized* in the stomach and are absorbed fairly well from this site, whereas weak bases are highly ionized in the stomach and are not significantly absorbed from the gastric surface. Alkalinization of the gastric environment by artificial means (simultaneous administration of alkaline or antacid drugs) would be expected to decrease the gastric absorption of weak acids and to increase that of weak bases. Strong acids and bases are generally poorly absorbed because of their high degree of ionization.

The small intestine serves as the major absorption site for drugs because of its suitable pH and the great surface area available for drug absorption along its approximately 20-foot length from the pylorus at the base of the stomach to the large intestine at the cecum. The pH of the lumen of the intestine is about 6.5 (Fig. 5.3), and both weakly acidic and weakly basic drugs are well absorbed from the intestinal surface, which behaves in the ionization and distribution of drugs between it and the plasma on the other side of the membrane as though its pH were about 5.3.

Rectal Route

Some drugs are administered rectally for their local effects and others for their systemic effects. Drugs given rectally may be administered as solutions, suppositories, or ointments. *Suppositories* are solid bodies of various weights and shapes intended for introduction into a body orifice (usually rectal, vaginal, or urethral) where they soften, melt, or dissolve; release their medication; and exert their drug effects. These effects simply may be the promotion of laxation (as with glycerin suppositories), the soothing of inflamed tissues (as with various commercial suppositories used to relieve the discomfort of hemorrhoids), or the promotion of systemic effects (as antinausea or anti-motion sickness). The composition of the suppository base, or carrier, can greatly influence the degree and rate of drug release and should be selected on an individual basis for each drug. The use of rectal ointments is generally limited to the treatment of local conditions. Rectal solutions are usually employed as enemas or cleansing solutions.

The rectum and the colon can absorb many soluble drugs. Rectal administration for systemic action may be preferred for drugs destroyed or inactivated by the environments of the stomach and intestines. The administration of drugs by the rectal route may also be indicated when the oral route is precluded because of vomiting or when the patient is unconscious or incapable of swallowing drugs safely without choking. Approximately 50% of a dose of drug absorbed from rectal administration is likely to bypass the liver, an important factor when considering orally administered drugs that are rapidly destroyed in the liver by the first-pass effect. On the negative side, compared with oral administration, rectal administration of drugs is inconvenient and offensive to some patients, and the absorption of drugs from the rectum is frequently irregular and difficult to predict.

Parenteral Route

The term *parenteral* is derived from the Greek words *para*, meaning beside, and *enteron*, meaning intestine, which together indicate something done outside of the intestine and not by way of the alimentary tract. A drug administered parenterally is one injected through the hollow of a fine needle into the body at various sites and to various depths. The three primary routes of parenteral administration are subcutaneous, intramuscular, and intravenous, although there are others, such as intracardiac and intraspinal.

Drugs destroyed or inactivated in the gastrointestinal tract or too poorly absorbed to provide satisfactory response may be parenterally administered. The parenteral route is also preferred when rapid absorption is essential, as in emergencies. Not only is absorption by the parenteral route faster than after oral administration but also the blood levels of drug that result are far more predictable, because little is lost after subcutaneous or intramuscular injection and virtually none by intravenous injection; this also generally permits the administration of smaller doses. The parenteral route of administration is especially useful in treating patients who are uncooperative, unconscious, or otherwise unable to accept oral medication.

One disadvantage of parenteral administration is that once the drug is injected, there is no retreat. That is, once the substance is in the tissues or bloodstream, removal of the drug warranted by an untoward or toxic effect or an inadvertent overdose is most difficult. By other means of administration, there is more time between drug administration and drug absorption, which becomes a safety factor by allowing for the extraction of unabsorbed drug (as by the induction of vomiting after an orally administered drug). Also, because of the strict sterility requirements for all injections, they are more expensive than are other dosage forms and require competent trained personnel for proper administration.

Dosage Forms Applicable

Pharmaceutically, most injectable preparations are either a sterile suspension or solution of a drug substance in water or in a suitable vegetable oil. Drugs in solution act more rapidly than do drugs in suspension, with an aqueous vehicle providing faster action in each instance than an oleaginous vehicle. As in other instances of drug absorption, a drug must be in solution to be absorbed, and a suspended drug must first submit to dissolution. Also, because body fluids are aqueous, they are more receptive to drugs in an aqueous vehicle than those in an oily one. For these reasons, the rate of drug absorption can be varied in parenteral products by selective combinations of drug state and supporting vehicle. For instance, a suspension of a drug in a vegetable oil is likely to be much more slowly absorbed than an aqueous solution of the same drug. Slow absorption means prolonged drug action, and when this is achieved through pharmaceutical means, the resulting preparation is referred to as a *depot* or *repository* injection, because it provides a storage reservoir of the drug substance within the body from which it is slowly removed into the systemic circulation. In this regard, even more sustained drug action may be achieved through the use of subcutaneous implantation of compressed tablets, termed pellets, that are only slowly dissolved from their site of implantation, releasing their medication at a fairly constant rate over several weeks to many months. The repository type of injection is mainly limited to the subcutaneous or intramuscular route. It is obvious that drugs injected intravenously do not encounter absorption barriers and thus produce only rapid drug effects. Preparations for intravenous injection must not interfere with the blood components or with circulation and therefore, with few exceptions, are aqueous solutions.

Subcutaneous Injections

The subcutaneous (hypodermic) administration of drugs entails injection through the skin into the loose subcutaneous tissue. Subcutaneous injections are prepared as aqueous solutions or as suspensions and are administered in relatively small volumes, 2 mL or less. Insulin is an example of a drug administered by the subcutaneous route. Subcutaneous injections are generally given in the forearm, upper arm, thigh, or buttocks. If the patient is to receive frequent injections, it is best to alternate injection sites to reduce tissue irritation. After injection, the drug comes into the immediate vicinity of blood capillaries and permeates them by diffusion or filtration. The capillary wall is an example of a membrane that behaves as a lipid pore barrier, with lipid-soluble substances penetrating the membrane at rates varying with their oil–water partition coefficients. Lipid-insoluble (generally more water-soluble) drugs penetrate the capillary membrane at rates that appear to be inversely related to their molecular size, with smaller molecules penetrating much more rapidly than larger ones. All substances, whether lipid soluble or not, cross the capillary membrane much more rapidly than other body membranes. The blood supply to the site of injection is an important factor in considering the rate of drug absorption; consequently, the closer capillaries are to the site of injection, the more prompt is the drug's entrance into the circulation. Also, the more the capillaries, the more surface area for absorption and the faster the rate of absorption. Some substances modify the rate of drug absorption from a subcutaneous site of injection. The addition of a vasoconstrictor to the injection formulation (or its prior injection) will generally diminish the rate of drug absorption by causing constriction of the blood vessels in the area of injection and thereby reducing blood flow and the capacity for absorption. This principle is used in the administration of local anesthetics by use of the vasoconstrictor epinephrine. Conversely, vasodilators may be used to enhance subcutaneous absorption by increasing blood flow to the area. Physical exercise can also influence the absorption of drug from an injection site. Diabetic patients who rotate subcutaneous injection sites and then do physical exercise such as jogging must realize that the onset of insulin activity may be influenced by the selected site of administration. Because of the movement of the leg and blood circulation to it during running, the absorption of insulin from a thigh injection site can be expected to be faster than from an abdominal injection site.

Intramuscular Injections

Intramuscular injections are performed deep into the skeletal muscles, generally the gluteal or lumbar muscles. The selected site is where the danger of hitting a nerve or blood vessel is minimal. Aqueous or oleaginous solutions or suspensions may be used intramuscularly. Certain drugs, because of their inherent low solubility, provide sustained drug action after an intramuscular injection. For instance, one deep intramuscular injection of a suspension of penicillin G benzathine results in effective blood levels of the drug for 7 to 10 days. The addition of the decanoate ester decreases the solubility of haloperidol and, consequently, extends haloperidol's half-life from 18 hours orally to 3 weeks by intramuscular injection, an advantage in antipsychotic drug therapy.

Drugs that are irritating to subcutaneous tissue are often administered intramuscularly. Also, greater volumes (2 to 5 mL) may be administered intramuscularly than subcutaneously. When a volume greater than 5 mL is to be injected subcutaneously, it is frequently administered in divided doses to two injection sites. Injection sites are best rotated when a patient is receiving repeated injections over time.

Intravenous Injections

In the intravenous administration of drugs, an aqueous solution is injected directly into the vein at a rate commensurate with efficiency, safety, comfort to the patient, and the desired duration of drug response. Drugs may be administered intravenously as a single, small-volume injection or as a large-volume slow intravenous drip infusion (as is common following surgery). Intravenous injection allows the desired blood level of drug to be achieved in an optimal and quantitative manner. Intravenous injections are usually made into the veins of the forearm and are especially useful in emergencies when immediate drug response is desired. It is essential that the drug be maintained in solution after injection and not be precipitated within the circulatory system, an event that might produce emboli. Because of a fear of the development of pulmonary embolism, oleaginous vehicles are not usually intravenously administered. However, an intravenous fat emulsion is used for patients receiving parenteral nutrition whose caloric requirements cannot be met by glucose. It may be administered either through a peripheral vein or a central venous catheter at a distinct rate to help prevent untoward reactions.

Intradermal Injections

Intradermal injections are administered into the corium of the skin, usually in volumes of about 0.1 mL. Common sites for the injection are the arm and the back. The injections are frequently performed as diagnostic measures, as in tuberculin and allergy testing.

Epicutaneous Route

Drugs are administered topically, or applied to the skin, for their action at the site of application or for systemic drug effects.

Drug absorption via the skin is enhanced if the drug substance is in solution, if it has a favorable lipid–water partition coefficient, and if it is not an electrolyte. Drugs that are absorbed enter the skin by way of the pores, sweat glands, hair follicles, sebaceous glands, and other anatomic structures of the skin's surface. Because blood capillaries lie just below the epidermal cells, a drug that penetrates the skin and is able to traverse the capillary wall finds ready access to the general circulation.

Among the few drugs applied to the skin surface for percutaneous absorption and systemic action are nitroglycerin (antianginal), testosterone (male hormone), oxybutynin (overactive bladder), methylphenidate (attention deficit hyperactivity disorder), rivastigmine (dementia), nicotine (smoking cessation), estradiol (estrogenic hormone), clonidine (antihypertensive), and scopolamine (antinausea, anti–motion sickness). Each of these drugs is available for use in a transdermal delivery system fabricated as an adhesive disk or patch that slowly releases the medication for percutaneous absorption. Additionally, nitroglycerin is available in an ointment for application to the skin for systemic absorption. Nitroglycerin is used therapeutically for ischemic heart disease, with the transdermal dosage forms becoming increasingly popular because of the benefit in patient compliance through their long-acting (24 hours) characteristics. The nitroglycerin patch is generally applied to the arm or chest, preferably in a hair-free or shaven area. The transdermal scopolamine system is also in the form of a patch to be applied to the skin, in this case behind the ear, for the prevention of nausea and vomiting associated with motion sickness. The commercial product is applied several hours before it is needed (as prior to an air or sea trip), and then where it releases its medication over 3 days. The concepts of transdermal therapeutic systems are discussed further in Chapter 11.

For the most part, pharmaceutical preparations applied to the skin are intended to serve some local action and as such are formulated to provide prolonged local contact with minimal absorption. Drugs applied to the skin for their local action include antiseptics, antifungal agents, anti-inflammatory agents, local anesthetic agents, skin emollients, and protectants against environmental conditions, such as the effects of the sun, wind, pests, and chemical irritants. For these purposes, drugs are most commonly administered in the form of ointments and related semisolid preparations such as creams and pastes, as solid dry powders or aerosol sprays, or as liquid preparations such as solutions and lotions.

Pharmaceutically, ointments, creams, and pastes are semisolid preparations in which the drug is contained in a suitable base (ointment base), which is itself semisolid and either hydrophilic or hydrophobic. These bases play an important role in the proper formulation of semisolid preparations, and there is no single base universally suitable as a carrier of all drug substances or for all therapeutic indications. The proper base for a drug must be determined individually to provide the desired drug release

rate, staying qualities after application, and texture. Briefly, *ointments* are simple mixtures of drug substances in an ointment base, whereas *creams* are semisolid emulsions less viscid and lighter than ointments. Creams are considered to have greater esthetic appeal for their nongreasy character, ability to vanish into the skin upon rubbing, and ability to absorb serous discharges from skin lesions. *Pastes* contain more solid materials than do ointments and are therefore stiffer and less penetrating. Pastes are usually employed for their protective action. Thus, when protective rather than therapeutic action is desired, the formulation pharmacist will favor a paste, but when therapeutic action is required, he will prefer ointments and creams. Commercially, many therapeutic agents are prepared in both ointment and cream form and are dispensed and used according to the particular preference of the patient and the prescribing practitioner.

Medicinal powders are intimate mixtures of medicinal substances usually in an inert base such as talcum powder or starch. Depending on the particle size of the resulting blend, the powder will have varying dusting and covering capabilities. In any case, the particle should be small enough to ensure against grittiness and consequent skin irritation. Powders are most frequently applied topically to relieve such conditions as diaper rash, chafing, and athlete's foot.

When topical application is desired in liquid form other than solution, lotions are most frequently employed. *Lotions* are emulsions or suspensions generally in an aqueous vehicle, although certain solutions have been designated as lotions because of either their appearance or application. Lotions may be preferred over semisolid preparations because of their nongreasy character and their increased spreadability over large areas of skin.

Ocular, Oral, Otic, and Nasal Routes

Drugs are frequently applied topically to the eye, ear, and mucous membranes of the nose, usually as ointments, suspensions, and solutions. Ophthalmic solutions and suspensions are sterile aqueous preparations with other ingredients essential to the safety and comfort of the patient. Ophthalmic ointments must be sterile and free of grit. Innovative new delivery systems for ophthalmic drugs continue to be investigated. One dosage form, the Ocusert, is an elliptical unit designed for continuous release of pilocarpine following placement in the cul-de-sac of the eye. Also, case reports of the ability of soft contact lenses to absorb drug from the eye have spawned research on soft contact lenses impregnated with drug. Most nasal preparations are solutions or suspensions administered by drops or as a fine mist. Research is directed toward the feasibility of nasal administration of insulin for diabetes mellitus. Ear preparations are usually viscid so that they have prolonged contact with the affected area. They may be employed simply to soften ear wax, to relieve an earache, or to combat an ear infection. Eye, ear, and nose preparations usually are not used for systemic effects, and although ophthalmic and otic preparations are not usually absorbed to any great extent, nasal preparations *may* be absorbed, and systemic effects after the intranasal application of solution are fairly common.

Other Routes

The lungs provide an excellent absorbing surface for the administration of gases and for aerosol mists of very minute particles of liquids or solids. The gas is usually oxygen, and the drugs are the common general anesthetics administered to patients entering surgery. The rich capillary area of the alveoli of the lungs, which in a man covers nearly a thousand square feet, provides rapid absorption and drug effects comparable in speed with those following an intravenous injection. In the case of drug particles, their size largely determines the depth to which they penetrate the alveolar regions and their solubility, the extent to which they are absorbed. After contact with the inner surface of the lungs, an insoluble drug particle is caught in the mucus and is moved up the pulmonary tree by ciliary action. Soluble drug particles that are approximately 0.5 to 1.0 mm in size reach the minute alveolar sacs and are most prompt and efficient in providing systemic effects. Particles smaller than 0.5 mm are expired to some extent, and thus, their absorption is not total but variable. Particles 1 to 10 mm effectively reach the terminal bronchioles and to some extent the alveolar ducts and are favored for local therapy. Therefore, in the pharmaceutical manufacture of aerosol sprays for inhalation therapy, the manufacturers not only must attain the proper drug particle size but also must ensure their uniformity for consistent penetration of the pulmonary tree and uniform effects.

In certain instances and for local effects, drugs are inserted into the vagina or the urethra. Drugs are usually presented to the vagina in tablet or other form, such as a suppository, ointment, emulsion foam, gel, or solution, and to the urethra as a suppository or solution. Systemic drug effects may result after vaginal or urethral application of drugs following absorption of the drug from the mucous membranes of these sites.

▌ FATE OF DRUG AFTER ABSORPTION

After absorption into the general circulation from any route of administration, a drug may become bound to blood proteins and delayed in its passage into the surrounding tissues. Many drug substances are highly bound to blood protein and others minimally bound. For instance, in the bloodstream, naproxen is 99% bound to plasma proteins, penicillin G is 60% bound, amoxicillin is only 20% bound, and minoxidil is unbound.

The degree of drug binding to plasma proteins is usually expressed as a percentage or as a fraction (termed *alpha*, or a) of the bound concentration (C_b) to the total concentration (C_t), bound plus unbound (C_u) drug:

$$\alpha = \frac{C_b}{C_u + C_b} = \frac{C_b}{C_t}$$

Thus, if one knows two of the three terms in the equation, the third may be calculated. Drugs having an alpha value above 0.9 are considered highly bound (90%); drugs with an alpha value below 0.2 are considered to be minimally (20% or less) protein bound. Table 5.8 presents approximate serum protein–binding characteristics for representative drugs in the blood under conditions associated with usual therapy. The drug–protein complex, which is reversible, involves albumin, although globulins also participate in the binding of drugs, particularly some of the hormones. The binding of drugs to biologic materials entails the formation of relatively weak bonds (e.g., van der Waals, hydrogen, and ionic bonds). The binding capacity of blood proteins is limited, and once they are saturated, additional drug absorbed into the bloodstream remains unbound unless bound drug is released, creating a vacant site for another drug molecule to attach. Any unbound drug is free to leave the bloodstream for tissues or cellular sites within the body.

Bound drug is neither exposed to the body's detoxification (metabolism) processes nor filtered through the renal glomeruli. Bound drug is therefore referred to as the

TABLE 5.8. Examples of Drug Binding to Plasma Proteins

Drug	Percent Bound
Naproxen (Naprosyn)	99
Carvedilol (Coreg)	98
Esomeprazole (Nexium)	97
Warfarin sodium (Coumadin)	97
Fluoxetine (Prozac)	95
Zolpidem (Ambien)	93
Duloxetine (Cymbalta)	90
Indomethacin (Indocin)	90
Rosuvastatin (Crestor)	88
Penicillin V (Veetids)	75
Nitroglycerin (Nitro-Bid)	60
Penicillin G potassium	60
Methotrexate	50
Methicillin (Staphcillin)	40
Ceftizoxime (Cefizox)	30
Ciprofloxacin (Cipro)	20–40
Digoxin (Lanoxin)	20–25
Amoxicillin (Amoxil)	20
Metronidazole (Flagyl)	20
Mercaptopurine (Purinethol)	19
Ranitidine (Zantac)	15
Gabapentin (Neurontin)	3
Lisinopril (Zestril)	0
Minoxidil (Loniten)	0

Approximate values based on conditions usually associated with drug therapy.

inactive portion in the blood, and unbound drug, with its ability to penetrate cells, is termed the *active* blood portion. The bound portion of drug serves as a reservoir or depot from which the drug is released as the free form when the level of free drug in the blood no longer is adequate to ensure protein saturation. The free drug may be only slowly released, which prolongs the drug's stay in the body. For this reason, a drug that is highly protein bound may remain in the body longer and require less frequent dosage than another drug that is only slightly protein bound and remains in the body for only a short period. Evidence suggests that the concentration of serum albumin decreases about 20% in the elderly. This may be clinically significant for drugs that bind strongly to albumin, for example, phenytoin, because if there is less albumin available to bind the drug, there will be a corresponding increase of the free drug in the body. Without a downward dosage adjustment in an elderly patient, there could be an increased incidence of adverse effects.

A drug's binding to blood proteins may be affected by the simultaneous presence of another drug or drugs. The additional drug or drugs may produce effects or duration of action quite dissimilar to that found when each is administered alone. Salicylates, for instance, decrease the binding capacity of thyroxin, the thyroid hormone, to proteins. Through this action, the displaced drugs become less protein bound, and their activity (and toxicity) may be increased. The intensity of a drug's pharmacologic response is related to the ratio of the bound drug to free active drug and to the therapeutic index of the drug. Warfarin sodium, an anticoagulant, is 97% bound to plasma protein, leaving 3% in free form to exert its effect. If a second drug, such as naproxen, which is strongly bound to plasma proteins, is administered and results in only 90% of the warfarin sodium being bound, 10% of warfarin sodium will be in the free form. Thus, the blood level of the free warfarin sodium (3% to 10%) will triple and possibly result in serious toxicity. The displacement of drugs from plasma protein sites is typical in the elderly, who normally take numerous medicines. Coupled with the aforementioned decrease in serum protein through the aging process, the addition of a highly protein-bound drug to an elderly patient's treatment regimen may pose significant problems if the patient is not monitored carefully for signs of toxicity.

In the same manner as they are bound to blood proteins, drugs may become bound to specific components of certain cells. Thus, drugs are not distributed uniformly among all cells of the body but rather tend to pass from the blood into the fluid bathing the tissues and may accumulate in certain cells according to their permeability and chemical and physical affinities. This affinity for certain body sites influences their action, for they may be brought into contact with reactive tissues (their *receptor sites*) or deposited in places where they are inactive. Many drugs, because of their affinity for and solubility in lipids, are deposited in fatty body tissue, creating a reservoir from which they are slowly released to other tissues.

Drug Metabolism or Biotransformation

Although some drugs are excreted from the body in their original form, many drugs undergo biotransformation prior to excretion. Biotransformation indicates the chemical changes to drugs within the body as they are metabolized and altered by various biochemical mechanisms. The biotransformation of a drug results in its conversion to one or more compounds that are more water soluble, more ionized, less capable of binding to proteins of the plasma and tissues, less capable of being stored in fat tissue, and less able to penetrate cell membranes, and thereby less active pharmacologically. Because of its new characteristics, a drug so transformed is rendered less toxic and is more readily excreted. It is for this reason that biotransformation is also commonly called detoxification or inactivation. (However, sometimes the metabolites are more active than the parent compound; see *prodrugs*, following.)

The exact metabolic processes (pathways) by which drugs are transformed are an active area of biomedical research. Much work has been done with the processes of animal degradation of drugs, and in many instances, the biotransformation in the animal is thought to parallel that in man. Four principal chemical reactions are involved in the metabolism of drugs: oxidation, reduction, hydrolysis, and conjugation. Most oxidation reactions are catalyzed by enzymes (oxidases) bound to the endoplasmic reticulum, a tubular system in liver cells. Only a small fraction of drugs are metabolized by reduction, through the action of reductases in the gut and liver. Esterases in the liver participate in the hydrolytic breakdown of drugs containing ester groups and amides. Glucuronide conjugation is the most common pathway for drug metabolism, through combination of the drug with glucuronic acid, forming ionized compounds that are easily eliminated via the urine (7). Other metabolic processes, including methylation and acylation conjugation reactions, occur with certain drugs to foster elimination.

In recent years, much interest has been shown in the metabolites of drug biotransformation. Certain metabolites may be as active as or even more active pharmacologically than the original compound. Occasionally, an active drug is converted into an active metabolite, which must be excreted as such or undergo further biotransformation to an inactive metabolite, for example, amitriptyline to nortriptyline. In other instances of drug therapy, an inactive parent compound, referred to as a *prodrug*, may be converted to an active therapeutic agent by chemical transformation in the body. An example is the prodrug enalapril (Vasotec), which after oral administration is hydrolyzed to enalaprilat, an active angiotensin-converting enzyme inhibitor used in the treatment of hypertension. Enalaprilat itself is poorly absorbed when taken orally (and thus the prodrug) but may be administered intravenously in aqueous solution. The use of these active metabolites as original drugs is a new area of investigation and a vast reservoir of potential therapeutic agents.

Several examples of biotransformations occurring within the body are as follows:

(1) Acetaminophen (active) $\xrightarrow{\text{conjugation}}$ Acetaminophen glucuronide (inactive)

(2) Amoxapine (active) $\xrightarrow{\text{oxidation}}$ 8-hydroxy-amoxapine (inactive)

(3) Procainamide (active) $\xrightarrow{\text{hydrolysis}}$ *p*-Aminobenzoic acid (inactive)

(4) Nitroglycerin (active) $\xrightarrow{\text{reduction}}$ 1 − 2 and 1 − 3 dinitroglycerol (inactive)

Some parent compounds undergo full, partial, or no biotransformation following administration. Lisinopril (Zestril), for example, does not undergo metabolism and is excreted unchanged in the urine. On the other hand, verapamil (Calan) metabolizes to at least 12 metabolites, the most prevalent of which is norverapamil. Norverapamil has 20% of the cardiovascular activity of the parent compound. Diltiazem (Cardizem) is partially metabolized (about 20%) to desacetyl diltiazem, which has 10% to 20% of the coronary vasodilator activity of the parent compound. Indomethacin (Indocin) is metabolized in part to desmethyl, desbenzoyl, and desmethyl–desbenzoyl metabolites. Propoxyphene napsylate (Darvon N) is metabolized to norpropoxyphene, which has less central nervous system depressant action than the parent compound but greater local anesthetic effects. Most metabolic transformations take place in the liver, with some drugs, including diltiazem and verapamil, undergoing extensive first-pass effects. Other drugs, such as terazosin (Hytrin), undergo minimal first-pass metabolism. The excretion of both drug and metabolites takes place primarily but to varying degrees via the urine and feces. For example, indomethacin and its metabolites are excreted primarily (60%) in the urine, with the remainder in the feces, whereas terazosin and its metabolites are excreted largely (60%) through the feces and the remainder in the urine.

Several factors influence drug metabolism. For example, there are marked differences between *species* in pathways of hepatic metabolism of a given drug. Species differences make it extremely difficult to extrapolate from one species to another, as with laboratory animals to humans. Furthermore, there are many examples of *interindividual variations* in hepatic metabolism of drugs within one species. Genetic factors affect the basal activity of the drug-metabolizing enzyme systems. Thus, there can be marked intersubject variation in rates of metabolism. Because of this variation, a physician must individualize therapy to maximize the chances for a constructive therapeutic outcome with minimal toxicity. Studies in humans have demonstrated that these differences have occurred within the cytochrome P-450 genetic codes for a family of isoenzymes responsible for drug metabolism.

Age of the patient is another significant factor in drug metabolism. Although pharmacokinetic calculations have not been able to develop a specific correlative relationship with age, it is known that the ability to metabolize drugs is low at the extremes of the age scale, that is, among the elderly and neonates. Liver blood flow is reduced by aging at about 1% per year beginning around age 30 (8). This decreased blood flow to the liver reduces the capacity for hepatic drug metabolism and elimination. For example, the half-life of chlordiazepoxide increases from about 6 hours at age 20 to about 36 hours at age 80. Furthermore, an immature hepatic system disallows the effective metabolism of drugs by the newborn or premature infant. As mentioned earlier, the half-life of theophylline ranges from 14 to 58 hours in the premature infant to 2.5 to 5 hours in young children aged 1 to 4 whose liver enzyme systems are mature.

Diet has also been demonstrated to modify the metabolism of some drugs. For example, the conversion of an asthmatic patient from a high- to a low-protein diet will increase the half-life of theophylline. It has also been demonstrated that the production of polycyclic hydrocarbons by the charcoal broiling of beef enhances the hepatic metabolism and shortens the plasma half-life of theophylline. It is conceivable that this effect also occurs with drugs that are metabolized in similar fashion to theophylline. Diet type, including starvation and intake of certain vegetables (brussels sprouts, cabbage, broccoli), has been shown to influence the metabolism of certain drugs. Coadministration of large quantities of grapefruit juice (at least 1 quart daily) may result in increased plasma levels of some of the HMG-CoA reductase inhibitors and increase the patient's risk of myopathy. Consequently, concurrent use of grapefruit juice should be avoided. Finally, exposure to other drugs or chemicals, such as pesticides, alcohol, and nicotine, and the presence of disease states, such as hepatitis, have all demonstrated an influence on drug metabolism and consequently the pharmacokinetic profile of certain drugs.

Excretion of Drugs

The excretion of drugs and their metabolites terminates their activity and presence in the body. They may be eliminated by various routes, with the kidney playing the dominant role by eliminating drugs via the urine. Drug excretion in the feces is also important, especially for drugs that are poorly absorbed and remain in the gastrointestinal tract after oral administration. Exit through the bile is significant only when reabsorption from the gastrointestinal tract is minimal. The lungs provide the exit for many volatile drugs through the expired breath. The sweat glands, saliva, and milk play only minor roles in drug elimination. However, if a drug gains access to the milk of a mother during lactation, it can easily exert its effects in the nursing infant. Drugs that do enter breast milk and may be passed on to nursing infants include theophylline, penicillin, reserpine, codeine, meperidine, barbiturates, diltiazem, and thiazide diuretics. It is generally good practice for the mother to abstain from taking medication until the infant is weaned. If she must take medication, she should abide by a dosage regimen and nursing schedule that permit her own therapy yet ensure the safety of her child. Not all drugs gain entrance into the milk; nevertheless, caution is advisable. A summary of drug safety in lactations, including biopharmaceutic parameters, calculation of infant exposure, and a listing of drugs and their risk assessment, may be found at the following Web site: http://www.medsafe.govt.nz/Profs/PUarticles/lactation.htm.

Manufacturers' package inserts contain product-specific information (usually in the section on precautions) on drug migration into breast milk.

The unnecessary use of medications during the early stages of pregnancy is likewise restricted by physicians, because certain drugs are known to cross the placental barrier and gain entrance to the tissues and blood of the fetus. Among the many drugs known to do so are all of the anesthetic gases, many barbiturates, sulfonamides, salicylates, and a number of other potent agents like quinine, meperidine, and morphine, the latter two being narcotic analgesics with great potential for addiction. In fact, it is fairly common for an infant to be born addicted because of the addiction of its mother and the passage of the drugs across the placental barrier.

The kidney, as the main organ for the elimination of drugs from the body, must be functioning adequately if drugs are to be efficiently eliminated. For instance, elimination of digoxin occurs largely through the kidney by first-order kinetics; that is, the quantity of digoxin eliminated at any time is proportional to the total body content. Renal excretion of digoxin is proportional to the glomerular filtration rate, which when normal results in a digoxin half-life that may range from 1.5 to 2 days. When the glomerular filtration rate is impaired or disrupted, however, as in an anuric patient, the elimination rate decreases. Consequently, the half-life of digoxin may be 4 to 6 days. Because of this prolongation of digoxin's half-life, the dosage of the drug must be decreased or the dosage interval prolonged. Otherwise, digoxin toxicity will occur. The degree of impairment can be estimated by measurements of glomerular filtration rates, most often by creatinine clearance (CrCL). Usually, however, this is not feasible, and the patient's serum creatinine value is used within appropriate pharmacokinetic equations to help determine a drug's dosage regimen.

Some drugs may be reabsorbed from the renal tubule even having been sent there for excretion. Because the rate of reabsorption is proportional to the concentration of drug in unionized form, it is possible to modify this rate by adjusting the pH of the urine. By acidifying the urine, as with the oral administration of ammonium chloride, or by alkalinizing it, as with the administration of sodium bicarbonate, one can increase or decrease the ionization of the drug and thereby alter its prospect of being reabsorbed. Alkalinization of the urine has been demonstrated to enhance the urinary excretion of weak acids such as salicylates, sulfonamides, and phenobarbital. The opposite effect can be achieved by acidifying the urine. Thus,

the duration of a drug's stay within the body may be markedly altered by changing the pH of the urine. Some foods, such as cranberry juice, can also acidify the urine and may alter drug excretion rates.

The urinary excretion of drugs may also be retarded by the concurrent administration of agents capable of inhibiting their tubular secretion. A well-known example is the use of probenecid to inhibit the tubular secretion of various types of penicillin, thereby reducing the frequency of dosage administrations usually necessary to maintain adequate therapeutic blood levels of the antibiotic drug. In this particular instance, the elevation of penicillin blood levels, by whatever route the antibiotic is administered, to twofold and even fourfold levels has been demonstrated by adjuvant therapy with probenecid. The effects are completely reversible upon withdrawal of the probenecid from concomitant therapy.

The fecal excretion of drugs appears to lag behind the rate of urinary excretion, partly because a day or so elapses before the feces reach the rectum. Drugs administered orally for local activity within the gastrointestinal tract and not absorbed will be eliminated completely via the feces. Unless a drug is particularly irritating to the gastrointestinal tract, there is generally no urgency about removing unabsorbable drugs from the system by means other than normal defecation. Some drugs that are only partially absorbed after oral administration will naturally be partly eliminated through the rectum.

PHARMACOKINETIC PRINCIPLES

This section introduces the concept of pharmacokinetics and how it interrelates the various processes that take place when one administers a drug to a patient, that is, ADME. It is not intended to be comprehensive, and thus, for further information about the subject, the reader is referred to other appropriate literature.

A problem encountered when one needs to determine a more accurate dosage of a drug or a more meaningful interpretation of a biologic response to a dose is the inability to determine the drug concentration at the active site in the body. Consequently, the concept of compartmental analysis is used to determine what has become of the drug as a function of time from the moment it is administered until it is no longer in the body. Pharmacokinetic analysis uses mathematical models to simplify or simulate the disposition of the drug in the body. The idea is to begin with a simple model and then modify as necessary. The principal assumption is that the human body may be represented by one or more *compartments* or pools in which a drug resides in a dynamic state for a short time. A compartment is a hypothetical space bound by an unspecified membrane across which drugs are transferred (Fig. 5.12). The transfer of drugs into and out of this compartment is indicated by arrows that point in the direction of drug movement into or out of the compartment. The rate at which a drug is transferred throughout the system is designated by a symbol that usually represents an

Where:
C_p is the drug concentration in plasma
V_d is the volume of the compartment or volume
    of distribution

FIGURE 5.12. A one-compartment system.

exponential rate constant. Typically, the letter K or k with numeric or alphanumeric subscripts is used.

Several assumptions are associated with modeling of drug behavior in the body. It is assumed that the volume of each compartment remains constant. Thus, an equation that describes the time course of the amount of drug in the compartment can be converted to an equation that depicts the time course of the drug concentration in the compartment by dividing both sides of the equation by the volume of the compartment. Second, it is assumed that once a drug enters the compartment, it is instantaneously and uniformly distributed throughout the entire compartment. Thus, it is assumed that a sampling of any one portion of the compartment will yield the drug concentration of the entire compartment.

In compartment models, it is assumed that drug passes freely into and out of compartments. Thus, these compartmental systems are known as open systems. Typically, drug transport between compartments follows first-order kinetics, wherein a constant fraction of drug is eliminated per unit of time and can be described by ordinary differential equations. In these linear systems, the time constants that describe the rate at which the plasma or blood concentration curve of a drug decays are independent of the dose, the volume of distribution, and the route of administration.

The simplest pharmacokinetic model is the single-compartment *open-model system* (Fig. 5.12). This model depicts the body as one compartment characterized by a certain volume of distribution (V_d) that remains constant. Each drug has its own distinct volume of distribution, and this can be influenced by factors including age and disease status. In this scheme, a drug can be instantaneously introduced into the compartment, that is, via rapid intravenous administration, or gradually, as with oral administration. In the former case, it is assumed that the drug distributes immediately to tissues and instantly attains equilibrium. In the latter case, the drug is absorbed at a certain rate and is characterized by the absorption rate constant K_a. Finally, the drug is eliminated from the compartment at a certain rate that is characterized by an elimination rate constant, K_{el}.

It is relevant at this point to consider the *volume of distribution*, V_d, a proportionality constant that refers to the volume into which the total amount of drug in the body must be uniformly distributed to provide the concentration of drug actually measured in plasma or blood. This term can be misleading because it does not represent a specific body fluid or volume. It is influenced by the plasma protein binding and tissue binding of a drug. These then influence the distribution of the drug between plasma water, extracellular fluid, intracellular fluid, and total body water. Furthermore, because a drug can partition between fat and water according to its unique partition coefficient, this can also influence the volume of distribution. Because of these phenomena, pharmacokineticists find it convenient to describe drug distribution in terms of compartmental models.

To determine the rate of drug transfer into and out of the compartment, plasma, serum, or blood samples are drawn at predetermined times after the drug is administered and analyzed for drug concentration. Once a sufficient number of experimental data points are determined, these are plotted on semilogarithmic paper, and an attempt is made to fit the experimental points with a smooth curve. Figure 5.13 depicts the plasma concentration–time profile for a hypothetical drug following rapid intravenous injection of a bolus dose of the drug with instantaneous distribution. For drugs whose distribution follows first-order one-compartment pharmacokinetics, a plot of the logarithm of the concentration of drug in the plasma (or blood) versus time will yield a straight line. The equation that describes the plasma decay curve is

$$C_p = C_p^0 e^{-K_{el}t}$$ **Equation 5.1**

where

K_{el} is the first-order rate of elimination of the drug from the body,

C_p is the concentration of the drug at a time equal to t, and

C_p^0 is the concentration of drug at time equal to zero, when all the drug administered has been absorbed but none has been removed from the body through elimination mechanisms, for example, metabolism and renal excretion.

The apparent first-order rate of elimination, K_{el}, is usually the sum of the rate constants of a number of individual processes, for example, metabolic transformation and renal excretion.

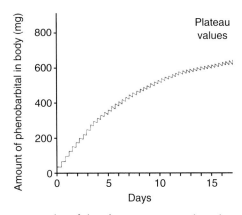

FIGURE 5.13. Plot of the plasma concentration–time data. (Adapted from Rowland M, Tozer TN. Clinical Pharmacokinetics. 2nd Ed. Philadelphia, PA: Lea & Febiger, 1989, with permission.)

For the purpose of pharmacokinetic calculation, it is simpler to convert Equation 5.1 to natural logs:

$$LnC_P = LnC_P^0 - K_{el}(t)$$ **Equation 5.2**

and then to log base$_{10}$:

$$LogC_P = LogC_P^0 - K_{el}(t)/2.303$$ **Equation 5.3**

Equation 5.3 is then thought of in terms of the Y-intercept form:

$$Y = b + mX$$
$$Log\ C_P = Log\ C_P^0 - K_{el}/2.303(t)$$

and interpreted as such in the semilogarithmic plot illustrated in Figure 5.14. Most drugs administered orally can be adequately described using a one-compartment model, whereas drugs administered by rapid intravenous infusion are usually best described by a two-compartment or three-compartment model system.

Assuming that a drug's volume of distribution is constant within this system, the total amount of drug in the body (Q_b) can be calculated from the following equation:

$$Q_b = \left[C_P^0 \right]\left[V_d \right]$$ **Equation 5.4**

Usually, C_P^0 is determined by extrapolating the drug concentration–time plot to time zero.

In this simple one-compartment system, it is assumed that the administered drug is confined to the plasma (or blood) and then excreted. Drugs that exhibit this behavior have small volumes of distribution. For example, a drug such as warfarin sodium, which is extensively bound to plasma albumin, will have a volume of distribution equivalent to that of plasma water, about 2.8 L in an average 70-kg adult. Some drugs, however, are initially

Where:
Q_c = Quantity of drug in central compartment
V_c = Volume of the central compartment
Q_p = Quantity of drug in peripheral compartment
V_p = Volume of the peripheral compartment

FIGURE 5.15. A two-compartment system.

distributed at somewhat different rates in various fluids and tissues. Consequently, these drugs' kinetic behavior can best be illustrated by considering an expansion of the one-compartment system to the *two-compartment model* (Fig. 5.15).

In the two-compartment system, a drug enters into and is instantaneously distributed throughout the central compartment. Its subsequent distribution into the second or peripheral compartment is slower. For simplicity, on the basis of blood perfusion and tissue–plasma partition coefficients for a given drug, various tissues and organs are considered together and designated either central compartment or peripheral compartment. The central compartment is usually considered to include the blood, the extracellular space, and organs with good blood perfusion, such as the lungs, liver, kidneys, and heart. The peripheral compartment usually comprises tissues and organs that are poorly perfused by blood, such as the skin, bone, and fat.

Figure 5.16 depicts the plasma drug concentration–time plot for a rapidly administered intravenous dose of a hypothetical drug that exhibits kinetic behavior exemplifying a two-compartment system. Note the initial steep decline of the plasma drug concentration curve. This typifies the distribution of the drug from the central compartment to the peripheral compartment. During this phase, the drug concentration in the plasma will decrease more rapidly than in the postdistributive or elimination phase. Whether this distributive phase is apparent depends on the timing of the plasma samples, particularly in the time immediately following administration. A distributive phase can be very short, a few minutes, or last for hours and even days.

A semilogarithmic plot of the plasma concentration versus time after rapid intravenous injection of a drug best described by a two-compartment model system can often be resolved into two linear components. This procedure can be performed by the method of residuals (or feathering), shown in Figure 5.16. In this procedure, a straight line is fitted through the tail of the original curve and extrapolated to the Y-axis (the value obtained is B). A plot is then

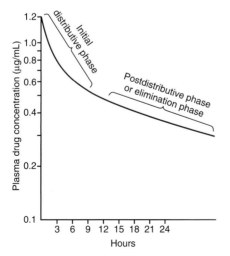

FIGURE 5.14. A semilogarithmic plot of plasma concentration versus time of an intravenous drug that follows first-order two-compartment pharmacokinetics.

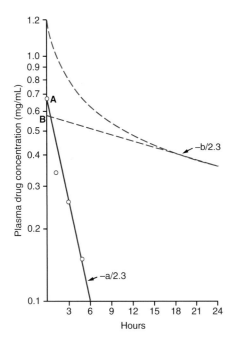

FIGURE 5.16. The logarithm of the drug concentration in plasma plotted versus time (*solid line*) after intravenous administration of a drug whose disposition can be described by a two-compartment model.

made of the absolute difference values of the original curve and the resultant extrapolated straight line. The slope of the feathered line (−a/2.303) and the extrapolated line (−b/2.303) and the intercepts, A and B, are determined. The following equation describes a two-compartment system:

$$C_p = Ae^{-at} + Be^{-bt} \qquad \textbf{Equation 5.5}$$

This is a two-exponential equation that describes the two-compartment system. In this scheme, the slope of the line, −a/2.303, obtained from feathering yields the distributive rate of the drug. The slope of the terminal linear phase or elimination phase, −b/2.303, describes the rate of loss of the drug from the body and usually is considered to be a reflection of the metabolic processes and renal elimination from the body. Appropriate pharmacokinetic formulas allow the clinician to calculate the various volumes of distribution and rates of distribution and elimination for drugs whose pharmacokinetic behavior is exemplified by the two-compartment system.

Half-Life

The half-life (t½) of a drug describes the time required for a drug's blood or plasma concentration to decrease by half. This fall in drug concentration is a reflection of metabolic processes and/or excretion. The biologic half-life of a drug in the blood may be determined graphically from a pharmacokinetic plot of a drug's blood concentration–time plot, typically after intravenous administration to a sample population. The half-life can also be mathematically

determined. Recall Equation 5.3 and rearrange the equation as follows:

$$\frac{K_{el}t}{2.303} = \text{Log } C_P^0 - \text{Log } C_P = \frac{\text{Log } C_P^0}{C_P} \qquad \textbf{Equation 5.6}$$

Then, if it assumed that C_p is equal to half of C_P^0

$$\frac{K_{el}t}{2.303} = \frac{\text{Log } C_P^0}{0.5C_P^0} = \text{Log } 2 \qquad \textbf{Equation 5.7}$$

Thus,

$$t_{1/2} = \frac{2.303 \, \text{Log} 2}{K_{el}} = \frac{0.693}{K_{el}} \qquad \textbf{Equation 5.8}$$

If this equation is rearranged, the half-life finds utility in the determination of drug elimination from the body, provided of course that the drug follows first-order kinetics. Rearranging the prior equation,

$$K_{el} = \frac{0.693}{t_{1/2}} \qquad \textbf{Equation 5.9}$$

First-order elimination rate constants are reported in time^{-1}, for example, minutes^{-1} or hours^{-1}. Thus, an elimination constant of a drug of 0.3 hour^{-1} indicates that 30% of the drug is eliminated per hour.

The half-life varies widely between drugs; for some, it may be a few minutes, whereas for others, it may be hours or even days (Table 5.9). Data on a drug's biologic half-life are useful in determining the most appropriate dosage regimen to achieve and maintain the desired blood level. These determinations usually result in recommended

TABLE 5.9. Some Elimination Half-Life Values

Drug Product	Elimination Half-Life[a]
Amoxicillin (Amoxil)	1 h
Cimetidine (Tagamet)	2 h
Digoxin (Lanoxin)	1.5–2 d
Diltiazem (Cardizem)	2.5 h
Esomeprazole (Nexium)	1–1.5 h
Ibuprofen (Motrin)	1.8–2 h
Nitroglycerin	3 min
Phenytoin sodium (Dilantin)	7–29 h
Propranolol HCl (Inderal)	4 h
Ranitidine (Zantac)	2.5–3 h
Ropinirole (Requip)	6 h
Rosuvastatin (Crestor)	19 h
Tadalafil (Cialis)	17.5 h
Tobramycin sulfate (Nebcin)	2 h
Zolpidem tartrate (Ambien)	2.6 h

[a]Mean, average, or value ranges taken from product information found in Physicians' Desk Reference. 65th Ed. Montvale, NJ: Thompson PDR, 2011. Half-life values may vary with patient characteristics (e.g., age, liver or renal function, smoking habits), dose levels, and routes of administration.

dosage schedules for a drug, such as every 4, 6, or 8 hours. Although these types of recommendations generally suit the requirements of most patients, they do not suit all patients. The most exceptional patients are those with reduced or impaired ability to metabolize or excrete drugs. These patients, most of whom have liver dysfunction or kidney disease, retain the administered drug in the blood or tissues for extended periods because of their decreased ability to eliminate the drug. The resulting extended biologic half-life of the drug generally necessitates an individualized dosage regimen calling for either less frequent administration than usual or the usual dosage schedule but a decrease in the amount of drug administered.

As mentioned previously, digoxin presents a good example of a drug having a half-life that is affected by the patient's pathologic condition. Digoxin is eliminated in the urine. Renal excretion of digoxin is proportional to glomerular filtration rate. In subjects with normal renal function, digoxin has a half-life of 1.5 to 2.0 days. In anuric patients (absence of urine formation), the half-life may be prolonged to 4 to 6 days. Theophylline's half-life also varies from population to population. In premature infants with immature liver enzyme systems in the cytochrome P-450 family, the half-life of theophylline ranges from 14 to 58 hours, whereas in children aged 1 to 4 whose liver enzyme systems are more mature, the theophylline half-life ranges from 2 to 5.5 hours. In adult nonsmokers, the half-life ranges from 6.1 to 12.8 hours, whereas in adult smokers, the average half-life of theophylline is 4.3 hours. The increase in theophylline clearance from the body among smokers is believed to be because of an induction of the hepatic metabolism of theophylline. The half-life of theophylline is decreased, and total body clearance is enhanced to such a degree in smokers that these individuals may actually require a 50% to 100% increase in theophylline dosage to produce effective therapeutic results. The time required to normalize the effect of smoking on theophylline metabolism in the body once the patient stops smoking may range from 3 months to 2 years. Because theophylline is metabolized in the liver, the half-life of theophylline will be extended in liver disease. For example, in one study of nine patients with decompensated cirrhosis, the average theophylline half-life was 32 hours.

The half-life of a drug in the bloodstream may also be affected by a change in the extent to which it is bound to blood protein or cellular components. Such a change in a drug's binding pattern may be brought about by the administration of a second drug having a greater affinity than the first drug for the same binding sites. The result is displacement of the first drug from these sites by the second drug and the sudden availability of free (unbound) drug, which may pass from the bloodstream to other body sites, including those concerned with its elimination. Displacement of one drug from its binding sites by another is generally viewed as an undesired event, because the amount of free drug resulting is greater than the level normally achieved during single-drug therapy and may result in untoward drug effects.

Concept of Clearance

The three main mechanisms by which a drug is removed or cleared from the body include (a) hepatic metabolism, that is, hepatic clearance, Cl^h, of a drug to either an active or inactive metabolite; (b) renal excretion, that is, renal clearance, Cl_r, of a drug unchanged in the urine; and (c) elimination of the drug into the bile and subsequently into the intestines for excretion in feces. An alternative way to express this removal or elimination from the body is to use total body clearance (Cl_B), which is defined as the fraction of the total volume of distribution that can be cleared per unit of time. Because most drugs undergo one or more of these processes, the total body clearance, Cl_B, of a drug is the sum of these clearances, usually hepatic, Cl_h, and renal, Cl_r. Clearance via the bile and feces is usually not significant for most drugs.

These processes of elimination work together, so a drug that is eliminated by renal excretion and hepatic biotransformation will have an overall rate of elimination. K_{el} is the sum of the renal excretion, k_u, and hepatic biotransformation, k_m. In the one-compartment model described earlier, total body clearance is the product of the volume of distribution, V_d, and the overall rate of elimination, K_{el}:

$$Cl_B = V_d \times k_{el}$$ **Equation 5.10**

But recall that K_{el} equals $0.693/t^{1/2}$. If this is substituted in Equation 5.10 and the half-life, $t^{1/2}$, solved for, the following equation is obtained:

$$t_{1/2} = \frac{0.693 V_d}{Cl_b}$$ **Equation 5.11**

Total body clearance is a function of one or more processes, so if a drug is eliminated from the body through hepatic biotransformation and renal clearance, Equation 5.11 becomes

$$t_{1/2} = \frac{0.693 V_d}{(Cl_b + Cl_r)}$$ **Equation 5.12**

Thus, a drug's half-life is directly proportional to the volume of distribution and inversely proportional to the total body clearance, which consists of hepatic and renal clearance. In infants and children, who exhibit larger volumes of distribution and have lower clearance values, most drugs have a longer half-life than in adults.

A decrease in the hepatic or renal clearance will prolong the half-life of a drug. This typically occurs in renal failure, and consequently, if one can estimate the percentage decrease in excretion due to renal failure, one can use Equation 5.11 to calculate the new half-life of the drug in the patient. Thus, an adjusted dosage regimen can be calculated to decrease the chance of drug toxicity.

Dosage Regimen Considerations

The previous chapter mentions factors that can influence the dosage of a drug. It is not easy to determine how much drug and how often to administer it for a desired therapeutic effect. There are two basic approaches to the development of dosage regimens. The first is the *empirical approach*, which entails administration of a drug in a certain quantity, noting the therapeutic response and modifying the amount and interval of dosage accordingly. Unfortunately, experience with administration of a drug usually starts with the first patient, and eventually, a sufficient number of patients receive the drug so that a fairly accurate prediction can be made. Besides the desired therapeutic effect, it is necessary to consider the occurrence and severity of side effects. Empirical therapy is usually employed when the drug concentration in serum or plasma does not reflect the concentration of drug at the receptor site in the body or the pharmacodynamic effect of the drug is not related (or correlated) with drug concentration at the receptor site. Empirical therapy is used for many anticancer drugs that demonstrate effects long after they have been excreted from the body. It is difficult to relate the serum level of these drugs with the desired therapeutic effect.

The second approach to the development of a dosage regimen is through the use of pharmacokinetics, or the *kinetic approach*. This approach is based on the assumption that the therapeutic and toxic effects of a drug are related to the amount of drug in the body or to the plasma (or serum) concentration of drug at the receptor site. Through careful pharmacokinetic evaluation of a drug's ADME after a single dose, the levels of drug attained from multiple dosing can be estimated. One can then determine the appropriateness of a dosage regimen to achieve a desired therapeutic concentration of drug in the body and evaluate the regimen according to therapeutic response.

Pharmacokinetics is but one of a number of factors that should be considered in the development of a dosage regimen. Table 5.10 illustrates a number of these. Certainly, an important factor is the inherent activity, that is, pharmacodynamics and toxicity. A second consideration is the pharmacokinetics of the drug, which are influenced by the

dosage form. The third factor focuses upon the patient to whom the drug will be given and encompasses the clinical state of the patient and how the patient will be managed. Finally, atypical factors may influence the dosage regimen. Collectively, all of these factors influence the dosage regimen.

The regimen of a drug may simply involve a single dose, as with pinworm medication, or may call for multiple doses. In the latter instance, the objective of pharmacokinetic dosing is to design a regimen that will continually maintain a drug's therapeutic serum or plasma concentration within the therapeutic index, that is, above the MEC but below the MTC.

Frequently, drugs are administered one to four times per day, most often in a fixed dose, for example, 75 mg three times daily after meals. As mentioned earlier, after a drug is administered, its level within the body varies because of the influence of all of the processes, ADME. A drug will accumulate in the body when the dosing interval is less than the time needed for the body to eliminate a single dose. Figure 5.17 illustrates the plasma concentration for a drug given by intravenous administration and oral administration. The 50-mg dose of this drug was given at a dosing interval of 8 hours. The drug has an elimination half-life of 12 hours. As one can see, with continued dosing, the drug concentration reaches a *steady-state* or *plateau* concentration. At this limit, the amount of drug lost per interval is replenished when the drug is dosed again. Consequently, the concentration of drug in the plasma or serum fluctuates. Thus, for certain patient types, it is optimal to target dosing so that the plateau concentration resides within the therapeutic index of a drug to maintain an MEC. For example, the asthmatic patient maintained on theophylline must have a serum concentration between 10 and 20 mg/mL. Otherwise, the patient may be susceptible to an asthma attack. Thus, when dosing the asthmatic patient, it is preferable

TABLE 5.10. Factors That Determine a Dosage Regimen

Activity, Toxicity			Pharmacokinetics
Minimum therapeutic dose			Absorption
Toxic dose			Distribution
Therapeutic index		Dosage Regimen	Metabolism
Side effects			Excretion
Dose–response relationships			

Clinical Factors			Other Factors
Clinical State of Patient	**Management of Therapy**		
Age, weight, urine pH	Multiple drug therapy		Tolerance–dependence
Condition being treated	Convenience of regimen		Pharmacogenetics–idiosyncrasy
Existence of other disease states	Compliance of patient		Drug interactions
			Lifestyle factors, for example, diet and recreational drug use

Reprinted from Rowland M, Tozer TN. Clinical Pharmacokinetics. 3rd Ed. Baltimore, MD: Lippincott Williams & Wilkins, 1995, with permission.

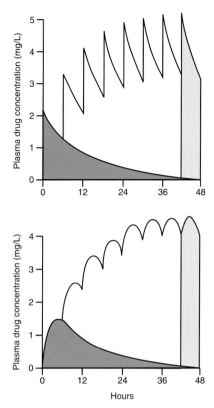

FIGURE 5.17. Plasma concentration of a drug given intravenously **(top)** and orally **(bottom)** on a fixed dose of 50 mg and fixed dosing interval of 8 hours. The half-life is 12 hours. The area under the plasma concentration–time curve during a dosing interval at steady state is equal to the total AUC for a single dose. The fluctuation of the concentration is diminished for oral administration (half-life of absorption is 1.4 hours), but the average steady-state concentration is the same as after intravenous administration, because f = 1. (Adapted from Rowland M, Tozer TN. Clinical Pharmacokinetics and Pharmacodynamics. 4th Ed. Baltimore, MD: Lippincott Williams & Wilkins, 2011, with permission.)

to give theophylline around the clock four times daily to sustain levels at least above the MEC. If this medicine is administered only every 4 hours during the waking hours, it is possible that the minimum concentration will fall below effective levels between the bedtime dose and the morning dose. Consequently, the patient may awaken in the middle of the night and have an asthma attack.

Patients can be monitored pharmacokinetically through appropriate plasma, serum, or blood samples, and some hospital pharmacies have implemented pharmacokinetic dosing services. The intent is to maximize drug efficacy, minimize toxicity, and keep health care costs at a minimum. Thus, complications associated with overdose are controlled, and known drug interactions, such as between smoking and theophylline, can be accommodated. In these services, once the physician prescribes a certain amount of drug and monitors the clinical response, it is the pharmacist who coordinates the appropriate sample time to determine drug concentration in the appropriate body

fluid. After the level of drug is attained, it is the pharmacist who interprets the result and consults with the physician regarding subsequent dosages.

Pharmacokinetic research has demonstrated that the determination of a patient's dosage regimen depends on numerous factors, and daily dose formulas exist for a number of drugs that must be administered on a routine maintenance schedule, for example, digoxin, procainamide, and theophylline. For certain drugs such as digoxin, which are not highly lipid soluble, it is preferable to use a patient's lean body weight (LBW) rather than total body weight (TBW) to provide a better estimate of the patient's volume of distribution. On the other hand, estimating a patient's CrCL for initial vancomycin dosing uses TBW according to Equation 5.13:

$$CrCL(male) \, mL/min = \frac{(140 - age) \times TBW(kg)}{72 \times Scr}$$

Equation 5.13

$$CrCL \, (female) \, mL/min = \\ = [0.85]\frac{(140 - age) \times TBW \, (kg)}{72 \times Scr}$$

Equation 5.14

Subsequent doses then must be calculated based on obtaining a trough vancomycin level 30 minutes before the next scheduled dose. In addition, the dosing interval (in hours) is based upon the patient's calculated CrCL (9).

Alternatively, even though pharmacokinetic dosing formulas may exist, one must be cognizant that patient factors may be more relevant. For example, with the geriatric patient, it is advisable to begin drug therapy with the lowest possible dose and increase the dosage as necessary in small increments to optimize the patient's clinical response. Then the patient should be monitored for drug efficacy and reevaluated periodically. Examples of bioanalytical research laboratories are demonstrated in Figures 5.18 and 5.19.

FIGURE 5.18. Computed gas chromatography with headspace injector. (Courtesy of ARL BioPharma, Inc. d/b/a Analytical Research Laboratories.)

FIGURE 5.19. Assay of product samples using high-performance liquid chromatography–mass spectroscopy. (Courtesy of ARL BioPharma, Inc d/b/a Analytical Research Laboratories.)

APPLYING THE PRINCIPLES AND CONCEPTS

GROUP ACTIVITIES

1. List the partition coefficients for erythromycin and its related chemical entities and predict comparable effectiveness when administered in a topical dosage form.
2. Create a listing of five prodrugs used therapeutically and describe the rationale for the use of each prodrug.
3. Select a drug available in various chemical moieties that dictate varying parenteral dosage forms and describe the effect of chemical formula on its onset of activity, duration of activity, etc., of the drug.
4. Given a serum concentration–time curve for a specific drug, determine the peak height concentration, the time of the peak concentration, and the serum (or blood or plasma) area under the curve.
5. Given a blood concentration *versus* time plot, perform various pharmacokinetic calculations.
6. Given comparative bioavailability data and cost information for identical drug products from different manufacturers, select a product for the hospital formulary and provide a rationale for your decision.
7. Make a listing of drug products whose brand names include the term "elixir" but have little or no Alcohol USP in their formulations.

INDIVIDUAL ACTIVITIES

1. Explain, with examples, how a drug's particle size influences its dissolution rate and solubility.
2. List four clinically available drugs that demonstrate either amorphous or crystalline forms, and describe the rationale for using a specific form for therapy.
3. Describe patient situations where one drug delivery approach would have advantages over another drug delivery approach.
4. Given a patient's data, calculate pharmacokinetic parameters.
5. Develop a listing of drugs dosed on peak and trough levels, and given patient data, demonstrate calculations for one such drug.
6. Given a patient case, select appropriate drug therapy, and determine an appropriate dosage regimen for the patient. Also, the selection of appropriate drug therapy should include flavor preference and discussion if a pediatric patient. Provide your rationale.

REFERENCES

1. Cogburn JN, Donovan MG, Schasteen CS. A model of human small intestinal absorptive cells 1: Transport barrier. Pharm Res 1991;8:210–216.

2. Christensen FN, et al. The use of gamma scintigraphy to follow the gastrointestinal transit of pharmaceutical formulations. J Pharm Pharmacol 1985;37:91–95.

3. Coupe AJ, Davis SS, Wilding IR. Variation in gastrointestinal transit of pharmaceutical dosage forms in healthy subjects. Pharm Res 1991;8:360–364.

4. Poole J, Owen G, Silverio J. Physiochemical factors influencing the absorption of the anhydrous and trihydrate forms of ampicillin. Curr Ther Res Clin Exp 1968;10:292–303.

5. Code of Federal Regulations, Title 21, Part 320. Bioavailability and Bioequivalence Requirements, 2012 (updated). Available at: http://www.accessdata.fda.gov/scripts/cdrh/cfdocs/cfcfr/CFRSearch.cfm?CFRPart. (Accessed July 23, 2020).

6. Chodos DJ, DiSanto AR. Basics of Bioavailability. Kalamazoo, MI: Upjohn, 1973.

7. Smith HJ. Process of drug handling by the body. Introduction to the Principles of Drug Design. 2nd Ed. London: Butterworth, 1988.

8. Cooper JW. Monitoring of drugs and hepatic status. Clinical Consult 1991;10(6):1991.

9. Vancomycin dosing and monitoring in adults. Available at: https://www.drugs.com/dosage/vancomycin.html (Accessed July 23, 2020).

SECTION THREE

Solid Dosage Forms and Solid Modified-Release Drug Delivery Systems

CHAPTER

6

Powders and Granules

CHAPTER AT A GLANCE Historical Use • Applications • Physicochemical Considerations • Mixing • Blending/Mixing Powders • Special Considerations • Powders as a Dosage Form • Granules • Quality Control • Packaging/Dispensing • Patient Counseling

OBJECTIVES

After reading this chapter, the student will be able to:

   Differentiate a powder from a granule

   Explain how a drug's powder particle size influences the pharmaceutical dosage forms that will be used to administer it

   Define micromeritics, the angle of repose, levigation, spatulation, and trituration

   Compare and contrast the various types of medicated powders, for example, bulk and divided

   Provide examples of medicated powders used in prescription and nonprescription products

   Differentiate between the fusion method and wet method for the preparation of effervescent granulated salts

INTRODUCTION

Most active and inactive pharmaceutical ingredients (APIs) occur in the solid state as amorphous powders or as crystals of various morphologic structures. The term "powder" has more than one connotation in pharmacy. It may be used to describe the physical form of a material, that is, a dry substance composed of finely divided particles. Or, it may be used to describe a type of pharmaceutical preparation, that is, a medicated powder intended for internal (i.e., oral powder) or external (i.e., topical powder) use. A powder is defined as a dosage form composed of a solid or mixture of solids reduced to a finely divided state and intended for internal or external use.

HISTORICAL USE

Originally, powders were found to be a convenient mode of administering drugs derived from hard vegetables such as roots (e.g., rhubarb), barks (e.g., cinchona), and woods (e.g., charcoal). As synthetic drugs were introduced, powders were used to administer insoluble drugs such as calomel, bismuth salts, mercury, and chalk.

Powders as a solid dosage form have been used historically as internal and external medications. For internal use, they can be taken orally, administered through the nose as snuffs, or blown into a body cavity as an insufflation. For external use, solid powders can be applied to compromised areas of the body. Powders have also been used to make solutions for topical and oral use and for use as douches. Such traditional applications and modes of administration of the dosage form continue today. Additional applications have also been developed; for example, powders containing a bioadhesive material can be applied to a specific body area such that the medication will adhere for a prolonged drug effect.

APPLICATIONS

Powders have qualities that make them an attractive dosage form for certain situations. Unlike a standardized capsule or tablet, powders enable a primary care provider to easily alter the quantity of medication for each dose. Powders can also aid in clinical studies of drug preparations because the dose can be so readily adjusted. Doses can be individually weighed and placed in powder papers, envelopes, or small vials/bottles ("Powder in a bottle" research studies are an example). In another example, infants and young children who cannot swallow tablets or capsules will accept powders that can be mixed with a formula or sprinkled in applesauce or some other appropriate food. Also, if a drug is too bulky to be prepared as a capsule or tablet, it may be suitable for a powder dosage form. Powders provide a rapid onset of action because they are readily dispersed, have a large surface area, and usually require only dissolution, not disintegration, before absorption.

Although the use of *medicated powders* per se in therapeutics is limited, the use of powdered substances in the preparation of other dosage forms is extensive. For example, powdered drugs may be blended with powdered fillers and other pharmaceutical ingredients to fabricate solid dosage forms as tablets and capsules; they may be dissolved or suspended in solvents or liquid vehicles to make various liquid dosage forms; or they may be incorporated into semisolid bases in the preparation of medicated ointments and creams.

Granules, which are prepared agglomerates of powdered materials, may be used per se for the medicinal value of their content, or they may be used for pharmaceutical purposes, as in making capsules and tablets, as described later in this and Chapters 7 and 8.

PHYSICOCHEMICAL CONSIDERATIONS

Particle Characteristics

Before their use in the preparation of pharmaceutical products, solid materials first are characterized to determine their chemical and physical features, including morphology, purity, solubility, flowability, stability, particle size, uniformity, and compatibility with any other formulation components (1). Drug and other materials commonly require chemical or pharmaceutical processing to imbue the features desired to enable both the efficient production of a finished dosage form and the optimum therapeutic efficacy. This usually includes the adjustment and control of a powder's particle size.

- *Particle size:* Generally, particles of uniform size are blended easier. One can visualize a mixture of large and small marbles and the difficulty involved in blending as the smaller marbles in this case tend to sink pushing the larger marbles to the surface. This is visually evident when baking if one takes a substance such as flour and shakes it back and forth and the larger particles rise to the surface. Common dosage forms and associated particle size ranges, in microns, include ophthalmic suspensions ($\leq$10), oral suspensions (10 to 50), parenteral suspensions (0.5 to 25), aerosols for the lung (1 to 5), tablets and capsules-immediate release ($\leq$50), topical aerosols (50 to 100), topical emulsions ($\leq$50), and topical suspensions (10 to 50).

- *Particle shape*: Spherical particles tend to be easier to mix as they will be transported more easily from areas of high concentration to lower concentrations. Needle-shape particles and cubic-shaped particles do not slide over each other as easily and tend to clog or stick together.
- *Particle density*: Higher-density, or heavier, particles tend to sink and less dense, or lighter, particles tend to rise. Consequently, when blending particles of different densities, care must be taken to ensure uniformity of mixing.
- *Electrostatic charge*: Static electricity tends to hamper blending and needs to be addressed. This can often be overcome by humidification of the work area or the inclusion (if appropriate) of a small quantity of sodium lauryl sulfate or similar material to neutralize the charges.
- *Adhering/repelling properties*: By their nature, some particles may tend to either adhere or repel each other, and the faster they are individually diluted with an inert substance or nonreactive material in the formulation, the easier it is to blend them.
- *Other characteristics*: Some substances, such as camphor, are slightly gummy in nature and need to be reduced in particle size (pulverization by intervention) and immediately mixed with an inert material in the formulation to aid in the overall blending process.

Particle Size and Analysis

The particles of pharmaceutical powders and granules may range from being extremely coarse, about 10 mm (1 cm) in diameter, to extremely fine, approaching colloidal dimensions of 1 μm or less. In order to characterize the particle size of a given powder, the *U.S. Pharmacopeia* (USP) uses these descriptive terms: very coarse, coarse, moderately coarse, fine, and very fine, which are related to the proportion of powder that is capable of passing through the openings of standard sieves of varying fineness in a specified period while being shaken, generally in a mechanical sieve shaker (2). Table 6.1 presents the standard sieve numbers and the openings in each, expressed in millimeters and in microns. Sieves for such pharmaceutical testing and measurement are generally made of wire cloth woven from brass, bronze, or other suitable wire. They are not coated or plated.

Powders of vegetable and animal origin drugs are officially defined as follows (2):

- Very coarse (No. 8): All particles pass through a No. 8 sieve, and not more than 20% pass through a No. 60 sieve.
- Coarse (No. 20): All particles pass through a No. 20 sieve, and not more than 40% pass through a No. 60 sieve.
- Moderately coarse (No. 40): All particles pass through a No. 40 sieve, and not more than 40% pass through a No. 80 sieve.
- Fine (No. 60): All particles pass through a No. 60 sieve, and not more than 40% pass through a No. 100 sieve.
- Very fine (No. 80): All particles pass through a No. 80 sieve. There is no limit to greater fineness.

TABLE 6.1. Opening of Standard Sieves

Sieve Number	Sieve Opening
2.0	9.50 mm
3.5	5.60 mm
4.0	4.75 mm
8.0	2.36 mm
10.0	2.00 mm
20.0	850.00 μm
30.0	600.00 μm
40.0	425.00 μm
50.0	300.00 μm
60.0	250.00 μm
70.0	212.00 μm
80.0	180.00 μm
100.0	150.00 μm
120.0	125.00 μm
200.0	75.00 μm
230.0	63.00 μm
270.0	53.00 μm
325.0	45.00 μm
400.0	38.00 μm

Source: USP 31–NF 26.

Granules typically fall within the range of 4- to 12-sieve size, although granulations of powders prepared in the 12- to 20-sieve range are sometimes used in tablet making. The particle size distribution impacts several aspects of drug product formulation and performance.

- Dissolution rate of particles intended to dissolve; drug micronization can increase the rate of drug dissolution and its bioavailability.
- Suspendability of particles intended to remain undissolved but uniformly dispersed in a liquid vehicle (e.g., fine dispersions have particles ~0.5 to 10 μm).
- Uniform distribution of a drug substance in a powder mixture or solid dosage form to ensure dose-to-dose content uniformity (3).
- Penetrability of particles intended to be inhaled for deposition deep in the respiratory tract (e.g., 1 to 5 μm) (4).
- Lack of grittiness of solid particles in dermal ointments, creams, and ophthalmic preparations (e.g., fine powders may be 50 to 100 μm in size).

A number of methods exist for the determination of particle size, including the following (Physical Pharmacy Capsule 6.1):

PHYSICAL PHARMACY CAPSULE **6.1** Micromeritics

Micromeritics is the science of small particles; a particle is any unit of matter having defined physical dimensions. It is important to study particles because most drug dosage forms are solids, solids are not static systems, the physical state of particles can be altered by physical manipulation, and particle characteristics can alter therapeutic effectiveness.

Micromeritics is the study of a number of characteristics, including particle size and size distribution, shape, angle of repose, porosity, true volume, bulk volume, apparent density, and bulkiness.

■ PARTICLE SIZE

A number of techniques can be used to determine particle size and size distributions. Particle size determinations are complicated by the fact that particles are not uniform in shape. Only two relatively simple examples are provided for a detailed calculation of the average particle size of a powder mixture. Other methods are generally discussed. The techniques used include the microscopic method and the sieving method.

The microscopic method can include not fewer than 200 particles in a single plane using a calibrated ocular on a microscope. Given the following data, what is the average diameter of the particles?

Size of Counted Particles (μm)	Middle Value μm "D"	No. of Particles Per Group "N"	"ND"
40–60	50	15	750
60–80	70	25	1,750
80–100	90	95	8,550
100–120	110	140	15,400
120–140	130	80	10,400
		$\sum n = 355$	$\sum nd = 36,850$

(continued)

(continued)

$$d_{av} = \frac{\Sigma nd}{\Sigma n} = \frac{36,850}{355} = 103.8\mu m$$

The sieving method entails using a set of U.S. standard sieves in the desired size range. A stack of sieves is arranged in order, the powder placed in the top sieve, the stack shaken, the quantity of the powder resting on each sieve weighed, and this calculation performed:

Sieve	Arithmetic Mean Opening (mm)	Weight Retained (g)	% Retained	% Retained × Mean Opening (mm)
20/40	0.630	15.5	14.3	9.009
40/60	0.335	25.8	23.7	7.939
60/80	0.214	48.3	44.4	9.502
80/100	0.163	15.6	14.3	2.330
100/120	0.137	3.5	3.3	0.452
		108.7	100.0	29.232

$$d_{av} = \frac{\Sigma(\%retained) \times (average\ size)}{100} = \frac{29,232}{100} = 0.2923\ mm$$

Another method of particle size determination entails sedimentation using the Andreasen pipette, a special cylindrical container from which a sample can be removed from the lower portion at selected intervals. The powder is dispersed in a nonsolvent in the pipette and agitated, and 20-mL samples are removed over time. Each 20-mL sample is dried and weighed. The particle diameters can be calculated from this equation:

$$d = \frac{18h\eta}{(\rho_i - \rho_e)gt}$$

where

d is the diameter of the particles,
h is the height of the liquid above the sampling tube orifice,
η is the viscosity of the suspending liquid,
$\rho_i - \rho_e$ is the density difference between the suspending liquid and the particles,
g is the gravitational constant, and
t is the time in seconds.

Other methods of particle size determinations include elutriation, centrifugation, permeation, adsorption, electronic sensing zone (the Coulter counter), and light obstruction. The last includes both standard light and laser methods. In general, the resulting average particle sizes by these techniques can provide the average particle size by weight (sieve method, light scattering, sedimentation method) and the average particle size by volume (light scattering, electronic sensing zone, light obstruction, air permeation, and even the optical microscope).

■ ANGLE OF REPOSE

The angle of repose is a relatively simple technique for estimating the flow properties of a powder. It can easily be determined by allowing a powder to flow through a funnel and fall freely onto a surface. The height and diameter of the resulting cone are measured, and the angle of repose is calculated from this equation:

$$\tan\theta = h/r$$

where

h is the height of the powder cone and
r is the radius of the powder cone.

■ EXAMPLE 1

A powder was poured through the funnel and formed a cone 3.3 cm high and 9 cm in diameter. What is the angle of repose?

$$\tan\theta = h/r = 3.3/4.5 = 0.73$$

$$arc\ tan\ 0.73 = 36.25°$$

(continued)

PHYSICAL PHARMACY CAPSULE **6.1** Micromeritics *(continued)*

Powders with a low angle of repose flow freely, and powders with a high angle of repose flow poorly. A number of factors, including shape and size, determine the flow properties of powders. Spherical particles flow better than needles. Very fine particles do not flow as freely as large particles. In general, particles in the size range of 250 to 2,000 mm flow freely if the shape is amenable. Particles in the size range of 75 to 250 mm may flow freely or cause problems, depending on shape and other factors. With most particles smaller than 100 mm, flow is a problem.

■ POROSITY, VOID, AND BULK VOLUME

If spheres and the different ways they pack together are used as an example, two possibilities arise. The closest packing may be rhombus–triangle, in which angles of 60 and 120 degrees are common. The space between the particles, the void, is about 0.26, resulting in porosity, as described later, of about 26%. Another packing, cubical, with the cubes packed at 90-degree angles to each other, may be considered. This results in a void of about 0.47 or a porosity of about 47%. This is the most open type of packing. If particles are not uniform, the smaller particles will slip into the void spaces between the larger particles and decrease the void areas.

Tapped density tester (Courtesy of Surasak_Photo/Shutterstock.)

Packing and flow are important, as they affect the size of the container required for packaging, the flow of granulations, the efficiency of the filling apparatus for making tablets and capsules, and the ease of working with the powders.

The characteristics used to describe powders include porosity, true volume, bulk volume, apparent density, true density, and bulkiness. The photo is a tapped density tester.

Porosity is

$$\text{Void} \times 100$$

This value should be determined experimentally by measuring the volume occupied by a selected weight of a powder, V_{bulk}. The true volume, V, of a powder is the space occupied by the powder exclusive of spaces greater than the intramolecular space.

Void can be defined as

$$\frac{V_{bulk} - V}{V_{bulk}}$$

therefore, porosity is

$$\frac{V_{bulk} - V}{V_{bulk}} \times 100$$

and the bulk volume is

$$\text{true volume} + \text{porosity}$$

■ APPARENT DENSITY, TRUE DENSITY, AND BULKINESS

The apparent density, $\rho\alpha$, is

$$\frac{\text{weight of the sample}}{V_{bulk}}$$

The true density, ρ, is

$$\frac{\text{weight of the sample}}{V}$$

The bulkiness, B, is the reciprocal of the apparent density,

$$B = 1/\rho_a$$

(continued)

(continued)

■ EXAMPLE 2

A selected powder has a true density (ρ) of 3.5 g/cc. Experimentally, 2.5 g of the powder measures 40 mL in a cylindrical graduate. Calculate the true volume, void, porosity, apparent density, and bulkiness.

True volume:

$$\text{Density} = \text{mass (weight)}/\text{volume}$$
$$\text{Volume} = \text{mass (weight)}/\text{density}$$
$$2.5 \text{ g}/(3./5 \text{ g/cc})0.715 \text{ cc}$$

Void:

$$\frac{V_{bulk} - V}{V_{bulk}} = \frac{40 \text{ mL} - 0.715 \text{ mL}}{40 \text{ mL}} = 0.982$$

Porosity:

$$\text{Void} \times 100 = 0.982 \times 100 = 98.2\%$$

Apparent density:

$$(\text{Pa}) = \frac{2.5 \text{ g}}{40 \text{ mL}} = 0.0625 \text{ g/mL}$$

Bulkiness:

$$1/\text{Pa} = \frac{1}{0.06265 (\text{g/mL})} = 16 \text{ mL/g}$$

Powders with a low apparent density and a large bulk volume are considered light, and those with a high apparent density and a small bulk volume are considered heavy. ■

- Sieving, in which particles are passed by mechanical shaking through a series of sieves of known and successively smaller size and the proportion of powder passing through or being withheld on each sieve is determined (range about 40 to 9,500 µm, depending upon sieve sizes) (2).
- Microscopy, in which sample particles are sized through the use of a calibrated grid background or other measuring device (range 0.2 to 100 µm).
- Sedimentation rate, in which particle size is determined by measuring the terminal settling velocity of particles through a liquid medium in a gravitational or centrifugal environment (range 0.8 to 300 µm). Stokes law allows calculation of particle size from sedimentation rate.
- Light energy diffraction or light scattering, in which particle size is determined by the reduction in light intensity reaching the sensor as the particle, dispersed in a liquid or gas, passes through the sensing zone (range 0.2 to 500 µm) (4). Laser scattering utilizes a He–Ne laser, silicon photo diode detectors, and an ultrasonic probe for particle dispersion (range 0.02 to 2,000 µm) (5).
- Laser holography, in which a pulsed laser is fired through an aerosolized particle spray and is photographed in three dimensions with a holographic camera, allowing the particles to be individually imaged and sized (range 1.4 to 100 µm) (6).
- Cascade impaction, which is based on the principle that a particle driven by an airstream will hit a surface in its path, provided its inertia is sufficient to overcome the drag force that tends to keep it in the airstream (7). Particles are separated into various size ranges by successively increasing the velocity of the airstream in which they are carried.
- Online methods for determining particle sizes during solid dosage form production are available (8).

These methods and others may be used for the analysis of particle size and shape. For some materials, a single method may be sufficient; however, a combination of methods is frequently preferred to provide greater certainty of size and shape parameters. Most commercial particle size analyzers are automated and linked with computers for data processing, distribution analysis, and printout.

The science of small particles is discussed further in Physical Pharmacy Capsule 6.1, Micromeritics. Physical Pharmacy Capsule 6.2, Particle Size Reduction, points out that a reduction in particle size increases the number of particles and the total surface area per gram of material.

PHYSICAL PHARMACY CAPSULE **6.2** Particle Size Reduction

Comminution, reduction of the particle size of a solid substance to a finer state, is used to facilitate crude drug extraction, increase the dissolution rates of a drug, aid in the formulation of pharmaceutically acceptable dosage forms, and enhance the absorption of drugs. The reduction in the particle size of a solid is accompanied by a great increase in the specific surface area of that substance. An example of the increase in the number of particles formed and the resulting surface area is as follows:

■ EXAMPLE

Increase in Number of Particles

If a powder consists of cubes 1 mm on edge and it is reduced to particles 10 mm on edge, what is the number of particles produced?

1. 1 mm equals 1,000 mm.
2. 1,000/10 mm = 100 pieces produced on each edge; that is, if the cube is sliced into 100 pieces on the X-axis, each 10 mm long, 100 pieces result.
3. If this is repeated on the Y- and Z-axes, the result is 100 × 100 × 100 = 1 million particles produced, each 10 mm on edge, for each original particle 1 mm on edge. This can also be written as $(10^2)^3 = 10^6$.

■ INCREASE IN SURFACE AREA

What increase in the surface area of the powder is produced by decreasing the particle size from 1 to 10 mm?

1. The 1-mm cube has six surfaces, each 1 mm on edge. Each face has a surface area of 1 mm^2. Because there are six faces, this is 6-mm^2 surface area per particle.
2. Each 10-mm cube has six surfaces, each 10 mm on edge. Each face has a surface area of 10 × 10 = 100 mm^2. Because there are six faces, this is 6 × 100 mm^2, or 600 mm^2 surface area per particle. Because 10^6 particles resulted from comminuting the 1-mm cube, each 10 mm on edge, the surface area now is 600 mm^2 × 10^6, or 6 × 10^8 mm^2.
3. To get everything in the same units for ease of comparison, convert the 6 × 10^8 mm^2 into square millimeters as follows.
4. Because there are 1,000 mm/mm, there must be 1,000^2, or 1 million mm^2/mm^2. This is more appropriately expressed as 10^6 mm^2,

$$\frac{6 \times 10^8 \, \mu m^2}{10^6 \, \mu m^2/mm^2} = 6 \times 10^2 \, mm^2$$

The surface areas have been increased from 6 to 600 mm^2 by the reduction in particle size of cubes 1 mm on edge to cubes 10 mm on edge, a 100-fold increase in surface area. This can have a significant increase in the rate of dissolution of a drug product. ■

Comminution of Drugs

On a small scale, the pharmacist reduces the size of chemical substances by grinding with a mortar and pestle. A finer grinding action is accomplished by using a mortar with a rough surface (as a porcelain mortar) than one with a smooth surface (as a glass mortar). Grinding a drug in a mortar to reduce its particle size is termed *trituration or comminution*. On a large scale, various types of mills and pulverizers may be used to reduce particle size. Figure 6.1 shows one such piece of equipment, a FitzMill comminuting machine with a product containment system. Rapidly moving blades in the comminuting chamber grind the material and particles fall through a screen into a collector when they have been reduced to the desired size dimension. The collection and containment system protects the environment from chemical dust, reduces product loss, and prevents product contamination.

Levigation is commonly used in small-scale preparation of ointments and suspensions to reduce the particle size and grittiness of the added powders. A mortar and pestle or an ointment tile may be used. A paste is formed by combining the powder and a small amount of liquid (the *levigating agent*) in which the powder is insoluble. The paste is then triturated, reducing the particle size. The levigated paste may then be added to the ointment base and the mixture made uniform and smooth by rubbing them together with a spatula on the ointment tile. A figure 8 track is commonly used to incorporate the materials. Mineral oil and glycerin are commonly used levigating agents.

FIGURE 6.1. Example of a FitzMill comminutor-sieve.

MIXING

Mixing is a unit operation involving the manipulation of a heterogeneous physical system with the goal of making it homogeneous. When two or more powdered substances are to be combined to form a "uniform" mixture, one must be aware of the characteristics of powders that affect blending, as follows:

Random Mixing

Generally, random mixing in compounding pharmacy involves a shuffling type unit operation process involving particle groups and even individual particles. Mixing is an energy-consuming process that produces a random distribution of particles. Some parameters affecting efficient mixing include the following:

1. Particle size, shape, density, cohesiveness, hygroscopicity, hardness, and size distribution
2. Mixer speed, time, batch quantity, and movement method
3. Segregation tendency of individual components based on density difference

Regarding mixtures, there are free-flowing mixtures, cohesive mixtures, and ordered mixtures.

Free-flowing mixtures suffer from the serious drawback of segregation of individual components during further processing in dosage form preparation. Particles can move easily and independently in a particular direction because of interparticulate forces. They should be handled with minimal shaking/bouncing, especially if not used immediately for filling capsules.

Cohesive mixtures are not free flowing; the individual agglomerates of particles must be repeatedly broken down

and allowed to redistribute within the system to ensure a satisfactorily mixed product. The extent of segregation may be less than that of free-flowing powders, but they will be more difficult to redistribute because of the formation of small agglomerates. Factors contributing to the formation of cohesive mixtures include moisture, electrostatic charges, Van der Waals forces, and solid bridges between the particles.

Mixing powders has gradually progressed from an empirical process to one that can be better controlled today to those that have an understanding of the dynamics of powder manipulation. What is desired is to move from Example 1 all the way to Example 4 and to maintain that distribution. However, something similar to Examples 2 and 3 generally results (X = drug; 0 = diluent).

Example 1	→	Example 2	→	Example 3	→	Example 4
00000000		X000XX00		XX0X00XX		X0X0X0X0
00000000		0XX000X0		0X00XX0X		0X0X0X0X
00000000		00X00XXX		00XX000X		X0X0X0X0
0000XXXX		00X0XX00		X000XX0X		0X0X0X0X
XXXXXXXX		00XXX0X0		X0XX000X		X0X0X0X0
XXXXXXXX		0XX0XX0X		0X00X0XX		0X0X0X0X
XXXXXXXX		XXXXX0X0		X00XX00X		X0X0X0X0

Examples 2 and 3 demonstrate why variation can occur when a powder blend is divided into individual doses. Actually, these variations can occur in the pharmaceutical industry as well as in extemporaneous compounding. This illustrates why it is important to have standard operating procedures for mixing steps in the pharmacy and they need to consider the different types of powdered ingredients and their characteristics.

Ordered Mixing

Ordered mixtures involve the mixing of a fine, micronized form with larger carrier particles. The small particles adhere tightly to the surface of the carrier particles. Ordered mixtures are formed by mechanical, adhesion, or coating forces so that the ordered unit consists of large particles and their associated adhered small particles that move as a unit within the mix. When particles of an ordered mix prepared with a water soluble carrier (e.g., mannitol or lactose) come into contact with water, the carrier dissolves and the active drug particles become surrounded with water and disperse as microscopic drug particles.

The concept of ordered mixing involves the mixing of small cohesive particles to a considerable degree of homogeneity. A basic principle is that fine particles will adhere, especially to larger particles; the adhesional forces involved may be electrostatic or surface tensional. In a random mix, each individual particle can move independently and randomly. In an ordered mix, the ordered "unit" moves as a whole, not the individual particles.

The surface area ratio, Rs, is a measurement of the quantity of particles of active drug that will adhere to the surfaces of the larger carrier particles, that is, the ratio of the projected surface of the adherent particles to the total external surface area of the carrier particles. The Rs value is defined as:

$$Rs = (API surface area covered on the carrier) / (Carrier total surface area)$$

An Rs = 1 is when the surface of the carrier particle is entirely covered with active drug particles. When the amount of active drug used is very high and the surface area is covered by a lot of the drug (the Rs value is high), then the dissolution rate is decreased.

The recommended value for dissolution rate enhancement is Rs ≤ 0.5. Generally, the dissolution rate decreases markedly at an Rs value as low as about 0.5 and that at values approaching or exceeding Rs = 1, the dissolution rate has decreased to such an extent that none of the advantages are realized. This is presumably because the surface particles prevent rapid penetration of the water to the underlying carrier substance and subsequent rapid dissolution.

The process of mixing cohesive, interacting particulate systems follows a "disorder to order" concept and probably occurs widely in actual systems. The requirements for ordered mixing are different from those required for random mixing. Ordered mixing requires larger carrier particle and smaller active drug particles.

If one of the constituents of a powder mix is added as a fine, often micronized form, then on mixing, the larger particles (carrier particles) may adsorb some of these very small particles on to active sites on their surface and these are held tenaciously. It is now recognized that ordered mixing is an important factor preventing the segregation of mixes of a drug with one or other of the direct compression bases. Ordered mixing is particularly useful in the manufacture of capsules and tablets containing potent materials because uniformity of mixture depends upon larger units, not smaller particles. The standard deviation of ordered mixtures tends to be very small.

Ordered mixing probably comes the closest to yielding the perfect mix and may be obtained by (*a*) mechanical means, (*b*) adhesion, and (*c*) coating. The major difference between the mechanical and adhesional and coated ordered mixing is the degree of force holding the ingredients in each type of the ordered units together.

Examples of "ordered" mixtures are dry blends of sucrose and antibiotics that can be reconstituted with water to provide antibiotic syrup formulations. Sorbitol can replace sucrose to prepare sucrose-free formulations for diabetic patients. During blending, a fine powder of an antibiotic is adsorbed onto the surface of coarse particles of sorbitol.

Another area where ordered mixtures are used is in powders for oral inhalation. These powders are most commonly binary ordered mixtures composed of micronized drugs and coarse carriers (often coarse lactose). One example is albuterol sulfate powder for oral inhalation. This product is a powdered mixture of microfine drug

(95% of particles having a diameter of 10 μm or less) and lactose and is contained in a hard gelatin capsule.

Preparation of ordered mixtures involves regular manufacturing/compounding equipment and methods. Particle size reduction to the desired size range for each of the ingredients is followed by blending processes for predetermined time periods to obtain an "ordered mixture." On a small scale, this may require up to 25 to 50 hours of mixing; on a larger scale, the time is decreased because of the mechanics involved and higher shear rates.

An illustration of an ordered mix would be as follows: when looking down on an individual, single carrier (0) particle with adhered smaller (x) particles cut in half (Example 1); next are complete particles looking at the carrier surface of an ordered mix with an Rs value of 0.25, 0.5, 0.75, and 1.0 (Examples 2 to 5).

Example 1	Example 2	Example 3	Example 4	Example 5
xxxxxxx	x000000x	x0x0x0x0	xxxx0xx0	xxxxxxxx
x000000x	0x0000x0	00xx00x0	0xxxxx0x	xxxxxxxx
x000000x	x000x000	x0x00x0	xxx00xxx	xxxxxxxx
x000000x	000x0x00	x00x0xx0	xx0xxx0x	xxxxxxxx
x000000x	0x00x000	0x00xx0x	0xxx0xxx	xxxxxxxx
x000000x	00x0000x	00xx00xx	0xx0xxxx	xxxxxxxx
x000000x	0x00x000	x00xx00x	xx0xxxx0	xxxxxxxx
xxxxxxx	0x0000x0	0x0x0x0x	00xxxxxx	xxxxxxxx

Example 1 shows the active drug particles adhered to the outer surface of the halved particle and the single carrier particle in the center. Example 2 contains a carrier particle that is 25% covered with active drug (x); Example 3 is 50% covered; Example 4 is 75% covered; and Example 5 is totally covered. Any additional drug would simply stack up on the already adhered particles or would remain free.

BLENDING/MIXING POWDERS

Manually

When two or more powdered substances are to be combined to form a uniform mixture, it is best to reduce the particle size of each powder individually before weighing and blending. Depending on the nature of the ingredients, the amount of powder, and the equipment, powders may be blended by spatulation, trituration, sifting, and tumbling.

Spatulation is blending small amounts of powders by movement of a spatula through them on a sheet of paper or an ointment tile. It is not suitable for large quantities of powders or for powders containing potent substances, because homogeneous blending is not as certain as other methods. Very little compression or compacting of the powder results from spatulation, which is especially suited to mixing solid substances that form *eutectic mixtures* (or liquefy) when in close and prolonged contact with one another (Table 6.2). To diminish contact, a powder prepared from such substances is commonly mixed in the presence of an

TABLE 6.2. Substances that Soften or Liquefy When Mixed

Acetanilide
Aminopyrine
Antipyrine
Aspirin
Benzocaine
Beta-naphthol
Camphor
Chloral hydrate
Lidocaine
Menthol
Phenacetin
Phenol
Phenyl salicylate
Prilocaine
Resorcinol
Salicylic acid
Thymol

inert diluent, such as light magnesium oxide or magnesium carbonate, to physically separate the troublesome agents.

Trituration may be employed both to comminute and to mix powders. If simple admixture is desired without the special need for comminution, the glass mortar is usually preferred. When a small amount of a potent substance is to be mixed with a large amount of diluent, the *geometric dilution* method is used to ensure the uniform distribution of the potent drug. This method is especially indicated when the potent substance and other ingredients are the same color and a visible sign of mixing is lacking. By this method, the potent drug is placed with an approximately equal volume of the diluent in a mortar and is mixed thoroughly by trituration. Then, a second portion of diluent equal in volume to the mixture is added and the trituration repeated. This process is continued by adding an equal volume of diluent to the powder mixture and repeating this until all of the diluent is incorporated. Some pharmacists add an inert colored powder to the diluent before mixing to permit visual inspection of the mixing process.

Powders may also be mixed by passing them through sifters like those used in the kitchen to sift flour. Sifting results in a light, fluffy product. This process is not acceptable for the incorporation of potent drugs into a diluent powder. Any process, like sifting, that generates airborne drug particles should be conducted in a dust containment hood to protect pharmacy personnel.

Another method of mixing powders is tumbling the powder in a rotating chamber. Special small-scale and large-scale motorized powder blenders mix powders by tumbling them (Figs. 6.2 to 6.5). Mixing by this process is thorough but time consuming. Such blenders are widely employed in industry, as are mixers that use motorized blades to blend powders in a large vessel.

FIGURE 6.2. Industrial-size solid-state processor or twin-shell blender used to mix solid particles. (Courtesy of Abbott Laboratories.)

Segregation is an undesirable separation of the different components of the blend. Segregation may occur by sifting or percolation, air entrapment (fluidization), and particle entrapment (dusting). Fine particles tend to sift or percolate through coarse particles and end up at the bottom of the container and actually "lift" the larger particles to the surface. Fine, aerated powders with differences in particle size or density may result in a striation pattern and may occur during powder transfer. Dusting occurs when the finer, lighter particles remain suspended in air longer and do not settle as quickly as the larger or denser particles. General guidelines to minimize or prevent segregation include (*a*) minimum number of transfer steps and drop heights; (*b*) control of dust generation; (*c*) control of fluidization of the powder; (*d*) slow fill/transfer rate; (*e*) appropriate venting; (*f*) use of a deflector, vane, or distributor; and (*g*) proper hopper design and operating valves (if present).

Mechanical

V-Blender: This method involves tumbling the powders in a rotating chamber designed to enhance the mixing process. Mixing by this process is thorough but can be time consuming; however, it can be done while performing other duties. The speed of the rotating chamber is such that the powders "tumble" over and over and do not

FIGURE 6.3. Ribbon blender used for mixing powders and preparing granulations. (Courtesy of ROSS Mixers.)

FIGURE 6.4. Laboratory-scale V-blender. (Courtesy of GlobePharma.)

simply slide down the side of the chamber. This type of blender is very widely used in industry on a large scale.

Triple V-Type Blender: This V-blender consists of three individual chambers attached to the blender power unit and allows up to three different blending processes to be conducted simultaneously.

Turbula Mixer: This blender is used to obtain a homogeneous mixing of powders with different specific weights and particle sizes. The powders can be mixed in their own closed container. The efficiency of this shaker–mixer is derived from the use of rotation, translation, and inversion. The mixing container is subjected to a three-dimensional movement that exposes the product to continuously changing, rhythmically pulsing motion.

As is evident, tumbling devices have numerous advantages. They are relatively easy to use, and the containers can, in some cases, be the ultimate dispensing container. These units revolve at about 40 rpm, which is about half the critical speed where the centrifugal force on the particles exceeds the pull of gravity so there are not complex

FIGURE 6.5. Laboratory-scale triple V-type blender. (Courtesy of GlobePharma.)

controls with which to adjust, etc. They do occupy approximately 4 to 9 sq ft of space on a workbench, but the benefits are many. The technology continues to evolve to produce uniform, homogenous mixtures of powders for dispensing or for additional processing. Demixing or powder segregation is related to particle size, particle density, drug–excipient interaction, and degree of agglomeration. The three primary mechanisms of segregation of powders involve percolation, vibration, and transportation.

Percolation can result from gravity causing small particles to move into voids between larger particles, because of large particle size differences.

Vibration causes small particles to move under the larger particles that are pushed to the surface and result in separation of differently sized particles.

Transportation of particle beds with the constant acceleration and deceleration results in separation. Similar changes occur when powders are poured in a pile. The heavier particles will roll to the outside, whereas the smaller particles locate in the center of the powder pile. The shape also is important during segregation.

Resonant Acoustic mixing technology uses low-frequency, high-intensity acoustic energy to create a uniform shear field throughout the entire mixing vessel, resulting in rapid fluidization (movement) and dispersion of the material. An oscillating mechanical driver creates motion in the mechanical system, which is then acoustically transferred to the material to be mixed; the system operates at resonance, and in this mode, there is a nearly complete exchange of energy between the mass elements and the spring elements in the mechanical system.

SPECIAL CONSIDERATIONS

Eutectics

Some powders may become sticky or pasty, or they may liquefy when mixed together, such as those listed in Table 6.2. To keep the powders dry, one can mix them with a bulky powder adsorbent such as light magnesium oxide or magnesium carbonate. Also, these powders should be triturated very lightly on a pill tile by using a spatula for mixing rather than a mortar and pestle. The latter will cause compression and make the problem worse. It may also be advisable to double wrap the papers. Mixing these powders with the bulky powders first and then performing a light blending can minimize the problem. Another approach is to first make the eutectic and then adsorb the paste or liquid that results onto a bulky powder. One also has the option of dispensing the ingredients separately. After preparation, the charts can be dispensed in a plastic bag.

Hygroscopic and Deliquescent Powders

Hygroscopic powders will absorb moisture from the air. Deliquescent powders will absorb moisture from the air to the extent that they will partially or wholly liquefy. These problems must be overcome for the powder to be acceptable

TABLE 6.3. Common Hygroscopic and Deliquescent Powders

Albuterol sulfate

Ammonium bromide

Ammonium chloride

Ammonium iodide

Aspartame

Bacitracin

Bismuth subnitrate

Calcium bromide

Calcium chloride

Carbomer

Carboxymethylcellulose sodium

Diphenhydramine HCl

Ephedrine sulfate

Histamine dihydrochloride

Hydrastine hydrochloride

Hydrastine sulfate

Hyoscyamine hydrobromide

Hyoscyamine sulfate

Hydroxyzine hydrochloride

Iron and ammonium citrate

Lithium bromide

Pepsin

Phenobarbital sodium

Physostigmine hydrobromide

Physostigmine hydrochloride

Physostigmine sulfate

Pilocarpine alkaloid

Potassium acetate

Potassium citrate

Sodium bromide

Sodium iodide

Sodium nitrate

Zinc chloride

TABLE 6.4. Common Efflorescent Powders

Alums

Atropine sulfate

Caffeine

Calcium lactate

Citric acid

Cocaine

Codeine

Codeine phosphate

Codeine sulfate

Ferrous sulfate

Morphine acetate

Quinine bisulfate

Quinine hydrobromide

Quinine hydrochloride

Scopolamine hydrobromide

Sodium acetate

Sodium carbonate (decahydrate)

Sodium phosphate

Strychnine sulfate

Terpin hydrate

to the patient and usable. The best approach is to dispense the ingredients in tight containers and incorporate a desiccant packet or capsule when necessary. The patient should be instructed to store the powder in a dry place in a tightly closed container. To lessen the extent of the problem, the compounding pharmacist can in some situations dilute the powder with an inert drying powder to reduce the amount of surface area exposed to the moisture. Common hygroscopic and deliquescent powders are listed in Table 6.3.

Efflorescent Powders

An *efflorescent powder* (Table 6.4) is a crystalline powder that contains water of hydration or crystallization. This water can be liberated either during manipulations or on exposure to a low-humidity environment. If this occurs, the powder will become sticky and pasty, or it may even liquefy. One approach to avoid this problem is to use an anhydrous salt form of the drug, keeping in mind the potency differential between its anhydrous form and its hydrated form. Another method is to include a drying bulky powder and to use a light, noncompacting method of mixing the powders.

Explosive Mixtures

Some combinations of powders (Table 6.5) may react violently when mixed together. Special precautions must be taken if it is necessary to prepare a formulation containing these mixtures.

Incorporation of Liquids

A liquid that is to be incorporated into a dry powder can be adsorbed onto an inert material (carrier) such as lactose or starch and then geometrically introduced into the bulk of the powder. Pasty material can be added to dry powder by mixing it with increasing quantities of the powder, which will dry out the paste. It is best to add some materials by preparing an alcoholic solution and spraying it evenly on the powder, which has been spread out on a pill tile. The alcohol, or another suitable solvent, should then be allowed to evaporate, leaving the ingredient uniformly dispersed. This method may be especially suitable for high-potency drugs or flavoring agents because it minimizes the possibility that clumps of active drug will develop in the powder blend.

TABLE 6.5. Common Oxidizing and Reducing Agents that May React Violently When Mixed

Oxidizing Agents	Reducing Agents
Bromine	Alcohol
Chlorates	Bisulfites
Chloric acid	Bromides
Chlorine	Charcoal
Chromates	Glycerin
Dichromates	Hydriodic acid
Ethyl nitrite spirit	Hypophosphites
Hydrogen peroxide	Hypophosphorous acid
Hypochlorites	Iodides
Hypochlorous acid	Lactose
Iodine	Nitrites (in some situations)
Nitrates	Organic substances (in general)
Nitric acid	Phosphorus
Nitrites	Sugar
Nitrohydrochloric acid	Sulfides
Nitrous acid	Sulfites
Perborates	Sulfur
Permanganates	Sulfurous acid
Permanganic acid	Tannic acid
Peroxides	Tannins
Potassium chlorate	Thiosulfates
Potassium dichromate	Volatile oils
Potassium nitrate	
Potassium permanganate	
Sodium peroxide	
Silver nitrate	
Silver oxide	
Silver salts	
Trinitrophenol	

▌ POWDERS AS A DOSAGE FORM

Some medicated powders are intended to be used internally and others, externally. Most powders for internal use are taken orally after mixing with water or in the case of infants in their infant formulas. Some powders are intended to be inhaled for local and systemic effects. Other dry powders are commercially packaged for constitution with a liquid solvent or vehicle, some for administration orally, others for use as an injection, and still others for use as a vaginal douche. Medicated powders for external use are dusted on the affected area from a sifter-type container or applied from a powder aerosol. Powders intended for external use should bear a label marked EXTERNAL USE ONLY or a similar label.

Medicated powders for oral use may be intended for local effects (e.g., laxatives) or systemic effects (e.g., analgesics) and may be preferred to counterpart tablets and capsules by patients who have difficulty swallowing solid dosage forms. The doses of some drugs are too bulky to be formed into tablets or capsules of convenient size, so they may be administered as powders. For administration, they can be mixed with a liquid or soft food. Powders taken orally for systemic use may be expected to result in faster rates of dissolution and absorption than solid dosage forms, because there is immediate contact with the gastric fluids; however, the actual advantage in terms of therapeutic response may be negligible or only minimal, depending on the drug release characteristics of the counterpart products. A primary disadvantage of the use of oral powders is the undesirable taste of the drug.

Some medications, notably antibiotics for children, are intended for oral administration as liquids but are relatively unstable in liquid form. They are provided to the pharmacist by the manufacturer as a dry powder or granule for constitution with a specified quantity of purified water at the time of dispensing. Under labeled conditions of storage, the resultant product remains stable for the prescribed period of use, generally up to 2 weeks. Example powders for oral administration include Benefiber, Goody's, and Questran. Sterile dry powders intended to be constituted with water or another suitable solvent prior to administration by injection are discussed in Chapter 15.

Composition

Properly prepared powders have a uniform, small particle size that has an elegant appearance. In general, powders are more stable than are liquid dosage forms and are rapidly soluble, enabling the drug to be absorbed quickly.

The properties of powders are related to the size and surface area of the particles. For example, large particles that are more dense tend to settle more rapidly than do small particles; particles that are more bulky will settle more slowly. This characteristic must be considered in mixing or storing and shipping, when powders of different particle size may become segregated. Another concern stems from the fact that powder dosage forms have a large surface area that is exposed to atmospheric conditions. Thus, powders should be dispensed in tight containers. Further, because powders of small particle size present a greater surface area to the atmosphere, they are more reactive in nature and can adsorb larger quantities of gases, such as carbon dioxide. However, if the powder has a smaller particle size, it can dissolve at a more rapid rate, unless adsorbed gases prevent the water from surrounding the individual particles and wetting them, thereby decreasing their wetting properties. An increase in surface free energy can increase the absolute solubility of the drug and have a positive effect on its bioequivalence.

Topical Powders

Topical powders should be free flowing and impalpable, that is, have a uniform, small particle size that will not irritate the skin when applied. Powders can be made impalpable by passing them through a No. 100-mesh or finer sieve. The powder should be prepared so that it adheres to the skin.

Highly sorptive powders should not be used for topical powders that are to be applied to oozing wounds, as a hard crust may form. A more hydrophobic, water-repellent powder will prevent loss of water from the skin and will not cake on the oozing surfaces. Talc, or any other naturally derived product that is to be used on open wounds, should first be sterilized to avoid an infection in the area.

Topical powders usually consist of a base or vehicle, such as cornstarch or talc; an adherent, such as magnesium stearate, calcium stearate, or zinc stearate, and possibly an active ingredient, along with an aromatic material. The powder should provide a large surface area, flow easily, and spread uniformly. The large surface area will aid in absorbing perspiration and give a cooling sensation to the skin. Examples include Zeasorb Super Absorbent, Gold Bond Body Powder, and WoundSeal Powder.

Insufflated Powders

Insufflated powders are finely divided powders that are intended to be applied in a body cavity, such as the ears, nose, vagina, tooth socket, or throat. When using an insufflator, or "puffer," the patient simply "puffs" the desired quantity of powder onto the affected area or into the cavity. This device is particularly appropriate for anti-infectives. Also, a moisture-activated adherent, such as Polyox, can be incorporated into the powder. Polyox is an ethylene oxide polymer with a high molecular weight that forms a viscous, mucoadhesive gel when in contact with moisture. The gel serves to provide a depot for long-term drug delivery spanning several hours.

Aerosol Powders

Some medicated powders are administered by inhalation with the aid of dry powder inhalers (DPIs), which deliver micronized particles of medication in metered quantities (Fig. 6.6). A DPI is a device used to administer an inhalation powder in a finely divided state suitable for oral inhalation by the patient. An inhalation powder is one used with a device that aerosolizes and delivers an accurately metered amount.

Most of these products are used in the treatment of asthma and other bronchial disorders that require distribution of medication deep in the lungs (Fig. 6.7). To accomplish this, the particle size of the micronized medication is prepared in the range of 1 to 6 μm in diameter. In addition to the therapeutic agent, these products contain inert propellants and pharmaceutical diluents, such as crystalline alpha-lactose monohydrate, to aid the formulation's flow properties and metering uniformity and to protect the powder from humidity (9). Powder blowers or insufflators (Fig. 6.8) may be used to deliver dry powders to various parts of the body, for example, the nose, throat, lung, and vagina. Depression of the device's rubber bulb causes turbulence of the powder in the vessel, forcing it out through the orifice in the tip.

FIGURE 6.6. Metered inhalation aerosol containing a micronized medicated powder and inert propellants. Each dose is delivered through the mouthpiece upon activation of the aerosol unit's valve.

Inhalation powders, commonly known as dry DPIs, consist of a mixture of APIs and typically the carrier; and all formulation components exist in a finely divided solid state packaged in a suitable container closure system. The dose is released from the packaging by a mechanism and is mobilized into a fine dispersion upon oral inhalation by the patient. The formulation may be packaged in premetered or device-metered units. Premetered DPIs contain a previously measured amount of formulation in individual units (e.g., capsules, blisters) that are inserted into the device before use. Premetered DPIs may also contain individual doses packaged in ordered multidose assemblies in the delivery system. Premetered DPIs include a mechanism designed to pierce the capsule or open the unit-dose container and allow mobilization and aerosolization of the powder by the patient inhaling through the integral mouthpiece. Device-metered DPIs have an internal reservoir that contains a

FIGURE 6.7. Relation of particle size to airway penetration. (Courtesy of Fisons Corporation.)

FIGURE 6.8. A general-purpose powder blower or insufflator. The powder is placed in the vessel. When the rubber bulb is depressed, internal turbulence disperses the powder and forces it from the orifice. Powders may be delivered to various body locations such as the nose, throat, tooth sockets, or skin. (Copyright © 2016 Medical Depot, Inc. dba Drive DeVilbiss Healthcare.)

sufficient quantity of formulation for multiple doses that are metered by the device during actuation by the patient. To facilitate dosing compliance, device-metered DPIs incorporate a dosing administration information mechanism, such as a dose counter or a dose indicator system.

Example Oral Inhalation Powders

Advair Diskus 100/50, 250/50, and 500/50 contains fluticasone propionate 100, 250, and 500 µg, respectively, along with salmeterol 50 µg in a powder for inhalation. Fluticasone propionate is a corticosteroid, and salmeterol xinafoate is a highly selective β_2-adrenergic bronchodilator. The Advair Diskus is a specially designed plastic device containing a double-foil blister strip of a powder formulation of fluticasone propionate and salmeterol xinafoate intended for oral inhalation only. Each blister in the device contains 100, 250, or 500 µg of microfine fluticasone propionate and 72.5 µg of microfine salmeterol xinafoate salt, the equivalent of 50 µg of salmeterol base, in 12.5 mg of formulation also containing lactose. Each blister contains one complete dose of medication. The blister is opened by activating the device, and the medication is dispersed into the airstream created by the patient inhaling through the mouthpiece (10).

Fluticasone propionate inhalation powder is available alone as Flovent Rotadisk 50, 100, and 250 µg marketed to be used with the Diskhaler inhalation device. Each double-foil Rotadisk contains four blisters; each blister contains 50, 100, or 250 µg of fluticasone propionate blended with lactose to a total weight of 25 mg per blister. When the Rotadisk is placed in the Diskhaler, a blister containing the medication is pierced, and the fluticasone propionate is dispersed into the airstream as with the Advair Diskus unit (11).

The Foradil Aerolizer is a capsule dosage form for oral inhalation only in the Aerolizer inhaler. The capsule contains a dry powder formulation of 12 µg of formoterol fumarate and 25 mg of lactose as a carrier. Formoterol fumarate is a long-acting selective β_2-adrenergic receptor agonist acting locally in the lung as a bronchodilator. To use this delivery system, the capsule is placed inside the well of the Aerolizer inhaler, and the capsule is pierced by pressing and releasing the buttons on the side of the device. The patient inhales rapidly and deeply through the mouthpiece, dispersing the formoterol fumarate formulation into the air for inhalation (12).

Zanamivir for inhalation (Relenza) is a neuraminidase inhibitor used to treat influenza. Relenza is packaged in Rotadisks and is administered using a Diskhaler, as previously described. For Relenza, the usual dose is two inhalations (one blister per inhalation) twice daily for 5 days; therefore, four blisters will be used each day. Relenza should be stored at room temperature; it is not a childproof container (13).

Bulk and Divided Powders

Medicated powders may be provided to the patient in bulk or may be divided into unit-of-use packages. Some powders are packaged by manufacturers, whereas others are prepared and packaged by the pharmacist.

Bulk Powders

Among the bulk powders available in prepackaged amounts are (*a*) antacids (e.g., sodium bicarbonate) and laxatives (e.g., psyllium [Metamucil]), which the patient takes by mixing with water or another beverages before swallowing; (*b*) douche powders (e.g., Massengill powder), dissolved in warm water by the patient for vaginal use; (*c*) medicated powders for external application to the skin, usually topical anti-infectives (e.g., bacitracin zinc and polymyxin B sulfate) or antifungals (e.g., tolnaftate); and (*d*) brewer's yeast powder containing B-complex vitamins and other nutritional supplements. In some cases, a small measuring scoop, spoon, or other device is dispensed with the powder for measuring the dose of the drug.

Dispensing powder medication in bulk quantities is limited to nonpotent substances. Powders containing substances that should be administered in controlled dosage are supplied to the patient in divided amounts in folded papers or packets. Patients should be educated about appropriate handling, storage, measurement, and preparation of bulk powder prescription and nonprescription products in addition to the customary counseling at the time of dispensing or purchase. Generally, these products are stored at room temperature in a clean, dry place. These products should be kept out of the reach of children and animals. Patients should be instructed how to measure the appropriate amount of the powder and be told the type of liquid or vehicle to use to deliver the medication consistent with package and/or physician instructions.

Divided Powders

After a powder has been properly blended (using the geometric dilution method for potent substances), it may be divided into individual dosing units based on the amount to be taken or used at a single time. Each divided portion of powder may be placed on a small piece of paper (Latin *chartula*; abbrev. chart.; powder paper) that is folded to enclose the medication. A number of commercially prepared premeasured products are available in folded papers or packets, including headache powders (e.g., BC powders), powdered laxatives (e.g., psyllium mucilloid, cholestyramine resin), and douche powders (e.g., Massengill powder packets).

Divided powders may be prepared by the pharmacist as follows. Depending on the potency of the drug substance, the pharmacist decides whether to weigh each portion of powder separately before enfolding in a paper or to approximate each portion by using the block-and-divide method. By the latter method, used only for nonpotent drugs, the pharmacist places the entire amount of the prepared powder on a flat surface such as a porcelain or glass plate, pill tile, or large sheet of paper and, with a large spatula, forms a rectangular or square block of the powder having a uniform depth. Then, using the spatula, the pharmacist cuts into the powder lengthwise and crosswise to delineate the appropriate number of smaller, uniform blocks, each representing a dose or unit of medication. Each of the smaller blocks is separated from the main block with the spatula, transferred to a powder paper, and wrapped.

The powder papers may be of any size convenient to hold the amount of powder required, but the most popular commercially available sizes are 2.75 × 3.75 inch, 3 × 4.5 inch, 3.75 × 5 inch, and 4.5 × 6 inch. The papers may be (*a*) simple bond paper; (*b*) vegetable parchment, a thin, semiopaque paper with limited moisture resistance; (*c*) glassine, a glazed, transparent paper, also with limited moisture resistance; and (*d*) waxed paper, a transparent waterproof paper. The selection of the type of paper is based primarily on the nature of the powder. If the powder contains hygroscopic or deliquescent materials, waterproof or waxed paper should be used. In practice, such powders are double wrapped in waxed paper, and then for esthetic appeal, they are wrapped in bond paper. Glassine and vegetable parchment papers may be used when only a limited barrier against moisture is necessary. Powders containing volatile components should be wrapped in waxed or glassine papers. Powders containing neither volatile components nor ingredients adversely affected by air or moisture are usually wrapped in a white bond paper.

A certain degree of expertise is required in the folding of a powder paper, and practice is required for proficiency. For the technique and details of folding powder papers, see the ninth edition of this text.

Today, compounded powder papers are rarely used on an outpatient, community practice basis. Their use is usually limited to institutional and research practice. Commercial drug products that are provided in this drug delivery form include polyethylene glycol 3350 (i.e., Mira-LAX), cholestyramine resin, pectin, L-glutamine, sodium phenylbutyrate, and wheat dextrin (i.e., Benefiber).

GRANULES

Granules are defined as a dosage form composed of dry aggregates of powder particles that may contain one or more APIs, with or without other ingredients. They may be swallowed as such, dispersed in food, or dissolved in water. Granules are frequently compacted into tablets or filled into capsules, with or without additional ingredients.

As indicated previously, *granules* are prepared agglomerates of smaller particles of powder. They are irregularly shaped but may be prepared to be spherical. They are usually in the 4- to 12-mesh sieve size range, although granules of various mesh sizes may be prepared depending upon their application.

Granules are prepared by wet methods and dry methods. There have been numerous technical innovations in wet granulation including steam granulation, moisture-activated dry granulation or moist granulation, thermal adhesion granulation, melt granulation, freeze granulation, foamed binder or foam granulation, and reverse wet granulation.

A common and basic wet method is to moisten the powder or powder mixture and then pass the resulting paste through a screen of the mesh size to produce the desired size of granules. The granules are placed on drying trays and are dried by air or under heat. The granules are periodically moved about on the drying trays to prevent adhesion into a large mass. Another type of wet method is fluid bed processing, in which particles are placed in a conical piece of equipment and are vigorously dispersed and suspended while a liquid excipient is sprayed on the particles and the product dried, forming granules or pellets of defined particle size (Figs. 6.9 and 6.10).

The dry granulation method may be performed in a couple of ways. By one method, the dry powder is passed through a roll compactor and then through a granulating machine (Fig. 6.11). A roll compactor, also called a roll press or roller compactor, processes a fine powder into dense sheets or forms by forcing it through two mechanically rotating metal rolls running counter to each other (10).

FIGURE 6.9. Granule prepared with fluid bed technology. (Courtesy of Glatt Air Techniques.)

FIGURE 6.10. Large oven for drying granulations. (Courtesy of O'Hara Technologies.)

The surface of the compacting rolls may be smooth or may have pocket indentations or corrugations that allow compaction of different forms and textures. The compacted powder is granulated to uniform particle size in a mechanical granulator. Powder compactors are generally combined in sequence in integrated compactor–granulation systems.

An alternative dry method, termed slugging, is the compression of a powder or powder mixture into large tablets or slugs on a compressing machine under 8,000 to 12,000 lb of pressure, depending on the physical characteristics of the powder. The slugs are generally flat faced and are about 2.5 cm (1 inch) in diameter (14). The slugs are granulated into the desired particle size, generally for use in the production of tablets. The dry process often results in the production of fines, that is, powder that has not agglomerated into granules. These fines are separated, collected, and reprocessed. The wet and dry granulation methods as they pertain to tablet making are discussed in greater detail in Chapter 8.

FIGURE 6.11. High-speed granulator–mixer. (Courtesy of Dmitry Kalinovsky/Shutterstock.)

Granules flow well compared to powders. For comparison, consider the pouring and flowing characteristics of granulated sugar and powdered sugar. Because of their flow properties, granulations are commonly used in tablet making to facilitate the free flow of material from the feeding container (or hopper) into the tablet presses.

Granules have other important characteristics. Because their surface area is less than that of a comparable volume of powder, granules are usually more stable to the effects of atmospheric humidity and are less likely to cake or harden upon standing. Granules also are more easily wetted by liquids than are certain light and fluffy powders (which tend to float on the surface) and are often preferred for dry products intended to be constituted into solutions or suspensions.

A number of commercial products containing antibiotic drugs that are unstable in aqueous solution are prepared as small granules for constitution by the pharmacist with purified water just prior to dispensing. The granules are prepared to contain not only the medicinal agent but also colorants, flavorants, and other pharmaceutical ingredients. Upon constitution, the resultant liquid has all of the desired medicinal and pharmaceutical features of a liquid pharmaceutical. Examples include Biaxin granules for oral suspension (clarithromycin, Abbott), Omnicef for oral suspension (cefdinir, Abbott), Augmentin ES-600 (amoxicillin/clavulanate potassium, GlaxoSmithKline), and Ceftin for oral suspension (cefuroxime axetil, GlaxoSmithKline).

Other types of granulated commercial products include Lactinex granules, a mixed culture of *Lactobacillus acidophilus* and *Lactobacillus bulgaricus* in 1-g packets used in the treatment of uncomplicated diarrhea and diarrhea due to antibiotic therapy. The granules are measured and mixed with water or other beverages, sprinkled on food, or eaten plain. Granulations of effervescent products may be compressed into tablet form, as Zantac EFFERdose tablets (GlaxoSmithKline). Effervescent granules and tablets are dissolved in water before use. The preparation of effervescent granulated salts is as follows.

Granular dosage forms are also used in veterinary medicine where they may be placed on top of or mixed with an animal's food. They are frequently provided with a measuring device to allow addition to feeds. The resultant mix facilitates dosing.

Effervescent Granulated Salts

An effervescent dosage form, frequently tablets or granules, contains ingredients that, when in contact with water, rapidly release carbon dioxide. The dosage form is dissolved or dispersed in water to initiate the effervescence prior to ingestion.

Effervescent salts are granules or coarse to very coarse powders containing a medicinal agent in a dry mixture usually composed of sodium bicarbonate, citric acid, and tartaric acid. When added to water, the acids and the base react to liberate carbon dioxide, resulting in effervescence. The resulting carbonated solution masks undesirable taste of any medicinal agent. Using granules or coarse particles of the mixed powders rather than small powder particles decreases the rate of solution and prevents violent and uncontrollable effervescence. Sudden and rapid effervescence could overflow the glass and leave little residual carbonation in the solution.

Using a combination of citric and tartaric acids rather than either acid alone avoids certain difficulties. When tartaric acid is used as the sole acid, the resulting granules readily lose their firmness and crumble. Citric acid alone results in a sticky mixture difficult to granulate.

A summary of the chemistry of effervescent granules may be found in Physical Pharmacy Capsule 6.3, Effervescent Granules.

Effervescent granules are prepared by two general methods: (*a*) the dry or fusion method and (*b*) the wet method.

PHYSICAL PHARMACY CAPSULE **6.3** Effervescent Granules

Granules are dosage forms that consist of particles ranging from about 4 to 10 mesh in size (4.76 to 2.00 mm), formed by moistening blended powders and passing through a screen or a special granulator. These moist granules are either air- or oven-dried. A special form of granules can be used to provide a pleasant vehicle for selected drug products, especially those with a bitter or salty taste. This special formulation, an effervescent granule, may consist of mixtures of citric acid and/or tartaric acid and/or sodium biphosphate combined with sodium bicarbonate.

■ EXAMPLE

R_x	
Active drug	500 mg/5 g tsp
In effervescent granule qs	120 g
Sig: Dissolve 1 teaspoonful in one-half glass of cool water, and drink. Repeat this every 8 hours.	

It is desired to dispense this as a granule, so that the patient will measure out a teaspoonful (5 g) dose, mix, and administer. Because each dose weighs 5 g and the prescription consists of 120 g, there are 24 doses. Each dose contains 0.5 g of the active drug, which comes to 12 g of the active drug for the entire prescription. This requires 120 g − 12 g = 108 g of effervescent vehicle. A good effervescent blend consists of both citric acid and tartaric acid (1:2 ratio), because the former is rather sticky and the latter produces a chalky, friable granule. It is necessary to calculate the amount of each ingredient required to prepare 108 g of the granulation.

■ CITRIC ACID

$$\underset{3\times84}{3NaHCO_3} + \underset{210}{C_6H_8O_7 \cdot H_2O} \rightarrow 4H_2O + 3CO_2 + Na_3C_6H_5O_7$$

Citric acid 1 g of citric acid (MW 210) reacts with 1.2 g of sodium bicarbonate (MW 84) as obtained from the following:

$$\frac{1}{210} = \frac{x}{3\times84}$$
$$x = 1.2\,g$$

■ TARTARIC ACID

$$\underset{2\times84}{2NaHCO_3} + \underset{150}{C_4H_6O_6} \rightarrow 2H_2O + 2CO_2 + Na_2C_4H_4O_6$$

Because it is desired to use a 1:2 ratio of citric acid to tartaric acid, 2 g (MW = 150) of tartaric acid reacts with sodium 2.24 g of bicarbonate according to the following calculation:

$$\frac{2}{150} = \frac{x}{2}\times84$$
$$x = 2.24\,g$$

(continued)

PHYSICAL PHARMACY CAPSULE **6.3** Effervescent Granules *(continued)*

Therefore, 1.2 g and 2.24 g of sodium bicarbonate are required to react with 1 + 2 g of the combination of citric acid and tartaric acid. Because it is desired to leave a small amount of the acids unreacted to enhance palatability and taste, of the required 3.44 g (2.24 g + 1.2 g), only 3.4 g of sodium bicarbonate will be used.

Therefore, the ratio of the effervescent ingredients is 1:2:3.4 for the citric acid/tartaric acid/sodium bicarbonate. Because the prescription requires 108 g of the effervescent mix, the quantity of each ingredient can be calculated as follows:

1 + 2 + 3.4 = 6.4
1/6.4 × 108 g = 16.875 g of citric acid
2/6.4 × 108 g = 33.750 g of tartaric acid
3.4/6.4 × 108 g = 57.375 g of sodium bicarbonate
Total = 108 g

The prescription will require 12 g of the active drug and 108 g of this effervescent vehicle.

$$d_{av} = \frac{\Sigma nd}{\Sigma n} = \frac{36,850}{355} = 103.8 \mu m \quad \blacksquare$$

Dry or Fusion Method

In the fusion method, the one molecule of water present in each molecule of citric acid acts as the binding agent for the powder mixture. Before mixing the powders, the citric acid crystals are powdered and then mixed with the other powders of the same sieve size to ensure uniformity of the mixture. The sieves and the mixing equipment should be made of stainless steel or other material resistant to the effect of the acids. The mixing of the powders is performed as rapidly as is practical, preferably in an environment of low humidity to avoid absorption of moisture and a premature chemical reaction. After mixing, the powder is placed on a suitable dish in an oven at 34°C to 40°C. During the heating process, an acid-resistant spatula is used to turn the powder. The heat releases the water of crystallization from the citric acid, which, in turn, dissolves a portion of the powder mixture, setting the chemical reaction and consequently releasing some carbon dioxide. This causes the softened mass of powder to become somewhat spongy, and when it has reached the proper consistency (as bread dough), it is removed from the oven and rubbed through a sieve to produce granules of the desired size. A No. 4 sieve produces large granules, a No. 8 sieve prepares medium-size granules, and a No. 10 sieve prepares small granules. The granules are dried at a temperature not exceeding 54°C and are immediately placed in containers and tightly sealed.

Wet Method

The wet method differs from the fusion method in that the source of binding agent is not the water of crystallization from the citric acid but the water added to alcohol as the moistening agent, forming the pliable mass for granulation. In this method, all of the powders may be anhydrous as long as water is added to the moistening liquid. Just enough liquid is added (in portions) to prepare a mass of proper consistency; then the granules are prepared and dried in the same manner as previously described.

▌ QUALITY CONTROL

Bulk Powders

The pharmacist should compare the final weight of the preparation with the theoretical weight. The powder should be examined for uniformity of color, particle size, flowability, and freedom from caking.

Divided Powders

For divided powders, the pharmacist should individually weigh the divided papers and then compare that weight with the theoretical weight. The packets should be checked to confirm uniformity.

▌ PACKAGING/DISPENSING

The powder mixture is packaged according to its use. Bulk oral powders can be packaged in glass, plastic, metal, or other containers that have a wide mouth to allow use of the powder measure. Divided powders, or powder papers, must be individually folded. Topical powders can be poured into sifter-top containers or powder shakers, and insufflations can be filled into plastic puffer units.

Granules for reconstitution may be packaged in unit-of-use containers or in containers with sufficient quantities to accommodate a typical course of therapy (frequently 10 days to 2 weeks with antibiotic products). Packaging should provide suitable protection from moisture; this is particularly true for effervescent granules. Granules may be stored under controlled room temperature conditions unless other conditions are specifically noted. Many granule products specify refrigerated storage following reconstitution and direct the patient to discard unused contents after a specified date that is based on the stability of the API in the reconstituted preparation.

Effervescent granules (and tablets) are to be labeled to indicate they are not be swallowed directly. Reconstitution of granules must ensure complete wetting of all ingredients and sufficient time and agitation to allow the soluble components to dissolve. Specific instructions for reconstitution provided by the manufacturer should be carefully followed.

| PATIENT COUNSELING |

POWDERS FOR RECONSTITUTION

(for suspensions) should be thoroughly mixed or shaken before use to resuspend the dispersed particulates. This is especially true of suspension preparations dosed from multiple-dose containers. For particularly viscous suspensions prone to air entrapment, instructions may advise the user how to shake the preparation to resuspend settled particles while minimizing air entrapment.

Counseling information for powders for reconstitution should include

1. Storage requirements according to the product label
2. Shake well or mix gently, as required, and
3. Discontinue after _____ date.

BULK ORAL POWDERS

Explain and demonstrate the exact technique for measuring the dose to be administered and the proper mode of administration.

- Should the powder be mixed with a liquid? If so, what liquid?
- Can it be premixed and stored for a day? A week?
- What happens if some water drops into the package containing the powder?
- Can the powder be mixed with food(s)? If so, which foods? Hot or cold?

BULK TOPICAL POWDERS

Explain and demonstrate the quantity of powder to apply and whether or not rubbing or patting the powder is recommended. Also, what to do if much of the powder falls off the skin?

Discuss patient safety and how to apply the powder in areas where children may be playing.

Discuss whether or not the skin needs to be dry and what to do if the skin is sweaty?

Keep container tightly closed and store it in the least humid environment available at room temperature.

PHARMACEUTICS CASE STUDY

SUBJECTIVE INFORMATION

A pharmaceutical manufacturer is planning to market a topical powder consisting of an antifungal agent in an inert powder vehicle. However, in the pilot plant scale-up, assay of the containers revealed that they did not have a uniform potency of the antifungal active ingredient. The current USP-NF monograph for a typical antifungal topical powder states that it is to contain not less than 90.0% and not more than 110.0% of the labeled amount of the active drug. This problem must be corrected before the product can proceed to full-scale manufacturing.

OBJECTIVE INFORMATION

The antifungal occurs as a white or nearly white crystalline powder with not more than a slight odor. It is only very slightly soluble in water and in ether and slightly soluble in alcohol. It has a true density in the range of 4.5 to 5.0 g/mL and an apparent density of 0.12 g/mL. It was sifted through a 40-mesh screen prior to blending.

The inert vehicle is talc that occurs as a very fine white or grayish-white crystalline powder. It is unctuous, adheres readily to the skin, and is free of grittiness. It is practically insoluble in dilute acids and alkalis, organic solvents, and water. It has a true density in the range of 2.7 to 2.8 and an apparent density of 0.05 g/mL. It has a specific surface area of 2.41 to 2.42 m²/g.

The powders are weighed and blended in a large V-blender. The powder is then moved to the hopper of a large packaging device. The machine vibrates significantly during packaging.

ASSESSMENT

It appears that the difference in the size and density of the two ingredients is sufficient to suggest a separation in the hopper of the packaging machine. The density of the antifungal is greater than that of the vehicle, and the particle size of the antifungal (40 mesh) is larger than that of the talc (very fine, ~ an 80-mesh powder). One would normally expect the finer powder to settle to the bottom, but because there is a difference in the density of these two powders, the antifungal appears to be settling. This would result in containers that would have varying amounts of the active drug.

PLAN

One approach to solving this problem is to reduce the particle size of the antifungal agent to be closer to that of the talc so their apparent densities are closer. Another possibility is to use a different packaging device with minimal vibration. Can you think of other reasonable approaches to solving this problem? ∎

CLINICAL CASE STUDY

SUBJECTIVE INFORMATION

CC: E.M. is an 86-year-old adult ambulatory male (AAM) who resides in a nursing home with complaints of pain in his right heel.

PMH:	HTN
	Hyperlipidemia
	Type II diabetes
Meds:	Hydrochlorothiazide 50 mg po q AM
	Enalapril 5 mg po bid
	Atorvastatin 10 mg po qhs
	Metformin 1,000 mg po bid
	Glyburide 5 mg po qd
	ASA 81 mg po qd
	Centrum 1 tablet po qd
PSH:	Tonsillectomy at age 10
FH:	Mother HTN, breast cancer, metastatic bone cancer
	Father hyperlipidemia, type II diabetes
SH:	(per KF)
	(–) Tobacco
	(–) EtOH
	(–) Illicit drugs
	(–) Caffeine
ALL:	NKDA

OBJECTIVE INFORMATION

BP: 125/78
HR: 72
Ht: 5'7"
Wt: 230 lb

Wound with a high volume of yellow slough and exudate on right heel area

ASSESSMENT

Decubitus ulcer

PLAN

Recommend Debrisan (dextranomer) beads twice a day. Sprinkle the beads onto the ulcer to 3-mm (~0.1-inch) thickness. To prevent maceration, apply a nonocclusive dressing, and seal on all four sides. Remove the beads before they become fully saturated by irrigating the wound with sterile water or normal saline using a syringe. Apply a new layer of beads while the area is still moist to prevent pain. Change the dressing before the beads become fully saturated. The number of changes per day will depend on the amount of exudate produced and will vary from one to three times a day. Also, it is suggested that for easier removal, the dressing be changed before it is completely dry. Avoid contact with the eyes. Contact the physician if the condition worsens or persists beyond 14 to 21 days. The patient's position should be frequently changed to prevent continuous pressure on any single part of the body. Avoid positioning the patient on the right heel. ■

APPLYING THE PRINCIPLES AND CONCEPTS

GROUP ACTIVITIES

1. Create a listing of oral prescription antibiotic products, including concentration of active ingredient(s), prepared as small powders for reconstitution.
2. Create a listing of oral nonprescription products, including concentration of active ingredient(s), prepared as small granules or powders for reconstitution by the consumer.
3. Locate a compounding formulation for a powder dosage form, and, using appropriate pharmaceutics terms (i.e., comminute, levigate, spatulate, powder, particle size), describe the steps in its preparation.
4. Create a listing of 10 prescription drug products, including concentration of active ingredient(s) and suggested dosage regimen, which are available as encapsulated granules that when opened can be added to food or drink prior to administration.

List three counseling points the pharmacist should provide the patient (or caregiver) when using these products.
5. Make a listing of conceivable ways a consumer/patient may misuse a medicated powder.

INDIVIDUAL ACTIVITIES

1. In layman's terms, explain the proper administration of a metered inhalation aerosol containing a micronized medicated powder with inert ingredients.
2. Give examples of situations where pharmacists will use spatulation, trituration, and levigation techniques in the practice of pharmacy.
3. List counseling points to discuss with a patient who has trouble swallowing and is picking up a prescription for Celebrex. Discuss the potential application of the Pill Glide for the patient.

4. Create a listing of 10 prescription medications, including concentration of active ingredient(s) and suggested dosage regimen, prepared as small granules for reconstitution, and discuss the demographics of patients most likely to utilize this dosage form.

5. Describe drawbacks associated with the use of topical powder dosage forms, and provide examples of other dosage forms that would overcome these drawbacks.

REFERENCES

1. Brittain HG. On the physical characterization of pharmaceutical solids. Pharm Technol 1997;21:100–108.
2. The United States Pharmacopeia–National Formulary. Current Ed. Rockville, MD: U.S. Pharmacopeial Convention.
3. Yalkowsky SH, Bolton S. Particle size and content uniformity. Pharm Res 1990;7:962–966.
4. Jager PD, DeStefano GA, McNamara DP. Particle-size measurement using right-angle light scattering. Pharm Technol 1993;17:102–110.
5. http://www.horiba.com/cz/scientific/products/particle-characterization/particle-size-analysis/details/la-960-laser-particle-size-analyzer-20235/. (Accessed July 23, 2020).
6. Gorman WG, Carroll FA. Aerosol particle-size determination using laser holography. Pharm Technol 1993;17:34–37.
7. Milosovich SM. Particle-size determination via cascade impaction. Pharm Technol 1992;16:82–86.
8. Närvänen T, Seppälä K, Antikainen O, et al. A new rapid on-line imaging method to determine particle size distribution of granules. AAPS Pharm Sci Tech 2008;9(1):282–287.
9. Hindle M, Byron PR. Size distribution control of raw materials for dry-powder inhalers using aerosizer with aero-dispenser. Pharm Technol 1995;19:64–78.
10. https://www.rxlist.com/advair-hfa-drug.htm. (Accessed July 23, 2020)
11. https://www.rxlist.com/flovent-drug.htm. (Accessed July 23, 2020)
12. https://www.rxlist.com/foradil-drug.htm. (Accessed July 23, 2020)
13. https://www.rxlist.com/relenza-drug.htm. (Accessed July 23, 2020)
14. Miller RW. Roller compaction technology. In: Parikh DM, ed. Handbook of Pharmaceutical Granulation Technology. New York, NY: Marcel Dekker, 1997:100–150.

7 Capsules

OBJECTIVES

After reading this chapter, the student will be able to:

   Differentiate between hard gelatin and soft gelatin capsules

   Compare and contrast advantages and disadvantages of hard gelatin and soft gelatin capsules

   List categories of inert ingredients, with examples, which are employed in the compounding or manufacture of capsules

   State USP compendial requirements for capsules

   Define and differentiate weight variation from content uniformity

   Describe appropriate techniques for compounding, inspecting, packaging, and storing capsules

▌ INTRODUCTION

When medications are to be administered orally to adults, capsules and tablets usually are preferred because they are conveniently carried, readily identified, and easily taken.

Consider the convenience of a patient carrying a day's, a week's, or a month's supply of capsules or tablets compared with equivalent doses of a liquid medication. With capsules and tablets, there is no need for spoons or other measuring devices, which may be inconvenient and may result in less than accurate dosing. Also, most capsules and tablets are tasteless when swallowed, which is not the case with oral liquid medication.

Numerous characteristics help to identify capsules and tablets, including the shapes and colors of capsules and tablets and the manufacturer's name and product code number commonly embossed or imprinted on their surface making them readily identifiable. This enhances communication between the patient and health care providers, assists patient compliance, and fosters safe and effective medication use.

Capsules and tablets are available for many medications in a variety of dosage strengths, providing flexibility

to the prescriber and accurate individualized dosage for the patient.

From a pharmaceutical standpoint, solid dosage forms are efficiently and productively manufactured; they are packaged and shipped by manufacturers at lower cost and with less breakage than comparable liquid forms. They are also more stable and have a longer shelf life than do their liquid counterparts.

As discussed later in this chapter, the pharmacist often uses empty hard gelatin capsules for extemporaneous compounding of prescriptions. On occasion, a pharmacist may use commercially available capsules and tablets as the *source* of a medicinal agent when it is not otherwise available. In these instances, the pharmacist must consider any excipients in the commercial product to ensure compatibility with the other ingredients in the compounded prescription. Capsules and tablets designed to provide modified drug release are discussed in Chapter 9.

Dosage forms that must be left intact include enteric-coated tablets, designed to pass through the stomach for drug release and absorption in the intestine; most extended-release dosage forms, designed to provide prolonged release of the medication; and sublingual or buccal tablets, formulated to dissolve under the tongue or in the mouth (1). If the patient cannot swallow an intact solid dosage form, an alternative product, such as a chewable tablet, instant dissolving tablet, oral liquid, oral or nasal inhalation solution, suppository, or injection, may be employed.

OVERVIEW OF CAPSULES

Capsules are solid dosage forms in which medicinal agents and/or inert substances are enclosed in a small shell of gelatin. Gelatin capsule shells may be *hard* or *soft*, depending on their composition. The shells may be composed of two pieces, a body and a cap, or they may be composed of a single piece. Two-piece capsules are commonly referred to as hard-shell capsules, and one-piece capsules are often referred to as soft-shell capsules. Most capsules are designed for oral administration. When no deliberate effort has been made to modify the API release rate, they are referred to as immediate release.

Most filled capsules are intended to be swallowed whole. However, it is fairly common in hospitals and extended care facilities for a caregiver to open capsules or crush tablets to mix with food or drink, especially for children or other patients unable to swallow solid dosage forms. This should be done only with the concurrence of the pharmacist, because the drug-release characteristics of certain dosage forms can be altered and can adversely affect the patient's welfare.

HARD GELATIN CAPSULES

Hard gelatin capsule shells are used in most commercial medicated capsules. They are also commonly employed in clinical drug trials to compare the effects of an investigational drug with those of another drug product or placebo. The community pharmacist also uses hard gelatin capsules in the extemporaneous compounding of prescriptions. The empty capsule shells are made of gelatin, sugar, and water (Fig. 7.1). As such, they can be clear, colorless, and essentially tasteless. They may be colored with

various FD&C and D&C dyes and made opaque by adding agents such as titanium dioxide. Most commercially available medicated capsules contain combinations of colorants and opaquants to make them distinctive, many with caps and bodies of different colors.

There are also vegetarian capsules which are cellulose-based and not made from animal by-products for vegetarian and vegan consumers. Vegetarian capsules have no known potential health risks and generally consist of hydroxypropyl methylcellulose (HPMC) and purified water. They contain no preservatives, gelatin, wheat, animal by-products or starch and are usually made from pure cellulose of either pine or poplar. They are fast dissolving and easily digestible as well as Kosher and Halal certified, GMO free, gluten free, and contain no preservatives.

There are also special capsule shells available for liquid fills, inhalation powders, hygroscopic drug fills as well as sodium lauryl sulfate-free capsules and opaque white capsules produced without titanium dioxide.

Gelatin is obtained by the partial hydrolysis of collagen obtained from the skin, white connective tissue, and bones of animals. In commerce, it is available in the form of a fine powder, a coarse powder, shreds, flakes, or sheets.

Gelatin is stable in air when dry but is subject to microbial decomposition when it becomes moist. Normally, hard gelatin capsules contain 13% to 16% of moisture (2). However, if stored in an environment of high humidity, additional moisture is absorbed by the capsules, and they may become distorted and lose their rigid shape. In an environment of extreme dryness, some of the moisture normally present in the gelatin capsules is lost, and the capsules may become brittle and crumble when handled. Therefore, it is desirable to maintain hard gelatin capsules in an environment free from excessive humidity or dryness.

Because moisture may be absorbed by gelatin capsules and may affect hygroscopic agents within, many capsules are packaged along with a small packet or cylinder of a desiccant material to protect against the absorption of atmospheric moisture. The desiccant materials most often used are dried silica gel, clay, and activated charcoal.

FIGURE 7.1. Diagram of a hard gelatin capsule manufacturing process.

Prolonged exposure to high humidity can affect in vitro capsule dissolution. Such changes have been observed in capsules containing tetracycline, chloramphenicol, and nitrofurantoin (3). Because such changes could forewarn of possible changes in bioavailability, capsules subjected to such stress conditions must be evaluated case by case (3).

Although gelatin is insoluble, it does soften in cold water through the absorption of water up to 10 times its weight of water. Some patients prefer to swallow a capsule wetted with water or saliva because a wetted capsule slides down the throat more readily than does a dry capsule. Gelatin is soluble in hot water and in warm gastric fluid; a gelatin capsule rapidly dissolves and exposes its contents. Gelatin, being a protein, is digested by proteolytic enzymes and absorbed.

A number of methods have been developed to track the passage of capsules and tablets through the gastrointestinal tract to map their transit time and drug-release patterns. Among these is gamma *scintigraphy*, a noninvasive procedure that entails the use of a gamma ray–emitting radiotracer incorporated into the formulation with a gamma camera coupled to a data recording system (4,5). The quantity of radiotracer added to allow gamma scintigraphy is small and does not compromise the usual in vivo characteristics of the dosage form being studied. When scintigraphy is combined with pharmacokinetic studies, the resultant *pharmacoscintigraphic* evaluation provides information about the transit and drug-release patterns of the dosage form as well as the rate of drug absorption from the various regions of the gastrointestinal tract (4). This method is particularly useful in (*a*) determining whether a correlation exists between in vitro and in vivo bioavailability for immediate-release products, (*b*) assessing the integrity and transit time of enteric-coated tablets through the stomach en route to the intestines, and (*c*) drug and dosage form evaluation in new product development (4,5). A separate technique uses a pH-sensitive nondigestible radiotelemetric device termed the Heidelberg capsule, the approximate size of a No. 0 gelatin capsule. It has been used as a *non*radioactive means to measure gastric pH, gastric residence time, and gastric emptying time

of solid dosage forms in fasting and nonfasting human subjects (6).

As discussed in Chapter 5, drug absorption from the gastrointestinal tract depends on a number of factors, including the solubility of the drug substance, the type of product formulation (i.e., immediate release, modified release, or enteric coated), the gastrointestinal contents, and intersubject differences in physiologic character and response.

The Manufacture of Hard Gelatin Capsule Shells

Hard gelatin capsule shells are manufactured in two sections, the capsule body and a shorter cap. The two parts overlap when joined, with the cap fitting snugly over the open end of the capsule body. Some capsule shells are designed to lock in place when closed. The shells are produced industrially by the mechanical dipping of pins or pegs of the desired shape and diameter into a temperature-controlled reservoir of melted gelatin mixture (Fig. 7.2). The pegs, made of manganese bronze, are affixed to plates, each capable of holding up to about 500 pegs. Each plate is mechanically lowered to the gelatin bath and the pegs submerged to the desired depth and maintained for the desired period to achieve the proper length and thickness of coating. Then the plate and the pegs are slowly lifted from the bath, and the gelatin is dried by a gentle flow of temperature- and humidity-controlled air. When dried, each capsule part is mechanically trimmed to the proper length and removed from the pegs, and the capsule bodies and caps are joined together. It is important that the thickness of the gelatin walls be strictly controlled so that the capsules' body and cap fit snugly to prevent disengagement. The pegs on which the caps are formed are slightly larger in diameter than the pegs on which the bodies are formed, allowing the telescoping of the caps over the bodies. In capsule shell production, there is a continuous dipping, drying, removing, and joining of capsules as the peg-containing plates rotate in and out of the gelatin bath. As noted earlier, capsule shells may be made distinctive by adding colorants and/or opaquants to the gelatin bath.

A manufacturer also may prepare distinctive-looking capsules by altering the usual rounded shape of the

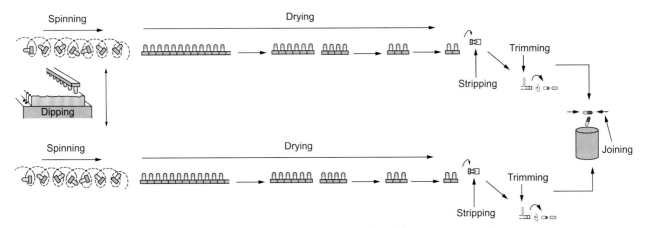

FIGURE 7.2. Dipping, spinning, drying, stripping, trimming, joining, and polishing empty capsules.

capsule-making pegs. By tapering the end of the body-producing peg while leaving the cap-making peg rounded, one manufacturer prepares capsules differentiated from those of other manufacturers (Pulvules, Eli Lilly). Another manufacturer uses capsules with the ends of both the bodies and caps highly tapered (Spansule Capsules, SmithKline Beecham). Yet another innovation in capsule shell design is the Snap-Fit, Coni-Snap, and Coni-Snap Supro hard gelatin capsules depicted in Figures 7.3 and 7.4. The original Snap-Fit construction enables the two halves of the capsule shells to be positively joined through locking grooves in the shell walls. The two grooves fit into each other and thus ensure reliable closing of the filled capsule. During the closing process, the capsule body is inserted into the cap. With the high-capacity filling rates of the modern capsule-filling machines (more than 180,000 capsules per hour), splitting (telescoping) and denting of the capsule shell occur with the slightest contact between the two rims when they are joined. This problem, which exists primarily with straight-walled capsule shells, led to the development of the Coni-Snap capsule, in which the rim of the capsule body is not straight but tapered slightly (Fig. 7.4). This reduces the risk of the capsule rims touching on joining and essentially eliminates the problem of splitting during large-scale filling operations. In the Coni-Snap Supro capsules, the upper capsule part extends so far over the lower part that only the rounded edge of the latter is visible (Fig. 7.4). Opening of such a filled capsule is difficult because the lower surface offers less gripping surface to

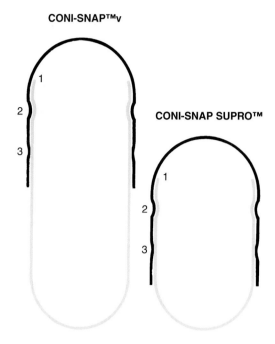

1. Tapered rim to avoid telescoping (CONI-SNAP™)

2. Grooves which lock the two halves together once the capsule has been filled (SNAP-FIT™ principle)

3. Indentations to prevent premature opening

FIGURE 7.4. Line drawings of the Coni-Snap and Coni-Snap Supro (*right*) capsules. The latter is designed to be smaller and to have the lower portion of the capsule shell concealed except for the rounded end. This makes separation of the two parts more difficult and contributes to capsule integrity. (Courtesy of Capsugel Division, Warner-Lambert.)

pull the two halves apart. This increases the security of the contents and the integrity of the capsule.

After filling, some manufacturers render their capsules tamper evident through various sealing techniques. These methods are discussed later in this section. Capsules and tablets also may be imprinted with the names or monograms of the manufacturer, the assigned national drug code number, and other markings making the product identifiable and distinguishable from other products.

Capsule Sizes

Empty gelatin capsules are manufactured in various lengths, diameters, and capacities. The size selected for use is determined by the amount of fill material to be encapsulated. The density and compressibility of the fill will largely determine to what extent it may be packed into a capsule shell (7) (Fig. 7.5). For estimation, a comparison may be made with powders of well-known features (Table 7.1) and an initial judgment made as to the approximate capsule size needed to hold a specific amount of material. However, the final determination may be largely the result of trial and error. For human use, empty capsules ranging in size from

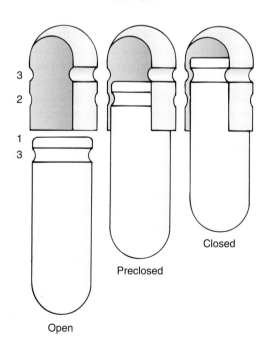

FIGURE 7.3. Line drawings of the Coni-Snap capsule in open, preclosed, and closed positions. The tapered rims (*1*) avoid telescoping; the indentations (*2*) prevent premature opening; and the grooves (*3*) lock the two capsule parts together after the capsule is filled. (Courtesy of Capsugel Division, Warner-Lambert.)

FIGURE 7.5. Capsule-filling machine. (Courtesy of Panatda Saengow/Shutterstock.)

000 (the largest) to 5 (the smallest) are commercially available (Fig. 7.6). Larger capsules are available for veterinary use.

For prescriptions requiring extemporaneous compounding, hard gelatin capsules permit a wide number of options for the physician. The pharmacist may compound capsules of a single medicinal agent or combination of agents at the precise dosage prescribed for the individual patient.

Preparation of Filled Hard Gelatin Capsules

The large-scale or small-scale preparation of filled hard gelatin capsules is divided into the following general steps:

1. Developing and preparing the formulation and selecting the capsule size
2. Filling the capsule shells
3. Capsule sealing (optional)
4. Cleaning and polishing the filled capsules

Developing the Formulation and Selecting the Capsule Size

In developing a capsule formulation, the goal is to prepare a capsule with accurate dosage, good bioavailability, ease of filling and production, stability, and elegance.

In dry formulations, the active and inactive components must be blended thoroughly to ensure a uniform powder mix for the fill. Care in blending is especially important for low-dose drugs, because lack of homogeneity in blending may result in significant therapeutic consequences. Preformulation studies are performed to determine whether all of the formulation's bulk powders may be effectively blended together as such or require reduction of particle size or any other processing to achieve homogeneity.

A diluent or filler may be added to the formulation to produce the proper capsule fill volume. Lactose, microcrystalline cellulose, and starch are commonly used for this purpose. In addition to providing bulk, these materials often provide cohesion to the powders, which is beneficial in the transfer of the powder blend into capsule shells (2). Disintegrants are frequently included in a capsule formulation to assist the breakup and distribution of the capsule's contents in the stomach. Among the disintegrants used are pregelatinized starch, croscarmellose, and sodium starch glycolate.

To achieve uniform drug distribution, it is advantageous if the density and particle size of the drug and nondrug components are similar. This is particularly important when a drug of low dosage is blended with other drugs or nondrug fill (8). When necessary, particle size may be reduced by *milling* to produce particles ranging from about 50 to 1,000 μm. Milled powders may be blended effectively for uniform distribution throughout a powder mix when the drug's dosage is 10 mg or greater (8). For drugs of lower dose or when smaller particles are required, *micronization* is employed. Depending on the materials and equipment used, micronization produces particles ranging from about 1 to 20 μm.

In preparing capsules on an industrial scale using high-speed automated equipment, the powder mix or granules must be free flowing to allow steady passage of the capsule fill from the hopper through the encapsulating equipment and into the capsule shells. The addition of a *lubricant* or *glidant* such as fumed silicon dioxide, magnesium stearate, calcium stearate, stearic acid, or talc (about 0.25% to 1%) to the powder mix enhances flow properties (2).

When magnesium stearate is used as the lubricant, the waterproofing characteristics of this water-insoluble material can retard penetration by the gastrointestinal fluids and delay drug dissolution and absorption. A surface-active agent, such as sodium lauryl sulfate, is used to facilitate wetting by the gastrointestinal fluids to overcome the problem (9). Even if a water-insoluble lubricant is used, after the gelatin capsule shell dissolves, gastrointestinal fluids must displace the air that surrounds the dry powder and penetrate the drug before it can be dispersed and dissolved. Powders of poorly soluble drugs have a tendency to resist such penetration. Disintegration agents in a capsule formulation facilitate the breakup and distribution of the capsule's contents.

TABLE 7.1. Approximate Capacity of Empty Gelatin Capsules

	Capsule Size							
	000	00	0	1	2	3	4	5
Volume (mL)	1.40	0.95	0.68	0.50	0.37	0.30	0.21	0.13
Drug Substance (mg)[a]								
Quinine sulfate	650	390	325	227	195	130	97	65
Sodium bicarbonate	1,430	975	715	510	390	325	260	130
Aspirin	1,040	650	520	325	260	195	162	97

[a]Amount may vary with the degree of pressure used in filling the capsules.

Empty Capsule Size										
Capsule Size	000	00E	00	0E	0	1	2	3	4	5
Empty Capsule Volume Capacity (mL)										
Capacity	1.37	1.00	0.90	0.78	0.68	0.48	0.36	0.27	0.20	0.13

FIGURE 7.6. Actual sizes of hard gelatin capsules.

Be it a lubricant, surfactant, disintegrating agent, or some other pharmaceutical excipient, formulation can influence the bioavailability of a drug substance and can account for differences in drug effects between two capsule products of the same medicinal substance. Pharmacists must be aware of this possibility when product interchange, for example, generic substitution, is considered.

Inserting tablets or small capsules into capsules is sometimes useful in the commercial production of capsules and in a pharmacist's extemporaneous preparation of capsules (Fig. 7.7). This may be done to separate chemically incompatible agents or to add premeasured amounts of potent drug substances. Rather than weighing a potent drug, a pharmacist may choose to insert a prefabricated tablet of the desired strength in each capsule. Other less potent agents and diluents may then be weighed and added. On an industrial scale, coated pellets designed for modified-release drug delivery are also commonly placed in capsule shells.

Gelatin capsules are unsuitable for aqueous liquids because water softens gelatin and distorts the capsules, resulting in leakage of the contents. However, some liquids, such as fixed or volatile oils, that do not interfere with the stability of the gelatin shells may be placed in locking gelatin capsules (or the capsules may be sealed with a solution of gelatin thinly coating the interface of the cap and body) to ensure retention of the liquid. Rather than placing a liquid as such in a capsule, the liquid may be mixed with an inert powder to make a wet mass or paste, which may then be placed in capsules in the usual manner (Fig. 7.7). *Eutectic mixtures* of drugs, or mixtures of agents that have a propensity to liquefy when admixed, may be mixed with a diluent or absorbent such as magnesium carbonate, kaolin, or light magnesium oxide to separate the interacting agents and to absorb any liquefied material that may form.

In large-scale capsule production, liquids are placed in *soft gelatin* capsules that are sealed during filling and manufacturing. Soft capsules are discussed later in this chapter.

In most instances, the amount of drug in a capsule is a single dose. When the usual dose of the drug is too large for a single capsule, two or more capsules may be required. The total amount of formula prepared is the amount necessary to fill the desired number of capsules. On an industrial scale, this means hundreds of thousands of capsules. In community practice, an individual prescription may call for preparation of a few to several hundred capsules. Any slight loss in fill material during preparation and capsule filling will not materially affect an industrial size batch, but in the community pharmacy, a slight loss of powder could result in an inadequate quantity to fill the last capsule. To ensure enough fill in the compounding of small numbers of capsules, the community pharmacist may calculate for the preparation of one or two more capsules than required to fill the prescription. However, this procedure must not be followed for capsules containing a controlled substance, because the amount of drug used and that called for in the prescription must strictly coincide.

The selection of the capsule size for a commercial product is done during product development. The choice is determined by requirements of the formulation, including the dose of the active ingredient and the density and compaction characteristics of the drug and other components. If the dose of the drug is inadequate to fill the volume of the capsule body, a diluent is added. Information on the density and compaction characteristics of a capsule's

1   **2**   **3**   **4**   **5**

FIGURE 7.7. Examples of fill in hard gelatin capsules. *1*, powder or granulate; *2*, pellet mixture; *3*, paste; *4*, capsule; and *5*, tablet. (Courtesy of Capsugel Division, Warner-Lambert.)

active and inactive components and comparison to other similar materials and prior experiences can serve as a guide in selecting capsule size (7).

Hard gelatin capsules are used to encapsulate about 65 mg to 1 g of powdered material. As shown in Table 7.1, the smallest capsule (No. 5) may be expected to hold 65 mg of powder or more, depending on the characteristics of the powder. Oftentimes, in the extemporaneous compounding of prescriptions, the best capsule size to use is determined by trial. Use of the smallest size capsule, properly filled, is preferred. A properly filled capsule should have its body filled with the drug mixture, not the cap. The cap is intended to fit snugly over the body to retain the contents.

An easy method to select the proper capsule is to weigh the ingredients for the required number of capsules to be prepared. Place the powders in a graduated cylinder, and obtain the volume occupied by the powders. Divide the volume by the number of capsules to be prepared, and this provides the volume that will be occupied by the powder for each capsule. Compare this volume (in mL) with the appropriate line of Table 7.1, and select the size that will accommodate the powder. If the capsule is too large, simply multiply the capsule size in volume by the number of capsules to be prepared to obtain the final volume of the powder that is required. Then add additional diluent to the graduated cylinder containing the other powders to the mark indicated for the total volume of powder required. For documentation, weigh the total powder blend and subtract the initial quantities that were weighed, and the quantity of additional diluent that was added will be obtained.

The following examples demonstrate the drug and nondrug contents of a few commercially available capsules:

Tetracycline Capsules

Active ingredient:	Tetracycline hydrochloride 250 mg
Filler:	Lactose
Lubricant/glidant:	Magnesium stearate
Capsule colorants:	FD&C Yellow No. 6, D&C Yellow No. 10, D&C Red No. 28, FD&C Blue No. 1
Capsule opaquant:	Titanium dioxide

Acetaminophen with Codeine Capsules

Active ingredients:	Acetaminophen 325 mg
	Codeine phosphate 30 mg
Disintegrant:	Sodium starch glycolate
Lubricant/glidants:	Magnesium stearate, stearic acid
Capsule colorants:	D&C Yellow No. 10, Edible Ink, FD&C Blue No. 1 (FD&C Green No. 3 and FD&C Red No. 40)

Diphenhydramine Hydrochloride Capsules

Active ingredient:	Diphenhydramine HCl 25 mg
Filler:	Confectioner's sugar
Lubricants/glidants:	Talc, colloidal silicon dioxide
Wetting agent:	Sodium lauryl sulfate
Capsule colorants:	FD&C Blue No. 1, FD&C Red No. 3
Capsule opaquant:	Titanium dioxide

Filling Hard Capsule Shells

When filling a small number of capsules in the pharmacy, the pharmacist may use the punch method. The pharmacist takes the precise number of empty capsules to be filled from the stock container. By counting the capsules as the initial step rather than taking a capsule from stock as each one is filled, the pharmacist guards against filling the wrong number of capsules and avoids contaminating the stock container with drug powder. The powder to be encapsulated is placed on a sheet of clean paper or on a glass or porcelain plate. Using the spatula, the powder mix is formed into a cake having a depth of approximately one-fourth to one-third the length of the capsule body. Then an empty capsule body is held between the thumb and forefinger and punched vertically into the powder cake repeatedly until filled. Some pharmacists wear surgical gloves (latex or other material) or finger cots to avoid handling the capsules with bare fingers. Because the amount of powder packed into a capsule depends on the degree of compression, the pharmacist should punch each capsule in the same manner and weigh the product after capping. When nonpotent materials are placed in capsules, the first filled capsule should be weighed (using an empty capsule of the same size on the opposite balance pan to counter the weight of the shell) to determine the capsule size to use and the degree of compaction to be used. After this determination, the other capsules should be prepared and weighed periodically to check the uniformity of the process. When potent drugs are being used, *each capsule* should be weighed after filling to ensure accuracy. Such weighings protect against uneven filling of capsules and premature exhaustion or underuse of the powder. After the body of a capsule has been filled and the cap placed on the body, the body may be squeezed or tapped gently to distribute some powder to the cap end to give the capsule a full appearance.

Granular material that does not lend itself to the punch method of filling capsules may be poured into each capsule from the powder paper on which it is weighed.

Pharmacists who prepare capsules on a regular or extensive basis may use a hand-operated filling machine (Fig. 7.8). The various types of machines have capacities ranging from 24 to 300 capsules and, when efficiently operated, are capable of producing about 200 to 2,000 capsules per hour. These are operated by weighing and mixing all the ingredients followed by thoroughly mixing. The required number of empty capsules is placed in the lower plate and the upper plate added followed by locking the capsules in the plates. The upper plate is removed separating the caps from the bodies of the capsules. The lower plate is loosened allowing the capsules to fall flush with the plate surface. A border dam is added to retain the powder in the area followed by the powder. The powder is moved around on the plate allowing the capsules to fill. It is generally necessary to use a tamper to aid in packing the powder in the capsules to allow more powder to be accommodated. After all the powder is filled in the capsule bodies,

FIGURE 7.8. Capsule hand-filling machine. (Courtesy of Medisca Inc.)

the plate with the capsule caps is then placed on the lower plate and the plates are pressed together. The upper plate is removed and all the capsules checked to confirm a good seal is made with all of them. The lower plate is removed and the capsules allowed to fall out of the plate onto a surface for examination.

Machines developed for industrial use automatically separate the caps from empty capsules, fill the bodies, scrape off the excess powder, replace the caps, seal the capsules as desired, and clean the outside of the filled capsules at up to 165,000 capsules per hour. The formulation must be such that the filled body contains the accurate drug dosage. This is verified through the use of automated in-process sampling and analysis (Figs. 7.9 and 7.10).

As described later, the USP requires adherence to standards for *content uniformity* and *weight variation* for capsules to ensure the accuracy of dosage units.

Special Capsules

A number of different special capsules can be prepared, including those filled with a semisolid mass or a liquid.

FIGURE 7.9. Automatic capsule-weighing machine. (Courtesy of CI Precision.)

Filling Capsules with a Semisolid Mass

Two common methods used to place semisolid materials into hard-gelatin capsules involve forming a cylinder or pouring a melt into the capsule shell.

Material that is sufficiently plastic can be rolled into a cylinder with a diameter slightly less than that of the inner diameter of the capsule in which it will be enclosed. The quantity of material desired is cut with a spatula or knife, with the length removed determining the weight of the material to be enclosed in the capsule shell. The pieces can be dusted with cornstarch and then inserted individually into the capsules.

If a material is too fluid, cornstarch or a similar material can be added to achieve a firmer consistency. The quantity to add can be determined empirically.

If the material is too firm to roll into a cylinder but its melting point is in a satisfactory temperature range, it can be melted until it is fluid and then poured into the bases of the gelatin capsules. After the capsules have cooled, the caps are replaced. When this technique is used, it is helpful to have a stand to hold the capsule bodies. A manual capsule machine can be used for this by loading the empty capsules, separating the capsule halves, filling the base and then replacing the caps on the bases followed by removal from the holder.

This method can also be used to enhance the bioavailability of drugs that are poorly soluble and exhibit bioavailability problems. In these cases, the drug is added to a melt of a material such as polyethylene glycol (PEG), which is very water soluble and is used to enhance the dissolution rate of some drugs. The mixture is heated and stirred until the powder is either melted or thoroughly mixed in the PEG. After the melt is cooled to just above the melting point of the PEG, it is poured into the capsule shells as described. When this method is used, the desired quantities can be measured using a pipette, syringe, or calibrated dropper to deliver the volume to the individual capsules. Excipients useful in formulating these preparations are shown in Table 7.2. An example formula is as follows:

Rx Estradiol 0.25 mg and Estrone 0.25 mg Semisolid-Fill Capsules

For 100 capsules

Estradiol	25 mg	Active
Estrone	25 mg	Active
Polyethylene glycol 1450	20 g	Diluent
Polyethylene glycol 3350	20 g	Diluent

1. Calculate the quantity of each ingredient required for the prescription.
2. Accurately weigh each ingredient.
3. Using geometric dilution, mix the estrogen powders.
4. Using low heat to about 60°C to 65°C, melt the PEGs.
5. Sprinkle on the estrogen powders and thoroughly mix.
6. Load a capsule machine, if available, with 100 No. 1 capsules and remove the caps.

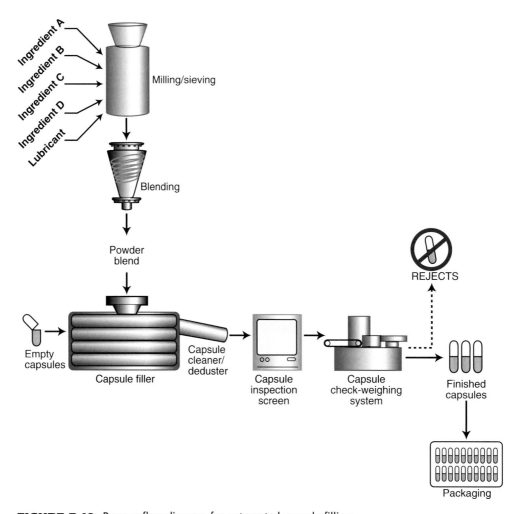

FIGURE 7.10. Process flow diagram for automated capsule filling.

7. To determine the volume of mixture to place in each capsule, perform the following steps:
   - Using a micropipette, place 330 μL of the estrogen–PEG melt into each of three capsule bases.
   - Weigh the three capsules and obtain the average weight for each.
   - Adjust the volume delivered, if necessary, to obtain capsules with a tared weight of 403 mg.
8. Place the required volume in each of the capsules, according to step 7.
9. Allow the mixture to harden and replace the caps on the capsules.
10. Check the weights of about 10 capsules for uniformity and accuracy.
11. Package and label.

Filling Liquids in Hard Gelatin Capsules

It may occasionally be necessary to prepare hard gelatin capsules containing liquid materials. This can be accomplished easily if the liquid material does not dissolve the gelatin and should work with alcoholic solutions, fixed oils or volatile oils, as gelatin is not soluble in these materials. It may be necessary to determine the solubility of the gelatin

in the liquid by experimentation. For filling, the liquid can be measured accurately using a pipette (micropipette) or a calibrated dropper and dropped into the capsule base, taking care not to touch the opening. For larger quantities to be prepared, the oil can be filled into the capsule bases using a standard capsule filling machine. The quantity of active material and diluent liquid are determined and measured. Table 7.3 lists the volumes of the various sizes of capsules. The capsules are placed into the machine and the caps separated from the bases. The thoroughly mixed liquid is then spread over the capsule bases and fills them uniformly to the top. For this procedure, it is necessary to determine the volume of material that will completely fill the base of the capsules. The capsule caps are then locked into place.

For best results, snap-lock type capsules should be used. If unavailable, however, regular capsules can be used and sealed.

Rx Progesterone 100 mg in Peanut Oil Capsules

For 100 capsules

Micronized progesterone	10 g	Active
Peanut oil	qs 30 mL	Diluent

TABLE 7.2. Excipients Used as Matrices for Semisolid Capsules

Vegetable Oils
Cottonseed
Maize
Nut
Olive
Soya
Hydrogenated Vegetable Oils
Castor
Coconut
Cottonseed
Palm
Soya
Vegetable Fats
Carnauba wax
Cocoa butter
Animal Fats
Beeswax
Lanolin
Spermaceti
Hydrocarbons
Paraffin
Fatty Alcohols
Cetyl
Lauryl
Stearyl
Fatty Acids
Lauryl
Myristic
Palmitic
Stearic
Esters
Ethyl oleate
Glycol stearates
Isopropyl myristate
Mixed Esters
Liquid
Labrafil
Miglyol 812
Solid
Suppocire
Witepsol

TABLE 7.3. Approximate Capacities of Capsules in Milliliters

Size	Milliliters
5	0.13
4	0.20
3	0.27
2	0.37
1	0.48
0	0.67
00	0.95
000	1.36
Veterinary Sizes	
10	30
11	15
12	7.5

Make progesterone 100 mg capsules.

1. Calculate the quantity of each ingredient required for the prescription.
2. Accurately weigh the progesterone.
3. Mix the progesterone with about 20 mL of peanut oil, in small portions.
4. Add sufficient peanut oil to make 30 mL and mix well.
5. Load a capsule machine with 100 No. 1 empty gelatin capsules.
6. Using a micropipette, add 300 μL of the mixture to each of the 100 capsules.
7. Remove the filled capsules from the capsule machine.
8. Package and label.

Capsule Sealing

As mentioned previously, some manufacturers make tamper-evident capsules by sealing the joint between the two capsule parts. One manufacturer makes distinctive-looking capsules by sealing them with a colored band of gelatin (Kapseals, Parke-Davis). If removed, the band cannot be restored without expert resealing with gelatin. Capsules may also be sealed through a heat-welding process that fuses the capsule cap to the body through the double wall thickness at their juncture (10). The process results in a distinctive ring around the capsule where heat welded. Still another process uses a liquid wetting agent that lowers the melting point in the contact areas of the capsule's cap and body and then thermally bonds the two parts using low temperatures (40°C to 45°C) (11). Industrial capsule-sealing machines are capable of producing 60,000 to 150,000 gelatin-banded, heat-welded, or thermally coupled capsules per hour (12). Figure 7.11 depicts a sealed hard gelatin capsule. Although it is difficult and tedious, extemporaneously prepared capsules may be sealed by lightly coating the inner surface of the cap with a warm gelatin solution immediately prior to placement on the filled capsule body.

CLEANING AND POLISHING CAPSULES

Small amounts of powder may adhere to the outside of capsules after filling. The powder may be bitter or otherwise unpalatable and should be removed before packaging

FIGURE 7.11. Z-Weld's gelatin seal fuses the two capsule halves to create a one-piece capsule that is tamper evident. (Courtesy of Raymond Automation.)

or dispensing. On a small scale, capsules may be cleaned individually or in small numbers by rubbing them with a clean gauze or cloth. On a large scale, many capsule-filling machines are affixed with a cleaning vacuum that removes any extraneous material from the capsules as they exit the equipment. Figure 7.12 shows industrial cleaning and polishing of filled hard capsules using a SaintyCo apparatus.

SOFT GELATIN CAPSULES

Soft gelatin capsules are made of gelatin to which glycerin or a polyhydric alcohol such as sorbitol has been added. Soft gelatin capsules, which contain more moisture than hard capsules, may have a preservative, such as methylparaben and/or propylparaben, to retard microbial growth. Soft gelatin capsules may be oblong, oval, or round. They may be single colored or two toned and may be imprinted with identifying markings. As with hard gelatin capsules, they may be prepared with opaquants to reduce transparency and render characteristic features to the capsule shell.

Soft gelatin capsules are used to encapsulate and hermetically seal liquids, suspensions, pasty materials, dry powders, and even preformed tablets. Soft gelatin capsules are pharmaceutically elegant and are easily swallowed.

Preparation of Soft Gelatin Capsules

Soft gelatin capsules may be prepared by the plate process, using a set of molds to form the capsules, or by the more efficient and productive rotary or reciprocating die processes by which they are produced, filled, and sealed in a continuous operation (Fig. 7.13) (13).

By the plate process, a warm sheet of plain or colored gelatin is placed on the bottom plate of the mold, and the medication-containing liquid is evenly poured on it. Then a second sheet of gelatin is carefully placed on top of the medication, and the top plate of the mold is put into place. Pressure is then applied to the mold to form, fill, and seal the capsules simultaneously. The capsules are removed and washed with a solvent harmless to the capsules.

Most soft gelatin capsules are prepared by the rotary die process, a method developed in 1933 by Robert P. Scherer. By this method, liquid gelatin flowing from an overhead tank is formed into two continuous ribbons by the rotary die machine and brought together between twin rotating

FIGURE 7.12. Hard-filled capsule cleaning and polishing machine.

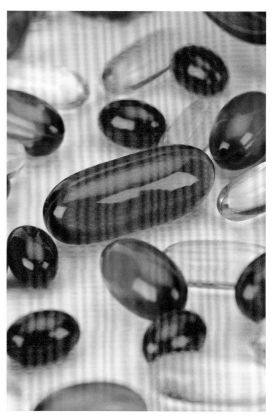

FIGURE 7.13. Examples of soft gelatin capsules. (Courtesy of Carlos Restrepo/Shutterstock.)

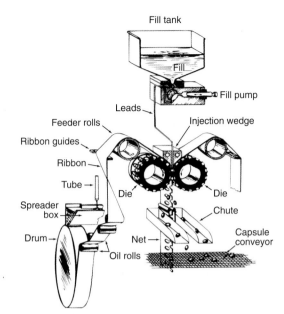

FIGURE 7.14. Rotary die process. (Courtesy of R.P. Scherer Corporation.)

dies (Fig. 7.14). At the same time, metered fill material is injected between the ribbons precisely at the moment that the dies form pockets of the gelatin ribbons. These pockets of fill-containing gelatin are sealed by pressure and heat and then severed from the ribbon. Use of ribbons of two different colors results in bicolored capsules.

The reciprocating die process is similar to the rotary process in that ribbons of gelatin are formed and used to encapsulate the fill, but it differs in the actual encapsulating process. The gelatin ribbons are fed between a set of vertical dies that continually open and close to form rows of pockets in the gelatin ribbons. These pockets are filled with the medication and are sealed, shaped, and cut out of the film as they progress through the machinery. As the capsules are cut from the ribbons, they fall into refrigerated tanks that prevent the capsules from adhering to one another.

Use of Soft Gelatin Capsules

Soft gelatin capsules are prepared to contain a variety of liquid, paste, and dry fills. Liquids that may be encapsulated into soft gelatin capsules include the following (13):

1. Water-immiscible volatile and nonvolatile liquids such as vegetable and aromatic oils, aromatic and aliphatic hydrocarbons, chlorinated hydrocarbons, ethers, esters, alcohols, and organic acids
2. Water-miscible nonvolatile liquids, such as PEGs, and nonionic surface-active agents, such as polysorbate 80
3. Water-miscible and relatively nonvolatile compounds such as propylene glycol and isopropyl alcohol, depending on factors such as concentration used and packaging conditions

Liquids that can easily migrate through the capsule shell are not suitable for soft gelatin capsules. These materials include water above 5% and low molecular weight

water-soluble and volatile organic compounds such as alcohols, ketones, acids, amines, and esters.

Solids may be encapsulated into soft gelatin capsules as solutions in a suitable liquid solvent, suspensions, dry powders, granules, pellets, or small tablets.

COMPENDIAL REQUIREMENTS FOR CAPSULES

Added Substances

Substances added to official preparations, including capsules, to enhance their stability, usefulness, or elegance or to facilitate their manufacture may be used only if they (14):

1. Are harmless in the quantities used
2. Do not exceed the minimum amounts required to provide their intended effect
3. Do not impair the product's bioavailability, therapeutic efficacy, or safety
4. Do not interfere with requisite compendial assays and tests

Containers for Dispensing Capsules

The USP lists specifications prescribing the type of container suitable for the repackaging or dispensing of each official capsule and tablet. Depending on the item, the container may be required to be *tight*, *well closed*, *light resistant*, and/or a combination of these.

Disintegration Test for Capsules

The disintegration test for hard and soft gelatin capsules follows the same procedure and uses the same apparatus described in the next chapter for uncoated tablets. The capsules are placed in the basket rack assembly, which is immersed 30 times per minute into a thermostatically controlled fluid at 37°C and observed over the time described in the individual monograph. To satisfy the test, the capsules disintegrate completely into a soft mass having no palpably firm core and only some fragments of the gelatin shell.

Dissolution Test for Capsules

The dissolution test for capsules uses the same apparatus, dissolution medium, and test as that for uncoated and plain-coated tablets described in Chapter 8. However, if the capsule shells interfere with the analysis, the contents of a specified number of capsules can be removed and the empty capsule shells are dissolved in the dissolution medium before proceeding with the sampling and chemical analysis. If the capsule floats on the surface of the dissolution fluid, a small, loose piece of nonreactive material, such as a few turns of a wire helix, may be attached to the dosage form to force it to sink to the bottom of the vessel.

Weight Variation

The uniformity of dosage units may be demonstrated by determining *weight variation* and/or *content uniformity*. The weight variation method is as follows.

Hard Capsules

Ten capsules are individually weighed and their contents removed. The emptied shells are individually weighed, and the net weight of the contents is calculated by subtraction. From the results of an assay performed as directed in the individual monograph, the content of the active ingredient in each of the capsules is determined.

Soft Capsules

The gross weight of 10 intact capsules is determined individually. Then each capsule is cut open, and the contents are removed by washing with a suitable solvent. The solvent is allowed to evaporate at room temperature over about 30 minutes, with precautions to avoid uptake or loss of moisture. The individual shells are weighed and the net contents calculated. From the results of the assay directed in the individual monograph, the content of the active ingredient in each of the capsules is determined.

Content Uniformity

Unless otherwise stated in the USP monograph for an individual capsule, the amount of active ingredient, determined by assay, is within the range of 85% to 115% of the label claim for 9 of 10 dosage units assayed, with no unit outside the range of 70% to 125% of the label claim. Additional tests are prescribed when two or three dosage units are outside of the desired range but within the stated extremes.

Content Labeling Requirement

All official capsules must be labeled to express the quantity of each active ingredient in each dosage unit.

Stability Testing

Stability testing of capsules is performed as described in Chapter 4 to determine the intrinsic stability of the active drug molecule and the influence of environmental factors such as temperature, humidity, light, formulative components, and the container and closure system. The battery of stress testing, long-term stability, and accelerated stability tests help determine the appropriate conditions for storage and the product's anticipated shelf life.

Moisture Permeation Test

The USP requires determination of the moisture permeation characteristics of single-unit and unit-dose containers to ensure their suitability for packaging capsules. The degree and rate of moisture penetration are determined by packaging the dosage unit together with a color-revealing desiccant pellet, exposing the packaged unit to known relative humidity over a specified time, observing the desiccant pellet for color change (indicating the absorption of moisture), and comparing the pretest and posttest weight of the packaged unit.

▌ OFFICIAL AND COMMERCIALLY AVAILABLE CAPSULES

Approximately 200 officially recognized medications in capsule form are listed in the USP. However, many times, this number of capsule products is available from various manufacturers for various drugs and in various dosage strengths.

Examples of official and commercially available medications in hard and soft gelatin capsules are presented in Tables 7.4 and 7.5.

TABLE 7.4. Examples of Some Official Capsules

Official Capsule	Representative Commercial Capsules	Strength (mg)	Category
Acyclovir	Various	200	Antiviral
Amoxicillin	Wymox (Wyeth-Ayerst)	250, 500	Antibacterial
Ampicillin	Omnipen (Wyeth-Ayerst)	250, 500	Antibacterial
Cephalexin	Keflex (Victory)	250, 333, 500, 750	Antibacterial
Diphenhydramine HCl	Benadryl (McNeil)	25	Antihistaminic
Docusate sodium	Various	250	Stool softener
Doxycycline hyclate	Vibramycin (Pfizer)	100	Antibacterial
Erythromycin estolate	Ilosone (Eli Lilly)	250	Antibacterial
Fluoxetine HCl	Various	10, 20, 40	Antidepressant
Flurazepam HCl	Various	15, 30	Hypnotic
Indomethacin	Indocin (Merck)	25, 50	Anti-inflammatory, antipyretic, analgesic
Loperamide HCl	Imodium (Janssen)	2	Antidiarrheal
Minocycline hydrochloride	Various	50, 75, 100	Antibacterial
Oxazepam	Various	10, 15, 30	Antianxiety
Paromomycin	Caraco Pharm Labs	250	Antiamoebic
Tetracycline HCl	Various	250, 500	Antibacterial
Vancomycin HCl	Vancocin (ViroPharma)	125, 250	Antibacterial
Zidovudine	Zidovudine (Aurobindo Pharma)	100	Antiretroviral

TABLE 7.5. Some Medications Commercially Prepared Into Soft Gelatin Capsules

Drug	Trade Name (Manufacturer)	Contents and Comments[a]
Acetazolamide	Diamox Sequels (Duramed)	Carbonic anhydrase inhibitor, slightly water-soluble powder. Contains coated pellets of sustained-release drug
Chloral hydrate	Various	Sedative–hypnotic
Cyclosporine	Sandimmune (Novartis)	Immunosuppressive, slightly water-soluble crystalline powder. Contains corn oil, polyoxyethylated glycolyzed glycerides
Cyclosporine	Neoral (Novartis)	Contains dehydrated alcohol; corn oil mono-, di-, and triglycerides; and polyoxyl 40 hydrogenated castor oil; forms microemulsion in contact with aqueous fluids for enhanced bioavailability
Docusate sodium	UDL	Stool softener–laxative
Ethosuximide	Zarontin (Parke–Davis)	Anticonvulsant, water-soluble powder. Contains polyethylene glycol 400
Ranitidine HCl	Zantac GELdose (Glaxo Wellcome)	Histamine H_2 receptor inhibitor, water-soluble granular powder in nonaqueous matrix of synthetic coconut oil, triglycerides

[a]Only a partial listing of the capsule contents is given. The soft capsule shells may also contain colorants, opaquants, preservatives, and other agents.

INSPECTING, COUNTING, PACKAGING, AND STORING CAPSULES

Capsules produced on a small or a large scale should be uniform in appearance. Visual or electronic inspection should be undertaken to detect any flaws in the integrity and appearance of the capsules. Defective capsules should be rejected. In commercial manufacture, Current Good Manufacturing Practice regulations require that if the number of production flaws is excessive, the cause must be investigated and documented and steps undertaken to correct the problem.

In the pharmacy, capsules may be counted manually or by automated equipment. Specially designed trays, such as the type depicted in Figure 7.15, are used for counting small numbers of solid dosage units. In using this tray, the pharmacist pours a supply of capsules or tablets from the bulk source onto the clean tray and, using the spatula, counts and sweeps the dosage units into the trough until the desired number is reached. Then the pharmacist closes the trough cover, picks up the tray, returns the uncounted dosage units to the bulk container by means of the lip at the back of the tray, places the prescription container at the opening of the trough, and carefully transfers the capsules or tablets into the container. With this method, the dosage units remain untouched by the pharmacist. To prevent batch-to-batch contamination, the tray must be wiped clean after each use because powder, particularly from uncoated tablets, may remain. In some community and hospital pharmacies, small automated counting and filling machines may be used as shown in Figure 7.16. Computer-based automated dispensing systems are also available that will fill, label, and check the drug using bar code or video systems.

On the industrial scale, solid dosage forms are counted by large automated pieces of equipment that count and transfer the desired number of dosage units into bulk containers. The containers are then mechanically capped, inspected visually or electronically, labeled, and inspected once more. Some filled containers are then placed in outer packaging cartons. An industrial counting and filling machine is shown in Figure 7.17. Capsules are packaged in glass or in plastic containers, some containing packets of a desiccant to prevent absorption of excessive moisture.

FIGURE 7.15. Pharmacy counting tray being used to count tablets.

FIGURE 7.16. Tablet/Capsule counting machine. (Courtesy of Molpix/Shutterstock.)

FIGURE 7.17. Capsule bottling-filling machine. (Courtesy of Shenzhen Penglai Industrial Corporation Ltd.)

FIGURE 7.19. Unit-dose packaging of tablets and capsules. The drug name and other information are imprinted on the backing portion of each unit. (Courtesy of Sergey Lavrentev/ Shutterstock.)

The unit-dose and strip packaging of solid dosage forms, particularly by pharmacies that service nursing homes and hospitals, provides sanitary handling of the medications, ease of identification, and security in accountability for medications. Typical small-scale strip packaging equipment and commercial unit-dose packages of capsules and tablets are presented in Figures 7.18 and 7.19, respectively. Capsules should be stored in tightly capped containers in a cool, dry place.

ORAL ADMINISTRATION OF SOLID DOSAGE FORMS

Solid dosage forms (capsules and tablets) for oral administration are best taken by placing the dose upon the tongue and swallowing it with a glassful of water or beverage, for example, milk, coffee, juice, and tea. Ingesting solid dosage forms with adequate amounts of fluid is important. Some patients attempt to swallow a tablet or capsule without water, but this can be dangerous because of the possibility that it will lodge in the esophagus. Esophageal ulceration can occur with dry ingestion of tablets and capsules, particularly taken just before bedtime. Among the drugs of greatest concern in this regard are alendronate sodium, aspirin, ferrous sulfate, any nonsteroidal anti-inflammatory drug, potassium chloride, and tetracycline antibiotics.

The proper administration of alendronate sodium tablets (Fosamax, Merck), for example, calls for the tablets to

FIGURE 7.18. Strip packaging machine for unit-dose packaging. (Courtesy of Packaging Machinery Associates.)

be taken with a full 6- or 8-ounce glass of plain water upon rising in the morning and at least half an hour before taking any food, beverage, or other medication to prevent local irritation of the esophagus and other upper gastrointestinal mucosa. The patient is also instructed not to recline for at least 30 minutes and until after the first food of the day is eaten because of the possibility that the drug will reflux into the esophagus.

In general, patients with gastroesophageal reflux disease must take their medications with adequate amounts of water and avoid reclining for at least an hour to avoid reflux.

The administration of oral medication in relation to meals is very important because the bioavailability and efficacy of certain drugs may be severely affected by food and certain drinks. For example, atorvastatin should not be administered with grapefruit juice because the juice inhibits the CYP3A4 isoenzyme resulting in a higher plasma concentration of atorvastatin. The pharmacist should know about such instances and counsel patients accordingly.

As mentioned earlier in this chapter, oral dosage forms with special coatings (e.g., enteric) or that are designed to provide controlled drug release, to preserve their drug-release features, must not be chewed, broken, or crushed.

When an ordinary tablet is crushed or a capsule opened to facilitate ease of administration, any unpleasant drug taste may be partially masked by mixing with custard, yogurt, rice pudding, other soft food, or fruit juice. The patient should be advised to consume the entire drug–food mixture to obtain the full dose, and to maintain stability, the drug should not be premixed and allowed to set.

If a patient cannot swallow a solid dosage form, the pharmacist can suggest a chewable or liquid form of the drug. If these are not available, an extemporaneously compounded liquid form may be prepared. Extemporaneous compounding involves a pharmacist preparing a dosage form suitable for an individual patient. There are numerous resources available for this very important and expanding part of pharmacy practice (15,16).

| PATIENT COUNSELING |

Take with a glass of water or other liquid (if instructed).

Discuss the frequency and onset of dose and what to do if a dose is missed.

Keep container tightly closed and store in the least humid environment available at room temperature.

Generally, capsule sizes Nos. 5 through 0 are not difficult to swallow in most cases; however, many patients can have difficulty swallowing No. 00 and No. 000 capsules. In such a case, a patient may be advised to place the capsule on the back of the tongue before drinking a liquid or to place the capsule in warm water for a few seconds before taking it, which makes it slide over the mucous membranes more easily. Also, a teaspoonful of a flavored candy gel can be placed in the mouth and swished around; the capsule is then placed into the mouth and easily swallowed. A pharmacist can also suggest alternatives such as smaller capsules or even a liquid preparation.

Routinely, explain whether or not to chew, crush or swallow the capsule whole. In some cases, a capsule may need to be mixed with a liquid or soft food for administration, especially to a small child.

PHARMACEUTICS CASE STUDY

SUBJECTIVE INFORMATION

You have received the following prescription:

Rx	
Diphenhydramine hydrochloride:	25 mg
Phenyltoloxamine citrate:	30 mg
Acetaminophen:	325 mg

Make No. 30

Sig: Caps i to ii po HS prn sleep

You need to determine the amounts of the ingredients and of lactose to use to make 30 capsules each of size 3, 1, or 0.

OBJECTIVE INFORMATION

Volume capacity of capsules

3: 0.3 mL

1: 0.5 mL

0: 0.67 mL

Tapped density of ingredients, excipients

Lactose:	950 mg/mL
Diphenhydramine hydrochloride:	800 mg/mL
Phenyltoloxamine citrate:	750 mg/mL
Acetaminophen:	850 mg/mL

ASSESSMENT

For each active ingredient, the amount required to make 30 capsules is

Diphenhydramine HCl:	750 mg
Phenyltoloxamine citrate:	900 mg
Acetaminophen:	9.75 g

DETERMINING THE AMOUNT OF LACTOSE REQUIRED: METHOD 1 USING NO. 1 CAPSULES

Fill five test capsules with each pure powder.

Weight of five empty No. 1 capsules: 400 mg

Weight of five No. 1 capsules full of lactose: 2.775 g

Weight of five No. 1 capsules full of diphenhydramine HCl: 2.4 g

Weight of five No. 1 capsules full of phenyltoloxamine citrate: 2.275 g

Weight of five No. 1 capsules full of acetaminophen: 2.525 g

Now average

Lactose: (2,775 − 400)/5 = 475 mg per capsule

Diphenhydramine HCl: (2,400 − 400)/5 = 400 mg per capsule

Phenyltoloxamine citrate: (2,275 − 400)/5 = 375 mg per capsule

Acetaminophen: (2,525 − 400)/5 = 425 mg per capsule

Percent of capsule filled by the required amounts of active ingredient

Diphenhydramine HCl: 25/400 × 100 = 6.25%

Phenyltoloxamine citrate: 30/375 × 100 = 8%

Acetaminophen: 325/425 × 100 = 76.47%

Total = 90.72%, so the remaining 9.28% of each capsule will be lactose. Therefore, we require a total of 0.0928 × 475 × 30 = 1.3 g approximately of lactose to make 30 No. 1 capsules. This calculation can be done in the same way for the No. 0 capsules, resulting in 6.15 g approximately of lactose required to make 30 No. 0 capsules. We cannot use No. 3 capsules for this prescription as only 255 mg of acetaminophen (and nothing else) will fit into a No. 3 capsule.

(continued)

PHARMACEUTICS CASE STUDY (continued)

DETERMINING THE AMOUNT OF LACTOSE REQUIRED: METHOD 2

Calculate the percentage of the volume of a No. 1 capsule that each active ingredient will occupy based on its tap density:

Diphenhydramine HCl: 25 mg/(800 mg/mL)/ 0.5 mL × 100 = 6.25%

Phenyltoloxamine citrate: 30 mg/(750 mg/mL)/ 0.5 mL × 100 = 8%

Acetaminophen: 325 mg/(850 mg/mL)/0.5 mL × 100 = 76.47%

Total = 90.72%, so the remaining 9.28% of each capsule will be lactose. The total amount of lactose required is

Lactose: 9.28/100 × 0.5 mL × (950 mg/mL) = 1.3 g approximately

PLAN

To make 30 No. 1 capsules, we will require

Diphenhydramine HCl:	750 mg
Phenyltoloxamine citrate:	900 mg
Acetaminophen:	9.75 g
Lactose:	1.3 g

To make 30 No. 0 capsules, we will require

Diphenhydramine HCl:	750 mg
Phenyltoloxamine citrate:	900 mg
Acetaminophen:	9.75 g
Lactose:	6.15 g

We cannot use No. 3 capsules for this prescription. ■

CLINICAL CASE STUDY

SUBJECTIVE INFORMATION

HPI: K.P. is a 12-year-old WF who is brought to the emergency department by her mother, who states that "she went unconscious for about a minute." Mother was teaching her to bake cookies when K.P. asked if there was something burning in the oven. She described the smell as being that of "gasoline." Mother did not pay much attention to the strange smell, at which time the patient started to "wiggle" both her hands and "smack her lips together." Mother also stated that she started to chew really hard without any food in her mouth. The episode of strange chewing and lip smacking lasted about a minute, after which K.P. appeared confused and disoriented for several minutes. Her mother recalls asking if something was wrong during the episode, but the patient was unable to respond. Immediately after the episode, mother anxiously drove her to the emergency department. Upon arrival, the patient was oriented to time, place, and people. She denies any nausea, vomiting, dizziness, or confusion. When asked about the episode, patient states that she does not recall what her mother described. Patient is otherwise well.

PMH: No hospitalizations since birth

Birth history: Mother was diagnosed with preeclampsia at 8.5 months. Mother denies any use of drugs and alcohol during pregnancy. K.P. was born at 39 weeks' gestational age. She was bottle-fed as an infant.

Developmental history: Not significant. Patient developed well according to age. Currently developmentally intact

Immunizations: Up-to-date

SH:	(−) EtOH
	(−) Tobacco
	(−) Caffeine
	(−) Illicit drugs

No siblings, lives with parents in Bloomingdale

FH: Mother with gestational diabetes × 12 years

Father with HTN × 2 years

Diet: Eats about five times a day, mostly snacks (i.e., fruit, granola bars). Does not like to eat breakfast or dinner. Lunch is her biggest meal of the day. Meals consist mostly of cooked vegetables and pasta. Does not like junk food. Does not follow any specific diet

All: NKDA

PTA: No meds

OBJECTIVE INFORMATION

Ht:	4'4"
Wt:	102 lb
T:	100.1
Na:	135 mmol/L
K:	4.5 mmol/L
Cl:	102 mmol/L
CO_2:	18 mmol/L
BUN:	3.0 mmol/L
SrCr:	65 mmol/L

(continued)

(continued)

Abnormal EEG findings consistent with complex partial seizures: pattern of spikes and slow waves with a frequency of two cycles per second.

ASSESSMENT

K.P. is a 12-year-old Caucasian female diagnosed with complex partial seizure per EEG and description of episode.

PLAN

1. Recommend extended-release carbamazepine (Carbatrol) 200 mg capsule by mouth twice daily. However, mother states that K.P. is unable to swallow capsules or tablets. Counsel the mother on gently opening the capsule at the seal, being careful not to break the capsule. Tell the mother to sprinkle the contents of the capsule into a small amount of food (e.g., a tablespoon of yogurt or applesauce) to ensure that all of the food with the drug is consumed. If contents are sprinkled in a large amount of food, the patient may not finish it all and hence may not receive the full dose of medication. This may lead to the medication not managing her seizures properly. As an alternative, counsel the mother about the use of the Pill Glide to enable the carbamazepine to be easily swallowed. Pill Glide is a lubricating spray for the throat that facilitates swallowing.

2. Teach the patient and the mother about the common side effects of carbamazepine (e.g., dizziness, fatigue, worsening of seizures, nausea, vomiting) that affect a small fraction of patients. Advise the patient and the mother to report any unusual side effects (e.g., unusual bleeding, bruising, jaundice, dark urine, sore throat, abdominal pain).

3. Teach the patient and the mother about signs and symptoms of seizures. Inform them that most complex seizures are followed by an aura, which may consist of a strange smell, taste, sound, or visual disturbance. For example, K.P. smelled something burning before she had the seizure. Other signs may include a feeling of fear or anxiety. Inform the patient and the mother of the tonic–clonic movements that usually follow the aura. Explain to the mother that loss of consciousness is common with this type of seizure. Also explain that the patient may appear confused for several minutes after the seizure.

4. Monitoring parameters: carbamazepine plasma levels, signs and symptoms of seizures, frequency of episodes, and side effects of the medication. Goals: Increased patient knowledge about the condition, no medication side effects, no second episode, and therapeutic carbamazepine levels (4 to 12 mg/mL). Make sure the patient and the mother understand the importance of follow-up physician visits and of exercising caution when purchasing nonprescription and herbal products (i.e., consult a pharmacist). ■

APPLYING THE PRINCIPLES AND CONCEPTS

GROUP ACTIVITIES

1. Compare the advantages and disadvantages of unit dose packaging versus capsules packaged in plastic bottle containers.
2. Create a listing of extemporaneous prescriptions that call for the creation of a capsule dosage form for a patient.
3. Create a listing of conceivable ways a consumer/patient may misuse a capsule dosage form.
4. List five counseling points for proper administration of solid dosage forms, for example, capsules.
5. Make a listing of factors that might make a patient apprehensive about taking a capsule dosage form. List the points of advice/counseling points and methods and devices that are available to overcome this apprehension.

6. Identify several patient populations who might have difficulty administering a solid dosage form, for example, capsules, and explain your examples.

INDIVIDUAL ACTIVITIES

1. Create a listing of liquid, oral prescription products, including the concentration of active ingredient(s), available in hard or soft gelatin capsules.
2. Create a listing of liquid, oral nonprescription products, including the concentration of active ingredient(s), available in hard or soft gelatin capsules.
3. Generate a listing of drug products that utilize active ingredients in a micronized powder form.
4. Select one USP drug monograph for a capsule dosage form and identify and describe its main components.

REFERENCES

1. http://www.ismp.org/tools/donotcrush.pdf. (Accessed July 24, 2020)
2. Jones BE. Hard gelatin capsules and the pharmaceutical formulator. Pharm Technol 1985;9:106–112.
3. Digenis A, Gold TB, Shah VP. Cross-linking of gelatin capsules and its relevance to their in vitro/in vivo performance. Dissolut Tech 1995;2:1.
4. Gardner D, Casper R, Leith F, et al. Noninvasive methodology for assessing regional drug absorption from the gastrointestinal tract. Pharm Technol 1997;21:82–89.
5. Wilding IR. Pharmacoscintigraphic evaluation of oral delivery systems, part I. Pharm Technol 1995;19:54–60.
6. Mojaverian P, Reynolds JC, Ouyang A, et al. Mechanism of gastric emptying of a nondisintegrating radiotelemetry capsule in man. Pharm Res 1991;8:97–100.
7. Nash RA. The "rule of sixes" for filling hard-shell gelatin capsules. Int J Pharm Compd 1997;1:40–41.

8. Zhang Y, Johnson KC. Effect of particle size on content uniformity of low-dose solid dosage forms. Int J Pharm 1997;154(2):179–183.

9. Caldwell HC. Dissolution of lithium and magnesium from lithium carbonate capsules containing magnesium stearate. J Pharm Sci 1974;63:770–773.

10. Etaseal. Windsor, ON: Capsule Technology International.

11. Licaps. Greenwood, SC: Capsugel Division of Warner-Lambert. Available at: http://www.capsugel.com/products/licaps.php. (Accessed July 24, 2020)

12. Quali-seal. Indianapolis, IN: Elanco Qualicaps, Eli Lilly.

13. Stanley JP. Soft gelatin capsules. In: Lachman L, Lieberman HA, Kanig JL, eds. The Theory and Practice of Industrial Pharmacy. 3rd Ed. Philadelphia, PA: Lea & Febiger, 1986:398–429.

14. The United States Pharmacopeia–National Formulary. Current Ed. Rockville, MD: U.S. Pharmacopeial Convention.

15. International Journal of Pharmaceutical Compounding. www.ijpc.com (Accessed May 20, 2021).

16. Allen LV Jr. The Art, Science, and Technology of Pharmaceutical Compounding. 5th Ed. Washington, DC: American Pharmaceutical Association, 2016.

8 Tablets

OBJECTIVES

After reading this chapter, the student will be able to:

1. Differentiate between the various types of tablet dosage forms
2. Compare and contrast advantages and disadvantages of the various types of tablet dosage forms
3. List categories of ingredients, with examples, which are employed in the manufacture of compressed tablets
4. State quality standards and USP compendial requirements for tablets
5. Define and differentiate weight variation from content uniformity
6. Describe appropriate techniques for inspecting, packaging, and storing tablets

▌INTRODUCTION

Tablets are solid dosage forms usually prepared with the aid of suitable pharmaceutical excipients. They may vary in size, shape, weight, hardness, thickness, disintegration, and dissolution characteristics and in other aspects, depending on their intended use and method of manufacture. Most tablets are used in the oral administration of drugs. Many of these are prepared with colorants and coatings of various types. Other tablets, such as those administered sublingually, buccally, or vaginally, are prepared to have features most applicable to their particular route of administration.

Tablets are prepared primarily by compression, with a limited number prepared by molding. Compressed tablets are manufactured with tablet machines capable of exerting great pressure in compacting the powdered or granulated material (Fig. 8.1A and B). Their shape and dimensions are determined by the use of various shaped punches and dies (Fig. 8.2). Molded tablets are prepared on a large scale by tablet machinery or on a small scale by manually forcing dampened powder material into a mold from which the formed tablet is then ejected and allowed to dry.

Some tablets are *scored*, or grooved, which allows them to be easily broken into two or more parts. This enables the patient to swallow smaller portions as may be desired, or when prescribed, it allows the tablet to be taken in reduced or divided dosage. Some tablets that are not scored are not intended to be broken or cut by the patient because they may have special coatings and/or drug-release features that would be compromised by altering the tablet's physical integrity.

▌TYPES OF TABLETS

The various types of tablets are described as follows.

Compressed Tablets

In addition to the medicinal agent or agents, compressed tablets usually contain a number of pharmaceutical excipients, including the following:

Diluents or *fillers*, which add the necessary bulk to a formulation to prepare tablets of the desired size

Binders or *adhesives*, which promote adhesion of the particles of the formulation, allowing a granulation to be prepared and maintaining the integrity of the final tablet

Disintegrants or *disintegrating agents*, which promote breakup of the tablets after administration to smaller particles for ready drug availability

MINIPRESS-II

FIGURE 8.1. **A:** Mini Tablet Press for development and small-scale production. (Courtesy of GlobePharma.) **B:** High-performance double rotary tablet press. (Courtesy of Chamunda Pharma Machinery Pvt. Ltd.)

Antiadherents, glidants, lubricants, or *lubricating agents,* which enhance the flow of the material into the tablet dies, minimize wear of the punches and dies, prevent fill material from sticking to the punches and dies, and produce tablets with a sheen

Miscellaneous adjuncts such as colorants and flavorants

After compression, tablets may be coated with various materials as described later. Tablets for oral, buccal, sublingual, or vaginal administration may be prepared by compression.

Multiple Compressed Tablets

Multiple compressed tablets are prepared by subjecting the fill material to more than a single compression. The result may be a multiple-layer tablet or a tablet within a tablet, the inner tablet being the *core* and the outer portion being

the *shell* (Fig. 8.3). Layered tablets are prepared by initial compaction of a portion of fill material in a die followed by additional fill material and compression to form two-layered or three-layered tablets, depending on the number of separate fills. Each layer may contain a different medicinal agent, separated for reasons of chemical or physical incompatibility, staged drug release, or simply the unique appearance of the layered tablet. Usually, each portion of fill is a different color to produce a distinctive-looking tablet. In preparation of tablets within tablets, special machines are required to place the preformed core tablet precisely within the die for application of surrounding fill material.

Sugarcoated Tablets

Compressed tablets may be coated with a colored or an uncolored sugar layer. The coating is water soluble and quickly dissolves after swallowing. The sugarcoat protects

FIGURE 8.2. Various punches and dies for the production of tablets. **A:** Multi-tip punches and dies. **B:** Single-tip punches and dies. (Courtesy of Natoli Engineering Company, Inc.)

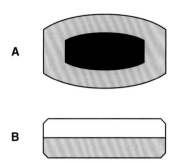

FIGURE 8.3. Multiple compressed tablets. **A:** A core of one drug and a shell of another. **B:** A layered tablet of two drugs.

the enclosed drug from the environment and provides a barrier to objectionable taste or odor. The sugarcoat also enhances the appearance of the compressed tablet and permits imprinting of identifying manufacturer's information. Among the disadvantages to sugarcoating tablets are the time and expertise required in the coating process and the increase in size, weight, and shipping costs. Sugarcoating may add 50% to the weight and bulk of the uncoated tablet.

Film-Coated Tablets

Film-coated tablets are compressed tablets coated with a thin layer of a polymer capable of forming a skinlike film. The film is usually colored and has the advantage over sugarcoatings in that it is more durable, less bulky, and less time-consuming to apply. By its composition, the coating is designed to rupture and expose the core tablet at the desired location in the gastrointestinal tract.

Gelatin-Coated Tablets

A recent innovation is the gelatin-coated tablet. The innovator product, the gelcap, is a capsule-shaped compressed tablet (Fig. 8.4) that allows the coated product to be about one-third smaller than a capsule filled with an equivalent amount of powder. The gelatin coating facilitates swallowing, and gelatin-coated tablets are more tamper evident than unsealed capsules. Examples include Tylenol Cold Multi-Symptom Daytime (McNeil Consumer).

FIGURE 8.4. Cutaway view of gelcap dosage form. (Courtesy of Steven Collins/Shutterstock.)

Enteric-Coated Tablets

Enteric-coated tablets have delayed-release features. They are designed to pass unchanged through the stomach to the intestines, where the tablets disintegrate and allow drug dissolution and absorption and/or effect. Enteric coatings are employed when the drug substance is destroyed by gastric acid or is particularly irritating to the gastric mucosa or when bypass of the stomach substantially enhances drug absorption. Examples include Ecotrin tablets and caplets (GlaxoSmithKline Beecham).

Buccal and Sublingual Tablets

Buccal and sublingual tablets are flat, oval tablets intended to be dissolved in the buccal pouch (*buccal tablets*) or beneath the tongue (*sublingual tablets*) for absorption through the oral mucosa. They enable oral absorption of drugs that are destroyed by the gastric juice and/or are poorly absorbed from the gastrointestinal tract. Buccal tablets are designed to erode slowly, whereas those for sublingual use (such as nitroglycerin [NTG]) dissolve promptly and provide rapid drug effects. *Lozenges* or *troches* are disc-shaped solid dosage forms containing a medicinal agent and generally a flavoring substance in a hard candy or sugar base. They are intended to be slowly dissolved in the oral cavity, usually for local effects, although some are formulated for systemic absorption. An example would be Mycelex troches (Bayer Consumer Care).

Chewable Tablets

Chewable tablets, which have a smooth, rapid disintegration when chewed or allowed to dissolve in the mouth, have a creamy base, usually of specially flavored and colored mannitol. Chewable tablets are especially useful for administration of large tablets to children and adults who have difficulty swallowing solid dosage forms. Examples include Pepcid AC chewable tablets (J&J Merck) and Rolaids chewable tablets (Pfizer Consumer Healthcare).

Effervescent Tablets

Effervescent tablets are prepared by compressing granular effervescent salts that release gas when in contact with water. These tablets generally contain medicinal substances that dissolve rapidly when added to water. The "bubble action" can assist in breaking up the tablets and enhancing the dissolution of the active drug. Examples include Alka-Seltzer Original tablets (Bayer Consumer Care) and Zantac EFFERdose (GlaxoSmithKline).

Molded Tablets

Certain tablets, such as tablet triturates, may be prepared by molding rather than by compression. The resultant tablets are very soft and soluble and are designed for rapid dissolution.

Tablet Triturates

Tablet triturates are small, usually cylindrical, molded, or compressed tablets containing small amounts of usually potent drugs. Today, only a few tablet triturate products are available commercially, with most of these produced by tablet compression. Because tablet triturates must be readily and completely soluble in water, only a minimal amount of pressure is applied during their manufacture. A combination of sucrose and lactose is usually the diluent. The few tablet triturates that remain are used sublingually, such as NTG tablets.

Pharmacists also employ tablet triturates in compounding. For example, triturates are inserted into capsules or dissolved in liquid to provide accurate amounts of potent drug substances.

Hypodermic Tablets

Hypodermic tablets are no longer available in the United States. They were originally used by physicians in extemporaneous preparation of parenteral solutions. The required number of tablets was dissolved in a suitable vehicle and sterilized, and the injection was performed. The tablets were a convenience, because they could be easily carried in the physician's medicine bag and injections prepared to meet the needs of the individual patients. However, the difficulty in achieving sterility and the availability of prefabricated injectable products, some in disposable syringes, have eliminated the need for hypodermic tablets.

Dispensing Tablets

Dispensing tablets are no longer in use. They might better have been termed *compounding tablets* because the pharmacist used them to compound prescriptions; they were *not* dispensed as such to the patient. The tablets contained large amounts of highly potent drug substances, so the pharmacist could rapidly obtain premeasured amounts for compounding multiple dosage units. These tablets had the dangerous potential of being inadvertently dispensed as such to patients.

Immediate-Release Tablets

Immediate-release tablets are designed to disintegrate and release their medication with no special rate-controlling features, such as special coatings and other techniques.

Rapidly Disintegrating or Dissolving Tablets

Rapid-release tablets (rapidly dissolving tablets or RDTs) are characterized by disintegrating or dissolving in the mouth within 1 minute, some within 10 seconds (e.g., Clarinex RediTabs [loratadine], Schering). Tablets of this type are designed for children and the elderly or for any patient who has difficulty in swallowing tablets. They liquefy on the tongue, and the patient swallows the liquid. A number of techniques are used to prepare these tablets, including lyophilization (e.g., Zydis, R.P. Scherer), soft direct compression (e.g., Wow-Tab, Yamanouchi Shaklee Pharma), and other methods (e.g., Quicksolv, Janssen). These tablets are prepared using very water-soluble excipients designed to wick water into the tablet for rapid

disintegration or dissolution. They have the stability characteristics of other solid dosage forms.

The original fast-dissolving tablets were molded tablets for sublingual use. They generally consisted of active drug and lactose moistened with an alcohol–water mixture to form a paste. The tablets were then molded, dried, and packaged. For use, they were simply placed under the tongue to provide a rapid onset of action for drugs such as NTG. Also, they have been used for drugs that are destroyed in the gastrointestinal tract, such as testosterone, administered sublingually for absorption to minimize the first-pass effect.

These RDTs are more convenient to carry and administer than an oral liquid. They are generally packaged in cards or bubble-type packaging with each individual tablet in its own cavity. As these tablets are often soft, the backing is peeled back to reveal the tablet where it is then removed, as opposed to attempting to press the tablet through the backing material as is common with standard compressed tablets. There are no standards that define an RDT, but one possibility is dissolution in the mouth within approximately 15 seconds; anything slower would not be categorized as rapidly dissolving.

Notwithstanding these advantages, there are a number of disadvantages and difficulties associated with formulating RDTs, including drug loading, taste masking, friability, manufacturing costs, and stability of the product. Taste masking can be accomplished by coating the drug particles with a Eudragit polymer prior to production that will not dissolve in the oral cavity but will in the stomach.

Drug loading is incorporation of the drug into the dosage form. Some RDTs are made as blanks to which a drug is postloaded, or added after the blank is made. Generally, the drug is in solution, often in an organic solvent (alcohol), and is added to the tablet, after which the solvent evaporates. It is also possible for the drug to be added as a dry powder electrostatically at this stage. Most drugs, however, are incorporated into the tablets during manufacturing.

Taste masking poses numerous challenges for RDTs. Because the drug product dissolves in the mouth, any taste of the drug must be covered, either by a flavoring technique or by microencapsulation or nanoencapsulation. The product also should not be gritty, which necessitates very small particle sizes if microencapsulation is used.

Friability, the tendency for particles to erode from the surface due to rubbing or mechanical impact, is an inherent problem in RDTs. For a product to dissolve instantly, it may be quite friable. Making it more firm and less friable may increase dissolution time. A balance generally must be achieved between friability and the speed of dissolution.

Lyophilized Foam

The first entry into the RDT field was the Zydis delivery system. The tablets are prepared by foaming a mixture of gelatin, one or more sugars, drug, and any other

FIGURE 8.5. A large-scale lyophilizer: ALUS™ Automatic Load and Unload Systems by GEA. (Courtesy of GEA Group.)

components and by pouring the foam into a mold. The mold also serves as the unit dose–dispensing package. The foam is lyophilized (Fig. 8.5), and the tablets in the mold are packaged. This system is the fastest disintegrating system on the market, as the tablets will dissolve on the tongue in a matter of a few seconds. One disadvantage of this method is that taste masking can be a problem, because the drug is incorporated during the formation of the tablet itself. Another difficulty is that these tablets are sometimes difficult to remove from the packaging, because they are soft and one should not press on the dosage unit to remove it but should peel off the material, exposing the tablet in its mold.

Claritin (loratadine) rapidly disintegrating tablets (RediTabs, Schering Corporation) contain 10 mg of micronized loratadine in a base containing citric acid, gelatin, mannitol, and mint flavor formed with the Zydis technology. It disintegrates within seconds after being placed on the tongue, with or without water. Claritin RediTabs have been shown to provide at least equivalent pharmacokinetic parameters to those of traditional tablets; in some cases, the RediTabs provided greater maximum concentration (C_{max}) and area under the curve values. Claritin RediTabs are blister-packaged tablets that should be stored in a dry place at 2°C to 25°C. They should be used within 6 months of opening the protective laminated foil pouch containing the blister cards; each foil pouch contains one blister card containing 10 individually sealed tablets (1). Other commercial products using this technology include the Maxalt-MLT (Merck), Zofran ODT (GlaxoSmithKline), Zyprexa Zydis (Eli Lilly) tablets, and Tylenol Meltaways Jr. (McNeil Consumer). It should be noted that the Clarinex RediTabs (desloratadine, Schering) use a different formulation principle than Claritin RediTabs, despite the same dosage form designation. The excipients consist of mannitol, microcrystalline cellulose, pregelatinized starch, sodium starch glycolate, magnesium stearate, butylated methacrylate copolymer, crospovidone, aspartame, citric acid, sodium bicarbonate, colloidal silicon dioxide, ferric oxide red, and tuttifrutti flavoring (2).

Compression

Another method of preparation is using standard tableting technology with a composition that will enhance fluid uptake and tablet disintegration and dissolution. For example, superdisintegrants incorporated with a small quantity of effervescent material will lead to intermediately fast disintegration. The tablets are compressed a little thinner than standard tablets to allow for a larger surface area exposed to the saliva in the mouth. Upon placement in the mouth, the disintegrant starts wicking water into the tablet. The effervescent materials start dissolving and aid in the breakup. This continues until the tablet has disintegrated.

An example product is the Dimetapp ND orally disintegrating tablet (nondrowsy allergy tablets; Wyeth Consumer Healthcare). These tablets contain loratadine 10 mg in a vehicle of artificial and natural flavor, aspartame, citric acid, colloidal silicon dioxide, corn syrup solids, crospovidone, magnesium stearate, mannitol, microcrystalline cellulose, modified food starch, and sodium bicarbonate (3).

One product using the DuraSolv and OraSolv technologies by Cima Labs is Tempra Quicklets containing acetaminophen 80 mg. These tablets also contain aspartame, citric acid, D&C Red No. 27 Lake, FD&C Blue No. 1 Lake, flavor, magnesium stearate, mannitol, potassium carbonate, silicon dioxide, and sodium bicarbonate. They are somewhat slower than the Zydis tablet, taking about 30 to 45 seconds, unless some tongue pressure is used. These tablets come in a firm molded plastic package to prevent breakage (4). Other commercial products using the same technology include the Alavert (Wyeth), NuLev FasTabs (Schwarz Pharma), Symax FasTabs (Capellon), Remeron SolTabs (Organon), Triaminic Softchews (Novartis Consumer Health), Abilify Discmelt (Otsuka America), Tylenol Meltaways (McNeil Consumer), and the Zomig ZMT (AstraZeneca).

The Flashtab technology by Ethypharm is used in Excedrin QuickTabs and an example of the Wowtab technology by Yamanouchi Pharma is the Benadryl Fastmelt.

Example Chewable Dispersible Tablets

Lamictal chewable dispersible tablets for oral administration contain 2, 5, or 25 mg of lamotrigine and the following inactive ingredients: black currant flavor, calcium carbonate, low-substituted hydroxypropyl cellulose, magnesium aluminum silicate, magnesium stearate, povidone, saccharin sodium, and sodium starch glycolate (5).

Lamotrigine is also available as standard swallow tablets for oral administration in strengths of 25, 100, 150, and 200 mg, also containing lactose, magnesium stearate, microcrystalline cellulose, povidone, sodium starch glycolate, and various coloring agents for the different strengths. Lamotrigine is an antiepileptic drug chemically unrelated to existing drugs in this therapeutic class. The swallow tablets should be swallowed whole, as chewing may leave a bitter taste. The chewable tablets may be swallowed whole, chewed, or mixed in water or diluted fruit juice. If they are chewed, a small amount of water or diluted fruit juice will aid in swallowing. If the tablet is to be dispersed before it is taken, it can be added to a small amount of liquid (one teaspoonful or sufficient to cover the medication in a glass or spoon), and approximately 1 minute later when the tablet is completely dispersed, it is mixed and administered immediately.

Didanosine (Videx) is available in three dosage forms: a chewable dispersible buffered tablet, buffered powder for oral solution, and a pediatric powder for oral solution (6). Videx is a synthetic purine nucleoside analog active against HIV. The chewable dispersible buffered tablets are for oral administration in strengths of 25, 50, 100, 150, and 200 mg. Each tablet is buffered with calcium carbonate and magnesium hydroxide. Also contained in the tablet matrix are aspartame, sorbitol, microcrystalline cellulose, Polyplasdone, mandarin orange flavor, and magnesium stearate.

Didanosine (2′,3′-dideoxyinosine) is unstable in acidic solutions; at a pH less than 3 at body temperature, 10% of didanosine decomposes to hypoxanthine in less than 2 minutes. This is the reason for the buffering agents in the chewable tablets and in one of the oral solutions. It is also available as an enteric-coated formulation (Videx EC delayed-release capsules) to protect it from the acidic contents of the stomach.

Because these tablets tend to be more fragile than standard compressed tablets, they are generally packaged in more sturdy materials to prevent damage.

Extended-Release Tablets

Extended-release tablets (sometimes called controlled-release tablets) are designed to release their medication in a predetermined manner over an extended period. They are discussed in Chapter 9.

Vaginal Tablets

Vaginal tablets, also called *vaginal inserts*, are uncoated, bullet-shaped, or ovoid tablets inserted into the vagina for local effects. They are prepared by compression and shaped to fit snugly on plastic inserter devices that accompany the product. They contain antibacterials for the treatment of nonspecific vaginitis caused by *Haemophilus vaginalis* or antifungals for the treatment of vulvovaginitis candidiasis caused by *Candida albicans* and related species.

▌ COMPRESSED TABLETS

The physical features of compressed tablets are well known: round, oblong, or unique in shape; thick or thin; large or small in diameter; flat or convex; unscored or *scored* (Fig. 8.6) in halves, thirds, or quadrants; engraved or imprinted with an identifying symbol and/or code number; coated or uncoated; colored or uncolored; and one, two, or three layered.

FIGURE 8.6. Packages of a drug product of different tablet strengths.

Tablet diameters and shapes are determined by the die and punches used in compression. The less concave the punches, the flatter the tablets; conversely, the more concave the punches, the more convex the resulting tablets (Fig. 8.7). Punches with raised impressions produce recessed impressions on the tablets; punches with recessed etchings produce tablets with raised impressions or monograms. Monograms may be placed on one or on both sides of a tablet, depending on the punches.

Quality Standards and Compendial Requirements

In addition to the apparent features of tablets, tablets must meet other physical specifications and quality standards. These include criteria for weight, weight variation, content uniformity, thickness, hardness, disintegration, and dissolution. These factors must be controlled during production (in-process controls) and verified after the production of each batch to ensure that established product quality standards are met (Fig. 8.8).

FIGURE 8.7. Contours of the punches determine the shape of the tablets. *From left to right*: flat face, shallow cup, standard cup, deep cup, and modified ball. (Courtesy of Cherry-Burrell Corporation.)

FIGURE 8.8. Quality control in the manufacturing of tablets. (Courtesy of Akank/Shutterstock.)

Tablet Weight and USP Weight Variation Test

The quantity of fill in the die of a tablet press determines the weight of the tablet. The volume of fill is adjusted with the first few tablets to yield the *desired weight and content*. For example, if a tablet is to contain 20 mg of a drug substance and if 100,000 tablets are to be produced, 2,000 g of drug is included in the formula. After the addition of the pharmaceutical additives, such as the diluent, disintegrant, lubricant, and binder, the formulation may weigh 20 kg, which means that each tablet must weigh 200 mg for 20 mg of drug to be present. Thus, the depth of fill in the tablet die must be adjusted to hold a volume of granulation weighing 200 mg. During production, sample tablets are periodically removed for visual inspection and automated physical measurement (Fig. 8.9).

The USP contains a test for determination of dosage form uniformity by *weight variation* for uncoated tablets (5). In the test, 10 tablets are weighed individually, and the average weight is calculated. The tablets are assayed, and the content of active ingredient in each of the 10 tablets is calculated assuming homogeneous drug distribution.

Content Uniformity

By the USP method, 10 dosage units are individually assayed for their content according to the method described in the individual monograph. Unless otherwise stated in the monograph, the requirements for content uniformity are met if the amount of active ingredient in each dosage unit lies within the range of 85% to 115% of the label claim and the standard deviation is less than 6%. If one or more dosage units do not meet these criteria, additional tests as prescribed in the USP are required (7).

Tablet Thickness

The thickness of a tablet is determined by the diameter of the die, the amount of fill permitted to enter the die, the compaction characteristics of the fill material, and the force or pressure applied during compression.

To produce tablets of uniform thickness during and between batch productions for the same formulation, care must be exercised to employ the same factors of fill, die, and pressure. The degree of pressure affects not only thickness but also hardness of the tablet; hardness is perhaps the more important criterion because it can affect disintegration and dissolution. Thus, for tablets of uniform thickness and hardness, it is doubly important to control pressure. Tablet thickness may be measured by hand gauge during production or by automated equipment (Figs. 8.10 to 8.12).

Tablet Hardness and Friability

It is fairly common for a tablet press to exert as little as 3,000 and as much as 40,000 lb of force in the production of tablets. Generally, the greater the pressure applied, the harder the tablets, although the characteristics of the granulation also have a bearing on hardness. Certain tablets, such as lozenges and buccal tablets, that are intended to dissolve slowly are intentionally made hard; other tablets, such as those for immediate drug release, are made soft.

FIGURE 8.9. Automatic balance that weighs product and prints statistics to determine compliance with USP weight variation requirements for tablets. (Courtesy of Mocon Modern Controls.)

FIGURE 8.10. Tablet thickness gauge. (Courtesy Digital Micrometers Ltd.)

FIGURE 8.11. Tablet thickness, diameter, and hardness testing instrument. (Courtesy of Vortex Sales Group.)

In general, tablets should be sufficiently hard to resist breaking during normal handling and yet soft enough to disintegrate properly after swallowing.

Special dedicated hardness testers (Fig. 8.13) or multifunctional systems (Fig. 8.12) are used to measure the degree of force (in kilograms, pounds, or in arbitrary units) required to break a tablet. A force of about 4 kg is considered the minimum requirement for a satisfactory tablet. Multifunctional automated equipment can determine weight, hardness, thickness, and diameter of the tablet.

A tablet's durability may be determined through the use of a *friabilator* (Fig. 8.14). This apparatus determines the tablet's *friability*, or tendency to crumble, by allowing it to roll and fall within the drum. The tablets are weighed before and after a specified number of rotations, and any weight loss is determined. Resistance to loss of weight

FIGURE 8.13. Tablet hardness tester. (Courtesy of ERWEKA GmbH.)

indicates the tablet's ability to withstand abrasion in handling, packaging, and shipment. A maximum weight loss of not more than 1% generally is considered acceptable for most products.

Tablet Disintegration

For the medicinal agent in a tablet to become fully available for absorption, the tablet must first disintegrate and discharge the drug to the body fluids for dissolution. Tablet disintegration also is important for tablets containing medicinal agents (such as antacids and antidiarrheals) that are not intended to be absorbed but rather to act locally within the gastrointestinal tract. In these instances, tablet

FIGURE 8.12. Automatic weight, hardness, thickness, and tablet diameter test instrument for quality control. Using a microprocessor and monitor for visualization, the instrument can test up to 20 samples at a time. (Courtesy of JB Pharmatron.)

FIGURE 8.14. Friabilator testing apparatus. (Courtesy of SOTAX.)

FIGURE 8.15. Tablet disintegration testing apparatus. (Courtesy of ARL Bio Pharma, Inc. d/b/a Analytical Research Laboratories.)

disintegration provides drug particles with an increased surface area for activity within the gastrointestinal tract.

All USP tablets must pass a test for disintegration, which is conducted in vitro using a testing apparatus such as the one shown in Figure 8.15. The apparatus consists of a basket and rack assembly containing six open-ended transparent tubes of USP-specified dimensions, held vertically upon a 10-mesh stainless steel wire screen. During testing, a tablet is placed in each of the six tubes of the basket, and through the use of a mechanical device, the basket is raised and lowered in the immersion fluid at 29 to 32 cycles per minute, the wire screen always below the level of the fluid. For uncoated tablets, buccal tablets, and sublingual tablets, water at about 37°C serves as the immersion fluid unless another fluid is specified in the individual monograph. For these tests, complete disintegration is defined as "that state in which any residue of the unit, except fragments of insoluble coating or capsule shell, remaining on the screen of the test apparatus is a soft mass having no palpably firm core" (7). Tablets must disintegrate within the times set forth in the individual monograph, usually 30 minutes, but varying from about 2 minutes for NTG tablets to up to 4 hours for buccal tablets. If one or more tablets fail to disintegrate, additional tests prescribed by the USP must be performed.

Enteric-coated tablets are similarly tested, except that the tablets are tested in simulated gastric fluid for 1 hour, after which no sign of disintegration, cracking, or softening must be seen. They are then actively immersed in the simulated intestinal fluid for the time stated in the individual monograph, during which time the tablets disintegrate completely for a positive test.

Tablet Dissolution

In vitro dissolution testing of solid dosage forms is important for a number of reasons (8):

1. It guides formulation and product development toward product optimization. Dissolution studies in the early stages of a product's development allow differentiation between formulations and correlations identified with in vivo bioavailability data.

2. Manufacturing may be monitored by dissolution testing as a component of the overall quality assurance program. The conduct of such testing from early product development through approval and commercial production ensures control of any variables of materials and processes that could affect dissolution and quality standards.

3. Consistent in vitro dissolution testing ensures bioequivalence from batch to batch. In assessing such bioequivalence, the U.S. Food and Drug Administration (FDA) allows manufacturers to examine scale-up batches of 10% of the proposed size of the actual production batch or 100,000 dosage units, whichever is greater.

4. It is a requirement for regulatory approval of marketing for products registered with the FDA and regulatory agencies of other countries. New Drug Applications (NDAs) submitted to the FDA contain in vitro dissolution data generally obtained from batches used in pivotal clinical and/or bioavailability studies and from human studies conducted during product development (9). Once the specifications are established in an approved NDA, they become official (USP) specifications for all subsequent batches and bioequivalent products.

The goal of in vitro dissolution testing is to provide a reasonable prediction of the product's in vivo bioavailability. The Biopharmaceutics Classification System (BCS) relates combinations of a drug's solubility (high or low) and its intestinal permeability (high or low) as a possible basis for predicting the likelihood of achieving a successful in vivo–in vitro correlation (IVIVC) (9,10). Using this system, drugs are placed into one of four categories as follows:

I	II
High solubility and high permeability	Low solubility and high permeability
III	IV
High solubility and low permeability	Low solubility and low permeability

For a high-solubility and high-permeability Category I drug, an IVIVC may be expected if the dissolution rate is slower than the rate of gastric emptying (the rate-limiting factor) (11). In the case of a low-solubility and high-permeability Category II drug, dissolution may be the rate-limiting step for absorption, and an IVIVC may be expected. In the case of a high-solubility and low-permeability Category III drug, permeability is the rate-controlling step, and only a limited IVIVC may be possible. In the case of a Category IV drug with low solubility and low permeability, significant problems are likely for oral drug delivery (9).

As noted previously, tablet disintegration is the important first step to the dissolution of the drug in a tablet. A number of formulation and manufacturing factors can affect the disintegration and dissolution of a tablet, including particle size of the drug substance; solubility and hygroscopicity of the formulation; type and concentration of the disintegrant, binder, and lubricant; manufacturing method, particularly the compactness of the granulation and compression force used in tableting; and any in-process variables (12). Together, these factors present a set of complex interrelated conditions that have a bearing on a product's dissolution characteristics. Therefore, batch-to-batch consistency is vitally important to establish dissolution test standards and controls for both materials and processes and to implement them during production and in final testing.

In addition to formulation and manufacturing controls, the method of dissolution testing must be controlled to minimize important variables such as paddle rotational speed, vibration, and disturbances by sampling probes. Dissolution testing for oral dosage forms has been a component of evaluating product quality in the USP since 1970, when only 12 monographs contained such a requirement. Today, the requirement is standard for tablets and capsules.

The USP includes seven apparatus designs for drug release and dissolution testing of immediate-release oral dosage forms, extended-release products, enteric-coated products, and transdermal drug delivery devices. Of primary interest here are USP Apparatus 1 and USP Apparatus 2, used principally for immediate-release solid oral dosage forms.

The equipment consists of (*a*) a variable-speed stirrer motor; (*b*) a cylindrical stainless steel basket on a stirrer shaft (USP Apparatus 1) or a paddle as the stirring element (USP Apparatus 2); (*c*) a 1,000-mL vessel of glass or other inert transparent material fitted with a cover having a center port for the shaft of the stirrer and three additional ports, two for removal of samples and one for a thermometer; and (*d*) a water bath to maintain the temperature of the dissolution medium in the vessel. For use of USP Apparatus 1, the dosage unit is placed inside the basket. For use of USP Apparatus 2, the dosage unit is placed in the vessel.

In each test, a volume of the dissolution medium (as stated in the individual monograph) is placed in the vessel and allowed to come to 37°C ± 0.5°C. Then, the stirrer is rotated at the speed specified, and at stated intervals, samples of the medium are withdrawn for chemical analysis of the proportion of drug dissolved. The tablet or capsule must meet the stated monograph requirement for rate of dissolution, for example, "not less than 85% of the labeled amount is dissolved in 30 minutes."

There is growing recognition that where inconsistencies in dissolution occur, they occur not between dosage units from the same production batch but rather between

FIGURE 8.16. Automated dissolution test system. (Courtesy of Agilent Technologies, Inc.)

batches or between products from different manufacturers, most likely because of the many factors of formulation, materials, and manufacturing pointed out earlier. However, because dosage units within a batch are generally not the problem, pooled dissolution testing has emerged. This process recognizes batch characteristics and allows pooled specimens to be tested. The pooled specimens may be sampled from the individual dissolution vessels in the apparatus or from multiple dosage units dissolved in a single vessel (13).

Sophisticated and highly automated equipment is continually being developed to provide high levels of quality assurance and control to dissolution testing (Figs. 8.16 and 8.17).

FIGURE 8.17. A modern computer laboratory for studies of drug dissolution from solid dosage forms. (Courtesy Surasak Petchang/Dreamstime.com.)

Compressed Tablet Manufacture

Compressed tablets may be made by three basic methods: *wet granulation*, *dry granulation*, and *direct compression*. Figure 8.18 presents schematic drawings of each method.

Most powdered medicinal agents require addition of excipients such as diluents, binders, disintegrants, and lubricants to provide the desired characteristics for tablet manufacture and efficacious use. One important requirement in tablet manufacture is that the drug mixture flows freely from the hopper of the tablet press into the dies to enable high-speed compression of the powder mix into tablets. Granulations of powders provide this free flow. Granulations also increase material density, improving powder compressibility during tablet formation.

Wet Granulation

Wet granulation is a widely employed method for the production of compressed tablets. The steps required are (*a*) weighing and blending the ingredients, (*b*) preparing a dampened powder or a damp mass, (*c*) screening the dampened powder or damp mass into pellets or granules, (*d*) drying the granulation, (*e*) sizing the granulation by dry screening, (*f*) adding lubricant and blending, and (*g*) forming tablets by compression.

Weighing and Blending

Specified quantities of active ingredient, diluent or filler, and disintegrating agent are mixed by mechanical powder blender or mixer until uniform.

Fillers include lactose, microcrystalline cellulose, starch, powdered sucrose, and calcium phosphate. The choice of filler usually is based on the experience of the manufacturer with the material, its relative cost, and its compatibility with the other formulation ingredients. For example, calcium salts must not be used as fillers with tetracycline antibiotics because of an interaction between the two agents that results in reduced tetracycline absorption from the gastrointestinal tract. Among the fillers most preferred are lactose, because of its solubility and compatibility, and microcrystalline cellulose, because of its easy compaction, compatibility, and consistent uniformity of supply (14).

Disintegrating agents include croscarmellose, corn and potato starches, sodium starch glycolate, sodium carboxymethylcellulose, polyvinylpyrrolidone (PVP), crospovidone, cation exchange resins, alginic acid, and other materials that swell or expand on exposure to moisture and effect the rupture or breakup of the tablet in the gastrointestinal tract. Croscarmellose (2%) and sodium starch glycolate (5%) are often preferred because of their high water uptake and rapid action. One commercial brand of sodium starch glycolate is reported to swell up to 300% of its volume in water (15). When starch is employed, 5% to 10% is usually suitable, but up to about 20% may be used to promote more rapid tablet disintegration. The total amount of disintegrant used is not always added in preparing the granulation. Often a portion (sometimes half) is reserved and added to the finished granulation prior to tablet formation. This results in double disintegration of the tablet. One portion assists in the breakup of the tablet into pieces, and the other portion assists in the breakup of the pieces into fine particles.

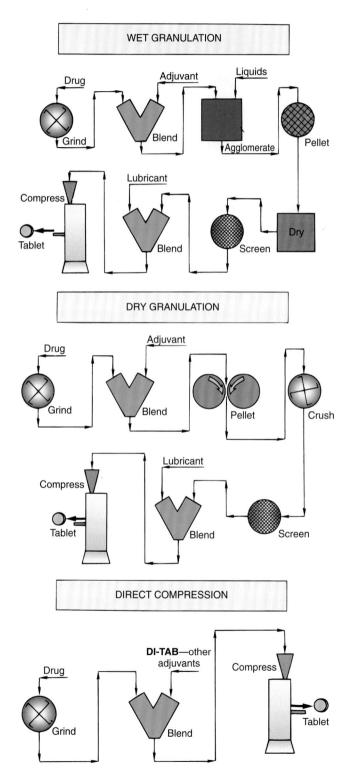

FIGURE 8.18. The three main methods for the preparation of tablets. (Courtesy of Stauffer Chemical Co.)

Preparing the Damp Mass

A liquid binder is added to the powder mixture to facilitate adhesion of the powder particles. Either a dampened powder formed into granules or a damp mass resembling dough is formed and used to prepare the granulation. A good binder results in appropriate tablet hardness and does not hinder the release of the drug from the tablet.

Among binding agents are solutions of povidone, an aqueous preparation of cornstarch (10% to 20%), glucose solution (25% to 50%), molasses, methylcellulose (3%), carboxymethylcellulose, and microcrystalline cellulose. If the drug substance is adversely affected by an aqueous binder, a nonaqueous solution, or dry binder, may be used. The amount of binding agent used is part of the operator's art; however, the resulting binder–powder mixture should compact when squeezed in the hand. The binding agent contributes to adhesion of the granules to one another and maintains the integrity of the tablet after compression. However, care must be exercised not to overwet or underwet the powder. Overwetting can result in granules that are too hard for proper tablet formation, and underwetting can result in tablets that are too soft and tend to crumble. When desired, a colorant or flavorant may be added to the binding agent to prepare a granulation with an added feature.

Screening the Damp Mass into Pellets or Granules

The dampened powder granules are screened, or the wet mass is pressed through a screen (usually 6 or 8 meshes) to prepare the granules. This may be done by hand or with special equipment that prepares the granules by extrusion through perforations in the apparatus. The resultant granules are spread evenly on large lined trays and dried to consistent weight or constant moisture content.

Drying the Granulation

Granules may be dried in thermostatically controlled ovens that constantly record the time, temperature, and humidity (Fig. 8.19).

Sizing the Granulation by Dry Screening

After drying, the granules are passed through a screen of a smaller mesh than that used to prepare the original granulation. The degree to which the granules are reduced depends on the size of the punches to be used. In general, the smaller the tablet to be produced, the smaller the granules. Screens of 12- to 20-mesh size are generally used for this purpose. Sizing of the granules is necessary so that the die cavities for tablet compression may be completely and rapidly filled by the free-flowing granulation. Voids or air spaces left by too large a granulation result in the production of uneven tablets.

Adding Lubricant and Blending

After dry screening, a dry lubricant is dusted over the spread-out granulation through a fine-mesh screen. Lubricants contribute to the preparation of compressed tablets

FIGURE 8.19. Temperature-controlled drying oven used in the preparation of granules and controlled-release beads. (Courtesy of Perrigo Company, plc Dublin, Ireland.)

in several ways: They improve the flow of the granulation in the hopper to the die cavity. They prevent adhesion of the tablet formulation to the punches and dies during compression. They reduce friction between the tablet and the die wall during the ejection of the tablet from the machine. They give a sheen to the finished tablet. Among the more commonly used lubricants are magnesium stearate, calcium stearate, stearic acid, talc, and sodium stearyl fumarate. Magnesium stearate is most used (14). The quantity of lubricant used varies from one operation to another but usually ranges from about 0.1% to 5% of the weight of the granulation.

All-in-One Granulation Methods

Technologic advances now allow the entire process of granulation to be completed in a continuous *fluid bed process*, using a single piece of equipment, the fluid bed granulator (Figs. 8.20 and 8.21).

The fluid bed granulator performs the following steps: (*a*) preblending the formulation powder, including active ingredients, fillers, and disintegrants, in a bed with fluidized air; (*b*) granulating the mixture by spraying onto the fluidized powder bed, a suitable liquid binder, such as an aqueous solution of acacia, hydroxypropyl cellulose, or povidone; and (*c*) drying the granulated product to the desired moisture content.

Another method, microwave vacuum processing, also allows the powders to be mixed, wetted, agglomerated, and dried within the confines of a single piece of equipment (Fig. 8.22). The wet mass is dried by gentle mixing, vacuum, and microwave. The use of the microwave reduces the drying time considerably, often by one-fourth.

FIGURE 8.20. Fluid bed granulator. (Courtesy of Glatt Air Techniques, Inc.)

The total batch production time is usually in the range of 90 minutes. After adding lubricants and screening, the batch is ready for tablet formation or capsule filling.

Dry Granulation

By the dry granulation method, the powder mixture is compacted in large pieces and subsequently broken down or sized into granules (Fig. 8.18). For this method, either the active ingredient or the diluent must have cohesive properties. Dry granulation is especially applicable to materials that cannot be prepared by wet granulation because they degrade in moisture or the elevated temperatures required for drying the granules.

FIGURE 8.22. Microwave vacuum processing equipment.

Slugging

After weighing and mixing the ingredients, the powder mixture is slugged, or compressed, into large flat tablets or pellets about 1 inch in diameter. The slugs are broken up by hand or by a mill (Fig. 8.23) and passed through a screen of desired mesh for sizing. Lubricant is added in the usual manner, and tablets are prepared by compression. Aspirin, which is hydrolyzed on exposure to moisture, may be prepared into tablets after slugging.

Roller Compaction

Instead of slugging, powder compactors may be used to increase the density of a powder by pressing it between rollers at 1 to 6 tons of pressure. The compacted material is broken up, sized, and lubricated, and tablets are prepared by compression in the usual manner. The *roller*

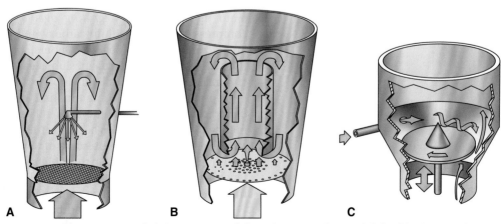

FIGURE 8.21. Top spray **(A)**, bottom spray **(B)**, and tangential spray **(C)** fluid bed coater designs.

FIGURE 8.23. The oscillating and rotating OscilloWitt sieve mill can be used to pulverize or granulate. (Courtesy Frewitt USA, Inc.)

compaction method is often preferred to slugging. Binding agents used in roller compaction formulations include methylcellulose or hydroxy methylcellulose (6% to 12%), which can produce good tablet hardness and friability (16).

Tableting of Granulation

There are a number of types of tablet presses or tableting machines, each varying in productivity but similar in basic function and operation. They all compress a tablet formulation within a steel die cavity by the pressure exerted by the movement of two steel punches, a lower punch and an upper punch (Fig. 8.24).

The operation of a single-punch tablet press describes the basic mechanical process. As the lower punch drops, the feed shoe filled with granulation from the hopper is positioned over and fills the die cavity. The feed shoe retracts,

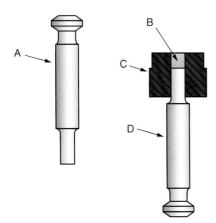

FIGURE 8.24. Punch and die set. *A*: Upper punch. *B*: Die cavity. *C*: Die. *D*: Lower punch. (Courtesy of Cherry-Burrell Corporation.)

scrapes away the excessive granulation, and levels the fill in the die cavity. The upper punch lowers and compresses the fill, forming the tablet. The upper punch retracts as the lower punch rises with the formed tablet to the precise level of the stage. The feed shoe moves over the die cavity, shoves the tablet aside, and once again fills the cavity with granulation to repeat the process. The tablets fall into a collection container. Samples of tablets are assayed and tested for the various quality standards described earlier.

Rotary tablet machines equipped with multiple punches and dies operate via continuous rotating movement of the punches. A single rotary press with 16 stations (16 sets of punches and dies) may produce up to 1,150 tablets per minute. Double rotary tablet presses with 27, 33, 37, 41, or 49 sets of punches and dies are capable of producing two tablets for each die. Some of these machines can produce 10,000 or more tablets per minute of operation (Fig. 8.25). For such high-speed production, induced die feeders are required to force the fill material into the dies to keep up with the rapidly moving punches (Fig. 8.26). A consequence of high-speed production is the increased occurrence of *lamination* (horizontal striations) and tablet *capping*, in which the top of the tablet separates from the whole because the fill material does not have enough time to bond after compression. Reduced speed remedies the problem (17).

Multiple-layer tablets are produced by multiple feed and multiple compression of fill material within a single die. Tablets with an inner core are prepared by machines with a special feed apparatus that places the core tablet precisely within the die for compression with surrounding fill.

Direct Compression Tableting

Some granular chemicals, like potassium chloride, possess free-flowing and cohesive properties that enable them to be compressed directly in a tablet machine without any need of granulation. For chemicals lacking this quality, special pharmaceutical excipients may be used to impart the necessary qualities for the production of tablets by direct compression. These excipients include *fillers*, such as spray-dried lactose, microcrystals of alpha-monohydrate lactose, sucrose–invert sugar–corn starch mixtures, microcrystalline cellulose, crystalline maltose, and dicalcium phosphate; *disintegrating agents*, such as direct compression starch, sodium carboxymethyl starch, cross-linked carboxymethylcellulose fibers, and cross-linked PVP; *lubricants*, such as magnesium stearate and talc; and *glidants*, such as fumed silicon dioxide.

Capping, splitting, or laminating of tablets during direct compression is sometimes related to air entrapment within the powder. When air is trapped, the resulting tablets expand when the pressure of tableting is released, resulting in splits or layers in the tablets. Forced or induced feeders can reduce air entrapment, making the fill powder more dense and amenable to compaction.

Capping also may be caused by punches that are not immaculately clean and perfectly smooth or by a granulation with too much fines or fine powder. Fine powder,

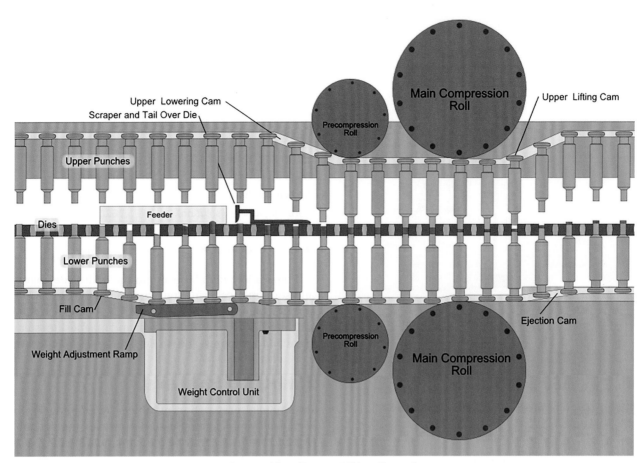

FIGURE 8.25. Rotapress rotary compression machine. (Source: Wikimedia.org.)

which results when a dried granulation is sized, is generally 10% to 20% of the weight of the granulation. Some fine powder is desired to fill the die cavity properly. However, an excess can lead to tablet softness and capping.

Tablets that have aged or been stored improperly also may exhibit splitting or other physical deformations (Fig. 8.27).

Tablet Dedusting

To remove traces of loose powder adhering to tablets following compression, the tablets are conveyed directly from the tableting machine to a deduster (Fig. 8.28). The compressed tablets may then be coated.

FIGURE 8.26. Induced die feeder. The standard gravity-fed open feed frame can be replaced with an induced die feeder, with which granulation is forced into the die by the rotary action of the agitator. (Courtesy of Cherry-Burrell Corporation.)

FIGURE 8.27. Tablets that have split either during production or on aging because of conditions of manufacture or storage. (Courtesy of Slashme at the English Wikipedia, via Wikimedia Commons.)

FIGURE 8.28. High-Speed Tablet Deduster. (Courtesy of Kraemer US, LLC.)

CHEWABLE TABLETS

Chewable tablets are pleasant-tasting tablets formulated to disintegrate smoothly in the mouth with or without chewing. They are prepared by wet granulation and compression, using only minimal degrees of pressure to produce a soft tablet. Generally, chewable tablets do not contain disintegrants, so patients must be counseled to chew the tablets thoroughly and not swallow them whole unless the product labeling specifically states otherwise.

Mannitol, a white crystalline hexahydric alcohol, is used as the excipient in most chewable tablets. Mannitol is about 70% as sweet as sucrose, with a cool feel in the mouth resulting from its negative heat of solution. Mannitol accounts for 50% or more of the weight of many chewable tablet formulations. Sometimes, other sweetening agents, such as sorbitol, lactose, dextrose, crystalline maltose, and glucose, may be substituted for part or all of the mannitol. Xylitol may be used in the preparation of sugar-free chewable tablets. Xylitol is sweeter than mannitol and has the desirable negative heat of solution that provides the cool mouth feel upon dissolution.

Lubricants and binders that do not detract from the texture or desired hardness of the tablet may be used. Colorants and tart or fruity flavorants are commonly employed to enhance the appeal of the tablets. Among the types of products prepared as chewable tablets are antacids (e.g., calcium carbonate), antibiotics (e.g., erythromycin), anti-infective agents (e.g., didanosine), anticonvulsants

(e.g., carbamazepine), vasodilators (e.g., isosorbide dinitrate), analgesics (e.g., acetaminophen), various vitamins, and cold–allergy combination tablets. Chewable tablets are particularly useful for children and adults who have difficulty swallowing other solid dosage forms.

The following is a formula for a typical chewable antacid tablet (18):

Per Tablet

Aluminum hydroxide	325.0 mg
Mannitol	812.0 mg
Sodium saccharin	0.4 mg
Sorbitol (10% w/v solution)	32.5 mg
Magnesium stearate	35.0 mg
Mint flavor concentrate	4.0 mg

Preparation: Blend the aluminum hydroxide, mannitol, and sodium saccharin. Prepare a wet granulation with the sorbitol solution. Dry at 49°C (120°F), and screen through a 12-mesh screen. Add the flavor and magnesium stearate, blend, and compress into tablets.

MOLDED TABLETS

Commercial preparation of tablets by molding has been replaced by tablet compression. However, molded tablets, or *tablet triturates*, may be prepared on a small laboratory scale as follows.

The mold is made of hard rubber, hard plastic, or metal. It has two parts, the upper part, or *die* portion, and the lower part, containing squat, flat *punches*. The die portion is a flat plate with the thickness of the tablets to be produced, with 50 to 200 uniformly drilled and evenly spaced circular holes (Fig. 8.29). The lower part of the mold has corresponding punches that fit the holes precisely. When the die is filled with material and placed atop the punches, the punches gently lift the fill material from the holes to rest upon the punches for drying.

The base for molded tablets is generally a mixture of finely powdered lactose with or without a portion of powdered sucrose (5% to 20%). The addition of sucrose results in less brittle tablets. In preparing the fill, the drug is mixed uniformly with the base by geometric dilution when potent drugs are used. The powder mixture is wetted with a 50% mixture of water and alcohol sufficient only to dampen the powder so that it may be compacted. The solvent action of the water on a portion of the lactose or lactose–sucrose base binds the powder mixture upon drying. The alcohol portion hastens drying.

The upper mold is placed on a clean flat glass surface and the damp mass added by a rubbing motion. When each opening is filled completely and smoothed, top and bottom, the mold is fitted on the punch portion of the mold and pressed down, leaving the tablets raised on the pegs to dry.

Before use, the mold should be calibrated for the fill material used because the densities of different formulas

FIGURE 8.29. Laboratory mold for preparation of tablet triturates. (From Elder DL. Practical Guide to Contemporary Pharmacy Practice and Compounding. 4th Ed. Philadelphia, PA: Wolters Kluwer, 2017.)

result in tablets of different weights. This may be done by preparing a test batch of the formula and weighing and recording the weight of the dry tablets. This weight is used in calculations for production quantities.

Molded tablets are intended to dissolve rapidly in the mouth. They do not contain disintegrants, lubricants, or coatings to slow their rate of dissolution. (A more complete discussion of the preparation of molded tablets and the

standardization of laboratory molds may be found on this book's companion Web site.)

TABLET COATING

Tablets are coated for a number of reasons, including to protect the medicinal agent against destructive exposure to air and/or humidity, to mask the taste of the drug, to provide special characteristics of drug release (e.g., enteric coatings), and to provide aesthetics or distinction to the product.

In a limited number of instances, tablets are coated to prevent inadvertent contact with the drug substance and the effects of drug absorption. For example, Proscar tablets (finasteride, Merck) are coated for just this reason. The drug is used by men in the treatment of benign prostatic hyperplasia. The labeling instructions warn that women who are pregnant or who may become pregnant should not come into contact with it. Drug contact can occur through handling broken tablets. If finasteride is absorbed by a woman who is pregnant with a male baby, the drug has the potential to adversely affect the developing male fetus.

The general methods involved in coating tablets are as follows.

Sugarcoating Tablets

The sugarcoating of tablets may be divided into the following steps: (*a*) waterproofing and sealing if needed, (*b*) subcoating, (*c*) smoothing and final rounding, (*d*) finishing and coloring if desired, and (*e*) polishing. The entire coating process is conducted in a series of mechanically operated acorn-shaped coating pans of galvanized iron, stainless steel, or copper. The pans, which are partially open in the front, have diameters ranging from about 1 to 4 feet and various capacities (Figs. 8.30 and 8.31). The smaller pans

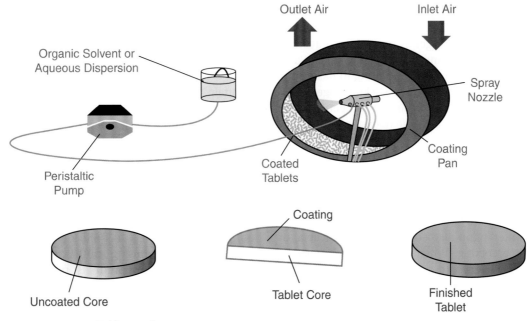

FIGURE 8.30. Tablet coating process.

FIGURE 8.31. Modern tablet-coating facility. (GCM© photo provided courtesy of Glatt Air Techniques, Inc.)

are used for experimental, developmental, and pilot plant operations and the larger pans for industrial production. The pans operate at about a 40-degree angle to contain the tablets while allowing the operator visual and manual access. During operation, the pan is mechanically rotated at moderate speeds, allowing the tablets to tumble over each other while making contact with the coating solutions, which are gently poured or sprayed onto the tablets. To allow gradual buildup of the coatings, the solutions are added in portions, with warm air blown in to hasten drying. Each coat is applied only after the previous coat has dried. Tablets intended to be coated are manufactured to be thin edged and highly convex to allow the coatings to form rounded rather than angular edges.

Waterproofing and Sealing Coats

For tablets containing components that may be adversely affected by moisture, one or more coats of a waterproofing substance, such as pharmaceutical shellac or a polymer (Eudragits and others), are applied to the compressed tablets before the subcoating application. The waterproofing solution (usually alcoholic) is gently poured or sprayed on the compressed tablets rotating in the coating pans. Warm air is blown into the pan during the coating to hasten the drying and to prevent tablets from sticking together. It should be noted that the Eudragits and other agents can be used to either taste-mask or alter the release of the drug(s) in the tablets.

Subcoating

After the tablets are waterproofed if needed, three to five subcoats of a sugar-based syrup are applied. This bonds the sugar coating to the tablet and provides rounding. The sucrose and water syrup also contains gelatin, acacia, or PVP to enhance coating. When the tablets are partially dry, they are sprinkled with a dusting powder, usually a mixture of powdered sugar and starch but sometimes talc, acacia, or precipitated chalk as well. Warm air is applied to the rolling tablets, and when they are dry, the process

FIGURE 8.32. Gauge used to measure coated tablets. (Courtesy Digital Micrometers Ltd.)

is repeated until the tablets are of the desired shape and size (Fig. 8.32). The subcoated tablets are then scooped out of the coating pan, and the excess powder is removed by gently shaking the tablets on a cloth screen.

Smoothing and Final Rounding

After the tablets are subcoated, 5 to 10 additional coatings of a thick syrup are applied to complete the rounding and smooth the coatings. This syrup is sucrose based, with or without additional components such as starch and calcium carbonate. As the syrup is applied, the operator moves his or her hand through the rolling tablets to distribute the syrup and to prevent the tablets from sticking to one another. A dusting powder is often used between syrup applications. Warm air is applied to hasten the drying time of each coat.

Finishing and Coloring

To attain final smoothness and the appropriate color to the tablets, several coats of a thin syrup containing the desired colorant are applied in the usual manner. This step is performed in a clean pan, free from previous coating materials.

Imprinting

Solid dosage forms may be passed through a special imprinting machine (Fig. 8.33) to impart identification codes and other distinctive symbols. By FDA regulation, effective in 1995, all solid dosage forms for human consumption, including both prescription-only and over-the-counter drug products, must be imprinted with product-specific identification codes. Some exemptions to this requirement are allowed: those used in clinical investigations, those that are extemporaneously compounded

FIGURE 8.33. Branding of coated compression tablets on a branding machine. (Courtesy of Ackley Machine Corporation.)

FIGURE 8.34. Coated, polished, and monogrammed tablets. (Courtesy of Wyeth-Ayerst Laboratories.)

in the course of pharmacy practice, radiopharmaceutical drug products, and products that, because of their size, shape, texture, or other physical characteristics, make imprinting technologically not feasible.

Technically, the imprint may be *debossed, embossed, engraved,* or printed on the surface with ink. *Debossed* means imprinted with a mark below the surface, *embossed* means imprinted with a mark raised above the surface, and *engraved* means imprinted with a code that is cut into the surface during production.

Polishing

Coated tablets may be polished in several ways. Special drum-shaped pans or ordinary coating pans lined with canvas or other cloth impregnated with carnauba wax and/or beeswax may be used to polish tablets as they tumble in the pan. Or, pieces of wax may be placed in a polishing pan, and the tablets allowed to tumble over the wax until the desired sheen is attained. A third method is light spraying of the tablets with wax dissolved in a nonaqueous solvent. Two or three coats of wax may be applied, depending upon the desired gloss. After each coat has been applied, the addition of a small amount of talc to the tumbling tablets contributes to their high luster (Fig. 8.34).

Film-Coating Tablets

The sugarcoating process, as described, not only is tedious, time-consuming, and specialized, requiring the expertise of highly skilled technicians, but also results in coated tablets that may be twice the size and weight of the original uncoated tablets. Also, sugarcoated tablets may vary slightly in size from batch to batch and within a batch. All of these factors are important considerations for a manufacturer. From a patient's point of view, large tablets are not as easily swallowed as are small tablets.

The film-coating process, which places a thin, skintight coating of a plastic-like material over the compressed tablet, was developed to produce coated tablets having essentially the same weight, shape, and size as the originally compressed tablet. Also, the coating is thin enough to reveal any identifying monograms embossed in the tablet during compression by the tablet punches. Film-coated tablets also are far more resistant to destruction by abrasion than are sugarcoated tablets. However, like sugarcoated tablets, the coating may be colored to make the tablets attractive and distinctive.

Film-coating solutions may be nonaqueous or aqueous. The nonaqueous solutions contain the following types of materials to provide the desired coating to the tablets:

1. A *film former* capable of producing smooth, thin films reproducible under conventional coating conditions and applicable to a variety of tablet shapes. Example: cellulose acetate phthalate
2. An *alloying substance* providing water solubility or permeability to the film to ensure penetration by body fluids and therapeutic availability of the drug. Example: polyethylene glycol
3. A *plasticizer* to produce flexibility and elasticity of the coating and thus provide durability. Example: castor oil
4. A *surfactant* to enhance spreadability of the film during application. Example: polyoxyethylene sorbitan derivatives
5. *Opaquants* and *colorants* to make the appearance of the coated tablets handsome and distinctive. Examples: opaquant, titanium dioxide; colorant, FD&C or D&C dyes
6. *Sweeteners, flavors,* and *aromas* to enhance the acceptability of the tablet by the patient. Examples: sweeteners, saccharin; flavors and aromas, vanillin
7. A *glossant* to provide luster to the tablets without a separate polishing operation. Example: beeswax
8. A *volatile solvent* to allow the spread of the other components over the tablets while allowing rapid evaporation to permit an effective yet speedy operation. Example: alcohol mixed with acetone

Tablets are film coated by application or spraying of the coating solution on the tablets in ordinary coating pans. The volatility of the solvent enables the film to adhere quickly to the surface of the tablets.

Because of both the expense of the volatile solvents used in the film-coating process and the environmental problem of the release of solvents, pharmaceutical manufacturers generally favor the use of aqueous solutions. One of the problems attendant to these, however, is slow evaporation of the water base compared to the volatile organic solvent–based solutions. One commercial water-based colloidal coating dispersion called Aquacoat (FMC Corporation) contains a 30% ethyl cellulose pseudolatex. Pseudolatex dispersions have a high solid content for greater coating ability and a relatively low viscosity. The low viscosity allows less water to be used in the coating dispersion, requiring less evaporation and reducing the likelihood that water will interfere with tablet formulation. In addition, the low viscosity permits greater coat penetration into the crevices of monogrammed or scored tablets. A plasticizer may be added to assist in the production of a dense, relatively impermeable film with high gloss and mechanical strength. Other aqueous film-coating products use cellulosic materials such as methylcellulose, hydroxypropyl cellulose, and hydroxypropyl methylcellulose as the film-forming polymer.

A typical aqueous film-coating formulation contains the following (19):

1. *Film-forming polymer* (7% to 18%). Examples: cellulose ether polymers such as hydroxypropyl methylcellulose, hydroxypropylcellulose, and methylcellulose
2. *Plasticizer* (0.5% to 2.0%). Examples: glycerin, propylene glycol, polyethylene glycol, diethyl phthalate, and dibutyl subacetate
3. *Colorant and opacifier* (2.5% to 8%). Examples: FD&C or D&C lakes and iron oxide pigments
4. *Vehicle* (water, to make 100%)

There are some problems attendant on aqueous film coating, including the appearance of small amounts (*picking*) or larger amounts (*peeling*) of film fragments flaking from the tablet surface, roughness of the tablet surface due to failure of spray droplets to coalesce (*orange peel effect*), an uneven distribution of color on the tablet surface (*mottling*), filling-in of the score line or indented logo on the tablet by the film (*bridging*), and disfiguration of the core tablet when subjected for too long to the coating solution (tablet *erosion*). The cause of each of these problems can be determined and the problem rectified through appropriate changes in formulation, equipment, technique, or process.

Enteric Coating

Enteric-coated solid dosage forms are intended to pass through the stomach intact to disintegrate and release their drug content for absorption along the intestines. The design of an enteric coating may be based on the transit time required for passage to the intestines and may be accomplished through coatings of sufficient thickness.

However, usually an enteric coating is based on factors of pH, resisting dissolution in the highly acid environment of the stomach but yielding to the less acid environment of the intestine. Some enteric coatings are designed to dissolve at pH 4.8 and greater.

Enteric-coating materials may be applied either to whole compressed tablets or to drug particles or granules used in the fabrication of tablets or capsules. The coatings may be applied in multiple portions to build a thick coating or as a thin film coat. The coating system may be aqueous or organic solvent based and effective so long as the coating material resists breakdown in the gastric fluid. Among the materials used in enteric coatings are pharmaceutical shellac, hydroxypropyl methylcellulose phthalate, polyvinyl acetate phthalate, diethyl phthalate, and cellulose acetate phthalate.

Fluid Bed or Air Suspension Coating

Fluid bed coating, which uses equipment of the type shown in Figure 8.35, is spray coating of powders, granules, beads, pellets, or tablets held in suspension by a column of air.

FIGURE 8.35. Vector/Freund Flo-Coater production system. A fluid bed system used to apply coatings to beads, granules, powders, and tablets. Capacity of models ranges from 5 to 700 kg. (Courtesy of Vector Corporation.)

FIGURE 8.36. Scanning electron microscope images of pharmaceutical granules coated through fluid bed technology. **A:** Layered and coated granule. **B:** Cross section of top-spray enteric-coated granule. (Courtesy of Glatt Air Techniques.)

Fluid bed processing equipment is multifunctional and may also be used in preparing tablet granulations.

In the Wurster process, named after its developer, the items to be coated are fed into a vertical cylinder and are supported by a column of air that enters from the bottom of the cylinder. Within the air stream, the solids rotate both vertically and horizontally. As the coating solution enters the system from the bottom, it is rapidly applied to the suspended, rotating solids, with rounding coats being applied in less than an hour with the assistance of warm air blasts released in the chamber.

In another type of fluid bed system, the coating solution is sprayed downward onto the particles to be coated as they are suspended by air from below. This method is commonly referred to as the *top-spray* method. This method provides greater capacity, up to 1,500 kg, than the other air suspension coating methods (20). Both the top-spray and bottom-spray methods may be employed using a modified apparatus used for fluid bed granulation. A third method, the *tangential-spray technique*, is used in rotary fluid bed coaters. The bottom-spray, top-spray, and tangential-spray methods are depicted in Figure 8.21. Electron microscope images of the results of this process are shown in Figure 8.36.

The three systems are increasingly used for application of aqueous or organic solvent–based polymer film coatings. The top-spray coating method is particularly recommended for taste masking, enteric release, and barrier films on particles or tablets. It is most effective when coatings are applied from aqueous solutions, latexes, or hot melts (17,18). The bottom-spray method is recommended for sustained-release and enteric-release products; the tangential method is used for layering coatings and for sustained-release and enteric-coated products (18).

Among the variables requiring control to produce the desired and consistent quality are equipment and the method of spraying (e.g., top, bottom, tangential), spray nozzle distance from spraying bed, droplet size, spray rate, spray pressure, volume of the air column, batch size, method and time for drying, and air temperature and moisture content in the processing compartment (18).

Compression Coating

In a manner similar to the preparation of multiple compressed tablets having an inner core and an outer shell of drug material, core tablets may be sugarcoated by compression. The coating material, in the form of a granulation or powder, is compressed onto a tablet core of drug with a special tablet press. Compression coating is an anhydrous operation and thus may be safely employed in the coating of tablets containing a drug that is labile to moisture. Compared to sugarcoating using pans, compression coating is more uniform and uses less coating material, resulting in tablets that are lighter, smaller, and easier to swallow and less expensive to package and ship.

Irrespective of the method used in coating, all tablets are visually or electronically inspected for physical imperfections (Fig. 8.37).

FIGURE 8.37. Checking for physical imperfections in coated tablets. (Courtesy of Sainty International Group/SaintyCo.)

IMPACT OF MANUFACTURING CHANGES ON SOLID DOSAGE FORMS

The quality and performance of a solid dosage form may be altered by changes in formulation or by changes in the method of manufacture.

The changes in formulation may arise from (a) the use of starting raw materials, including both the active ingredient and pharmaceutical excipients, that have different chemical or physical characteristics (e.g., solubility or particle size) than the standards set for the original components; (b) the use of different pharmaceutical excipients (e.g., magnesium stearate instead of calcium stearate as the lubricant); (c) the use of different quantities of the same excipients in a formulation (e.g., use of a more concentrated wet tablet binder); or (d) the addition of a new excipient to a formulation (e.g., a revised tablet-coating formula).

The changes in the method of manufacture may be (a) use of processing or manufacturing equipment of a different design; (b) a change in the steps or order in the process or method of manufacture (e.g., different mixing times); (c) different in-process controls, quality tests, or assay methods; (d) production of different batch sizes; (e) employment of different product reprocessing procedures; or (f) employment of a different manufacturing site.

Changes such as these may be proposed or implemented during the product development stage, during scale-up of product manufacture before NDA approval, or after NDA approval and product marketing. In all instances, it is critical to assess any effects of the change in meeting the proposed or established standards for product quality (e.g., dissolution rate and bioavailability). It is necessary for a manufacturer to document the change, validate its effect, and provide the necessary information to the FDA. Some changes are considered minor (e.g., a change in tablet color) and do not affect product quality; they do not require prior FDA approval. Other changes that may affect product quality and performance (e.g., use of a substantially different quantity or grade of an excipient or use of a piece of manufacturing equipment that changes the methodology of manufacture) require prior FDA approval (21).

OFFICIAL AND COMMERCIALLY AVAILABLE TABLETS

There are hundreds of tablets recognized by the USP and literally thousands of commercially available tablet products from virtually all pharmaceutical manufacturers, in most therapeutic categories and in various dosage strengths. Examples of a limited number of these are presented in Table 8.1.

PACKAGING AND STORING TABLETS

Tablets are stored in tight containers, in places of low humidity, and protected from extremes in temperature. Products that are prone to decomposition by moisture generally are packaged with a desiccant packet. Drugs that are adversely affected by light are packaged in light-resistant containers. With a few exceptions, tablets that are properly stored will remain stable for several years or more.

In dispensing tablets, the pharmacist is well advised to use a similar type of container as provided by the manufacturer of the product. The patient is well advised to keep the drug in the container dispensed. Storage conditions, as recommended for the particular product, should be maintained by the pharmacist and patient alike and expiration dates observed.

The pharmacist should be aware also that the hardness of certain tablets may change upon aging, usually resulting in a decrease in the disintegration and dissolution rates of the product. The increase in tablet hardness can frequently be attributed to the increased adhesion of the binding agent and other formulative components within the tablet. Examples of increased tablet hardening with age have been reported for a number of drugs, including aluminum hydroxide, sodium salicylate, and phenylbutazone (22).

In tablets containing volatile drugs, such as NTG, the drug may migrate between tablets in the container, resulting in a lack of uniformity among the tablets (23). Also, packing materials, such as cotton and rayon, in contact with NTG tablets may absorb varying amounts of NTG, reducing potency of the tablets (24). The USP directs that NTG tablets be preserved in tight containers, preferably of glass, at controlled room temperature. Also, migration within tablets can occur resulting in unequal distribution within a single tablet; this can be problematic if the tablet is scored and designed to be broken in half where the two halves may not contain equal portions of the drug. Storage of a container next to a heat source may result in greater loss or movement of the volatile drug in the portion of the bottle closest to the heat. Some third-party payors require the dispensing of higher strength tablets with the patient to divide them prior to administration to decrease costs. In addition to the difficulties just mentioned, it is troublesome for many patients to split tablets into two equal halves.

The USP further directs that NTG tablets be dispensed in the original unopened container, labeled with the following statement directed to the patient. "Warning: to prevent loss of potency, keep these tablets in the original container or in a supplemental NTG container specifically labeled as being suitable for NTG tablets. Close tightly immediately after use" (4).

The pharmacist also should caution patients about handling medication when it poses a risk. For example, as noted earlier, finasteride tablets are taken by men to treat benign prostatic hyperplasia. Finasteride has the potential to harm a male fetus if absorbed by a pregnant woman

TABLE 8.1. Examples of Official Tablets

Official Tablet	Representative Commercial Products	Strength (mg)	Category
Acetaminophen	Tylenol (McNeil)	325, 500	Analgesic, antipyretic
Acyclovir	Zovirax (Valeant)	400, 800	Antiviral
Allopurinol	Zyloprim (Faro Pharmaceuticals)	100, 300	Antigout and antiurolithic
Amitriptyline HCl	Endep (Roche)	10, 25, 50, 75, 100, 150	Antidepressant
Carbamazepine	Tegretol (Novartis)	200	Anticonvulsant
Chlorambucil	Leukeran (GlaxoSmithKline)	2	Antineoplastic
Cimetidine	Tagamet (GlaxoSmithKline)	200, 300, 400, 800	Histamine H_2 receptor antagonist
Ciprofloxacin	Cipro (Schering-Plough)	100, 250, 500, 750	Antibacterial
Conjugated estrogens	Premarin (Wyeth-Ayerst)	0.3, 0.45, 0.625, 0.9, 1.25, 2.5	Estrogen
Diazepam	Valium (Roche)	2, 5, 10	Sedative, skeletal muscle relaxant
Digoxin	Lanoxin (GlaxoSmithKline)	0.125, 0.25	Cardiotonic
Enalapril	Vasotec (Biovail)	2.5, 5, 10, 20	Antihypertensive
Furosemide	Lasix (Aventis)	20, 40, 80	Diuretic, antihypertensive
Griseofulvin	Various	250, 500	Antifungal
Haloperidol	Haldol (McNeil)	0.5, 1, 2, 5, 10, 20	Tranquilizer
Ibuprofen	Motrin (McNeil Consumer Healthcare)	400, 600, 800	Analgesic and antipyretic
Levothyroxine sodium	Synthroid (Abbott)	0.025, 0.05, 0.075, 0.088, 0.1, 0.122, 0.125, 0.137, 0.15, 0.2, 0.3	Thyroid hormone
Loratadine	Claritin (Schering-Plough)	10	Antihistamine
Meperidine HCl	Demerol (Sanofi-Synthelabo)	50, 100	Narcotic analgesic
Methyldopa	Aldomet (Merck)	125, 250, 500	Antihypertensive
Nitroglycerin	Nitrostat (Parke-Davis)	0.3, 0.4, 0.6	Antianginal
Penicillin V	Pen-Vee-K (Wyeth)	250, 500	Anti-infective
Propranolol	Inderal (Wyeth-Ayerst)	10, 20, 40, 60, 80	Antianginal, antiarrhythmic, antihypertensive
Terbutaline sulfate	Various	2.5, 5	Antiasthmatic
Verapamil HCl	Calan (Searle)	40, 80, 120	Antihypertensive
Warfarin sodium	Coumadin (Bristol-Myers Squibb)	1, 2, 2.5, 4, 5, 6, 7.5, 10	Anticoagulant

either through direct contact with finasteride or possibly through semen. Therefore, a woman who is pregnant or who may become pregnant should not handle finasteride tablets or come into contact with finasteride powder. In addition, when the male patient's sexual partner is pregnant or may become pregnant, the patient should avoid exposure of his partner to semen or should discontinue the use of this drug.

Finally, RDTs tend to be softer than regular compressed immediate-release tablets and require special packaging. An example is shown in Figure 8.38.

OTHER SOLID DOSAGE FORMS FOR ORAL ADMINISTRATION

Lozenges (Troches)

Lozenges (troches) are solid oral dosage forms that are designed to dissolve or disintegrate slowly in the mouth. They contain one or more active drugs that are slowly released from the flavored and sweetened base. They are used for both local and systemic action. Typically, the active drugs include antiseptics, analgesics, decongestants, antitussives, and antibiotics. Some molded lozenges may also be called cough drops or pastilles.

Lozenges can be made by compression or molding. Compressed lozenges are made using a tablet machine and large, flat punches. The machine is operated at a high degree of compression to produce lozenges that are harder than ordinary tablets so that they dissolve or disintegrate slowly in the mouth. Medicinal substances that are heat stable may be molded into hard sugar candy lozenges by candy-making machines that process a warm, highly concentrated, flavored syrup as the base and form the lozenges by molding and drying.

Lozenges can be made using sugars such as sucrose and dextrose or can be "sugar-free" in a formulation generally based on sorbitol or mannitol. To slow the rate of

FIGURE 8.38. Rapidly dissolving/melting tablet. (Loratadine Orally Disintegrating Tablets—Dimetapp ND.)

dissolution, polyethylene glycols and hypromellose are sometimes added. Compressed lozenges are made with excipients that may include a filler, binder, sweetening agent, flavoring agent, and lubricant and are prepared similar to conventional tablets. They can also be prepared by formulating a paste, cutting or stamping, and drying. Also, they can be prepared by forcing dampened powders under low pressure into mold cavities, ejecting them, and allowing them to dry.

Lollipops

Fentanyl Actiq (Cephalon) is a raspberry lollipop that is a sugar-based lozenge on a stick and contains fentanyl citrate. It has an off-white color, and the stick bears a large Rx mark. Actiq is the first product specifically designed to aid in controlling breakthrough pain in cancer patients. It is indicated only for the management of breakthrough cancer pain in patients with malignancies who are already taking and are tolerant to opioids. Breakthrough cancer pain occurs in about 50% of cancer pain patients and is a component of chronic cancer pain that is particularly difficult to treat because of its severity, rapid onset, and frequent unpredictability. The lollipop provides almost immediate relief as the drug starts being absorbed in the mouth and starts to work within minutes; its effects last for only about 15 minutes, but that is usually long enough to relieve the breakthrough pain. The concern about this product being accidentally used by children is addressed by special packaging that requires scissors to open (1).

Pellets

Pellets are dosage forms that are composed of small, solid particles of uniform shape sometimes called beads. Typically, pellets are nearly spherical, but that is not a

requirement. They may be administered orally or parenterally. They can be used to provide physical separation for chemically or physically incompatible materials, extended release of an active pharmaceutical ingredient (API), or delayed release to protect an acid-labile API from degradation in the stomach or to protect stomach tissues from irritation. Pellet dosage forms can be formulated as single or multiple entities. Oral pellets are usually placed within hard gelatin capsules for administration. The size range of the pellets is governed by the constraints of the volume of commonly used capsules (typically size no. 1 or no. 0). Typically, pellets for oral use fall within a size range of 710 μm to 2.36 mm.

For delayed release, pellets are prepared by applying a coating in various numbers of layers.

Pellets are typically manufactured by wet extrusion processes followed by spheronization, by wet or dry coating processes, or by compression. Pellets prepared by wet coating involve the application of successive coatings onto nonpareil seeds; this process may be carried out in a fluid bed processing equipment. The manufacture of pellets by compression is largely restricted to the production for subcutaneous implantation as it can be done in an aseptic processing environment. Coacervation techniques can be used for coating and will generally produce coated particles that are smaller than those produced by other techniques.

Bolus Tablets

Bolus tablets are large, usually elongated tablets intended for administration to large animals. Conventional tableting processes can be used to manufacture bolus tablets, but higher compression forces may be necessary because of their larger size.

Pills

By definition, pills are small, round solid dosage forms containing a medicinal agent and intended to be administered orally. Although the manufacture and administration of pills were at one time quite prevalent, today pills have been replaced by compressed tablets and capsules. Pills are distinguished from tablets as they are usually prepared by a wet massing and molding technique, whereas tablets are typically formed by compression.

Excipients are selected for pills based on their ability to produce a firm and plastic mass. The API is triturated with powdered excipients using geometric dilution to obtain a uniform mixture. Liquid excipients are added to bind and provide plasticity to the mass, which is formed by kneading. The firmness and plasticity are required for the mass to be worked and retain the produced shape. A cylindrical pill pipe is produced and then cut into individual lengths corresponding to the intended size/dose. These short cylinders are then rolled to form the final spherical shape. Small machines/devices are available that can automate this process.

PATIENT COUNSELING

TABLETS

1. Take with a glass of water or other liquid (if instructed).
2. Explain whether to chew, crush, or swallow whole.
3. Discuss the frequency and onset of dose.
4. Explain what to do if a dose is missed.
5. Store in the least humid environment available at room temperature.

CHEWABLE TABLETS

1. Chew the tablet thoroughly before swallowing.
2. Swallow all the contents and saliva to get the full dose.
3. Confirm the frequency and timing of use.
4. Store in the least humid environment available at room temperature.

SUBLINGUAL TABLETS

1. Place the tablet under the tongue.
2. Do not chew or swallow the tablet.
3. Allow to dissolve and remain in the mouth for a time to be absorbed.
4. Avoid drinking or eating for several minutes until the drug has been absorbed.
5. Confirm the frequency and timing of use.
6. Store in the least humid environment available at room temperature.

BUCCAL TABLETS

1. Place the tablet between the cheek and the gum.
2. Do not chew or swallow the tablet.
3. Allow time to dissolve or for the drug to be released.
4. Confirm if the tablet should be removed or if it will dissolve and erode away.

5. Rotate the site of application to minimize irritation.
6. Confirm the frequency and timing of use.
7. Store in the least humid environment available at room temperature.

ORALLY DISINTEGRATING TABLETS

1. Open the single dose/use container with dry hands by peeling back the foil layer. Do not push the tablet through the foil as it may be fragile and crush.
2. Remove the tablet from the blister and place in the mouth.
3. The tablet will disintegrate quickly in the saliva so it can be easily swallowed without drinking a liquid.
4. Store in the least humid environment available at room temperature.

LOZENGES

Hard Lozenges

1. Explain that a hard lozenge is designed to provide a slow, continuous release of the drug over a prolonged period of time and should not be chewed but allowed to slowly dissolve.
2. Store in the least humid environment available at room temperature.

Soft and Chewable Lozenges

1. They should be taken only as directed and should not be considered candy. Keep out of the reach of children.
2. Store in the least humid environment available at room temperature.

PHARMACEUTICS CASE STUDY

SUBJECTIVE INFORMATION

A pharmaceutical manufacturer has developed a formula for an antihistamine compressed tablet. During the initial run, the tablets were found to be too friable. What can be done?

OBJECTIVE INFORMATION

The formula for the tablet is as follows:

Antihistamine	50 mg
Directly compressible lactose	150 mg
Magnesium stearate	10 mg
Starch	100 mg
Talc	25 mg

The tablet is to be compressed, so it has the following characteristics:

Description	8-mm white biconvex bisected tablet
Weight	335 mg
Hardness	8 kg
Dissolution	Medium: 0.01 N Hydrochloric acid, 500 mL Apparatus 2: 50 rpm Time: 30 minutes

Following the initial run, hardness testing reveals that the tablet's hardness is only 6.5 kg.

(continued)

PHARMACEUTICS CASE STUDY *(continued)*

ASSESSMENT

The tablet's hardness must be increased to meet specifications. There are a couple of different approaches to accomplishing this:

1. Increase the pressure of the upper punch of the tableting machine.
2. Add a tablet binder such as pregelatinized starch, acacia, or methylcellulose. Some or all of the

starch in the tablet formula could be replaced by pregelatinized starch, as it will serve all of the functions of regular starch (diluent, dissolution enhancer, etc.) plus serve as a tablet binder.

PLAN

Adjust the tableting machine, and increase the pressure of the upper punch. Sometimes, the simplest solutions are the best. ■

CLINICAL CASE STUDY

SUBJECTIVE INFORMATION

HPI:	F.L. is a 46-year-old AAM brought to the emergency department (ER) by his wife with chief complaint of "chest pain." His spouse states that F.L. began to feel constant pain in his chest while watching television. The pain radiated to his left arm and back. Spouse noticed excessive sweating on his forehead as he started to "gasp for breath." Immediately, she brought him to the ER. At the ER, F.L. describes pain as the "worst pain of his life" and feels like "an elephant's foot is pressuring into my chest." The patient was brought into the ER within an hour of onset of symptoms. F.L. denies any previous episodes of chest pain, sweating, weakness, shortness of breath, syncope, nausea, or vomiting. The patient denies any previous episodes of pain on exertion. He rates pain intensity as 10/10.
PMH:	HTN × 12 years
	Type II diabetes × 2 years
PSH:	Lasik eye surgery, 2002
SH:	(−) EtOH: quit drinking in 1996
	(−) Tobacco: quit smoking in 1996
	(−) Caffeine
	(−) Illicit drugs: "none, never"
	Patient lives in Hanover Park with wife and one daughter and one son, no pets
	Has own business, works at home
FH:	Father died of an asthma attack at 67 y/o
	Mother died of a myocardial infarction (MI) at 59 y/o
Sister:	Asthma

Diet:	Eats three times a day and two or three snacks a day. Denies following any low-fat, low-cholesterol, or low-salt diet. On a low-sugar diet and states that he follows it. Eats fast food at least twice a week. Snacks consist mostly of chips, cookies, and salsa.
Exer:	Pt states, "I don't have time to exercise. I've got a business and a family to handle." The extent of patient's exercise is walking up and down the stairs when he needs to get around the house.
All:	NKDA
PTA:	Lisinopril (Zestril) 40 mg po qhs for HTN
	Felodipine (Plendil) 10 mg po qd for HTN
	Glyburide/metformin (Glucovance)—2.5/500 mg po tid for type II diabetes

ADHERENCE

The patient states that he adheres to all his medications. He uses a pillbox to help remind him. He checks his blood glucose levels three times a day, alternating before and after meals.

OBJECTIVE INFORMATION

Ht:	5'8"	**Wt:**	185 lb
Pain:	10/10	**BP:**	112/80
Na:	140 mmol/L	**K:**	4.0 mmol/L
Cl:	100 mmol/L	**CO$_2$:**	24 mmol/L
BUN:	4.0 mmol/L	**SrCr:**	70 mmol/L
HgA$_{1c}$:	7	**CK:**	30
Last Accu-Checks:			After breakfast, 9:30 AM: 151 After lunch, 1:00 PM: 155 After dinner, 7:00 PM: 141

(continued)

(continued)

ASSESSMENT

The patient is a 46-year-old AAM with a PMH of controlled HTN and type II diabetes who has had his first MI. The patient is at increased risk for MI because of HTN, diabetes, and significant family history. Though the patient adheres to his medication regimen, he does not adhere to a healthy diet and exercise plan, which may increase his chances of experiencing a similar episode in the future.

PLAN

1. Recommend sustained-release NTG Nitro-Bid 2.5-mg capsules once a day on an empty stomach with a full glass of water, either 30 minutes before or an hour after meals. Instruct the patient to take the medication the same time each day and to swallow the capsule whole. If the patient misses a dose, he should take it as soon as he remembers unless the next scheduled dose is within 2 hours; in that case, he should skip the missed dose and take only the next dose.
2. Recommend sublingual NTG NitroQuick 0.30-mg (1/200 g) tablets. Instruct the patient to use the sublingual tablet at the first sign of attack. Instruct the patient to wet the tablet with saliva and place under the tongue or between the gums or in cheek until the tablet dissolves. Do not swallow the tablet. Effects of NTG should be felt within 2 minutes, lasting for up to 30 minutes. If symptoms do not resolve within 5 minutes of the first dose, repeat with a second sublingual tablet. Again, wait 5 minutes, and use a third sublingual tablet if symptoms persist. Call for emergency assistance (911) if symptoms continue after three doses of NTG. Inform the patient to keep and store sublingual tablets in original glass container, keep them away from heat or light, and keep the bottle tightly closed after use.
3. Counsel the patient on common side effects of NTG, such as headache, dizziness, drowsiness, and low blood pressure. Recommend acetaminophen (e.g., Tylenol) for relief of headache. Tell the patient to avoid alcoholic beverages and medications containing alcohol while using NTG, as their concurrent use may cause severe hypotension and cardiovascular difficulties. Inform the patient that the use of sildenafil (Viagra) is dangerous and should be avoided while using this medication as it may increase the blood pressure–lowering effect of NTG. Instruct the patient to check expiration dates of tablets regularly because therapeutic effectiveness of NTG may decrease in tablets older than 6 months. Consult physician before stopping the use of NTG because abrupt discontinuation may cause severe chest pain.
4. Educate the spouse and the patient to recognize the signs and symptoms of a heart attack (e.g., excessive sweating, chest pain, jaw or back pain). Explain that a "silent" MI can occur without any symptoms. Further education on the condition and how it may be managed and prevented may benefit this patient. Stress the importance of lifestyle changes such as exercise and dietary modifications (e.g., low-fat, low-salt, low-cholesterol diet). Have the patient consult physician before embarking on an exercise regimen. An exercise regimen may include exercising at least three or four times a week for 15 to 30 minutes or as tolerated by the patient.
5. Monitoring parameters: BP, signs and symptoms of heart attack, frequency of episodes, and side effects of the medication. Goal: Increased patient knowledge of the condition, improved adherence to diet and exercise regimen, no medication side effects, and no second episode. Make sure the patient understands the importance of follow-up physician visits and exercising caution when purchasing nonprescription and herbal products (i.e., consult a pharmacist). ∎

APPLYING THE PRINCIPLES AND CONCEPTS

GROUP ACTIVITIES

1. Compare the advantages and disadvantages of unit dose packaging *versus* tablets packaged in plastic bottle containers.
2. Create a listing of extemporaneous prescriptions that provide the pharmacist an opportunity to use a tablet dosage form in its preparation.
3. Create a listing of conceivable ways a consumer/patient may misuse a tablet dosage form.
4. List five counseling points for proper administration of solid dosage forms, for example, tablets.
5. Make a listing of factors that might make a patient apprehensive about taking a tablet dosage form. List points of advice/counseling points to overcome this apprehension.
6. Identify several patient populations who might have difficulty administering a tablet dosage form, and explain your reasoning.

INDIVIDUAL ACTIVITIES

1. Create a table of oral, chewable tablets, including amount of active ingredient(s), indication, contra-indication, adverse effects/precautions, and dosage.
2. Create a listing of trademarked tablet dosage forms that have unique characteristics, for example, size, shape, and color, and describe/detail those features.
3. Generate a listing of tablet drug products that utilize (an) active ingredient(s) in a micronized powder form.
4. From the primary literature, find a clinical study demonstrating a comparison between a sustained-release tablet product and a compressed tablet for clinical effectiveness, and determine which one would be preferred in terms of patient acceptance, patient adherence, bioequivalence, and cost. Explain the rationale for your decision.
5. Select one USP drug monograph for an official tablet dosage form, and identify and describe its main components.

REFERENCES

1. Available at: http://www.drugs.com/mtm/claritin-reditab.html. (Accessed July 25, 2020)

2. Physicians' Desk Reference. 70th Ed. Montvale, NJ: Medical Economics, 2016:1216–1220.

3. Product Package. Dimetapp ND. Madison, NJ: Wyeth Consumer Healthcare.

4. Package Insert. Tempra Quicklets. New York, NY: Bristol-Myers Products.

5. Physicians' Desk Reference. 70th Ed. Montvale, NJ: Thomson PDR, 2016:1001–1015.

6. Product Information. Available at: www.rxlist.com/videx-drug.htm. (Accessed July 25, 2020)

7. The United States Pharmacopeia–National Formulary. Current Ed. Rockville, MD: U.S. Pharmacopeial Convention.

8. Hanson R, Gray V. Handbook of Dissolution Testing. 3rd Ed. Hockessin, DE: Dissolution Technologies, Inc., 2004.

9. Guidance for Industry: Dissolution Testing of Immediate Release Solid Oral Dosage Forms. Rockville, MD: FDA/CDER, 2007.

10. Amidon GL, Lennernas H, Shah VP, et al. A theoretical basis for a biopharmaceutic drug classification: The correlation of in vitro drug product dissolution and in vivo bioavailability. Pharm Res 1995;12:413–420.

11. Swarbrick J. In vitro dissolution, drug bioavailability, and the spiral of science. Pharm Technol 1997;21:68–72.

12. Chowhan ZT. Factors affecting dissolution of drugs and their stability upon aging in solid dosage forms. Pharm Technol 1994;18:60–73.

13. Hanson R, Swartz ME, Jarnutowski RJ. Pooled dissolution testing: A primer. Dissolution Technol 1998;5:15–17.

14. Shangraw RF, Demarest DA. A survey of current industrial practices in the formulation and manufacture of tablets and capsules. Pharm Technol 1993;17:32–44.

15. Explotab. Patterson, NY: Mendell, Penmwest Co., 1992.

16. METHOCEL as a Granulation Binding Agent for Immediate-release Tablet and Capsule Products. Wilmington, DE: Dow Chemical, 1996.

17. Loeffler GF, Ebey GC. Pharmaceutical tablet compression tooling. In: Lieberman HA, Lachman L, Schwartz JB, eds. Pharmaceutical Dosage Forms: Tablets. Volume 2. 2nd Ed. New York, NY: Marcel Dekker, Inc., 1990.

18. Atlas Mannitol. USP Tablet Excipient. Wilmington, DE: ICI Americas, 1973.

19. McGinity JW, ed. Aqueous Polymeric Coatings for Pharmaceutical Dosage Forms. 2nd Ed. New York, NY: Marcel Dekker, Inc., 1997.

20. Ghebre-Sellassie I, ed. Pharmaceutical Pelletization Technology. New York, NY: Marcel Dekker, Inc., 1989.

21. Lucisano LJ, Franz RM. FDA proposed guidance for chemistry, manufacturing, and control changes for immediate-release solid dosage forms: A review and industrial perspective. Pharm Technol 1995;19:30–44.

22. Barrett D, Fell JT. Effect of aging on physical properties of phenylbutazone tablets. J Pharm Sci 1975;64:335.

23. Page DP, Carson NA, Buhr CA, et al. Stability study of nitroglycerin sublingual tablets. J Pharm Sci 1975;64:140.

24. Fusari SA. Nitroglycerin sublingual tablets I: Stability of conventional tablets. J Pharm Sci 1973;62:122.

9 Solid Oral Modified-Release Dosage Forms and Drug Delivery Systems

CHAPTER AT A GLANCE The Rationale for Extended-Release Pharmaceuticals • Terminology • Extended-Release Oral Dosage Forms • Delayed-Release Oral Dosage Forms • USP Requirements and FDA Guidance for Modified-Release Dosage Forms • Clinical Considerations in the Use of Oral Modified-Release Dosage Forms • Packaging and Storing Modified-Release Tablets and Capsules • Patient Counseling

OBJECTIVES

After reading this chapter, the student will be able to:

1. Differentiate between the various types of modified-release dosage forms

2. Compare and contrast advantages and disadvantages of the various types of modified-release dosage forms

3. List physical–chemical characteristics of drugs that make them candidates for an extended-release dosage form

4. Explain microencapsulation, embedding, ion exchange, and osmotic pump as these apply to modified-release dosage forms

5. Describe how the in vitro and in vivo drug release from an extended-release/delayed-release oral dosage form will differ from an oral, film-coated tablet

6. List applicable criteria to the development of in vitro–in vivo correlations to the development of oral, extended-release products

▌ INTRODUCTION

This chapter describes solid oral dosage forms and drug delivery systems that, by virtue of formulation and product design, have modified drug-release features. U.S. prescription drug sales rose to 300.3 billion in 2009, an increase of 1.8% over the previous year (1). There are two primary driving forces behind this market, namely, patient-related factors and market-driven factors (2). The patient-related factors are discussed later in the chapter. The life cycle of a drug includes introduction of the new molecular entity, initial product introduction, and, later, possibly a new patent or patents obtained by the introduction of controlled-release formulations of the existing immediate-release products. This and the addition of new therapeutic indications for these products provide an attractive financial option for pharmaceutical companies. Example products include Augmentin XR (GlaxoSmithKline) and Cipro XR (Bayer) (2).

In contrast to conventional (immediate-release) forms, modified-release products provide either delayed release or extended release (ER) of drug. Most *delayed-release* products are enteric-coated tablets or capsules designed to pass through the stomach unaltered, later to release their medication within the intestinal tract. As noted in the previous chapter, enteric coatings are used either to protect a substance from destruction by gastric fluids or to reduce stomach distress caused by irritating drugs. *Extended-release* products are designed to release their medication in a *controlled* manner, at a predetermined rate, duration, and location to achieve and maintain optimum therapeutic blood levels of drug.

Most modified-release products are orally administered tablets and capsules, and therefore, these dosage forms are emphasized in this chapter. However, some other modified-release dosage forms and drug delivery systems are also described, including ocular, parenteral, subdermal, and vaginal products. Transdermal patches, which provide rate-controlled drug delivery, are touched on here and discussed at length in Chapter 11.

THE RATIONALE FOR EXTENDED-RELEASE PHARMACEUTICALS

Some drugs are inherently long lasting and require only once-a-day oral dosing to sustain adequate drug blood levels and the desired therapeutic effect. These drugs are formulated in the conventional manner in immediate-release dosage forms. However, many other drugs are not inherently long lasting and require multiple daily dosing to achieve the desired therapeutic results.

Multiple daily dosing is inconvenient for the patient and can result in missed doses, made-up doses, and noncompliance with the regimen. When conventional immediate-release dosage forms are taken on schedule and more than once daily, they cause sequential therapeutic blood level peaks and valleys (troughs) associated with the taking of each dose (Fig. 9.1). However, when doses are *not* administered on schedule, the resulting peaks and valleys reflect less than optimum drug therapy. For example, if doses are administered too frequently, minimum toxic concentrations of drug may be reached, with toxic side effects resulting. If doses are missed, periods of subtherapeutic drug blood levels or those below the minimum effective concentration may result, with no benefit to the patient.

Extended-release tablets and capsules are commonly taken only once or twice daily, compared with counterpart conventional forms that may have to be taken three or four times daily to achieve the same therapeutic effect. Typically, extended-release products provide an immediate release of drug that promptly produces the desired therapeutic effect, followed by gradual release of additional amounts of drug to maintain this effect over a predetermined period (Fig. 9.2). The sustained plasma drug levels provided by extended-release products oftentimes eliminate the need for night dosing, which benefits not only the

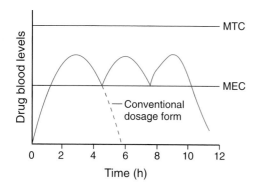

FIGURE 9.1. Hypothetical drug blood level–time curves for a conventional solid dosage form and a multiple-action product. MEC, minimum effective concentration; MTC, minimum toxic concentration.

FIGURE 9.2. Hypothetical drug blood level–time curves for a conventional solid dosage form and a controlled-release product. MEC, minimum effective concentration; MTC, minimum toxic concentration.

patient but the caregiver as well (3–5). For nonoral rate-controlled drug delivery systems, the drug-release pattern ranges in duration from 24 hours for most transdermal patches to 3 months for the estradiol vaginal ring insert (Estring, Pharmacia).

Some advantages of extended-release systems are given in Table 9.1. Some disadvantages are the loss of flexibility in adjusting the drug dose and/or dosage regimen and a risk of sudden and total drug release, or dose dumping, due to a failure or inappropriate use of technology.

TERMINOLOGY

Drug products that provide extended or sustained release (SR) first appeared as a major new class of dosage form in the late 1940s and early 1950s (6). Over the years, many terms (and abbreviations), such as *sustained release* (*SR*), *sustained action* (*SA*), *prolonged action* (*PA*), *controlled release* (*CR*), *extended release* (*ER*), *timed release* (*TR*), and *long acting* (*LA*), have been used by manufacturers to describe product types and features. Although these terms often have been used interchangeably, individual products bearing these descriptions may differ in design and performance and must be examined individually to ascertain their respective features. For the most part, these terms are used to describe orally administered dosage forms, whereas the term *rate-controlled delivery* is applied to certain types of drug delivery systems in which the rate of delivery is controlled by features of the device rather than by physiologic or environmental conditions like gastrointestinal pH or drug transit time through the gastrointestinal tract.

Modified Release

In recent years, *modified release* has come into general use to describe dosage forms having drug-release features based on time, course, and/or location that are designed to accomplish therapeutic or convenience objectives not offered by conventional or immediate-release forms (4,7).

TABLE 9.1. Advantages of Extended-Release Dosage Forms over Conventional Forms

Advantage	Explanation
Less fluctuation in drug blood levels	Controlling rate of release eliminates peaks and valleys of blood levels.
Less frequent administration	Extended-release products frequently deliver more than a single dose, hence may be taken less often than conventional forms.
Enhanced convenience and compliance	With less frequency of dosing, a patient is less apt to neglect taking a dose; also greater convenience with day and night administration.
Reduction in adverse side effects	Because of fewer blood level peaks outside therapeutic range and into toxic range, adverse side effects are less frequent.
Reduction in overall health care costs	Although initial cost of extended-release dosage forms may be greater than for conventional forms, overall cost of treatment may be less because of enhanced therapeutic benefit, fewer side effects, and reduced time for health care personnel to dispense and administer drugs and monitor patients.

The *U.S. Pharmacopeia* (USP) differentiates modified-release forms as *extended release* and *delayed release* (8).

Extended Release

The U.S. Food and Drug Administration (FDA) defines an extended-release dosage form as one that allows a reduction in dosing frequency from that necessitated by a conventional dosage form, such as a solution or an immediate-release dosage form (4,9).

Delayed Release

A delayed-release dosage form is designed to release the drug at a time other than promptly after administration. The delay may be time based or based on the influence of environmental conditions, like gastrointestinal pH. Delayed release can be accomplished either by coating or using specially prepared capsules such as Vcaps Enteric, which consist of cellulosic enteric derivatives (HPMCAS, HPMC).

Repeat Action

Repeat-action forms usually contain two single doses of medication, one for immediate release and the second for delayed release. Two-layer tablets, for example, may be prepared with one layer of drug for immediate release with the second layer designed to release drug later either as a second dose or in an extended-release manner.

Targeted Release

Targeted release describes drug release directed toward isolating or concentrating a drug in a body region, tissue, or site for absorption or for drug action.

▌EXTENDED-RELEASE ORAL DOSAGE FORMS

Not all drugs are suited for formulation into extended-release products and not all medical conditions require treatment with such a product. The drug and the therapeutic indication must be considered jointly in determining whether or not to develop an extended-release dosage form.

Drug Candidates for Extended-Release Products

To be a successful extended-release product, the drug must be released from the dosage form at a predetermined rate, dissolved in the gastrointestinal fluids, maintained at sufficient gastrointestinal residence time, and absorbed at a rate that will replace the amount of drug being metabolized and excreted.

In general, the drugs best suited for incorporation into an extended-release product have the following characteristics:

- *They exhibit neither very slow nor very fast rates of absorption and excretion.* Drugs with slow rates of absorption and excretion are usually inherently LA, and it is not necessary to prepare them in extended-release forms. Drugs with very short half-lives, that is, less than 2 hours, are poor candidates for ER because of the large quantities of drug required for such a formulation. Also, drugs that act by affecting enzyme systems may be longer acting than indicated by their quantitative half-lives because of residual effects and recovery of the diminished biosystem (10).
- *They are uniformly absorbed from the gastrointestinal tract.* Drugs prepared in extended-release forms must have good aqueous solubility and maintain adequate residence time in the gastrointestinal tract. Drugs absorbed poorly or at varying and unpredictable rates are not good candidates for extended-release products.
- *They are administered in relatively small doses.* Drugs with large single doses frequently are not suitable for ER because the tablet or capsule needed to maintain a sustained therapeutic blood level of the drug would be too large for the patient to swallow easily.
- *They possess a good margin of safety.* The most widely used measure of the margin of a drug's safety is its therapeutic index, that is, the median toxic dose divided by the median effective dose. For very potent drugs, the

therapeutic index may be narrow or very small. The larger the therapeutic index, the safer the drug. Drugs that are administered in very small doses or possess very narrow therapeutic indices are poor candidates for formulation into extended-release formulations because of technologic limitations of precise control over release rates and the risk of dose dumping because of a product defect. Patient misuse (e.g., chewing dosage unit) also could result in toxic drug levels.

- *They are used in the treatment of chronic rather than acute conditions.* Drugs for acute conditions require greater adjustment of the dosage by the physician than that provided by extended-release products.

Extended-Release Technology for Oral Dosage Forms

For orally administered dosage forms, extended drug action is achieved by affecting the rate at which the drug is released from the dosage form and/or by slowing the transit time of the dosage form through the gastrointestinal tract (4).

The rate of drug release from solid dosage forms may be modified by the technologies described next, which in general are based on (*a*) modifying drug dissolution by controlling access of biologic fluids to the drug through the use of barrier coatings, (*b*) controlling drug diffusion rates from dosage forms, and (*c*) chemical reaction or interaction between the drug substance or its pharmaceutical barrier and site-specific biologic fluids.

Coated Beads, Granules, and Microspheres

In these systems, the drug is distributed onto beads, pellets, granules, or other particulate systems. Using conventional pan coating or air suspension coating, a solution of the drug substance is placed on small inert nonpareil seeds or beads made of sugar and starch or on microcrystalline cellulose spheres. The nonpareil seeds are most often in the range of 425 to 850 mm, whereas the microcrystalline cellulose spheres range from 170 to 600 mm. The microcrystalline spheres are considered more durable during production than sugar-based cores (11).

If the dose of the drug is large, the starting granules of material may be composed of the drug itself. Some of these granules may remain uncoated to provide immediate drug release. Other granules (about two-thirds to three-fourths) receive varying coats of a lipid material like beeswax,

carnauba wax, glyceryl monostearate, or cetyl alcohol or a cellulosic material like ethylcellulose. Then, granules of different coating thicknesses are blended to achieve a mix having the desired drug-release characteristics. The coating material may be colored to distinguish granules or beads of different coating thicknesses (by depth of color) and to provide distinctiveness to the product. When properly blended, the granules may be placed in capsules or formed into tablets. Various commercial aqueous coating systems use ethylcellulose and plasticizer as the coating material (e.g., Aquacoat [FMC Corporation] and Surelease [Colorcon]) (12,13). Aqueous coating systems eliminate the hazards and environmental concerns associated with organic solvent–based systems.

The variation in the thickness of the coats and in the type of coating material used affects the rate at which body fluids penetrate the coating to dissolve the drug. Naturally, the thicker the coat, the more the resistance to penetration and the more delayed will be drug release and dissolution. Typically, the coated beads are about 1 mm in diameter. They are combined to have three or four release groups among the more than 100 beads contained in the dosing unit (10). This provides the different desired rates of sustained or ER and the targeting of the coated beads to the desired segments of the gastrointestinal tract. An example of this type of dosage form is the Spansule (SmithKline Beecham) capsule shown in Figure 9.3.

Multitablet System

Small spheroid compressed tablets 3 to 4 mm in diameter may be prepared to have varying drug-release characteristics. They then may be placed in gelatin capsule shells to provide the desired pattern of drug release (14). Each capsule may contain 8 to 10 minitablets, some uncoated for immediate release and others coated for extended drug release.

Microencapsulated Drug

Microencapsulation is a process by which solids, liquids, or even gases may be enclosed in microscopic particles by formation of thin coatings of wall material around the substance. The process had its origin in the late 1930s as a cleaner substitute for carbon paper and carbon ribbons as sought by the business machine industry. The ultimate development in the 1950s of reproduction paper and ribbons that contained dyes in tiny gelatin capsules released on impact by a typewriter key or the pressure of a pen or

FIGURE 9.3. The Spansule capsule showing the hard gelatin capsule containing hundreds of tiny pellets for sustained drug release and rupture of one of the pellets as occurs in the gastric fluid. (Courtesy of SmithKline Beecham.)

pencil was the stimulus for the development of a host of microencapsulated materials, including drugs. Gelatin is a common wall-forming material, and synthetic polymers, such as polyvinyl alcohol, ethylcellulose, polyvinyl chloride, and other materials, also may be used.

The typical encapsulation process usually begins with dissolving the wall material, say gelatin, in water. The material to be encapsulated is added and the two-phase mixture thoroughly stirred. With the material to be encapsulated broken up to the desired particle size, a solution of a second material, usually acacia, is added. This additive material concentrates the gelatin (polymer) into tiny liquid droplets. These droplets (the *coacervate*) form a film or coat around the particles of the substance to be encapsulated as a consequence of the extremely low interfacial tension of the residual water or solvent in the wall material so that a continuous tight film coating remains on the particle (Fig. 9.4). The final dry microcapsules are free-flowing discrete particles of coated material. The wall material usually constitutes 2% to 20% of the total particle weight. Different rates of drug release may be obtained by changing the ratio of core to wall, the polymer used for the coating, and the method of microencapsulation (15).

One of the advantages of microencapsulation is that the administered dose of a drug is subdivided into small units that are spread over a large area of the gastrointestinal tract, which may enhance absorption by diminishing local drug concentration (15). An example of a drug commercially available in a microencapsulated extended-release dosage form is potassium chloride (Micro-K Extencaps, Wyeth).

Embedding Drug in Slowly Eroding or Hydrophilic Matrix System

The drug substance is combined and made into granules with an excipient material that slowly erodes in body

fluids, progressively releasing the drug for absorption. When these granules are mixed with granules of drug prepared without the excipient, the uncombined granules provide the immediate effect and the drug–excipient granules provide extended action. The granule mix may be formulated as tablets or capsules for oral delivery.

Hydrophilic cellulose polymers are commonly used as the excipient base in tablet matrix systems. The effectiveness of these hydrophilic matrix systems is based on the successive processes of hydration of the cellulosic polymer, gel formation on the polymer's surface, tablet erosion, and the subsequent and continuous release of drug. Hydroxypropyl methylcellulose (HPMC), a free-flowing powder, is commonly used to provide the hydrophilic matrix. Tablets are prepared by thoroughly distributing HPMC in the formulation, preparing the granules by wet granulation or roller compaction, and manufacturing the tablets by compression (16).

After ingestion, the tablet is wetted by gastric fluid, and the polymer begins to hydrate. A gel layer forms around surface of the tablet, and an initial quantity of drug is exposed and released. As water permeates further into the tablet, the thickness of the gel layer increases and soluble drug diffuses through the gel layer. As the outer layer becomes fully hydrated, it erodes from the tablet core. If the drug is insoluble, it is released as such with the eroding gel layer. Thus, the rate of drug release is controlled by diffusion and tablet erosion (17).

For a successful hydrophilic matrix system, the polymer must form a gelatinous layer rapidly enough to protect the inner core of the tablet from disintegrating too rapidly after ingestion. As the proportion of polymer in a formulation increases, so does the viscosity of the gel, with a resultant decrease in the rate of drug diffusion and drug release (17). In general, 20% of HPMC results in satisfactory rates of release for an extended-release tablet formulation. However, as with all formulations, consideration must be given to the possible effects of other formulation ingredients, including fillers, tablet binders, and disintegrants. An example of a proprietary product using a hydrophilic matrix base of HPMC for extended drug release is Oramorph SR tablets (AllPharma), which contains morphine sulfate.

When hydrophilic matrix formulations are used in the preparation of extended-release capsules, the same concept applies. When the capsule is ingested, water penetrates the capsule shell, comes in contact with the fill, hydrates the outer layer of powder, and forms a gelatinous plug from which the drug content diffuses gradually over time as hydration continues and the gelatinous plug dissolves.

Manufacturers may prepare two-layer tablets, with one layer containing the uncombined drug for immediate release and the other layer having the drug embedded in a hydrophilic matrix for ER. Three-layer tablets may be similarly prepared, with both outer layers containing the drug for immediate release. Some commercial tablets are prepared with an inner core containing the extended-release portion of drug and an outer shell enclosing the core and containing drug for immediate release.

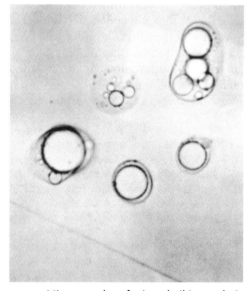

FIGURE 9.4. Microcapsules of mineral oil in a gelatin–acacia coacervate.

Embedding Drug in Inert Plastic Matrix

The drug is granulated with an inert plastic material such as polyethylene, polyvinyl acetate, or polymethacrylate, and the granulation is compressed into tablets. The drug is slowly released from the inert plastic matrix by diffusion. The compression creates the matrix or plastic form that retains its shape during leaching of the drug and during its passage through the alimentary tract. An immediate-release portion of drug may be compressed onto the surface of the tablet. The inert tablet matrix, expended of drug, is excreted with the feces. The historical example of a dosage form of this type is the Gradumet (Abbott).

Complex Formation

Some drug substances, when chemically combined with certain other chemical agents, form complexes that may be only slowly soluble in body fluids, depending on the pH of the environment. This slow dissolution rate provides the ER of the drug. Salts of tannic acid, tannates, provide this quality in a variety of proprietary products by the trade name Rynatan (Wallace) (10).

Ion-Exchange Resins

A solution of a cationic drug may be passed through a column containing an ion-exchange resin, forming a complex by displacing a less tightly bound ion, such as H^+ or Na^+. The resin–drug complex is washed and may be tableted, encapsulated, or suspended in an aqueous vehicle. The release of the drug depends on the pH and electrolyte concentration in the gastrointestinal tract. Release is greater in the acidity of the stomach than in the less acidic environment of the small intestine. Examples of drug products of this type include hydrocodone polistirex and chlorpheniramine polistirex suspension (Tussionex Pennkinetic extended-release suspension [CellTech]) and phentermine resin capsules (Ionamin capsules [CellTech]).

The mechanism of action of drug release from ion-exchange resins may be depicted as follows:

In the Stomach.

1. Drug resinate + HCl $\rightleftharpoons$ acidic resin
   + drug hydrochloride

2. Resin salt + HCl $\rightleftharpoons$ resin chloride
   + acidic drug

In the Intestine.

1. Drug resinate + NaCl $\rightleftharpoons$ sodium resinate
   + drug hydrochloride

2. Resin salt + NaCl $\rightleftharpoons$ resin chloride
   + sodium salt of drug

This system incorporates three ER technologies in a single product: a polymer barrier coating and bead technology in addition to the ion-exchange mechanism. The initial dose comes from an uncoated portion and the remainder from the coated beads. The coating does not dissolve, and release is extended over 12 hours by ionic exchange. The drug-containing polymer particles are minute and may be suspended to produce a liquid with extended-release characteristics as well as solid dosage forms.

Osmotic Pump

The pioneer *oral osmotic* pump drug delivery system is the *OROS* system developed by Alza. The system is composed of a core tablet surrounded by a semipermeable membrane coating having a 0.4-mm-diameter hole produced by laser beam (Fig. 9.5). The core tablet has two layers, one containing the drug (the active layer) and the other containing a polymeric osmotic agent (the push layer). The system operates on the principle of osmotic pressure.

When the tablet is swallowed, water from the patient's stomach diffuses through the semipermeable membrane via osmosis into the core tablet, dissolving or suspending the drug. As pressure increases in the osmotic layer, it pumps the drug solution out of the delivery orifice on the side of the tablet. Only the drug solution (not the undissolved drug) is capable of passing through the hole in the tablet. The system is designed such that only a few drops of water are drawn into the tablet each hour. The rate of inflow of water and the function of the tablet depend on an osmotic gradient between the contents of the two-layer core and the fluid in the gastrointestinal tract. Drug delivery is essentially constant as long as the osmotic gradient

FIGURE 9.5. **A:** Elementary OROS (oral release osmotic system) osmotic pump drug delivery system. **B:** Push–pull osmotic system.

remains constant. The drug-release rate may be altered by changing the surface area, thickness or composition of the membrane, and/or diameter of the drug-release orifice. The drug-release rate is not affected by gastrointestinal acidity, alkalinity, fed conditions, or gastrointestinal motility. The biologically inert components of the tablet remain intact during gastrointestinal transit and are eliminated in the feces as an insoluble shell.

This type of osmotic system, termed the *gastrointestinal therapeutic system* (GITS [Pfizer]), is employed in the manufacture of Glucotrol XL ER tablets and Procardia XL ER tablets. Another example of the osmotic system is the *controlled-onset extended release* (COER [Searle]) system used in Covera-HS tablets, in which initial drug is released 4 to 5 hours after tablet ingestion. The delay in drug release is effected by a slowly solubilized coated layer between the active drug core and the outer semipermeable membrane.

Repeat-Action Tablets

Repeat-action tablets are prepared so that an initial dose of drug is released immediately and a second dose follows later. The tablets may be prepared with the immediate-release dose in the tablet's outer shell or coating and the second dose in the tablet's inner core, separated by a slowly permeable barrier coating. In general, the drug from the inner core is exposed to body fluids and released 4 to 6 hours after administration. An example of this type of product is Repetabs (Schering). Repeat-action dosage forms are best suited for treatment of chronic conditions requiring repeated dosing. The drugs should have low dosage and fairly rapid rates of absorption and excretion.

DELAYED-RELEASE ORAL DOSAGE FORMS

The release of a drug from an oral dosage form may be intentionally delayed until it reaches the intestines for several reasons. The purpose may be to protect a drug destroyed by gastric fluids, to reduce gastric distress caused by drugs particularly irritating to the stomach, or to facilitate gastrointestinal transit for drugs that are better absorbed from the intestines. As stated previously, capsules and tablets specially coated to remain intact in the stomach and to yield their ingredients in the intestines are termed *enteric coated*. The enteric coating may be pH dependent, breaking down in the less acidic environment of the intestine; time dependent, eroding by moisture over time during gastrointestinal transit; or enzyme dependent, deteriorating as a result of the hydrolysis–catalyzing action of intestinal enzymes. Among the many agents used for enteric coating of tablets and capsules are fats, fatty acids, waxes, shellac, and cellulose acetate phthalate.

Examples of modified-release tablets and capsules official in the USP are presented in Table 9.2, and examples of proprietary modified-release oral dosage forms are

---

TABLE 9.2. Modified-Release Tablets and Capsules Official in the USP

Delayed Release

Aspirin delayed-release tablets

Dirithromycin delayed-release tablets

Doxycycline hyclate delayed-release capsules

Erythromycin delayed-release capsules

Oxybutynin chloride extended-release tablets

Oxtriphylline delayed-release tablets

Extended Release

Aspirin extended-release tablets

Bupropion hydrochloride extended-release tablets

Diltiazem hydrochloride extended-release capsules

Disopyramide phosphate extended-release capsules

Indomethacin extended-release capsules

Isosorbide dinitrate extended-release tablets and capsules

Lithium carbonate extended-release tablets

Oxtriphylline extended-release tablets

Potassium chloride extended-release tablets

Phenytoin sodium extended-release capsules

Procainamide hydrochloride extended-release tablets

Propranolol hydrochloride extended-release capsules

Quinidine gluconate extended-release tablets

Theophylline extended-release capsules

---

presented in Table 9.3. Table 9.4 is a summary of release mechanisms and commercial examples.

USP REQUIREMENTS AND FDA GUIDANCE FOR MODIFIED-RELEASE DOSAGE FORMS

The USP contains general chapters and specific tests to determine the drug-release capabilities of extended-release and delayed-release tablets and capsules (8).

Drug Release

The USP test for drug release for extended-release and delayed-release articles is based on drug dissolution from the dosage unit against elapsed test time (Fig. 9.6). Descriptions of the various test apparatus and procedures may be found in the USP Chapter <724> (8). The individual monographs contain specific criteria for compliance with the test and the apparatus and test procedures to be used. For example, for aspirin extended-release tablets, the USP requires the following aspirin dissolution rate to meet the stated drug-release test:

Time (Hours)	Percent of Dose Dissolved
1.0	15%–40%
2.0	25%–60%
4.0	35%–75%
8.0	Not <70%

TABLE 9.3. Proprietary Modified-Release Oral Dosage Forms

Drug Product and Manufacturer	Dosage Form Characteristics
Delayed Release	
E-Mycin (erythromycin) delayed-release tablets (Knoll)	Tablets enteric coated with cellulose acetate phthalate, carnauba wax, and cellulose polymers. Use: antibiotic
Erythromycin delayed-release capsules (Abbott)	Capsules contain enteric-coated pellets of erythromycin base. Use: antibiotic
Asacol (mesalamine) delayed-release tablets (Procter & Gamble)	Tablets coated with Eudragit S (methacrylic acid copolymer B), a resin that bypasses the stomach and dissolves in the ileum and beyond. Use: treat ulcerative colitis
Prilosec (omeprazole) delayed-release capsules (AstraZeneca)	Enteric-coated granules of omeprazole placed in capsules. Omeprazole is acid labile and is degraded by gastric acid. Use: treatment of duodenal ulcer
Extended-Release Coated Particles and Beads	
Toprol-XL (metoprolol succinate) tablets (AstraZeneca)	Drug pellets coated with cellulose polymers compressed into tablets. Use: treatment of hypertension
Indocin SR (indomethacin) capsules (Merck)	Coated pellets for SR. Formulation includes polyvinyl acetate–crotonic acid copolymer and HPMC. Use: analgesic, anti-inflammatory
Compazine (prochlorperazine) Spansule capsules (SmithKline Beecham)	Coated pellets in capsule formulated to release initial dose promptly with additional drug for prolonged release. Use: antinausea, antivomiting
Adderall XR (amphetamines) capsules (Shire US Inc.)	Encapsulated sugar spheres coated with drug and HPMC and methacrylic acid copolymer providing a double-pulsed delivery. Use: attention deficit disorder
Extended-Release Inert Matrix	
Procanbid (procainamide HCl) tablets (Monarch)	Extended-release tablets with a core tablet of a nonerodible wax matrix coated with cellulose polymers. Use: an antiarrhythmic
Extended-Release Hydrophilic/Eroding Matrix	
Depakote ER (divalproex sodium) extended-release tablets (Abbott)	Drug is dispersed and compressed in a hypromellose and microcrystalline cellulose matrix. Use: antiepileptic
Quinidex (quinidine sulfate) tablets (Robins)	Extended-release provided by hydrophilic matrix that swells and slowly erodes. Use: antiarrhythmic
Oramorph SR (morphine sulfate) tablets (AllPharma)	Sustained-release hydrophilic matrix system, based on polymer HPMC. Use: analgesic for severe pain
Extended-Release Microencapsulated	
K-Dur microburst release system (potassium chloride) tablets (Key)	Immediately dispersing drug microencapsulated with ethylcellulose and hydroxypropyl cellulose. Use: potassium depletion
Effexor XR (venlafaxine hydrochloride) capsules cellulose, ethylcellulose, and hypromellose resulting in once a day	Drug dispersed in spheroids and coated. Polymers used include (Wyeth) administration that is not pH dependent. Use: antidepressant
Extended-Release Osmotic	
Glucotrol XL (glipizide) tablets (Pfizer)	Controlled-release GITS[a] osmotic system. Ingredients include polyethylene oxide, hydroxypropyl cellulose, and cellulose acetate. Use: antihyperglycemic
Covera-HS (verapamil HCl) tablets (Searle)	A COER[b] osmotic system. Use: antihypertensive, antianginal

[a]Gastrointestinal therapeutic system.
[b]Controlled onset, ER.

Uniformity of Dosage Units

Modified-release tablets and capsules must meet the USP standard for uniformity as described in Chapter 8 for conventional dosage units. Uniformity of dosage units may be demonstrated by either of two methods, weight variation or content uniformity, as described in USP Chapter <905> (8).

In Vitro–In Vivo Correlations

In vitro–in vivo relationships (IVIVRs) or in vitro–in vivo correlations (IVIVCs) are critical to the development of oral extended-release products. Assessing IVICRs is important throughout product development, clinical evaluation, submission of an application for FDA approval for marketing, and during postapproval for any proposed formulation or manufacturing changes (18).

In 1997, the FDA published a guidance document, *Extended Release Oral Dosage Forms: Development, Evaluation, and Application of* In Vitro/In Vivo *Correlations* (9). It provides guidance to sponsors of new drug applications and abbreviated new drug applications for extended-release oral products. The guidance provides methods of (*a*) developing an IVIVC and evaluating its predictability,

TABLE 9.4. Summary of Release Mechanisms and Commercial Examples

Type	Release Mechanism	Commercial Example
Hydrophilic matrix	Dissolution/diffusion	Oramorph SR, Seroquel XR, Opana ER, Paxil CR, Glucophage XR, TheoChron
Inert matrix	Diffusion	Fero-Gradumet, Oxycontin, Slow K
Microparticulate reservoir	Diffusion	Micro-K Extencaps, Klor-Con tablets, Dilacor XR, Luvox CR, Coreg CR, Amrix ER, Focalin XR, Metadate CD, Cardizem CD, Avinza
Hybrid microparticulate reservoir in matrix	Diffusion	Cardizem LA, Toprol XL
Single reservoir	Diffusion	Ultram ER
Osmotic tablets	Osmotic pressure	Glucotrol XL, Procardia XL, Concerta, Covera HS, Tegretol XR, Invega, Ditropan XL
Ion exchange	pH or ion displacement	Tussionex capsules, Tussionex suspension, Paxil suspension, Delsym suspension

(*b*) using an IVIVC to establish dissolution specifications, and (*c*) applying an IVIVC as a surrogate for in vivo bioequivalence when it is necessary to document bioequivalence during the approval process or during postapproval for certain formulation or manufacturing changes.

Three categories of IVIVCs are included in the document:

- *Level A*: A predictive mathematical model for the relationship between the entire in vitro dissolution and release time course and the entire in vivo response time course, for example, the time course of plasma drug concentration or amount of drug absorbed. This is the most common type of correlation submitted.
- *Level B*: A predictive mathematical model of the relationship between summary parameters that characterize the in vitro and in vivo time courses, for example, models that relate the mean in vitro dissolution time to the mean in vivo dissolution time, the mean in vitro dissolution time to the mean residence time in vivo, or the in vitro dissolution rate constant to the absorption rate constant.

- *Level C*: A predictive mathematical model of the relationship between the amount dissolved in vitro at a particular time (or the time required for in vitro dissolution of a fixed percent of the dose, e.g., T_{50}) and a summary parameter that characterizes the in vivo time course (e.g., maximum concentration [C_{max}] or area under the curve). The level of IVIVCs may be useful in the early stages of formulation development when pilot formulations are being selected.

The most common process for developing an IVIVC model (level A) is to (*a*) develop formulations with different release rates (e.g., slow, fast, and intermediate) or a single-release rate if dissolution is independent of condition, (*b*) obtain in vitro dissolution profiles and in vivo plasma concentration profiles for these formulations, and (*c*) estimate the in vivo absorption or dissolution time course for each formulation and subject using appropriate mathematical approaches.

Among the criteria applicable to the development of IVIVCs are the following (9):

- In determining in vitro dissolution, USP dissolution apparatus, type I (basket) or type II (paddle), is preferred,

} pH 7.5 like distal ileum

} pH 7.2 like proximal ileum

} pH 6.8 like lower small intestines

} pH 4.5 like upper small intestines

} pH 1.2 like stomach

FIGURE 9.6. Dissolution apparatus for determining dissolution characteristics of modified-release products.

although type III (reciprocating cylinder) or type IV (flow-through cell) may be applicable in some instances.

- An aqueous medium with a pH not exceeding 6.8 is preferred as the medium for dissolution studies. For poorly soluble drugs, a surfactant (e.g., 1% sodium lauryl sulfate) may be added.
- The dissolution profiles of at least 12 individual dosage units from each lot should be determined.
- For in vivo studies, human subjects are used in the fasted state unless the drug is not well tolerated, in which case the studies may be conducted in the fed state. Acceptable data sets have been shown to be generated with use of 6 to 36 human subjects.
- Crossover studies are preferred, but parallel studies or cross-study analysis may be acceptable using a common reference treatment product, such as an intravenous solution, an aqueous oral solution, or an immediate-release product.

Labeling

The USP indicates labeling requirements for modified-release dosage form articles in addition to general labeling requirements. The requirements are specific to the monograph article. For example, the label of aspirin delayed-release tablets must state that *the tablets are enteric coated*, whereas the labeling for theophylline extended-release capsules must indicate *whether the product is intended for dosing every 12 or 24 hours and state with which* in vitro *drug-release test the product complies* (seven tests are described in the monograph, each with different drug-release times and tolerances).

CLINICAL CONSIDERATIONS IN THE USE OF ORAL MODIFIED-RELEASE DOSAGE FORMS

Patients should be advised of the dose and dosing frequency of modified drug-release products and instructed not to use them interchangeably or concomitantly with immediate-release forms of the same drug. Patients stabilized on a modified-release product should not be changed to an immediate-release product without consideration of any existing blood level concentrations of the drug. Also, once stabilized, patients should not be changed to another extended-release product unless there is assurance of equivalent bioavailability. A different product can result in a marked shift in the patient's drug blood level because of differences in drug-release characteristics.

Patients should be advised that modified-release tablets and capsules should not be crushed or chewed, because such action compromises their drug-release features (19). Patients being fed by enteral nutrition through a nasogastric tube may receive conventional or modified-release medication. For example, coated pellets from inside capsules simply may be mixed with water and poured down the feeding tube (20). Similarly, modified-release tablets and capsules should not generally be used as the source of a drug to prepare other dosage forms, that is, pediatric oral liquids.

Patients and caregivers should be advised that nonerodible plastic matrix shells and osmotic tablets remain intact throughout gastrointestinal transit and the empty shells or ghosts from osmotic tablets may be seen in the stool. The patient should be assured of the normalcy of this event and that drug absorption has taken place (4).

PACKAGING AND STORING MODIFIED-RELEASE TABLETS AND CAPSULES

Modified-release tablets and capsules are packaged and stored in the same manner as conventional products as discussed in Chapters 7 and 8.

PATIENT COUNSELING

DELAYED-RELEASE SOLIDS

1. Take with a glass of water or acidic juice (apple, orange, etc.).
2. Take on an empty stomach if applicable 30 minutes before a meal. Proton pump inhibitors need to empty from the stomach to the small intestine to be released and be effective as they may degrade in the acid content of the stomach.
3. Generally, food does not significantly affect the bioavailability of delayed-release tablets and capsules used for maintenance therapy.
4. Do not chew or crush.
5. Confirm the onset, frequency, and storage of the medication with the patient.
6. Store in the least humid environment available at room temperature.

EXTENDED-RELEASE SOLIDS

1. Take with a glass of water or acidic juice (apple, orange, etc.).
2. Food generally does not affect the bioavailability of extended-release tablets and capsules.
3. Explain whether or not the dosage form can be cut or halved.
4. Do not chew or crush.
5. Nonerodible dosage form "ghosts" or residues may appear in the stool.
6. Confirm the onset, frequency, and storage for the drug. This is not a rapid-onset form of the drug even though there is often an immediate-release component.
7. Store in a low humidity environment at room temperature.

PHARMACEUTICS CASE STUDY

SUBJECTIVE INFORMATION

You work in a small but growing pharmaceutical company producing extended-release tablets. Sales have been good, and the pressure is on to increase production by 20% per day. The only way you can accomplish this is to increase the speed at which your rotary machines work, because you are running three shifts of 8 hours each. When you increase the speed of your machine and start production, you start getting reports that the tablets do not produce the proper extended-release dissolution profile and they are not of the proper hardness. Also, the tablets are less potent and weigh less than that specified. No other adjustments have been made to the machine other than to increase the speed. What will you do?

OBJECTIVE INFORMATION

Your machines are 36-station rotary tablet presses using gravity feed. You produce the tablets, which are oblong, with a hydrophilic matrix system and an oblong punch and die. The optimal speed was established during the scale-up phase of product development and has been used for the past 18 months with no problems.

ASSESSMENT

The production of tablets must follow a well-defined set of conditions. If not, the final product may not have the desired characteristics of hardness, disintegration, dissolution, friability, and appearance. It appears that the increase in speed is not allowing the powder blend sufficient time to flow by gravity into the tablet dies, as the increased speed causes the die to pass under the powder feed apparatus faster than before. This results in less powder per tablet in the die, and when they are compressed, the resulting tablets are not as firm; when subjected to a dissolution test, the result is a more rapid release of the drug. This also explains the lighter tablets and the lower quantity of active drug per tablet.

PLAN

There are two options here: first, decrease the rate of speed to that at which the production was validated, and second, consider a force-feed system to move the powder into the dies faster. The latter option requires validation of the equipment under the new conditions. A third option may be the most reasonable and that is to purchase additional machines. ■

CLINICAL CASE STUDY

SUBJECTIVE INFORMATION

CC: K.F. is a 9-year-old WM who arrives at the pediatric clinic with his mother. The mother states that K.F. talks excessively, interrupts others when they speak, rarely follows her directions, and frequently runs around the house. The mother also states that she has heard from the teacher that he leaves the classroom in the middle of the class, often blurts out answers before questions have been completed, has a difficult time waiting his turn (e.g., in the lunchroom), is "fidgety," rarely follows directions or pays attention, and turns in incomplete homework assignments. His teacher has also told the mother that he frequently distracts the other students at school. The mother states, "I would like your help. But I do not want him to be put on a medicine where he has to take it more than once a day because I might forget to give it to him. Also, I do not want him taking any medicine to school."
HPI: The mother states that K.F. has been "this way" since he was 6 years old. However, it is now at the point where he does not complete any of his tasks (e.g., making his bed, doing his homework) and his grades are "slipping." His latest report card showed "many Cs and Ds."
PMH: Otitis media, 4 weeks ago

Meds: Zithromax suspension, finished it about 3 weeks ago
OTC Meds: K.F. and his mother deny K.F.'s use of vitamins, herbals, or any other supplements.
PSH: None

FH:	Mother, DM type II since age 29
SH:	(per K.F.)
	(–) Tobacco
	(–) EtOH
	(–) Illicit drugs
	(+) Caffeine: loves Mountain Dew, drinks a couple of cans (~2 to 3) per day

Exercise, daily activities: Goes to school from 8 AM to 3 PM; after school, likes to watch TV, in-line skate, and play basketball
Timing of meals: Breakfast at 7:30 AM, lunch at noon, snack at 3:30 PM, and dinner at 6:30 PM
Diet: Chips, candy, peanut butter and jelly sandwiches, pasta, and two or three cans of Mountain Dew per day
Bedtime: 9:30 to 10:30 PM
Siblings: None

(continued)

CLINICAL CASE STUDY *(continued)*

Mother and father are both accountants, and each works approximately 40 hours per week. They have been married for 11 years.

ALL: NKDA

OBJECTIVE INFORMATION

9-year-old WM

Ht: 4'2"	Wt: 71 lb		
BP: 119/75	P: 70	T: 98.6°F	RR: 15
Pain:	None		

The mother presents K.F.'s last report card with grades Cs and Ds along with notes from K.F.'s teacher about his behavior.

ASSESSMENT

ADHD, combined type

PLAN

Recommend extended-release methylphenidate HCl (i.e., Concerta) 18 mg by mouth once a day with breakfast and a full glass of water, milk, or juice at 7:30 AM (to aid with adherence). Inform the mother that the prescription has to be dispensed to her within 7 days after the date it is issued. Concerta has a rapid onset of action to help K.F. focus in the morning at school and a long duration of action, which will be useful during and after school for homework.

Counsel the mother on possible side effects, such as insomnia, loss of appetite, and weight loss. Inform K.F.'s mother also about a possible decrease in rate of height growth (not final height). Advise her not to administer it after school if her son misses a dose of the drug in the morning.

Wait until the next morning for the next dose. Do not double the dose the next day. Inform the mother that this product is prepared in a nonabsorbable shell, which means that the empty shell may or may not be observed in the stool. So if K.F. notices something that resembles a tablet in the stool and mentions it to his mother, she can tell him not to worry; the medicine is working. As methylphenidate is a class II drug, the mother should understand the necessity to secure a new prescription from the physician for every cycle of therapy. This can be done when K.F. returns to the physician's office for routine monitoring (e.g., blood pressure, pulse, height, weight, encountered side effects).

Counsel K.F. and his mother that he should take the tablet with a full glass of water or juice. He should swallow the tablet whole and not to chew it. Discuss the change in medication dosage forms for children when they convert from liquid dosage forms to solid dosage forms and the apprehension that may be involved. K.F. and his mother should know that there is no conclusive evidence regarding sugar dietary intake and its effect on ADHD. However, if K.F.'s mother believes that K.F.'s symptoms are worse with sugary foods or drinks, these should be minimized and decreased from his diet. It is given that the caffeinated soft drink (i.e., Mountain Dew) should be changed for a caffeine-free soft drink. No caffeinated beverages should be ingested by K.F. after 6 PM.

Goal: Resolution of symptoms (e.g., improved attention, less fidgeting), improvement in grades, and no side effects from Concerta. Also, K.F.'s mother should be referred to a child psychologist who can provide K.F.'s needed behavioral therapy.

www.concerta.net

www.add.org

www.adhd.com ∎

| APPLYING THE PRINCIPLES AND CONCEPTS |

GROUP ACTIVITIES

1. Compare the advantages and disadvantages of modified-release dosage forms to conventional oral dosage forms.
2. Create a listing of conceivable ways a consumer/patient might misuse a modified-release dosage form.
3. List five counseling points for proper administration of solid modified-release dosage forms, and provide a rationale for each counseling point.
4. Referring to the USP <724>, select three individual drug monographs containing specific criteria for compliance with the test and the apparatus and test procedures to be used, and state the reasons for any differences that exist among the three monographs.

5. Create a listing, including active ingredient(s), of 10 modified-release dosage form products whose names imply a modified-release product.

INDIVIDUAL ACTIVITIES

1. Create a table of modified-release dosage form products including amount of active ingredient(s), indication, contraindication, adverse effects/precautions, and dosage.
2. Create a listing of trademarked modified-release dosage forms that possess unique characteristics, for example, size, shape, and color, and describe/detail those features.
3. Generate a listing of drugs whose physical–chemical characteristics make them a candidate for incorporation into a modified-release dosage form.

4. From the primary literature, find a clinical study demonstrating a comparison between a modified-release tablet product and a compressed tablet for clinical effectiveness, and determine which one would be preferred in terms of patient acceptance, patient adherence, bioequivalence, and cost. Explain the rationale for your decision.

5. Select one USP drug monograph for an official modified-release tablet dosage form, and identify and describe its main components.

REFERENCES

1. Available at: http://www.reuters.com/article/2010/04/01/us-drug-sales-idUSTRE6303CU20100401. (Accessed July 25, 2020)
2. Das NG, Das SK. Controlled-release of oral dosage forms. Formulation, Fill Finish (Suppl Pharm Technol) 2003;27:10–16.
3. Rogers JD, Kwan KC. Pharmacokinetic requirements for controlled-release dosage forms. In: Urquhart J, ed. Controlled-Release Pharmaceuticals. Washington, DC: Academy of Pharmaceutical Sciences, American Pharmaceutical Association, 1979:95–119.
4. Bogner RH. Bioavailability and bioequivalence of extended-release oral dosage forms. US Pharm 1997;22(Suppl):3–12.
5. Madan PL. Sustained-release drug delivery systems, part II: Preformulation considerations. Pharm Manuf 1985;2:41–45.
6. Madan PL. Sustained-release drug delivery systems, part I: An overview. Pharm Manuf 1985;2:23–27.
7. AAPS/FDA Workshop Committee. Scale-up of oral extended-release dosage forms. Pharm Technol 1995;19:46–54.
8. United States Pharmacopeia–National Formulary. Current Ed. Rockville, MD: U.S. Pharmacopeial Convention.
9. Guidance for industry. Extended Release Oral Dosage Forms: Development, Evaluation, and Application of In Vitro/In Vivo Correlations. Rockville, MD: Center for Drug Evaluation and Research, Food & Drug Administration, 1997.
10. Madan PL. Sustained release dosage forms. US Pharm 1990;15:39–50.
11. Celphere Microcrystalline Cellulose Spheres. Philadelphia, PA: FMC Corporation, 1996.
12. Aquacoat Aqueous Polymeric Dispersion. Philadelphia, PA: FMC Corporation, 1996.
13. Surelease Aqueous Controlled Release Coating System. West Point, PA: Colorcon, 2006.
14. Butler J, Cumming I, Brown J, et al. A novel multiunit controlled-release system. Pharm Technol 1998;22:122–138.
15. Yazici E, Oner L, Kas HS, et al. Phenytoin sodium microcapsules: Bench scale formulation, process characterization and release kinetics. Pharm Dev Technol 1996;1:175–183.
16. Sheskey PJ, Cabelka TD, Robb RT, et al. Use of roller compaction in the preparation of controlled-release hydrophilic matrix tablets containing methylcellulose and hydroxypropyl methylcellulose polymers. Pharm Technol 1994;18:132–150.
17. Formulating for Controlled Release with Methocel Premium Cellulose Ethers. Midland, MI: Dow Chemical, 1995.
18. Devane J, Butler J. The impact of in vitro-in vivo relationships on product development. Pharm Technol 1997;21:146–159.
19. Available at: http://www.ismp.org/tools/donotcrush.pdf. (Accessed July 25, 2020)
20. Beckwith MC, Barton RG, Graves C. A guide to drug therapy in patients with enteral feeding tubes: Dosage form selection and administration methods. Hosp Pharm 1997;32:57–64.

SECTION FOUR

Semisolid Dosage Forms and Transdermal Systems

CHAPTER

10

Ointments, Creams, and Gels

CHAPTER AT A GLANCE Ointments • Selection of the Appropriate Base • Compendial Requirements for Ointments • Creams • Gels • Transdermal Preparations • Miscellaneous Semisolid Preparations: Pastes, Plasters, and Glycerogelatins • Features and Uses of Dermatologic Preparations • Features and Uses of Ophthalmic Ointments and Gels • Features and Uses of Nasal Ointments and Gels • Features and Uses of Rectal Preparations • Features and Uses of Vaginal Preparations • Drug Release from Semisolid Dosage Forms • Patient Counseling

OBJECTIVES

After reading this chapter, the student will be able to:

Differentiate between the various types of semisolid bases on the basis of physical and chemical properties

List the criteria for the selection of a semisolid base to treat a topical affliction

Describe the methods to incorporate (an) active ingredient(s) into a semisolid base

Explain the difference between an ointment, a cream, and a gel

Compare and contrast an ophthalmic ointment base and a topical ointment base for application to the skin

List advantages and disadvantages of administering drugs rectally and vaginally

List counseling points the pharmacist should share with the patient for each of the routes of administration used for topical product application

▌INTRODUCTION

The skin is a highly complex organ that regulates heat and water loss from the body while preventing the ingress of noxious chemicals or microorganisms. It is about 10% of the body mass and covers about 1.7 m² in the average adult male. It is large and accessible and provides a reasonable site to administer therapeutic agents for both local and systemic effects; it is also highly efficient at "self-repairing" and is designed to "keep the insides in and the outsides out!"

Ointments, creams, and gels are semisolid dosage forms intended for topical application. They may be applied to the skin, placed on the surface of the eye, or used nasally, vaginally, or rectally. Most of these preparations are used for the effects of the therapeutic agents they contain. The unmedicated ones are used for their physical effects as protectants or lubricants.

Topical preparations are used for both local and systemic effects; a "topical" drug (active pharmaceutical ingredient [API]) dosage form would be one that is designed to deliver the drug into the skin in treating skin disorders where the skin is the target organ. Systemic drug absorption should always be considered when using topical products if the patient is pregnant or nursing, because drugs can enter the fetal blood supply and breast milk and be transferred to the fetus or nursing infant.

Topical applications can be designed for either local effects or systemic absorption. The following distinction is an important one with regard to dermatologic applications. A *topical dermatological* product is designed to deliver drug *into* the skin in treating dermal disorders, *with the skin as the target organ*. A *transdermal* product is designed to deliver drugs *through* the skin (*percutaneous absorption*) to the general circulation for systemic effects, *with the skin not being the target organ* (1).

OINTMENTS

Ointments are semisolid preparations intended for external application to the skin or mucous membranes. Ointments may be medicated or not. Unmedicated ointments are used for the physical effects they provide as protectants, emollients, or lubricants. *Ointment bases*, as described, may be used for their physical effects or as vehicles for medicated ointments.

Ointment Bases

Ointment bases are generally classified by the U.S. Pharmacopeia (USP) (2) into four groups: (*a*) oleaginous bases, (*b*) absorption bases, (*c*) water-removable bases, and (*d*) water-soluble bases.

Oleaginous Bases

Oleaginous bases are also termed *hydrocarbon bases*. On application to the skin, they have an emollient effect, protect against the escape of moisture, are effective as occlusive dressings, can remain on the skin for long periods without drying out, and, because of their immiscibility with water, are difficult to wash off. Water and aqueous preparations may be incorporated, but only in small amounts and with some difficulty. Petrolatum, white petrolatum, white ointment, and yellow ointment are examples of hydrocarbon ointment bases.

When powdered substances are to be incorporated into hydrocarbon bases, liquid petrolatum (mineral oil) may be used as the levigating agent.

Petrolatum, USP, is a purified mixture of semisolid hydrocarbons obtained from petroleum. It is an unctuous mass, varying in color from yellowish to light amber. It melts at 38°C to 60°C and may be used alone or in combination with other agents as an ointment base. Petrolatum is also known as yellow petrolatum and petroleum jelly. A commercial product is Vaseline (Chesebrough–Ponds).

White Petrolatum, USP, is a purified mixture of semisolid hydrocarbons from petroleum that has been wholly or nearly decolorized. It is used for the same purpose as petrolatum, but because of its lighter color, it is considered more esthetically pleasing by some pharmacists and patients. White petrolatum is also known as white petroleum jelly. A commercial product is White Vaseline (Chesebrough–Ponds).

Yellow Ointment, USP. This ointment has the following formula for the preparation of 1,000 g:

Yellow wax:	50 g
Petrolatum:	950 g

Yellow wax is the purified wax obtained from the honeycomb of the bee *Apis mellifera*. The ointment is prepared by melting the yellow wax on a water bath, adding the petrolatum until the mixture is uniform, and then cooling and stirring until congealed. Also called simple ointment, it has a slightly greater viscosity than plain petrolatum.

White Ointment, USP. This ointment differs from yellow ointment by substitution of white wax (bleached and purified yellow wax) and white petrolatum in the formula.

Absorption Bases

Absorption bases are of two types: (*a*) those that *permit* the incorporation of aqueous solutions resulting in the formation of water-in-oil (W/O) emulsions (e.g., *hydrophilic petrolatum*) and (*b*) those that *are* W/O emulsions (syn: *emulsion bases*) that permit the incorporation of additional quantities of aqueous solutions (e.g., lanolin). These bases may be used as emollients, although they do not provide the degree of occlusion afforded by the oleaginous bases. Absorption bases are not easily removed from the skin with water washing, because the external phase of the emulsion is oleaginous. Absorption bases are useful as pharmaceutical adjuncts to incorporate small volumes of aqueous solutions into hydrocarbon bases. This is accomplished by incorporating the aqueous solution into the absorption base and then incorporating this mixture into the hydrocarbon base.

Hydrophilic Petrolatum, USP, has the following formula for the preparation of 1,000 g:

Cholesterol:	30 g
Stearyl alcohol:	30 g
White wax:	80 g
White petrolatum:	860 g

It is prepared by melting the stearyl alcohol and white wax on a steam bath, adding the cholesterol with stirring until dissolved, adding the white petrolatum, and allowing the mixture to cool while stirring until congealed.

Commercial products, Aquaphor and Aquabase, variations of hydrophilic petrolatum, have the capacity to absorb up to three times their weight in water and are useful to help incorporate a water-soluble drug, for example, tobramycin sulfate, into an oleaginous ointment base. This concept is used in the preparation of ophthalmic ointments. Eucerin is a 50% W/O emulsion.

Lanolin, USP (anhydrous lanolin), obtained from the wool of sheep (*Ovis aries*), is a purified waxlike substance that has been cleaned, deodorized, and decolorized. It contains not more than 0.25% water. Additional water may be incorporated into lanolin by mixing. *Modified Lanolin, USP*, is lanolin processed to reduce the contents of free lanolin alcohols and any detergent and pesticide residues.

Water-Removable Bases

Water-removable bases are oil-in-water emulsions commonly called creams. Because the external phase of the emulsion is aqueous, they are easily washed from skin and are often called water-washable bases. They may be diluted with water or aqueous solutions. They can absorb serous discharges. Hydrophilic ointment, USP, is an example of this type of base.

Hydrophilic Ointment, USP, has the following formula for 1,000 g:

Ingredient	Amount (g)
Methylparaben:	0.25
Propylparaben:	0.15
Sodium lauryl sulfate:	10.00
Propylene glycol:	120.00
Stearyl alcohol:	250.00
White petrolatum:	250.00
Purified water:	370.00

The stearyl alcohol and white petrolatum are melted together at about 75°C. The other agents, dissolved in the purified water, are added with stirring until the mixture congeals. Sodium lauryl sulfate is the emulsifying agent, with the stearyl alcohol and white petrolatum constituting the oleaginous phase of the emulsion and the other ingredients the aqueous phase. Methylparaben and propylparaben are antimicrobial preservatives.

Water-Soluble Bases

Water-soluble bases do not contain oleaginous components. They are completely water washable and often referred to as greaseless. Because they soften greatly with the addition of water, large amounts of aqueous solutions are not effectively incorporated into these bases. They mostly are used for incorporation of solid substances. Polyethylene glycol (PEG) ointment, NF, is the prototype example of a water-soluble base.

Polyethylene Glycol Ointment, NF, PEG is a polymer of ethylene oxide and water represented by the formula $H(OCH_2CH_2)_nOH$, in which n represents the average number of oxyethylene groups. The numeric designations associated with PEGs refer to the average molecular weight of the polymer. PEGs having average molecular weight below 600 are clear, colorless liquids; those with molecular weight above 1,000 are waxlike white materials; and those with molecular weight in between are semisolids. The greater the molecular weight, the greater the viscosity. The NF lists the viscosity of PEGs ranging from average molecular weight of 200 to 8,000.

The general formula for preparation of 1,000 g of PEG ointment is as follows:

PEG 3350:	400 g
PEG 400:	600 g

Combining PEG 3350, a solid, with PEG 400, a liquid, results in a very pliable semisolid ointment. If a firmer ointment is desired, the formula may be altered to contain up to equal parts of the two ingredients. When aqueous solutions are to be incorporated into the base, substitution of 50 g of PEG 3350 with an equal amount of stearyl alcohol is advantageous in rendering the final product firmer.

SELECTION OF THE APPROPRIATE BASE

Selection of the base to use in the formulation of an ointment depends on careful assessment of a number of factors, including the following:

- Desired release rate of the drug substance from the ointment base
- Desirability of topical or percutaneous drug absorption
- Desirability of occlusion of moisture from the skin
- Stability of the drug in the ointment base
- Effect, if any, of the drug on the consistency or other features of the ointment base
- Desire for a base easily removed by washing with water
- Characteristics of the surface to which it is applied

For example, an ointment is generally applied to dry, scaly skin; a cream is applied to weeping or oozing surfaces; and a lotion is applied to intertriginous areas or where friction may occur, as between the thighs or under the armpit. The base that provides the best combination of the most desired attributes should be selected.

Preparation of Ointments

Ointments are prepared by two general methods, (*a*) incorporation and (*b*) fusion, depending primarily on the nature of the ingredients.

Incorporation

The components are mixed until a uniform preparation is attained (Fig. 10.1). On a small scale, as in extemporaneous compounding, the pharmacist may mix the components using a mortar and pestle, or a spatula may be used to rub the ingredients together on an ointment slab (a large glass or porcelain plate or pill tile). Some pharmacists use nonabsorbent parchment paper to cover the working surface; being disposable, the paper eliminates cleaning the ointment slab. If using an ointment parchment pad, it is

FIGURE 10.1. Mixing tanks for ointments, creams, and gels. (Courtesy of Dmitry Kalinovsky/Shutterstock.)

best to not allow too long a contact of the ointment with the parchment, as it may soften and tear.

Others will use an ointment mill, an electronic mortar and pestle, or a device called an "Unguator," which allows a pharmacist to place the ingredients in a plastic ointment jar with a special lid that allows for a mixing blade to be used to mix the ingredients in the dispensing container. These devices can be controlled manually or via computer software. See Figures 10.2 to 10.4.

Incorporation of Solids. When preparing an ointment by spatulation, the pharmacist works the ointment with a stainless steel spatula having a long, broad blade and periodically removes the accumulation of ointment on the large spatula with a smaller one. If the components of an ointment react with metal (as does iodine), hard rubber or silicone spatulas may be used. The ointment is prepared by thoroughly rubbing and working the components together on the hard surface until the product is smooth and uniform. The ointment base is placed on one side of the working surface and the powdered components, previously reduced to fine powders and thoroughly blended in a mortar, on the other side. A small portion of the powder is mixed with a portion of the base until uniform.

FIGURE 10.3. Example mixing spindles for use with the Unguator electronic mortar and pestle. (Courtesy of Health Engineering Systems.)

Geometric dilution is continued until all portions of the powder and base are combined and thoroughly and uniformly blended.

It often is desirable to reduce the particle size of a powder or crystalline material before incorporation into the ointment base so the final product will not be gritty. This may be done by *levigating* or mixing the solid material in a vehicle in which it is insoluble to make a smooth dispersion. The levigating agent (e.g., mineral oil for bases in which oils are the external phase or glycerin for bases in which water is the external phase) should be physically and chemically compatible with the drug and base. The levigating agent should be about equal in volume to the solid material. A mortar and pestle are used for levigation. This allows both reduction of particle size and dispersion of the substance in the vehicle. After levigation, the dispersion is incorporated into the ointment base by spatulation or with the mortar and pestle until the product is uniform.

Solids soluble in a common solvent that will affect neither the stability of the drug nor the efficacy of the product may first be dissolved in that solvent (e.g., water or alcohol) and the solution added to the ointment base by spatulation or in a mortar and pestle. The mortar and pestle method is preferred when large volumes of liquid

FIGURE 10.2. Unguator Model B-R Electronic mortar and pestle. (Courtesy of Health Engineering Systems.)

FIGURE 10.4. Containers for use with the Unguator electronic mortar and pestle system. The mixing actually occurs within the container that is also used as the dispensing container. They have a "push-up" bottom, and the cap is removed to allow the material to be delivered. (Courtesy of Health Engineering Systems.)

are added, because the liquid is more captive than on an ointment slab.

For incorporating a gummy material that cannot be ground or levigated to an impalpable size, such as camphor, pulverization by intervention can be used. The material is dissolved in a solvent and spread out on the pill tile. The solvent is allowed to evaporate, leaving a thin film of the material onto which the other ingredient or ingredients are spread. The material is then worked into the ingredients by trituration with a spatula.

Incorporation of Liquids. Liquid substances or solutions of drugs, as described above, are added to an ointment only after due consideration of an ointment base's capacity to accept the volume required. For example, as noted previously, only very small amounts of an aqueous solution may be incorporated into an oleaginous ointment, whereas hydrophilic ointment bases readily accept aqueous solutions. When it is necessary to add an aqueous preparation to a hydro*phobic* base, the solution first may be incorporated into a minimum amount of a hydro*philic* base and then that mixture added to the hydrophobic base. However, all bases, even if hydrophilic, have their limits to retain liquids, beyond which they become too soft or semiliquid.

Alcoholic solutions of small volume may be added easily to oleaginous vehicles or emulsion bases. Natural balsams, such as Peru balsam, are usually mixed with an equal portion of castor oil before incorporation into a base. This reduces the surface tension of the balsam and allows even distribution of the balsam throughout the base.

Ointment or roller mills can be used to force coarsely formed ointments through stainless steel or ceramic rollers to produce ointments uniform in composition, smooth in texture, and free of entrapped air bubbles (Fig. 10.5). Small ointment mills also find use in product development laboratories and in small-batch manufacture or compounding.

FIGURE 10.5. Ointment roller mill. (Courtesy of EXAKT Technologies, Inc.)

Fusion

By the fusion method, all or some of the components of an ointment are combined by being melted together and cooled with constant stirring until congealed. Components not melted are added to the congealing mixture as it is being cooled and stirred. Naturally, heat-labile substances and any volatile components are added last, when the temperature of the mixture is low enough not to cause decomposition or volatilization of the components. Substances may be added to the congealing mixture as solutions or as insoluble powders levigated with a portion of the base. On a small scale, fusion may be conducted in a porcelain dish or glass beaker. On a large scale, it is carried out in large steam-jacketed kettles. Once congealed, the ointment may be passed through an ointment mill (in large-scale manufacture) or rubbed with a spatula or in a mortar to ensure a uniform texture.

Medicated ointments and ointment bases containing components such as beeswax, paraffin, stearyl alcohol, and high molecular weight PEGs, which do not lend themselves well to mixture by incorporation, are prepared by fusion. By this general process, the materials with the highest melting points are heated to the lowest required temperature to produce a melt. The additional materials are added with constant stirring during cooling of the melt until the mixture is congealed. In this way, not all of the components are subjected to the highest temperature. Alternative methods entail melting the component with the lowest melting point first and adding the remaining components in order of their melting points or simply melting all of the components together under slowly increasing temperature. By these methods, a lower temperature is usually sufficient to achieve fusion because of the solvent action exerted by the first melted components on the others.

In preparation of ointments having an emulsion base, the method of manufacture often involves both melting and emulsification. The water-immiscible components such as the oil and waxes are melted together in a steam bath to about 70°C to 75°C. Meantime, an aqueous solution of the heat-stable, water-soluble components is prepared and heated to the same temperature as the oleaginous components. Then, the aqueous solution is slowly added, with mechanical stirring, to the melted oleaginous mixture. The temperature is maintained for 5 to 10 minutes, and the mixture is slowly cooled and stirred until congealed. If the aqueous solution is not at the same temperature as the oleaginous melt, some of the waxes will solidify on addition of the colder aqueous solution to the melted mixture.

▌ COMPENDIAL REQUIREMENTS FOR OINTMENTS

Ointments and other semisolid dosage forms must meet USP tests for *microbial content, minimum fill, packaging, storage, and labeling* (2). As discussed later in this chapter, ophthalmic ointments must also meet tests for *sterility* and *metal particles* content.

Microbial Content

With the exception of ophthalmic preparations, topical applications are not required to be sterile. They must, however, meet acceptable standards for microbial content, and preparations prone to microbial growth must contain antimicrobial preservatives. Preparations that contain water tend to support microbial growth to a greater extent than water-free preparations. Among the antimicrobial preservatives used to inhibit microbial growth in topical preparations are methylparaben, propylparaben, phenols, benzoic acid, sorbic acid, and quaternary ammonium salts.

Microbial limits are stated for certain articles in the USP. For example, Betamethasone Valerate Ointment, USP, must *meet the requirements of the tests for absence of Staphylococcus aureus and Pseudomonas aeruginosa*. These particular microbes have special importance in dermatologic preparations because of their capacity to infect the skin, which, for patients being treated for a skin condition, is already compromised.

In the USP chapter <1111> Microbiological Examination of Nonsterile Pharmaceutical Products: Acceptance Criteria for Pharmaceutical Preparations and Substances for Pharmaceutical Use, microbial limits on substances and various dosage forms are given; in USP chapter <1115> Bioburden Control of Nonsterile Drug Substances and Products, emphasis is placed on strict adherence to environmental control and application of good manufacturing practices to minimize both the type and the number of microorganisms in unsterilized pharmaceutical products (2). The latter chapter involves the testing of raw materials, use of acceptable water, in-process controls, and final product testing. The USP states that certain products should be routinely tested for microorganisms because of the way they are used. Thus, dermatologic products should be examined for *P. aeruginosa* and *S. aureus*, and those intended for rectal, urethral, or vaginal use should be tested for yeasts and molds, common offenders at these sites of application.

Minimum Fill

The USP's *minimum fill* test is determination of the net weight or volume of the contents of filled containers to ensure proper contents compared with the labeled amount.

Packaging, Storage, and Labeling

Ointments and other semisolid preparations are packaged either in large-mouth ointment jars or in metal or plastic tubes. Semisolid preparations must be stored in well-closed containers to protect against contamination and in a cool place to protect against product separation in heat. When required, light-sensitive preparations are packaged in opaque or light-resistant containers.

In addition to the usual labeling requirements for pharmaceutical products, the USP directs the labeling for certain ointments and creams including proper storage conditions, dosing, and administration.

Additional Standards

In addition to the USP requirements, manufacturers often examine semisolid preparations for viscosity and for in vitro drug release to ensure within-lot and lot-to-lot uniformity (3,4). In vitro drug release tests include diffusion cell studies to determine the drug's release profile from the semisolid product.

■ CREAMS

Pharmaceutical *creams* are semisolid preparations containing one or more medicinal agents dissolved or dispersed in either a water-in-oil (W/O) emulsion or an oil-in-water (O/W) emulsion or in another type of water-washable base. The so-called vanishing creams are oil-in-water emulsions containing large percentages of water and stearic acid or other oleaginous components. After application of the cream, the water evaporates, leaving behind a thin residual film of the stearic acid or other oleaginous component. Chapter 14 discusses the types of emulsions, their physical characteristics, and the method of manufacture.

Creams find primary application in topical skin products and in products used on mucous membranes, such as rectally and vaginally. Many patients and physicians prefer creams to ointments because they are easier to spread and remove. Pharmaceutical manufacturers frequently manufacture topical preparations of a drug in both cream and ointment bases to satisfy the preference of the patient and physician.

Creams have a relatively soft, spreadable consistency; an example of a W/O cream is cold cream, and an example of an O/W cream is hydrophilic ointment. Creams are generally described as either nonwashable or washable, reflecting that an emulsion with an aqueous external continuous phase (O/W) is more easily removed than one with a nonaqueous external phase (W/O emulsion). When the term "cream" is used without further qualification, a water-washable formulation is generally inferred.

Preparation of Creams

Creams may be formulated from a variety of oils, both mineral and vegetable, and from fatty alcohols, fatty acids, and fatty esters. The solid excipients are melted at the time of preparation. Emulsifying agents include nonionic surfactants, detergents, and soaps. Soaps are usually formed from a fatty acid in the oil phase hydrolyzed by a base dissolved in the aqueous phase in situ during the preparation of creams.

Preparation usually involves separating the formula components into two portions: lipid and aqueous.

The lipid portion contains all water-insoluble components and the aqueous portion the water-soluble components. Both phases are heated to a temperature above the melting point of the highest melting component. The phases then are mixed, and the mixture is stirred until reaching ambient temperature or the mixture has congealed. Mixing generally is continued during the cooling process to promote uniformity. Traditionally, the aqueous phase is added to the lipid phase, but comparable results have been obtained with the reverse procedure. High-shear homogenization may be employed to reduce particle or droplet size and improve the physical stability of the resultant dosage form.

The APIs can be added to the phase in which it is soluble at the beginning of the process, or it can be added after the cream is prepared by a suitable dispersion process such as levigation or milling with a roller mill. Creams usually require the addition of a preservative(s) unless they are compounded immediately prior to use and intended to be consumed in a relatively short period of time.

GELS

Gels (sometimes called jellies) are semisolid systems consisting of dispersions of small or large molecules in an aqueous liquid vehicle rendered jellylike by the addition of a *gelling agent*. Among the gelling agents used are synthetic macromolecules, such as carbomer 934; cellulose derivatives, such as carboxymethylcellulose or hydroxypropyl methylcellulose; and natural gums, such as tragacanth. Carbomers are high molecular weight water-soluble polymers of acrylic acid cross-linked with allyl ethers of sucrose and/or pentaerythritol. Their viscosity depends on their polymeric composition. The NF contains monographs for six such polymers, carbomers 910, 934, 934P, 940, 941, and 1342. They are used as gelling agents at concentrations of 0.5% to 2.0% in water. Carbomer 940 yields the highest viscosity, between 40,000 and 60,000 centipoises as a 0.5% aqueous dispersion.

Single-phase gels are gels in which the macromolecules are uniformly distributed throughout a liquid with no apparent boundaries between the dispersed macromolecules and the liquid. A gel mass consisting of floccules of small distinct particles is termed a *two-phase* system, often referred to as a *magma*. Milk of magnesia (or magnesia magma), which consists of a gelatinous precipitate of magnesium hydroxide, is such a system. Gels may thicken on standing, forming a thixotrope, and must be shaken before use to liquefy the gel and enable pouring.

In addition to the gelling agent and water, gels may be formulated to contain a drug substance, solvents, such as alcohol and/or propylene glycol; antimicrobial preservatives, such as methylparaben and propylparaben or chlorhexidine gluconate; and stabilizers, such as edetate

disodium. Medicated gels may be prepared for administration by various routes, including the skin, the eye, the nose, the vagina, and the rectum.

AndroGel 1.62% for topical use is a clear, colorless gel containing testosterone; it also contains Carbopol 980, ethyl alcohol, isopropyl myristate, purified water, and sodium hydroxide. It is an androgen indicated for replacement therapy in adult males for conditions associated with a deficiency or absence of endogenous testosterone. It delivers about 20 mg of testosterone per pump actuation applied topically once daily in the morning to the shoulders and upper arms (5).

Gels can be administered by the topical oromucosal routes. Antibiotic-containing gels can be administered by teat infusion in veterinary medicine to treat mastitis.

Preparation of Gels

Gels formed with large organic molecules may be formed by dispersing the molecule in the continuous phase (e.g., by heating starch), by cross-linking the dispersed molecules by changing the pH (as for carbomers), or by reducing the continuous phase (as for jellies formed with sucrose).

Care should be taken to ensure uniformity of the APIs by dispersing them by vigorous mixing or milling or by shaking if the preparation is less viscous.

Packaging and Storage

Gels should be stored in tight containers to prevent water loss. Avoid freezing gels.

TRANSDERMAL PREPARATIONS

Recent years have seen an increase in the number of topical ointments, creams, and gels designed to deliver a drug systemically. This is often accomplished by addition of penetration enhancers to the topical vehicle. Penetration enhancers include dimethyl sulfoxide (DMSO), ethanol, propylene glycol, glycerin, PEG, urea, dimethylacetamide (DMA), sodium lauryl sulfate, poloxamers, Spans, Tweens, lecithin, terpenes, and many others. However, sometimes, the difference between topical and transdermal delivery becomes "blurred" (see Physical Pharmacy Capsule 10.1, Clinical Pharmaceutics—The Blurred Line Between "Topical" and "Transdermal" Delivery).

A transdermal preparation commonly compounded is Pluronic lecithin organogel. It consists of a Pluronic (poloxamer) F127 gel (usually 20% or 30% concentration) mixed at a ratio of approximately 1:5 with a mixture of equal parts of isopropyl palmitate and lecithin. This gel vehicle aids in rapid penetration of many active drugs through the skin. There are also several commercial bases intended to provide transdermal delivery for compounded preparations.

PHYSICAL PHARMACY CAPSULE **10.1** Clinical Pharmaceutics— The Blurred Line Between "Topical" and "Transdermal"

The skin is a highly complex organ that regulates heat and water loss from the body while preventing the ingress of noxious chemicals or microorganisms. It is about 10% of the body mass and covers about 1.7 m² in the average person. It is large and accessible and provides a reasonable site to administer therapeutic agents for both local and systemic effects; it is also highly efficient at "self-repairing" and is designed to "keep the insides in and the outsides out!"

The USP <1151> Glossary defines "topical" as "a route of administration characterized by application to the outer surface of the body." It does not define "transdermal" but does define a "transdermal system." The chapter states that "Ointments are semisolid preparations intended for external application to the skin or mucous membranes. APIs delivered in ointments are intended for local action or for systemic absorption."

Pharmaceutics textbooks and specialized reference books state:

"Topical preparations are used for both local and systemic effects. Systemic drug absorption should always be considered if the patient is pregnant or nursing...."

"Topical applications can be designed for either local effects or systemic absorption."

Also, we read the following:

"The following distinction is an important one with regard to dermatologic applications. A *topical* dermatological product is designed to deliver drug into the skin in treating dermal disorders, with the *skin as the target organ*. A *transdermal* product is designed to deliver drugs through the skin (percutaneous absorption) to the general circulation for system effects, with the *skin not being the target organ*." As is evident, there are differences in these two terms with clinical implications. This generally involves the way the terms are used, especially the term "topical."

"Topical" can be used in much the same manner as "oral," "parenteral," "inhalation," etc., where the general route of administration is intended, as described in USP <1151> Pharmaceutical Dosage Forms. This would be the Tier One: Route of Administration level in Figure 1: Compendial Taxonomy for Pharmaceutical Dosage Forms.

"Topical" and "transdermal" can be considered as subcategories of "Topical Route of Administration" at the level of "Tier Two: Dosage Form and Physical Properties" and refer to the "extent, if any, of absorption" of the active drug. To complete the taxonomy, the remaining levels are "Tier Three: Type of Release Pattern" and "Tier Four: Comprehensive Testing Strategy." Our emphasis here will be on the intended site of action of the contained drug. Nondrug (no API) containing "topicals" would generally be for emollient, hydrating effects and would usually be "topical."

A "topical" drug (API) dosage form would be one that is designed to deliver the drug into the skin in treating skin disorders where the skin is the target organ.

A "transdermal" drug (API) dosage form would be one that is designed to deliver drugs through the skin (percutaneous absorption) to the general circulation for systemic effects. In this case, the skin is NOT the target organ but merely the route the drug must pass to reach the circulatory system.

Now, we will compare the differences in composition of "topicals" and "transdermals."

The following "general" table of compositions may help in differentiation of formulations with penetrating ability:

Ingredient Category	Topical	Transdermal
Vehicle	Yes	Yes
Solvents	Yes	Yes
Preservative	Yes	Yes
Stiffening agent	Yes	Yes
Gelling agent	Yes	Yes
pH adjustment	Yes	Yes
Humectant	Yes	Yes
Penetration enhancer	No	Yes
Liposomes	No	Yes

(continued)

PHYSICAL PHARMACY CAPSULE **10.1** Clinical Pharmaceutics—
The Blurred Line Between "Topical" and "Transdermal" *(continued)*

There may be some extent of transdermal penetration in almost any dosage form applied topically, even an aqueous solution. However, as is evident, the presence of a penetration enhancer and liposome formation can result in greater penetration when properly formulated. Example penetration enhancers include the following:

Water
Dimethyl sulfoxide (DMSO)
Dimethylacetamide (DMA)
Dimethylformamide (DMF)
Azone (Laurocapram)
Pyrrolidones
Fatty acids (lauric acid, oleic acid, linoleic, linolenic)
Ethanol, propylene glycol
Surfactants (anionic and nonionic)
Urea
Terpenes (essential oils)
Phospholipids
Others ■

MISCELLANEOUS SEMISOLID PREPARATIONS: PASTES, PLASTERS, AND GLYCEROGELATINS

Pastes

Pastes are semisolid preparations intended for application to the skin. They generally contain a larger proportion of solid material (such as 25%) than ointments and therefore are stiffer.

Pastes can be prepared in the same manner as ointments, by direct mixing or the use of heat to soften the base prior to incorporating the solids, which have been comminuted and sieved. However, when a levigating agent is to be used to render the powdered component smooth, a portion of the base is often used rather than a liquid, which would soften the paste.

Because of the stiffness of pastes, they remain in place after application and are effectively employed to absorb serous secretions. Because of their stiffness and impenetrability, pastes are not suited for application to hairy parts of the body.

Among the few pastes in use today is zinc oxide paste (Lassar's Plain Zinc Paste), which is prepared by mixing 25% each of zinc oxide and starch with white petrolatum. The product is very firm and is better able to protect the skin and absorb secretions than is zinc oxide ointment.

Plasters

Plasters are solid or semisolid adhesive masses spread on a backing of paper, fabric, moleskin, or plastic. The adhesive material is a rubber base or a synthetic resin. Plasters are applied to the skin to provide prolonged contact at the site. Unmedicated plasters provide protection or mechanical support at the site of application. Adhesive tape used to

be official under the title adhesive plaster, the use of this material being well known.

Medicated plasters provide effects at the site of application. They may be cut to size to conform to the surface to be covered. Among the few plasters in use today is salicylic acid plaster used on the toes for the removal of corns. The horny layers of skin are removed by the keratolytic action of salicylic acid. The concentration of salicylic acid used in commercial corn plasters ranges from 10% to 40%.

Glycerogelatins

Glycerogelatins are plastic masses containing gelatin (15%), glycerin (40%), water (35%), and an added medicinal substance (10%), such as zinc oxide. They are prepared by first softening the gelatin in the water for about 10 minutes, heating on a steam bath until the gelatin is dissolved, adding the medicinal substance mixed with the glycerin, and allowing the mixture to cool with stirring until congealed.

Glycerogelatins are applied to the skin for the long term. They are melted before application, cooled to slightly above body temperature, and applied to the affected area with a fine brush. Following application, the glycerogelatin hardens, is usually covered with a bandage, and is allowed to remain in place for weeks. The most recent official glycerogelatin was zinc gelatin, used in the treatment of varicose ulcers. It was also known as zinc gelatin boot because of its ability to form a pressure bandage.

Packaging Semisolid Preparations

Topical dermatologic products are packaged in jars, tubes, or syringes, whereas ophthalmic, nasal, vaginal, and rectal semisolid products are almost always packaged in tubes or syringes.

Ointment jars are made of clear or opaque glass or plastic. Some are colored green, amber, or blue. Opaque jars, used for light-sensitive products, are porcelain white, dark green, or amber. Commercially available empty ointment jars vary in size from about 0.5 oz to 1 lb.

In commercial manufacture and packaging of topical products, the jars and tubes are first tested for compatibility and stability for the intended product. This includes stability testing of filled containers at room temperatures (e.g., 20°C) as well as under accelerated stability testing conditions (e.g., 40°C and 50°C).

Tubes used to package topical pharmaceutical products are gaining in popularity. They are light in weight, relatively inexpensive, convenient for use, and compatible with most formulative components, and they provide greater protection against external contamination and environmental conditions than jars (6).

Ointment tubes are made of aluminum or plastic. When the ointment is to be used for ophthalmic, rectal, vaginal, aural, or nasal application, they are packaged with special applicator tips. Tubes of aluminum generally are coated with an epoxy resin, vinyl, or lacquer to eliminate any interactions between the contents and the tube. Plastic tubes are made of high- or low-density polyethylene (HDPE or LDPE) or a blend of each, polypropylene (PP), polyethylene terephthalate (PET), and various plastic, foil, and/or paper laminates, sometimes 10 layers thick.

Each type of plastic offers special features and advantages. For example, LDPE is soft and resilient, and it provides a good moisture barrier. HDPE provides a superior moisture barrier but is less resilient. PP has a high level of heat resistance, and PET offers transparency and a high degree of product chemical compatibility. Laminates provide an excellent moisture barrier because of the foil content, high durability, and product compatibility (5). These qualities and flexibility make plastic and plastic laminate tubes preferable to metal tubes for packaging of pharmaceuticals.

The cylindrical bodies of plastic tubes are made by extrusion and then joined to the shoulder, neck, and tip piece, which is made by molding. Most multiple-dose tubes used for pharmaceuticals have conventional, continuous thread closures. Single-dose tubes may be prepared with a tearaway tip. Metered-dose, tamper-evident, and child-resistant closures are available (6). Standard sizes of empty tubes have capacities of 1.5, 2, 3.5, 5, 15, 30, 45, 60, and 120 g (7). Ointments, creams, and gels are most frequently packaged in 5-, 15-, and 30-g tubes.

Ophthalmic ointments typically are packaged in small aluminum or collapsible plastic tubes holding 3.5 g (about 0.125 oz) of ointment, as shown in Figure 17.4. The tubes, which are sterilized before being aseptically filled, are fitted with narrow gauge tips, which permit extrusion and placement of narrow bands of ointment on the inner margin of the eyelid, the usual site of application.

Compounded ointments are commonly dispensed in either syringes for injection or syringes for oral use. The advantages include the exclusion of air from the system and the ability to accurately measure each dose, especially for transdermal applications.

Filling Ointment Jars

Ointment jars are filled on a small scale in the pharmacy by carefully transferring the weighed amount of ointment into the jar with a spatula. The ointment is packed on the bottom and along the sides of the jar, avoiding entrapment of air. The jar size should allow the ointment to reach near the top of the jar but not so high as to touch the lid when closed. Ointments prepared by fusion may be poured directly into the ointment jar to congeal in it. This must be done cautiously to prevent stratification of the components. In large-scale manufacture of ointments, pressure fillers force the specified amount of ointment into the jars.

Filling Ointment Tubes

Tubes are filled from the open back end of the tube, opposite from the cap end (Fig. 10.6). Ointments prepared by fusion may be poured while still soft but viscous directly into the tubes with caution to prevent stratification of the components. On a small scale, as in the extemporaneous filling of an ointment in the pharmacy, the tube may be filled manually (Fig. 10.7) or with a small-scale filling machine (Fig. 10.8). The filled tube is closed and sealed. As depicted in Figure 10.7, manual filling of an ointment tube requires a number of steps: (*a*) The prepared ointment, placed on waxed or parchment paper and rolled into a cylindrical shape, is inserted into the open end of the tube and pushed forward as far as allowed. (*b*) With a spatula pressing against the lower portion of the tube and making a crease below the ointment fill, the paper is slowly removed, leaving the ointment in the tube. (*c*) The bottom of the tube is flattened, folded, and sealed with a crimping tool or clip.

Tubes can also be filled using a "caulking-gun" system where the semisolid is filled into the chamber and the product is delivered into the tube. The tubes can then be

FIGURE 10.6. Tube-filling machine for ointments, creams, and gels. (Courtesy of CapsulCN International Co., Ltd.)

FIGURE 10.7. Steps in the manual filling of ointment, cream, and gel tubes.

heat sealed using a heat-sealing crimper for a nice, professional appearance.

Industrially, automatic filling, closing, crimping, and labeling machines are used for large-scale tube packaging of semisolid pharmaceuticals (Fig. 10.6). Depending on the model, machines have the capacity to fill about 1,000 to 6,000 tubes per hour (6–8). Rotary machines have four stations for tube feeding, cleaning, filling, and closing. Plastic and laminate tubes are closed and sealed by heat and crimping. Metal tubes are sealed by folding and crimping with or without a vinyl, latex, or lacquer sealant (6).

Electronic mortars and pestles can be used to prepare an ointment, cream, or gel in the dispensing container. The ingredients are placed in the container and the cap, which has a stirring rod and blade assembly put in place. The unit can be programmed for thorough mixing using different speeds and up and down rates until the product is uniform. The rod is removed and the cap replaced with a dispensing cap. For administration, the bottom of the ointment jar is moved up, forcing the product out of the orifice in the dispensing cap. The small orifice cap is replaced for a tight seal. This system provides greater efficiency as compared to manual ointment preparation by reducing the

FIGURE 10.8. A small-scale filling machine for ointment, cream, and gel tubes. (Courtesy of Itsanan/Shutterstock.)

number of manipulations, reducing the time required for compounding and clean-up between products, and eliminating the loss of product during preparation.

Filling Syringes

Syringes can be filled either by drawing the semisolid into the barrel using the plunger (it may be necessary to soften the preparation by gentle heating first) or by removing the plunger and filling through the back end of the syringe. The plunger can then be reinserted. (This can be accomplished by placing a straightened paper clip down the inside of the barrel and inserting the plunger. The paper clip allows the escape of air until the plunger contacts the ointment. The paper clip can then be removed, and the seal formed by the plunger is reestablished.)

FEATURES AND USES OF DERMATOLOGIC PREPARATIONS

Among the dosage forms used in the topical treatment of conditions and diseases of the skin are ointments, creams, gels, pastes, and plasters. Other dosage forms include solutions, powders, and transdermal drug delivery systems, discussed elsewhere in this text. Oral therapy also may be used for skin conditions, as in the treatment of poison ivy with prednisone.

In treating skin diseases, the drug in a medicated application should *penetrate* and be *retained* in the skin for a while. Drug penetration into the skin depends on a number of factors, including the physicochemical properties of the medicinal substance, the characteristics of the pharmaceutical vehicle, and the condition of skin itself. Normal unbroken skin acts as a natural barrier, limiting both the rate and degree of drug penetration.

The skin is divided histologically into the stratum corneum (the outer layer), the living epidermis, and the dermis, collectively a laminate of barriers protecting against permeation by external agents and loss of water from the body. Blood capillaries and nerve fibers rise from the subcutaneous fat into the dermis and up to the epidermis. Sebaceous glands, sweat glands, and hair follicles originating in the dermis and subcutaneous layers rise to the skin's surface (Fig. 10.9). The stratum corneum is the desquamating horny layer, a 10- to 15-mm-thick layer of flat, partially desiccated, dead epidermal cells (9,10). The stratum corneum is composed of approximately 40% protein (mainly keratin) and 40% water, with the balance being lipid, principally as triglycerides, free fatty acids, cholesterol, and phospholipids. On the surface is the acid mantle, a thin emulsified film composed of a complex mixture of sebum, sweat, and desquamating epidermal cells.

The acid mantle varies in composition, thickness, and continuity as a result of differences in the proportion of sebum and sweat produced and the extent of their removal through washing and sweat evaporation. It offers little resistance to drug penetration. Hair follicles and gland

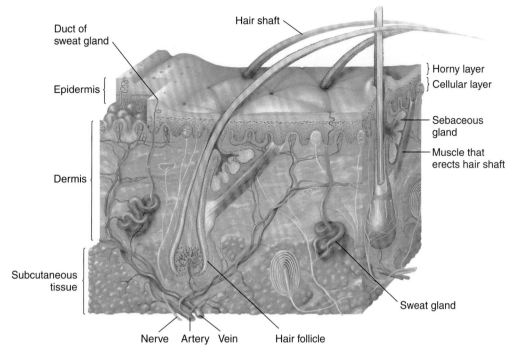

FIGURE 10.9. Stratified organization of the skin. (Reprinted from Anatomical Chart Company, with permission.)

ducts can provide entry for drug molecules, but because their relative surface area is so minute compared to the total epidermis, they are minor factors in drug absorption.

The stratum corneum, being keratinized tissue, behaves as a semipermeable membrane, and drug molecules can penetrate by passive diffusion. The rate of drug movement across this skin layer depends on the drug concentration in the vehicle, its aqueous solubility, and the oil–water partition coefficient between the stratum corneum and the product's vehicle (11). Substances with both aqueous and lipid solubility characteristics are good candidates for diffusion through the stratum corneum. Once through the stratum corneum, drug molecules may pass through the deeper epidermal tissues and into the dermis. If the drug reaches the vascularized dermal layer, it becomes available for absorption into the general circulation.

Whereas drug blood levels achieved by transdermal delivery systems may be measured and equated against desired therapeutic effects, the same is not true for topical *non*systemic dermatologic products. For topical products, the therapeutically effective drug concentration in the skin is not known, so treatment is based on qualitative measures, with clinical efficacy often varying between patients and products.

Differences in emollient and occlusive effects and ease of application and removal between products are factors of the base used and product type. As noted earlier, oleaginous bases provide greater occlusion and emollient effects than do hydrophilic or water-washable bases. Pastes offer even greater occlusion and are more effective than ointments at absorbing serous discharge. Creams, usually oil-in-water emulsions, spread more easily than

ointments and are easier to remove. Water-soluble bases are nongreasy and are easily removed.

Unless otherwise directed, before applying a dermatologic product, the patient should thoroughly clean the affected area with soap and water and dry by patting with a soft cloth. In most instances, a thin layer of medication should be applied to the affected area and spread evenly using gentle pressure with the fingertips. Typically, about 1 to 3 mg of ointment or cream is applied per square centimeter of skin (1). Unless there is a specified need for an occlusive dressing to protect the area from excessive contact or contaminants, a bandage should not be used. After application, the hands should be thoroughly washed. Additional clinical information is provided in Physical Pharmacy Capsule 10.2, Clinical Pharmaceutics—Quantity to Apply, Skin Types, and Thermodynamic Properties.

Upon dispensing a prescription or over-the-counter (OTC) product, the pharmacist should be certain that the patient understands the proper method of administration, frequency and duration of use, special warnings (such as those related to pregnancy or nursing), therapeutic goals and anticipated outcomes, signs of adverse response, allergic sensitivity reactions or treatment failure, and reasons to discontinue treatment and seek further professional guidance.

The patient should be advised if symptoms persist or irritation develops, use of the product should be discontinued, and a physician or pharmacist should be consulted. It is fairly common for patients to have an allergic response, such as a skin rash, to a topical product as a result of sensitivity to the medicinal agent or pharmaceutical ingredient. An alternative product that does not contain the suspected offending agent may be substituted to solve the problem.

PHYSICAL PHARMACY CAPSULE **10.2** Clinical Pharmaceutics—Quantity to Apply, Skin Types, and Thermodynamic Properties

■ HOW MUCH SHOULD BE APPLIED?

Generally, 0.5 g of a preparation will treat two palms of an adult. General guidelines are given in the following table but must be used with caution because of patient variables and the area to be covered:

Site	Approx. Quantity (g)[a]
Face	1
Neck	1
Trunk (one side)	3
Arm	1.5
Hand (including fingers)	0.5
Palm	0.25
Leg	3
Foot	1
Entire body	20–30

[a]From Williams AC. Transdermal and Topical Drug Delivery. London: Pharmaceutical Press, 2003:195–196.

The above numbers apply to a "typical" patient with a total BSA of about 1.8 m². Also, if the preparation is fluid, it tends to cover more area easier. This table is a reasonable guide for creams, gels, ointments, and pastes.

The following provides information on the use of formulations for different skin types and situations.

Skin Types	Preparations
Normal to oily	Ointments, pastes, and gels
Normal to dry	Lotions
Dry	Creams
Hairy	Lotions, gels, and sprays
Intertriginous areas	Creams and lotions

Situations	Preparations
Wet, vesicular, weeping lesions	Creams, lotions, and gels
Dry, thickened scaly lesions	Ointments and pastes

The statement is often heard that "Formulation is more important than concentration." Well, what is the optimum drug concentration for efficient drug delivery through the skin? It is when the vehicle is saturated with the drug. There are very few cases in which the drug is so poorly soluble in the vehicle that rapid depletion of the drug in the formulation occurs. When the drug is in excess (suspended in the vehicle), as the dissolved drug moves from the vehicle into the skin, then it is replaced in solution by some of the suspended drug to maintain a saturated state.

Thermodynamic activity of the dissolved drug molecules is what drives the drug across the skin, not the total drug concentration, so adding higher and higher concentrations of drug is wasteful and does not add to the drug effect. In other words, "More is not always better." There are examples where commercial products have decreased drug concentration and maintained clinical equivalence.

Proper use of (a) penetration enhancers within the formulation, (b) drug concentration, (c) overall vehicle acceptability and effectiveness, (d) area covered, and (e) maintenance of skin health and hydration and other factors can lead to effective clinical results. Keep in mind that "More is not always better" and can lead to untoward effects in some patients. "Smart formulation development" may be less expensive for the patient and provide better patient care.

"What drugs are delivered to and through the skin?"

For topical administration, a large variety of agents are used, both in broken skin and where the skin barrier is intact. Classes of agents include anesthetics, antiacne agents, antibacterials, antifungals, antiparasitics, antiseptics/cleaners, antivirals, coal tar, corticosteroids, cytotoxic agents, dithranol, phototherapy drugs, retinoids, and vitamin D analogs.

(continued)

(continued)

For transdermal administration, generally, the best candidates are low molecular weight (300 to 500) potent lipophilic molecules with a relatively wide therapeutic window. The candidates also need to have suitable aqueous solubility (>100 µg/mL) and a log partition coefficient (octanol/water) in the range of 1 to 3.5. Generally, a reasonably good candidate will have a flux, or transport from the skin into the blood, in the vicinity of 1 mg/cm²/d. As an example, if 10 cm² is covered, then about 10 mg of drug could be delivered per day. Using this value of 1 mg/cm²/d, one can get an approximation of the maximum achievable dose for the drug. It is also best to keep in mind that the first-pass effect is avoided and the transdermal dose may be lower than the corresponding oral dose for some drugs. ∎

Examples of dermatologic ointments, creams, and gels are presented in Table 10.1 (ointments and creams by therapeutic categories) and Table 10.2 (gels by active ingredient).

▌FEATURES AND USES OF OPHTHALMIC OINTMENTS AND GELS

Among the dosage forms used in the topical treatment of conditions and diseases of the eye are ointments and gels.

Other ophthalmic dosage forms used topically include solutions, suspensions, and inserts, discussed elsewhere in this text. Systemic therapy also may be undertaken, as in the use of diuretics in the adjunctive treatment of glaucoma.

The application of medication to the eye or conjunctival sac affects the surface of the eye and underlying tissues as the drug penetrates. The major route by which drugs enter the eye is simple diffusion via the cornea. For drugs that are poorly absorbed by the cornea, the conjunctiva and sclera provide an alternate route (12). The cornea is a three-layered structure with a lipophilic epithelial layer,

TABLE 10.1. Dermatologic Ointments and Creams by Therapeutic Category

Preparation	Corresponding Commercial Product	Usual Strength of Active Ingredient	Use
Adrenocortical Steroids			
Alclometasone dipropionate cream and ointment	Aclovate Cream and Ointment (PharmaDerm)	0.05% cream and ointment	Relief of inflammatory dermatoses
Fluocinolone acetonide cream and ointment	Fluonid (Allergan)	0.025% cream and ointment	Relief of inflammatory dermatoses
Hydrocortisone acetate cream and ointment	Cortaid Cream and Ointment (J&J Consumer)	0.5% and 1%	Relief of inflammatory dermatoses
Triamcinolone acetonide cream and ointment	Aristocort A Cream and Ointment (Fujisawa Healthcare)	0.1% ointment; 0.1%, 0.025%, and 0.5% cream	Relief of inflammatory dermatoses
Adrenocorticoid–Antifungal Combination			
Betamethasone and clotrimazole cream	Lotrisone Cream (Schering)	0.05% betamethasone and 1% clotrimazole	Relief and treatment of inflammatory pruritic manifestations that may be complicated by fungal overgrowth
Analgesic			
Capsaicin cream	Zostrix Cream (Health Care Products)	0.025%	Relief of arthritic pain
Antiacne			
Tretinoin cream	Retin-A (Ortho)	0.025%, 0.05%, and 0.1%	Derivative of vitamin A for topical treatment of acne vulgaris
Antianginal			
Nitroglycerin ointment	Nitro-Bid Ointment (Savage)	2%	Reduces workload of heart by smooth muscle relaxation of peripheral arteries and veins
Antibacterial/Anti-infectives			
Gentamicin sulfate cream and ointment	Garamycin Cream and Ointment (Schering)	0.1%	Local treatment of skin infections by susceptible microorganisms

(continued)

TABLE 10.1. Dermatologic Ointments and Creams by Therapeutic Category *(continued)*

Preparation	Corresponding Commercial Product	Usual Strength of Active Ingredient	Use
Mupirocin calcium cream	Bactroban Cream (GlaxoSmithKline)	2%	Treatment of secondarily infected skin lesions because of susceptible strains of *S. aureus* and *Streptococcus pyogenes*
			Oil-in-water–based emulsion
Mupirocin calcium ointment	Bactroban Nasal Ointment (GlaxoSmithKline)	2%	Indicated for eradication of nasal colonization of methicillin-resistant *S. aureus*
			Petrolatum-based vehicle
Mupirocin ointment	Bactroban Ointment (GlaxoSmithKline)	2%	Vehicle of water-miscible polyethylene glycols
Nystatin cream	Mycostatin Cream (Bristol-Myers Squibb)	100,000 U/g	Local treatment of skin infections by susceptible microorganisms
Polymyxin B sulfate, bacitracin zinc, and neomycin ointment	Neosporin Ointment (Johnson & Johnson)	5,000 U/g polymyxin B; 400 U/g bacitracin zinc; 3.5 mg/g neomycin	Treatment of minor cuts and scrapes
Retapamulin ointment	Altabax Ointment (GlaxoSmithKline)	1%	Treatment of impetigo
Antifungals			
Butenafine HCl cream	Mentax Cream (Mylan)	1%	Treatment of dermatologic infection and tinea versicolor because of *Malassezia furfur*
Miconazole nitrate cream	Monistat-Derm Cream (Personal Products)	2%	Cutaneous candidiasis and tinea infections of *Trichophyton* spp.
Tolnaftate cream	Tinactin Cream (Schering-Plough)	1%	Topical treatment of tinea pedis, tinea cruris, tinea corporis, and tinea manuum
Antineoplastic			
Fluorouracil cream	Efudex Cream (Valeant Pharmaceuticals)	5%	Treatment of multiple actinic and solar keratoses
Antipruritic, Analgesic			
Lidocaine ointment	Xylocaine Ointment (APP Pharmaceutical)	2.5%	Relief of pain, itching of minor skin irritation, and insect bites
Astringent, Protectant			
Zinc oxide ointment	Desitin Ointment (Pfizer)	40%	Topical astringent, protective in skin conditions such as diaper rash
Depigmenting Agents			
Hydroquinone cream	Eldopaque Cream (ICN)	4%	Temporary bleaching of skin with freckles, old age spots, and chloasma
Scabicide			
Crotamiton cream	Eurax Cream (Bristol-Myers Squibb)	10%	Eradication of scabies and symptomatic treatment of pruritus

a hydrophilic stromal layer, and a less lipophilic endothelial layer on the inside (12). Drug penetration depends on a drug's ability to traverse these three layers. Lipophilic drugs are more capable of penetration than hydrophilic compounds (12).

In general, ocular ophthalmic drug penetration is limited by the short residence time on the surface of the eye because of rapid removal by tearing and other natural mechanisms, the small surface area of the cornea for drug absorption, and the cornea's natural resistance to drug penetration (12). Compared with ophthalmic solutions, ophthalmic ointments and gels provide extended residence time on the surface of the eye, increasing the duration of their surface effects and bioavailability for absorption into the ocular tissues. Ophthalmic ointments are cleared from the eye as slowly as 0.5% per minute, compared with solutions, which can lose up to 16% of their volume per minute (13,14).

The ointment base selected for an ophthalmic ointment must not be irritating to the eye and must permit the diffusion of the medicinal substance throughout the secretions bathing the eye. Ointment bases used for ophthalmics should have a softening point close to body temperature, both for comfort and for drug release. Most often,

TABLE 10.2. Examples of Topical Gels

Active Ingredient	Proprietary Product	Gelling Agent	Route and Use
Acetic acid	Aci-Jel (Ortho-McNeil)	Tragacanth and acacia	Vaginal: restoration and maintenance of acidity
Becaplermin	Regranex Gel (Johnson & Johnson)	Sodium CMC	Dermatologic: recombinant human platelet–derived growth factor; promotes healing of diabetic ulcers of lower extremity
Benzoyl peroxide	Desquam-X Gel (Westwood-Squibb)	Carbomer 940	Dermatologic: acne vulgaris
Bexarotene	Targretin 1% Gel (Eisai)	Hydroxypropyl cellulose	Dermatologic: cutaneous T-cell lymphoma
Clindamycin	Cleocin T Topical Gel (Pfizer)	Carbomer 934P	Dermatologic: acne vulgaris
Clobetasol propionate	Temovate Gel (PharmaDerm)	Carbomer 934P	Dermatologic: antipruritic
Cyanocobalamin	Nascobal (Strativa Pharmaceuticals)	Methylcellulose	Nasal: hematologic
Desoximetasone	Topicort Gel (Taro)	Carbomer 940	Dermatologic: anti-inflammatory and antipruritic
Metronidazole	MetroGel Vaginal (Galderma)	Carbomer 934P	Vaginal: bacterial vaginosis
Podofilox	Condylox Gel (Watson)	Hydroxypropyl cellulose	Rectal: anogenital warts
Progesterone	Crinone Gel (Watson)	Carbomer 934P	Vaginal: bioadhesive gel for progesterone supplementation and replacement
Timolol maleate	Timoptic-XE (Aton Pharma)	Gelrite gellan gum	Ophthalmic gel-forming solution used in treatment of elevated intraocular pressure
Tretinoin	Retin-A Gel (Ortho)	Hydroxypropyl cellulose	Dermatologic: acne vulgaris

mixtures of white petrolatum and liquid petrolatum (mineral oil) are used as the base in medicated and unmedicated (lubricating) ophthalmic ointments. Sometimes, a water-absorbing agent such as lanolin is added. A gel base of PEG and mineral oil is also used; this form permits water and water-insoluble drugs to be retained within the base.

Medicinal agents are added to an ointment base either as a solution or as a finely micronized powder. The ointment is made uniform and smooth by fine milling.

In addition to the previously stated quality standards for ointments, ophthalmic ointments must meet the USP *sterility tests* and the test for *metal particles in ophthalmic ointments*. Rendering an ophthalmic ointment sterile requires special technique and processing. For a number of reasons, the terminal sterilization of a finished ointment by standard methods may be problematic. Steam sterilization or ethylene oxide methods are ineffective because neither is capable of penetrating the ointment base. Although dry heat sterilization can penetrate the ointment base, the high heat required may pose a threat to the stability of the drug substance and introduces the possibility of separating the ointment base from the other components (15). Because of these difficulties, terminal sterilization generally is not undertaken. Rather, strict methods of aseptic processing are employed as each drug and nondrug component is rendered sterile and then aseptically weighed and incorporated in a final product that meets the sterility requirement (15). When an antimicrobial preservative is needed, among those used are methylparaben (0.05%) and propylparaben (0.01%) combinations, phenylmercuric

acetate (0.0008%), chlorobutanol (0.5%), and benzalkonium chloride (0.008%).

The USP test for metal particles is microscopic examination of a heat-melted ophthalmic ointment. Detected metal particles are counted and measured by a calibrated eyepiece micrometer disk. The requirements are met if the total number of particles 50 mm or larger from ten product tubes does not exceed 50 and if not more than one tube contains more than eight such particles (2).

The USP directs that ophthalmic ointments must be packaged in collapsible ointment tubes. These tubes have an elongated narrow tip to facilitate application of a narrow band of ointment to the eye. Use of a collapsible tube reduces the chance for contamination of the product, as air would be drawn back into the product if the tube rebounded to its original round shape after application. It also eliminates air and minimizes oxidative deterioration.

In preparation to apply an ointment to the eye, the patient's or caregiver's hands should be washed and dried thoroughly. Then, the ointment tube is held between the thumb and forefinger and the tip placed near the eyelid without touching it. The patient's head should be tilted back, and with the index finger of the opposite hand, the lower eyelid of the affected eye should be gently pulled downward. The tip of the ointment tube should be held slightly above the inside portion of the sack between the lower eyelid and eyeball. Without touching the tip to any part of the eye, a thin ribbon of ointment, approximately 0.25 to 0.5 inch, should be placed along the inside of the lower lid. The patient should face down and slowly close the eye for a few seconds. Then, any excess ointment should be wiped from the eyelids and lashes with a clean tissue. To facilitate the procedure, a patient may sit in front of a mirror with elbows stabilized or have another person administer the ointment. After use, the ointment must be capped quickly and tightly.

The patient should be advised that blurred vision will occur as the ointment spreads over the eye and not to be alarmed. If the ointment is to be administered only once daily, it is often preferable to do so at bedtime, when vision impairment will be inconsequential.

It is important to emphasize to the patient that ocular products if handled improperly can become contaminated by bacteria that cause ocular infections, which may lead to serious consequences. Thus, every effort must be made to avoid touching the tip of the tube to the eye, eyelid, fingertip, or any other surface, and the ointment should be used by only one person. Examples of ophthalmic ointments and gels are presented in Table 10.3.

FEATURES AND USES OF NASAL OINTMENTS AND GELS

Among the dosage forms used in the topical treatment of the nasal mucosa are ointments and gels. Other dosage forms include inhalants, solutions, and suspensions, discussed elsewhere in this text.

The nose is a respiratory organ, a passageway for air to the lungs. Its surface is coated with a continuous thin layer of mucus produced by subepithelial mucous glands. The ciliated epithelium of the nasal passage facilitates the movement of the mucous layer. The mucus contains lysozyme, glycoproteins, and immunoglobulins that act against bacteria and protect against their entry into the lungs. The ciliary action and the sneeze reflex add further defense against entry (16).

Drugs introduced into the nasal passage are primarily for local effects on the mucous membranes and underlying tissues (e.g., nasal decongestants). However, drug absorption to the general circulation does occur through the rich blood supply feeding the nasal lining. The nasal route of administration is also used for the systemic absorption of a number of drugs, including butorphanol tartrate (Stadol NS, Bristol-Myers Squibb), an analgesic; cyanocobalamin (Nascobal Gel, Schwartz), a hematopoietic; nafarelin acetate (Synarel, Searle) for the treatment of endometriosis; and nicotine (Nicotrol NS, McNeil) as an adjunct in smoking cessation. In addition, the nasal route holds great promise for the administration of insulin, vaccines, and a number of other polypeptides and proteins.

Cyanocobalamin (Nascobal Gel) for intranasal administration is used in the treatment of vitamin B_{12} deficiency, including pernicious anemia. It is self-administered as a nasal gel. Generally, 0.1 mL of the gel, containing 500 mg of cyanocobalamin, is administered intranasally once weekly. The cyanocobalamin is effectively absorbed through the nasal mucosa to produce therapeutic blood levels (17).

FEATURES AND USES OF RECTAL PREPARATIONS

Among the dosage forms used in the topical treatment of anorectal conditions are ointments, gels, creams, and creamlike aerosol foams. Other dosage forms are solutions (for enema or irrigation) and suppositories, discussed elsewhere in this text.

Ointments, creams, and gels are used for topical application to the perianal area and for insertion within the

TABLE 10.3. Examples of Ophthalmic Ointments

Ointment	Commercial Product	Active Ingredient	Category
Chloramphenicol ophthalmic	Chloromycetin Ophthalmic Ointment (Parke-Davis)	1%	Antibacterial antibiotic
Dexamethasone sodium phosphate ophthalmic	Decadron Phosphate Ophthalmic Ointment (Merck)	0.05%	Anti-inflammatory adrenocortical steroid
Gentamicin sulfate ophthalmic	Garamycin Ophthalmic Ointment (Schering)	0.3%	Antibacterial antibiotic
Isoflurophate ophthalmic	Floropryl Sterile Ophthalmic Ointment (Merck)	0.025%	Cholinesterase inhibitor
Polymyxin B–bacitracin ophthalmic	Polysporin Ophthalmic Ointment (Pfizer)	Per gram: polymyxin B sulfate, 10,000 U; bacitracin zinc, 500 U	Antimicrobial
Polymyxin B–bacitracin–neomycin ophthalmic	Neosporin Ophthalmic Ointment (Johnson & Johnson)	Per gram: polymyxin B sulfate, 10,000 U; bacitracin, zinc, 400 U; neomycin sulfate, 3.5 mg	Antimicrobial
Sulfacetamide sodium ophthalmic	Sodium Sulamyd Ophthalmic Ointment (Schering–Plough)	10% and 30%	Antibacterial
Tobramycin ophthalmic	Tobrex Ophthalmic Ointment (Alcon)	0.3%	Antibacterial antibiotic
Vidarabine ophthalmic	Vira-A Ophthalmic Ointment (Monarch)	3%	Antiviral

anal canal. They largely are used to treat local conditions of anorectal pruritus, inflammation, and the pain and discomfort associated with hemorrhoids. The drugs include astringents (e.g., zinc oxide), protectants and lubricants (e.g., cocoa butter, lanolin), local anesthetics (e.g., pramoxine HCl), antipruritics, anti-inflammatory agents (e.g., hydrocortisone), and antiepileptics (diazepam).

The perianal area is the skin immediately surrounding the anus. The anal canal is approximately 3 cm long and connects to the rectum. Both the anal canal and rectum have mucosal linings. Healthy perianal skin and the mucosa act as barriers to infection.

Substances applied rectally may be absorbed by diffusion into the general circulation via the network of three hemorrhoidal arteries and accompanying veins in the anal canal (18). The rectal route *is* used for systemic absorption of therapeutic levels of certain drugs (e.g., prochlorperazine as suppositories) when the oral route is unsatisfactory, as during vomiting. However, systemic effects from ointments and creams intended for local action are usually limited by the insolubility of certain agents (e.g., zinc oxide) and absorption of only subtherapeutic amounts of soluble drugs in the formulation.

The bases used in anorectal ointments and creams include combinations of PEG 300 and 3350, emulsion cream bases using cetyl alcohol and cetyl esters wax, and white petrolatum and mineral oil. When antimicrobial preservatives are required, methylparaben, propylparaben, benzyl alcohol, and butylated hydroxyanisole are frequently used.

Before applying rectal ointments and creams to the perianal skin, the affected area should be cleansed and dried by gentle patting with toilet tissue. Then, a portion of the ointment or cream is placed on a tissue, and a thin film is gently spread over the affected area. Products having a water-washable base are easier to spread and remove after application and tend to stain clothing less than the products having an oleaginous base.

FIGURE 10.10. Rectal ointment with perforated inserter/applicator tip.

Rectal ointments and creams are packaged with special perforated plastic tips for products to be administered into the anus, primarily in the treatment of the pain and inflammation associated with hemorrhoids (Fig. 10.10). Before use, the rectal tip should be thoroughly cleaned, screwed onto the ointment tube in place of the cap, and lubricated with mineral oil or a lubricating jelly. With the patient lying down on the back or side or in an otherwise comfortable position, the rectal tip is slowly and carefully inserted part way into the anus. Squeezing the tube forces medication through the perforations in the rectal tip and releases it to the inner lining of the anus. The tip is then slowly removed from the anus and any excess ointment or cream removed from the perianal area. The rectal tip should be cleaned thoroughly, the closure cap replaced on the tube, and the hands washed.

Rectal aerosol foam products (e.g., Proctofoam-HC, Schwarz) also are accompanied by applicators to facilitate administration. The applicator is attached to the aerosol container and filled with a measured dose of product. The applicator is then inserted into the anus and the product delivered by pushing the plunger of the applicator. After removal, the applicator and the patient's hands should be thoroughly washed.

Patients should be instructed on the proper use of the product dispensed and, in case of rectal bleeding, advised to seek additional medical advice. Examples of rectal ointments and creams are presented in Table 10.4.

TABLE 10.4. Examples of Rectal and Vaginal Creams and Ointments

Commercial Preparation	Active Ingredients	Product Type	Primary Use
Rectal			
Anusol (Salix)	Starch	Ointment	Hemorrhoid treatment
Tronolane (Monticello)	Pramoxine HCl	Cream	Hemorrhoidal analgesic and antipruritic
Vaginal			
Mycelex-7 (Ortho-McNeil)	Clotrimazole	Cream	Antifungal
AVC (Novavax)	Sulfanilamide	Cream	Vulvovaginitis (*C. albicans*)
Cleocin (Pfizer)	Clindamycin PO_4	Cream	Bacterial vaginosis
Terazol 7 (Ortho-McNeil)	Terconazole	Cream	Antifungal (*C. albicans*)
Ogen (Pharmacia)	Estropipate	Cream	Estrogenic for vulvar and vaginal atrophy
Premarin (Wyeth-Ayerst)	Conjugated estrogens	Cream	Atrophic vaginitis and kraurosis vulvae

FEATURES AND USES OF VAGINAL PREPARATIONS

Among the dosage forms used in the topical treatment of conditions and diseases of the vulvovaginal area are ointments, creams, creamlike foams, and gels. Other dosage forms include vaginal inserts, transdermal drug delivery systems, and oral forms, discussed elsewhere in this text.

The vaginal surface is lined with squamous epithelium cells and mucus produced by various underlying glands. Topical products are used to treat vulvovaginal infections, vaginitis, conditions of endometrial atrophy, and for contraception with spermatocidal agents.

The usual pathogenic organisms of vulvovaginal infections and vaginitis are *Trichomonas vaginalis*, *Candida* (*Monilia*) *albicans*, and *Haemophilus vaginalis*. Among the anti-infective agents are nystatin, clotrimazole, miconazole, clindamycin, and sulfonamides. Endometrial atrophy may be treated locally with the hormones dienestrol and progesterone, which are used to restore the vaginal mucosa to its normal state. Contraceptive preparations containing spermicidal agents such as nonoxynol-9 and octoxynol are used alone or in combination with a cervical diaphragm.

As noted previously, because products intended for use in the vulvovaginal area come into direct contact with tissues prone to infection, it is important these products be manufactured and tested to be free of offending microorganisms, yeasts, and molds. Because gels are especially subject to bacterial growth, most vaginal gels are preserved with antimicrobial agents.

Ointments, creams, and gels for vaginal use are packaged in tubes and vaginal foams in aerosol canisters. Although some preparations are applied externally to the vulva (e.g., Mycelex-7 Vaginal Cream, Ortho-McNeil), most are intended to be delivered to the vagina by means of applicator tips that accompany the products (Fig. 10.11).

In treating external vulvar conditions, the patient squeezes a small amount of product onto the fingers or tissue and gently spreads it over the affected area. For intravaginal treatment, the patient uses a plastic applicator, some of which are prefilled and disposable and others reusable and filled by the patient immediately prior to use.

To fill the applicator, the closure cap is removed from the tube, the applicator screwed on in its place, and the tube gently squeezed until the applicator is filled and the plunger rises to its marked stopping point. The filled applicator is unscrewed from the tube and replaced by the cap. Inserting intravaginal products is best accomplished with the patient lying on her back or in an otherwise comfortable position. The applicator barrel is firmly grasped and inserted into the vagina as far as possible without causing discomfort. The plunger is depressed until it stops, releasing the medication in the vagina. The applicator is carefully withdrawn for washing and ultimately discarding. The patient should be instructed to wash her hands thoroughly after use.

Aerosol foams are used intravaginally in the same general manner. The aerosol package contains an inserter device, which, when attached to the canister, may be filled with foam. The filled inserter is placed in the vagina and the product delivered by pushing the plunger. Vaginal foams are oil-in-water emulsions resembling light creams. They are water miscible and nongreasy. The patient should be instructed to wash her hands thoroughly after use.

When once-a-day administration is prescribed, it is best done at bedtime for reasons of medication retention, avoidance of daytime leakage, and lessened soiling of clothing. Creams with water-washable bases are preferred to oleaginous ointments. Patients who are pregnant must not use intravaginal products except with their doctor's approval and supervision. Tampons are not to be used during intravaginal treatment.

Unmedicated lubricant jellies are used by physicians in rectal, urethral, and vaginal examinations. All products should be tightly closed when not in use to prevent contamination. If left unsealed, gels and jellies are particularly prone to dry out. Examples of vaginal ointments, creams, and gels are presented in Tables 10.2 and 10.4.

DRUG RELEASE FROM SEMISOLID DOSAGE FORMS

Semisolid dosage forms are used for either topical/local or systemic effects. If the purpose is to deliver a drug to the surface of the skin or to be absorbed into the systemic circulation, it must be capable of being released from the vehicle in a reproducible way. Additional information on formulation considerations is detailed in Physical Pharmacy Capsule 10.3, Clinical Pharmaceutics—Formulating for Successful Transdermal/Topical Delivery. Also, in some practice situations, pharmacists are called upon to dilute creams or gels for specific patients. This is discussed in Physical Pharmacy Capsule 10.4, Clinical Pharmaceutics—Dilution of Creams and Gels.

For uniformity of the same product from batch to batch as well as for release of the drug for absorption, it is critical that the rate of release of the drug be reproducibly determined. In vitro release testing is recommended by the FDA as a measure of "product sameness" during scale-up and postapproval changes for semisolids (SUPAC-SS).

Semisolid dosage forms can produce distinct difficulties in the development of in vitro models because of the physicochemical properties of formulations and the specific physiological environment in which they must

FIGURE 10.11. Vaginal cream with inserter.

PHYSICAL PHARMACY CAPSULE **10.3** Clinical Pharmaceutics— "Formulating for Successful Transdermal/Topical Delivery"

You have been assigned the task of formulating for a successful transdermal/topical preparation. Obviously, not all drugs are suitable for application to the skin; however, many are suitable and the list seems to be getting longer as we are seeing more and more manufactured as well as compounded transdermal/topical products/ preparations. Let's look at some general guidelines.

■ SELECT AN APPROPRIATE DRUG

Passive drug delivery seems to be appropriate for small molecules with good lipophilicity and adequate aqueous solubility. Generally, one looks at 300 to 500 Da and a log partition coefficient (octanol/water) in the range of 1 to 3.5 and an aqueous solubility in excess of 100 µg/mL. A reasonable drug would have a "flux" in the range of about 1 mg/cm^2/d so covering an area of about 10 cm^2 would deliver about 10 mg/d. One must keep in mind that first-pass hepatic metabolism is avoided so dosing may not necessarily follow oral dosing regimens.

■ DRUG FLUX CONSIDERATIONS

These data are sometimes available from published studies. If not, an estimate can be obtained using the Potts and Guy equation:

$$\log K_p = 0.71 \times \log P_{(oct/water)} - 0.0061 \times MW - 2.74$$

where K_p is the permeability coefficient (cm/h) through the stratum corneum, $P_{(oct/water)}$ is the octanol/water partition coefficient of the permeant, and MW is the molecular weight of the drug.

■ MAINTAIN SATURATION FOR MAXIMUM DELIVERY

The driving force for permeation is the thermodynamic activity of the API in the vehicle. Maximum flux is generally obtained with the drug saturated in the vehicle. So the drug should be at its solubility limit at about 32°C. Drug depletion over time resulting in nonsaturated can be addressed by adding a slight excess of drug in a suspended state.

■ POSSIBLY IMPROVE DRUG FLUX USING FORMULATION MANIPULATION

Vehicles that aid in skin hydration and solvents that also contain penetration enhancing properties can improve drug flux. Also, specific penetration enhancing excipients can be added to formulation to enhance flux and the amount of drug delivered through the skin. There are many excipients that can be used but should be selected after considering compatibility and stability issues.

■ A VOLATILE/EVAPORATING VEHICLE CAN INCREASE FINITE DOSE DELIVERY

The use of a vehicle/solvent that is volatile and evaporates after application to the skin will enhance drug concentration by producing a supersaturated solution on the skin surface and also may serve to modify the stratum corneum to aid drug passage. These vehicles may not be advisable for open lesions but tend to work well on intact skin. The "push" across the stratum corneum often results in a reservoir buildup of the drug for prolonged release.

■ AFTER PENETRATING THE SKIN, THE DRUG MOLECULE TENDS TO CONTINUE MOVING FOLLOWING A CONCENTRATION GRADIENT OR AN ACTIVE PROCESS

In the treatment of many skin disorders, it is desirable for the drug to stay just below the skin surface with little or no drug entering into the systemic circulation. Localizing or targeting drugs to specific skin regions or layers is not currently feasible; however, there are a couple of approaches that can be considered. Placing the drug in a liposomal carrier may help hold the drug closer to the surface and may even result in the liposomes entering hair follicles for prolonged release of the drug. Also, the use of a solvent that will aid in rapid penetration to form a reservoir and alter the penetration capabilities of the surrounding tissue may result in holding the drug at the surface. Last, the use of occlusive lipid vehicles may result in a slow partitioning of the drug into the superficial layers. ■

PHYSICAL PHARMACY CAPSULE 10.4 Clinical Pharmaceutics—"Dilution of Creams and Gels"

Numerous topical and transdermal products are available in different strengths and formulations. Corticosteroids are formulated in lotions, pastes, gels, creams, and ointments in various strengths. It is sometimes necessary to reduce the dose used by either diluting the formulation or applying less to the involved area. Normally, dilution of creams and gels is not recommended because the stability of the formulation may be compromised and there may be a risk of microbial contamination that may need to be considered if the formulations are applied to broken skin. Even though many creams and gels contain preservatives, the dilution of these may reduce the concentration of the preservative to less than that needed to be effective.

Despite these considerations, it is sometimes necessary to dilute a cream or gel. If so, one may consider limiting the dilution to no more than 1 in 10 and to not use any heat or not use excessive heat (keep less than ~50°C) in the process. If dilution is required, the "diluent" should be a similar cream or gel (or ointment vehicle as appropriate for ointment products) that is easily miscible with the formulation and one that is preserved, etc. Diluents may include oil-in-water creams, water-in-oil creams, gels, PEG-based semisolids, etc., as appropriate. Patient characteristics should be considered for allergies, etc., in selecting the diluent.

In summary, dilution of topicals and transdermals is not recommended but sometimes is necessary. If done, it should be done appropriately with due consideration to the diluent characteristics and patient requirements. ∎

release their API. It is important to validate a release test before using it; it must be reproducible and reliable. Even though it is not a measure of bioavailability, the test must be capable of detecting changes in drug release characteristics from the finished product. Changes in these release characteristics may alter the biological performance of the drug in the dosage form.

Drug release measurements for ointments, creams, and gels have been in the literature for years. Formerly, the semisolid dosage form was placed in direct contact with a receptor fluid. Today, generally, a Franz diffusion cell is used where the semisolid dosage form is placed on a membrane that is situated on top of a receptor chamber containing a receptor solution. The drug is released from the dosage form and passes through the membrane into the receptor solution where it is sampled and analyzed for content. The results are plotted as the concentration of the drug in the receptor fluid versus time. The rates of drug release can be calculated and compared.

PATIENT COUNSELING

ALL OINTMENTS, CREAMS, AND GELS

1. Generally, only a thin film of an ointment or a cream should be applied.
2. Unless otherwise instructed, remove a sufficient quantity from the container, apply it, and gently rub it into the affected area.
3. Leave the drug undisturbed for sufficient time to take effect.
4. If the area is to be covered with clothing, use a protective pad to prevent the preparation from being removed by the clothing.
5. If advised, continue using the preparation for a short while after the symptom or injury has been resolved.
6. Unless otherwise indicated, ointments, creams, and pastes should be stored at room temperature away from children, heat, and direct sunlight.
7. Percutaneous absorption may vary with the site of application.
8. Explain the importance of using the recommended site and rotating locations within that site. Rotating locations is important to allow the skin to regain its normal permeability after being occluded and to prevent skin irritation. Skin sites may be reused after 1 week.
9. Application should be to clean, dry skin and not to oily, irritated, inflamed, broken, or callused skin.
10. Use of skin lotions or body creams should be avoided at the application site because they can affect skin hydration and can alter the partition coefficient between the drug and the skin.
11. The drug should be placed at a site that will not subject it to being rubbed off by clothing or movement (as the belt line) or onto another person or pet.
12. Care should be taken not to rub the eyes or touch the mouth during handling of the product.
13. If the patient exhibits sensitivity or intolerance to the drug or if undue skin irritation results, contact your pharmacist or physician.
14. A plastic, disposable glove can be worn during application. Otherwise, hands must be washed before and after the application to remove any medication from the hands.

OINTMENTS

1. Wash and dry hands.
2. Confirm that the surface where the medication is to be applied is clean and dry.
3. Apply a thin layer of medication to the skin.
4. If directed, apply a breathable covering. Otherwise, leave it open. Do not apply an occlusive dressing (Saran Wrap or other plastic film) unless specifically directed by the physician.
5. For measuring the quantity to be applied, it may be expressed as a specific length or "ribbon" when dispensed in a tube. If in a jar, it can be expressed as a visual quantity using a tongue depressor, ice cream stick, or other device. If dispensed in a syringe, it can be expressed as a volume in milliliters (mLs).
6. Removal of ointments and pastes requires warm water, soap, and some mechanical action.
7. For creams and ointments, the proper application may differ depending on the dosage form, active ingredients, and desired therapeutic outcomes.

CREAMS

1. Wash and dry hands.
2. Confirm that the surface where the medication is to be applied is clean and dry.
3. Apply a thin layer of medication to the skin.
4. If directed, apply a breathable covering. Otherwise, leave it open. Do not apply an occlusive dressing (Saran Wrap or other plastic film) unless specifically directed by the physician.
5. For measuring the quantity to be applied, it may be expressed as a specific length or "ribbon" when dispensed in a tube. If in a jar, it can be expressed as a visual quantity using a depressor, ice cream stick, or other device. If dispensed in a syringe or dispenser (Topi-CLICK), it can be expressed as a volume in milliliters (mLs).
6. Explain that some of the drug intended for local effect will be absorbed systemically and is capable of causing side effects.
7. Creams (o/w) can be removed relatively easily by using warm water and, if necessary, soap. Creams (w/o) may take soap and warm water and some mild mechanical action.
8. For creams and ointments, the proper application may differ depending on the dosage form, active ingredients, and desired therapeutic outcomes.

PASTES

1. Pastes may be placed on an area but not rubbed in, because of their viscosity.
2. Pastes are usually used for a protectant effect and should not be removed until indicated.
3. Removal of ointments and pastes requires warm water, soap, and some mechanical action.

GELS

1. Wash and dry hands.
2. Confirm that the surface where the medication is to be applied is clean and dry.
3. Apply a thin layer of medication to the skin.
4. If directed, apply a breathable covering. Otherwise, leave it open. Do not apply an occlusive dressing (Saran Wrap or other plastic film) unless specifically directed by the physician.
5. For measuring the quantity to be applied, it may be expressed as a specific length of "ribbon" when dispensed in a tube. If in a jar, it can be expressed as a visual quantity using a depressor, ice cream stick, or other device. If dispensed in a syringe, it can be expressed as a volume in milliliters (mLs).
6. Explain that some of the drug intended for local effect will be absorbed systemically and is capable of causing side effects.
7. Keep the package tightly closed when not in use.

ADMINISTERING RECTAL CREAMS AND FOAMS

1. Wash hands and rectal area and pat dry. Preferably, use a disposable plastic glove.
2. Remove the cap of the ointment and attach the applicator tip or shake the foam canister and attach the applicator to its opening.
3. Fill the applicator with the designated dose or explain the quantity to be administered.
4. If desired, lubricate the applicator with a small quantity of the ointment, lubricating jelly, or petrolatum prior to insertion.
5. Lie on the left side with the left leg extended and the right leg bent.
6. Gently insert the applicator and administer the dose into the rectum.
7. Clean the applicator tip or applicator with soap and warm water and allow to dry.
8. Remove and dispose of the glove if used; wash and dry hands again.
9. The onset of action is reasonably rapid for local treatments (30 minutes to 2 hours).

ADMINISTERING VAGINAL DOSAGE FORMS— GENERAL

1. A sanitary pad may be used to prevent the medication from soiling clothing or sleepwear.
2. Administration at bedtime is preferred.
3. Vaginal medications can be used during menstruation (except for birth control vaginal rings).

ADMINISTERING VAGINAL CREAMS

1. Wash and dry hands and the vaginal area.
2. Vaginal creams and gels come with applicators. The applicator is intended to screw onto the threads of the medication tube. The medication tube may require penetration using the tube cap with a pointed end.

3. Fill the applicator tube to the indicated line for the correct dose.
4. Stand or lie on the back and insert the applicator high in the upper part of the vagina. Use the plunger to push the cream or gel out of the applicator.
5. Clean the applicator with soap and warm water and allow to dry.
6. Wash and dry hands again.

PASTES AND GELS FOR ORAL CAVITY USE—NOT TO BE SWALLOWED AS A BOLUS

1. Demonstrate the size of the dose in whatever means it is to be measured.
2. Explain the frequency of use.
3. To avoid excess swallowing, administer after meals and at bedtime.

ORAL FILMS FOR ORAL CAVITY USE—NOT TO BE SWALLOWED WHOLE

1. Confirm the number of units to apply.
2. Confirm the frequency of use.

3. To avoid excess swallowing, administer after meals and at bedtime.
4. Confirm if the unit should be removed or if it will dissolve and/or erode away.
5. If treating local conditions, the application site is not rotated.
6. If for treating systemically, the site of application should be rotated to minimize irritation.

ADMINISTERING OPHTHALMIC OINTMENTS AND GELS

1. Ointments will blur vision because they may not be miscible with tears, so administration prior to sleep is best to avoid disruption of normal activities.
2. Wash hands first.
3. Apply the prescribed "ribbon" of ointment or gel to the formed pouch in the lower eyelid.
4. Close the eye to spread the drug over the eye.
5. Administer liquid eye drops before ointments or gels, if prescribed.
6. Wait 10 minutes after drops are administered before administering ointments or gels to the same eye.

PHARMACEUTICS CASE STUDY

SUBJECTIVE INFORMATION

You have received the following prescription:

Rx:	
Sulfur:	2 g
Salicylic acid:	2 g
Calamine:	5 g
Urea:	2 g
Hydrophilic petrolatum qs:	100 g

After you prepared the prescription, you observed it to be a granular ointment that is not appropriate for dispensing because it feels very coarse.

OBJECTIVE INFORMATION

In preparing the ointment, you weighed sublimed sulfur 2 g, salicylic acid 2 g, calamine 5 g, and urea 2 g and mixed the powders together on a pill tile using a spatula. However, you had difficulty with the sulfur, which seemed to be difficult to comminute and blend. Finally, you added the hydrophilic petrolatum and obtained a light pink, quite granular ointment.

Sulfur produces electrostatic charges when mixed on a pill tile using a spatula. It is official as the precipitated sulfur, a very fine powder, and sublimed sulfur, a fine powder. It is practically insoluble in water. Salicylic acid occurs as white crystals, usually in fine needles or a fluffy, white, crystalline powder, and is slightly soluble in water and freely soluble in alcohol. Calamine is a fine pink

powder that is insoluble in water. Urea occurs as a white, crystalline powder and freely soluble in water. It is made up of zinc oxide with a small proportion of ferric oxide.

ASSESSMENT

Particle size reduction of sulfur is best accomplished using a levigating agent compatible with the base, in this case, hydrophilic petrolatum. Salicylic acid and calamine should pose no real problem in incorporation. Urea can be dissolved, if desired, in a small quantity of water (because it has a solubility of 1 g in 1.5 mL of water, it would take ~3 mL of water to dissolve it) and incorporated into the ointment, or it can be levigated with a small amount of mineral oil prior to incorporation if an anhydrous preparation is desired.

PLAN

In this case, an anhydrous preparation is desired, so the precipitated sulfur is levigated with about 2 to 3 mL of mineral oil. The urea is levigated with about 2 to 3 mL of mineral oil. The salicylic acid is comminuted to a fine powder, as is the calamine; the two powders are mixed together. The sulfur and urea mixtures are combined and the hydrophilic petrolatum incorporated geometrically. Following this, the salicylic acid and calamine powders are incorporated geometrically and the final preparation thoroughly mixed. This procedure produces a slightly thinner vehicle after the sulfur with urea in mineral oil is incorporated, which makes it easier to incorporate the additional powders. The preparation is then packaged and labeled. ■

CLINICAL CASE STUDY

A.R. is a 22-year-old WF who comes into the pharmacy complaining of a painful sunburn. She states she spent most of yesterday "on the beach with friends" and says she did not use any sunscreen, even though she does occasionally when exposed to the sun. A.R. admits she did not realize the extent of her sunburn until about 4 hours after her fun on the beach, at which time she began to have pain, chills, and fatigue. Now, she is also itching. When asked, she says she does not have any blisters on her burned skin. When asked if this has happened to her before, A.R. confides she has had sunburns similar to this about once a summer for approximately the past 5 years. When asked about her pain based on a scale of 1 to 10, she rates her pain as an 8.

PMH:	Sunburns many times throughout her life
	Moderate acne
	Freckles easily; fair complexioned
	Red hair
	None significant otherwise
SH:	None contributory
FH:	Mother (–)
	Father (–)
	Grandfather (+) for melanoma
ALL:	NKDA
MEDS:	Ortho Tri-Cyclen, 1 tablet po qd
	Differin Gel, apply thin layer hs

PHARMACEUTICAL CARE PLAN

S: Burning, painful, reddened skin, and first-degree burn

General fatigue

Chills

Pain 8/10

Itching

O: Bright red skin on the face, neck, shoulders, arms, and legs without any evidence of blistering

A: The patient is a 22-year-old WF with a PMH of sunburns and moderate acne. The patient is at increased risk for sunburns d/t her history of freckling, fair skin, red hair, current medications, and the frequency of past burns. In addition to these characteristics, her FH of melanoma increases her risk of future sunburns and skin cancer.

P: 1. Recommend an oral OTC analgesic to relieve the pain of sunburn. There are many choices, and product selection often depends on personal preferences. Any NSAID (e.g., ibuprofen 200 to 400 mg q4h to q6h prn pain not to exceed 1,200 mg/d, naproxen 200 mg q12h prn pain, aspirin 325 to 650 mg q3h to q4h prn not to exceed 4 g/d, or acetaminophen 325 to 650 mg q4h to q6h prn not to exceed 4 g/d) would be a good choice. The patient should understand to take these as recommended with a full glass of water and to continue taking them until the pain abates.

2. Applying a clean cloth soaked in cool tap water or taking a cool bath for 10 to 30 minutes will also help to alleviate pain. One can also recommend a topical anesthetic to aid in relieving pain, such as Solarcaine Aloe Extra Burn Relief Cream, Gel, or Spray. A.R. should be instructed that topical anesthetics should not be used more often than three or four times daily and continuous pain relief cannot be obtained with these agents. Before and after applying the product, the patient should wash her hands.

3. A W/O topical lotion can provide protection and moisture. These factors are important for sunburned skin because the goal is to replenish skin moisture lost to the sun and protect it from drying out further, which can lead to more irritation and itching. A lotion that could be recommended is Keri. A.R. should apply liberally as needed; however, she should avoid her face, because this lotion contains mineral oil, which may exacerbate her acne. Because this lotion has a W/O base, the patient should be told it will be necessary to use soap and water to remove it.

4. Counsel A.R. on her current medications, especially because the medications she is using for acne may have played a role in developing the sunburn (i.e., photosensitivity). A.R. should also be told that exposure to the sun can exacerbate her acne. A.R. should avoid excessive sun exposure, especially for the next few weeks, because the skin should have time to heal and will be more susceptible to sunburn during this time. The patient should also be counseled on her many risk factors for skin cancer, including fair skin, red hair, a history of freckling, family history of melanoma, and the frequency of past burns. In the future, A.R. should completely avoid sun exposure. Because this may be unrealistic, she should be told to use a hat and clothing while in the sun to decrease the amount of skin exposed to the sun. If she believes she cannot comply with these suggestions, she should, at least, use a W/O-based sunscreen with an SPF of 30. This will also provide water resistance.

5. Monitoring: The patient should reassess her sunburn in another 24 hours, because the full extent of skin damage may not be initially apparent until 24 to 48 hours after exposure. If she notices any breaks in the skin and/or pain persists or increases, she should seek medical attention from a primary care provider. ■

APPLYING THE PRINCIPLES AND CONCEPTS

GROUP ACTIVITIES

1. Obtain three topical extemporaneous prescriptions for each of the four various types of ointment bases and outline a procedure to prepare each.
2. Create a listing of conceivable ways a consumer/patient might misuse a topical semisolid dosage form.
3. List five counseling points for proper administration of a topical semisolid dosage form and provide a rationale for each counseling point.
4. Determine how the preparation of an ophthalmic ointment differs from that of a rectal ointment.

INDIVIDUAL ACTIVITIES

1. Identify three topical diseases where each of the four various types of ointment bases might be employed to deliver (an) active ingredient(s).

2. Identify three drugs whose topical concentration differs for the treatment of a specific topical affliction.
3. Develop a procedure to incorporate a water-soluble drug, for example, gentamicin sulfate, into an oleaginous ophthalmic ointment base, for example, white petrolatum.
4. List five drugs used topically that are available in ointment, cream, and gel dosage forms and identify conceivable disease states for which each is used.
5. (*a*) A physician asks you to prepare 30 g of betamethasone valerate ointment 0.01% for a pediatric patient. Examine the product formulation and propose two bases you could use to compound the ointment. (*b*) List three other topical products that represent different types of ointment bases. For each product, list an appropriate base that should be used if you were called on to dilute the product for a patient.

REFERENCES

1. Osborne DW, Amann AH. Topical Drug Delivery Formulations. New York, NY: Marcel Dekker, Inc., 1990.
2. U.S. Pharmacopeial Convention. United States Pharmacopeia–National Formulary. Current Ed. Rockville, MD: Author, Current edition.
3. Corbo M, Schulz TW, Wong GK, et al. Development and validation of in vitro release testing methods for semisolid formulations. Pharm Technol 1993;17:112–128.
4. Shah VP, Elkins J, Hanus J, et al. In vitro release of hydrocortisone from topical preparations and automated procedure. Pharm Res 1991;8:55–63.
5. Androgel package insert. Abbott laboratories, 2011.
6. Forcinio H. Tubes: The ideal packaging for semisolid products. Pharm Technol 1998;22:32–36.
7. Montebello Packaging, 124 Madison Street, Oak Park, IL. Available at: http://www.montebellopkg.com. (Accessed July 27, 2020)
8. MG America, Inc., 31 Kulick Rd., Fairfield, NJ. Available at: http://www.mgamerica.com. (Accessed July 27, 2020)
9. Potts RO, Buy RH. Mechanisms of Transdermal Drug Delivery. New York, NY: Marcel Dekker, Inc., 1997.
10. Smith EW, Maibach HI, eds. Percutaneous Penetration Enhancers. New York, NY: CRC Press, 1995.
11. Surber C, Wilhelm KP, Hori M, et al. Optimization of topical therapy: Partitioning of drugs into stratum corneum. Pharm Res 1990;7:1320–1324.
12. Lee VHL. Mechanisms and facilitation of corneal drug penetration. J Control Release 1990;11:79–90.
13. Allen LV Jr. Compounding ophthalmic preparations. Int J Pharm Compd 1998;2:184–188.
14. Fiscella RG, Jensen MK. Ophthalmic disorders. In: Handbook of Nonprescription Drugs. 17th Ed. Washington, DC: American Pharmaceutical Association, 2012:509–530.
15. Lee JY. Sterilization control and validation for topical ointments. Pharm Technol 1992;16:104–110.
16. Scolaro KL. Disorders related to cold and allergy. In: Handbook of Nonprescription Drugs. 17th Ed. Washington, DC: American Pharmaceutical Association, 2012:179–204.
17. Product Information. Available at: www.nascobal.com. (Accessed July 27, 2020)
18. Chan C. Anorectal disorders. In: Handbook of Nonprescription Drugs. 17th Ed. Washington, DC: American Pharmaceutical Association, 2012:299–312.

Transdermals and Transdermal Drug Delivery Systems

CHAPTER AT A GLANCE Factors Affecting Percutaneous Absorption
• Percutaneous Absorption Enhancers • Percutaneous Absorption Models
• Design Features of Transdermal Drug Delivery Systems • Advantages and
Disadvantages of TDDSs • Examples of Transdermal Drug Delivery Systems
• General Clinical Considerations in the Use of Transdermals and TDDSs
• Patches (Not Systems) • Tapes • Examples of Transdermal Preparations
• Patient Counseling

OBJECTIVES

After reading this chapter, the student will be able to:

1. Explain the physical–chemical properties of drugs that determine their ability to be incorporated into a transdermal dosage form

2. Describe physiological factors of the skin that influence percutaneous absorption

3. Define a chemical permeation enhancer and describe physical methods used to facilitate the percutaneous absorption of drugs

4. Differentiate between the various types of systems used for transdermal delivery

5. List the advantages and the disadvantages of transdermal delivery of drugs compared to other forms of drug delivery

6. Provide examples of drugs that are delivered transdermally, and list precautions associated with their use

7. Describe important counseling information to share with a patient prescribed a drug to be administered in a transdermal drug delivery system

INTRODUCTION

Transdermal drug delivery systems (TDDSs) facilitate the passage of therapeutic quantities of drug substances through the skin and into the general circulation for their systemic effects. In 1965, Stoughton first conceived of the *percutaneous absorption* of drug substances (1). The first transdermal system, Transderm Scop (Baxter), was approved by the U.S. Food and Drug Administration (FDA) in 1979 for prevention of nausea and vomiting associated with travel, particularly at sea.

Evidence of percutaneous drug absorption may be found through measurable blood levels of the drug, detectable excretion of the drug and/or its metabolites in the urine, and clinical response of the patient to the therapy. With transdermal drug delivery, the blood concentration needed to achieve therapeutic efficacy may be determined by comparative analysis of the patient's response to drug blood levels. For transdermal drug delivery, it is considered ideal for the drug to migrate through the skin to the underlying blood supply without buildup in the dermal layers (2). This is in direct contrast to the types of topical dosage forms discussed in the previous chapter, in which drug residence in the skin, the target organ, is desired.

As discussed in the previous chapter, the skin is composed of the stratum corneum (the outer layer), the living epidermis, and the dermis, which together provide the skin's barrier layers to penetration by external agents (see Fig. 10.9). The film that covers the stratum corneum is composed of sebum and sweat, but because of its varied composition and lack of continuity, it is not a significant factor in drug penetration, nor are the hair follicles and sweat and sebaceous gland ducts, which constitute only a minor proportion of the skin's surface.

Percutaneous absorption of a drug generally results from direct penetration of the drug through the stratum corneum, a 10- to 15-μm-thick layer of flat, partially desiccated nonliving tissue (3,4). The stratum corneum is composed of approximately 40% protein (mainly keratin) and 40% water, with the balance being lipid, principally as triglycerides, free fatty acids, cholesterol, and phospholipids. The lipid content is concentrated in the extracellular phase of the stratum corneum and forms to a large extent the membrane surrounding the cells. Because a drug's major route of penetration is through the intercellular channels, the lipid component is considered an important determinant in the first step of absorption (5). Once through the stratum corneum, drug molecules may pass through the deeper epidermal tissues and into the dermis. When the drug reaches the vascularized dermal layer, it becomes available for absorption into the general circulation.

The stratum corneum, being keratinized tissue, behaves as a semipermeable artificial membrane, and drug molecules penetrate by passive diffusion. It is the major rate-limiting barrier to transdermal drug transport (6). Over most of the body, the stratum corneum has 15 to 25 layers of flattened corneocytes with an overall thickness of about 10 μm (6). The rate of drug movement across this layer depends on its concentration in the vehicle, its aqueous solubility, and the oil–water partition coefficient between the stratum corneum and the vehicle (7). Substances with both aqueous and lipid solubility characteristics are good candidates for diffusion through the stratum corneum, epidermis, and dermis.

FACTORS AFFECTING PERCUTANEOUS ABSORPTION

Not all drug substances are suitable for transdermal delivery. Among the factors playing a part in percutaneous absorption are the physical and chemical properties of the drug, including its molecular weight, solubility, partitioning coefficient and dissociation constant (pK_a), the nature of the carrier vehicle, and the condition of the skin. Although general statements applicable to all possible combinations of drug, vehicle, and skin condition are difficult to draw, most research findings may be summarized as follows (2–11):

1. Drug concentration is an important factor. Generally, the amount of drug percutaneously absorbed per unit of surface area per time interval increases with an increase in the concentration of the drug in the TDDS.
2. The larger the area of application (the larger the TDDS), the more drug is absorbed.
3. The drug should have a greater physicochemical attraction to the skin than to the vehicle so that the drug will leave the vehicle in favor of the skin. Some solubility of the drug in both lipid and water is thought to be essential for effective percutaneous absorption. In essence, the aqueous solubility of a drug determines the concentration presented to the absorption site, and the partition coefficient influences the rate of transport across

the absorption site. Generally, drugs penetrate the skin better in their unionized form. Nonpolar drugs tend to cross the cell barrier through the lipid-rich regions (transcellular route), whereas the polar drugs favor transport between cells (intercellular route) (6). For example, erythromycin base demonstrates better percutaneous absorption than does erythromycin ethyl succinate.

4. Drugs with molecular weights of 100 to 800 and adequate lipid and aqueous solubility can permeate skin. The ideal molecular weight of a drug for transdermal drug delivery is believed to be 400 or less.
5. Hydration of the skin generally favors percutaneous absorption. The TDDS acts as an occlusive moisture barrier through which sweat cannot pass, increasing skin hydration.
6. Water from the formulation will be absorbed into the skin but will only have transient effects on hydration.
7. Occlusive properties increase the hydration and permeability of the stratum corneum.
8. Percutaneous absorption appears to be greater when the TDDS is applied to a site with a thin horny layer than with a thick one.
9. Generally, the longer the medicated application is permitted to remain in contact with the skin, the greater is the total drug absorption.
10. Select a vehicle, or base, that will dissolve the drug and select a form of the drug that will dissolve in the base. In the case of two-phase systems water-in-oil and oil-in-water emulsions, there must be an appreciable amount dissolved in the continuous phase.
11. Use of a cosolvent ingredient with polarity similar to the stratum corneum enhances partitioning of the drug and cosolvent into the stratum corneum.
12. Penetration enhancers may be required to enhance the mobility of large molecular weight drugs.

These general statements apply to the skin in the normal state. Skin that is abraded or cut permits drugs to gain direct access to the subcutaneous tissues and the capillary network, defeating the function of the TDDS. Table 11.1 is a "general" table of compositions that may help in differentiation of formulations with penetrating ability.

TABLE 11.1. General Compositions of Topical Versus Transdermal Formulations

Ingredient Category	Topical	Transdermal
Vehicle	Yes	Yes
Solvents	Yes	Yes
Preservatives	Yes	Yes
Stiffening agents	Yes	Yes
Gelling agent	Yes	Yes
pH adjustment	Yes	Yes
Humectant	Yes	Yes
Penetration enhancer	No	Yes
Liposomes	No	Yes

PERCUTANEOUS ABSORPTION ENHANCERS

There is great interest among pharmaceutical scientists to develop chemical permeation enhancers and physical methods that can increase percutaneous absorption of therapeutic agents.

Chemical Enhancers

By definition, a chemical skin penetration enhancer *increases skin permeability by reversibly damaging or altering the physicochemical nature of the stratum corneum to reduce its diffusional resistance* (12). Among the alterations are increased hydration of the stratum corneum, a change in the structure of the lipids and lipoproteins in the intercellular channels through solvent action or denaturation, or both (4,13–17).

Some drugs have an inherent capacity to permeate the skin without chemical enhancers. However, when this is not the case, chemical permeation enhancers may render an otherwise impenetrable substance useful in transdermal drug delivery (17). More than 275 chemical compounds have been cited in the literature as skin penetration enhancers; they include acetone, azone, dimethylacetamide, dimethylformamide, dimethyl sulfoxide, ethanol, oleic acid, polyethylene glycol, propylene glycol, and sodium lauryl sulfate (13–15). The selection of a permeation enhancer should be based not only on its efficacy in enhancing skin permeation but also on its dermal toxicity (low) and its physicochemical and biologic compatibility with the system's other components (16).

Iontophoresis and Sonophoresis

In addition to chemical means, some physical methods are being used to enhance transdermal drug delivery and penetration, namely, iontophoresis and sonophoresis (6,15,18–23). *Iontophoresis* is delivery of a charged chemical compound across the skin membrane using an electrical field. A number of drugs have been the subject of iontophoretic studies; they include lidocaine (18); dexamethasone; amino acids, peptides, and insulin (19,20); verapamil (6); and propranolol (21). There is particular interest to develop alternative routes for delivery of biologically active peptides. At present, these agents are delivered by injection because of their rapid metabolism and poor absorption after oral delivery. They are also poorly absorbed by the transdermal route because of their large molecular size and ionic character and the general impenetrability of the skin (20). However, iontophoresis-enhanced transdermal delivery has shown some promise as a means of peptide and protein administration.

Sonophoresis, or high-frequency ultrasound, is also being studied as a means to enhance transdermal drug delivery (22,23). Among the agents examined are hydrocortisone, lidocaine, and salicylic acid in such formulations as gels, creams, and lotions. It is thought that high-frequency ultrasound can influence the integrity of the stratum corneum and thus affect its penetrability.

PERCUTANEOUS ABSORPTION MODELS

Skin permeability and percutaneous absorption have been the subject of numerous studies to define the underlying principles and to optimize transdermal drug delivery. Although many experimental methods and models have been used, they tend to fall into one of two categories, in vivo or in vitro.

In Vivo Studies

In vivo skin penetration studies may be undertaken for one or more of the following purposes (24):

1. To verify and quantify the cutaneous bioavailability of a topically applied drug
2. To verify and quantify the systemic bioavailability of a transdermal drug
3. To establish bioequivalence of different topical formulations of the same drug substance
4. To determine the incidence and degree of systemic toxicologic risk following topical application of a specific drug or drug product
5. To relate resultant blood levels of drug in human to systemic therapeutic effects

The most relevant studies are performed in humans; however, animal models may be used insofar as they may be effective as predictors of human response. Animal models include the weanling pig, rhesus monkey, and hairless mouse or rat (24,25). Biologic samples used in drug penetration and drug absorption studies include skin sections, venous blood from the application site, blood from the systemic circulation, and excreta (urine, feces, and expired air) (24–28).

In Vitro Studies

Skin permeation may be tested in vitro using various skin tissues (human or animal whole skin, dermis, or epidermis) in a diffusion cell (29). In vitro penetration studies using human skin are limited because of difficulties of procurement, storage, expense, and variation in permeation (30). Excised animal skins may also vary in quality and permeation. Animal skins are much more permeable than human skin. One alternative that has been shown to be effective is shed snakeskin (*Elaphe obsoleta*, black rat snake), which is nonliving, pure stratum corneum, hairless, and similar to human skin but slightly less permeable (30,31). Also, the product Living Skin Equivalent Testskin (Organogenesis, Inc.) was developed as an alternative for dermal absorption studies. The material is an organotypic coculture of human dermal fibroblasts in a collagen-containing matrix and a stratified epidermis composed of human epidermal keratinocytes. The material may be used in cell culture studies or in standard diffusion cells.

Diffusion cell systems are employed in vitro to quantify the release rates of drugs from topical preparations (32). In these systems, skin membranes or synthetic membranes may be employed as barriers to the flow of drug and vehicle

FIGURE 11.1. Typical side-by-side diffusion cell setup used for permeability/diffusion studies. A membrane or skin can be placed in the holder in the center. There are three ports on each side for sampling; one can be used to insert an electrode for iontophoresis studies. Each half cell has an inlet and outlet for constant temperature water to circulate.

to simulate the biologic system. The typical diffusion cell has two chambers, one on each side of the test diffusion membrane (Figs. 11.1 to 11.3). A temperature-controlled solution of the drug is placed in one chamber and a receptor solution in the other chamber. When skin is used as the test membrane, it separates the two solutions. Drug

FIGURE 11.2. Typical Franz diffusion cell. The donor cell is on top, and the upper and lower chambers are separated by either a membrane or skin. A solution or semisolid containing the drug is placed in the upper cell and a receiver solution in the lower cell. The angle tube on the right is for sampling and fluid replacement. The two ports on the left consist of an inlet and outlet where constant temperature water can be circulated.

FIGURE 11.3. A microdiffusion cell for working with very low quantities of drugs and solutions.

diffusion through the skin may be determined by periodic sampling and assay of the drug content in the receptor solution. The skin may also be analyzed for drug content to show permeation rates and/or retention in the skin (29).

The *United States Pharmacopeia* (USP) describes the apparatus and procedure to determine dissolution (release) of medication from a transdermal delivery system and provides an acceptance table to which the product must conform to meet the monograph standard for a given article (33). Commercial systems use transdermal diffusion cells and automatic sampling systems to determine the release rates of drugs from transdermal systems (34). In USP 43/NF 38, there are four official transdermal systems; clonidine, estradiol, rotigotine, and nicotine.

DESIGN FEATURES OF TRANSDERMAL DRUG DELIVERY SYSTEMS

TDDSs (also often called transdermal patches) are designed to support the passage of drug substances from the surface of the skin through its various layers and into the systemic circulation. Examples of the configuration and composition of TDDSs are described in the text, presented in Table 11.2, and shown in Figures 11.4 to 11.7. Figures 11.8 to 11.10 depict the manufacture of TDDSs. Technically, TDDSs may be categorized into two types, monolithic and membrane-controlled systems.

TABLE 11.2. Examples of Transdermal Drug Delivery Systems (35–44)

Therapeutic Agent	TDDS	Design, Contents	Comments
Clonidine	Catapres-TTS (Boehringer Ingelheim)	Four-layer patch: (*a*) backing of pigmented polyester film; (*b*) reservoir of clonidine, mineral oil, polyisobutylene, colloidal silicon dioxide; (*c*) microporous polypropylene membrane–controlling rate of delivery; (*d*) adhesive formulation of agents	Transdermal therapeutic system to deliver therapeutic dose of antihypertensive drug at constant rate for 7 d. TDDS generally applied to hairless or shaven area of upper arm or torso
Estradiol	Estraderm (Novartis)	Four-layer patch: (*a*) transparent polyester film; (*b*) reservoir of estradiol, alcohol gelled with hydroxypropyl cellulose; (*c*) ethylene–vinyl acetate copolymer membrane; (*d*) adhesive formulation of light mineral oil, polyisobutylene	Transdermal system to release 17β-estradiol continuously. Patch is generally applied to the trunk, including abdomen and buttocks, alternating sites, twice weekly over a 3-wk cycle with dosage frequency adjusted as required
	Vivelle (Novartis)	Three-layer patch: (*a*) translucent ethylene–vinyl alcohol copolymer film; (*b*) estradiol in matrix of medical adhesive of polyisobutylene, ethylene–vinyl acetate copolymer; (*c*) polyester release liner, removed prior to application	Use and application similar to Estraderm TDDS
	Climara (Bayer Healthcare)	Three-layer system: (*a*) translucent polyethylene film; (*b*) acrylate adhesive matrix containing estradiol; (*c*) protective liner of siliconized or fluoropolymer-coated polyester film, removed prior to use	Use and application similar to Estraderm TDDS. System may be applied weekly
Fentanyl	Duragesic (Janssen)	Four-layer patch: (*a*) backing layer of polyester film; (*b*) reservoir of fentanyl, alcohol gelled with hydroxyethyl cellulose; (*c*) rate-controlling ethylene–vinyl acetate copolymer membrane; (*d*) fentanyl-containing silicone adhesive	Transdermal therapeutic system providing continuous 72-h systemic delivery of potent opioid analgesic; indicated in patients with chronic pain requiring opioid analgesia
Nicotine	Habitrol (Basel Pharma)	Multilayer round patch: (*a*) aluminized backing film; (*b*) pressure-sensitive acrylate adhesive; (*c*) methacrylic acid copolymer solution of nicotine dispersed in pad of nonwoven viscose, cotton; (*d*) acrylate adhesive layer; (*e*) protective aluminized release liner that overlies adhesive layer, removed prior to use	Transdermal therapeutic systems providing continuous release, systemic delivery of nicotine to aid smoking cessation. Patches vary somewhat in nicotine content and dosing schedules
	NicoDerm CQ (Glaxo SmithKline)	Multilayer rectangular patch: (*a*) occlusive backing of polyethylene, aluminum, polyester, ethylene–vinyl acetate copolymer; (*b*) reservoir of nicotine in ethylene–vinyl acetate copolymer matrix; (*c*) rate-controlling polyethylene membrane; (*d*) polyisobutylene adhesive; (*e*) protective liner, removed prior to application	
	Nicotrol (Pharmacia)	Multilayer rectangular patch: (*a*) outer backing of laminated polyester film; (*b*) rate-controlling adhesive, nonwoven material, nicotine; (*c*) disposable liner, removed prior to use	
	Prostep (Wyeth)	Multilayer round patch: (*a*) beige foam tape, acrylate adhesive; (*b*) backing foil, gelatin, low-density polyethylene coating; (*c*) nicotine gel matrix; (*d*) protective foil with well; (*e*) release liner, removed prior to use	
Nitroglycerin	Deponit (UCB)	Three-layer system: (*a*) covering foil; (*b*) nitroglycerin matrix with polyisobutylene adhesive, plasticizer, release membrane; (*c*) protective foil, removed before use	
Nitroglycerin	Nitro-Dur (Key)	Nitroglycerin in gel-like matrix of glycerin water, lactose, polyvinyl alcohol, povidone, sodium citrate sealed in polyester, foil, polyethylene laminate	
Nitroglycerin	Transderm-Nitro (Summit)	Four-layer patch: (*a*) backing layer of aluminized plastic; (*b*) reservoir of nitroglycerin adsorbed on lactose, colloidal silicon dioxide, silicone medical fluid; (*c*) ethylene–vinyl acetate copolymer membrane; (*d*) silicone adhesive	

(continued)

TABLE 11.2. Examples of Transdermal Drug Delivery Systems (35–44) (*continued*)

Therapeutic Agent	TDDS	Design, Contents	Comments
Scopolamine	Transderm Scop (Baxter)	Four-layer patch: (*a*) backing layer of aluminized polyester film; (*b*) reservoir of scopolamine, mineral oil, polyisobutylene; (*c*) microporous polypropylene membrane for rate delivery of scopolamine; (*d*) adhesive of polyisobutylene, mineral oil, scopolamine	Continuous release of drug over 3 d to prevent nausea and vomiting of motion sickness. Patch is placed behind the ear. For repeated administration, the first patch is removed and second placed behind the other ear. Also approved to prevent nausea of certain anesthetics and analgesics used in surgery
Testosterone	Testoderm (Alza)	Three-layer patch: (*a*) backing layer of PET; (*b*) matrix film layer of testosterone, ethylene–vinyl acetate copolymer; (*c*) adhesive strips of polyisobutylene, colloidal silicon dioxide	Patch is placed on scrotum in treatment of testosterone deficiency
	Androderm (Watson)	Five-layer patch: (*a*) backing film of ethylene–vinyl acetate copolymer, polyester laminate; (*b*) reservoir of testosterone, alcohol, glycerin, glyceryl monooleate, methyl laurate gelled with acrylic acid copolymer; (*c*) microporous polyethylene membrane; (*d*) acrylic adhesive; (*e*) adhesive polyester laminate	Patch is placed on back, abdomen, upper arms, or thighs for treatment of testosterone deficiency

FIGURE 11.4. Four-layer therapeutic transdermal system showing the continuous and controlled amount of medication released from the system, permeating the skin, and entering the systemic circulation.

FIGURE 11.6. Nitro-Dur Transdermal Infusion System: Construction of the product. (Courtesy of Key Pharmaceuticals.)

FIGURE 11.5. The Transderm-Nitro Transdermal Therapeutic System (Summit). The patch delivers nitroglycerin through the skin directly into the bloodstream for 24 hours. Transderm-Nitro is used to treat and prevent angina. The system consists of a water-resistant backing layer, a reservoir of nitroglycerin, followed by a semipermeable membrane to control precisely and predictably the release of medicine, and an adhesive layer to hold the system onto the skin. The adhesive layer also contains an initial priming dose of nitroglycerin to ensure prompt release and absorption of the medication. (Courtesy of Summit Pharmaceuticals, Novartis.)

- 1) Film backing
- 2) Drug/adhesive layer
- 3) Protective liner

FIGURE 11.7. Two-layer TDDS, showing removal of the protective liner prior to application.

Monolithic systems incorporate a drug matrix layer between the backing and the frontal layers (Fig. 11.4). The drug matrix layer is composed of a polymeric material in which the drug is dispersed. The polymer matrix controls the rate at which the drug is released for percutaneous absorption. The matrix may be of two types, either with or without an excess of drug with regard to its equilibrium solubility and steady-state concentration gradient at the stratum corneum (21,45). In types having no excess, drug is available to maintain the saturation of the stratum corneum only as long as the level of drug in the device exceeds the solubility limit of the stratum corneum. As the concentration of drug in the device diminishes below the skin's saturation limit, the rate of drug transport from device to skin declines (45). In systems with excess drug in the matrix, a drug reserve is present to ensure continued saturation at the stratum corneum. In these instances, the rate of drug decline is less than in the type having no reserve.

In the preparation of monolithic systems, the drug and the polymer are dissolved or blended together, cast as the matrix, and dried (21). The gelled matrix may be produced in sheet or cylindrical form, with individual dosage units cut and assembled between the backing and frontal layers. Most TDDSs are designed to contain an excess of drug and thus have drug-releasing capacity beyond the time frame recommended for replacement. This ensures continuous drug availability and absorption as used TDDSs are replaced on schedule with fresh ones.

Membrane-controlled transdermal systems are designed to contain a drug reservoir, or pouch, usually in liquid or gel form; a rate-controlling membrane; and backing, adhesive, and protecting layers (Fig. 11.5).

Transderm-Nitro (Summit) and Transderm Scop (Baxter) are examples of this technology. Membrane-controlled systems have the advantage over monolithic systems in that as long as the drug solution in the reservoir remains saturated, the release rate of drug through the controlling membrane remains constant (21,22). In membrane systems, a small quantity of drug is frequently placed in the adhesive layer to initiate prompt drug absorption and pharmacotherapeutic effects on skin placement. Membrane-controlled systems may be prepared by preconstructing the delivery unit, filling the drug reservoir, and sealing or by lamination, a continuous process of construction, dosing, and sealing (Figs. 11.8 to 11.10).

In summary, either the drug delivery device or the skin may serve as the rate-controlling mechanism. If the drug is delivered to the stratum corneum at a rate less than the absorption capacity, the *device* is the controlling factor; if the drug is delivered to the skin area to saturation, the *skin* is the controlling factor. Thus, the rate of drug transport in all TDDSs, monolithic and membrane, is controlled by either artificial or natural (skin) membranes.

TDDSs may be constructed of a number of layers, including (*a*) an occlusive backing membrane to protect the system from environmental entry and from loss of drug

Adhesive layer

Rate-controlling membrane

Drug reservoir

Backing layer

FIGURE 11.9. Transdermal system reservoir containing a measured dose of drug in a matrix and a rate-controlling membrane.

FIGURE 11.8. Transdermal drug delivery adhesive coating line at ProSolus, Inc. (Courtesy of ProSolus, Inc.)

FIGURE 11.10. Equipment used in cutting and packaging transdermal drug delivery patches. Delta ModTech® transdermal manufacturing line. (Courtesy of Delta ModTech.)

from the system or moisture from the skin; (*b*) a drug reservoir or matrix system to store and release the drug at the skin site; (*c*) a release liner, which is removed before application and enables drug release; and (*d*) an adhesive layer to maintain contact with the skin after application. Two types of adhesive layers, the peripheral adhesive and the face adhesive, can be used. The peripheral adhesive contains adhesive around the outer edge of the TDDS, usually in a wide strip surrounding the active drug portion. The face adhesive, which covers the entire face of the TDDS, is very common. TDDSs are packaged in individual sealed packets to preserve and protect them until use.

The backing layer must be occlusive to retain skin moisture and hydrate the site of application, enabling increased drug penetration. Preferred backing materials are approximately 2 to 3 mm thick and have a low moisture vapor transmission rate, less than about 20 g/m² in 24 hours (46).

Transparent or pigmented films of polypropylene, polyethylene, and polyolefin are in use in TDDSs as backing liners.

The adhesive layer must be pressure sensitive, providing the ability to adhere to the skin with minimal pressure and remain in place for the intended period of wear. The adhesive should be nonirritating, allow easy peel-off after use, permit unimpeded drug flux to the skin, and be compatible with all other system components. The adhesive material is usually safety tested for skin compatibility, including tests for irritation, sensitivity, and cytotoxicity (47). In some TDDSs, the adhesive layer contains the drug. Polybutyl acrylate is commonly used as the adhesive in TDDSs. The drug release membranes are commonly made of polyethylene, with microporous structures of varying pore sizes to fit the desired specifications of the particular transdermal system.

Included among the design objectives of TDDSs are the following (2,8,45,48,49):

1. Deliver the drug to the skin for percutaneous absorption at therapeutic levels at an optimal rate
2. Contain medicinal agents having the necessary physicochemical characteristics to release from the system and partition into the stratum corneum
3. Occlude the skin to ensure one-way flux of the drug into the stratum corneum
4. Have a therapeutic advantage over other dosage forms and drug delivery systems
5. Not irritate or sensitize the skin
6. Adhere well to the patient's skin and have size, appearance, and site placement that encourage acceptance

See Physical Pharmacy Capsule 11.1 Formulating for Successful Transdermal/Topical Delivery for some example steps involved to produce an effective product.

PHYSICAL PHARMACY CAPSULE 11.1 Formulating for Successful Transdermal/Topical Delivery

The following are some example steps in formulating a successful transdermal/topical preparation. Obviously, not all drugs are suitable for application to the skin; however, many are suitable, and the list seems to be getting longer as we are seeing more and more manufactured as well as compounded transdermal/topical products/preparations. Let's look at some general guidelines.

1. Select an Appropriate Drug
   Passive drug delivery seems to be appropriate for small molecules with good lipophilicity and adequate aqueous solubility. Generally, one looks at 300 to 500 Da and a log partition coefficient (octanol/water) in the range of 1 to 3.5 and an aqueous solubility in excess of 100 µg/mL. A reasonable drug would have a "flux" in the range of about 1 mg/cm²/d so covering an area of about 10 cm² would deliver about 10 mg/d. One must keep in mind that first-pass hepatic metabolism is avoided, so dosing may not necessarily follow oral dosing regimens.

(continued)

2. Drug Flux Considerations

These data are sometimes available from published studies. If not, an estimate can be obtained using the Potts and Guy equation:

$$\text{Log } k_p = 0.71 \log P_{(oct/water)} - 0.0061 \text{ MW} - 2.74$$

Where K_p is the permeability coefficient (cm/h) through the stratum corneum, $P_{(oct/water)}$ is the octanol/water partition coefficient of the permeant, and MW is the molecular weight of the drug.

3. Maintain Saturation for Maximum Delivery

The driving force for permeation is the thermodynamic activity of the API in the vehicle. Maximum flux is generally obtained with the drug saturated in the vehicle. So, the drug should be at its solubility limit at about 32°C. Drug depletion over time resulting in nonsaturation can be addressed by adding a slight excess of drug in a suspended state.

4. Possibly Improve Drug Flux Using Formulation Manipulation

Vehicles that aid in skin hydration and solvents that also contain penetration-enhancing properties can improve drug flux. Also, specific penetration-enhancing excipients can be added to formulation to enhance flux and the amount of drug delivered through the skin. There are many excipients that can be used but should be selected after considering compatibility and stability issues.

5. A Volatile/Evaporating Vehicle Can Increase Finite Dose Delivery

The use of a vehicle/solvent that is volatile and evaporates after application to the skin will enhance drug concentration by producing a supersaturated solution and also may serve to modify the stratum corneum to aid drug passage. These vehicles may not be advisable for open lesions but tend to work well on intact skin. The "push" across the stratum corneum often results in a reservoir buildup of the drug for prolonged release.

6. After Penetrating the Skin, the Drug Molecule Tends to Continue Moving Following a Concentration Gradient or an Active Process

In the treatment of many skin disorders, it is desirable for the drug to stay just below the skin surface with little or no drug entering into the systemic circulation. Localizing or targeting drugs to specific skin regions or layers is not currently feasible; however, there are a couple of approaches that can be considered. Placing the drug in a liposomal carrier may help hold the drug closer to the surface and may even result in the liposomes entering hair follicles for prolonged release of the drug. Also, the use of a solvent that will aid in rapid penetration to form a reservoir and alter the penetration capabilities of the surrounding tissue may result in holding the drug at the surface. Last, the use of occlusive lipid vehicles may result in a slow partitioning of the drug into the superficial layers. ∎

ADVANTAGES AND DISADVANTAGES OF TDDSs

Among the advantages of TDDSs are the following:

1. They can avoid gastrointestinal drug absorption difficulties caused by gastrointestinal pH, enzymatic activity, and drug interactions with food, drink, and other orally administered drugs.

2. They can substitute for oral administration of medication when that route is unsuitable, as with vomiting and diarrhea.

3. They avoid the *first-pass effect*, that is, the initial pass of a drug substance through the systemic and portal circulation following gastrointestinal absorption, possibly decreasing the required daily dose for many drugs.

4. They are noninvasive, avoiding the inconvenience of parenteral therapy.

5. They provide extended therapy with a single application, improving compliance over other dosage forms requiring more frequent dose administration.

6. The activity of drugs having a short half-life is extended through the reservoir of drug in the therapeutic delivery system and its controlled release.

7. Drug therapy may be terminated rapidly by removal of the application from the surface of the skin.

8. They are easily and rapidly identified in emergencies (e.g., unresponsive, unconscious, or comatose patient) because of their physical presence, features, and identifying markings.

The disadvantages of TDDSs are as follows:

1. Only relatively potent drugs are suitable candidates for transdermal delivery because of the natural limits of drug entry imposed by the skin's impermeability.

2. Some patients develop contact dermatitis at the site of application from one or more of the system components, necessitating discontinuation.

EXAMPLES OF TRANSDERMAL DRUG DELIVERY SYSTEMS

The following sections briefly describe some of the TDDSs in use. Table 11.1 describes the specific design components of representative examples of these systems.

Transdermal Scopolamine

As noted at the outset of this chapter, transdermal scopolamine was the first TDDS to receive FDA approval. Scopolamine, a belladonna alkaloid, is used to prevent travel-related motion sickness and the nausea and vomiting that result from the use of certain anesthetics and analgesics used in surgery.

The Transderm Scop system is a circular flat patch 0.2 mm thick and 2.5 cm^2 in area (35). It is a four-layer system described in Table 11.1. The TDDS contains 1.5 mg of scopolamine and is designed to deliver approximately 1 mg of scopolamine at an approximately constant rate to the systemic circulation over the 3-day lifetime of the system. An initial priming dose of 200 µg of scopolamine in the adhesive layer of the system saturates the skin binding sites and rapidly brings the plasma concentration to the required steady-state level. The continuous release of scopolamine through the rate-controlling microporous membrane maintains the plasma level constant. The rate of release is less than the skin's capability for absorption, so the membrane, not the skin, controls the delivery of the drug into the circulation.

The patch is worn in a hairless area behind the ear. Because of the small size of the patch, the system is unobtrusive, convenient, and well accepted by the patient. The TDDS is applied at least 4 hours before the antinausea effect is required. Only one disk should be worn at a time and may be kept in place for up to 3 days. If continued treatment is required, a fresh disk is placed behind the other ear and the other removed. The most common side effects are dryness of the mouth and drowsiness. Particularly in the geriatric population, use also may interfere with orientation, cognition, and memory. The TDDS is not intended for use in children and should be used with caution during pregnancy.

Transdermal Nitroglycerin

A number of nitroglycerin-containing TDDSs have been developed, including Minitran (3M Pharmaceuticals), Nitro-Dur (Key), Transderm-Nitro (Summit), and Nitrodisc (Roberts). The design of each of these systems is briefly described in Table 11.1. Each of these products maintains nitroglycerin drug delivery for 24 hours after application. Tolerance, however, is a major factor limiting the effectiveness of these systems when used continuously for more than 12 hours per day. Hence, an appropriate dosing schedule would include a daily "patch on" period of 12 to 14 hours and a "patch off" period of 10 to 12 hours.

Nitroglycerin patches are used widely in the prophylactic treatment of angina. It has a relatively low dose, short plasma half-life, and is rapidly transported through skin, making it an excellent drug for transdermal delivery. It is rapidly metabolized by the liver when taken orally; this first-pass effect is bypassed by the transdermal route. The controlled rate of nitroglycerin absorption from a TDDS is intended to maintain moderate plasma levels and prevent angina attacks. Nitroglycerin sublingual products, on the other hand, achieve much higher plasma levels and are intended to stop an angina attack after it has started. The higher plasma levels are associated with greater intensity of side effects.

The various nitroglycerin TDDSs control the rate of drug delivery through a membrane and/or controlled release from the matrix or reservoir. When a TDDS is applied to the skin, nitroglycerin is absorbed continuously, resulting in active drug reaching the target organs (heart, extremities) before inactivation by the liver. Only a portion of the total nitroglycerin in the system is delivered over the usual 24-hour use period; the remainder serves as the thermodynamic energy source to release the drug and remains in the system. For example, in the Deponit TDDS (UCB), only 15% of the nitroglycerin content is delivered after 12 hours of use (36).

The rate of drug release depends on the system. In the Transderm-Nitro system, nitroglycerin 0.02 mg is delivered per hour for every square centimeter of patch, whereas in the Deponit system, each square centimeter delivers approximately 0.013 mg of nitroglycerin per hour (36,37). Systems of various surface areas and nitroglycerin content are provided to accommodate individual patients' requirements. Because of different release rates, these systems cannot be used interchangeably by a patient.

The Nitro-Dur matrix is in a highly kinetic equilibrium state (38). Dissolved nitroglycerin molecules are constantly exchanging with adsorbed nitroglycerin molecules bound to the surfaces of the suspended lactose crystals. Sufficient nitroglycerin is adsorbed to the lactose in each matrix to maintain nitroglycerin in the fluid phase (aqueous glycerol) at a stable but saturated level (5 mg nitroglycerin/cm^2 matrix). When the matrix is applied to the skin, nitroglycerin molecules migrate by diffusion from solution in the matrix to solution in the skin. To make up for the molecules lost to the body, the equilibrium in the matrix shifts such that more molecules of nitroglycerin leave the crystals than are adsorbed from solution. When balance is restored, the solution is again saturated. Thus, the crystals of lactose act as a reservoir of drug to maintain drug saturation in the fluid phase. The Nitro-Dur matrix in turn acts as a saturated reservoir for diffusive drug input through the skin (38).

Not all nitroglycerin systems have the same construction. For example, the Transderm-Nitro TDDS is a four-layer drug pouch system, as described in Table 11.1 and depicted in Figure 11.5, whereas the Deponit TDDS is a thin two-layer matrix system resembling that shown in Figure 11.7.

Patients should be given explicit instructions regarding the use of Nitroglycerin Transdermal Systems. Generally, these TDDSs are placed on the chest, back, upper arms, or shoulders (Fig. 11.11). The site should be free of hair, clean, and dry so that the patch adheres without difficulty. The use of the extremities below the knee or elbow is discouraged, as are the areas that are abraded or have lesions or cuts. The patient should understand that physical exercise and elevated ambient temperatures, such as in a sauna, may increase the absorption of nitroglycerin.

FIGURE 11.11. A Nitroglycerin Transdermal System that will deliver 0.4 mg/h (18 cm²) at a constant and predetermined rate through the skin directly into the bloodstream.

Transdermal Clonidine

The first transdermal system for hypertension, Catapres-TTS (clonidine *t*ransdermal *t*herapeutic *s*ystem, Boehringer Ingelheim), was marketed in 1985. Clonidine lends itself to transdermal delivery because of its lipid solubility, high volume of distribution, and therapeutic effectiveness in low plasma concentrations. The TDDS provides controlled release of clonidine for 7 days. The product is a four-layer patch as described in Table 11.1.

Catapres-TTS is available in several sizes, with the amount of drug released proportional to the patch size. To ensure constant release over the 7-day use period, the drug content is greater than the total amount of drug delivered. The energy of drug release derives from the concentration gradient between a saturated solution of drug in the TDDS and the much lower concentration prevailing in the skin. Clonidine flows in the direction of lower concentration at a constant rate controlled by a membrane (39).

The system is applied to a hairless area of intact skin on the upper outer arm or chest. After application, clonidine in the adhesive layer saturates the skin site. Then clonidine from the reservoir begins to flow through the rate-controlling membrane and the skin to the systemic circulation. Therapeutic plasma clonidine levels are achieved 2 to 3 days after initial application. Application of a new system to a fresh skin site at weekly intervals maintains therapeutic plasma concentrations. If the patch is removed and not replaced with a new system, therapeutic plasma clonidine levels will persist for about 8 hours and then decline slowly over several days. Over this period, blood pressure returns gradually to pretreatment levels. If the patient has local skin irritation before 7 days of use, the system may be removed and replaced with a new one applied on a fresh skin site (39).

Transdermal Nicotine

Nicotine TDDSs are used as adjuncts (e.g., along with counseling) in smoking cessation programs. They have been shown to be an effective aid in quitting smoking when used according to product-recommended strategies (50). In a blinded study, users of nicotine TDDSs are more than twice as likely to quit smoking as individuals wearing a placebo patch (50). Example products include NicoDerm CQ (GlaxoSmithKline), Nicotrol (Pharmacia), and Prostep (Wyeth).

The nicotine TDDSs provide sustained blood levels of nicotine as nicotine replacement therapy to help the patient establish and sustain remission from smoking (51). Motivation to quit smoking is enhanced through the reduction of withdrawal symptoms and by partially satisfying the nicotine craving and desired sensory feelings provided by smoking (51).

The commercially available patches contain 7 to 21 mg of nicotine for daily application during the course of treatment ranging from about 6 to 12 weeks. Different treatment regimens are used for light versus heavy smokers. Examples of nicotine TDDSs are described in Table 11.1. A nicotine TDDS usually is applied to the arm or upper front torso, with patients advised not to smoke when wearing the system. The TDDS is replaced daily, with sites alternated. Some of the nicotine replacement programs provide a gradual reduction in nicotine dosage (patch strength) during the treatment program. Used TDDSs should be discarded properly because the retained nicotine is poisonous to children and pets.

Transdermal Estradiol

The estrogen estradiol has been developed for transdermal delivery. The Estraderm (Novartis) TDDS delivers 17β-estradiol through a rate-limiting membrane continuously upon application to intact skin (40). Two systems (10 or 20 cm²) provide delivery of 0.05 or 0.1 mg estradiol per day. Estraderm is a four-layer TDDS as described in Table 11.1.

Estradiol is indicated for the treatment of moderate to severe vasomotor symptoms associated with menopause, female hypogonadism, female castration, primary ovarian failure, and atrophic conditions caused by deficient endogenous estrogen production, such as atrophic vaginitis and kraurosis vulvae.

Orally administered estradiol is rapidly metabolized by the liver to estrone and its conjugates, giving rise to higher circulating levels of estrone than estradiol. In contrast, the skin metabolizes estradiol only to a small extent. Therefore, transdermal administration produces therapeutic serum levels of estradiol with lower circulating levels of estrone and estrone conjugates than does oral therapy and requires a smaller total dose. Research results show that postmenopausal women receiving either transdermal or oral therapy will obtain the desired therapeutic effects, that is, lower gonadotropin levels, lower percentages of vaginal parabasal cells, decreased excretion of calcium, and lower ratio of calcium to creatinine, from both dosage forms. Studies have also demonstrated that systemic side effects from oral estrogens can be reduced by using the transdermal dosage form. Because estradiol has a short half-life (about 1 hour), transdermal administration allows a rapid decline in blood levels after the transdermal system is removed, as in a cycling regimen (40).

Therapy is usually administered on a cycling schedule (3 weeks of therapy followed by 1 week without), especially in women who have not undergone a hysterectomy. The transdermal system is applied to a clean, dry area of the skin on the trunk of the body, either the abdomen or upper quadrant of the buttocks. The patch should not be applied to the waistline because tight clothing may damage or dislodge it.

The Vivelle (Novartis) and Climara (Bayer Healthcare) estradiol TDDSs are two-layer matrix systems described in Table 11.1 and resembling that shown in Figure 11.7. The estradiol is contained in the adhesive layer (41,42). These systems are used in the same general manner as Estraderm TDDS; however, some of these systems are applied every 7 days.

Climara Pro Transdermal System (Bayer Healthcare) contains both estradiol and levonorgestrel in an adhesive-based matrix transdermal patch. The 22-cm^2 patch contains 4.5 mg estradiol and 11.39 mg of levonorgestrel; it delivers a daily dose of 0.045 mg of estradiol and 0.015 mg of levonorgestrel.

Transdermal Contraceptive System

The Ortho Evra (norelgestromin, ethinyl estradiol; Ortho-McNeil) Transdermal System is a combination contraceptive patch with a contact surface area of 20 cm^2; it contains 6 mg of norelgestromin and 0.75 mg of ethyl estradiol. It is released at a rate of norelgestromin 150 µg and ethinyl estradiol 20 µg into the blood stream every 24 hours. One patch is applied for 7 days for a total of 21 days per cycle, followed by 7 patch-free days per cycle.

The Ortho Evra is a thin matrix-type transdermal contraceptive patch consisting of three layers, including a two-ply backing layer composed of beige flexible film of low-density polyethylene and a polyester inner ply. The middle layer contains polyisobutylene and polybutene adhesive, crospovidone, nonwoven polyester fabric, and lauryl lactate as inactive components; the norelgestromin and ethinyl estradiol are in this layer. The third layer is the release liner that protects the adhesive layer during storage and is removed just prior to application. It is a transparent polyethylene terephthalate (PET) film with a polydimethylsiloxane coating on the side that is in contact with the middle layer.

Transdermal Testosterone

The testosterone transdermal systems Testoderm (Alza) and Androderm (Watson) are available with various delivery rates as hormone replacement therapy in men who have an absence or deficiency of testosterone (43,44).

The Testoderm TDDS is a two-layer system as described in Table 11.1. For optimal absorption, it is applied to clean, dry scrotal skin that has been dry shaved. Scrotal skin is reported to be at least five times as permeable to testosterone as other skin sites (43). The TDDS is placed on the scrotum by stretching the scrotal skin with one hand and pressing the adhesive side of the TDDS against the skin with the other hand, holding it in place for about 10 seconds. The TDDS is applied daily, usually in the morning to mimic endogenous testosterone release (52). Optimum serum levels are reached within 2 to 4 hours after application. The patch is worn 22 to 24 hours daily for 6 to 8 weeks.

The Androderm TDDS is designed to be applied nightly to a clean, dry, unabraded area of the skin of the back, abdomen, upper arms, or thighs. It should not be applied to the scrotum (44). The five-layer system is described in Table 11.1.

Transdermal Methylphenidate

Transdermal methylphenidate (Daytrana, Shire) is an adhesive-based matrix transdermal system applied to intact skin. The methylphenidate is dispersed in acrylic adhesive that is dispersed in a silicone adhesive. The composition per unit area is identical in all dosage strengths, and the total dose delivered is dependent on the patch size and wear time. It is available as 10-, 15-, 20-, and 30-mg patches nominally delivering the indicated dose over a 9-hour period. The 10-mg patch actually contains 27.5 mg of the drug, the 15-mg patch contains 41.3 mg, the 20-mg patch contains 55 mg, and the 30-mg patch contains 82.5 mg of the drug. After 9 hours, the patch is to be removed, folded in on itself (adhesive to adhesive), and appropriately discarded (52). There is a dose titration schedule that should be followed initially until the individualized final dosage and wear time are determined.

Usually, methylphenidate is indicated for attention deficit hyperactivity disorder in children. The advantage of the transdermal patch is that it can be applied in the morning 2 hours prior to the time the effect is needed, that is, at school, and removed later in the day after school. This obviates the need for oral medication to be administered during the day and trips to the school nurse's office. The patch should not be worn for more than 9 hours per day.

Other Transdermal Therapeutic Systems

Other transdermal therapeutic systems include the Oxytrol (oxybutynin chloride transdermal system, Watson), and additional drugs under study for use in TDDSs include diltiazem, isosorbide dinitrate, propranolol, nifedipine, mepindolol, and verapamil (cardiovascular agents);

levonorgestrel with estradiol for hormonal contraception; physostigmine and xanomeline for Alzheimer disease therapy; naltrexone and methadone for substance addiction; buspirone for anxiety; bupropion for smoking cessation; and papaverine for male impotence.

GENERAL CLINICAL CONSIDERATIONS IN THE USE OF TRANSDERMALS AND TDDSs

The patient should be advised of the following general guidelines along with product-specific instructions in the use of TDDSs (53,54) and quantities of transdermal gels to be applied to the body in Table 11.3.

1. Percutaneous absorption may vary with the site of application. The preferred general application site is stated in the package insert for each product. The patient should be advised of the importance of using the recommended site and rotating locations within that site. Rotating locations is important to allow the skin beneath a patch to regain its normal permeability after being occluded and to prevent skin irritation. Skin sites may be reused after a week.

2. TDDSs should be applied to clean, dry skin that is relatively free of hair and not oily, irritated, inflamed, broken, or callused. Wet or moist skin can accelerate drug permeation beyond the intended rate. Oily skin can impair adhesion of the patch. If hair is present at the intended site, it should be carefully cut; it should not be wet-shaved nor should a depilatory agent be used, because the latter can remove the outermost layers of the stratum corneum and affect the rate and extent of drug permeation.

3. Use of skin lotion should be avoided at the application site because lotions affect skin hydration and can alter the partition coefficient between the drug and the skin. Lotions may also make it difficult for the patch to adhere to the skin.

4. TDDSs should not be physically altered by cutting (as in an attempt to reduce the dose) because this destroys the integrity of the system.

5. A TDDS should be removed from its protective package, with care not to tear or cut into the unit. The protective backing should be removed to expose the adhesive layer with care not to touch the adhesive surface (which sometimes contains drug) to the fingertips. The TDDS should be pressed firmly against the skin site with the heel of the hand for about 10 seconds to ensure uniform contact and adhesion.

6. A TDDS should be placed at a site that will not subject it to being rubbed off by clothing or movement (as the belt line). TDDSs generally may be left on when showering, bathing, or swimming. Should a TDDS prematurely dislodge, an attempt may be made to reapply it or it may be replaced with a fresh system, the replacement being worn for a full period before it is replaced.

7. A TDDS should be worn for the full period stated in the product's instructions. Following that period, it should be removed and replaced with a fresh system as directed.

8. The patient or caregiver should be instructed to cleanse the hands thoroughly before and after applying a TDDS. Care should be taken not to rub the eyes or touch the mouth during handling of the system.

9. If the patient exhibits sensitivity or intolerance to a TDDS or if undue skin irritation results, the patient should seek reevaluation.

10. Upon removal, a used TDDS should be folded in half with the adhesive layer together so that it cannot be reused. The used patch, which contains residual drug, should be placed in the replacement patch's pouch and discarded in a manner safe to children and pets.

TABLE 11.3. Example Quantities of a Preparation for Application to a Patient (Consider Other Variables When Interpreting This Table)

Site	Approximate Quantity (g)
Face	1
Neck	1
Trunk (one side)	3
Arm	1.5
Hand (including fingers)	0.5
Palm (each)	0.25
Leg	3
Foot	1
Entire body	20–30

PATCHES (NOT SYSTEMS)

The Lidoderm (lidocaine; Endo) 5% patch consists of an adhesive material containing 5% lidocaine, which is applied to a nonwoven polyester felt backing and covered with a PET film release liner. The release liner is removed just prior to application. The patch is 10 × 14 cm, and each patch contains 700 mg of lidocaine in an aqueous base. The base contains dihydroxyaluminum aminoacetate, disodium edentate, gelatin, glycerin, kaolin, methylparaben, polyacrylic acid, polyvinyl alcohol, propylene glycol, propylparaben, sodium carboxymethylcellulose, sodium polyacrylate, D-sorbitol, tartaric acid, and urea. This product is indicated to treat postherpetic neuralgia. The patch is applied to intact skin to cover the most painful area. Depending upon the directions for use, the patient can apply up to three patches, only once for up to

12 hours within a 24-hour period. This patch may be cut with scissors into a smaller size prior to the removal of the release liner. The patient should wash his/her hands prior to and after handling the lidocaine patch and should avoid eye contact. After removal, the patch should be immediately disposed of, and in such a way as to avoid accidental exposure to children and animals. Lidoderm is not a transdermal product because the site of action is the skin immediately underneath the patch.

TAPES

A tape is a dosage form that is suitable for delivering drugs to the skin. It consists of a drug that is impregnated into a flexible, durable woven fabric or extruded synthetic material that is coated with an adhesive agent. Typically, the drug is present in the dry state. The adhesive layer is designed to retain the tape securely in place without the aid of additional bandaging. Tapes are not designed to control the release rate of the druglike transdermal patches. The active drug content is expressed as an amount per surface area with respect to the tape surface exposed to the skin. The use of an occlusive dressing over the tape enhances the rate and extent of delivery of the drug to deeper layers of the skin and may result in greater systemic absorption of the drug.

For administration, a portion of the tape slightly larger than the area to be treated is cut and removed from the backing paper. It should not be applied to folds in the skin but rather to a smooth skin surface. It should be applied to dry skin. An example product is shown in Figure 11.12.

EXAMPLES OF TRANSDERMAL PREPARATIONS

There are numerous transdermal products on the market that are commercially manufactured and many that are routinely compounded, as follows:

FIGURE 11.12. Cordran Tape commercial product.

Rx	Amitriptyline hydrochloride 2% in Pluronic Lecithin Organogel (PLO)		
	Amitriptyline hydrochloride		2 g
	Ethanol, 95%		5 mL
	Lecithin/isopropyl palmitate solution		22 mL
	Pluronic F-127 20% gel	qs	100 mL

Mix the amitriptyline hydrochloride with the alcohol to form a smooth paste. Add the lecithin:isopropyl palmitate solution and mix well. Add sufficient Pluronic F-127 gel to volume and mix well. Package and label.

Rx	Capsaicin 0.05% and Ketamine Hydrochloride 2% in PLO Gel		
	Capsaicin		50 mg
	Ketamine hydrochloride		2 g
	Ethanol, 95%		5 mL
	Lecithin/isopropyl palmitate solution		22 mL
	Pluronic F-127 20% gel	qs	100 mL

Mix the capsaicin and the ketamine hydrochloride with the alcohol to form a smooth paste. Add the lecithin:isopropyl palmitate solution and mix well. Add sufficient Pluronic F-127 gel to volume and mix well. Package and label.

PATIENT COUNSELING

Administering and Removing Patches

1. Wash the area where the patch is to be applied thoroughly with soap and warm water and pat dry.
2. If patches are to be replaced and used over a time period, rotate the application sites.
3. Explain the lag-time before the drug effect of the patch is noticed by a patient.
4. Remember to remove the old patch before applying a new one.
5. For disposal, after removal, fold the patch in half with the adhesive side in so it will seal closed and discard appropriately so that children cannot access. Do NOT flush.
6. Generally, bathing, showering, and swimming will not affect the patch, but it is best to avoid scrubbing the area.

PHARMACEUTICS CASE STUDY

SUBJECTIVE INFORMATION

Working at a large transdermal drug delivery company, you have been given the responsibility of developing an analgesic drug delivery system for use in patients with moderate to severe chronic pain. After development of several prototypes, one is selected that delivers the drug at a rapid rate for the first 12 hours and then at a zero-order rate over the next 36 hours. In clinical trials, however, patients who tended to sweat excessively had to use a new patch about every 6 to 12 hours, as the previous patch would not adhere. They were instructed that if the patch would not adhere after repeated attempts to reapply it, it was to be removed and a new patch applied. These patients had central nervous system depression and respiratory depression as compared to patients who could use a single patch over the 48-hour period. The patients who had to replace the patch early also had blood levels in the toxic range for the drug.

OBJECTIVE INFORMATION

The release rate of the TDDS was designed to provide a rapid onset of action by providing a high rate of drug transfer after application of the patch from the drug in the adhesive. This high rate of drug flux occurred with repeated application of each new patch. The analgesic

drug is highly lipophilic, and a very low dose (microgram range) is all that is required.

ASSESSMENT

There was an initial loading dose of the drug in the adhesive layer and a combination of penetration enhancers in the matrix of the TDDS, including alcohol. The lipophilic nature of the drug apparently resulted in a depot effect of the drug in the fatty tissue of the skin. The drug rapidly moved from the adhesive layer and was followed by the movement of active drug in solution in the alcohol and other penetration enhancers. After the alcohol was depleted in the TDDS matrix, the flux of drug slowed to a near-zero-order release.

PLAN

Available options include changing the formulation and adding a label caution statement. Changing the formulation would require extensive changes and new in vitro, animal, and clinical studies. A labeling statement could warn against application of a new patch for a preselected time period, such as approximately 12 hours after removal of a patch that would not adhere if it had been applied for less than 24 hours. This would allow for a depletion of the drug buildup in the skin. ■

CLINICAL CASE STUDY

A.R. is a 20-year-old BF who comes into the pharmacy with concerns because she has missed the last two birth control tablets in the 2nd week of her cycle. She says, "It's so hard to remember to take the pill every night." She is a student at a local junior college, and her irregular work schedule seems to be the major contributing factor to her lack of adherence. She expresses concern about the possibility of becoming pregnant and asks for your advice.

PMH:	Noncontributory
SH:	(+) Smoker (~1 PPD)
	Exercises 3 days per week
FH:	Father (+) DM type 2
	Grandmother (+) ovarian cancer
MEDS:	Ibuprofen 400 mg po prn cramps
	Ortho Tri-Cyclen 1 tablet po qd

PHARMACEUTICAL CARE PLAN

S: Lack of adherence to birth control pill regimen

O: Smoker

Grandmother (+) ovarian cancer

Father (+) DM type 2

A: A.R. is a 20-year-old BF with a history of lack of adherence to her oral contraceptive regimen. She is a student with an irregular schedule. A.R. smokes about a pack of cigarettes per day and has a family history of diabetes mellitus and ovarian cancer.

P: 1. Suggest to the patient that she contact her physician to change her prescription from an oral contraceptive tablet to a transdermal birth control patch, Ortho Evra.

(continued)

CLINICAL CASE STUDY *(continued)*

2. Assuming that the physician concurs and prescribes Ortho Evra, inform the patient that the patch is applied once a week for 3 consecutive weeks, followed by 1 week that is patch free. This should help her compliance because she will have to remember to change the patch only once weekly. However, it will be good to have her write a reminder down somewhere to change the patch on the same day each week.

   She should not write the date on the patch. It is important for A.R. to know that she should remove the old patch before applying the new patch.
3. When changing over from her oral contraceptive tablet to the TDDS, she should understand to apply the first patch on the first day of her menstrual period. The patch can be applied to her abdomen, buttocks, upper torso (front or back, except the breasts), and upper outer arm. The patient can rotate the placement of the patch to a different location each week. However, this is not necessary.
4. The patch is to be applied to clean, dry skin. There should be no body lotion or oils on the skin where the patch will be applied. A.R. can shower, bathe, exercise, and swim while the patch is in place. If the patch gets loose or falls off <24 hours after application, the patient can reapply it or get a replacement patch at the pharmacy. If a replacement patch is applied, the patient must replace it with the next patch on the original patch change day. However, if it is beyond 24 hours since the initial application of that patch, the patient must start her cycle all over. That is, the patient will start a new 4-week cycle with a new patch change day. In that case, the patient must use backup contraceptive measures, such as condom, spermicide, or diaphragm, for the first week.

5. The patient should be made aware that smoking increases her risk of heart problems, such as blood clots, stroke, and heart attacks, when using a hormonal contraceptive product. A.R. should be encouraged to quit smoking. If the patient agrees that she would like to quit, be prepared to suggest a local wellness program where she can get help and support. Most importantly, to have an opportunity to quit smoking, she has to make a firm commitment to want to stop smoking.
6. Monitoring: Because the patient has a family history of ovarian cancer, she should be strongly encouraged to have annual Pap smears. In addition, the patient should be advised to continue to exercise regularly and increase her frequency to 4 or 5 days per week. An increase in exercise and a well-balanced diet will be advantageous in the prevention of diabetes mellitus type 2, as her family demonstrates a history of this disease. ■

APPLYING THE PRINCIPLES AND CONCEPTS

GROUP ACTIVITIES

1. Compare and contrast transdermal drug delivery to other forms of drug delivery.
2. Compare and contrast the official USP monographs of the clonidine transdermal system and the nicotine transdermal system.
3. Describe special handling, storage, and disposal precautions a patient must take when using a transdermal delivery system.
4. List five counseling points for proper administration of a transdermal nitroglycerin system.
5. Create a listing of conceivable ways a consumer/patient might misuse a TDDS.

INDIVIDUAL ACTIVITIES

1. Create a table of six transdermal products including amount of active ingredient(s), indication, contraindication, adverse effects/precautions, and dosage.
2. Generate a listing of drugs whose physical–chemical characteristics make them a candidate for incorporation into a transdermal dosage form. Hint: start with drugs that have a low oral dose or have high first-pass metabolism.
3. From the primary literature, find a clinical drug study demonstrating a comparison between a transdermal delivery system and another route of delivery for the drug in terms of clinical effectiveness, and determine which delivery system would be preferred in terms of patient acceptance, patient adherence, bioequivalence, and cost. Explain the rationale for your decision.

REFERENCES

1. Stoughton RD. Percutaneous absorption. Toxicol Appl Pharmacol 1965;7:1–8.
2. Black CD. Transdermal drug delivery systems. US Pharma 1982;1:49.
3. Osborne DW, Amann AH. Topical Drug Delivery Formulations. New York, NY: Marcel Dekker Inc., 1990.
4. Walters KA. Percutaneous absorption and transdermal therapy. Pharm Technol 1986;10:30–42.

5. Hadgraft J. Structure activity relationships and percutaneous absorption. J Control Release 1991;25:221–226.

6. Ghosh TK, Banga AK. Methods of enhancement of transdermal drug delivery, part I: Physical and biochemical approaches. Pharm Technol 1993;17:72–98.

7. Surber C, Wilhelm KP, Hori M, et al. Optimization of topical therapy: Partitioning of drugs into stratum corneum. Pharm Res 1990;7:1320–1324.

8. Cleary GW. Transdermal Concepts and Perspectives. Miami, FL: Key Pharmaceuticals, 1982.

9. Melendres JL, Bucks DA, Camel E, et al. In vivo percutaneous absorption of hydrocortisone: Multiple-application dosing in man. Pharm Res 1992;9:1164.

10. Smith EW, Maibach HI, eds. Percutaneous Penetration Enhancers. New York, NY: CRC Press, 1995.

11. Idson B. Percutaneous absorption. J Pharm Sci 1975;64:901–924.

12. Shah VP, Peck CC, Williams RL. Skin penetration enhancement: Clinical pharmacological and regulatory considerations. In: Walters KA, Hadgraft J, eds. Pharmaceutical Skin Penetration Enhancement. New York, NY: Marcel-Dekker, 1993.

13. Osborne DW, Henke JJ. Skin penetration enhancers cited in the technical literature. Pharm Technol 1997;21:50–66.

14. Idson B. Percutaneous absorption enhancers. Drug Cosmetic Ind 1985;137:30.

15. Rolf D. Chemical and physical methods of enhancing transdermal drug delivery. Pharm Technol 1988;12:130–139.

16. Ghosh TK, Banga AK. Methods of enhancement of transdermal drug delivery, part IIA: Chemical permeation enhancers. Pharm Technol 1993;17:62–90.

17. Ghosh TK, Banga AK. Methods of enhancement of transdermal drug delivery, part IIB: Chemical permeation enhancers. Pharm Technol 1993;17:68–76.

18. Riviere JE, Monteiro-Riviere NA, Inman AO. Determination of lidocaine concentrations in skin after transdermal iontophoresis: Effects of vasoactive drugs. Pharm Res 1992;9:211–219.

19. Green PG, Hinz RS, Cullander C, et al. Iontophoretic delivery of amino acids and amino acid derivatives across the skin in vitro. Pharm Res 1991;8:1113–1120.

20. Choi HK, Flynn GL, Amidon GL. Transdermal delivery of bioactive peptides: The effect of n-decylmethyl sulfoxide, pH, and inhibitors on enkephalin metabolism and transport. Pharm Res 1990;7:1099–1106.

21. D'Emanuele A, Staniforth JN. An electrically modulated drug delivery device III: Factors affecting drug stability during electrophoresis. Pharm Res 1992;9:312–315.

22. Bommannan D, Okuyama H, Stauffer P, et al. Sonophoresis I: The use of high-frequency ultrasound to enhance transdermal drug delivery. Pharm Res 1992;9:559–564.

23. Bommannan D, Menon GK, Okuyama H, et al. Sonophoresis II: Examination of the mechanism(s) of ultrasound-enhanced transdermal drug delivery. Pharm Res 1992;9:1043–1047.

24. Shah VP, Flynn GL, Guy RH, et al. In vivo percutaneous penetration/absorption. Pharm Res 1991;8:1071–1075.

25. Bronaugh RL, Stewart RF, Congdon ER. Methods for in vitro percutaneous absorption studies II. Animal models for human skin. Toxicol Appl Pharmacol 1982;62:481–488.

26. Nugent FJ, Wood JA. Methods for the study of percutaneous absorption. Can J Pharm Sci 1980;15:1–7.

27. Addicks W, Weiner N, Flynn G, et al. Topical drug delivery from thin applications: Theoretical predictions and experimental results. Pharm Res 1990;7(10):1048–1054.

28. Kushla GP, Zatz JL. Evaluation of a noninvasive method for monitoring percutaneous absorption of lidocaine in vivo. Pharm Res 1990;7:1033–1037.

29. Chaisson D. Dissolution performance testing of transdermal systems. Dissolution Technol 1995;2:8–11.

30. Itoh T, Magavi R, Casady RL, et al. A method to predict the percutaneous permeability of various compounds: Shed snake skin as a model membrane. Pharm Res 1990;7:1302–1306.

31. Itoh T, Wasinger L, Turunen TM, et al. Effects of transdermal penetration enhancers on the permeability of shed snakeskin. Pharm Res 1992;9:1168–1172.

32. Rolland A, Demichelis G, Jamoulle JC, et al. Influence of formulation, receptor fluid, and occlusion on in vitro drug release from topical dosage forms, using an automated flow-through diffusion cell. Pharm Res 1992;9:82–86.

33. United States Pharmacopeia–National Formulary. Current Ed. Rockville, MD: U.S. Pharmacopeial Convention.

34. Microette Transdermal Diffusion Cell Autosampling System. Chatsworth, CA: Hanson Research, 1992.

35. Transderm-Scop Transdermal Therapeutic System: Professional Literature. Summit, NJ: Novartis Consumer Pharmaceuticals, 2010.

36. Deponit Nitroglycerin Transdermal Delivery System: Professional Literature. Milwaukee, WI: Schwarz Pharma, 2006.

37. Transderm-Nitro Transdermal Therapeutic System: Professional Literature. East Hanover, NJ: Novartis Pharmaceuticals, 2006.

38. Nitro-Dur Transdermal Infusion System: Professional Literature. Kenilworth, NJ: Key Pharmaceuticals, 2004.

39. Catapres-TTS: Professional Literature. Ridgefield, CT: Boehringer Ingelheim Pharmaceuticals, 2008.

40. Estraderm Estradiol Transdermal System: Professional Literature. East Hanover, NJ: Novartis Pharmaceuticals, 2005.

41. Vivelle Estradiol Transdermal System: Professional Literature. East Hanover, NJ: Novartis Pharmaceuticals, 2004.

42. Climara Estradiol Transdermal System: Professional Literature. Wayne, NJ: Bayer Healthcare, 2009.

43. Testoderm Testosterone Transdermal System: Professional Literature. Palo Alto, CA: Alza Pharmaceuticals, 2005.

44. Androderm Testosterone Transdermal System: Professional Literature. Corona, CA: Watson Pharmaceuticals, 2006.

45. Good WR. Transdermal drug-delivery systems. Med Device Diagnost Ind 1986;8:37–42.

46. Godbey KL. Development of a novel transdermal drug delivery backing film with a low moisture vapor transmission rate. Pharm Technol 1997;21:98–107.

47. 3M Transdermal Drug Delivery Components. St. Paul, MN: 3M, 1996.

48. Fara JW. Short- and long-term transdermal drug delivery systems. In: Drug Delivery Systems. Springfield, OR: Aster, 1983:33–40.

49. Shaw JE, Chadrasekaran SK. Controlled topical delivery of drugs of systemic action. Drug Metab Rev 1978;8:223.

50. Fiore MC, Smith SS, Jorenby DE, et al. The effectiveness of the nicotine patch for smoking cessation. JAMA 1994;271:1940–1947.

51. Wongwiwatthananukit S, Jack HM, Popovich NG. Smoking cessation, part 2: Pharmacologic approaches. J Am Pharm Assoc 1998;38:339–353.

52. Levien T, Baker DE. Reviews of transdermal testosterone and liposomal doxorubicin. Hosp Pharm 1996;31:973–988.

53. Black CD. A Pharmacist's Guide to the Use of Transdermal Medication. Washington, DC: American Pharmaceutical Association, 1996.

54. Berba J, Banakar U. Clinical efficacy of current transdermal drug delivery systems: A retrospective evaluation. Am Pharm 1990;NS30:33–41.

SECTION FIVE

Suppositories, Inserts, and Medication Sticks

Suppositories, Inserts, and Medication Sticks

CHAPTER AT A GLANCE Suppositories • Uses and Applications • Some Factors of Drug Absorption from Rectal Suppositories • Suppository Bases • Formulation Variables • Preparation of Suppositories • Manufacturing Suppositories • Quality Control • Packaging and Storage • Stability • Rectal Suppositories • Urethral Suppositories • Vaginal Inserts • Vaginal Inserts (Tablets) • Medication Sticks • Special Types of Suppositories • Clinical Considerations • Patient Counseling

OBJECTIVES

After reading this chapter, the student will be able to:

Compare and contrast various suppository, insert, and stick dosage forms in terms of physical appearance, size, and shape

Describe the advantages and disadvantages of suppository, insert, and stick drug delivery versus oral drug delivery

Identify and explain physiologic factors that influence the drug absorption from rectal suppository and vaginal/urethral insert administration

Identify and explain the physicochemical factors of the drug and suppository/insert base as these influence absorption

Compare and contrast the various classes of suppository/insert/stick bases

Describe the three methods of suppository/insert/stick preparation

Generate a listing of key counseling points a pharmacist should share with the patient prescribed a drug in a suppository/insert/stick drug delivery system

▌SUPPOSITORIES

The use of rectal suppositories has been documented since the civilization of Ancient Egypt, but in modern society, suppositories have not gained the level of acceptability, respect, and usage as most other dosage forms. However, much work has been conducted in recent years as evidenced by the literature citations; in the past 50 years, there have been over 4,000 citations in Medline (1). Even though much work has been done in Europe, in the United States, and elsewhere, there continues to be a tendency away from rectal delivery for routine administration of drugs. Urethral administration of suppositories has become more acceptable with urethral suppositories in the treatment of male erectile dysfunction (Muse-Vivus).

Suppositories are used more routinely in southern European countries and in Latin American countries, as compared to northern European and Anglo-Saxon countries. In the United States, less than 1% of drugs are formulated as suppositories; in Germany, it may be as high as 5% (2). In the past 5 to 10 years in the United States, progesterone vaginal inserts have become much more widely used by postmenopausal women. Hormone replacement therapy in postmenopausal women using bioidentical hormones, or those that are identical to those hormones produced by the body as compared to synthetic or semisynthetic hormones, is more popular in the treatment of postmenopausal symptoms (flushing, night sweats, mood swings, etc.) (3).

Although suppositories are not very popular as a mode of administering drugs, this dosage form will probably always have a place in medicine. Suppositories generally have been employed for three reasons:

1. To promote defecation
2. To introduce drugs into the body
3. To treat anorectal diseases

Rectal administration is not often the first route of choice, but it becomes a good alternative when the oral route is inadvisable. Relatively low cost and lack of technical difficulties make rectal drug administration attractive when compared to parenteral therapy. The downside of rectal administration includes the esthetics and stigma of violating the patient's dignity; these, along with potential rectal irritation due to frequent administration and difficulty in titrating a correct dose due to limited strengths of commercial suppositories, pose some challenges.

In treating hospice patients, rectally administered medications are essential in palliative medicine. Properly selected drugs and suppository vehicles can enhance the quality of life of these patients. A suppository is also an excellent dosage form for those patients to whom one does not want to administer numerous injections daily. They are also a dosage form that can be administered to avoid nausea and vomiting caused by certain medications upon oral administration, and it is a dosage form that can often result in a fast onset of action (4). Compounding pharmacists often view suppositories as a way to meet individual patient needs when other routes of administration are not really appropriate. This is especially true for pediatric and hospice patients (4).

Definitions

A suppository is a solid dosage form in which one or more active pharmaceutical ingredients (APIs) are dispersed in a suitable base and molded or otherwise formed into a suitable shape for insertion into the rectum to provide local or systemic effect. Upon administration, suppositories melt, soften, or dissolve and exert local or systemic effects. The derivation of the word *suppository* is from the Latin *supponere*, meaning "to place under," as derived from *sub* (under) and *ponere* (to place) (4). Thus, suppositories are meant both linguistically and therapeutically to be placed under the body, as into the rectum.

An insert is a solid dosage form that is inserted into a naturally occurring (nonsurgical) body cavity other than the mouth or rectum, including the vagina and urethra.

Medication sticks are a convenient form for administering topical drugs. Their development is interesting because it involves the history of cosmetics, which parallels human history.

Suppository, Insert, and Stick Shapes

Suppositories have various shapes and weights; the shape and size of a suppository must be such that it can be easily inserted into the intended orifice without causing undue distension, and once inserted, it must be retained for the appropriate period. Rectal suppositories are inserted with the fingers, but certain vaginal inserts (and tablets prepared by compression) may be inserted high in the tract with the aid of an appliance.

Rectal suppositories are usually about 32 mm (1.5 inch) long, are cylindrical, and have one or both ends tapered. Some rectal suppositories are shaped like a bullet, a torpedo, or the little finger. Depending on the density of the base and the medicaments in the suppository, the weight may vary. Adult rectal suppositories weigh about 2 g when cocoa butter (theobroma oil) is employed as the base. Rectal suppositories for use by infants and children are about half the weight and size of the adult suppositories and assume a more pencil-like shape.

Vaginal inserts, formerly called suppositories *or pessaries*, are usually globular, oviform, or cone shaped and weigh about 5 g when cocoa butter is the base. However, depending on the base and the manufacturer's product, the weights of vaginal inserts may vary widely.

Urethral inserts, also called bougies, are slender, pencil-shaped suppositories intended for insertion into the male or female urethra. Male urethral suppositories may be 3 to 6 mm in diameter and approximately 140 mm long, although this may vary. When cocoa butter is employed as the base, these suppositories weigh about 4 g. Female urethral suppositories are about half the length and weight of the male urethral suppository, being about 70 mm long and weighing about 2 g when made of cocoa butter.

Medication sticks are cylindrical in shape and generally range from 5 to 25 g. They are generally packaged in an applicator tube for topical administration, and the applicator can be adjusted to continually expose new, fresh stick from inside the tube.

❚ USES AND APPLICATIONS

Examples of commonly used official suppositories and inserts are presented in Figure 12.1 and Tables 12.1 to 12.3. It is now well accepted that many active ingredients can be administered rectally and achieve therapeutic blood levels. Some medications are best administered by this route, whereas others can be if needed.

Suppositories containing drugs such as aspirin and opiates for pain, ergotamine tartrate for treating migraine headaches, and many other drugs for other uses are commonly used as suppositories. These drugs are intended to be absorbed into the general circulation to provide systemic drug effects. Other examples of suppositories given for systemic results include diazepam, metronidazole, progesterone, aminophylline, morphine, prochlorperazine, chlorpromazine, thiethylperazine, indomethacin, diclofenac, ketoprofen, naproxen, and ondansetron.

The advantages of rectal administration include the following:

1. First-pass effect: Avoiding, at least partially, the first-pass effect that may result in higher blood levels for those drugs subject to extensive first-pass metabolism upon oral administration.

FIGURE 12.1. **A:** Close-up of a commercial adult rectal suppository. (Courtesy of Eric Schulz, English Wikipedia.) **B:** An example of a commercial pediatric rectal suppository. (Courtesy of C.B. Fleet Company, Inc.)

A

B

2. Drug stability: Avoiding the breakdown of certain drugs that are susceptible to gastric degradation.
3. Large-dose drugs: Ability to administer somewhat larger doses of drugs than using oral administration.
4. Irritating drugs: Ability to administer drugs that may have an irritating effect on the oral or gastrointestinal mucosa when administered orally.
5. Unpleasant tasting or smelling drugs: Ability to administer unpleasant tasting or smelling drugs whose oral administration is limited.
6. In children, the rectal route is especially useful. An ill child may refuse oral medication and may fear injections.
7. In patients experiencing nausea and vomiting or when the patient is unconscious.
8. The presence of disease of the upper gastrointestinal tract that may interfere with drug absorption.
9. Objectionable taste or odor of a drug (especially important in children).
10. Achievement of a rapid drug effect systemically (as an alternate to injection).

Rectal administration provides for a rapid and, in many cases, extensive absorption of the active ingredient. The rapidity, intensity, and duration of action are three parameters that must be considered during formulation for rectal administration and, in many cases, can be altered to meet the needs of the individual patient.

The disadvantages of suppositories and the reasons given for the infrequent use of suppositories include the following.

1. A perceived lack of flexibility regarding dosage of commercially available suppositories resulting in underuse and a lack of availability.
2. If suppositories are made on demand, they may be expensive.
3. Suppositories as a dosage form are safe, but they exhibit variable effectiveness, depending upon many factors to be discussed later, including the pathology of the anorectal lesions.
4. Different formulations of a drug with a narrow therapeutic margin, such as aminophylline, cannot be interchanged without risk of toxicity.
5. The "bullet-shaped" suppository after insertion can leave the anorectal site and ascend to the rectosigmoid and descending colon. Hence, one may consider that suppositories with this shape possibly should not be used at bedtime.
6. Defecation may interrupt the absorption process of the drug; this may especially occur if the drug is irritating.

TABLE 12.1. Examples of Rectal Suppositories

Suppository	Commercial Product	Active Constituent	Type of Effect	Category and Comments
Bisacodyl	Dulcolax (Boehringer Ingelheim)	10 mg	Local	Cathartic. Base: hydrogenated vegetable oil
Hydrocortisone	Anusol-HC (Salix)	25 mg	Local	Pruritus ani, inflamed hemorrhoids, other inflammatory conditions of the anorectum. Base: hydrogenated glycerides
Hydromorphone	Dilaudid (Purdue Pharma)	3 mg	Systemic	Analgesic. Base: cocoa butter with silicon dioxide
Indomethacin	Indocin (Iroko)	50 mg	Systemic	Anti-inflammatory. Base: polyethylene glycols
Mesalamine	Canasa (Axcan Scandipharm)	500 mg	Local	Anti-inflammatory. Base: hard fat
Promethazine HCl	Phenergan (Wyeth)	12.5, 25 mg	Systemic	Antihistamine, antiemetic, sedative: used to manage allergic conditions; preoperative or postoperative sedation or nausea and vomiting; motion sickness. Base: cocoa butter, white wax

TABLE 12.2. Examples of Vaginal Inserts and Tablets

Product (Manufacturer)	Active Constituents	Category and Comments
Cleocin inserts (Pfizer)	Clindamycin phosphate 100 mg	Bacterial vaginosis
Monistat 7 inserts (Personal products)	Miconazole nitrate 100 mg	Antifungal for local vulvovaginal candidiasis (moniliasis)
Semicid vaginal contraceptive inserts (Whitehall-Robins)	Nonoxynol 9 100 mg	Nonsystemic reversible birth control
Encare contraceptive inserts (Blairex Laboratories)	Nonoxynol 9 100 mg	Nonsystemic reversible birth control

7. The absorbing surface area of the rectum is much smaller than that of the small intestine.

8. The fluid content of the rectum is much less than that of the small intestine, which may affect dissolution rate, etc.

9. There is the possibility of degradation of some drugs by the microflora present in the rectum.

10. The dose of a drug required for rectal administration may be greater than or less than the dose of the same drug given orally. This can be dependent upon such factors as the constitution and condition of the patient, the physicochemical nature of the drug and its ability to traverse the physiologic barriers to absorption, and the nature of the suppository vehicle and its capacity to release the drug and make it available for absorption.

11. The factors that affect the rectal absorption of a drug administered in the form of a suppository may be divided into two main groups: (*a*) anatomic and physiologic factors and (*b*) physicochemical factors of the drug and the base.

TABLE 12.3. Official Suppositories and Inserts in the USP

Acetaminophen

Aminophylline

Aspirin

Bisacodyl

Chlorpromazine

Ergotamine tartrate and caffeine

Glycerin

Indomethacin

Miconazole nitrate vaginal

Morphine sulfate

Nystatin vaginal

Oxymorphone hydrochloride

Prochlorperazine

Progesterone vaginal

Promethazine hydrochloride

Thiethylperazine maleate

Local Action

Once inserted, the suppository base melts, softens, or dissolves, distributing its medicaments to the tissues of the region. These medicaments may be intended for retention within the cavity for local effects, or they may be intended to be absorbed for systemic effects. Rectal suppositories intended for local action are most frequently used to relieve constipation or the pain, irritation, itching, and inflammation associated with hemorrhoids or other anorectal conditions. Antihemorrhoidal suppositories frequently contain a number of components, including local anesthetics, vasoconstrictors, astringents, analgesics, soothing emollients, and protective agents. A popular laxative, glycerin suppositories promote laxation by local irritation of the mucous membranes, probably by the dehydrating effect of the glycerin on those membranes. Vaginal suppositories or inserts intended for local effects are employed mainly as contraceptives, as antiseptics in feminine hygiene, and as specific agents to combat an invading pathogen. Most commonly, the drugs used are nonoxynol 9 for contraception, trichomonacides to combat vaginitis caused by *Trichomonas vaginalis*, antifungals to treat *Candida* (*Monilia*) *albicans*, and anti-infectives/antibiotics directed at other microorganisms. Urethral suppositories may be antibacterial or a local anesthetic preparative for a urethral examination.

Sticks are commonly used for local effect and include hydration/emollient, antibacterial, sunscreen, antipruritic, and other uses.

Systemic Action

For systemic effects, the mucous membranes of the rectum and vagina permit the absorption of many soluble drugs. Although the rectum is used frequently as the site for the systemic absorption of drugs, the vagina is not as frequently used for this purpose.

Examples of drugs administered rectally in the form of suppositories for their systemic effects include (*a*) prochlorperazine and chlorpromazine for the relief of nausea and vomiting and as a tranquilizer; (*b*) morphine and oxymorphone for opioid analgesia; (*c*) ergotamine tartrate for the relief of migraine syndrome; (*d*) indomethacin, a nonsteroidal anti-inflammatory analgesic and antipyretic; and (*e*) ondansetron for the relief of nausea and vomiting.

■ SOME FACTORS OF DRUG ABSORPTION FROM RECTAL SUPPOSITORIES

The dose of a drug administered rectally may be greater than or less than the dose of the same drug given orally, depending on such factors as the constitution of the patient, the physicochemical nature of the drug and its ability to traverse the physiologic barriers to absorption, and the nature of the suppository vehicle and its capacity to release the drug and make it available for absorption.

Table 12.4 contains a list of some drugs that are absorbed better rectally as compared to orally, some that are absorbed better orally as compared to rectally, and some cases where the oral and rectal doses are comparable. In some cases, the doses are different, for example, lincomycin or chloral hydrate requires four times the dose rectally as compared to orally, and empirically, phenytoin requires about three times the dose rectally as compared to orally.

Physiological Factors and Drug Effect

Among the physiologic factors that affect drug absorption from the rectum are the circulation route, colonic contents, and the pH and lack of buffering capacity of the rectal fluids.

Circulation Route

Unlike drugs absorbed after oral administration, drugs absorbed rectally can bypass the portal circulation during their first pass into the general circulation. This enables drugs that are otherwise destroyed in the liver to exert systemic effects. The lower hemorrhoidal veins surrounding the colon receive the absorbed drug and initiate its circulation throughout the body, bypassing the liver. Lymphatic circulation also assists in the absorption of rectally administered drugs.

TABLE 12.4. Examples of Drugs with Different Optimal Routes of Administration

Absorbed better rectally than orally	Sodium salicylate
	Chloral hydrate
	Methylene blue
	Atropine, morphine
Absorbed better orally than rectally	Iodides
	Tetracycline hydrochloride
	Sodium penicillin G
Oral and rectal absorptions comparable	Sulfanilamide in a glycerinated gelatin base
	Prednisone

From Allen LV Jr. Suppositories. London, UK: Pharmaceutical Press, 2008:52.

pH and Lack of Buffering Capacity of the Rectal Fluids

The pH of the rectal fluid is generally in the range of 7.2 to 7.4, and it has negligible buffer capacity. The form in which the drug is administered will not generally be chemically changed by the rectal environment; therefore, the pH of the medium may be determined by the characteristics of the drug.

Rectal The last few inches of the large intestine constitute the rectum, terminating at the anus. The rectum contains three types of hemorrhoidal veins:

• Superior hemorrhoidal vein
• Middle hemorrhoidal vein
• Inferior hemorrhoidal vein

These veins act by transporting the active principle absorbed in the rectum to the blood system either directly by means of iliac veins and the vena cava (inferior and middle hemorrhoidal veins) or indirectly by means of the portal vein and the liver (superior hemorrhoidal vein).

The three hemorrhoidal veins are linked by an anastomosis network. Because it is not really possible to predict the position or exact location of the suppository in the rectum, it is not really possible to predict exactly which way the active principle will be transported. It may be preferably by one pathway or another or a combination. However, it is generally accepted that at least 50% to 70% of the active ingredients administered rectally take the direct pathway, thus bypassing the liver and avoiding the first-pass effect. There is also the possibility of absorption into the lymphatic vessels that should not be dismissed, but may be minimal.

Vaginal The vagina is a specialized organ whose primary function is reproduction. It is a highly elastic muscular tube, located between the urethra and the rectum. It has three tissue layers: epithelial tissue, loose connective tissue, and muscle tissue. The upper, middle, and lower vaginal sections have separate blood supplies. Branches of the uterine arteries supply blood to the upper vagina; the inferior vesical arteries supply blood to the middle portion of the vagina, and the hemorrhoidal and internal pudendal arteries feed into the lower vagina. Blood is returned through the venous plexus to the hemorrhoidal, pudendal, and uterine veins and then to the hypogastric veins. The pH of the vagina is in the range of about 4 to 4.5. It is moistened and cleansed daily by secretions that also serve to lubricate the vaginal tract. Normal vaginal discharge consists of about 1.5 g of vaginal fluid daily. This fluid occurs as an odorless, clear or white, and viscous or sticky fluid. This normal physiologic fluid consists of endocervical mucus, serum transudate from vaginal capillary beds, endogenous vaginal flora, and epithelial cells.

Urethra The urethral epithelium begins as transitional cells as it exits the bladder. Further along the urethra, there are stratified columnar cells and then stratified squamous cells near the external meatus (exit hole). There are small mucus-secreting urethral glands that help protect the epithelium from the corrosive urine. The female urethra is supplied by blood vessels called the internal pudendal and vaginal arteries. The male urethra is supplied by the inferior vesical and middle rectal arteries. The veins follow these blood vessels. The nerve supply is via the pudendal nerve.

Colonic Content

When systemic effects are desired from the administration of a medicated suppository, greater absorption may be expected from a rectum that is void than from one that is distended with fecal matter. A drug will obviously have greater opportunity to make contact with the absorbing surface of the rectum and colon in the absence of fecal matter. Therefore, when deemed desirable, an evacuant enema may be administered and allowed to act before the administration of a suppository of a drug to be absorbed. Other conditions such as diarrhea, colonic obstruction due to tumorous growths, and tissue dehydration can all influence the rate and degree of drug absorption from the rectal site.

Physicochemical Factors and Drug Effect

Physicochemical factors include such properties as the relative solubility of the drug in lipid and in water and the particle size of a dispersed drug. Physicochemical factors of the base include its ability to melt, soften, or dissolve at body temperature; its ability to release the drug substance; and its hydrophilic or hydrophobic character.

Lipid–Water Solubility

The lipid–water partition coefficient of a drug (discussed in Chapter 4) is an important consideration in the selection of the suppository base and in anticipating drug release from that base. A lipophilic drug that is distributed in a fatty suppository base in low concentration has less tendency to escape to the surrounding aqueous fluids than does a hydrophilic substance in a fatty base. Water-soluble bases—for example, polyethylene glycols (PEGs)—that dissolve in the anorectal fluids release for absorption water-soluble and oil-soluble drugs. Naturally, the more drug a base contains, the more drug will be available for absorption. However, if the concentration of a drug in the intestinal lumen is above the drug's solubility, the rate of absorption is not changed by a further increase in the concentration of the drug.

Particle Size

For undissolved drugs in a suppository, the size of the drug particle will influence its rate of dissolution and its availability for absorption. As indicated many times previously, the smaller the particle, the greater the surface area, the more readily the dissolution of the particle, and the greater the chance for rapid absorption.

Whenever the active principle has a limited water solubility, the use of finely divided products (high specific surface area) often leads to an appreciable absorption improvement. This is especially important for suppositories because the volume available for drug dissolution is very small. Here, as well as in oral medication absorption, the rate of absorption is influenced by the solubilization rate, which in turn is related to the particle size of the active principle.

It is preferable to avoid a too fine particle size, especially for high-dose drugs, because excessively small particles can raise the viscosity of the melted formulation and cause difficulties in flow during production.

▌ SUPPOSITORY BASES

Analogous to the ointment bases, suppository bases play an important role in the release of the medication they hold and, therefore, in the availability of the drug. Of course, one of the first requisites for a suppository base is that it should remain solid at room temperature but soften, melt, or dissolve readily at body temperature so that the drug is fully available soon after insertion. Certain bases are more efficient in drug release than others. For instance, cocoa butter (theobroma oil) melts quickly at body temperature, but because it is immiscible with body fluids, fat-soluble drugs tend to remain in the oil and have little tendency to enter the aqueous physiologic fluids. For water-soluble drugs in cocoa butter, the reverse is usually true and good release results. Fat-soluble drugs seem to be released more readily from bases of glycerinated gelatin or PEG, both of which dissolve slowly in body fluids. When irritation or inflammation is to be relieved, as in the treatment of anorectal disorders, cocoa butter appears to be the superior base because of its emollient or soothing, spreading action.

Nature of the Base

As previously discussed, the base must be capable of melting, softening, or dissolving to release its drug for absorption. If the base interacts with the drug to inhibit its release, drug absorption will be impaired or even prevented. Also, if the base irritates the mucous membranes of the rectum, it may initiate a colonic response and prompt a bowel movement, eliminating the prospect of complete drug release and absorption.

Because of the possibility of chemical and/or physical interactions between the medicinal agent and the suppository base, which may affect the stability and/or bioavailability of the drug, the absence of any drug interaction between the two agents should be ascertained before or during formulation.

Long-acting or slow-release suppositories have also been prepared. Morphine sulfate in slow-release suppositories is prepared in a base that includes a material such as alginic acid, which will prolong the release of the drug over several hours (5,6).

Classification of Bases

For most purposes, it is convenient to classify suppository bases according to their physical characteristics into two main categories and a third miscellaneous group: (*a*) fatty or oleaginous bases, (*b*) water-soluble or water-miscible bases, and (*c*) miscellaneous bases, generally combinations of lipophilic and hydrophilic substances.

A suppository base should be physically and chemically stable, nonirritating, nontoxic, nonsensitizing, chemically and physiologically inert, compatible with a variety of drugs, stable during storage, and esthetically acceptable (free from objectionable odor and a pleasing appearance). It should contract slightly on cooling to release itself from the mold with requiring mold lubricants, has wetting and emulsifying properties, has a high water number, and can be manufactured by molding by hand, machine, compression, or extrusion. It should melt or dissolve in rectal fluids and should not bind or otherwise interfere with the release or absorption of drug substances.

Other desirable characteristics depend upon the drugs to be added. For example, bases with higher melting points can be used to incorporate drugs that generally lower the melting points of the base (e.g., camphor, chloral hydrate, menthol, phenol, thymol, and volatile oils) or to formulate suppositories for use in tropical climates. Bases with lower melting points can be used when adding materials that will raise the melting points or when adding large amounts of solids. Examples of different types of suppository bases and their melting ranges are shown in Table 12.5. Additional characteristics of importance in selecting a suppository base can include the following: acid value, iodine value, saponification value, and hydroxyl value (7).

Fatty or Oleaginous Bases

Fatty bases are perhaps the most frequently employed suppository bases, principally because cocoa butter is a member of this group of substances. Among the other fatty or oleaginous materials used in suppository bases are many hydrogenated fatty acids of vegetable oils, such as palm kernel oil and cottonseed oil. Also, fat-based compounds containing compounds of glycerin with the higher molecular weight fatty acids, such as palmitic and stearic acids,

may be found in fatty bases. Glyceryl monostearate and glyceryl monopalmitate, are examples of this type of agent. The bases in many commercial products employ varied combinations of these types of materials to achieve the desired hardness under conditions of shipment and storage and the desired quality of submitting to the temperature of the body to release their medicaments. Some bases are prepared with the fatty materials emulsified or with an emulsifying agent present to prompt emulsification when the suppository makes contact with the aqueous body fluids. These types of bases are arbitrarily placed in the third, or miscellaneous, group of bases.

Cocoa Butter, NF, is the fat obtained from the roasted seed of *Theobroma cacao*. At room temperature, it is a yellowish-white solid having a faint, agreeable chocolate-like odor. Chemically, it is a triglyceride (combination of glycerin and one or different fatty acids) primarily of oleopalmitostearin and oleodistearin. Because cocoa butter melts at 30°C to 36°C (86°F to 97°F), it is an ideal suppository base, melting just below body temperature and yet maintaining its solidity at usual room temperatures. However, because of its triglyceride content, cocoa butter exhibits marked *polymorphism* or existence in several crystalline forms. Because of this, when cocoa butter is hastily or carelessly melted at a temperature greatly exceeding the minimum required temperature and is then quickly chilled, the result is a metastable crystalline form (alpha crystals) with a melting point much lower than that of the original cocoa butter. In fact, the melting point may be so low that the cocoa butter will not solidify at room temperature. However, because the crystalline form is a metastable condition, there is a slow transition to the more stable *beta* form of crystals having the greater stability and a higher melting point. This transition may require several days. Consequently, if suppositories that have been prepared by melting cocoa butter for the base do not harden soon after molding, they will be useless to the patient and a loss of time, materials, and prestige to the pharmacist. Cocoa butter must be slowly and evenly melted, preferably over a bath of warm water, to avoid formation of the unstable crystalline form and ensure retention in the liquid of the more stable *beta* crystals that will constitute nuclei upon which the congealing may occur during chilling of the liquid.

TABLE 12.5. Melting Ranges of some Suppository Bases

Base	Composition	Melting Range (°C)
Cocoa butter	Mixed triglycerides of oleic, palmitic, and stearic acids	34–35
Fattibase	Triglycerides from palm, palm kernel, and coconut oils with self-emulsifying glyceryl monostearate and polyoxyl stearate	35.5–37
Polybase	A homogeneous blend of PEGs and polysorbate 80	60–71
Suppocire OSI	Eutectic mixtures of mono-, di-, and triglycerides derived from natural vegetable oils, each type having slightly different properties	33–35
Wecobee W	Triglycerides derived from coconut oil	31.7–32.8
Witepsol H15	Triglycerides of saturated fatty acids C12–C18 with varied portions of the corresponding partial glycerides	33–35

Substances such as phenol and chloral hydrate have a tendency to lower the melting point of cocoa butter. If the melting point is low enough that it is not feasible to prepare a solid suppository using cocoa butter alone as the base, solidifying agents like cetyl esters wax (about 20%) or beeswax (about 4%) may be melted with the cocoa butter to compensate for the softening effect of the added substance. However, the addition of hardening agents must not be so excessive as to prevent the base from melting in the body, nor must the waxy material interfere with the therapeutic agent in any way so as to alter the efficacy of the product.

Other bases in this category include commercial products such as Fattibase (triglycerides from palm, palm kernel, and coconut oils with self-emulsifying glyceryl monostearate and polyoxyl stearate), the Wecobee bases (triglycerides derived from coconut oil), and Witepsol bases (triglycerides of saturated fatty acids C12–C18 with varied portions of the corresponding partial glycerides).

Water-Soluble and Water-Miscible Bases

The main members of this group are glycerinated gelatin and PEGs. Glycerinated gelatin suppositories may be prepared by dissolving granular gelatin (20%) in glycerin (70%) and adding water or a solution or suspension of the medication (10%). A glycerinated gelatin base is most frequently used in the preparation of vaginal suppositories, with which prolonged local action of the medicinal agent is usually desired. The glycerinated gelatin base is slower to soften and mix with the physiologic fluids than is cocoa butter and therefore provides a slower release.

Because glycerinated gelatin–based suppositories have a tendency to absorb moisture as a result of the hygroscopic nature of glycerin, they must be protected from atmospheric moisture if they are to maintain their shape and consistency. Also as a result of the hygroscopicity of the glycerin, the suppository may have a dehydrating effect and irritate the tissues upon insertion. The water in the formula for the suppositories minimizes this action; however, if necessary, the suppositories may be moistened with water prior to insertion to reduce the initial tendency of the base to draw water from the mucous membranes and irritate the tissues.

Urethral suppositories may be prepared from a glycerinated gelatin base of a formula somewhat different from the one indicated earlier. For urethral suppositories, the gelatin constitutes about 60% of the weight of the formula, the glycerin about 20%, and the medicated aqueous portion about 20%. Urethral suppositories of glycerinated gelatin are much more easily inserted than are those with a cocoa butter base owing to the brittleness of cocoa butter and its rapid softening at body temperature.

Various combinations of these PEGs may be combined by fusion, using two or more of the various types to achieve a suppository base of the desired consistency and characteristics. PEGs are polymers of ethylene oxide and water prepared to various chain lengths, molecular weights, and physical states. They are available in a number of molecular weight ranges, the most commonly used being PEG 300, 400, 600, 1,000, 1,500, 1,540, 3,350, 4,000, 6,000, and 8,000. The numeric designations refer to the average molecular weight of each of the polymers. PEGs having average molecular weights of 300, 400, and 600 are clear, colorless liquids. Those having average molecular weights of greater than 1,000 are waxlike white solids whose hardness increases with an increase in the molecular weight. Melting ranges, for example, PEGs, are PEG 300 (−15°C to 18°C), PEG 1000 (37°C to 40°C), PEG 3350 (54°C to 58°C), and PEG 8000 (60°C to 63°C).

Pharmacists have been called on in recent years to prepare progesterone vaginal suppositories extemporaneously. These suppositories, used in premenstrual syndrome, are commonly molded with either a PEG base or a fatty acid base. Formulas for these suppositories are presented later in this chapter.

PEG suppositories do not melt at body temperature but rather dissolve slowly in the body's fluids. Therefore, the base need not be formulated to melt at body temperature. Thus, it is possible, in fact routine, to prepare suppositories from PEG mixtures having melting points considerably higher than body temperature. This property permits a slower release of the medication from the base once the suppository has been inserted and permits convenient storage of these suppositories without need for refrigeration and without danger of their softening excessively in warm weather. Further, their solid nature permits slow insertion without fear that they will melt in the fingertips (as cocoa butter suppositories sometimes do). Because they do not melt at body temperature but mix with mucous secretions upon dissolution, PEG-based suppositories do not leak from the orifice, as do many cocoa butter–based suppositories. PEG suppositories that do not contain at least 20% water should be dipped in water just before use to avoid irritation of the mucous membranes after insertion. This procedure prevents moisture being drawn from the tissues after insertion and the stinging sensation.

Poloxamers (Pluronics) are water-soluble, block copolymers with a wide range of uses. Pluronics L44, L62, L64, and F68 are potential suppository bases. The poloxamers have practically no odor or taste. They have surfactant properties and may solubilize some drugs in the rectal fluid. This property can help solid drugs dissolve more quickly in vivo. An example of an aspirin suppository using a poloxamer base uses the following formula:

Pluronic F68	6.00 g
Pluronic L44	7.00 mL
Aspirin	1.02 g

To prepare, the poloxamers were placed in a beaker on a water bath and heated until they melted. The aspirin was added and the mixture stirred until uniform. The solution is placed in a mold and allowed to cool, and the suppositories are removed. The authors summarized that the Pluronic-base aspirin suppository should be further tested in clinical situations (8).

FORMULATION VARIABLES

Formulation variables that are generally considered include (*a*) the nature and form of the active principle (esters, salts, complexes, etc.); (*b*) the physical state, particle dimensions, and the specific surface of the product; (*c*) the solubility of the drug in various bases; (*d*) the presence or absence of adjuvants added to the active principle; (*e*) the nature and type of dosage form in which the active principle is incorporated; and (*f*) pharmaceutical procedures used in the preparation of the dosage form.

Active drugs have a number of physical characteristics. In suppositories, those of interest involve the drug's physical state, particle size, solubility, dielectric constant, and bulk density. Some of these have been discussed in detail in other chapters.

Physical State

An active drug can be a solid, liquid, or semisolid in nature. For solids, the drug's particle size may be very important, especially if the drug is not very water soluble; the increase in surface area resulting from decreased particle size can serve to enhance its activity. For liquids, it is necessary to take up the liquid into the suppository base using one of several techniques such as forming an emulsion, adding a drying powder, or adding a suitable thickening agent when the liquid is mixed with the suppository base. For the semisolids or paste-type drugs, it can be either mixed with a solid that will serve to thicken the drug prior to mixing with the base or mixed with the base to which a thickener is added.

Particle Size

If a drug is readily soluble, the influence of particle size may be minimal. For highly water-soluble drugs, the tendency will be to dissolve and migrate to the rectal mucosa. For poorly water-soluble drugs, the dissolution rate will be slower, and a reduction in particle size may increase the rate of dissolution by exposing a greater surface area. This can also be affected by the nature of the suppository base.

Solubility

Increased solubility of the active ingredient in the base can improve product homogeneity; however, it may also delay the release of the active if there is too great an affinity of the drug for the suppository vehicle.

If the active ingredient is insoluble in the base, as is the case when a "suspension" or "emulsion" is formed, this poses different problems. It is necessary to maintain homogeneity of the total mixture; this can usually be obtained by constant agitation of the mixture during processing and filling. Oftentimes, it is best to select a temperature just above the melting point of the suppository mixture where the mixture is thick but still pourable.

Viscosity

Viscosity considerations are also important in the preparation of the suppositories and the release of the drug. If the viscosity of a base is low, it may be necessary to add a suspending agent such as silica gel to ensure that the drug is uniformly dispersed until solidification occurs. When preparing the suppository, the pharmacist should stir the melt constantly and keep it at the lowest possible temperature to maintain a high viscosity. After the suppository has been administered, the release rate of the drug may be slowed if the viscosity of the base is very high. This is because the viscosity causes the drug to diffuse more slowly through the base to reach the mucosal membrane for absorption.

Brittleness

Brittle suppositories can be difficult to handle, wrap, and use. Cocoa butter suppositories are usually not brittle unless the percentage of solids present is high. In general, brittleness results when the percentage of nonbase materials exceeds about 30%. Synthetic fat bases with high stearate concentrations or those that are highly hydrogenated are typically more brittle. Shock cooling also causes fat and cocoa butter suppositories to crack. This condition can be prevented by ensuring that the temperature of the mold is as close to the temperature of the melted base as possible. Suppositories should not be placed in a freezer, which also causes shock cooling.

Volume Contraction

Bases, excipients, and active ingredients generally occupy less space at lower temperatures than at higher temperatures. When preparing a suppository, the pharmacist pours hot melt into a mold and allows the melt to cool. During this cooling process, the melt has a tendency to contract in size. This makes it easier to release the suppository from the mold, but it may also produce a cavity or deep indentation at the back, or open end, of the mold. Such a cavity is undesirable and can be prevented if the melt is permitted to approach its congealing temperature immediately before it is poured into the mold. It is advisable to pour a small amount of excess melt at the open end of the mold to allow for the slight contraction during cooling. Scraping with a blade or spatula dipped in warm water will remove the excess after solidification, but care must be taken not to remove the metal from the mold. The heated instrument can also be used to smooth out the back of the suppository.

Drug Release Rates

General approximate drug release rates as they relate to the drug and base characteristics are summarized as follows:

Drug: Base Characteristics	Approximate Drug Release Rate
Oil-soluble drug: Oily base	Slow release; poor escaping tendency
Water-soluble drug: Oily base	Rapid release
Oil-soluble drug: Water-miscible base	Moderate release
Water-miscible drug: Water-miscible base	Moderate release; based on diffusion; all water soluble

Special Problems

Some active drugs are more difficult to incorporate in a base and require additional preparation steps. Before vegetable extracts are added, they can be moistened by levigation with a small amount of melted base. This makes it easier to distribute the active drug throughout the base.

Hard, crystalline materials can be incorporated either by pulverizing them to a fine state or by dissolving them in a small quantity of solvent, which is then taken up into the base. An aqueous solvent and a PEG base are appropriate for water-soluble materials. Alternatively, if the material is water soluble and an oily base must be used, wool fat could be used to take up the solution for incorporation into the suppository base.

When liquid ingredients are mixed with an inert powder such as starch, they become less fluid, which makes them easier to handle. The suppository produced will thus hold together better.

There are several ways of incorporating excess powder into a suppository base, depending on the base used. If the base is oil miscible, one can add a few drops of a bland oil like mineral oil. When excess powder is incorporated into water-soluble bases, the pharmacist can vary the ratio of low to high melting point ingredients. For example, because additional powders will make the suppository harder, using a higher percentage of a PEG having a low molecular weight would result in a suppository of the proper character.

A number of ingredients are incompatible with PEG bases, including benzocaine, iodochlorhydroxyquin, sulfonamides, ichthammol, aspirin, silver salts, and tannic acid. Other materials reported to have a tendency to crystallize out of PEG include sodium barbital, salicylic acid, and camphor. PEG-based suppositories may be irritating to some patients. Suppositories prepared with PEG should not be stored or dispensed in a polystyrene prescription vial, as the PEG will adversely interact with polystyrene. All PEG suppositories should be dispensed in glass or cardboard containers.

Triglyceride-type bases can sometimes accept up to about 50% glycerin without much difficulty. Some solids may be dissolved in water or solidified with Aerosil (nanoparticulate silicon dioxide) prior to incorporation. Fluid extracts can be incorporated at about 35°C to 38°C into an emulsifiable triglyceride base. Ichthammol and Peru balsam can be mixed with an equal amount of castor oil prior to incorporation. Essential oils can be incorporated without difficulty in small amounts. Larger amounts may result in lowering the melting point of the suppository, so a higher melting point suppository base may be required. Because of the volatile nature of the essential oils, they must be incorporated at the lowest possible temperature. Inert materials, such as lactose, magnesium carbonate of highly dispersed silicon dioxide, can be used to sorb the essential oils prior to incorporation. Lipophilic drugs with melting points higher than that of the base can be incorporated by suspending these drugs in PEG 200 to 400 to a total amount of about 10%, based on the amount of triglyceride base used. Fat bloom (a whitish discoloration) that can occur on the surface of suppositories can be minimized by the addition of lecithin to the suppository base.

PREPARATION OF SUPPOSITORIES

Suppositories are prepared by two methods: (*a*) *molding* from a melt and (*b*) *hand rolling* and *shaping*. The method most frequently employed both on a small scale and on an industrial scale is molding.

Molding

The steps in molding include (*a*) melting the base, (*b*) incorporating any required medicaments, (*c*) pouring the melt into molds, (*d*) allowing the melt to cool and congeal into suppositories, and (*e*) removing the formed suppositories from the mold. Cocoa butter, glycerinated gelatin, PEG, and most other bases are suitable for preparation by molding.

Suppository Molds

Commercially available molds can produce individual or large numbers of suppositories of various shapes and sizes. Individual plastic molds may be obtained to form a single suppository. Other molds, such as those most commonly found in the community pharmacy, are capable of producing 6, 12, or more suppositories in a single operation (Fig. 12.2). Industrial molds produce hundreds of suppositories from a single batch (Figs. 12.3 and 12.4).

Molds in common use today are made from stainless steel, aluminum, brass, or plastic. The molds, which separate into sections, generally longitudinally, are opened for cleaning before and after preparation of a batch of suppositories, closed when the melt is poured, and opened again to remove the cold, molded suppositories. Care must be exercised in cleaning the molds, as any scratches on the molding surfaces will take away from the desired smoothness of the suppositories. Plastic molds are especially prone to scratching.

FIGURE 12.2. Adjustable suppository mold capable of producing up to 100 torpedo-shaped suppositories in a single molding. (Courtesy of Gallipot, Inc.)

FIGURE 12.3. Large heated tanks for preparation of the melt in commercial production of suppositories by molding. (Courtesy of Wyeth-Ayerst Laboratories.)

Although satisfactory reusable and disposable molds are commercially available for preparation of rectal, vaginal, and urethral suppositories, if necessary, temporary molds may be successfully formed by pressing heavy aluminum foil about an object having the shape of the desired suppository, then carefully removing the object, and filling the shaped foil with the melt. For instance, glass stirring rods may be used to form molds for urethral suppositories, round pencils or pens may be used to form molds for rectal suppositories, and any cone-shaped object may be used to form vaginal suppositories.

Lubrication of the Mold

Depending on the formulation, suppository molds may require lubrication before the melt is poured to facilitate clean and easy removal of the molded suppositories. Lubrication is seldom necessary when the base is cocoa

FIGURE 12.4. Automated large-scale production of molded suppositories prepared and packaged in strips. (BP-2 suppository filler courtesy of Dott. Bonapace—Italy.)

butter or PEG, as these materials contract sufficiently on cooling to separate from the inner surfaces and allow easy removal. Lubrication is usually necessary with glycerinated gelatin. A thin coating of mineral oil applied with the finger to the molding surfaces usually suffices. However, no material that might irritate the mucous membranes should be employed as a mold lubricant.

Calibration of the Mold

Each individual mold is capable of holding a specific volume of material in each of its openings. Because of the difference in the densities of the materials, if the base is cocoa butter, the weight of the suppositories will differ from the weight of suppositories prepared in the same mold with a base of PEGs. Similarly, any added medicinal agent alters the density of the base, and the weight of the resulting suppository differs from that of those prepared with base material alone.

The pharmacist should calibrate each suppository mold for the usual base (generally cocoa butter and a PEG base) so as to prepare medicated suppositories each having the proper quantity of medicaments.

The first step in calibration of a mold is to prepare molded suppositories from base material alone. After removal from the mold, the suppositories are weighed, and the total weight and average weight of each suppository are recorded (for the particular base used). To determine the volume of the mold, the suppositories are carefully melted in a calibrated beaker, and the volume of the melt is determined for the total number as well as for the average of one suppository.

Determination of the Amount of Base Required

In the prescription for medicated suppositories to be prepared extemporaneously by the pharmacist, the prescribing physician indicates the amount of medicinal substance desired in each suppository but leaves the amount of base to the discretion of the pharmacist. Generally, in preparing such prescriptions, the pharmacist calculates the amounts of materials needed for the preparation of one or two more suppositories than the number prescribed to compensate for the inevitable loss of some material and to ensure having enough material.

In determining the amount of base to be incorporated with the medicaments, the pharmacist must be certain that the required amount of drug is provided in each suppository. Because the volume of the mold is known (from the determined volume of the melted suppositories formed from the base), the volume of the drug substances subtracted from the total volume of the mold will give the volume of base required. If the added amounts of medicaments are slight, they may be considered to be negligible, and no deduction from the total volume of base may be deemed necessary. However, if considerable quantities of other substances are to be used, the volumes of these materials are important and should be used to calculate the amount of base actually required to fill the mold. The total volume of these materials is subtracted from the volume of the mold, and the appropriate amount of base is added. Because the bases are solid at room temperature, the volume of base may be converted to weight from the density of the material. For example, if 12 mL of cocoa butter is required to fill a suppository mold and if the medicaments in the formula have a collective volume of 2.8 mL, 9.2 mL of cocoa butter will be required. By multiplying 9.2 mL times the density of cocoa butter, 0.86 g/mL, it may be calculated that 7.9 g of cocoa butter will be required. After adjusting for the preparation of an extra suppository or two, the calculated amount is weighed.

Another method for determination of the amount of base in the preparation of medicated suppositories requires the following steps: (*a*) weigh the active ingredient for the preparation of a single suppository; (*b*) dissolve it or mix it (depending on its solubility in the base) with a portion of melted base insufficient to fill one cavity of the mold and add the mixture to a cavity; (*c*) add additional melted base to the cavity to fill it completely; (*d*) allow the suppository to congeal and harden; and (*e*) remove the suppository from the mold and weigh it. The weight of the active ingredients subtracted from the weight of the suppository yields the weight of the base. This amount of base multiplied by the number of suppositories to be prepared in the mold is the total amount of base required.

A third method is to place all of the required medicaments for the preparation of the total number of suppositories (including one extra) in a calibrated beaker, add a portion of the melted base, and incorporate the drug substances. Then add sufficient melted base to reach the required volume of mixture based on the original calibration of the volume of the mold.

A summary of density calculations for molding of suppositories is found in Physical Pharmacy Capsule 12.1.

Preparing and Pouring the Melt

Using the least possible heat, the weighed suppository base material is melted, generally over a water bath, because not a great deal of heat is required. A porcelain casserole, that is, a dish with a pouring lip and a handle, is perhaps the best utensil, because it later permits convenient pouring of the melt into the cavities of the mold. Usually, medicinal substances are incorporated into a portion of the melted base by mixing on a glass or porcelain tile with a spatula. After incorporation, this material is stirred into the remaining base, which has been allowed to cool almost to its congealing point. Any volatile materials or heat-labile substances should be incorporated at this point with thorough stirring.

The melt is poured carefully and continuously into each cavity of the mold, which has been previously equilibrated to room temperature. If any undissolved or suspended materials in the mixture are denser than the base, so that they have a tendency to settle, constant stirring, even during pouring, is required, else the last filled cavity will contain a disproportionate share of the undissolved materials. The solid materials remain suspended if the pouring is performed just above the congealing point and not when the base is too fluid. If the melt is not near the congealing point when poured, the solids may settle within each cavity of the mold to reside at the tips of the suppositories, with the result that the suppositories may be broken when removed from the mold. Alternatively, a small quantity of silica gel (about 25 mg per suppository) can be incorporated into the formula to aid in keeping the active drug suspended. In filling each suppository cavity, the pouring must be continuous to prevent *layering*, which may lead to a product easily broken on handling. To ensure a completely filled mold upon congealing, the melt is poured excessively over each opening, actually rising above the level of the mold. The excessive material may form a continuous ribbon along the top of the mold above the cavities. This use of extra suppository material prevents formation of recessed dips in the ends of the suppositories

PHYSICAL PHARMACY CAPSULE **12.1** Density (Dose Replacement) Calculations for Suppositories

In preparation of suppositories, it is generally assumed that if the quantity of active drug is less than 100 mg, then the volume occupied by the powder is insignificant and need not be considered. This is usually based on a 2-g suppository weight. Obviously, if a suppository mold of less than 2 g is used, the powder volume may need to be considered.

The density factors of various bases and drugs need to be known to determine the proper weights of the ingredients to be used. Density factors relative to cocoa butter have been determined. If the density factor of a base is not known, it is simply calculated as the ratio of the blank weight of the base and cocoa butter. Density factors for a selected number of ingredients are shown in the below table.

(continued)

PHYSICAL PHARMACY CAPSULE **12.1** Density (Dose Replacement) Calculations for Suppositories *(continued)*

Alum	1.7	Morphine HCl	1.6
Aminophylline	1.1	Opium	1.4
Aspirin	1.3	Paraffin	1.0
Barbital	1.2	Peruvian balsam	1.1
Belladonna extract	1.3	Phenobarbital	1.2
Benzoic acid	1.5	Phenol	0.9
Bismuth carbonate	4.5	Potassium bromide	2.2
Bismuth salicylate	4.5	Potassium iodide	4.5
Bismuth subgallate	2.7	Procaine	1.2
Bismuth subnitrate	6.0	Quinine HCl	1.2
Boric acid	1.5	Resorcinol	1.4
Castor oil	1.0	Sodium bromide	2.3
Chloral hydrate	1.3	Spermaceti	1.0
Cocaine HCl	1.3	Sulfathiazole	1.6
Digitalis leaf	1.6	Tannic acid	1.6
Glycerin	1.6	White wax	1.0
Ichthammol	1.1	Witch hazel fluid extract	1.1
Iodoform	4.0	Zinc oxide	4.0
Menthol	0.7	Zinc sulfate	2.8

Three methods of calculating the quantity of base that the active medication will occupy and the quantities of ingredients required are illustrated here: (*a*) dosage replacement factor, (*b*) density factor, and (*c*) occupied volume methods.

Determination of the Dosage Replacement Factor Method

$$f = \frac{\left[100(E-G)\right]}{\left[(G)(X)\right]} + 1$$

where

E is the weight of the pure base suppositories, and
G is the weight of suppositories with X% of the active ingredient.

Cocoa butter is arbitrarily assigned a value of 1 as the standard base. Examples of other dosage replacement factors are shown in the below table.

Balsam of Peru	0.83	Phenol	0.9
Bismuth subgallate	0.37	Procaine HCl	0.8
Bismuth subnitrate	0.33	Quinine HCl	0.83
Boric acid	0.67	Resorcin	0.71
Camphor	1.49	Silver protein, mild	0.61
Castor oil	1.00	Spermaceti	1.0
Chloral hydrate	0.67	White or yellow wax	1.0
Ichthammol	0.91	Zinc oxide	0.15–0.25
Phenobarbital	0.81		

(continued)

■ EXAMPLE 1

Prepare a suppository containing 100 mg of phenobarbital (f = 0.81) using cocoa butter as the base. The weight of the pure cocoa butter suppository is 2.0 g. Because 100 mg of phenobarbital is to be contained in an approximately 2.0-g suppository, it will be about 5% phenobarbital. What will be the total weight of each suppository?

$$0.81 = \frac{[100(2-G)]}{[(G)(5)]+1} = 2.019$$

■ DETERMINATION OF DENSITY FACTOR METHOD

1. Determine the average blank weight, A, per mold using the suppository base of interest.
2. Weigh the quantity of suppository base necessary for 10 suppositories.
3. Weigh 1.0 g of medication. The weight of medication per suppository, B, is equal to 1 g/10 supp = 0.1 g/supp.
4. Melt the suppository base and incorporate the medication, mix, pour into molds, cool, trim, and remove from the molds.
5. Weigh the 10 suppositories and determine the average weight (C).
6. Determine the density factor as follows:

$$\text{Density factor} = \frac{B}{A - C + B}$$

where

A is the average weight of blank,
B is the weight of medication per suppository, and
C is the average weight of medicated suppository.

7. Take the weight of the medication required for each suppository and divide by the density factor of the medication to find the replacement value of the suppository base.
8. Subtract this quantity from the blank suppository weight.
9. Multiply by the number of suppositories required to obtain the quantity of base required for the prescription.
10. Multiply the weight of drug per suppository by the number of suppositories required to obtain the quantity of active drug required for the prescription.

■ EXAMPLE 2

Prepare 12 acetaminophen 300 mg suppositories using cocoa butter. The average weight of the cocoa butter blank is 2 g, and the average weight of the medicated suppository is 1.8 g.

$$DF = \frac{0.3}{2 - 1.8 + 0.3} = 0.6$$

From step 7: (0.3 g)/0.6 = 0.5 (the replacement value of the base)
From step 8: 2.0 − 0.5 g = 1.5 g
From step 9: 12 × 1.5 g = 18 g cocoa butter required
From step 10: 12 × 0.3 g = 3.6 g acetaminophen

■ DETERMINATION OF OCCUPIED VOLUME METHOD

1. Determine the average weight per mold (blank) using the designated base.
2. Weigh out enough base for 12 suppositories.
3. Divide the density of the active drug by the density of the base to obtain a ratio.
4. Divide the total weight of active drug required for the total number of suppositories by the ratio obtained in step 3. This will give the amount of base displaced by the active drug.
5. Subtract the amount obtained in step 4 from the total weight of the prescription (number of suppositories multiplied by the weight of the blanks) to obtain the weight of base required.
6. Multiply the weight of active drug per suppository times the number of suppositories to be prepared to obtain the quantity of active drug required.

(continued)

PHYSICAL PHARMACY CAPSULE **12.1** Density (Dose Replacement) Calculations for Suppositories *(continued)*

■ EXAMPLE 3

Prepare 10 suppositories, each containing 200 mg of a drug with a density of 3.0. The base has a density of 0.9, and a prepared blank weighs 2.0 g. Using the determination of occupied volume method, prepare the requested suppositories.

From step 1: The average weight per mold is 2.0 g.
From step 2: The quantity required for 10 suppositories is 2 × 10 g = 20 g.
From step 3: The density ratio is 3.0/0.9 = 3.3.
From step 4: The amount of suppository base displaced by the active drug is 2.0 g/3.3 = 0.6 g.
From step 5: The weight of the base required is 20 − 0.6 g = 19.4 g.
From step 6: The quantity of active drug required is 0.2 × 10 g = 2.0 g.

The required weight of the base is 19.4 g, and the weight of the active drug is 2 g. ■

and justifies preparation of extra melt. When solidified, the excess material is evenly scraped off of the top of the mold with a spatula warmed by dipping into a beaker of warm water; this will make a smooth surface on the back of the suppository during trimming. The filled mold is usually placed in the refrigerator to hasten hardening.

When the suppositories are hard, the mold is removed from the refrigerator and allowed to come to room temperature. Then the sections of the mold are separated, and the suppositories are dislodged, with pressure being exerted principally on their ends and only if needed on the tips. Generally, little or no pressure is required, and the suppositories simply fall out of the mold when it is opened.

An example formula for a compounded ABHR suppository used for nausea and vomiting associated with chemotherapy is as follows:

Ativan (lorazepam)	0.5 mg
Benadryl (diphenhydramine HCl)	25 mg
Haldol (haloperidol)	0.5 mg
Reglan (metoclopramide)	10 mg
Fatty acid base	2.25 g

Melt the fatty acid base at about 50°C. Slowly and with stirring, sprinkle the powders on the surface of the melted base and mix well. Remove from heat and cool until still fluid and pourable. Pour into a suitable mold. Cool and trim, if necessary. Package and label.

Hand Rolling and Shaping

With ready availability of suppository molds of accommodating shapes and sizes, there is little requirement for today's pharmacist to shape suppositories by hand. Hand rolling and shaping is a historic part of the art of the pharmacist; a description of it may be found in the third edition of this text or in pharmacy compounding texts.

■ MANUFACTURING SUPPOSITORIES

Manufactured suppositories are generally prepared by the melt fusion method. Commercially automated equipment for melt fusion is available to continually produce large quantities of finished suppositories per hour. See Figures 12.3 and 12.4.

The automated equipment for preparing suppositories has provided an efficient method for manufacturing large quantities of suppositories in a relatively short time. This equipment allows for a single continuous manufacturing process. The process starts with two main components, the packaging shell material and the molten bulk drug product.

The primary packaging of suppositories in the automated process is composed of five distinct stages. The stages include forming, dosing, cooling, sealing, and finishing. These stages are completed in a continuous process, at rates that can reach 30,000 suppositories per hour.

The forming process determines the shape and volume of the mold. It begins with two rolls of material. The film is heated between a set of dies. After the film is heated, it is transferred to the next station where it is blow molded into shape. The sides of the film are sealed as air is blown in between the heated film. The cavity is created, while the top remains open for dosing of the product.

Once the shells are formed, they move to the dosing station. The empty shells are aligned with the nozzles of the dosing pump, and the molten product is dosed into the empty shells. For high-speed machines, multiple cavities can be dosed at one time. This can be accomplished with an accuracy of ±0.01 g, depending on the product and equipment.

Filled shells are moved to the cooling tunnels. The cooling tunnels reduce temperature of the molten mass in the shells. This allows the product to solidify in the shells. Cooling tunnels blow chilled air around the molds. The cooling is controlled by the time the suppositories spend in the tunnels and the temperature of the tunnels.

Once the solidified suppositories leave the cooling tunnel, they move to the *sealing* area where the open top of the mold is closed. This process is accomplished by reheating the top edge of the film above the solidified suppository. After passing the shells through a series of reheating jaws, the molds move to sealing jaws. Sealing jaws are cooled with chilled water. The cooled jaws press the plastic film together and seal them. Also, during this phase, it is possible to press the lot code and expiration date into the seal area for each individual suppository. Once the suppositories are sealed, the finishing touches can be completed.

The *finishing* of the suppositories includes perforating, notching, and cutting the molds into the appropriate count strips. The cutting of the strip length allows for the suppositories to be placed in the final cartons for distribution.

QUALITY CONTROL

Quality control procedures listed in the USP/NF for manufactured suppositories and inserts include identification, assay, and, in some cases, loss on drying, disintegration, and dissolution. Also, stability considerations in dispensing practice for suppositories include observation for excessive softening and oil stains on packaging (9). Compounded suppositories can be checked for calculations of theoretical and actual weight and weight variation, color, hardness, surface texture, and overall appearance.

PACKAGING AND STORAGE

Glycerin suppositories and glycerinated gelatin suppositories are packaged in tightly closed glass containers to prevent a change in moisture content. Suppositories prepared from a cocoa butter base are usually individually wrapped or otherwise separated in compartmented boxes to prevent contact and adhesion. Suppositories containing light-sensitive drugs are individually wrapped in an opaque material such as a metallic foil. In fact, most commercial suppositories are individually wrapped in either foil or plastic. Some are packaged in a continuous strip, separated by tearing along perforations. Suppositories are also commonly packaged in slide boxes or in plastic boxes.

Because suppositories are adversely affected by heat, it is necessary to maintain them in a cool place. Cocoa butter suppositories must be stored below 30°C (86°F) and preferably in a refrigerator (2°C to 8°C or 36°F to 46°F). Glycerinated gelatin suppositories can be stored at controlled room temperature (20°C to 25°C or 68°F to 77°F). Suppositories made from a base of PEG may be stored at usual room temperatures.

Suppositories stored in high humidity may absorb moisture and tend to become spongy, whereas suppositories stored in places of extreme dryness may lose moisture and become brittle.

STABILITY

Pharmacists should avoid ingredients and conditions that could result in excessive physical deterioration or chemical decomposition of drug preparations, especially when compounding.

Physical Stability

Listed in Table 12.6 are the major modifications of suppository characteristics because of natural aging, as well as the causes. Physical observation can generally detect physical stability problems, including softening, hardening, drying, cracking, separation, polymorphs when melting range is affected, and one can often detect the odor of rancidity.

Chemical Stability

In working with suppositories, the majority will be anhydrous, so the presence of water is not really an issue. However, in some cases, water may be present to help incorporate the drug into the base, or it may be present as part of the hydrated form of the drug components' crystalline structure. Also, if emulsions or suspensions are incorporated into suppositories, water may be present. Last, some suppositories may be hygroscopic and absorb water from the atmosphere. Consequently, some of the issues related to instability in water will also be discussed here.

In suppositories, the following reactions and conditions can result in loss of active drug content and may not provide obvious visual or olfactory evidence of their occurrence: hydrolysis, epimerization, decarboxylation, dehydration, oxidation, photochemical decomposition, pH effect, solid state stability, temperature, and microbiological considerations.

TABLE 12.6. Major Changes in Suppository Characteristics Due to Natural Aging and the Causes

Modifications	Causes	Examples
Odor	Fungal contamination	Suppositories with vegetable extracts
Color	Discoloration because of oxidation	Suppositories with tartrazine yellow aqueous solution
Shape	Incorrect temperature during storage	Suppositories with essential oils
Surface condition	Whitening	Suppositories with vegetable extracts or caffeine base suppositories
Weight	Loss of volatile substances	Suppositories with camphor, menthol, etc.

Microbiological Stability

Most suppository formulations do not contain preservatives or antioxidants because water is usually excluded from the formulations. However, in the event water is present or the formulation may support the growth of microorganisms, an appropriate preservative may be indicated.

Beyond-Use Dating for Compounded Suppositories

There are numerous suppositories that are routinely compounded. The completed compounded suppositories are generally considered dry or nonaqueous and thus provide a stable dosage form as long as they are protected from moisture and heat. According to USP general Chapter <795> Pharmacy Compounding—Nonsterile Preparations, these preparations should have a beyond-use date of 25% of the time remaining on the expiration date if the compounded preparation is made using a manufactured product as the source of the active drug, or 6 months, whichever is earlier. If the product is prepared from USP/NF ingredients, a beyond-use date of 6 months is appropriate, unless evidence is available to support other dating.

If the stability of a compounded water-containing preparation is unknown and there are no other supporting data for an alternate beyond-use date, then a beyond-use date of 14 days when stored in a refrigerator can be used.

Expiration Dating for Manufactured Suppositories

To ensure that a drug product meets applicable standards of identity, strength, quality, and purity at the time of use, a commercially manufactured suppository must bear an expiration date determined by appropriate stability testing. Exempt from this requirement are homeopathic drug products, allergenic extracts, and investigational new drugs providing the latter meet the standards established during preclinical and clinical studies.

As previously mentioned, excessive softening is the major indication of instability in suppositories, although some suppositories may dry out and harden or shrivel. Evidence of oil stains on packaging material should warn the pharmacist to examine individual suppositories more closely by removing any foil covering. As a general rule (although there are exceptions), suppositories should be stored in a refrigerator.

Informing and Educating the Patient

As a final step in meeting responsibility for the stability of drugs dispensed, the pharmacist is obligated to inform the patient about the proper storage conditions (e.g., in a cool, dry place—not in the bathroom) for both prescription and nonprescription products and to suggest a reasonable estimate of the time after which the medication should be discarded. When beyond-use dates are applied, the pharmacist should emphasize to the patient that the dates are applicable only when proper storage conditions are observed. Patients should be encouraged to clean out their drug storage cabinets periodically.

RECTAL SUPPOSITORIES

Examples of rectal suppositories are presented in Table 12.1. As noted earlier, drugs like aspirin given for pain; ergotamine tartrate for treating migraine headaches; theophylline as a smooth muscle relaxant in treating asthma; and chlorpromazine and prochlorperazine, which act as antiemetics and tranquilizers, are intended to be absorbed into the general circulation to provide systemic effects. The rectal route of administration is especially useful if the patient is unwilling or unable to take medication by mouth.

Suppositories are also intended to provide local action within the perianal area. Local anesthetic suppositories are commonly employed to relieve *pruritus ani* of various causes and the pain sometimes associated with hemorrhoids. Many commercial hemorrhoidal suppositories contain a number of medicinal agents, including astringents, protectives, anesthetics, lubricants, and others, intended to relieve the discomfort of the condition. Cathartic suppositories are contact-type agents that act directly on the colonic mucosa to produce normal peristalsis. Because the contact action is restricted to the colon, the motility of the small intestine is not appreciably affected. Cathartic suppositories are more rapid acting than orally administered medication. Suppositories of bisacodyl are usually effective within 15 minutes to an hour and glycerin suppositories usually within a few minutes following insertion.

Some commercially prepared suppositories are available for both adult and pediatric use. The difference is in the shape and drug content. Pediatric suppositories are narrower and pencil shaped than the typical bullet-shaped adult suppository. Glycerin suppositories are commonly available in each type.

A formula for glycerin suppositories is as follows:

Glycerin	91 g
Sodium stearate	9 g
Purified water	5 g
To make about	105 g

In preparation of this suppository, the glycerin is heated in a suitable container to about 50°C (120°F). Then the sodium stearate is dissolved with stirring in the hot glycerin, the purified water added, and the mixture immediately poured into the suppository mold. It is recommended that if the mold is metal, it also be heated prior to addition of the glycerin mixture. After cooling to solidification, the suppositories are removed. This formula will prepare about 50 adult suppositories. Approximately the same formulation is used in pharmaceutical and cosmetic stick products, such as deodorants and antiperspirants.

Glycerin, a hygroscopic material, contributes to the laxative effect of the suppository by drawing water from the intestine and from its irritant action on the mucous lining. The sodium stearate, a soap, is the solidifying agent and may also contribute to the laxative action. Because of the hygroscopic nature of glycerin, the suppositories attract moisture and should be maintained in tight containers, preferably at temperatures below 25°C (77°F).

URETHRAL SUPPOSITORIES

Suppositories for urethral administration tend to be thinner and tapered, often about 5 mm in diameter. They have been used in the treatment of local infections, and a much smaller urethral suppository has been introduced for the administration of alprostadil in the treatment of erectile dysfunction.

Compounding Urethral Suppositories

In addition to a urethral mold, a straw or thin glass tube can be used as the mold when preparing urethral suppositories. A 1-mL tuberculin syringe can also be used if the lower portion of the barrel is cut off (a pencil sharpener works well for this). The urethral suppository can be removed from the syringe barrel by inserting the plunger and forcing out the suppository after slight warming. A large-diameter needle, attached to the syringe filled with the suppository melt, will aid in transferring the product into the 1-mL tuberculin syringe.

The MUSE (alprostadil) urethral microsuppository (Vivus, Inc.) is a single-use medicated transurethral system for the delivery of alprostadil to the male urethra. The drug is suspended in a PEG 1450 excipient and is formed into a medicated pellet, or microsuppository, measuring 1.4 mm in diameter and 3 or 6 mm in length. Available strengths are 125, 250, 500, and 1,000 µg. The microsuppository resides in the tip of a translucent hollow applicator. It is administered by inserting the applicator tip into the urethra after urination. The pellet is delivered by depressing the applicator button. The PEG 1450 vehicle will dissolve in the available fluid, releasing the drug for absorption. The applicator system is composed of medical grade polypropylene; each system is individually foil packaged. The MUSE microsuppository is indicated for the treatment of erectile dysfunction.

VAGINAL INSERTS

Examples of vaginal inserts (which includes vaginal tablets) are presented in Table 12.2. These preparations are employed principally to combat infections in the female genitourinary tract and to restore the vaginal mucosa to its normal state and for contraception. The usual pathogenic organisms are *T. vaginalis*, *C.* (*Monilia*) *albicans* or other species, and *Haemophilus vaginalis*. Among the anti-infective agents in commercial vaginal preparations are nystatin, clotrimazole, butoconazole nitrate, terconazole, and miconazole (antifungals) and triple sulfas, sulfanilamide, povidone–iodine, clindamycin phosphate, metronidazole, and oxytetracycline (antibacterials). Nonoxynol 9, a spermicide, is employed for vaginal contraception. Estrogenic

substances such as dienestrol are found in vaginal preparations to restore the vaginal mucosa to its normal state.

The most commonly used base for vaginal inserts consists of combinations of the various molecular weight PEGs. To this base are frequently added surfactants and preservative agents, commonly the parabens. Many vaginal inserts and other types of vaginal dosage forms are buffered to an acid pH usually about 4.5, consistent with the normal vagina. This acidity discourages pathogenic organisms and provides a favorable environment for eventual recolonization by the acid-producing bacilli normally found in the vagina.

The PEG-based vaginal suppositories are water miscible and are generally sufficiently firm for the patient to handle and insert without great difficulty. However, to make the task easier, many manufacturers provide plastic insertion devices that are used to hold the suppository or tablet for proper placement within the vagina (Fig. 12.5).

As noted earlier, pharmacists frequently are called on to prepare progesterone vaginal suppositories. Formulas for extemporaneous preparation of these suppositories have been presented in the professional literature. Micronized progesterone powder is used in a base of PEG, although, in some formulas, cocoa butter is employed. The suppositories are prepared by adding the progesterone to a melt of the base and molding. Some representative formulas are as follows:

Rx

Progesterone, micronized	qs	qs	qs
Polyethylene glycol 400	60%	—	—
Polyethylene glycol 8000	40%	—	—
Polyethylene glycol 1000	—	75%	—
Polyethylene glycol 3350	—	25%	—
Cocoa butter	—	—	100%

The amount of progesterone per suppository usually ranges from 25 to 600 mg. The suppositories are used in treating luteal phase defect, premenstrual syndrome, and

FIGURE 12.5. Dosage forms used intravaginally, including suppositories (*top* and *middle*), vaginal inserts packaged in foil (*bottom*), vaginal cream, and corresponding insert devices.

luteal phase spotting and in preparation of the endometrium for implantation.

The pharmacist should share several helpful hints with a woman who is about to use a vaginal suppository. She should first be told to read the instructions with the product. Throughout the course of therapy, the suppository should be inserted high into the vagina with the provided applicator. The patient should not discontinue therapy when the symptoms abate. Furthermore, she should notify her physician if burning, irritation, or any signs of an allergic reaction occur. When vaginal inserts (i.e., compressed tablets) are prescribed, the pharmacist should instruct the woman to dip the tablet into water quickly before insertion. Because these dosage forms are usually administered at bedtime and can be somewhat messy if formulated into an oleaginous base, the pharmacist should suggest that the woman wear a sanitary napkin to protect her nightwear and bed linens.

VAGINAL INSERTS (TABLETS)

Vaginal inserts (tablets) are widely used today as they are easy to manufacture, more stable, and less messy than cocoa butter or PEG suppositories. They are usually ovoid and are accompanied in their packaging with a plastic inserter, a device for easy placement of the tablet within the vagina. They are prepared by tablet compression and are commonly formulated to contain lactose as the base or filler, a disintegrating agent such as starch, a dispersing agent such as polyvinylpyrrolidone, and a tablet lubricant such as magnesium stearate. They are intended to disintegrate within the vagina, releasing their medication. Examples are presented in Table 12.2.

Some vaginal inserts are gelatin capsules containing medication to be released intravaginally. Capsules may also be used rectally, especially to administer medication to children unwilling or unable to tolerate the drug orally. Capsule insertion into the rectum can be facilitated by first lightly wetting the capsule with water. Holes may be punched into these capsules prior to moistening and insertion to facilitate fluid movement into the capsule if desired. Drugs are absorbed from the rectum, but frequently at unpredictable rates and in varying amounts, as previously noted. Drugs that do not dissolve rapidly and that irritate mucous membranes should not be placed in direct contact with such membranes.

MEDICATION STICKS

Although cosmetics are viewed as preparations aimed at improving a person's appearance, many cosmetic preparations can serve as either medications or drug vehicle bases. Some formulations that have been introduced and improved for cosmetic use—powders, sticks, gels, solutions, suspensions, pastes, ointments, and oils—are widely used in the pharmaceutical sciences.

The medication stick, a fairly recent dosage form, is used for both cosmetic and medical purposes. Examples include styptic pencils and lip balm sticks (ChapStick), which became available in the early 1940s. Today, medication sticks provide pharmacists, patients, and primary care providers with a unique, convenient, relatively stable, easy-to-prepare dosage form for the topical delivery of drugs. The use of this form will probably continue to grow.

Medication sticks are prepared similar to suppositories except that the melt is poured into the administering device, or tube. For application, the stick is pushed up from the bottom or using a screw-type device to raise the stick.

Melting bases include the bases used to prepare soft opaque and soft clear sticks. These bases, which will soften and melt at body temperatures, include cocoa butter, petrolatum, waxes, PEGs, and the like. Active drugs can include any agent that can be applied directly to a specific skin site or over a larger area of skin to relieve such discomforts as muscle sprains and arthritis. Penetration enhancers (e.g., glycerin, propylene glycol, alcohol, and surfactants) can increase the amount of transdermal drug delivery. Using waxes, oils, or plain polymers such as PEGs alone achieves a topical effect. Melting bases can be further divided into opaque and clear. Opaque bases include waxes, oils, PEGs, and the like, whereas clear bases include sodium stearate/glycerin mixtures.

Sticks are a convenient form for administering topical medications. They come in different sizes and shapes, are readily transportable, and can be applied directly to the affected site of the body. Sticks can be easily compounded by using different materials to produce topical or systemic effects. Medications and other ingredients that have been incorporated into sticks include local anesthetics, sunscreens, oncology drugs, antivirals, and antibiotics. Sticks containing antibiotics, antivirals, and oncology agents are usually packaged in 5-g tubes, whereas sticks containing local anesthetics are usually packaged in 1- or 2-oz tubes.

The medication in a soft stick is applied by raising the stick above the tube level and simply rubbing it onto the skin, where it softens and flows easily onto the affected area. The medication usually cannot be seen on the skin. When a hard stick is applied, the tip of the stick is moistened and then touched to the affected area. The crystalline powder used to prepare the stick can leave a white residue on the skin.

Patient Counseling

When counseling a patient about the use of medication sticks, the pharmacist must take into account the active drug and the method of application. In general, the patient should be told to apply the stick only to the involved area and not to the surrounding skin. In addition, the patient should apply the medication liberally over the area but only as needed. The surface of the stick should be cleaned with a clean tissue after each use, and, to avoid transmitting infection, the product should not be shared with others.

Sample Formulations

Acyclovir Lip Balm

Acyclovir 200 mg capsules (tab)	6
Polyethylene glycol base (Polybase)	25 g

These formulas can be modified by incorporating lidocaine, PABA, or other ingredients as needed.

Formula

1. Weigh or measure the ingredients.
2. Heat the PEG base to about 55°C.
3. Empty the acyclovir capsules into a mortar and reduce the particle size to a fine powder.
4. Add these powders to the melted base and mix thoroughly.
5. Cool to just above the melting point of the preparation, until it starts to thicken.
6. While stirring, pour into the lip balm molds or tubes.

Analgesic Medication Stick

Methyl salicylate	35 g
Menthol	15 g
Sodium stearate	13 g
Purified water	12 mL
Propylene glycol	25 g

1. Weigh or measure the ingredients.
2. Gently heat and melt the sodium stearate.
3. Mix the purified water with the propylene glycol and add to the melted sodium stearate.
4. Mix thoroughly, remove from heat, and allow the base to cool slightly.
5. Dissolve the menthol in the methyl salicylate; add this solution to the base and mix thoroughly.
6. As the preparation begins to thicken, continue to mix and pour into either 5- or 20-g stick containers.
7. Allow to harden at room temperature.

SPECIAL TYPES OF SUPPOSITORIES

There has been a lot of work done in the development of altered release suppository dosage forms, both long-acting and slow-release suppositories (4,5). Morphine sulfate in slow-release suppositories is prepared by compounding pharmacists. The base includes a material such as alginic acid, which will prolong the release of the drug over several hours. Speeding up or slowing down the release and prolonging the action of the incorporated drug in suppositories have been investigated using various coatings, emulsions, hydrogels, layering, matrices of different substances, hollow-type suppositories, nanoparticles, osmotic release, micellar solutions, thermoreversible liquid suppositories, xerogel suppositories, and others.

CLINICAL CONSIDERATIONS

The pharmacist should relate several helpful items of information about the proper use of suppositories. If they must be stored in the refrigerator, suppositories should be allowed to warm to room temperature before insertion. The patient should be advised to rub cocoa butter suppositories gently with the fingers to melt the surface to provide lubrication for insertion. Glycerinated gelatin or PEG suppositories should be moistened with water to enhance lubrication. If the PEG suppository formulation does not contain at least 20% water, dipping it into water just prior to insertion prevents moisture from being drawn from rectal tissues after insertion and decreases subsequent irritation. The shape of the suppository determines how it will be inserted. Bullet-shaped rectal suppositories should be inserted point-end first. When the patient is instructed to use one-half suppository, the patient should be told to cut the suppository in half lengthwise with a clean razor blade. Most suppositories are dispensed in paper, foil, or plastic wrappings, and the patient must be instructed to completely remove the wrapping before insertion. Depending upon the medication, purpose of the suppository, and associated factors, the administration of an enema prior to a suppository may increase the absorption of the drug. Also, the patient should be provided information on proper disposal of suppositories and inserts. Additional information on inserting rectal suppositories and informed consent has been published and may be useful for patient counseling (10).

PATIENT COUNSELING

ADMINISTERING RECTAL SUPPOSITORIES

1. Wash hands and rectal area and pat dry.
2. A disposable glove can be used if desired.
3. Instruct the patient on the proper insertion of the suppository, how far to insert it, and how long to remain inactive after insertion. An example of the

consultation related to administration of a suppository may be as follows:

- Position the patient on the left side with the upper leg flexed.
- Lubricate the suppository with a water-soluble lubricant or a small amount of water, if needed.

- For ages 12 and older and adults, insert the suppository about a finger-length into the rectum; for ages less than 12, insert a shorter length depending upon the age of the patient. Gently insert the suppository at an angle toward the umbilicus, so the suppository is placed against the rectal wall for absorption, rather than being left in the canal or pushed into a mass of stool.
- After the finger is withdrawn, hold the buttocks together until the urge to expel has ceased.

4. Wash and dry hands again or if a glove is used, remove and dispose of the glove and wash and dry hands again.
5. Onset of action may be 30 minutes to 2 hours.
6. Some suppositories require refrigeration and some may be stored at room temperature.

ADMINISTERING VAGINAL DOSAGE FORMS—GENERAL

1. A sanitary pad may be used to prevent the medication from soiling clothing or sleepwear.
2. Administration at bedtime is preferred.
3. Vaginal medications can be used during menstruation (except for birth control vaginal rings).

ADMINISTERING VAGINAL SUPPOSITORIES OR VAGINAL TABLETS

1. Wash and dry hands and the vaginal area.
2. Vaginal suppositories and tablets are packaged with applicators.
3. Place the unit into the open end of the applicator.
4. Stand or lie on the back and insert the tablet or suppository high in the upper part of the vagina. Use the plunger to push the unit out of the applicator.
5. Remove and clean the applicator with soap and warm water and allow to dry.
6. Wash and dry hands again.

MEDICATION STICKS

1. Explain about the active drug and the method of application.
2. Generally, apply the stick only to the involved area and not to the surrounding skin.
3. Apply the medication liberally over the area but only as needed.
4. After each use, clean the surface of the stick with a clean tissue.
5. To avoid transmitting infection, do not share with others.

PHARMACEUTICS CASE STUDY

SUBJECTIVE INFORMATION

A colleague calls you and asks for help concerning a prescription that was recently compounded. A teenage boy with epilepsy brought in a prescription for diazepam 10 mg suppositories, and your colleague filled it using a compounded preparation that had been used in the past. However, the boy has been to the emergency room twice now with uncontrolled seizures, even after using the suppositories in an effort to bring the seizures under control. His parents have returned to the pharmacy with questions concerning the use of these suppositories. What should you tell your colleague?

OBJECTIVE INFORMATION

When questioned about the formulation for the suppositories, your colleague provides the following:

For 10 suppositories:

Diazepam powder, USP	100.0 mg
Cocoa butter	19.9 g
Mix and mold	

ASSESSMENT

The use of cocoa butter (a fatty acid base) in the formulation for diazepam suppositories may be the problem, because diazepam is a fat-soluble drug. As a result, the drug may remain dissolved in the vehicle and not be released from the dosage form rapidly enough to control the boy's seizures; the tendency for diazepam to diffuse from the lipid suppository base to the aqueous mucosal secretions is low. The use of a water-soluble base such as polyethylene glycol (PEG) may be a better choice. Another possibility is to use a hollow suppository with a diazepam solution in the cavity.

PLAN

Recommend reformulation of the suppositories using PEG as the base. ■

CLINICAL CASE STUDY

SUBJECTIVE INFORMATION

HPI:	J.R. is a 32-year-old Hispanic female who presents to the oncology clinic for a follow-up visit 4 days after being discharged from the hospital. At that time, she received her first cycle of cyclophosphamide, doxorubicin, vincristine, and prednisone (CHOP) chemotherapy for her newly diagnosed large B-cell lymphoma. During the administration of CHOP, the patient started a regimen of two antiemetic medications, Compazine 10 mg by mouth every 6 hours as needed and lorazepam 2 mg intravenously every 6 hours as needed, to control her chemotherapy-induced nausea and vomiting (N&V). Upon discharge from the hospital, she was also given a prescription for prochlorperazine 10 mg tablets by mouth every 6 hours as needed for any N&V she might have at home. However, this morning J.R. is complaining of "feeling sick to her stomach" for the past 2 days, and she states, "Yesterday I threw up three times." She took her prochlorperazine tablets. However, twice after taking them, she threw them up, and she simply "feels too nauseous now to take anything by mouth." Upon questioning, the patient denies any fever, chills, hematemesis (i.e., bloody vomitus), and diarrhea and otherwise is without complaints except for feeling "a little tired after the chemo."
PMH:	Large B-cell lymphoma iron deficiency anemia
PSH:	None
MEDS:	CHOP regimen (each cycle is 21 days long): Cyclophosphamide 750 mg/m^2 IV on day 1 Doxorubicin 50 mg/m^2 IV on day 1 Vincristine 1.4 mg/m^2 IV on day 1 100 mg po on days 1 to 5 Compazine 10 mg tablets po q6h prn N&V Ferrous sulfate 325 mg tablets po tid Tylenol 650 mg tablets po q6h prn pain
Allergies:	NKDA
SH:	(–) Alcohol (–) Tobacco (–) Illicit drugs Pt came to the United States from Mexico 2 years ago
FH:	Sister with cancer died at age 36

PHARMACEUTICAL CARE PLAN

S:	Chemotherapy-induced N&V uncontrolled by prochlorperazine
O: Vital Signs:	Temp 36.0°C, pulse 87, BP 117/76 Na 143, Cl 105, BUN 12, Glu 129 K 3.9, CO$_2$ 30, Cr 0.8
A:	A 32-year-old woman with chemotherapy-induced N&V uncontrolled by oral prochlorperazine. Pt is at risk for continued N&V because of the emetogenic potential of the CHOP regimen. Specifically, cyclophosphamide is associated with delayed-onset N&V that can last up to 6 or 7 days after the administration of chemotherapy. Also, J.R. has other characteristics, for example, female, <50 years of age, that increase her risk of N&V.
P:	Because J.R. cannot take her medication by mouth, the rectal route of administration would be useful for her. Prochlorperazine is available as rectal suppositories, and the recommended dosage for adults for N&V is 25 mg rectally twice daily. J.R. should be counseled to use her prochlorperazine suppositories as needed for N&V. J.R. should be told that it is not necessary to store the suppositories in the refrigerator. However, they should be kept away from heat. If they are kept in the refrigerator, they should be warmed to room temperature for 5 to 10 minutes before use. Counsel J.R. on the proper administration technique. She should be instructed to remove the foil wrapping before insertion. Advise her to moisten the suppositories with some water to provide lubrication for insertion. Specific instructions are to use her finger to insert the suppository into the rectum about 1 inch and hold the suppository in place for a few moments. Afterward, the patient should thoroughly wash her hands and then resume her normal activities. Explain to J.R. the common side effects associated with prochlorperazine use: sedation, restlessness, blurred vision, constipation, dizziness, and dry mouth. Caution J.R. about performing activities that require alertness: driving a car, using machinery. Instruct J.R. to avoid alcoholic beverages and prolonged exposure to sunlight because prochlorperazine may cause skin photosensitivity. J.R. should be monitored for resolution of her N&V. Also, monitor her for any complaint of abnormal body movements associated with long-term prochlorperazine use, such as extrapyramidal dyskinesias and tardive dyskinesia. ∎

APPLYING THE PRINCIPLES AND CONCEPTS

GROUP ACTIVITIES

1. Compare and contrast suppository and insert dosage forms in terms of physical appearance, size, and shape.
2. Compare and contrast pharmacist counseling directions to a patient prescribed a cocoa butter-based suppository product and a water-soluble-based suppository product.
3. Develop a listing of drugs in suppository dosage forms for inclusion into a hospital formulary system and indicate the rationale for their inclusion on the list.
4. Develop a listing of conceivable ways a patient might misuse a drug to be administered in a rectal suppository dosage form.
5. Describe special handling, storage, and disposal precautions a patient must take when prescribed a drug in a suppository dosage form.
6. Compile examples of prescriptions written for the extemporaneous preparation of a suppository delivery system.

INDIVIDUAL ACTIVITIES

1. Create a table of six vaginal insert products including amount of active ingredient(s), indication, contraindication, adverse effects/precautions, and dosage.
2. Generate a listing of drugs whose physical–chemical characteristics make them a candidate for incorporation into a suppository dosage form. Predict which type of base would be most appropriate for each drug.
3. List five clinical situations where the administration of a suppository or insert dosage form might be preferred over oral administration.
4. List five reasons a patient might be reluctant to use a suppository dosage form and how you might counsel them to overcome each concern.
5. List five counseling points for proper administration of a specific rectal suppository or vaginal insert.
6. From the primary literature, locate a clinical drug study demonstrating a comparison between a rectal suppository delivery system and another route of delivery for the drug in terms of clinical effectiveness and determine which delivery system would be preferred in terms of patient acceptance, patient adherence, bioequivalence, and cost. Explain the rationale for your decision.

REFERENCES

1. Available at: http://www.ncbi.nlm.nih.gov/entrez/query.fcgi. (Accessed July 27, 2020)
2. Gold M, VePuri M, Block LH. Suppository development and production. In: Lieberman HA, Rieger MM, Banker GS, eds. Pharmaceutical Dosage Forms: Disperse Systems. Vol. 2. New York, NY: Marcel Dekker, 1996:447–496.
3. Gillson GR, Zava DT. A perspective on HRT for women: Picking up the pieces after the women's health initiative trial, Part I. Int J Pharm Compd 2003;7:250–256.
4. Guillot BR, Lombard AP, eds. Le Suppositoire. Paris, France: Maloine S.A., 1973:6–7.
5. Kawashima S, Nishiura N, Noguchi T, et al. Studies on sustained-release suppositories. 1. Effect of alginic acid addition on rectal absorption of bacampicillin in rabbits. Chem Pharm Bull (Tokyo) 1989;37:766–770.
6. Morgan DJ, McCormick Y, Cosolo W, et al. Prolonged release of morphine alkaloid from a lipophilic suppository base in vitro and in vivo. Int J Clin Pharmacol Ther Toxicol 1991;30:576–581.
7. Jenkins GL, Christian JE, Hager GP. Quantitative Pharmaceutical Chemistry. 5th Ed. New York, NY: McGraw-Hill, 1957:269–288.
8. Neville J, Swafford WB. Pluronics as a suppository base. Am J Pharm Sci Support Public Health 1960;132:301–303.
9. United States Pharmacopeia–National Formulary. Current Ed. Rockville, MD: U.S. Pharmacopeial Convention.
10. Allen LV Jr. Suppositories. London, UK: Pharmaceutical Press, 2008:177–178.

SECTION SIX

Liquid Dosage Forms

Solutions

CHAPTER AT A GLANCE Solubility • Some Solvents for Liquid Preparations • Preparation of Solutions • Cosolvents • Mixing Oral Liquids • Oral Solutions and Preparations for Oral Solution • Syrups • Elixirs • Tinctures • Proper Administration and Use of Liquid Peroral Dosage Forms • Topical Solutions and Tinctures • Vaginal and Rectal Solutions • Topical Tinctures • Topical Oral (Dental) Solutions • Miscellaneous Solutions • Nonaqueous Solutions • Extraction Methods for Preparing Solutions • Patient Counseling

OBJECTIVES

After reading this chapter, the student will be able to:

1. Define the various types of oral and topical liquid dosage forms
2. List the advantages and disadvantages of using liquid dosage forms in extemporaneous compounded prescriptions and in patient therapy
3. Compare and contrast liquid dosage forms to solid oral dosage forms
4. Define solubility and describe how different factors increase or decrease solute solubility in a given solvent
5. Evaluate and select a proper solvent and delivery system for a given solute, purpose, and/or patient population

INTRODUCTION

In physicochemical terms, solutions may be prepared from any combination of a solid, liquid, and gas, the three states of matter. For example, a solid solute may be dissolved in another solid, a liquid, or a gas, and the same being true for a liquid solute and for a gas; nine types of homogeneous mixtures are possible. In pharmacy, however, interest in solutions is for the most part limited to preparations of a solid, a liquid, and less frequently a gas solute in a liquid solvent.

In pharmaceutical terms, solutions are "liquid preparations that contain one or more chemical substances dissolved in a suitable solvent or mixture of mutually miscible solvents" (1). Because of a particular pharmaceutical solution's use, it may be classified as oral, otic, ophthalmic, or topical. Still other solutions, because of their composition or use, may be classified as other dosage forms. For example, aqueous solutions containing a sugar are classified as

syrups (even though some syrups may contain some alcohol), sweetened hydroalcoholic (combinations of water and ethanol) solutions are termed elixirs, and solutions of aromatic materials are termed spirits if the solvent is alcoholic or aromatic waters if the solvent is aqueous. Solutions prepared by extracting active constituents from crude drugs are termed tinctures or fluidextracts, depending on their method of preparation and concentration. Tinctures may also be solutions of chemical substances dissolved in alcohol or in a hydroalcoholic solvent. Certain solutions prepared to be sterile and pyrogen-free and intended for parenteral administration are classified as injections. Although other examples could be cited, it is apparent that a solution, as a distinct type of pharmaceutical preparation, is much further defined than the physicochemical definition of the term solution.

Oral solutions, syrups, elixirs, spirits, and tinctures are prepared and used for the specific effects of the medicinal agents they carry. In these preparations, the medicinal agents are intended to provide systemic effects. The fact that they are administered in solution form usually means that they are soluble in aqueous systems and their absorption from the gastrointestinal tract into the systemic circulation may be expected to occur more rapidly than from suspension or solid dosage forms of the same medicinal agent.

Solutes other than the medicinal agent are usually present in orally administered solutions. These additional agents are frequently included to provide color, flavor, sweetness, or stability. In formulating or compounding a pharmaceutical solution, the pharmacist must use information on the solubility and stability of each solute with regard to the solvent or solvent system. Combinations of medicinal or pharmaceutical agents that will result in chemical and/or physical interactions affecting the therapeutic quality or pharmaceutical stability of the product must be avoided.

For single-solute solutions and especially for multiple-solute solutions, the pharmacist must be aware of the solubility characteristics of the solutes and the features of the common pharmaceutical solvents. Each chemical agent has its own solubility in a given solvent. For many medicinal agents, their solubilities in the usual solvents are stated in the *U.S. Pharmacopeia–National Formulary* (USP–NF) as well as in other reference books.

SOLUBILITY

Attractive forces between atoms lead to the formation of molecules and ions. The intermolecular forces, which are developed between like molecules, are responsible for the physical state (solid, liquid, or gas) of the substance under given conditions, such as temperature and pressure. Under ordinary conditions, most organic compounds, and thus most drug substances, form molecular solids.

When molecules interact, attractive and repulsive forces are in effect. The attractive forces cause the molecules to cohere, whereas the repulsive forces prevent molecular interpenetration and destruction. When the attractive and repulsive forces are equal, the potential energy between two molecules is minimal, and the system is most stable.

Dipolar molecules frequently tend to align themselves with other dipolar molecules so that the negative pole of one molecule points toward the positive pole of the other. Large groups of molecules may be associated through these weak attractions, known as dipole–dipole or van der Waals forces. Other attractions also occur between polar and nonpolar molecules and ions. These include ion-dipole forces and hydrogen bonding. The latter is of particular interest. Because of small size and large electrostatic field, the hydrogen atom can move in close to an electronegative atom, forming an electrostatic type of association, a hydrogen bond or a hydrogen bridge. Hydrogen bonding involves strongly electronegative atoms such as oxygen, nitrogen, and fluorine. Such a bond exists in water, represented by the dotted lines.

Water

Hydrogen bonds also exist between some alcohol molecules, esters, carboxylic acids, aldehydes, and polypeptides.

When a solute dissolves, the substance's intermolecular forces of attraction must be overcome by forces of attraction between the solute and the solvent molecules. This entails breaking the solute–solute forces and the solvent–solvent forces to achieve the solute–solvent attraction.

The solubility of an agent in a particular solvent indicates the maximum concentration to which a solution may be prepared with that agent and that solvent. When a solvent at a given temperature has dissolved all of the solute possible, it is said to be saturated. To emphasize the possible variation in solubility between two chemical agents and, therefore, in the amounts of each required to prepare a saturated solution, two official aqueous saturated solutions are cited as examples, Calcium Hydroxide Topical Solution, USP, and Potassium Iodide Oral Solution, USP. The first solution, prepared by agitating an excess amount of calcium hydroxide with purified water, contains only about 140 mg of dissolved solute per 100 mL of the solution at 25°C, whereas potassium iodide solution contains about 100 g of solute per 100 mL of the solution, more than 700 times as much solute as in the calcium hydroxide topical solution. Thus, the maximum possible concentration to which a pharmacist may prepare a solution varies greatly and depends in part on the chemical constitution of the solute. Through selection of a different solubilizing agent or a different chemical salt form of the medicinal agent, alteration of the pH of a solution, or substitution in part or in whole of the solvent, a pharmacist can, in certain instances, dissolve greater quantities of a solute than would otherwise be possible. For example, iodine granules are soluble in water only to the extent of 1 g in about 3,000 mL. Using only these two agents, the maximum concentration possible would be approximately 0.03% of iodine. However, through the use of an aqueous solution of potassium iodide or sodium iodide as the solvent, much larger amounts of iodine may be dissolved as the result of the formation of a water-soluble complex with the iodide salt. This reaction is taken advantage of, for example, in Iodine Topical Solution, USP, prepared to contain about 2% iodine and 2.4% sodium iodide.

Temperature is an important factor in determining the solubility of a drug and in preparing its solution. Most chemicals absorb heat when they are dissolved and are said to have a positive heat of solution, resulting in increased solubility with an increase in temperature. A few chemicals have a negative heat of solution and exhibit a decrease in solubility with a rise in temperature. Other factors in addition to temperature affect solubility. These include the various chemical and other physical properties of the solute and the solvent, pressure, the pH of the solution, the state of subdivision of the solute, and the physical agitation applied to the solution as it dissolves. The solubility of a pure chemical substance at a given temperature and pressure is constant; however, its rate of solution, that is, the speed at which it dissolves, depends on the particle size of the substance and the extent of agitation. The finer the powder, the greater the surface area, which comes in contact with the solvent, and the more rapid the dissolving process. Also, the greater the agitation, the more unsaturated solvent passes over the drug and the faster the formation of the solution.

The solubility of a substance in a given solvent may be determined by preparing a saturated solution of it at a specific temperature and by determining by chemical analysis the amount of chemical dissolved in a given weight of solution. The amount of solvent required to dissolve the amount of solute can be determined by a simple calculation. The solubility may then be expressed as grams of solute dissolving in milliliters of solvent, for example, "1 g of sodium chloride dissolves in 2.8 mL of water." When the exact solubility has not been determined, general expressions of relative solubility may be used. These terms are defined in the USP and presented in Table 13.1 (1).

Many of the important organic medicinal agents are either weak acids or weak bases, and their solubility depends on a large measure on the pH of the solvent. These drugs react with either strong acids or strong bases to form water-soluble salts. For instance, the weak bases, including many of the alkaloids (atropine, codeine, and morphine), antihistamines (diphenhydramine and pro-

methazine), local anesthetics (cocaine, procaine, and tetracaine), and other important drugs, are not very water soluble, but they are soluble in dilute solutions of acids. Pharmaceutical manufacturers have prepared many acid salts of these organic bases to enable the preparation of aqueous solutions. However, if the pH of the aqueous solution of these salts is changed by the addition of alkali, the free base may separate from solution unless it has adequate solubility in water. Organic medicinals that are weak acids include the barbiturate drugs (e.g., phenobarbital) and the sulfonamides (e.g., sulfadiazine and sulfacetamide). These and other weak acids form water-soluble salts in basic solution and may separate from solution by a lowering of the pH. Table 13.2 presents the comparative solubilities of some typical examples of weak acids and weak bases and their salts.

Although there are no exact rules for unerringly predicting the solubility of a chemical agent in a particular liquid, experienced pharmaceutical chemists can estimate the general solubility of a chemical compound based on its molecular structure and functional groups. The information gathered on a great number of individual chemical compounds has led to the characterization of the solubilities of groups of compounds, and though there may be an occasional inaccuracy with respect to an individual member of a group of compounds, the generalizations nonetheless are useful. As demonstrated by the data in Table 13.2 and other similar data, salts of organic compounds are more soluble in water than are the corresponding organic bases. Conversely, the organic bases are more soluble in organic solvents, including alcohol, than are the corresponding salt forms. Perhaps the most widely written guideline for the prediction of solubility is "like dissolves like," meaning a solvent having a chemical structure most

TABLE 13.1. Relative Terms of Solubility

Descriptive Term	Parts of Solvent Required for 1 Part of Solute
Very soluble	<1
Freely soluble	1–10
Soluble	10–30
Sparingly soluble	30–100
Slightly soluble	100–1,000
Very slightly soluble	1,000–10,000
Practically insoluble or insoluble	>10,000

Pure Water Handbook. 2nd Ed. Minnetonka, MN: Osmonics, 1997.

TABLE 13.2. Water and Alcohol Solubilities of Some Weak Acids, Weak Bases, and Their Salts

Drug	(Milliliters of Solvent Required to Dissolve 1 g of Drug)	
	Water	Alcohol
Atropine	455.0	2
Atropine sulfate	0.5	5
Codeine	120.0	2
Codeine sulfate	30.0	1,280
Codeine phosphate	2.5	325
Morphine	5,000.0	210
Morphine sulfate	16.0	565
Phenobarbital	1,000.0	8
Phenobarbital sodium	1.0	10
Procaine	200.0	10–30
Procaine hydrochloride	1.0	15
Sulfadiazine	13,000.0	30–100
Sodium sulfadiazine	2.0	100–1,000

TABLE 13.3. Solubilities of Selected Organic Compounds in Water as a Demonstration of Chemical Structure–Solubility Relationship

Compound	Formula		Milliliters of Water Required to Dissolve 1 g of Compound
Benzene	C_6H_6		1,430.0
Benzoic acid	C_6H_5COOH		275.0
Benzyl alcohol	$C_6H_5CH_2OH$		25.0
Phenol	C_6H_5OH		15.0
Pyrocatechol	$C_6H_4(OH)_2$		2.3
Pyrogallol	$C_6H_3(OH)_3$		1.7
Carbon tetrachloride	CCl_4		2,000.0
Chloroform	$CHCl_3$		200.0
Methylene chloride	CH_2Cl_2		50.0

similar to that of the intended solute will be most likely to dissolve it. Thus, organic compounds are more soluble in organic solvents than in water. Organic compounds may, however, be somewhat water soluble if they contain polar groups capable of forming hydrogen bonds with water. In fact, the greater the number of polar groups present, the greater will likely be the organic compound's solubility in water. Polar groups include OH, CHO, COH, CHOH, CH_2OH, COOH, NO_2, CO, NH_2, and SO_3H. The introduction of halogen atoms into a molecule tends to decrease water solubility because of an increase in the molecular

weight of the compound without a proportionate increase in polarity. An increase in the molecular weight of an organic compound without a change in polarity reduces solubility in water. Table 13.3 demonstrates some of these generalities with specific chemical examples.

As with organic compounds, the pharmacist is aware of some general patterns of solubility that apply to inorganic compounds. For instance, most salts of monovalent cations, for example, sodium, potassium, and ammonium, are water soluble, whereas divalent cations, for example, calcium, magnesium, and barium, usually form water-soluble compounds with nitrate, acetate, and chloride anions but not with carbonate, phosphate, or hydroxide anions. To be sure, certain combinations of anion and cation seem to be similar in makeup but do not have similar solubility characteristics. For instance, magnesium sulfate (Epsom salt) is soluble, but calcium sulfate is only slightly soluble; barium sulfate is very insoluble (1 g dissolves in about 400,000 mL of water) and is used as an opaque medium for x-ray observation of the intestinal tract, but barium sulfide and barium sulfite are more soluble, and their oral use can result in poisoning; and mercurous chloride (HgCl) is insoluble and was formerly used as a cathartic, but mercuric chloride ($HgCl_2$) is soluble in water and is a deadly poison if taken internally. In many instances, solubilities of drugs and their differentiation from other drugs are critical to the pharmacist for avoidance of compounding failures or therapeutic disasters.

The ability of a solvent to dissolve organic as well as inorganic solutes depends on its effectiveness in overcoming the electronic forces that hold the atoms of the solute together and the corresponding lack of resolute on the part of the atoms themselves to resist the solvent action. During dissolution, the molecules of the solvent and the solute become uniformly mixed, and cohesive forces of the atoms are replaced by new forces as a result of the attraction of the solute and solvent molecules for one another.

The student may find the following general rules of solubility useful.

Inorganic Molecules

1. If both the cation and anion of an ionic compound are monovalent, the solute–solute attractive forces are usually easily overcome, and therefore, these compounds are generally water soluble (e.g., NaCl, LiBr, KI, NH_4NO_3, and $NaNO_2$).
2. If only one of the two ions in an ionic compound is monovalent, the solute–solute interactions are also usually easily overcome and the compounds are water soluble (e.g., $BaCl_2$, MgI_2, Na_2SO_4, and Na_3PO_4).
3. If both the cation and anion are multivalent, the solute–solute interaction may be too great to be overcome by the solute–solvent interaction, and the compound may have poor water solubility (e.g., $CaSO_4$, $BaSO_4$, and $BiPO_4$; exceptions: $ZnSO_4$, $FeSO_4$).
4. Common salts of alkali metals (e.g., Na, K, Li, Cs, and Rb) are usually water soluble (exception: Li_2CO_3).

5. Ammonium and quaternary ammonium salts are water soluble.
6. Nitrates, nitrites, acetates, chlorates, and lactates are generally water soluble (exceptions: silver and mercurous acetate).
7. Sulfates, sulfites, and thiosulfates are generally water soluble (exceptions: calcium and barium salts).
8. Chlorides, bromides, and iodides are water soluble (exceptions: salts of silver and mercurous ions).
9. Acid salts corresponding to an insoluble salt will be more water soluble than the original salt.
10. Hydroxides and oxides of compounds other than alkali metal cations and the ammonium ion are generally water insoluble.
11. Sulfides are water insoluble except for their alkali metal salts.
12. Phosphates, carbonates, silicates, borates, and hypochlorites are water insoluble except for their alkali metal salts and ammonium salts.

Organic Molecules

1. Molecules having one polar functional group are usually soluble to total chain lengths of five carbons.
2. Molecules having branched chains are more soluble than the corresponding straight-chain compound.
3. Water solubility decreases with an increase in molecular weight.
4. Increased structural similarity between solute and solvent is accompanied by increased solubility.

It is the pharmacist's knowledge of the chemical characteristics of drugs that permits the selection of the proper solvent for a particular solute. However, in addition to the factors of solubility, the selection is based on such additional characteristics as clarity, low toxicity, viscosity, compatibility with other formulative ingredients, chemical inertness, palatability, odor, color, and economy. In most instances, especially for solutions to be taken orally, used intranasally, used ophthalmically, or injected, water is the preferred solvent because it comes closer to meeting these criteria than other solvents. When water is used as the primary solvent, commonly an auxiliary solvent is also employed to augment the solvent action of water or to contribute to a product's chemical or physical stability. Alcohol, glycerin, and propylene glycol, perhaps the most widely used auxiliary solvents, have been quite effective in contributing to the desired characteristics of pharmaceutical solutions and in maintaining their stability.

Other solvents, such as acetone, ethyl oxide, and isopropyl alcohol, are too toxic to be permitted in pharmaceutical preparations to be taken internally, but they are useful as reagent solvents in organic chemistry and in the preparatory stages of drug development, as in the extraction or removal of active constituents from medicinal plants. For purposes such as this, certain solvents are officially recognized in the compendia. A number of fixed oils, such as corn oil, cottonseed oil, peanut oil, and sesame oil, are useful solvents, particularly in the preparation of oleaginous injections, and are recognized in the official compendia for this purpose.

SOME SOLVENTS FOR LIQUID PREPARATIONS

The following agents find use as solvents in the preparation of solutions.

Alcohol, USP: Ethyl Alcohol, Ethanol, C_2H_5OH

Next to water, alcohol is the most useful solvent in pharmacy. It is used as a primary solvent for many organic compounds. Together with water, it forms a hydroalcoholic mixture that dissolves both alcohol-soluble and water-soluble substances, a feature especially useful in the extraction of active constituents from crude drugs. By varying the proportion of the two agents, the active constituents may be selectively dissolved and extracted or allowed to remain behind, according to their particular solubility characteristics in the menstruum. Alcohol, USP, is 94.9% to 96.0% C_2H_5OH by volume (i.e., v/v) when determined at 15.56°C, the U.S. government's standard temperature for alcohol determinations. Dehydrated Alcohol, USP, also called absolute alcohol, contains not less than 99.5% C_2H_5OH by volume and is used when an essentially water-free alcohol is desired.

Alcohol has been well recognized as a solvent and excipient in the formulation of oral pharmaceutical products. Certain drugs are insoluble in water and must be dissolved in an alternative vehicle. Alcohol is often preferred because of its miscibility with water and its ability to dissolve many water-insoluble ingredients, including drug substances, flavorants, and antimicrobial preservatives. Alcohol is frequently used with other solvents, such as glycols and glycerin, to reduce the amount of alcohol required. It is also used in liquid products as an antimicrobial preservative alone or with parabens, benzoates, sorbates, and other agents.

However, aside from its pharmaceutical advantages as a solvent and a preservative, concern has been expressed over the undesired pharmacologic and potential toxic effects of alcohol when ingested in pharmaceutical products, particularly by children. Thus, the U.S. Food and Drug Administration (FDA) has proposed that insofar as possible manufacturers of over-the-counter (OTC) oral drug products restrict the use of alcohol and include appropriate warnings in the labeling. For OTC oral products intended for children under 6 years of age, the recommended alcohol content limit is 0.5%; for products intended for children 6 to 12 years of age, the recommended limit is 5%; and for products recommended for children over 12 years of age and for adults, the recommended limit is 10%.

Diluted Alcohol, NF

Diluted Alcohol, NF, is prepared by mixing equal volumes of Alcohol, USP, and Purified Water, USP. The final volume of such mixtures is not the sum of the individual volumes of the two components because the liquids contract upon mixing; the final volume is generally about 3% less than what would otherwise be expected. Thus, when 50 mL of each component is combined, the resulting product measures approximately 97 mL. It is for this reason that the strength of Diluted Alcohol, NF, is not exactly half that of the more concentrated alcohol but slightly greater, approximately 49%. Diluted alcohol is a useful hydroalcoholic solvent in various pharmaceutical processes and preparations.

Rubbing Alcohol

Rubbing alcohol contains about 70% ethyl alcohol by volume, the remainder consisting of water, denaturants with or without color additives and perfume oils, and stabilizers. Each 100 mL must contain not less than 355 mg of sucrose octaacetate or 1.4 mg of denatonium benzoate, bitter substances that discourage accidental or abusive oral ingestion. According to the Internal Revenue Service, U.S. Treasury Department, the denaturant employed in rubbing alcohol is formula 23-H, which is composed of 8 parts by volume of acetone, 1.5 parts by volume of methyl isobutyl ketone, and 100 parts by volume of ethyl alcohol. The use of this denaturant mixture makes the separation of ethyl alcohol from the denaturants virtually impossible with ordinary distillation apparatus. This discourages the illegal removal for use as a beverage of the alcoholic content of rubbing alcohol.

The product is volatile and flammable and should be stored in a tight container remote from fire. It is employed as a rubefacient externally and as a soothing rub for bed-ridden patients, a germicide for instruments, and a skin cleanser prior to injection. It is also used as a vehicle for topical preparations. Synonym: alcohol rubbing compound.

Glycerin, USP (Glycerol), $CH_2OH \cdot CHOH \cdot CH_2OH$

Glycerin is a clear syrupy liquid with a sweet taste. It is miscible with both water and alcohol. As a solvent, it is comparable with alcohol, but because of its viscosity, solutes are slowly soluble in it unless it is rendered less viscous by heating. Glycerin has preservative qualities and is often used as a stabilizer and as an auxiliary solvent in conjunction with water or alcohol. It is used in many internal preparations.

Isopropyl Rubbing Alcohol

Isopropyl rubbing alcohol is about 70% by volume isopropyl alcohol, the remainder consisting of water with or without color additives, stabilizers, and perfume oils. It is used externally as a rubefacient and soothing rub and as a vehicle for topical products. This preparation and a commercially available 91% isopropyl alcohol solution are commonly employed by diabetic patients in preparing needles and syringes for hypodermic injections of insulin and for disinfecting the skin.

Propylene Glycol, USP, $CH_3CH(OH)CH_2OH$

Propylene glycol, a viscous liquid, is miscible with water and alcohol. It is a useful solvent with a wide range of applications and is frequently substituted for glycerin in modern pharmaceutical formulations.

Purified Water, USP, H_2O

Naturally occurring water exerts its solvent effect on most substances it contacts and, thus, is impure, containing varying amounts of dissolved inorganic salts, usually sodium, potassium, calcium, magnesium, and iron; chlorides; sulfates; and bicarbonates, along with dissolved and undissolved organic matter and microorganisms. Water found in most cities and towns where water is purified for drinking usually contains less than 0.1% of total solids, determined by evaporating a 100-mL sample to dryness and weighing the residue (which weighs <100 mg). Drinking water must meet the U.S. Public Health Service regulations with respect to bacteriologic purity. Acceptable drinking water should be clear, colorless, odorless, and neutral or only slightly acidic or alkaline, the deviation from neutral being due to the nature of the dissolved solids and gases (carbon dioxide contributing to the acidity and ammonia to the alkalinity of water).

Ordinary drinking water from the tap is not acceptable for the manufacture of most aqueous pharmaceutical preparations or for the extemporaneous compounding of prescriptions because of the possible chemical incompatibilities between dissolved solids and the medicinal agents being added. Signs of such incompatibilities are precipitation, discoloration, and occasionally effervescence. Its use is permitted in washing, in extraction of crude vegetable drugs, in preparation of certain products for external use, and when the difference between tap water and purified water is of no consequence. Naturally, when large volumes of water are required to clean pharmaceutical machinery and equipment, tap water may be economically employed so long as a residue of solids is prevented by using purified water as the final rinse or by wiping the water dry with a meticulously clean cloth.

Purified Water, USP, is obtained by distillation, ion exchange treatment, reverse osmosis, or other suitable process. It is prepared from water complying with the federal Environmental Protection Agency with respect to drinking water. Purified Water, USP, has fewer solid impurities than does ordinary drinking water. When evaporated to dryness, it must not yield more than 0.001% of residue (1 mg of solids per 100 mL of water). Thus, purified water has only 1% as much dissolved solids as tap water. Purified Water, USP, is intended for use in the preparation of aqueous dosage forms except those intended for parenteral administration (injections). Water for Injection, USP; Bacteriostatic Water for Injection, USP; or Sterile Water for Injection, USP, is used for injections. These are discussed in Chapter 15.

The main methods used in the preparation of purified water are distillation, ion exchange, and reverse osmosis; these methods are described briefly next.

Distillation Method

Many stills in various sizes and styles with capacities ranging from about 0.5 to 100 gallons of distillate per hour are available to prepare purified water. Generally, the first portion of aqueous distillate (about the first 10% to 20%) must be discarded because it contains many foreign volatile substances usually found in urban drinking water, the usual starting material. Also, the last portion of water (about 10% of the original volume of water) remaining in the distillation apparatus must be discarded and not subjected to further distillation because distillation to dryness would undoubtedly result in decomposition of the remaining solid impurities to volatile substances that would distill and contaminate the previously collected portion of distillate.

Ion Exchange Method

On a large or small scale, ion exchange for the preparation of purified water offers a number of advantages over distillation. For one thing, the requirement of heat is eliminated and with it, the costly and troublesome maintenance frequently encountered in the operation of the more complex distillation apparatus. Because of the simpler equipment and the nature of the method, ion exchange permits ease of operation, minimal maintenance, and a more mobile facility. Many pharmacies and small laboratories that purchase large volumes of distilled water from commercial suppliers for use in their work would no doubt benefit financially and in convenience through the installation of an ion exchange demineralizer in the work area.

The ion exchange equipment in use today generally passes water through a column of cation and anion exchangers consisting of water-insoluble synthetic polymerized phenolic, carboxylic, amino, or sulfonated resins of high molecular weight. These resins are mainly of two types: (*a*) the cations, or acid exchangers, which permit the exchange of the cations in solution (in the tap water) with hydrogen ion from the resin, and (*b*) the anions, or base exchange resins, which permit the removal of anions. These two processes are successively or simultaneously employed to remove cations and anions from water. The processes are indicated as follows, with M^+ indicating the metal or cation (as Na^+) and the X^- indicating the anion (as Cl^-).

Cation exchange:

$$H - resin + M^+ + X^- + H_2O \rightarrow$$
$$M - resin + H^+ + X^- + H_2O \ (pure)$$

Anion exchange:

$$Resin - NH_2 + H^+ + X^- + H_2O \rightarrow$$
$$Resin - NH_2 \cdot HX + H_2O \ (pure)$$

Water purified in this manner, referred to as demineralized or deionized water, may be used in any pharmaceutical preparation or prescription calling for distilled water.

Reverse Osmosis

Reverse osmosis is one of the processes referred to in the industry as cross-flow (or tangential flow) membrane filtration (2). In this process, a pressurized stream of water is passed parallel to the inner side of a filter membrane core. A portion of the feed water, or influent, permeates the membrane as filtrate, while the balance of the water sweeps tangentially along the membrane to exit the system without being filtered. The filtered portion is called the permeate because it has permeated the membrane. The water that has passed through the system is called the concentrate because it contains the concentrated contaminants rejected by the membrane. Whereas in osmosis, the flow through a semipermeable membrane is from a less concentrated solution to a more concentrated solution, the flow in this cross-flow system is from a more concentrated to a less concentrated solution, thus the term reverse osmosis. Depending on their pore size, cross-flow filter membranes can remove particles defined in the range of microfiltration (0.1 to 2 μm, e.g., bacteria), ultrafiltration (0.01 to 0.1 μm, e.g., virus), nanofiltration (0.001 to 0.01 μm, e.g., organic compounds in the molecular weight range of 300 to 1,000), and reverse osmosis (particles <0.001 μm). Reverse osmosis removes virtually all viruses, bacteria, pyrogens, and organic molecules and 90% to 99% of ions (2).

PREPARATION OF SOLUTIONS

Most pharmaceutical solutions are unsaturated with solute. Thus, the amounts of solute to be dissolved are usually well below the capacity of the volume of solvent employed. The strengths of pharmaceutical preparations are usually expressed in terms of percent strength, although for very dilute preparations, expressions of ratio strength may be used. These expressions and examples are shown in Table 13.4.

The symbol % used without qualification (as with w/v, v/v, or w/w) means percent weight in volume for solutions or suspensions of solids in liquids, percent weight in volume for solutions of gases in liquids, percent volume in volume for solutions of liquids in liquids, and weight in weight for mixtures of solids and semisolids.

Some chemical agents in a given solvent require an extended time to dissolve. To hasten dissolution, a pharmacist may employ one of several techniques, such as applying heat, reducing the particle size of the solute,

TABLE 13.4. Common Methods of Expressing the Strengths of Pharmaceutical Preparations

Expression	Abbreviated Expression	Meaning and Example
Percent weight in volume	% w/v	Grams of constituent in 100 mL of preparation (e.g., 1% w/v = 1 g constituent in 100 mL preparation)
Percent volume in volume	% v/v	Milliliters of constituent in 100 mL of preparation (e.g., 1% v/v 1 mL constituent in 100 mL preparation)
Percent weight in weight	% w/w	Grams of constituent in 100 g of preparation (e.g., 1% w/w = 1 g constituent in 100 g preparation)
Ratio of strength to weight in volume	–:— w/v	Grams of constituent in stated milliliters of preparation (e.g., 1:1,000 w/v = 1 g constituent in 1,000 mL preparation)
Ratio of strength to volume in volume	–:— v/v	Milliliters of constituent in milliliters of preparation (e.g., 1:1,000 v/v = 1 mL constituent in 1,000 mL preparation)
Ratio of strength to weight in weight	–:— w/w	Grams of constituent in stated number of grams of preparation (e.g., 1:1,000 w/w = 1 g constituent in 1,000 g preparation)

using a solubilizing agent, and/or subjecting the ingredients to vigorous agitation. Most chemical agents are more soluble at elevated temperatures than at room temperature or below because an endothermic reaction between the solute and the solvent uses the energy of the heat to enhance dissolution. However, elevated temperatures cannot be maintained for pharmaceuticals, and the net effect of heat is simply an increase in the rate of solution rather than an increase in solubility. An increased rate is satisfactory to the pharmacist because most solutions are unsaturated anyway and do not require a concentration of solute above the normal capacity of the solvent at room temperature. Pharmacists are reluctant to use heat to facilitate solution, and when they do, they are careful not to exceed the minimally required temperature, for many medicinal agents are destroyed at elevated temperatures and the advantage of rapid solution may be completely offset by drug deterioration. If volatile solutes are to be dissolved or if the solvent is volatile (as is alcohol), the heat would encourage the loss of these agents to the atmosphere and must therefore be avoided. Pharmacists are aware that certain chemical agents, particularly calcium salts, undergo exothermic reactions as they dissolve and give off heat. For such materials, the use of heat would actually discourage the formation of a solution. The best pharmaceutical example of this type of chemical is calcium hydroxide, which is used in the preparation of Calcium Hydroxide Topical Solution, USP. Calcium hydroxide is soluble in water to the extent of 140 mg/100 mL of solution at 25°C (about 77°F) and 170 mg/100 mL of solution at 15°C (about 59°F). Obviously, the temperature at which the solution is prepared or stored can affect the concentration of the resultant solution.

In addition to or instead of raising the temperature of the solvent to increase the rate of solution, a pharmacist may choose to decrease the particle size of the solute. This may be accomplished by comminution (grinding a solid to a fine state of subdivision) with a mortar and pestle on a small scale or industrial micronizer on a larger scale. The reduced particle size increases the surface area of the solute. If the powder is placed in a suitable vessel (e.g., a beaker, graduated cylinder, bottle) with a portion of the solvent and is stirred or shaken, as suited to the container, the rate of solution may be increased by the continued circulation of fresh solvent to the drug's surface and the constant removal of newly formed solution from the drug's surface.

Most solutions are prepared by simple mixing of the solutes with the solvent. On an industrial scale, solutions are prepared in large mixing vessels with ports for mechanical stirrers (Fig. 13.1). When heat is desired, thermostatically controlled mixing tanks may be used.

COSOLVENTS

When the aqueous solubility of a drug is considerably below its therapeutic dose, a mixture of solvents is often added to achieve sufficiently high solubility, unless a suspension or emulsion dosage form is being prepared. If a drug is not sufficiently water soluble, then either a mixture of solvents or a cosolvent system can be used to increase

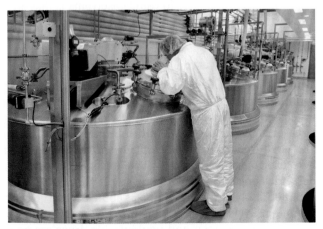

FIGURE 13.1. Large-scale pharmaceutical mixing vessels. (Courtesy of NavinTar/Shutterstock.)

the solubility of a poorly water-soluble compound. Cosolvents can increase the solubility of a nonpolar drug up to several orders of magnitude compared to its plain and unaltered water solubility. This is significant for a formulation where it may be necessary to substantially increase the solubility of the drug.

Cosolvents are solvents used in conjunction with primary solvents and are used to increase drug solubility; they are generally organic in nature but have a reasonable degree of solubility or miscibility in water. The addition of a solvent with lower polarity (lower DC) than water makes the combined "solvent" less water-like, improving solubility of drugs with less polar nature.

The DC approach is based upon the fact that the poor solubility of drugs in water results from a great difference in the polarity of the two components, water being of high polarity and the drug with low polarity. The addition of a cosolvent with a polarity less than that of water reduces the difference between the polarity of the drug and water cosolvent system and improves solubility.

Cosolvents can change the overall solvent property resulting in a change in the rate and order of the degradation reaction of the drug. For drugs that undergo hydrolysis, an advantage to using a cosolvent is to reduce the degradation rate of the drug by reducing the concentration of water in the formulation resulting in enhancing the chemical stability of the drug in its liquid state. Also, a cosolvent may enhance the stability of a drug by making a less suitable environment for the transition state of the reactants; providing the transition state is more polar than the reactants.

Another advantage is that with both parenteral and oral administration, a drug in solution is more readily bioavailable as compared to solid dosage forms. However, cosolvents used in a dosage form must meet certain criteria, including nontoxicity, compatibility with the formulation, compatibility with the blood (for parenterals). They must also be nonsensitizing, nonirritating, and physically and chemically stable and inert. Hydrophilic cosolvents (ethanol, propylene glycol, polyethylene glycol 300 and 400) can be used in lipid-based oral formulations to improve solubilization. One advantage to using cosolvents is that after administration, the cosolvents remain in the local area to aid in preventing drug precipitation, etc.

Dielectric Constant

Generally, the "dielectric constant" (DC, ε) has been used as an aid in developing cosolvent systems. The DC is a dimensionless parameter since it is a ratio of the capacitance of a condenser filled with the material of interest compared to a vacuum. More polar solvents have larger dielectric constants, and less polar solvents have smaller dielectric constants. The DC for water is about 80.4, ethanol is about 24.3, propylene glycol is about 32, and glycerin is about 47. Most poorly soluble drugs have DC values of less than 20. Nonpolar and nonionizable drugs are good candidates for cosolvent systems.

The optimal cosolvent system usually should have a dielectric constant similar to the solute being dissolved. Consider water versus pentane. Polar solvents such as water (ε = 80.4) dissolve ionic solutes and polar substances, whereas nonpolar solvents such as pentane (ε = 1.8) cannot. Pentane can dissolve nonpolar substances like oils and fats, however, but water cannot.

The DC of a mixture of two or more solvents is approximately equal to the weighted average of the individual solvents, allowing the calculation of a reasonable estimate of a defined mixture as based on the simplified Onsager-Kirkwood equation:

$$DC = \sum \left(\text{Solvent A fraction} \times \text{DC of Solvent A} \right) \\ + \left(\text{Solvent B fraction} \times \text{DC of Solvent B} \right)$$

This equation is adequate for solvent mixtures that behave as ideal solutions, but most solvent mixtures exhibit a degree of intermolecular association so the "ε" value calculated would lead to a deviation from the experimental data. It does, however, provide a reasonable estimate. Another variable is that when volumes are used to determine the fraction, when two solvents are mixed, the individual volumes do not always add up to the total expected volume due to hydrogen bonding; ethanol mixed with water is a good example.

Consider in general, as an example, a cosolvent system where the drug is semipolar and the solvent is polar. Generally, semipolar drugs have parabolic log solubility curves, and the peak is where the best mixture of cosolvent and water is best for maximum solubilization of the drug.

- For a semipolar drug, the addition of more nonpolar cosolvent results in a decrease in the drugs solubility.
- For polar drugs, the cosolvent tends to decrease the solubility of the drug.

Also, when the cosolvent is less polar than water:

- For a nonpolar drug, there is an increase in solubility with increasing cosolvent content.
- For a polar drug, there is a decrease in solubility with the addition of cosolvent.

Cosolvents increase drug solubility by altering the DC and hydrogen bonding capability of the vehicle and by providing a hydrophobic microenvironment. Generally, nonpolar solvents have a DC of 1 to 20, semipolar 20 to 50, and polar greater than 50, as shown in Table 13.1.

As an example calculation, let's look at the following situation:

If a 30% ethanol (DC 24.3) in water (DC 80.4) preparation is required for a drug delivery system, what is an estimate of the DC of the 30% ethanol in water mixture:

$$0.30 \times 24.3 + 0.70 \times 80.4 = 63.6.$$

When this mixture is actually experimentally determined, it is 59.5; this shows this estimation method is sufficiently close for this application. As previously mentioned, the variation in results may be partially contributed to the hydrogen bonding activity between water and ethanol.

An early example of the use of cosolvents is Phenobarbital Elixir, USP, which utilized a cosolvent system of alcohol, glycerin, and water.

A current example of the use of cosolvents is the following compounded formula:

Rx Beclomethasone Dipropionate Topical Solution

Beclomethasone dipropionate	150 mg
Absolute alcohol	70 mL
0.9% Sodium chloride solution qs	120 mL

Some practical tips when working with cosolvent systems include the following:

- When working with cosolvent systems, it is generally advisable to add the API to the cosolvent first and then slowly add the water with mixing. This will maintain as high a cosolvent concentration as possible as the water is slowly added. Do not add the cosolvent phase to the water phase as the initial portions of the cosolvent solution may precipitate out the drug due to rapid dilution with the water.
- When compounding topical foams, solvents and cosolvents are the primary constituents as the API is generally present in a much lower concentration and one consideration is the selection of a cosolvent that will not break the foam or prevent or minimize its formation upon application.
- Ethanol is a more efficient cosolvent than glycerin as it is less polar.
- Adding an organic cosolvent to water makes the solvating environment less polar, resulting in a more favorable mixing (solvation) of a hydrophobic solute in the liquid phase.
- Generally, the more hydrophobic the solute, the greater the solubilizing effect produced by an organic cosolvent that is less polar than water.

When formulation development involves poorly water-soluble drugs, the use of cosolvent(s) is a simple and common approach. Solubilized formulations are especially appropriate for pediatric and geriatric patients as well as adults with swallowing difficulties. Limitations with using cosolvents include taste (alcohol, propylene glycol) and adverse physiological effects (alcohol, benzyl alcohol). The DC calculations may be useful in determining the ratios of selected cosolvents to be used with the primary solvent, water. Some common solvents and cosolvents and their DC include the following:

TABLE 1 Dielectric Constants of Some Common Solvents And Cosolvents

Solvent or Cosolvent	DC (ε)
Water	80.4
Glycerin	47.0
Ethanol	24.3
Acetone	20.7
Isopropyl alcohol	18.3
Acetic acid	6.2
Diethyl ether	4.3
Olive oil	3.1
Pentane	1.8

MIXING ORAL LIQUIDS

Mixing is a unit operation; it is the process of thoroughly combining different materials to produce a homogeneous product. Mixing and blending are very demanding as the final product depends upon how well and completely the process is accomplished. "Blending" is a process of combining materials and is a relatively gentle process compared to "mixing." Mixing of liquids includes dissolving solids and semisolids in liquids and mixing liquids in liquids; all these processes can involve both nonsterile and sterile products.

As will be further discussed in Chapter 14, fluids are generally classified as newtonian or nonnewtonian, depending on the relationship between their shear rates and the applied stress. Newtonian fluids are generally easier to mix than nonnewtonian. Shear forces are generated by interactions between moving fluids and the surfaces over which they flow during mixing.

The nature of the liquid(s) to be blended determines the equipment used for mixing; single-phase blending tends to involve low-shear, high-flow mixers to cause liquid engulfment, whereas multiphase mixing generally requires the use of high-shear, low-flow mixers to create droplets of one liquid in another. Liquid–liquid mixers operate in laminar, turbulent, or transitional flow regimens. Turbulent or transitional mixing is frequently conducted with turbines or impellers; laminar mixing is conducted with helical ribbon or anchor mixers. Mixing immiscible liquids often necessitates different equipment than is used for single-phase blending.

Mixing mechanisms for fluids involve four different categories: bulk transport, turbulent flow, laminar flow, and molecular diffusion. Generally, more than one of these processes is occurring in most mixing situations.

1. *Bulk transport* involves the movement of a relatively large portion of material being mixed from one location to another location. For it to be effective, it must result in a rearrangement or permutation of the various portions of the materials to be mixed, usually accomplished using paddles, blades, or other devices with the mixer to move adjacent volumes of the fluid

in different directions, resulting in shuffling the system in three dimensions. (Examples include mixing liquids using paddle-type mixers and the addition of a drug to a large volume parenteral [LVP] in a plastic container mixed by kneading.)

2. *Turbulent mixing* is a direct result of turbulent fluid flow, which is characterized by a random fluctuation of the fluid velocity at any given point within the system. Generally, turbulence involves a fluid having different instantaneous velocities at different locations at the same instant in time (syringe-to-syringe mixtures; syringe additions to LVP glass containers and bags; also using some magnetic stirrers, Lightnin'-type mixers).

3. *Laminar mixing* is frequently encountered when highly viscous fluids are being processed and can also occur if stirring is relatively gentle and may exist adjacent to stationary surfaces in vessels in which the flow is predominantly turbulent. When two dissimilar fluids are mixed using laminar flow, the shear generated stretches the interface between them and a "mixer" folds them back upon themselves and the process continues resulting in mixing (magnetic stirrers).

4. *Molecular diffusion* is the primary mechanism responsible for mixing at the molecular level; it can result from thermal motion of the molecules. Also, the concentration gradient at the original boundary is a decreasing function of time and approaches zero as mixing approaches completion. Diffusion mixing is a mechanism where two different fluids come together and is a relatively slow process. It can occur when adding one liquid to another and letting it set for a time. (An example would be adding water to propylene glycol or glycerin and letting it set. It also occurs after adding syringe contents to bags, in the outer areas of paddle mixing, etc.)

Time is important in any mixing process, and the time required must be determined to bring about acceptable uniformity, completeness, or "goodness of mixing." Y-site mixing, T junctions, and three-way intersections and other designs can be used to enhance the interfacial area between the two fluids. Twisting channels can also assist the two fluids to mix, including multilayered devices where the fluids will corkscrew, loop, or flow around obstructions and wavy devices where the channel will constrict and flare out; also, channels with features on the walls like notches or grooves have been used.

Selection of appropriate equipment for mixing involves consideration of the physical properties of the materials to be mixed, that is, density, viscosity, and miscibility. Also, a "mixer" is not just a generic production/compounding tool but a critical and decisive piece of equipment that helps determine the quality of the final preparation. Mixers generally involve an "impeller" and are of two types, axial and radial, depending upon the angle that the impeller/agitator blade makes with the plane of impeller rotation.

Axial flow impeller is the impeller blade that makes an angle of less than 90 degrees with the plane of impeller rotation, resulting in the flow occurring along the axis of the impeller (parallel to the impeller shaft). Examples include a marine propeller and a pitched blade turbine.

Radial flow impeller is where the impeller blade is parallel to the axis of the impeller, resulting in discharging flow along the impeller radius in distinct patterns. Examples include a flat blade turbine and paddle.

Mixing in a compounding pharmacy is often achieved using magnetic stirrers, simple shaking by hand, stirring rods and beakers, and Lightnin'-type mixers. Magnetic stir bars are radial flow mixers that induce solid body rotation in the fluid being mixed. This is acceptable on a small scale as the vessels are small and mixing generally occurs rapidly. A variety of stir bar configurations are available, but because of the small size and low fluid viscosity of the fluid, it is possible to use one configuration for nearly all mixing tasks. One peculiarity of magnetic stir bar mixing is that the stir bar rests on the bottom of the vessel instead of being located up near the center. The impellers in Lightnin'-type mixers can be placed almost anywhere within the system to obtain optimum mixing in the shortest time.

The quality of mixtures is ultimately judged on the basis of some measure of the random distribution of their components, that is, uniformity throughout the batch, and can be referred to as the "goodness of mixing." It should be evident that the uniformity of the finished preparation is dependent upon each mixing step involved in the procedure.

ORAL SOLUTIONS AND PREPARATIONS FOR ORAL SOLUTION

Most solutions intended for oral administration contain flavorants and colorants to make the medication more attractive and palatable. When needed, they may also contain stabilizers to maintain the chemical and physical stability of the medicinal agents and preservatives to prevent the growth of microorganisms in the solution. The formulation pharmacist must be wary of chemical interactions between the various components of a solution that may alter the preparation's stability and/or potency. For instance, esters of *p*-hydroxybenzoic acid (methyl-, ethyl-, propyl-, and butylparabens), frequently used preservatives in oral preparations, have a tendency to partition into certain flavoring oils (3). This partitioning effect could reduce the effective concentration of the preservatives in the aqueous medium of a pharmaceutical product below the level needed for preservative action.

Liquid pharmaceuticals for oral administration are usually formulated such that the patient receives the usual dose of the medication in a conveniently administered volume, as 5 (one teaspoonful), 10, or 15 mL (one tablespoonful). A few solutions have unusually large doses, for example, Magnesium Citrate Oral Solution, USP, with a usual adult dose of 200 mL. On the other hand, many solutions for children are given by drop with a calibrated dropper usually furnished by the manufacturer in the product package.

Dry Mixtures for Solution

A number of medicinal agents, particularly certain antibiotics, for example, penicillin V, have insufficient stability in aqueous solution to meet extended shelf life periods. Thus, commercial manufacturers of these products provide them to the pharmacist in dry powder or granule form for reconstitution with a prescribed amount of purified water immediately before dispensing to the patient. The dry powder mixture contains all of the formulative components, including drug, flavorant, colorant, buffers, and others, except for the solvent. Once reconstituted by the pharmacist, the solution remains stable when stored in the refrigerator for the labeled period, usually 7 to 14 days, depending on the preparation. This is a sufficient period for the patient to complete the regimen usually prescribed. However, in case the medication remains after the patient completes the course of therapy, the patient should be instructed to discard the remaining portion, which would be unfit for use at a later time.

Examples of dry powder mixtures intended for reconstitution to oral solutions are the following:

- Cloxacillin Sodium for Oral Solution, USP (Teva), an anti-infective antibiotic
- Penicillin V Potassium for Oral Solution, USP (Veetids, Geneva), an anti-infective antibiotic
- Potassium Chloride for Oral Solution, USP (K-LOR, Abbott), a potassium supplement

Oral Solutions

The pharmacist may be called on to dispense a commercially prepared oral solution; dilute the concentration of a solution, as in the preparation of a pediatric form of an adult product; prepare a solution by reconstituting a dry powder mixture; or extemporaneously compound an oral solution from bulk ingredients.

In each instance, the pharmacist should be sufficiently knowledgeable about the dispensed product to expertly advise the patient of the proper use, dosage, method of administration, and storage of the product. Knowledge of the solubility and stability characteristics of the medicinal agents and the solvents employed in the commercial products is useful to the pharmacist for informing the patient of the advisability of mixing the solution with juice, milk, or other beverage upon administration. Information regarding the solvents used in each commercial product appears on the product label and in the accompanying package insert. Table 13.5 presents examples of some oral solutions. Some solutions of special pharmaceutical interest are described later in this chapter.

TABLE 13.5. Examples of Oral Solutions by Category

Oral Solution	Representative Commercial Products	Concentration of Commercial Product	Comments
Antidepressants			
Escitalopram oxalate	Lexapro (Forest)	1 mg/mL	For major depressive disorder
Fluoxetine HCl	Prozac Liquid (Dista)	20 mg fluoxetine/5 mL	For depression, obsessive–compulsive disorder
Antinauseant			
Ondansetron HCl	Zofran Oral Solution (GlaxoSmithKline)	4 mg/5 mL	For prevention of nausea and vomiting due to cancer-related therapies
Antiperistaltic			
Diphenoxylate HCl, atropine sulfate	Lomotil Liquid (Pfizer)	2.5 mg diphenoxylate HCl, 0.025 mg atropine sulfate/5 mL	For diarrhea. Diphenoxylate is related structurally and pharmacologically to the opioid meperidine. Atropine sulfate in subtherapeutic amounts discourages (by virtue of side effects) deliberate overdosage
Loperamide HCl	Imodium A-D Liquid (Ortho-McNeil)	1 mg loperamide HCl/5 mL	For diarrhea in adults and children aged 6 y and older. Structurally related to haloperidol
Antipsychotics			
Haloperidol	Haloperidol Oral Solution	2 mg haloperidol/mL	Primarily for severe neuropsychiatric conditions when oral medication is preferred and tablets and capsules are impractical. Concentrated solutions used by adding desired amount of concentrate by calibrated dropper to soup or a beverage
Perphenazine	Perphenazine Oral Solution	16 mg perphenazine/5 mL	
Antiretroviral			
Emtricitabine	Emtriva (Gilead)	10 mg/mL	Indicated, in combination with other antiretrovirals, for the treatment of HIV-1 infections

(Continued)

TABLE 13.5. Examples of Oral Solutions by Category (*Continued*)

Oral Solution	Representative Commercial Products	Concentration of Commercial Product	Comments
Bronchodilator			
Theophylline	Theophylline Oral Solution (Roxane)	80 mg theophylline/15 mL	Alcohol-free solution for the treatment of bronchial asthma and reversible bronchospasm associated with chronic bronchitis and emphysema
Cathartics			
Magnesium Citrate, USP		Magnesium citrate equivalent to 1.55–1.9 g/100 mL magnesium oxide	Discussed in text
Sodium phosphate	Phospho-Soda (Fleet)	2.4 g monobasic sodium phosphate, 0.9 g dibasic sodium phosphate/5 mL	Works as a laxative within 1 h taken before meals or overnight taken at bedtime. Usual dose is 10–20 mL, best diluted in half glass of water and followed with full glass of water
Corticosteroid			
Prednisolone sodium phosphate	Pediapred Oral Solution (USB)	5 mg prednisolone (as sodium phosphate)/5 mL	Synthetic adrenocortical steroid with mainly glucocorticoid properties indicated for endocrine, rheumatic, collagen, allergic, and other disorders
Dementia			
Memantine HCl	Namenda Oral Solution (Forest)	2 mg/mL	Treatment of moderate to severe dementia of the Alzheimer type
Dental Caries Protectant			
Sodium fluoride	Pediaflor Drops (Ross)	0.5 mg/mL	Prophylaxis of dental caries; for use when community water supply is inadequately fluoridated
Electrolyte Replenisher			
Potassium chloride	Kaochlor 10% Liquid (Pharmacia)	20 mEq KCl/15 mL in flavored aqueous vehicle	For hypopotassemia (low blood level of potassium). Condition may be prompted by severe or chronic diarrhea, low dietary intake of potassium, increased renal excretion of potassium, or other causes. Solution is diluted with water or fruit juice
Fecal Softener			
Docusate sodium	Colace Syrup (Purdue)	10 mg docusate sodium/mL	Usually 50–200 mg measured by calibrated dropper, mixed with milk, fruit juice, or other liquid to mask the taste. Softens fecal mass by lowering the surface tension, permitting normal bowel habits, particularly in geriatric, pediatric, cardiac, obstetric, and surgical patients. Taken for several days or until the bowel movements are normal
Hematinic			
Ferrous sulfate	Fer-In-Sol Drops (Mead Johnson Nutritional)	15 mg/0.6 mL	For prevention and treatment of iron deficiency anemias. Usual prophylactic dose 0.3 or 0.6 mL, measured by calibrated dropper, mixed with water or juice. Dosage form intended primarily for infants and children
Histamine H2 Antagonist			
Cimetidine HCl	Tagamet HCl Liquid (GlaxoSmithKline Consumer)	300 mg/5 mL	For peptic ulcer disease, pathologic hypersecretory conditions, for example, Zollinger-Ellison syndrome
Immunosuppressant			
Cyclosporine	Sandimmune Oral Solution (Novartis) Neoral Oral Solution (Novartis)	100 mg/mL	For prophylaxis of organ rejection
Opioid Agonist Analgesic			
Methadone HCl	Methadone HCl (Roxane)	1 or 2 mg/mL	For relief of severe pain; detoxification, maintenance treatment of opioid addiction
Vitamin D			
Ergocalciferol	Calciferol Drops (Schwartz)	8,000 U/mL	Water-insoluble ergocalciferol (vitamin D_2) in propylene glycol. Usual prophylactic dose is about 400 U; therapeutic dose may be as high as 200,000–500,000 U daily in treating rickets

Oral Rehydration Solutions

Rapid fluid loss associated with diarrhea can lead to dehydration and ultimately death in some patients, particularly infants. More than 5 million children younger than 4 years of age die of diarrhea each year worldwide (4). Diarrhea is characterized by an increased frequency of loose, watery stools, and because of the rapid fluid loss, dehydration can be an outcome. During diarrhea, the small intestine secretes far more than the normal amount of fluid and electrolytes, and this simply exceeds the ability of the large intestine to reabsorb it. This fluid loss, which occurs mostly from the body's extracellular fluid compartment, can lead to a progressive loss of blood volume culminating in hypovolemic shock.

Diarrhea is a normal physiologic body response to rid itself of a noxious or toxic substance, such as rotavirus or *Escherichia coli*. Thus, the treatment approach is to allow the diarrhea to proceed and not to terminate it too quickly but promptly replace the lost fluid and electrolytes to prevent dehydration. The loss of fluid during diarrhea is accompanied by depletion of sodium, potassium, and bicarbonate ions; if severe, the loss can result in acidosis, hyperpnea, and vomiting as well as hypovolemic shock. If continuous, bouts of vomiting and diarrhea can cause malnutrition as well. Consequently, the goal is to replace lost fecal water with an oral rehydration solution and use nutritional foods, such as soybean formula and bran.

Oral rehydration solutions are usually effective in treatment of patients with mild volume depletion, 5% to 10% of body weight. These are available OTC and are relatively inexpensive, and their use has diminished the incidence of complications associated with parenterally administered electrolyte solutions. Therapy with these solutions is based on the observation that glucose is actively absorbed from the small intestine, even during bouts of diarrhea. This active transport of glucose is advantageous because it is coupled with sodium absorption. Almost in domino fashion, sodium absorption promotes anion absorption, which in turn promotes water absorption to short-circuit dehydration. To produce maximal absorption of sodium and water, studies have demonstrated that the optimal concentrations of glucose and sodium in an isotonic solution are 110 mM (2%) glucose and 60 mEq/L of sodium ion, respectively. Bicarbonate and/or citrate ions are also included in these solutions to help correct the metabolic acidosis caused by diarrhea and dehydration.

A liter of typical oral rehydration solution contains 45 mEq Na^+, 20 mEq K^+, 35 mEq Cl^-, 30 mEq citrate, and 25 g dextrose. These formulations are available in liquid or powder packet form for reconstitution. It is important that the user add the specific amount of water needed to prepare the powder forms. Furthermore, these products should not be mixed with or given with other electrolyte-containing liquids, such as milk or fruit juices. Otherwise, there is no method to calculate how much electrolyte the patient actually received. Commercial ready-to-use oral electrolyte solutions to prevent dehydration or achieve rehydration include Pedialyte Solution (Ross) and Rehydralyte Solution (Ross). These products also contain dextrose or glucose. Infalyte Oral Solution (Bristol-Myers Squibb) contains electrolytes in a syrup of rice solids. The rice-based formula produces a lower osmotic effect than the dextrose- or glucose-based formulas and is thought to be more effective in reducing stool output and shortening the duration of diarrhea. The success of the commercial solutions is based on the physiologic design of the formulation.

Oral Colonic Lavage Solution

Traditionally, preparation of the bowel for procedures such as a colonoscopy consisted of administration of a clear liquid diet for 24 to 48 hours preceding the procedure, administration of an oral laxative such as magnesium citrate or bisacodyl the night before, and a cleansing enema administered 2 to 4 hours prior to the procedure. Typically, to circumvent hospitalization of the patient the night before the procedure, patients were allowed to perform this regimen at home. However, although the results have been satisfactory, that is, the bowel is cleared for the procedure, poor compliance with and acceptance of this regimen can cause problems during the procedure. Furthermore, additive effects of malnutrition and poor oral intake prior to the procedure can cause more patient problems.

Consequently, an alternative method to prepare the gastrointestinal tract has been devised. This procedure requires less time and dietary restriction and obviates the cleansing enemas. This method entails oral administration of a balanced solution of electrolytes with polyethylene glycol (PEG-3350-Electrolyte Solution), that is, Colyte (Alaven Pharmaceuticals). Before dispensing it to the patient, the pharmacist reconstitutes this powder with water, creating an iso-osmotic solution having a mildly salty taste. The PEG acts as an osmotic agent in the gastrointestinal tract, and the balanced electrolyte concentration results in virtually no net absorption or secretion of ions. Thus, a large volume of this solution can be administered without a significant change in water or electrolyte balance.

The formulation of this oral colonic lavage solution is as follows:

PEG-3350	240.00 g
Sodium sulfate	22.72 g
Sodium bicarbonate	6.72 g
Sodium chloride	5.84 g
Potassium chloride	2.98 g

In 4,000 mL disposable container

The recommended adult dose of this product is 4 L of solution before the gastrointestinal procedure. The patient is instructed to drink 240 mL of solution every 10 minutes until about 4 L is consumed. The patient is advised to drink each portion quickly rather than sipping it continuously. Usually, the first bowel movement will occur within 1 hour. Several regimens are used, and one method is to schedule patients for a midmorning procedure, allowing the patient 3 hours for drinking and a 1-hour waiting period to complete bowel evacuation.

To date, this approach to bowel evacuation has been associated with a low incidence of side effects (primarily nausea, transient abdominal fullness, bloating, and occasionally cramps and vomiting). Ideally, the patient should not have taken any food 3 to 4 hours before beginning to take the solution. In no case should solid foods be taken by the patient for at least 2 hours before the solution is administered. No foods except clear liquids are permitted after this product is administered and prior to the examination. The product must be stored in the refrigerator after reconstitution, and this aids somewhat in decreasing the salty taste of the product.

PEG-ES solutions are employed for unlabeled use in the management of acute iron overdose in children.

Magnesium Citrate Oral Solution

Magnesium citrate oral solution is a colorless to slightly yellow clear effervescent liquid having a sweet, acidulous taste and a lemon flavor. It is commonly referred to as citrate or as citrate of magnesia. It is required to contain an amount of magnesium citrate equivalent to 1.55 to 1.9 g of magnesium oxide in each 100 mL.

The solution is prepared by reacting official magnesium carbonate with an excess of citric acid (Equation 13.1), flavoring and sweetening the solution with lemon oil and syrup, filtering with talc, and then carbonating it by the addition of either potassium or sodium bicarbonate (Equation 13.2). The solution may be further carbonated by the use of carbon dioxide under pressure:

$$(MgCO_3)_4 \cdot Mg(OH)_2 + 5H_3C_6H_5O_7 \rightarrow$$
$$5MgHC_6H_5O_7 + 4CO_2 + 6H_2O \qquad \textbf{Equation 13.1}$$

$$3KHCO_3 + H_3C_6H_5O_7 \rightarrow$$
$$K_3C_6H_5O_7 + 3CO_2 + 3H_2O \qquad \textbf{Equation 13.2}$$

The solution provides an excellent medium for the growth of molds, and any mold spores present during the manufacture of the solution must be killed if the preparation is to remain stable. For this reason, during the preparation of the solution, the liquid is heated to boiling (prior to carbonation); boiled water is employed to bring the solution to its proper volume; and boiling water is used to rinse the final container. The final solution may be sterilized.

The solution is employed as a saline cathartic, with the citric acid, lemon oil, syrup, carbonation, and the low temperature of the refrigerated solution all contributing to the patient's acceptance of the large volume of medication. For many patients, it is a pleasant way of taking an otherwise bitter saline cathartic.

Sodium Citrate and Citric Acid Oral Solution

This official solution contains sodium citrate 100 mg and citric acid 67 mg in each milliliter of aqueous solution. The solution is administered orally in doses of 10 to 30 mL as frequently as four times daily as a systemic alkalinizer. Systemic alkalinization is useful for patients for whom long-term maintenance of an alkaline urine is desirable, such as those with uric acid and cystine calculi of the urinary tract. The solution is also a useful adjuvant when administered with uricosuric agents in gout therapy because urates tend to crystallize out of an acid urine.

SYRUPS

Syrups are concentrated aqueous preparations of a sugar or sugar substitute with or without flavoring agents and medicinal substances. Syrups containing flavoring agents but not medicinal substances are called nonmedicated or flavored vehicles (syrups). Some official, previously official, and commercially available nonmedicated syrups are presented in Table 13.6. These syrups are intended to serve as pleasant-tasting vehicles for medicinal substances to be added in the extemporaneous compounding of prescriptions or in the preparation of a standard formula for a medicated syrup, which is a syrup containing a therapeutic agent. Because of the inability of some children and elderly people to swallow solid dosage forms, it is fairly common today for a pharmacist to be asked to prepare an oral liquid dosage form of a medication available in the pharmacy only as tablets or capsules. In these instances, drug solubility, stability, and bioavailability must be considered case by case (5,6). The liquid dosage form selected for compounding may be a solution or a suspension, depending on the chemical and physical characteristics of the particular drug and its solid dosage form. Vehicles are commercially available for this purpose (6).

Medicated syrups are commercially prepared from the starting materials, that is, by combining each of the individual components of the syrup, such as sucrose, purified water, flavoring agents, coloring agents, the therapeutic agent, and other necessary and desirable ingredients. Naturally, medicated syrups are employed in therapeutics for the value of the medicinal agent present in the syrup.

Syrups provide a pleasant means of administering a liquid form of a disagreeable-tasting drug. They are particularly effective in the administration of drugs to youngsters, because their pleasant taste usually dissipates any reluctance on the part of the child to take the medicine. The fact that syrups contain little or no alcohol adds to their favor among parents.

Any water-soluble drug that is stable in aqueous solution may be added to a flavored syrup. However, care must be exercised to ensure compatibility between the drug substance and the other formulative components of the syrup. Also, certain flavored syrups have an acidic medium, whereas others may be neutral or slightly basic,

TABLE 13.6. Examples of Nonmedicated Syrups (Vehicles)

Syrup	Comments
Cherry syrup	Sucrose-based syrup with cherry juice about 47% by volume. Tart fruit flavor is attractive to most patients, and acidic pH makes it useful as a vehicle for drugs requiring an acid medium
Cocoa syrup	Suspension of cocoa powder in aqueous vehicle sweetened and thickened with sucrose, liquid glucose, glycerin; flavored with vanilla, sodium chloride. Particularly effective in administering bitter-tasting drugs to children
Humco Flavor Blend	A uniquely formulated, flavored suspending vehicle combining both flavored vehicle and suspending vehicle forming a sweet, buffered vehicle for oral use
Humco Flavor Plus	A suspending vehicle for use in preparing nonsoluble aqueous dosage forms; buffered to an acidic pH and preserved
Humco Flavor Sweet	A flavored syrup vehicle for compounding oral delivery preparations either used alone or combined with suspending agents. Contains buffers and preservatives
Humco Flavor Sweet SF	A sugar-free version of Humco Flavor Sweet
Humco Flavored Syrups	Flavored syrup vehicles used to mask the taste of medications; suitable for ionic and hydrophilic additives
Humco Syrpalta	A tasty syrup vehicle without added color for use where palatability is desired
Humco Syrpalta Red	A tasty syrup vehicle for use where palatability is desired
Humco Versa Free	A dye-, flavor-, paraben-, sugar-, saccharin-, and aspartame-free syrup resulting in fewer allergic reactions. Virtually no aftertaste
Humco Versa Plus	A dye-, flavor-, paraben-, sugar-, saccharin-, and aspartame-free syrup resulting in fewer allergic reactions. Virtually no aftertaste. Suspending agent
Orange syrup	Sucrose-based syrup uses sweet orange peel tincture, citric acid as the source of flavor and tartness. Resembles orange juice in taste; good vehicle for drugs stable in acidic medium
Ora-Sweet, Ora-Sweet SF	Commercial vehicles for extemporaneous compounding of (Paddock Laboratories) syrups. Both have a pH of 4–4.5 and are alcohol-free. Ora-Sweet SF is sugar-free
Ora-Blend	A preblended combination of Ora-Sweet and Ora-Plus (1:1) and Ora-Sweet SF and Ora-Plus (1:1)
PCCA Acacia Syrup	A sweet, demulcent suspending vehicle with a mild vanilla flavor
PCCA Fixed Oil Suspension Vehicle	Add the active drug, sweetener, and flavor. The sweetener and flavor must be oil soluble
PCCA-Plus Oral Suspending Vehicle	A preserved, buffered vehicle with demulcent qualities
PCCA Sweet SF	A sugar-free syrup containing sorbitol and can be used in diabetic patients as well as others
PCCA Syrup	A syrup vehicle with less sucrose than Syrup NF
Raspberry syrup	Sucrose-based syrup with raspberry juice about 48% by volume. Pleasant-flavored vehicle to disguise salty or sour taste of saline medicaments
SyrSpend SF Alka	An alkaline suspension vehicle with a pH of about 7.0, when reconstituted as directed. It is low osmolality (<50 mOsmol), pleasant-tasting, sugar-free, alkaline medium available in unflavored and cherry formulas
SyrSpend SF Suspension Vehicle	A low osmolality suspending vehicle using modified starch technology. It is buffered at pH 4.2; it is sugar-free and paraben-free; it is available in unflavored, cherry, and grape formulations
SyrSpend Syrup	85% sucrose in purified water. Simple syrup may be used as the basis for flavored or medicated syrups

and the proper selection must be made to ensure the stability of any added medicinal agent. Perhaps the most frequently found types of medications administered as medicated syrups are antitussive agents and antihistamines. This is not to imply that other types of drugs are not formulated into syrups; a variety of medicinal substances can be found in syrup form and among the many commercial products. Examples of medicated syrups are presented in Table 13.7.

Components of Syrups

Most syrups contain the following components in addition to the purified water and any medicinal agents present: (*a*) the sugar, usually sucrose, or sugar substitute used to provide sweetness and viscosity; (*b*) antimicrobial preservatives; (*c*) flavorants; and (*d*) colorants. Also, many types of syrups, especially those prepared commercially, contain special solvents (including alcohol), solubilizing agents, thickeners, or stabilizers.

TABLE 13.7. Examples of Medicated Syrups by Category

Syrup	Representative Commercial Products	Concentration of Commercial Product[a]	Comments
Analgesic			
Meperidine HCl	Demerol Syrup (Sanofi-Synthelabo)	50 mg/5 mL	Opioid analgesic for the relief of moderate to severe pain, adjunct to general anesthesia
Anticholinergics			
Dicyclomine HCl	Various	10 mg/5 mL	Adjunctive therapy in the treatment of peptic ulcer
Oxybutynin chloride	Various	5 mg/5 mL	Relief of symptoms with voiding in patients with uninhibited neurogenic and reflex neurogenic bladder
Antiemetics			
Chlorpromazine HCl	Thorazine Syrup (GlaxoSmithKline)	10 mg HCl/5 mL	Control of nausea and vomiting
Dimenhydrinate	Children's Dramamine Liquid (Pharmacia)	12.5 mg/5 mL	Control of nausea, vomiting, motion sickness
Prochlorperazine edisylate	Various	5 mg/5 mL	Control of nausea and vomiting
Promethazine HCl	Various	6.25, 25 mg/5 mL	Control of nausea, vomiting, motion sickness, allergic reactions
Anticonvulsant			
Sodium valproate	Depakene Syrup (Abbott)	250 mg as sodium salt/5 mL	Sole or adjunctive therapy in simple (petit mal), complex absence seizure disorders
Antihistamines			
Chlorpheniramine maleate	Chlor-Trimeton Allergy Syrup (Schering-Plough)	2 mg/5 mL	For prevention, treatment of allergic reactions
Desloratadine	Clarinex Syrup (Schering)	0.5 mg/1 mL	For relief of nasal and nonnasal symptoms of allergic rhinitis and urticaria
Hydroxyzine HCl	Atarax Syrup (Roerig)	10 mg/5 mL	
Antipsychotic			
Citalopram hydrobromide	Various	10 mg/5 mL	For depression
Lithium citrate	Various	8 mEq/5 mL	Management of psychotic disorders
Risperidone	Risperdal (Janssen)	1 mg/mL	For treatment of schizophrenia
Antitussives			
Dextromethorphan	Benylin Adult Cough and Various	15 mg/5 mL	For relief of cough
Diphenhydramine	Benadryl Allergy Liquid Medication (McNeil) and Various	12.5 mg/5 mL	For control of coughs due to colds or allergy
Antiviral			
Amantadine HCl	Symmetrel Syrup (Endo)	50 mg/5 mL	Prevention of respiratory infections caused by A2 (Asian) viral strains. Treatment of idiopathic Parkinson disease
Lamivudine	Epivir Oral Solution (GlaxoSmithKline)	10 mg/mL	Treatment of HIV
Ritonavir	Norvir (Abbott)	80 mg/mL	Treatment of HIV
Bronchodilators			
Albuterol sulfate	Proventil Syrup (Schering) Ventolin Syrup (Schering)	2 mg/5 mL	Relief of bronchospasm of obstructive airway disease; prevention of exercise-induced bronchospasm
Metaproterenol sulfate	Alupent Syrup (Boehringer Ingelheim)	10 mg/5 mL	
Cathartic			
Lactulose	Chronulac Syrup (Hoechst)	10 g/15 mL	15–30 mL qd as laxative

TABLE 13.7. Examples of Medicated Syrups by Category (*Continued*)

Syrup	Representative Commercial Products	Concentration of Commercial Product[a]	Comments
Cholinergic			
Pyridostigmine bromide	Mestinon Syrup (ICN Pharmaceuticals)	60 mg/5 mL	Treatment of myasthenia gravis
Decongestant			
Pseudoephedrine hydrochloride	Sudafed Children's Nondrowsy (Pfizer Consumer)	15 mg/5 mL	Temporary relief of nasal congestion of common cold, hay fever, upper respiratory allergies, sinusitis
Emetic			
Ipecac	Various	21 mg ether-soluble alkaloids of ipecac/15 mL	To induce vomiting in poisoning. Dose of 15 mL may be repeated in 20 min if vomiting does not occur. If after the second dose vomiting does not occur, the stomach should be emptied by gastric lavage
Expectorant			
Guaifenesin	Various	100 mg/5 mL	For symptomatic relief of respiratory conditions associated with cough and bronchial congestion
Fecal Softener			
Docusate sodium	Colace Syrup (Purdue)	20 mg/5 mL	Stool softener by surface action
Gastrointestinal Stimulant			
Metoclopramide	Various	5 mg/5 mL	Relief of symptoms of diabetic gastroparesis (gastric stasis) and gastroesophageal reflux
H2 receptor antagonist ranitidine HCl	Zantac Syrup (GlaxoSmithKline)	15 mg/mL	Treatment of duodenal ulcers and GERD
Hemostatic			
Aminocaproic acid	Amicar Syrup (Xanodyne)	1.25 g/5 mL	Treatment of excessive bleeding from systemic hyperfibrinolysis, urinary fibrinolysis
Hypnotic Sedative			
Chloral hydrate	Chloral Hydrate Syrup (Pharmaceutical Associates)	250 mg/5 mL	Sedative at 250 mg; hypnotic to induce sleep at 500 mg. Alcoholic beverages should be avoided. Usually diluted with water or some other beverage

[a]A usual single dose unless otherwise stated.

Sucrose- and Non–Sucrose-Based Syrups

Sucrose is the sugar most frequently employed in syrups, although in special circumstances, it may be replaced in whole or in part by other sugars or substances such as sorbitol, glycerin, and propylene glycol. In some instances, all glycogenetic substances (materials converted to glucose in the body), including the agents mentioned earlier, are replaced by nonglycogenetic substances, such as methylcellulose or hydroxyethylcellulose. These two materials are not hydrolyzed and absorbed into the bloodstream, and their use results in an excellent syrup-like vehicle for medications intended for use by diabetic patients and others whose diet must be controlled and restricted to nonglycogenetic substances. The viscosity resulting from the use of these cellulose derivatives is much like that of a sucrose syrup. The addition of one or more artificial sweeteners usually produces an excellent facsimile of a true syrup.

The characteristic body that the sucrose and alternative agents seek to impart to the syrup is essentially the result of attaining the proper viscosity. This quality, together with the sweetness and flavorants, results in a type of pharmaceutical preparation that masks the taste of added medicinal agents.

When the syrup is swallowed, only a portion of the dissolved drug actually makes contact with the taste buds, the remainder of the drug being carried past them and down the throat in the viscous syrup. This type of physical concealment of the taste is not possible for a solution of a drug in an unthickened, mobile aqueous preparation. In the case of antitussive syrups, the thick, sweet syrup has a soothing effect on the irritated tissues of the throat as it passes over them.

Most syrups contain a high proportion of sucrose, usually 60% to 80%, not only because of the desirable sweetness and viscosity of such solutions but also because of their inherent stability in contrast to the unstable character of dilute sucrose solutions. The aqueous sugar medium of dilute sucrose solutions is an efficient nutrient medium for the growth of microorganisms, particularly yeasts and molds. On the other hand, concentrated sugar solutions are quite resistant to microbial growth because of the unavailability of the water required for the growth of microorganisms. This aspect of syrups is best demonstrated by the simplest of all syrups, Syrup, NF, also called simple syrup. It is prepared by dissolving 85 g of sucrose in enough purified water to make 100 mL of syrup. The resulting preparation generally requires no additional preservation if it is to be used soon; in the official syrup, preservatives are added if the syrup is to be stored. When properly prepared and maintained, the syrup is inherently stable and resistant to the growth of microorganisms. An examination of this syrup reveals its concentrated nature and the relative absence of water for microbial growth. Syrup has a specific gravity of about 1.313, which means that each 100 mL of syrup weighs 131.3 g. Because 85 g of sucrose is present, the difference between 85 and 131.3 g, or 46.3 g, represents the weight of the purified water. Thus, 46.3 g, or mL, of purified water is used to dissolve 85 g of sucrose. The solubility of sucrose in water is 1 g in 0.5 mL of water; therefore, to dissolve 85 g of sucrose, about 42.5 mL of water would be required. Thus, only a very slight excess of water (about 3.8 mL per 100 mL of syrup) is employed in the preparation of syrup. Although not enough to be particularly amenable to the growth of microorganisms, the slight excess of water permits the syrup to remain physically stable in varying temperatures. If the syrup were completely saturated with sucrose, in cool storage, some sucrose might crystallize from solution and, by acting as nuclei, initiate a type of chain reaction that would result in separation of an amount of sucrose disproportionate to its solubility at the storage temperature. The syrup would then be very much unsaturated and probably suitable for microbial growth. As formulated, the official syrup is stable and resistant to crystallization and microbial growth. However, many of the other official syrups and a host of commercial syrups are not intended to be as nearly saturated as Syrup, NF, and therefore must employ added preservative agents to prevent microbial growth and to ensure their stability during their period of use and storage.

As noted earlier, sucrose-based syrup may be substituted in whole or in part by other agents in the preparation of medicated syrups. A solution of a polyol, such as sorbitol, or a mixture of polyols, such as sorbitol and glycerin, is commonly used. Sorbitol Solution, USP, which contains 64% by weight of the polyhydric alcohol sorbitol, is employed as shown in the following example formulations for medicated syrups (7):

Antihistamine Syrup

Chlorpheniramine maleate (Active)	0.4 g
Glycerin (Cosolvent and Sweetener)	25.0 mL
Syrup (Cosolvent and Sweetener)	83.0 mL
Sorbitol solution (Cosolvent and Sweetener)	282.0 mL
Sodium benzoate (Preservative)	1.0 g
Alcohol (Cosolvent and Preservative)	60.0 mL
Color and flavor	qs
Purified water, to make (Solvent)	1,000.0 mL

Ferrous Sulfate Syrup

Ferrous sulfate (Active)	135.0 g
Citric acid (pH Adjustment, Tartness for flavor)	12.0 g
Sorbitol solution (Cosolvent and Sweetener)	350.0 mL
Glycerin (Cosolvent and Sweetener)	50.0 mL
Sodium benzoate (Preservative)	1.0 g
Flavor	qs
Purified water, to make (Solvent)	1,000.0 mL

Acetaminophen Syrup

Acetaminophen (Active)	24.0 g
Benzoic acid (Preservative)	1.0 g
Disodium calcium EDTA (Chelating Agent)	1.0 g
Propylene glycol (Cosolvent)	150.0 mL
Alcohol (Cosolvent and Preservative)	150.0 mL
Saccharin sodium (Sweetener)	1.8 g
Purified water (Solvent–Vehicle)	200.0 mL
Flavor	qs
Sorbitol solution, to make (Cosolvent, Sweetener, Vehicle)	1,000.0 mL

Cough and Cold Syrup

Dextromethorphan hydrobromide (Active)	2.0 g
Guaifenesin (Active)	10.0 g
Chlorpheniramine maleate (Active)	0.2 g
Phenylephrine hydrochloride (Active)	1.0 g
Sodium benzoate (Preservative)	1.0 g
Saccharin sodium (Sweetener)	1.9 g
Citric acid (pH Adjustment and Tartness for flavor)	1.0 g
Sodium chloride (Flavor enhancer)	5.2 g
Alcohol (Cosolvent and Preservative)	50.0 mL
Sorbitol solution (Cosolvent and Sweetener)	324.0 mL
Syrup (Cosolvent and Sweetener)	132.0 mL
Liquid glucose (Cosolvent and Sweetener)	44.0 mL
Glycerin (Cosolvent and Sweetener)	50.0 mL
Color	qs
Flavor	qs
Purified water, to make (Solvent and Vehicle)	1,000.0 mL

All materials used in the extemporaneous compounding and manufacturing of pharmaceuticals should be of USP–NF quality and obtained from FDA-approved sources.

Antimicrobial Preservative

The amount of a preservative required to protect a syrup against microbial growth varies with the proportion of water available for growth, the nature and inherent preservative activity of some formulative materials (e.g., many flavoring oils that are inherently sterile and possess antimicrobial activity), and the capability of the preservative itself. Among the preservatives commonly used in syrups with the usually effective concentrations are benzoic acid 0.1% to 0.2%, sodium benzoate 0.1% to 0.2%, and various combinations of methylparabens, propylparabens, and butylparabens totaling about 0.1%. Frequently, alcohol is used in syrups to assist in dissolving the alcohol-soluble ingredients, but normally, it is not present in the final product in amounts that would be considered to be adequate for preservation (15% to 20%). See Physical Pharmacy Capsule 13.1, Preservation of Syrups.

PHYSICAL PHARMACY CAPSULE **13.1** Preservation of Syrups

Syrups can be preserved by (a) storage at low temperature; (b) adding preservatives such as glycerin, benzoic acid, sodium benzoate, methylparaben, or alcohol in the formulation; or (c) the maintenance of a high concentration of sucrose as a part of the formulation. High sucrose concentrations will usually protect an oral liquid dosage form from growth of most microorganisms. A problem arises, however, when pharmacists must add other ingredients to syrups that can result in a decrease in the sucrose concentration. This may cause a loss of the preservative effectiveness of the sucrose. This can be overcome, however, by calculating the quantity of a preservative (such as alcohol) to add to the formula to maintain the preservative effectiveness of the final product.

■ EXAMPLE

Rx active drug	5 mL volume occupied
Other drug solids	3 mL volume occupied
Glycerin	15 mL
Sucrose	25 g
Ethanol	95% qs
Purified water qs	100 mL

How much alcohol would be required to preserve this prescription? We will use the free-water method to calculate the quantity of alcohol required.

Simple syrup contains 85 g sucrose per 100 mL of solution, which weighs 131.3 g (specific gravity, 1.313). It takes 46.3 mL of water to prepare the solution (131.3 − 85 = 46.3), and the sucrose occupies a volume of (100 − 46.3 = 53.7) 53.7 mL.

1. Because this solution is preserved, 85 g of sucrose preserves 46.3 mL of water, and 1 g of sucrose preserves 0.54 mL of water. With 25 g of sucrose present, the amount of water preserved is

$$25 \times 0.54 = 13.5 \text{ mL}$$

2. Because 85 g of sucrose occupies a volume of 53.7 mL, 1 g of sucrose will occupy a volume of 0.63 mL. The volume occupied by the sucrose in this prescription is

$$25 \times 0.63 = 15.75 \text{ mL}$$

3. The active drug and other solids occupy 8 mL (5 + 3) volume.
4. Each mL of glycerin can preserve an equivalent quantity of volume (2 × 15 = 30), so 30 mL would be preserved.
5. The volume taken care of so far is 13.5 + 15.75 + 8 + 30 = 67.25 mL. The quantity of free water remaining is

$$100 - 67.25 = 32.75 \text{ mL}$$

6. Because it requires about 18% alcohol to preserve the water,

$$0.18 \times 32.75 = 5.9 \text{ mL of alcohol (100\%)}$$

would be required.
7. If 95% ethanol is used, 5.9/0.95 = 6.21 mL would be required.

To prepare the prescription, about 6.21 mL of 95% ethanol can be added with sufficient purified water to make 100 mL of the final solution. ■

Flavorant

Most syrups are flavored with synthetic flavorants or with naturally occurring materials, such as volatile oils (e.g., orange oil), vanillin, and others, to render the syrup pleasant tasting. Because syrups are aqueous preparations, these flavorants must be water soluble. However, sometimes a small amount of alcohol is added to a syrup to ensure the continued solution of a poorly water-soluble flavorant. Commercial flavoring systems (FLAVORx) may also be considered and used.

Colorant

To enhance the appeal of the syrup, a coloring agent that correlates with the flavorant employed (i.e., green with mint, brown with chocolate) is used. Generally, the colorant is water soluble, nonreactive with the other syrup components, and color stable at the pH range and under the intensity of light that the syrup is likely to encounter during its shelf life.

Preparation of Syrups

Syrups are most frequently prepared by one of four general methods, depending on the physical and chemical characteristics of the ingredients. Broadly stated, these methods are (a) solution of the ingredients with the aid of heat, (b) solution of the ingredients by agitation without the use of heat or the simple admixture of liquid components, (c) addition of sucrose to a prepared medicated liquid or to a flavored liquid, and (d) percolation of either the source of the medicating substance or the sucrose. Sometimes a syrup is prepared by more than one of these methods, and the selection may simply be a matter of preference on the part of the pharmacist. Many of the official syrups have no officially designated method of preparation.

Solution with the Aid of Heat

Syrups are prepared by this method when it is desired to prepare the syrup as quickly as possible and when the syrup's components are not damaged or volatilized by heat. In this method, the sugar is generally added to the purified water, and heat is applied until the sugar is dissolved. Then, other heat-stable components are added to the hot syrup, the mixture is allowed to cool, and its volume is adjusted to the proper level by the addition of purified water. If heat-labile agents or volatile substances, such as volatile flavoring oils and alcohol, are to be added, they are generally added to the syrup after the sugar is dissolved by heat, and the solution is rapidly cooled to room temperature.

The use of heat facilitates rapid solution of the sugar and certain other components of syrups; however, caution must be exercised against becoming impatient and using excessive heat. Sucrose, a disaccharide, may be hydrolyzed into monosaccharides, dextrose (glucose), and fructose (levulose). This hydrolytic reaction is called inversion, and the combination of the two monosaccharide products is invert sugar. When heat is applied in the preparation of a sucrose syrup, some inversion of the sucrose is almost certain. The speed of inversion is greatly increased by the presence of acids, the hydrogen ion acting as a catalyst to the reaction. Should inversion occur, the sweetness of the syrup is altered because invert sugar is sweeter than sucrose, and the normally colorless syrup darkens because of the effect of heat on the levulose portion of the invert sugar. When the syrup is greatly overheated, it becomes amber colored as the sucrose caramelizes. Syrups so decomposed are more susceptible to fermentation and to microbial growth than the stable, undecomposed syrups. Because of the prospect of decomposition by heat, syrups cannot be sterilized by autoclaving. The use of boiled purified water in the preparation of a syrup can enhance its permanency, and the addition of preservative agents,

when permitted, can protect it during its shelf life. Storage in a tight container is a requirement for all syrups.

Solution by Agitation Without the Aid of Heat

To avoid heat-induced inversion of sucrose, a syrup may be prepared without heat by agitation. On a small scale, sucrose and other formulative agents may be dissolved in purified water by placing the ingredients in a vessel larger than the volume of syrup to be prepared, permitting thorough agitation of the mixture. This process is more time-consuming than the use of heat, but the product has maximum stability. Huge glass-lined or stainless steel tanks with mechanical stirrers or agitators are employed in large-scale preparation of syrups.

Sometimes, simple syrup or some other nonmedicated syrup, rather than sucrose, is employed as the sweetening agent and vehicle. In that case, other liquids that are soluble in the syrup or miscible with it may be added and thoroughly mixed to form a uniform product. When solid agents are to be added to a syrup, it is best to dissolve them in minimal amount of purified water and incorporate the resulting solution into the syrup. When solid substances are added directly to a syrup, they dissolve slowly because the viscous nature of the syrup does not permit the solid substance to distribute readily throughout the syrup to the available solvent and also because a limited amount of available water is present in concentrated syrups.

Addition of Sucrose to a Medicated Liquid or to a Flavored Liquid

Occasionally, a medicated liquid, such as a tincture or fluidextract, is employed as the source of medication in the preparation of a syrup. Many such tinctures and fluidextracts contain alcohol-soluble constituents and are prepared with alcoholic or hydroalcoholic vehicles. If the alcohol-soluble components are desired medicinal agents, some means of rendering them water soluble is employed. However, if the alcohol-soluble components are undesirable or unnecessary components of the corresponding syrup, they are generally removed by mixing the tincture or fluidextract with water, allowing the mixture to stand until separation of the water-insoluble agents is complete, and filtering them from the mixture. The filtrate is the medicated liquid to which the sucrose is added in preparation of the syrup. If the tincture or fluidextract is miscible with aqueous preparations, it may be added directly to simple syrup or to a flavored syrup.

Percolation

In the percolation method, either sucrose may be percolated to prepare the syrup or the source of the medicinal component may be percolated to form an extractive to which sucrose or syrup may be added. This latter method really is two separate procedures: first the preparation of the extractive of the drug and then the preparation of the syrup.

An example of a syrup prepared by percolation is ipecac syrup, which is prepared by adding glycerin and syrup to an extractive of powdered ipecac obtained by percolation. The drug ipecac, which consists of the dried rhizome and roots of *Cephaëlis ipecacuanha*, contains the medicinally active alkaloids emetine, cephaline, and psychotrine. These alkaloids are extracted from the powdered ipecac by percolation with a hydroalcoholic solvent.

The syrup is categorized as an emetic with a usual dose of 15 mL. This amount of syrup is commonly used in the management of poisoning in children when evacuation of the stomach contents is desirable. About 80% of children given this dose will vomit within half an hour. For a household emetic in the event of poisoning, 1-oz bottles of the syrup are sold without a prescription. Ipecac syrup also has some application as a nauseant expectorant in doses smaller than the emetic dose.

Evidence indicates that many bulimics—most commonly young women in their late teens to early 30s—use the syrup of ipecac to bring on attacks of vomiting in an attempt to lose weight (8). Pharmacists must be aware of this misuse of the syrup of ipecac and warn these individuals because one of the active ingredients in the syrup is emetine. With continual use of the syrup, emetine builds up toxic levels within the body tissues and can do irreversible damage to the heart muscles in 3 to 4 months, resulting in symptoms mimicking a heart attack. Shortness of breath is the most common symptom in patients who misuse the syrup of ipecac, but some persons describe low blood pressure–related symptoms and irregularities of heartbeat.

ELIXIRS

Elixirs are clear, sweetened hydroalcoholic solutions intended for oral use and are usually flavored to enhance their palatability. Nonmedicated elixirs are employed as vehicles, and medicated elixirs are used for the therapeutic effect of the medicinal substances they contain. Compared with syrups, elixirs are usually less sweet and less viscous because they contain a lower proportion of sugar and consequently are less effective than syrups in masking the taste of medicinal substances. However, because of their hydroalcoholic character, elixirs are better able than aqueous syrups to maintain both water-soluble and alcohol-soluble components in solution. Also, because of their stable characteristics and the ease with which they are prepared (by simple solution), from a manufacturing standpoint, elixirs are preferred to syrups.

The proportion of alcohol in elixirs varies widely because the individual components of the elixirs have different water and alcohol solubility characteristics. Each elixir requires a specific blend of alcohol and water to maintain all of the components in solution. Naturally, for elixirs containing agents with poor water solubility, the proportion of alcohol required is greater than for elixirs prepared from components having good water solubility. In addition to alcohol and water, other solvents, such as glycerin and propylene glycol, are frequently employed in elixirs as adjunctive solvents.

Although many elixirs are sweetened with sucrose or with a sucrose syrup, some use sorbitol, glycerin, and/or artificial sweeteners. Elixirs having a high alcoholic content usually use an artificial sweetener, such as saccharin, which is required only in small amounts, rather than sucrose, which is only slightly soluble in alcohol and requires greater quantities for equivalent sweetness.

All elixirs contain flavorings to increase their palatability, and most elixirs have coloring agents to enhance their appearance. Elixirs containing more than 10% to 12% of alcohol are usually self-preserving and do not require the addition of an antimicrobial agent.

Although the USP monographs for medicated elixirs provide standards, they do not generally provide official formulas. Formulations are left up to the individual manufacturers. Example formulations for some medicated elixirs are as follows (7):

Phenobarbital Elixir

Phenobarbital (Active)	4.0 g
Orange oil (Flavor)	0.25 mL
Propylene glycol (Cosolvent)	100.0 mL
Alcohol (Cosolvent and Preservative)	200.0 mL
Sorbitol solution (Cosolvent and Sweetener)	600.0 mL
Color	qs
Purified water, to make (Solvent and Vehicle)	1,000.0 mL

Theophylline Elixir

Theophylline (Active)	5.3 g
Citric acid (pH Adjustment and Tartness for flavor)	10.0 g
Liquid glucose (Cosolvent and Sweetener)	44.0 g
Syrup (Cosolvent and Sweetener)	132.0 mL
Glycerin (Cosolvent and Sweetener)	50.0 mL
Sorbitol solution (Cosolvent and Sweetener)	324.0 mL
Alcohol (Cosolvent and Preservative)	200.0 mL
Saccharin sodium (Sweetener)	5.0 g
Lemon oil (Flavor)	0.5 g
FD&C Yellow No. 5 (Color)	0.1 g
Purified water, to make (Solvent and Vehicle)	1,000.0 mL

Medicated elixirs are formulated so that a patient receives the usual adult dose of the drug in a convenient measure of elixir. For most elixirs, one or two teaspoonfuls (5 or 10 mL) provide the usual adult dose of the drug. One advantage of elixirs over their counterpart drugs in solid dosage forms is the flexibility and ease of dosage administration to patients who have difficulty swallowing solid forms.

A disadvantage of elixirs for children and for adults who choose to avoid alcohol is their alcoholic content. The reader may wish to refer to the discussion of alcohol as a solvent earlier in this chapter for FDA-recommended limits on alcohol content for OTC oral products.

Because of their usual content of volatile oils and alcohol, elixirs should be stored in tight, light-resistant containers and protected from excessive heat.

Preparation of Elixirs

Elixirs are usually prepared by simple solution with agitation and/or by admixture of two or more liquid ingredients. Alcohol-soluble and water-soluble components are generally dissolved separately in alcohol and in purified water, respectively. Then the aqueous solution is added to the alcoholic solution, rather than the reverse, to maintain the highest possible alcoholic strength at all times so that minimal separation of the alcohol-soluble components occurs. When the two solutions are completely mixed, the mixture is made to the volume with the specified solvent or vehicle. Frequently, the final mixture will be cloudy, principally because of separation of some of the flavoring oils by the reduced alcoholic concentration. If this occurs, the elixir is usually permitted to stand for a prescribed number of hours to ensure saturation of the hydroalcoholic solvent and to permit the oil globules to coalesce so that they may be more easily removed by filtration. Talc, a frequent filter aid in the preparation of elixirs, absorbs the excessive amounts of oils and therefore assists in their removal from the solution. The presence of glycerin, syrup, sorbitol, and propylene glycol in elixirs generally contributes to the solvent effect of the hydroalcoholic vehicle, assists in the dissolution of the solute, and enhances the stability of the preparation. However, the presence of these materials adds to the viscosity of the elixir and slows the rate of filtration.

Nonmedicated Elixirs

Nonmedicated elixirs may be useful to the pharmacist in the extemporaneous filling of prescriptions involving (a) the addition of a therapeutic agent to a pleasant-tasting vehicle and (b) dilution of an existing medicated elixir. In selecting a liquid vehicle for a drug substance, the pharmacist should be concerned with the solubility and stability of the drug substance in water and alcohol. If a hydroalcoholic vehicle is selected, the proportion of alcohol should be only slightly above the amount needed to effect and maintain the drug's solution. When a pharmacist is called on to dilute an existing medicated elixir, the nonmedicated elixir he or she selects as the diluent should have approximately the same alcoholic concentration as the elixir being diluted. Also, the flavor and color characteristics of the diluent should not be in conflict with those of the medicated elixir, and all components should be chemically and physically compatible.

In years past, when pharmacists were called on more frequently than today to compound prescriptions, the three most commonly used nonmedicated elixirs were aromatic elixir, compound benzaldehyde elixir, and isoalcoholic elixir.

Medicated Elixirs

As noted previously, medicated elixirs are employed for the therapeutic benefit of the medicinal agent. Most official and commercial elixirs contain a single therapeutic agent. The main advantage of having only a single therapeutic agent is that the dosage of that single drug may be increased or decreased by simply taking more or less of the elixir, whereas when two or more therapeutic agents are present in the same preparation, it is impossible to increase or decrease the dose of one without an automatic and corresponding adjustment in the dose of the other, which may not be desired. Thus, for patients required to take more than a single medication, many physicians prefer them to take separate preparations of each drug so that if an adjustment in the dosage of one is desired, it may be accomplished without the concomitant adjustment of the other. Table 13.8 presents some examples of medicated elixirs. Some of these are briefly discussed next.

Antihistamine Elixirs

As indicated in Table 13.8, antihistamines are useful primarily in the symptomatic relief of certain allergic disorders. They suppress symptoms caused by histamine, one of the chemical agents released during the antigen–antibody reaction of the allergic response. Although only minor differences exist in the properties of most antihistamines, one or another may be preferred by a prescriber because of experience in managing a specific type of allergic reaction. A prescriber's preference may also be based on the incidence of adverse effects that may be expected to occur. The incidence and severity of these effects do vary somewhat with the drug and the dose. The most common untoward effect is sedation, and patients taking antihistamines should be warned against engaging in activities requiring mental alertness, such as driving an automobile or tractor or operating machinery. Other common adverse effects include dryness of the nose, throat, and mouth; dizziness; and disturbed concentration. Among the most sedating antihistamines are diphenhydramine and doxylamine. In fact, diphenhydramine is used as a sleep aid in numerous OTC products for its ability to cause drowsiness.

Most antihistaminic agents are basic amines. By forming salts through interaction with acid, the compounds are rendered water soluble. These salt forms are used in elixirs, so the elixirs of the antihistamines are not required to contain a large proportion of alcohol. Because the acid salts of the antihistamines are used, the pH of these elixirs is on the acid side and must remain so if the drugs are to remain freely soluble in water. A pharmacist should keep this in mind when using one of these elixirs to compound a prescription with other components.

Barbiturate Sedative and Hypnotic Elixirs

The barbiturates are sedative and hypnotic agents that are used to produce various degrees of central nervous system depression. As the dose of these drugs is increased, the effects go from sedation to hypnosis to respiratory depression, the last being the cause of death in fatal barbiturate overdosage.

TABLE 13.8. Examples of Medicated Elixirs by Category

Elixir	Representative Commercial Products	Usual Adult Dose/Volume of Commercial Elixir	Comments
Adrenocortical Steroid			
Dexamethasone	Dexamethasone Elixir	500 mg/5 mL	Synthetic analog of hydrocortisone, about 30 times more potent. Commercial elixir is packaged with a calibrated dropper for accurate measurement of small doses; intended primarily for children; also has utility for adults with trouble swallowing tablets. Used for many indications: rheumatoid arthritis, skin diseases, allergies, inflammatory conditions. Commercial product contains 5% alcohol.
Analgesic, Antipyretic			
Acetaminophen	Children's Tylenol Elixir (McNeil)	160 mg/5 mL	Reduction of pain and lowering of fever particularly in patients sensitive to or unable to take aspirin. Elixir is especially useful for pediatric patients and is alcohol-free.
Anticholinergic, Antispasmodic			
Hyoscyamine sulfate	Levsin Elixir	0.125 mg/5 mL	Used to control gastric secretion, visceral spasm, hypermotility, abdominal cramps. Commercial product contains 20% alcohol.
Antihistamine			
Diphenhydramine HCl	Diphenhydramine HCl Elixir	12.5 mg/5 mL	Antihistamines are used for a variety of allergic reactions, for example, perennial and seasonal allergic rhinitis, vasomotor rhinitis, allergic skin manifestations of urticaria, and reactions to insect bites. Commercial product contains 5.6% alcohol.
Antipsychotic			
Fluphenazine HCl	Fluphenazine HCl Elixir (Pharmaceutical Associates)	2.5 mg/5 mL	Management of psychotic disorders.
Cardiotonic			
Digoxin	Various	50 mg/mL	Among other effects, increases the force of myocardial contraction. Used in congestive heart failure, atrial fibrillation, other cardiac conditions. Commercial product contains 10% alcohol.
Sedatives, Hypnotics			
Butabarbital sodium	Butisol Sodium Elixir (Medpointe)	30 mg/5 mL	In low dosage, sedatives; in higher dosage, hypnotics. Butabarbital sodium elixir contains 7% alcohol; phenobarbital elixir contains 14% alcohol.
Phenobarbital	Various	20 mg/5 mL	

Barbiturates are administered in small doses in the daytime as sedatives to reduce restlessness and emotional tension. The appropriate dose for this purpose is the amount that alleviates anxiety or tension but does not produce drowsiness or lethargy. Greater doses of the barbiturates may be given before bedtime as hypnotics to relieve insomnia.

Barbiturates have been classified according to the duration of their hypnotic effects, that is, long-acting, intermediate-acting, short-acting, or ultrashort-acting agents. The long-acting barbiturates, including phenobarbital, are considered most useful in maintaining daytime sedation and in treating some convulsive states and least useful as hypnotics. The intermediate-acting barbiturates include amobarbital; they are used primarily for short-term daytime sedation and are effective in treating insomnia. The barbiturates classified as short-acting include secobarbital; they are used similarly to the intermediate-acting barbiturates. The ultrashort-acting barbiturates, including thiopental, are given intravenously to induce anesthesia.

The most common untoward effects in patients taking barbiturates are drowsiness and lethargy. Large doses may produce residual sedation resembling the hangover following alcohol intoxication. Prolonged use of barbiturates may lead to psychic or physical dependence. This dependence, in susceptible individuals, leads to compulsive abuse of the drug with severe withdrawal symptoms following abstinence. In heavy chronic users, abrupt withdrawal may lead to convulsions, to delirium, and occasionally to coma and death. Some pharmaceutical aspects of phenobarbital elixir are presented below.

Phenobarbital Elixir

Phenobarbital elixir is formulated to contain phenobarbital 0.4%, which provides about 20 mg of drug per teaspoonful (5 mL) of elixir. The elixir is commonly flavored with orange oil, colored red with an FDA-approved colorant, and sweetened with syrup. The official elixir contains about 14% alcohol, which is used to dissolve the phenobarbital. However, this amount is almost the very minimum required to keep the phenobarbital in solution. Therefore, glycerin is often added to enhance the solubility of phenobarbital.

Phenobarbital is a long-acting barbiturate with a duration of action of about 4 to 6 hours, a usual adult dose as a sedative of about 30 mg and a hypnotic dose of about 100 mg. The strength of the elixir permits convenient adjustment of dosage to achieve the proper degree of sedation in the treatment of infants, children, and certain adults. The elixir is commercially available from a variety of manufacturers under its nonproprietary name.

Digoxin Elixir

No official method of preparation is indicated for Digoxin Elixir, USP; however, it is required to contain 4.5 to 5.25 mg of digoxin per 100 mL of elixir, or about 0.25 mg/5 mL teaspoonful. The usual oral adult dose of digoxin as a cardiotonic agent is about 1.5 mg on initial therapy and about 0.5 mg for maintenance therapy.

Digoxin is a cardiotonic glycoside obtained from the leaves of *Digitalis lanata*. It is a white crystalline powder that is insoluble in water but soluble in dilute alcohol solutions. The official elixir contains about 10% alcohol. Digoxin is poisonous, and its dose must be carefully determined and administered to each individual patient. Adults generally take digoxin tablets rather than the elixir, which must be measured by the highly variable household teaspoon. The elixir is generally employed for children, and the commercial product available for this purpose is packaged with a calibrated dropper to facilitate accurate dosing.

Digoxin is one of many drugs available in more than a single dosage form. The prescriber frequently has the choice of a solid dosage form—a tablet or capsule—or a liquid. The advantages of each have been noted previously, but it is important to point out again that drugs administered in different dosage forms may exhibit different bioavailability characteristics, with varying patterns of drug release and rates and extents of absorption. Such differences have been noted for digoxin between tablets from different manufacturers and between tablets and oral liquid forms. Figure 13.2 shows the differences noted in one study of the serum digoxin levels following administration of 0.5 mg of digoxin by oral tablet and oral solution having an elixir-like vehicle. It can be readily observed that the serum digoxin levels following administration of the oral solution were considerably greater than from the oral tablet.

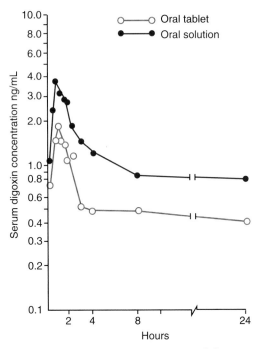

FIGURE 13.2. Serum digoxin concentrations following administration of digoxin 0.5 mg by oral tablet and elixir-like oral solution. (Adapted from Huffman DH, Azarnoff DL. Absorption of orally given digoxin preparations. JAMA 1972;222:957, with permission. Copyright © 2010 American Medical Association. All rights reserved.)

A patient taking a drug known to exhibit bioavailability problems and whose therapeutic dosage regimen has been successfully established with a particular drug product should not be changed to another product.

TINCTURES

Tinctures are alcoholic or hydroalcoholic solutions prepared from vegetable materials or from chemical substances. They vary in method of preparation, strength of the active ingredient, alcoholic content, and intended use in medicine or pharmacy. When they are prepared from chemical substances (e.g., iodine, thimerosal), tinctures are prepared by simple solution of the chemical agent in the solvent.

Depending on the preparation, tinctures contain alcohol in amounts ranging from approximately 15% to 80%. The alcohol content protects against microbial growth and keeps the alcohol-soluble extractives in solution. In addition to alcohol, other solvents, such as glycerin, may be employed. The solvent mix of each tincture is important in maintaining the integrity of the product. Tinctures cannot be mixed successfully with liquids too diverse in solvent character because the solute may precipitate. For example, compound benzoin tincture, prepared with alcohol as the sole menstruum, contains alcohol-soluble principles that are immediately precipitated from solution upon addition of water.

Because of the alcoholic content, tinctures must be tightly stoppered and not exposed to excessive temperatures. Also, because many of the constituents found in tinctures undergo a photochemical change upon exposure to light, many tinctures must be stored in light-resistant containers and protected from sunlight.

Medicated tinctures taken orally include Paregoric, USP, or camphorated tincture of opium. Usually, patients requiring oral medication nowadays prefer to take a tablet or capsule or a pleasant-tasting elixir or syrup. Tinctures have a rather high alcoholic content, and some physicians and patients alike prefer other forms of medication. Opium Tincture, USP, or laudanum, is much more potent than paregoric, and the two should not be confused. Opium Tincture contains 10% opium (which equates to 1% morphine), and camphorated tincture of opium contains 0.4% opium (which equates to 0.04% morphine). Any prescription for either one should be carefully evaluated and the dose checked and confirmed.

∎ PROPER ADMINISTRATION AND USE OF LIQUID PERORAL DOSAGE FORMS

Most of the dosage forms discussed in this chapter are to be administered by mouth. Conveniently, these can be measured in a teaspoon or tablespoon, depending on the desired dosage. Preferably, however, these medicines should be measured out in calibrated devices for administration. These devices ensure that the correct dose will be received, and household flatware can vary dramatically in the volume delivered. Even though these are liquids, it is recommended that the patient follow the administration of the liquid dosage form with a glassful of water.

The pharmacist must be careful in the selection of liquid products, given the patient's history and other concurrent medicines. For example, some syrups contain sucrose or another sugar, and the pharmacist must recall that such syrups would not be suitable for use in an oral prescription intended for a diabetic patient. Similarly, a product that is formulated as an elixir or syrup containing alcohol would not be suitable for a patient who receives concurrent medicines that possess an Antabuse-like activity; the patient may get violently ill from the concurrent ingestion of alcohol. Metronidazole and chlorpropamide have been implicated to cause this reaction when mixed with alcohol. Furthermore, if the patient is receiving another drug that causes drowsiness, the pharmacist must consult the prescribing physician to determine whether the prescribed elixir could be harmful to the patient.

∎ TOPICAL SOLUTIONS AND TINCTURES

Generally, the topical solutions employ an aqueous vehicle, whereas the topical tinctures characteristically employ an alcoholic vehicle. As required, cosolvents or adjuncts to enhance stability or the solubility of the solute are employed.

Most topical solutions and tinctures are prepared by simple dissolving. However, certain solutions are prepared by chemical reaction; these, in particular, are discussed later in this section. Of the tinctures for topical use, one, compound benzoin tincture, is prepared by maceration of the natural components in the solvent; the others are prepared by simple solution.

Because of the nature of the active constituents or the solvents, many topical solutions and tinctures are self-preserved. Those that are not may contain suitable preservatives. Topical solutions and tinctures should be packaged in containers that make them convenient to use. Those that are used in small volume, such as the anti-infectives, are usually packaged in glass or plastic bottles with an applicator tip as a part of the cap assembly or in plastic squeeze bottles that deliver the medication in drops. Many of the anti-infective solutions and tinctures contain a dye to delineate the area of application to the skin. In contrast to aqueous solutions, when the alcoholic tinctures are applied to abraded or broken skin, they sting.

Sprays

Sprays may be defined as aqueous or oleaginous solutions in the form of coarse droplets or as finely divided solids to be applied topically, most usually to the nasopharyngeal tract or to the skin. Many commercial sprays are used intranasally to relieve nasal congestion and inflammation and to combat infection and contain antihistamines, sympathomimetic agents, and antibiotic substances. Because of the noninvasive nature and quickness with which nasal sprays can deliver medication systemically, in the future, several drugs that typically have been administered by other routes may be taken nasally. Most notably, insulin and glucagon may be administered in this fashion. It has been demonstrated that the administration of glucagon via a nasal spray can relieve hypoglycemic symptoms within 7 minutes, a definite advantage over conventional emergency intravenous glucose or intramuscular glucagon.

Other sprays that are employed against sunburn and heat burn contain local anesthetics, antiseptics, skin protectants, and antipruritics. Throat sprays containing antiseptics, deodorants, and flavorants may be effectively employed to relieve conditions such as halitosis, sore throat, and laryngitis. Other sprays treat athlete's foot and other fungal infections. Numerous other medicinal and cosmetic uses of sprays are commonly available in pharmacies.

To break up a solution into small particles so that it may be effectively sprayed or to facilitate the spraying of a powder, several mechanical devices are commonly employed. The plastic spray bottle, gently squeezed to issue a spray of its contents, is familiar to most. It is commonly used for nasal decongestant sprays as well as cosmetically, especially for body deodorant products. Recently, one-way

FIGURE 13.3. A common type of atomizer for spray administration of liquid medication. (From Walls R, Murphy M. Manual of Emergency Airway Management. 4th Ed. Philadelphia, PA: Lippincott Williams & Wilkins, 2012.)

pump sprays have been developed to deliver medication into the nose. These sprays are used for both prescription, such as Nasalide (Syntex), and nonprescription, such as Nostrilla (Boehringer Ingelheim), medicines. The advantage of these over conventional sprays is that the design prevents drawback contamination of nasal fluids into the bottle after administration, a definite advantage for someone trying to cope with viruses associated with the common cold. Pharmacists are familiar with medicinal atomizers, which emit medication in the form of fine droplets (Fig. 13.3). One type of atomizer has a rubber bulb at the end of the apparatus, which when squeezed causes a flow of air, some of which enters the glass reservoir and some of which exits from the opposite end of the system. The air forced into the reservoir causes the liquid to rise in a small dip tube, forcing the solution up and into the stream of air exiting the system. The air and the solution are forced through a jet opening, and the liquid is broken up into a spray, the droplets being carried by the airstream. In other similar apparatus, the stream of air caused by the depression of the bulb does not enter the reservoir of solution but passes swiftly over it, creating a pressure change and sucking the liquid into the dip tube and into the airstream, in which it exits the system. Examples of solutions and tinctures intended for application to the skin are presented in Tables 13.9 and 13.10. As shown in these tables, most of these preparations are used as anti-infective agents. All medications intended for external use should be clearly labeled FOR EXTERNAL USE ONLY and kept out of the reach of children. In addition to their listing in Table 13.9, the following topical solutions are discussed because of their particular pharmaceutical interest.

Aluminum Acetate Topical Solution

Aluminum acetate is colorless and has a faint acetous odor and a sweetish, astringent taste. It is widely applied topically as an astringent wash or wet dressing after dilution with 10 to 40 parts of water. It is frequently used in various types of dermatologic lotions, creams, and pastes. Commercial premeasured tablets and packets of powders are available for preparation of this solution. Synonym: Burow solution.

Aluminum Subacetate Topical Solution

The requirement for the amount of acetic acid differentiates aluminum acetate topical solution from aluminum subacetate topical solution. In the subacetate solution, the ratio of aluminum oxide to acetic acid is 1:2.35, whereas in the acetate solution, the ratio is 1:3.52. Aluminum subacetate topical solution, the stronger of the two, is used in preparation of aluminum acetate topical solution. Aluminum acetate topical solution, diluted first with 20 to 40 parts of water, is used externally as an astringent wash and wet dressing (modified Burow solution).

Calcium Hydroxide Topical Solution

Calcium hydroxide topical solution, commonly called limewater, must contain not less than 140 mg of $Ca(OH)_2$ in each 100 mL of solution. Calcium hydroxide is less soluble in hot than in cold water, and cool purified water is the solvent. The solution is intended to be saturated with solute, and to ensure saturation, an excess of calcium hydroxide, 300 mg for each 100 mL of solution to be prepared, is agitated with the purified water, vigorously and repeatedly, for 1 hour. After this time, the excess calcium hydroxide is allowed to settle to the bottom of the container. This permits the solution to remain saturated should a portion of the dissolved solute at the solution's surface react with the carbon dioxide of the air to form insoluble calcium carbonate:

$$Ca(OH)_2 + CO_2 \rightarrow CaCO_3 + H_2O$$

The calcium carbonate settles to the bottom of the container and, by appearance, is indistinguishable from the remaining excess of calcium hydroxide. The calcium hydroxide reserve dissolves as calcium is removed from the solution in the form of the carbonate, and in this way, it continually maintains the saturation of the solution. After the solution stands for an appreciable length of time, the undissolved material at the bottom of the container is composed of varying proportions of calcium hydroxide and calcium carbonate. Because of the uncertainty of the residue's composition, one may not prepare additional quantities of calcium hydroxide solution by adding more purified water.

The solution should be stored in well-filled, tightly stoppered containers to deter the absorption of carbon dioxide and should be kept in a cool place to maintain an adequate concentration of dissolved solute. Only the clear supernatant liquid is dispensed. This is best accomplished by the use of a siphon with care not to entrain the residue.

The solution is categorized as an astringent. For this purpose, it is generally employed in combination with other ingredients in dermatologic solutions and lotions to be applied topically. Synonyms: limewater, liquor calcis.

Coal Tar Topical Solution

Coal tar topical solution is an alcoholic solution containing 20% coal tar and 5% polysorbate 80. It is prepared by

TABLE 13.9. Examples of Solutions Applied to the Skin

Solution	Corresponding Commercial Solution	Active Constituent in Commercial Product	Vehicle	Category and Comments
Aluminum acetate	—	5%	Aqueous	Astringent
Aluminum subacetate	—	~2.45% aluminum oxide, 5.8% acetic acid	Aqueous	Astringent
Calcium hydroxide (limewater)	—	0.14%	Aqueous	Astringent
Chlorhexidine gluconate	Hibiclens Skin Cleanser (Molnlycke)	4%		Skin wound and general skin cleanser, surgical scrub, preoperative skin preparation. Effective for gram-positive and gram-negative bacteria such as *Pseudomonas aeruginosa*
Clindamycin phosphate	Cleocin T Topical Solution (Pfizer)	1%	Isopropyl alcohol, water	Treatment of acne vulgaris
Clotrimazole	Lotrimin Solution (Schering-Plough)	1%	PEG 400	Antifungal
Coal tar (liquor carbonis detergens; LCD)	—	20%	Alcohol	Antieczematic; antipsoriatic
Erythromycin	Erymax Topical Solution (Allergan)	2%	Polyethylene glycol/acetone/alcohol	Treatment of acne vulgaris
Fluocinolone acetonide	Synalar Topical Solution (E. Fougera)	0.01%	Propylene glycol	Adrenocortical steroid (topical anti-inflammatory)
Fluorouracil	Efudex Topical Solution (Valeant Pharmaceuticals)	2, 5%	Propylene glycol	Antineoplastic (actinic keratoses)
Hydrogen peroxide	—	3%	Aqueous	Topical anti-infective
Hydroquinone	Melanex Topical Solution (Neutrogena Dermatologics)	3%	Water, alcohol, propylene glycol	Temporary bleaching of hyperpigmented skin, for example, chloasma, melasma
Ketoconazole	Nizoral A-D (McNeil)	1%	Water	Treatment of dandruff
Minoxidil	Rogaine Topical Solution (Pfizer Consumer Health)	2, 5%	Alcohol, water, propylene glycol	Long-term topical treatment of male pattern baldness by stimulating hair regrowth
Povidone–iodine	Betadine Solution (Purdue)	7.5, 10%	Aqueous	Topical anti-infective
Tolnaftate	Tinactin Solution (Schering-Plough)	1%	Polyethylene glycol	Topical antifungal
Undecylenic acid	Gordochom Solution (Gordon Laboratories)	25%	Oil base	Topical antifungal

TABLE 13.10. Examples of Tinctures Applied to the Skin

Tincture	Percent Active Constituent in Commercial Tincture	Vehicle	Category and Comments
Green soap tincture	65%	Alcohol	Detergent. Also contains 2% lavender oil as perfume
Iodine tincture	2%	Alcohol, water	Topical anti-infective
Compound benzoin tincture	10% benzoin; 2% aloe; 8% storax; 4% Tolu balsam	Alcohol	Topical protectant. Prepared by maceration in alcohol
Podophyllin	Podocon-25	Benzoin tincture	Removal of soft genital warts

mixing the coal tar with two and a half times its weight of washed sand, adding the polysorbate 80 and most of the alcohol, and then macerating the mixture for 7 days in a closed vessel with frequent agitation followed by filtration and adjustment to the proper volume with alcohol. The final content is 81% to 86% ethyl alcohol.

Coal tar is a nearly black viscous liquid having a characteristic naphthalene-like odor and a sharp, burning taste. It is the tar obtained as a by-product during the destructive distillation of bituminous coal. It is slightly soluble in water and partially soluble in most organic solvents, including alcohol. In the preparation of the official solution, the coal tar is mixed with the sand to distribute it mechanically and create a large surface area of tar exposed to the solvent action of the alcohol. During the maceration, or soaking, the alcohol-soluble components of the tar dissolve, leaving the undissolved portion clinging to the sand. Filtration removes the sand and the insoluble tar components from the solution. The container in which the solution was prepared should be rinsed with alcohol, and the washings should be passed through the filter paper in the adjustment of the final volume of the solution.

In the extemporaneous compounding of prescriptions and in the therapeutic application of this preparation to the skin, the solution is frequently mixed with aqueous preparations or simply diluted with water. Because coal tar is only slightly soluble in water, it would separate from the solution were it not for the polysorbate 80 in the preparation. This agent, commercially available as Tween 80 (ICI Americas) and as other brand name products, is an oily liquid that is a nonionic surfactant. It is quite effective in dispersing the water-insoluble components of coal tar upon admixture with an aqueous preparation.

Coal tar is a local antieczematic used in external treatment of a wide variety of chronic skin conditions after dilution with about nine volumes of water or in combination with other agents in various lotions, ointments, or solutions. Synonyms: liquor carbonis detergens; liquor picis carbonis; LCD.

Hydrogen Peroxide Topical Solution

Hydrogen peroxide topical solution contains 2.5% to 3.5% (w/v) hydrogen peroxide, or H_2O_2. Suitable preservatives, totaling not more than 0.05%, may be added.

One method of preparation uses the action of either phosphoric or sulfuric acid on barium peroxide:

$$BaO_2 + H_2SO_4 \rightarrow BaSO_4 + H_2O_2$$

Another method uses electrolytic oxidation of a cold solution of concentrated sulfuric acid to form persulfuric acid, which when hydrolyzed liberates hydrogen peroxide:

$$2H_2SO_4 \rightarrow H_2S_2O_8 + H_2$$

$$H_2S_2O_8 + 2H_2O \rightarrow 2H_2SO_4 + H_2O_2$$

A solution prepared by this method usually contains about 30% hydrogen peroxide and is capable of liberating 100 times its volume of oxygen. A solution of this strength is commonly referred to as 100-volume peroxide. The dilute solution, which contains about 3% hydrogen peroxide and liberates 10 times its volume of oxygen, may be prepared from the concentrated solution.

The solution is a clear, colorless liquid that may be odorless or have the odor of ozone. It usually deteriorates upon long standing, forming oxygen and water. Preservative agents, such as acetanilide, have been found to retard decomposition. Decomposition is enhanced by light and by heat, and for this reason, the solution should be preserved in tight, light-resistant containers, preferably at a temperature not exceeding 35°C (95°F). The solution is also decomposed by practically all organic matter and other reducing agents and reacts with oxidizing agents to liberate oxygen and water; metals, alkalis, and other agents can catalyze its decomposition.

Hydrogen peroxide solution is categorized as a local anti-infective for use topically on the skin and mucous membranes. Its germicidal activity is based on the release of nascent oxygen on contact with the tissues. However, because of the short duration of this release, the chief value of the preparation in the reduction of infection is probably its ability to cleanse wounds by mechanical action through the bubbling and frothing caused by the release of oxygen. It is also used to disinfect aseptic working environments. Synonym: peroxide.

Chlorhexidine Gluconate Solution

Since 1957, chlorhexidine gluconate has been employed extensively as a broad-spectrum antiseptic in clinical and veterinarian medicine. Its spectrum encompasses gram-positive and gram-negative bacteria, including *Pseudomonas aeruginosa*. In a concentration of 4% (Hibiclens, Molnlycke Health Care Inc.), it is used as a surgical scrub, hand wash, and skin wound and general skin cleanser. Procedures are established for all of these purposes to maximize the effectiveness of the chlorhexidine. Experience has demonstrated that irritation, dermatitis, and photosensitivity associated with topical use of chlorhexidine are rare.

In 1987, the FDA and the Council of Dental Therapeutics of the American Dental Association approved chlorhexidine gluconate 0.12% (Peridex, Procter & Gamble) as the first prescription-only antiplaque, antigingivitis drug with antimicrobial activity. Microbiologic sampling of plaque has shown a reduction of aerobic and anaerobic bacteria ranging from 54% to 97% through 6 months of use when it is used as a mouth rinse. The oral rinse should be used twice daily for 30 seconds, morning and night, after tooth brushing. Usually, a 15-mL dose of undiluted solution is used and expectorated after rinsing. The most common side effect of chlorhexidine is the formation of an extrinsic yellow-brown stain on the teeth and tongue after only a few days of use. The amount of stain depends on the concentration of chlorhexidine and individual susceptibility. Increased consumption of tannin-containing substances, such as tea, red wine, and port wine, will increase the level of discoloration. The developed stain can be periodically removed with dental prophylaxis.

Povidone–Iodine Topical Solution

The agent povidone–iodine is a chemical complex of iodine with polyvinylpyrrolidone, the latter agent being a polymer having an average molecular weight of about 40,000. The povidone–iodine complex contains approximately 10% available iodine and slowly releases it when applied to the skin.

The preparation is employed topically as a surgical scrub and nonirritating antiseptic solution, with its effectiveness directly attributable to the presence and release of iodine from the complex. Commercial product: Betadine Solution (Purdue).

Thimerosal Topical Solution

Thimerosal is a water-soluble organic mercurial antibacterial agent used topically for its bacteriostatic and mild fungistatic properties. It is used mainly to disinfect skin prior to surgery and as a first aid application to wounds and abrasions. It has been applied to the eye, nose, throat, and urethra in dilutions of 1:5,000. It is also used as a preservative for various pharmaceutical preparations, including many vaccines and other biologic products.

Thimerosal topical solution contains 0.1% thimerosal. Also present are ethylenediamine solution and sodium borate to maintain the alkalinity (usually pH 9.8 to 10.3) required for the solution's stability. Monoethanolamine is used as an additional stabilizer. The solution is affected by light and must be maintained in light-resistant containers. Commercial product: Merthiolate Solution (Lilly).

Medicated Soaps and Shampoo Solutions

Medicated soaps and shampoos are liquid or solid preparations intended for topical application to the skin or scalp followed by subsequent rinsing with water. They are solution, emulsion, or surface-active products that readily form emulsions or foams upon the addition of water followed by rubbing. Incorporation of active pharmaceutical ingredients (APIs) in the soaps and shampoos combines the cleansing/degreasing abilities of the vehicle and facilitates the topical application of the API to affected areas of the body. The surface-active properties of the vehicle facilitate contact of the API with the skin or scalp. Medicated soap and shampoo formulations frequently contain antimicrobial agents to protect against bacteria, yeast, and mold contamination.

▌ VAGINAL AND RECTAL SOLUTIONS

Vaginal Douches

Solutions may be prepared from powders as indicated earlier or from liquid solutions or liquid concentrates. In using liquid concentrates, the patient is instructed to add the prescribed amount of concentrate (usually a

FIGURE 13.4. Products for vaginal use, including solution concentrates, powder, and aerosol foam with insert device.

teaspoonful or capful) to a certain amount of warm water (frequently a quart). The resultant solution contains the appropriate amount of chemical agents in proper strength. The agents are similar to the ones described for douche powders. Examples are shown in Figure 13.4.

Powders are used to prepare solutions for vaginal douche, that is, for irrigation cleansing of the vagina. The powders themselves may be prepared and packaged in bulk or as unit packages. A unit package is designed to contain the appropriate amount of powder to prepare the specified volume of douche solution. The bulk powders are used by the teaspoonful or tablespoonful in preparation of the desired solution. The user simply adds the prescribed amount of powder to the appropriate volume of warm water and stirs until dissolved. Among the components of douche powders are the following:

1. Boric acid or sodium borate
2. Astringents, for example, potassium, alum, ammonium alum, and zinc sulfate
3. Antimicrobials, for example, oxyquinoline sulfate and povidone–iodine
4. Quaternary ammonium compounds, for example, benzethonium chloride
5. Detergents, for example, sodium lauryl sulfate
6. Oxidizing agents, for example, sodium perborate
7. Salts, for example, sodium citrate and sodium chloride
8. Aromatics, for example, menthol, thymol, eucalyptol, methyl salicylate, and phenol

Douche powders are used for their hygienic effects. A few douche powders containing specific therapeutic anti-infective agents such as those mentioned in the discussion of vaginal suppositories are used against monilial and trichomonal infections.

Retention Enemas

A number of solutions are administered rectally for local effects (e.g., hydrocortisone) or for systemic absorption (e.g., aminophylline). In the case of aminophylline, rectal administration minimizes the undesirable gastrointestinal reactions associated with oral therapy. Clinically effective blood levels of the agents are usually obtained within 30 minutes following rectal instillation. Corticosteroids are administered as retention enemas or continuous drip as adjunctive treatment of some patients with ulcerative colitis.

Evacuation Enemas

Rectal enemas are used to cleanse the bowel. Commercially, many enemas are available in disposable plastic squeeze bottles containing a premeasured amount of enema solution. The agents are solutions of sodium phosphate and sodium biphosphate, glycerin and docusate potassium, and light mineral oil.

Instruction from a pharmacist is advantageous to ensure that the patient correctly uses these products. The patient should be advised to gently insert the tip of the product with steady pressure and be told that it is not absolutely necessary to squeeze all of the contents out of the disposable plastic bottle. The patient should be told that the product will most probably work within 5 to 10 minutes.

▌ TOPICAL TINCTURES

Examples of tinctures for topical application to the skin are presented in Table 13.10. Those of particular pharmaceutical interest are discussed briefly as follows.

Iodine Tincture

Iodine tincture is prepared by dissolving 2% iodine crystals and 2.4% sodium iodide in an amount of alcohol equal to half the volume of tincture to be prepared and diluting the solution to volume with sufficient purified water. The sodium iodide reacts with the iodine to form sodium triiodide:

$$I_2 + NaI \leftrightarrow NaI_3$$

This reaction prevents formation of ethyl iodide from the interaction between iodine and alcohol, which would result in the loss of the antibacterial activity of the tincture. An added benefit of the triiodide form of iodine is its water solubility, which is important should the tincture, which contains between 44% and 50% alcohol, be diluted with water during use.

The tincture is a popular local anti-infective agent applied to the skin in general household first aid. The reddish-brown color, which produces a stain on the skin, is useful in delineating the application over the affected skin area. The tincture should be stored in a tight container to prevent loss of alcohol.

Compound Benzoin Tincture

Compound benzoin tincture is prepared by maceration in alcohol of 10% benzoin and lesser amounts of aloe, storax, and Tolu balsam totaling about 24% of starting material. The drug mixture is best macerated in a wide-mouthed container because it is difficult to introduce storax, a sticky semiliquid material, into a narrow-mouthed container. Generally, it is advisable to weigh the storax in the container in which it will be macerated to avoid possible loss through a transfer of the material from one container to another.

The tincture is categorized as a protectant. It is used to protect and toughen skin in the treatment of bedsores, ulcers, cracked nipples, and fissures of the lips and anus. It is also commonly used as an inhalant in bronchitis and other respiratory conditions, one teaspoonful commonly being added to a pint of boiling water. The volatile components of the tincture travel with the steam vapor and are inhaled by the patient. Because of the incompatibility of the alcoholic tincture and water, the mixture produces a milky product with some separation of resinous material. Alcohol or acetone may be used as necessary to remove the residue from the vaporizer after use.

Compound tincture of benzoin serves as a delivery vehicle of podophyllum in the treatment of venereal warts. It is important that podophyllum not be systemically absorbed because it can cause peripheral neuropathy characterized by paresthesias, loss of sensation, and loss of deep tendon reflexes in the extremities, in addition to neuropathy of the central nervous system including lethargy, confusion, and coma. Second, the podophyllum is teratogenic and should be administered to a pregnant woman only when the risk–benefit ratio is extremely low. Thus, the nonocclusive compound tincture of benzoin is preferred to the occlusive flexible collodion.

Compound benzoin tincture is best stored in tight, light-resistant containers. Exposure to direct sunlight or to excessive heat should be avoided.

The tincture originated in the 15th or 16th century and, through the years, probably has acquired more synonyms than any other official preparation. A few of these are friar's balsam, Turlington drops, Persian balsam, Swedish balsam, Jerusalem balsam, Wade drops, and Turlington balsam of life.

Thimerosal Tincture

The same general remarks about thimerosal topical solution apply to thimerosal tincture except that sodium chloride and sodium borate are absent from the tincture and the vehicle of the tincture is water, acetone, and about 50% alcohol. A number of metals, notably copper, cause decomposition of the tincture, and for this reason, it must be manufactured and stored in glass or suitably resistant containers. Monoethanolamine and ethylenediamine are used as stabilizers in the official solution and tincture and are thought to be effective because of their chelating action on traces of metallic impurities that may be present at the time of preparation or may later gain access to the preparation.

The commercial preparation is colored orange-red and has greenish fluorescence. The red stain it leaves on the skin defines the area of application. It is a commonly used household antiseptic for application to abrasions and cuts and also in the preparation of patients for surgery.

TOPICAL ORAL (DENTAL) SOLUTIONS

A variety of medicinal substances are employed topically in the mouth for a number of purposes and in a wide range of dosage forms. Among the drugs and preparations included in this group are the following:

- Benzocaine: Topical anesthetic. Indicated for temporary relief of pain, soreness, and irritation in the mouth associated with teething, orthodontic appliances, new or poorly fitting dentures, and canker sores.
- Camphorated parachlorophenol: Dental anti-infective. A eutectic liquid composed of 65% camphor and 35% parachlorophenol, used in dentistry for sterilization of deep root canals.
- Carbamide peroxide topical solution: Dental anti-infective. Acts as a chemomechanical cleansing and debriding agent through the release of bubbling oxygen. The commercial product (Gly-Oxide Liquid, GlaxoSmithKline) contains 10% carbamide in flavored anhydrous glycerin.
- Cetylpyridinium chloride solution and cetylpyridinium chloride lozenges: Local anti-infective. Commercial counterparts (Cepacol Mouthwash/Gargle and Cepacol Lozenges; Combe) contain 1:2,000 w/v and 1:1,500 w/v of cetylpyridinium chloride, respectively. Used primarily as a freshening mouth cleanser. Lozenges have benzyl alcohol as a local anesthetic in soothing throat irritations.
- Erythrosine sodium topical solution and erythrosine sodium soluble tablets: Diagnostic aid (dental disclosing agent). Solution applied to the teeth to reveal plaque left by inadequate brushing. Tablets chewed for the same purpose and are not to be swallowed.
- Eugenol: Dental analgesic. Applied topically to dental cavities and dental protectives. Eugenol is a pale yellow liquid having an aromatic odor of clove and a spicy taste.
- Lidocaine oral spray: Topical dental anesthetic. Applied through metered spray at 10 mg per spray; 20 mg per quadrant of gingiva and oral mucosa is usually employed (Xylocaine Oral Spray, AstraZeneca).
- Nystatin oral suspension: Antifungal. May be employed for oral fungal infections by retaining in the mouth as long as possible before swallowing.
- Saliva substitutes: Electrolytes in a carboxymethylcellulose base. They are indicated for relief of dry mouth and throat in xerostomia.
- Sodium fluoride oral solution and sodium fluoride tablets: Dental caries prophylactic. Solution applied to the teeth; or when drinking water does not contain adequate fluoride, a dilute solution may be swallowed. Tablets containing sodium fluoride 1.1 or 2.2 mg are chewed or swallowed as required.
- Sodium fluoride and phosphoric acid gel and sodium fluoride and phosphoric acid topical solution: Dental caries prophylactic. Gel and solution applied to the teeth; each contains 1.23% of fluoride ion and 1% of phosphoric acid. Triamcinolone acetonide dental paste—topical anti-inflammatory agent. Applied to the oral mucous membranes as a 0.1% paste.
- Zinc oxide–eugenol mixture: Temporary filling mix.

In addition to these drugs and preparations, a host of other products for oral use are commercially available. Some of these products, such as teething lotions and toothache drops, are medicated, whereas others are used for hygienic purposes, such as dentifrices, denture products, and many of the mouthwashes. Among the variety of products are a like variety of physical forms—solutions, emulsions, ointments, pastes, aerosols, and so on, with the manufacture of each following the general procedures outlined in this text. One type of dosage form for oral use, the lozenge, has not been previously described.

MISCELLANEOUS SOLUTIONS

Aromatic Waters

Aromatic waters are clear, aqueous solutions saturated with volatile oils or other aromatic or volatile substances. Aromatic waters are no longer in widespread use. In years past, aromatic waters were prepared from a number of volatile substances, including orange flower oil, peppermint oil, rose oil, anise oil, spearmint oil, wintergreen oil, camphor, and chloroform. Naturally, the odors and tastes of aromatic waters are of the volatile substances from which they are prepared.

Most of the aromatic substances in the preparation of aromatic waters have very low solubility in water, and even though the water may be saturated, its concentration of aromatic material is still rather small. Aromatic waters may be used for perfuming and/or flavoring.

Diluted Acids

Diluted acids are aqueous solutions prepared by diluting the corresponding concentrated acids with purified water. The strength of a diluted acid is generally expressed on a percent weight-to-volume (% w/v) basis, that is, the weight in grams of solute per 100 mL of solution, whereas the strength of a concentrated acid is generally expressed in terms of percent weight to weight (% w/w), which indicates the number of grams of solute per 100 g of solution. To prepare a diluted acid from a concentrated one, it is necessary first to calculate the amount of solute required in the diluted product. Then the amount of concentrated acid required to supply the needed amount of solute can be determined.

To illustrate, concentrated hydrochloric acid contains not less than 35 g and not more than 38 g of solute (absolute HCl) per 100 g of acid and therefore is considered to be, on the average, 36.5% w/w in strength. Diluted hydrochloric acid contains 9.5 to 10.5 g of solute per 100 mL of solution and is therefore considered to be approximately 10% w/v in strength. If one wished to prepare 100 mL of the diluted acid from the concentrated acid, one would require 10 g of solute. The amount of concentrated HCl required to supply this amount of solute may be calculated by the following proportion:

$$\frac{36.5\,\text{g (solute)}}{100\,\text{g (conc. acid)}} = \frac{10\,\text{g (solute)}}{x\,\text{(g conc. acid)}}$$

Solving for x:

$$36.5x = 1,000\,\text{g}$$
$$x = 27.39\,\text{g (conc. acid)}$$

Thus, 27.39 g of concentrated acid is required to supply 10 g of solute needed for the preparation of 100 mL of the diluted acid. Although the required amount of concentrated acid may be accurately weighed, it is a cumbersome task, and as a rule, pharmacists prefer to measure liquids by volume. Therefore, in the preparation of diluted acids, the calculations are generally carried one step further to determine the volume of concentrated acid that corresponds to the calculated weight. Because this additional step requires the use of the concentrated acid's specific gravity, a brief review of specific gravity seems appropriate.

By definition, specific gravity is a ratio, expressed decimally, of the weight of a substance to the weight of an equal volume of a standard, both substances having the same temperature or the temperature of each being known. Water is used as the standard for liquids and solids and hydrogen or air for gases. In pharmacy, specific gravity calculations mainly involve liquids and solids, and water is an excellent choice for a standard because it is readily available and easily purified.

At 4°C, the density of water is 1 g/cc. Because the USP states that 1 mL may be considered the equivalent of 1 cc, in pharmacy, water is assumed to weigh 1 g/mL. By the following equation used to calculate specific gravity, a substance having a density the same as water would have a specific gravity of 1.0:

$$\text{spgr} = \frac{\text{weight of a substance}}{\text{weight of an equal volume of water}}$$

In solving this equation, the same units of weight must be used in each part of the ratio. These units cancel out, and the ratio is expressed decimally.

Specific gravity indicates the ratio of the weight of a substance to that of an equal volume of water. For example, 10 mL of a liquid weighs 20 g. An equal volume of water weighs 10 g, and the ratio in the equation is 20:10, yielding a specific gravity of 2.0. This indicates that the liquid is twice as heavy as water in equal volume. By the same

token, a liquid having a specific gravity of 0.5 is half as heavy as water; a liquid with a specific gravity of 0.8 is eight-tenths as heavy as water and so on.

If both the volume of a liquid and its specific gravity are known, its weight may be calculated. For instance, if concentrated hydrochloric acid has a specific gravity of 1.17, it is that number times as heavy as water, and 100 mL of the acid would weigh 1.17 times as much as 100 mL of water. Because 100 mL of water weighs 100 g, 100 mL of the acid weighs 1.17 times that, or 117 g.

If one knows the weight of a liquid and its specific gravity, the volume of the liquid may be determined. For example, a liquid that is twice as heavy as water has a specific gravity of 2.0 and occupies half the volume that an equal weight of water occupies. If one has 100 g of this liquid and substitutes in the equation as indicated next, the volume of the liquid can be arrived at

$$2.0 = \frac{100\,\text{g}}{\text{weight of an equal volume of water}}$$

$$\text{weight of an equal volume of water} = \frac{100\,\text{g}}{2.0}$$
$$= 50\,\text{g}$$

Because 50 g is the weight of an equal volume of water, it follows that the water must measure 50 mL. Because the volume of the water is an equal volume to the other liquid, that liquid must also measure 50 mL.

The volume represented by 27.39 g of the concentrated hydrochloric acid may be similarly determined by dividing the weight of the concentrated acid by its specific gravity and equating the weight of an equal volume of water to the volume of the acid:

$$\frac{27.39\,\text{g}}{1.17} = 23.41\,\text{mg, weight of an equal volume of water}$$

Thus, because 23.41 g of water measures 23.41 mL and it is equal in volume to the concentrated acid, the latter also measures 23.41 mL, and this is the amount required to prepare 100 mL of the 10% w/v diluted acid.

Once the aforementioned is thoroughly understood, the following simplified formula can be used to calculate the amount of a concentrated acid required in the preparation of a specific volume of the corresponding diluted acid:

$$\frac{\substack{\text{Percentage strength} \\ \text{(w/v) of diluted acid}} \times \substack{\text{Volume of diluted} \\ \text{acid to be prepared}}}{\substack{\text{Percentage strength of} \\ \text{concentrated acid (w/w)}} \times \substack{\text{Specific gravity of} \\ \text{concentrated acid}}}$$
$$= \text{volume of concentrated acid to use}$$

Recalculating the preparation of 100 mL of diluted hydrochloric acid from the concentrated acid gives the following:

$$\frac{10 \times 100\,\text{mL}}{36.5 \times 1.17} = 23.41\,\text{mL of concentrated acid to use}$$

Most diluted acids have a strength of 10%w/v, with the exception of diluted acetic acid, which is 6%w/v. The strengths of these acids are commensurate with the concentrations generally used for medicinal or pharmaceutical purposes. The concentrations of the corresponding concentrated acids vary widely from one acid to another, depending on various properties of the solute such as solubility, stability, and ease of preparation. For instance, concentrated sulfuric acid is generally between 95% and 98%w/w, nitric acid between 69% and 71%w/w, and concentrated phosphoric acid between 85% and 88%w/w. As a result, the amounts of each concentrated acid required to prepare the corresponding diluted acid vary widely and must be calculated on an individual basis.

There is very little use of diluted acids in medicine today. However, because of its antibacterial effects, acetic acid finds application as a 1% solution in surgical dressings, as an irrigating solution to the bladder in 0.25% concentration, and as a spermatocidal in some proprietary contraceptive preparations.

Spirits

Spirits are alcoholic or hydroalcoholic solutions of volatile substances. Generally, the alcoholic concentration of spirits is rather high, usually over 60%. Because of the greater solubility of aromatic or volatile substances in alcohol than in water, spirits can contain a greater concentration of these materials than the corresponding aromatic waters. When mixed with water or with an aqueous preparation, the volatile substances present in spirits generally separate from the solution and form a milky preparation.

Spirits may be used pharmaceutically as flavoring agents and medicinally for the therapeutic value of the aromatic solute. As flavoring agents, they are used to impart the flavor of their solute to other pharmaceutical preparations. For medicinal purposes, spirits may be taken orally, applied externally, or used by inhalation, depending upon the particular preparation. When taken orally, they are generally mixed with a portion of water to reduce the pungency of the spirit. Depending on the materials, spirits may be prepared by simple solution, solution by maceration, or distillation. The spirits most recently official in the USP–NF are aromatic ammonia spirit, camphor spirit, compound orange spirit, and peppermint spirit.

▌ NONAQUEOUS SOLUTIONS

Liniments

Liniments are alcoholic or oleaginous solutions or emulsions of various medicinal substances intended to be rubbed on the skin. Liniments with an alcoholic or hydroalcoholic vehicle are useful when rubefacient, counterirritant, or penetrating action is desired; oleaginous liniments are employed primarily when massage is desired. By their nature, oleaginous liniments are less irritating to the skin than alcoholic liniments. Liniments are not applied to skin areas that are broken or bruised because excessive irritation might result. The vehicle for a liniment should therefore be selected for the type of action desired (rubefacient, counterirritant, or massage) and also on the solubility of the desired components in the various solvents. For oleaginous liniments, the solvent may be a fixed oil such as almond oil, peanut oil, sesame oil, or cottonseed oil or a volatile substance such as wintergreen oil or turpentine, or it may be a combination of fixed and volatile oils.

All liniments should bear a label indicating that they are suitable only for external use and must never be taken internally. Liniments that are emulsions or that contain insoluble matter must be shaken thoroughly before use to ensure even distribution of the dispersed phase, and these preparations should be labeled SHAKE WELL. Liniments should be stored in tight containers. Depending on their individual ingredients, liniments are prepared in the same manner as solutions, emulsions, or suspensions, as the case may warrant.

Collodions

Collodions are liquid preparations composed of pyroxylin dissolved in a solvent mixture usually composed of alcohol and ether with or without added medicinal substances. Pyroxylin (i.e., nitrocellulose, soluble gun cotton, collodion cotton), obtained by the action of a mixture of nitric and sulfuric acids on cotton, consists chiefly of cellulose tetranitrate. It has the appearance of raw cotton when dry but is harsh to the touch. It is frequently available commercially moistened with about 30% alcohol or other similar solvent.

One part of pyroxylin is slowly but completely soluble in 25 parts of a mixture of 3 volumes of ether and 1 volume of alcohol. It is also soluble in acetone and glacial acetic acid. Pyroxylin is precipitated from solution in these solvents upon the addition of water. Pyroxylin, like collodions, is exceedingly flammable and must be stored away from flame in well-closed containers, protected from light.

Collodions are intended for external use. When applied to the skin with a fine camel's hair brush or glass applicator, the solvent rapidly evaporates, leaving a filmy residue of pyroxylin. This provides an occlusive protective coating to the skin, and when the collodion is medicated, it leaves a thin layer of that medication firmly placed against the skin. Naturally, collodions must be applied to dry tissues to adhere to the skin's surface. The products must be clearly labeled "for external use only" or with words of similar effect.

Collodion

Collodion is a clear or slightly opalescent viscous liquid prepared by dissolving pyroxylin (4%w/v) in a 3:1 mixture of ether and alcohol. The resulting solution is highly volatile and flammable and should be preserved in a tight container remote from fire at a temperature not exceeding 30°C.

The product is capable of forming a protective film on application to the skin and the volatilization of the solvent. The film is useful in holding the edges of an incised wound together. However, its presence on the skin is uncomfortable because of its inflexible nature. The following product, which is flexible, has a greater appeal when a pliable film is acceptable.

Flexible Collodion

Flexible collodion is prepared by adding 2% camphor and 3% castor oil to collodion. The castor oil renders the product flexible, permitting its comfortable use over skin areas that are normally moved, such as joints, fingers, and toes. The camphor makes the product waterproof. Physicians frequently apply the coating over bandages or stitched incisions to make them waterproof and to protect them from external stress.

Salicylic Acid Collodion

Salicylic acid collodion is a 10% solution of salicylic acid in flexible collodion. It is used for its keratolytic effects, especially in the removal of corns from the toes. Patients who use such products should be advised about their proper use. The product should be applied one drop at a time on the corn or wart, allowing time to dry before the next drop is added. Because salicylic acid can irritate normal, healthy skin, every attempt must be made to ensure application directly on the corn or wart. A useful preventive measure is to line the adjacent healthy skin with some white petrolatum prior to application of the product. Proper tightening and storage of the product after use are absolutely necessary because of the volatility of the vehicle.

EXTRACTION METHODS FOR PREPARING SOLUTIONS

Certain pharmaceutical preparations are prepared by extraction, that is, by withdrawal of desired constituents from crude drugs through the use of selected solvents in which the desired constituents are soluble. Crude drugs are vegetable or animal drugs that have undergone no other processes than collection, cleaning, and drying. Because each crude drug contains a number of constituents that may be soluble in a given solvent, the products of extraction, termed extractives, do not contain just a single constituent but rather varying constituents, depending on the drug used and the conditions of the extraction. Tinctures, fluidextracts, and extracts are the pharmaceutical products most commonly prepared from extractives.

Plant materials are composed of heterogeneous mixtures of constituents, some of which are pharmacologically active and others pharmacologically inactive and considered inert. Among the varied plant constituents are sugars, starches, mucilages, proteins, albumins, pectins, cellulose, gums, inorganic salts, fixed and volatile oils, resins, tannins, coloring materials, and a number of very active constituents such as alkaloids and glycosides.

The solvent systems used in extraction are selected on the basis of their capacity to dissolve the maximum amount of desired active constituents and the minimum amount of undesired constituents.

In many instances, the active constituents of a plant drug are of the same general chemical type, have similar solubility characteristics, and can be simultaneously extracted with a single solvent or a single solvent mixture. Extraction concentrates the active constituents of a crude drug and removes from it the extraneous matter. In drug extraction, the solvent or solvent mixture is referred to as the menstruum, and the plant residue, which is exhausted of active constituents, is termed the marc.

The selection of the menstruum to use in the extraction of a crude drug is based primarily on its ability to dissolve the active constituents. Although water and alcohol and to a lesser extent glycerin are probably the most frequently employed solvents in drug extraction, acetic acid and organic solvents like ether may be used for special purposes.

Because of its ready availability, cheapness, and good solvent action for many plant constituents, water has some use in drug extraction, particularly in combination with other solvents. However, as a sole solvent, it has many disadvantages and is infrequently used alone. For one thing, most active plant constituents are complex organic chemical compounds that are less soluble in water than in alcohol. Although water has a great solvent action on such plant constituents as sugars, gums, starches, coloring principles, and tannins, most of these are not particularly desirable components of an extracted preparation. Water also tends to extract plant principles that separate upon standing in the extractive, leaving an undesired residue. Finally, unless preserved, aqueous preparations serve as excellent growth media for molds, yeasts, and bacteria. When water alone is employed as the menstruum, alcohol is frequently added to the extractive or to the final preparation as an antimicrobial preservative.

Hydroalcoholic mixtures are perhaps the most versatile and most widely employed menstrua. They combine the solvent effects of both water and alcohol, and the complete miscibility of these two agents permits flexible combining of the two agents to form solvent mixtures most suited to the extraction of the active principles from a particular drug. A hydroalcoholic menstruum generally provides inherent protection against microbial contamination and helps to prevent the separation of extracted material on standing. Alcohol is used alone as a menstruum only when necessary because it is more expensive than hydroalcoholic mixtures.

Glycerin, a good solvent for many plant substances, is occasionally employed as a cosolvent with water or alcoholic menstrua because of its ability to extract and then prevent inert materials from precipitating upon standing. It is especially useful in this regard in preventing separation of tannin and tannin oxidation products in extractives. Because glycerin has preservative action, depending on its concentration in the final product, it may contribute to the stability of a pharmaceutical extractive.

Methods of Extraction

The principal methods of drug extraction are maceration and percolation. Generally, the method of extraction selected for a given drug depends on several factors, including the nature of the crude drug, its adaptability to each of the various extraction methods, and the interest in obtaining complete or nearly complete extraction of the drug.

Frequently, a combination of maceration and percolation is actually employed in the extraction of a crude drug. The drug is macerated first to soften the plant tissues and to dissolve much of the active constituents, and percolation separates the extractive from the marc.

Maceration

The term maceration comes from the Latin *macerare*, meaning to soak. It is a process in which the properly comminuted drug is permitted to soak in the menstruum until the cellular structure is softened and penetrated by the menstruum and the soluble constituents are dissolved.

In the maceration process, the drug to be extracted is generally placed in a wide-mouthed container with the prescribed menstruum, the vessel is stoppered tightly, and the contents are agitated repeatedly over a period usually ranging from 2 to 14 days. The agitation permits the repeated flow of fresh solvent over the entire surface area of the comminuted drug. An alternative to repeated shaking is to place the drug in a porous cloth bag that is tied and suspended in the upper portion of the menstruum, much the same as a tea bag is suspended in water to make a cup of tea. As the soluble constituents dissolve in the menstruum, they tend to settle to the bottom because of an increase in the specific gravity of the liquid due to its added weight. Occasional dipping of the drug bag may facilitate the speed of the extraction. The extractive is separated from the marc by expressing the bag of drug and washing it with additional fresh menstruum, the washings being added to the extractive. If the maceration is performed with the drug loose, the marc may be removed by straining and/or filtration, with the marc being washed free of extractive by the additional passage of menstruum through the strainer or filter into the total extractive.

For drugs containing little or no cellular material, such as benzoin, aloe, and Tolu, which dissolve almost completely in the menstruum, maceration is the most efficient method of extraction.

Maceration is usually conducted at a temperature of 15°C to 20°C for 3 days or until the soluble matter is dissolved.

Percolation

The term *percolation*, from the Latin *per*, meaning through, and *colare*, meaning to strain, may be described generally as a process in which a comminuted drug is extracted of its soluble constituents by the slow passage of a suitable solvent through a column of the drug. The drug is packed in a special extraction apparatus termed a percolator, with the collected extractive called the percolate. Most drug extractions are performed by percolation, a process whereby coffee is routinely prepared.

In the process of percolation, the flow of the menstruum over the drug column is generally downward to the exit orifice, drawn by the force of gravity as well as the weight of the column of liquid. In certain specialized and more sophisticated percolation apparatus, additional pressure on the column is exerted with positive air pressure at the inlet and suction at the outlet or exit.

Percolators for drug extraction vary greatly as to their shape, capacities, composition, and, most important, utility. Percolators employed in the large-scale industrial preparation of extractives are generally stainless steel or glass-lined metal vessels that vary greatly in size and in operation. Percolators used to extract leaves, for instance, may be 6 to 8 feet in diameter and 12 to 18 feet high. Other vegetable parts like seeds that are greater in density than leaves and would pack too tightly in percolators of such large dimensions are extracted in much smaller percolators. Some special industrial percolators are designed to percolate with hot menstrua; in others, pressure is used to force the menstruum through the drug columns.

Percolation on a small scale generally involves the use of glass percolators of various shapes for extraction of small amounts (perhaps up to 1,000 g) of crude drug. The shapes of percolators in common laboratory and small-scale use are (*a*) cylindrical, with little, if any, taper except for the lower orifice; (*b*) roundish, but with a definite taper downward; and (*c*) conical, or funnel shaped. Each type has a special utility in drug extraction.

The cylindrical percolator is particularly suited to the complete extraction of drugs with a minimal expenditure of menstruum. By the passage of the menstruum over the drug contained in a high, narrow column (rather than in a lower, wider column), each drug particle is more repeatedly exposed to the passing solvent. A funnel-shaped percolator is useful for drugs that swell a great deal during maceration, because the large upper surface permits expansion of the drug column with little risk of a too tightly packed column or breakage of a glass percolator.

Example Preparations Prepared by Extraction Processes

Fluidextracts

Fluidextracts are liquid preparations of vegetable drugs prepared by percolation. They contain alcohol as a solvent, preservative, or both and are made so that each milliliter contains the therapeutic constituents of 1 g of the standard drug that it represents. Because of their concentrated nature, many fluidextracts are considered too potent to be safely self-administered, and their use per se is almost nonexistent in medical practice. Also, many fluidextracts are simply too bitter tasting or otherwise unpalatable to be accepted by the patient. Therefore, most fluidextracts today are either modified by the addition of flavoring or sweetening agents before use or used as the drug source of other liquid dosage forms, such as syrups.

Extracts

Extracts are concentrated preparations of vegetable or animal drugs obtained by removal of the active constituents of the respective drugs with suitable menstrua, evaporation of all or nearly all of the solvent, and adjustment of the residual masses or powders to the prescribed standards.

Extracts are potent preparations, usually between two and six times as potent on a weight basis as the crude drug. They contain primarily the active constituents of the crude drug, with a great portion of the inactive constituents and structural components of the crude drug having been removed. Their function is to provide in small amounts and in convenient, stable physical form the medicinal activity and character of the bulkier plants that they represent. As such, they have use in product formulation.

In the manufacture of most extracts, percolation is employed to remove the active constituents from the drug, with the percolates generally being reduced in volume by distillation under reduced pressure to reduce the degree of heat and to protect the drug substances against thermal decomposition. The extent of removal of the solvent determines the final physical character of the extract. Extracts are made in three forms: (*a*) semiliquid extracts or those of a syrupy consistency prepared without the intent of removing all or even most of the menstruum, (*b*) pilular or solid extracts of a plastic consistency prepared with nearly all of the menstruum removed, and (*c*) powdered extracts prepared to be dry by the removal of all of the menstruum insofar as is feasible or practical. Pilular and powdered extracts differ only by the slight amount of remaining solvent in the former preparation, but each has its pharmaceutical advantage because of its physical form. For instance, the pilular extract is preferred in compounding a plastic dosage form such as an ointment or paste or one in which a pliable material facilitates compounding, whereas the powdered form is preferred in the compounding of such dosage forms as powders, capsules, and tablets.

PHARMACEUTICS CASE STUDY

SUBJECTIVE INFORMATION

You have been given the responsibility of formulating a new oral solution containing a nasal decongestant (phenylephrine) and cough suppressant (dextromethorphan) for treating the symptoms of a cold or influenza. The oral solution should have a reasonably pleasant taste and appearance, be stable and preserved, and contain a suitable dose combination so that one or two teaspoonfuls can be used per administration to a 6- to 12-year-old child.

OBJECTIVE INFORMATION

Phenylephrine hydrochloride ($C_9H_{13}NO_2 \cdot HCl$), molecular weight 203.67, is the salt form selected for this drug. Phenylephrine hydrochloride occurs as white or nearly white odorless crystals with a bitter taste. It melts at 140°C to 145°C (284°F to 293°F). It is freely soluble in water and in alcohol. It is stable in aqueous solution below pH 7. Above pH 7, degradation occurs apparently involving the side chain, with loss of the secondary amine function; the phenolic group remains intact. The presence of heavy metals, especially copper, can catalyze the decomposition. It has two dissociation constant (pK_a) values, one at 8.77 and one at 9.84.

Dextromethorphan ($C_{18}H_{25}NO$, MW 271.40) is a practically white to slightly yellow odorless crystalline powder that melts at 109.5°C to 112.5°C (229°F to 234.5°F). It is practically insoluble in water. Dextromethorphan hydrobromide ($C_{18}H_{25}NO \cdot HBr \cdot H_2O$, MW 370.32) occurs as practically white crystals or crystalline powder with a faint odor and a melting range of 124°C to 126°C (255°F to 259°F). It is freely soluble in alcohol. It is stable in aqueous and hydroalcoholic solutions.

ASSESSMENT

The two drugs should be soluble and stable in a slightly acidic oral solution consisting of water and alcohol. The vehicle should be slightly thickened by a viscosity-increasing additive; it also should be sweetened and flavored. These drugs are bitter, so a flavor that will help mask the bitterness must be selected. The addition of a small amount of menthol may also be considered as a flavor enhancer. An appropriate preservative must be selected.

PLAN

An aqueous solution consisting of water, alcohol (low concentration, such as 5%), and glycerin (10%) adjusted to a pH in the range of 4 to 5 should be reasonable. Sucrose can be added as a sweetener (40%) and also for its viscosity-enhancing effect. It can be further thickened with methylcellulose (0.5%) or other cellulose polymer commonly used in oral liquids. A small amount of sorbitol (10%) will help give a smooth mouth feel and minimize cap lock of the container. Several flavor combinations can work, but raspberry and marshmallow work nicely to cover the bitter tastes of drugs. A blend of 0.05% methylparaben and 0.02% propylparaben can be added as a preservative. The addition of about 0.25% menthol will further enhance the flavoring and also impart an additional aromatic effect. ∎

CLINICAL CASE STUDY

HPI: Late one evening at the local pharmacy, the pharmacist notices a woman searching aimlessly in the nonprescription medication aisle. In hopes of being able to help this customer, the pharmacist approaches the woman and asks if he can help her find anything. The woman replies, "My husband and I are taking a family vacation to Florida tomorrow, and my son gets sick to his stomach when he flies. I was trying to find something that he could take for motion sickness." After asking the woman a few questions, the pharmacist discovers that her 5-year-old son is quite finicky and will not take tablets, including chewables. The pharmacist recalls a similar situation from a while back for which he compounded an oral solution of dimenhydrinate (Dramamine), and he asked the woman if this would be a suitable option for her son. The woman expressed much gratitude and asked the pharmacist if he could have the solution ready for her by the morning. The pharmacist said that would be fine, and he obtained the following information about her son, J.M.

PMH:	Motion sickness
	Recurrent ear infections
SH:	None
FH:	Mother (–)
	Father (+) for hypertension
ALL:	NKDA
MEDS:	None

PHARMACEUTICAL CARE PLAN

S: Mother states that her "finicky" son will not take oral tablets, including chewables.

O: Dimenhydrinate, a common nonprescription medication used for motion sickness, is no longer available in liquid form.

A: J.M. is a 5-year-old WM who has motion sickness on airplanes, and his family is leaving on vacation in the morning. Because the patient will not take tablets, the pharmacist plans to compound an oral solution of dimenhydrinate. The patient does not have any present medical conditions or a medication history that would contraindicate the use of dimenhydrinate.

P: 1. The pharmacist decides that to make the compound, he must first review information on the solubility and stability of dimenhydrinate. To do so, he consults Remington (9), where he reads that dimenhydrinate is "slightly soluble in water and freely soluble in alcohol and chloroform."

2. Although the pharmacist has prepared this solution before, he does not remember exactly how he did so. He does, however, remember that in the **U.S. Pharmacist** journal, there is a monthly Contemporary Compounding section, which he thinks may be useful. He scans the journal archives in the pharmacy until he finds the article "Oral Solution Stops Motion Sickness" (10). He secures the appropriate issue and reads the article to review how to prepare the dimenhydrinate solution.

3. Following the methods for preparation outlined in this article, the pharmacist prepares the compound from the following formula:

4. **Rx:**
Dimenhydrinate 12.5 mg/5 mL oral solution
Dimenhydrinate 250 mg
Glycerin qs
Ora-Plus 50 mL
Ora-Sweet or Ora-Sweet SF qs 100 mL

5. As the article suggests, the pharmacist packages the solution in a tight, light-resistant container. In addition, he labels the bottle take only as directed, keep out of the reach of children, may cause drowsiness, and contents should be discarded (6 months from the date of preparation).

6. The pharmacist is working the next morning, so he plans to counsel the woman on her son's medication at that time. Based on the dimenhydrinate package directions, a 5-year-old child should take one-quarter to one-half of a tablet every 6–8 hours, not to exceed one and a half tablets in 24 hours or as directed by a doctor. Each manufactured tablet contains dimenhydrinate 50 mg, and the compounded oral solution contains dimenhydrinate 12.5 mg/5 mL. Thus, the pharmacist should instruct the woman to give J.M. 1–2 teaspoonfuls by mouth every 6–8 hours, not to exceed 5 teaspoonfuls every 24 hours.

   Because dimenhydrinate's onset of action is approximately 30 minutes, the pharmacist recommends that J.M. take the first dose about 30 minutes prior to the flight departure.

7. In addition to dosage information, the pharmacist counsels the mother on the possible side effects. The most common is drowsiness, which should prove useful in this situation. Other adverse effects include a dry mouth and constipation. However, these can be relieved or prevented by drinking plenty of fluid.

8. Finally, the pharmacist reminds the mother that the solution may be stored at refrigerated temperature until the beyond-use date. After that time, any remaining contents should be discarded. The pharmacist also gives her the directions from the dimenhydrinate package along with the remaining tablets so that the patient and his family have the important product information that should accompany the medication (9,10).■

PATIENT COUNSELING

SOLUTIONS AND OTHER ORAL LIQUIDS

1. Explain and demonstrate how to measure the dose of a liquid preparation and how to administer it, using a measuring device (spoon, cup, syringe, etc.).
2. Explain whether or not to shake and on replacing and tightening the cap, and storing the preparation properly, including keeping it out of the reach of children.
3. Explain how to check the preparation for physical stability and to return it if signs of instability are noted.
4. Instruct on how to store the medication as well as how to dispose of preparations that have reached their expiration or beyond-use date.
5. If a suspension or emulsion, shake well before taking. If difficult to re-suspend, contact the pharmacist.
6. Explain the frequency and onset of dose.
7. Explain what to do if a dose is missed.

ADMINISTERING RECTAL ENEMAS

1. Wash the hands and rectal area and pat dry. Use gloves if desired.
2. Some enemas may require dilution prior to administration. If so, dilute as indicated.
3. Shake the liquid well.
4. Assemble or uncap the applicator tip and lubricate with petrolatum or lubricating jelly as desired.
5. Explain the following to the patient regarding actual administration.

   - Lie on the left side with the left leg extended and the right leg bent for balance; this allows delivery of the liquid into the sigmoid colon. A towel can be used if desired.
   - Gently insert the applicator tip fully into the rectum with the tip aimed toward the navel.
   - Tilt the bottle as needed so the applicator nozzle is aimed toward the back and instill slowly. If uncomfortable, slow down the instillation of the liquid.
   - Retain the enema for the prescribed length of time. The buttocks may need to be held closed to prevent the solution from being expelled prematurely.
   - Wash and dry hands again.

APPLYING THE PRINCIPLES AND CONCEPTS

GROUP ACTIVITIES

1. Compare and contrast the useful properties of various solvents used in liquid dosage forms.
2. Name medicinal preparations that utilize each of the following solvents: ethyl alcohol, diluted alcohol, rubbing alcohol, glycerin, isopropyl alcohol, propylene glycol, and purified water.
3. Consult the FDA Center for Drug Evaluation and Research's Data Standards Manual Web site and distinguish which dosage forms are liquid formulations.
4. Discuss pertinent patient counseling points regarding each liquid dosage form.
5. Define the following and explain benefits for use and contraindications for use of syrups, elixirs, topical solutions, tinctures, and fluidextracts.
6. Amass a number of extemporaneous compounded prescriptions, which use liquids within their formulation.
7. List specific patient circumstances and therapeutic circumstances where alcoholic liquid dosage forms would be contraindicated.
8. Describe common indications for oral solutions and how these liquid formulations have improved patient medication adherence.

INDIVIDUAL ACTIVITIES

1. Name a prescription or nonprescription product that utilizes each of the following solvents: Alcohol USP, diluted alcohol, rubbing alcohol, glycerin, isopropyl rubbing alcohol, propylene glycol, and purified water.
2. Identify two advantages of purifying water with the ion exchange method versus the distillation method.
   a. Describe two methods utilized to increase the rate of solute dissolution in a given solvent, and provide an example of each.
3. List the four main components of syrups and the role each play in the final formulation.
4. Construct a table of the four general methods utilized in preparing syrups, including advantages and disadvantages of each method.
5. Identify the role of nonmedicated elixirs and what components the pharmacist should be aware of in selecting an appropriate vehicle.
6. Compare and contrast aqueous solutions from nonaqueous solutions.
7. List the factors that determine the appropriate method of drug extraction.
8. Explain how the final dosage form can be determined by the process of extraction.
9. Find the chemical structure of four common drugs in the Description section of the package insert. Characterize their polarity and probably water solubility using the guidelines in this chapter.

REFERENCES

1. United States Pharmacopeia–National Formulary. Current Ed. Rockville, MD: U.S. Pharmacopeial Convention.
2. Pure Water Handbook. 2nd Ed. Minnetonka, MN: Osmonics, 1997.
3. Chemburkar PB, Joslin RS. Effect of flavoring oils on preservative concentrations in oral liquid dosage forms. J Pharm Sci 1975;64:414–441.
4. Gossel TA. Oral rehydration solutions. US Pharm 1987;12:90–98.
5. Handbook on Extemporaneous Formulations. Bethesda, MD: American Society of Hospital Pharmacists, 1987.
6. Pesko LJ. Compounding: Oral liquids. Am Druggist 1993;208:49.
7. Allen LV Jr. The Art, Science and Technology of Pharmaceutical Compounding. 4th Ed. Washington, DC: American Pharmaceutical Association, 2012.
8. Murphy D. Ipecac misuse by bulimics: APhA launches educational campaign. Am Pharm 1985;NS25:264–265.
9. Allen LV Jr. Remington: The Science and Practice of Pharmacy. 22nd Ed. London, UK: Pharmaceutical Press, 2012:1401.
10. Allen LV Jr. Oral solution stops motion sickness. US Pharm 2002;Aug:64–65.

Disperse Systems

CHAPTER AT A GLANCE Suspensions • Emulsions • Gels and Magmas
• Proper Administration and Use of Disperse Systems • Aerosols • Types of
Aerosols • Foams • Preparation of Foams • Patient Counseling

OBJECTIVES

After reading this chapter, the student will be able to:

Differentiate between a suspension, an emulsion, a gel, and a magma

Compare and contrast the different disperse systems, and list advantages and disadvantages of each system

Compare and contrast the following emulsification theories: surface tension, oriented wedge, and interfacial film

Define and differentiate the following terms from one another: lyophobic, lyophilic, hydrophobic, hydrophilic, amphiphilic, imbibition, swelling, syneresis, thixotropy, and xerogel

Evaluate and select a proper disperse system and delivery method for a given purpose, patient population, and/or patient circumstance

▌ INTRODUCTION

This chapter includes the main types of liquid preparations containing undissolved or immiscible drug distributed throughout a vehicle. In these preparations, the substance distributed is referred to as the *dispersed phase*, and the vehicle is termed the *dispersing phase* or *dispersion medium*. Together, they produce a *dispersed or disperse system.*

The particles of the dispersed phase are usually solid materials that are insoluble in the dispersion medium. In the case of emulsions, the dispersed phase is a liquid that is neither soluble nor miscible with the liquid of the dispersing phase. Emulsification results in the dispersion of liquid drug as fine droplets throughout the dispersing phase. In the case of an aerosol, the dispersed phase may be small air bubbles throughout a solution or an emulsion. Dispersions also consist of droplets of a liquid (solution or suspension) in air.

The particles of the dispersed phase vary widely in size, from large particles visible to the naked eye down to particles of colloidal dimension, falling between 1.0 nm and 0.5 μm. A discussion on the difference between particles and molecules is provided in Physical Pharmacy Capsule 14.1.

Dispersions containing coarse particles, usually 10 to 50 μm, are referred to as *coarse dispersions*; they include the *suspensions* and *emulsions*. Dispersions containing particles of smaller size are termed *fine dispersions* (0.5 to 10 μm) and, if the particles are in the colloidal range, *colloidal dispersions*. *Magmas* and *gels* are fine dispersions.

Largely because of their greater size, particles in a coarse dispersion have a greater tendency to separate from the dispersion medium than do the particles of a fine dispersion. Most solids in dispersion tend to settle to the bottom of the container because of their greater density than the dispersion medium, whereas most emulsified liquids for oral use are oils, which are generally less dense than the aqueous medium in which they are dispersed, so they tend to rise toward the top of the preparation. Complete and uniform redistribution of the dispersed phase is essential to the accurate administration of uniform doses. For a properly prepared dispersion, this should be accomplished by moderate agitation of the container.

The focus of this chapter is on dispersions of drugs administered orally or topically. The same basic pharmaceutical characteristics apply to dispersion systems administered by other routes. Included among these are

PHYSICAL PHARMACY CAPSULE **14.1** Particles Versus Molecules

Particles of drug substances can actually range from an aggregation of two or more molecules to millions of molecules. The term "particle" should not be confused with "molecule." The molecule is the smallest unit of any chemical compound that possesses all the native properties of that compound. Particles consist of numerous molecules, generally in a solid state (but can be liquid or gaseous). Dissolution is the solid to liquid transformation that converts solid drug particles to individual, dissolved liquid molecules. Even the smallest invisible drug particle contains billions of molecules. Most nonprotein or small molecule organic drugs have formula weights ranging from 150 to 500.

■ EXAMPLE

Let's look at how many molecules may be present in a 1-ng particle of ibuprofen with a formula weight of 206:

$$\frac{(1\,ng)(1\,g)(6.02 \times 10^{23}\,molecules)}{(particle)(1 \times 10^9)(206\,g)(Mole)} = 2.923 \times 10^{12}\,molecules$$

This illustrates that a 1-ng invisible particle will contain 2,923,000,000,000 molecules. ■

ophthalmic and otic suspensions and sterile suspensions for injection, covered in Chapters 15 and 17, respectively.

SUSPENSIONS

Suspensions may be defined as preparations containing finely divided drug particles (the *suspensoid*) distributed somewhat uniformly throughout a vehicle in which the drug exhibits a minimum degree of solubility. Some suspensions are available in ready-to-use form, that is, already distributed through a liquid vehicle with or without stabilizers and other additives (Fig. 14.1). Other preparations are available as dry powders intended for suspension in liquid vehicles. Generally, this type of product is a powder mixture containing the drug and suitable suspending and dispersing agents to be diluted and agitated with a specified quantity of vehicle, most often purified water. Drugs that are unstable if maintained for extended periods in the presence of an aqueous vehicle (e.g., many antibiotic drugs) are most frequently supplied as dry powder mixtures for reconstitution at the time of dispensing. This type of preparation is designated in the USP by a title of the form "for Oral Suspension." Figure 14.2 shows an example of a dry powder for suspension. Prepared suspensions not requiring reconstitution at the time of dispensing are simply designated as "Oral Suspension."

Reasons for Suspensions

There are several reasons for preparing suspensions. For example, certain drugs are chemically unstable in solution but stable when suspended. In this instance, the suspension ensures chemical stability while permitting liquid therapy. For many patients, the liquid form is preferred

FIGURE 14.1. Commercial oral suspension.

FIGURE 14.2. Commercial antibiotic preparation for oral suspension. *Left*, dry powder mixture. *Right*, suspension after reconstitution with the specified amount of purified water.

to the solid form of the same drug because of the ease of swallowing liquids and the flexibility in administration of a range of doses. This is particularly advantageous for infants, children, and the elderly. The disadvantage of a disagreeable taste of certain drugs in solution form is overcome when the drug is administered as undissolved particles of an oral suspension. In fact, chemical forms of certain poor-tasting drugs have been specifically developed for their insolubility in a desired vehicle for the sole purpose of preparing a palatable liquid dosage form. For example, erythromycin estolate is a less water-soluble ester form of erythromycin and is used to prepare a palatable liquid dosage form of erythromycin, the result being Erythromycin Estolate Oral Suspension, USP. Use of insoluble forms of drugs in suspensions greatly reduces the difficult taste-masking problems of developmental pharmacists, and selection of the flavorants to be used in a given suspension may be based on taste preference rather than on a particular flavorant's ability to mask an unpleasant taste. For the most part, oral suspensions are aqueous preparations with the vehicle flavored and sweetened to suit the anticipated taste preferences of the intended patient.

Features Desired in a Pharmaceutical Suspension

There are many considerations in the development and preparation of a pharmaceutically elegant suspension. In addition to therapeutic efficacy, chemical stability of the components of the formulation, physical stability of the preparation, and aesthetic appeal of the preparation—desirable qualities in all pharmaceutical preparations—a few other features apply more specifically to the pharmaceutical suspension:

1. A properly prepared pharmaceutical suspension should settle slowly and should be readily redispersed upon gentle shaking of the container.

2. The particle size of the suspensoid should remain fairly constant throughout long periods of undisturbed standing.
3. The suspension should pour readily and evenly from its container.

These main features of a suspension, which depend on the nature of the dispersed phase, the dispersion medium, and pharmaceutical adjuncts, will be discussed briefly.

Sedimentation Rate of the Particles of a Suspension

The various factors involved in the rate of settling of the particles of a suspension are embodied in the equation of Stokes law, which is presented in the Physical Pharmacy Capsule 14.2.

The Stokes equation was derived for an ideal situation in which uniform, perfectly spherical particles in a very dilute suspension settle without producing turbulence, without colliding with other particles of the suspensoid, and without chemical or physical attraction or affinity for the dispersion medium. Obviously, the Stokes equation does not apply precisely to the usual pharmaceutical suspension in which the suspensoid is irregularly shaped and of various particle diameters, in which the fall of the particles *does* result in both turbulence and collision, and also in which the particles may have some affinity for the suspension medium. However, the basic concepts of the equation do give a valid indication of the factors that are important to suspension of the particles and a clue to the possible adjustments that can be made to a formulation to decrease the rate of sedimentation.

From the equation, it is apparent that the velocity of fall of a suspended particle is greater for larger particles than it is for smaller particles, all other factors remaining constant. Reducing the particle size of the dispersed phase produces a slower *rate* of descent of the particles. Also, the greater the density of the particles, the greater the rate of descent, provided the density of the vehicle is not altered. Because aqueous vehicles are used in pharmaceutical oral suspensions, the density of the particles is generally greater than that of the vehicle, a desirable feature. If the particles were less dense than the vehicle, they would tend to float, and floating particles would be quite difficult to distribute uniformly in the vehicle. The rate of sedimentation may be appreciably reduced by increasing the viscosity of the dispersion medium, and within limits of practicality, this may be done. However, a product having too high a viscosity is not generally desirable because it pours with difficulty and it is equally difficult to redisperse the suspensoid. Therefore, if the viscosity of a suspension is increased, it is done so only to a modest extent to avoid these difficulties.

The viscosity characteristics of a suspension may be altered not only by the vehicle used but also by the solid content. As the proportion of solid particles in a suspension increases, so does the viscosity. The viscosity of a

PHYSICAL PHARMACY CAPSULE 14.2 Sedimentation Rate and Stokes Equation

Stokes equation:

$$\frac{dx}{dt} = \frac{d^2 (\rho_i - \rho_e) g}{18\eta}$$

where

dx/dt is the rate of settling,
d is the diameter of the particles,
ρ_i is the density of the particle,
ρ_e is the density of the medium,
g is the gravitational constant, and
η is the viscosity of the medium.

A number of factors can be adjusted to enhance the physical stability of a suspension, including the diameter of the particles and the density and viscosity of the medium. The effect of changing these is illustrated in the following example.

■ EXAMPLE

A powder has a density of 1.3 g/mL and an average particle diameter of 2.5 μm (assuming the particles to be spheres). According to the Stokes equation, this powder will settle in water (viscosity of 1 cP assumed) at this rate:

$$\frac{(2.5 \times 10^{-4})^2 (1.3 - 1.0)(980)}{18 \times 0.01} = 1.02 \times 10^{-4} \, cm/s$$

If the particle size of the powder is reduced to 0.25 μm and water is still used as the dispersion medium, the powder will now settle at this rate:

$$\frac{(2.5 \times 10^{-5})^2 (1.3 - 1.0)(980)}{18 \times 0.01} = 1.02 \times 10^{-6} \, cm/s$$

As is evident, a decrease in particle size by a factor of 10 results in a reduction in the rate of settling by a factor of 100. This enhanced effect is a result of the d factor in the Stokes equation being squared.

If a different dispersion medium, such as glycerin, is used in place of water, a further decrease in settling will result. Glycerin has a density of 1.25 g/mL and a viscosity of 400 cP. The larger particle size powder (2.5 μm) will settle at this rate:

$$\frac{(2.5 \times 10^{-5})^2 (1.3 - 1.25)(980)}{18 \times 4} = 4.25 \times 10^{-10} \, cm/s$$

The smaller particle size (0.25 μm) powder will now settle at this rate:

$$\frac{(2.5 \times 10^{-5})^2 (1.3 - 1.25)(980)}{18 \times 4} = 4.25 \times 10^{-10} \, cm/s$$

A summary of these results is shown in the following table:

Condition	Rate of Settling (cm/s)
2.5 μm powder in water	1.02×10^{-4}
0.25 μm powder in water	1.02×10^{-6}
2.5 μm powder in glycerin	4.25×10^{-8}
0.25 μm powder in glycerin	4.25×10^{-10}

As is evident from this table, a change in dispersion medium results in the greatest change in the rate of settling of particles. Particle size reduction also can contribute significantly to suspension stability. These factors are important in the formulation of physically stable suspensions. ■

pharmaceutical preparation may be determined through the use of a viscometer, such as a Brookfield viscometer, which measures viscosity by the force required to rotate a spindle in the fluid being tested (Fig. 14.3).

For the most part, the physical stability of a pharmaceutical suspension appears to be most appropriately adjusted by an alteration in the dispersed phase rather than through great changes in the dispersion medium. In most instances, the dispersion medium supports the adjusted dispersed phase. These adjustments are concerned mainly with particle size, uniformity of particle size, and separation of the particles so that they are not likely to become greatly larger or to form a solid cake upon standing.

Physical Features of the Dispersed Phase of a Suspension

Probably the most important single consideration in a discussion of suspensions is the size of the particles. In most good pharmaceutical suspensions, the particle diameter is 1 to 50 μm.

Generally, particle size reduction is accomplished by dry milling prior to incorporation of the dispersed phase into the dispersion medium. One of the most rapid, convenient, and inexpensive methods of producing fine drug powders of about 10 to 50 μm size is *micropulverization*. Micropulverizers are high-speed attrition or impact mills that are efficient in reducing powders to the size acceptable for most oral and topical suspensions. For still finer particles, under 10 μm, *fluid energy* grinding, sometimes

referred to as *jet milling* or *micronizing*, is quite effective. By this process, the shearing action of high-velocity compressed airstreams on the particles in a confined space produces the desired ultrafine or micronized particles. The particles to be micronized are swept into violent turbulence by the sonic and supersonic velocities of the airstreams. The particles are accelerated to high velocities and collide with one another, resulting in fragmentation. This method may be employed when the particles are intended for parenteral or ophthalmic suspensions. Particles of extremely small dimensions may also be produced by *spray drying*. A spray dryer is a cone-shaped apparatus into which a solution of a drug is sprayed and the small solution droplets are rapidly dried by a current of warm, dry air circulating in the cone. The resulting dry powder is collected. It is not possible for a pharmacist to achieve the same degree of particle size reduction with such comminuting equipment as the mortar and pestle. However, many micronized drugs are commercially available to the pharmacist in bulk, such as progesterone.

As shown by the Stokes equation, the reduction in the particle size of a suspensoid is beneficial to the stability of the suspension because the rate of sedimentation of the solid particles is reduced as the particles are decreased in size. The reduction in particle size produces slow, more uniform rates of settling. However, one should avoid reducing the particle size too much because fine particles have a tendency to form a compact cake upon settling to the bottom of the container. The result may be that the cake resists breakup with shaking and, especially during

FIGURE 14.3. The Brookfield viscometer. (Courtesy of Brookfield Engineering Laboratories.)

prolonged storage, forms rigid aggregates of particles that are larger and less suspendable than the original suspensoid. The particle shape of the suspensoid can also affect caking and product stability. It has been shown that symmetrical barrel-shaped particles of calcium carbonate produced more stable suspensions than did asymmetrical needle-shaped particles of the same agent. The needle-shaped particles formed a tenacious sediment cake on standing that could not be redistributed, whereas the barrel-shaped particles did not cake upon standing (1).

To avoid formation of a cake, it is necessary to prevent agglomeration of the particles into larger crystals or into masses. One common method of preventing rigid cohesion of small particles of a suspension is intentional formation of a less rigid or loose aggregation of the particles held together by comparatively weak particle-to-particle bonds. Such an aggregation of particles is termed a *floc* or a *floccule*, with flocculated particles forming a type of lattice that resists complete settling (although flocs settle more rapidly than do fine, individual particles) and thus are less prone to compaction than unflocculated particles. The flocs settle to form a higher sediment volume than unflocculated particles, the loose structure of which permits the aggregates to break up easily and distribute readily with a small amount of agitation.

There are several methods of preparing flocculated suspensions, the choice depending on the type of drug and the type of product desired. For instance, in the preparation of an oral suspension of a drug, clays such as diluted bentonite magma are commonly employed as the flocculating agent. The structure of the bentonite magma and of other clays used for this purpose also assists the suspension by helping to support the floc once formed. When clays are unsuitable as agents, as in a parenteral suspension, frequently a floc of the dispersed phase can be produced by an alteration in the pH of the preparation (generally to the region of minimum drug solubility). Electrolytes can also act as flocculating agents, apparently by reducing the electrical barrier between the particles of the suspensoid and forming a bridge so as to link them together. The carefully determined concentration of nonionic and ionic surface-active agents (surfactants) can also induce flocculation of particles in suspension and increase the sedimentation volume.

Dispersion Medium

Oftentimes, as with highly flocculated suspensions, the particles of a suspension settle too rapidly to be consistent with what might be termed a pharmaceutically elegant preparation. The rapid settling hinders accurate measurement of dosage and, from an aesthetic point of view, produces too unsightly a supernatant layer. In many commercial suspensions, suspending agents are added to the dispersion medium to lend it structure. Carboxymethylcellulose (CMC), methylcellulose, microcrystalline cellulose, polyvinylpyrrolidone, xanthan gum, and bentonite are a few of the agents employed to thicken the dispersion medium and help suspend the suspensoid. When polymeric substances and hydrophilic colloids are used as suspending agents, appropriate tests must be performed to show that the agent does not interfere with availability of the drug. These materials can bind certain medicinal agents, rendering them unavailable or only slowly available for therapeutic function. Also, the amount of the suspending agent must not be such to render the suspension too viscous to agitate (to distribute the *suspensoid*) or to pour. The study of flow characteristics is rheology. A summary of the concepts of rheology is found in Physical Pharmacy Capsule 14.3.

PHYSICAL PHARMACY CAPSULE **14.3** Rheology

*R*heology, the study of flow, addresses the viscosity characteristics of powders, fluids, and semisolids. Materials are divided into two general categories, newtonian and nonnewtonian, depending on their flow characteristics. Newtonian flow is characterized by constant viscosity, regardless of the shear rates applied. Nonnewtonian flow is characterized by a change in viscosity characteristics with increasing shear rates. Nonnewtonian flow includes plastic, pseudoplastic, and dilatant flow.

The Newton law of flow relates parallel layers of liquid: with the bottom layer fixed, when a force is placed on the top layer, the top plane moves at constant velocity, and each lower layer moves with a velocity directly proportional to its distance from the stationary bottom layer. The velocity gradient, or rate of shear (dv/dr), is the difference of velocity dv between two planes of liquid separated by the distance dr. The force (F'/A) applied to the top layer that is required to result in flow (rate of shear, G) is called the shearing stress (F). The relationship can be expressed:

$$\frac{F'}{A} = \eta \frac{dv}{dr}$$

(continued)

PHYSICAL PHARMACY CAPSULE **14.3** Rheology *(continued)*

where η is the viscosity coefficient or viscosity. This relationship is often written:

$$\eta = \frac{F}{G}$$

where

F = F'/A and
G = dv/dr.

The higher the viscosity of a liquid, the greater the shearing stress required to produce a certain rate of shear. A plot of F versus G yields a rheogram. A newtonian fluid will plot as a straight line with the slope of the line being η. The unit of viscosity is the *poise*, the shearing force required to produce a velocity of 1 cm/s between two parallel planes of liquid, each 1 cm² in area and separated by a distance of 1 cm. The most convenient unit to use is the centipoise, or cP (equivalent to 0.01 poise).

These basic concepts can be illustrated in the following two graphs.

■ EXAMPLE 1

What is the shear rate when an oil is rubbed into the skin with a relative rate of motion between the fingers and the skin of about 10 cm/s and the film thickness is about 0.02 cm?

$$G = \frac{10 \text{ cm/s}}{0.02} = 500 \text{ s}^{-1}$$

The viscosity of newtonian materials can be easily determined using a capillary viscometer, such as the Ostwald pipette, and the following relationship:

$$\eta' = ktd$$

where

η' is viscosity;
k is a coefficient, including such factors as the radius and length of the capillary, volume of the liquid flowing, pressure head, and so on;
t is time; and
d is density of the material.

The official compendia, the USP and NF, use kinematic viscosity, the absolute viscosity divided by the density of the liquid, as follows:

$$\text{Kinematic viscosity} = \eta'/\rho$$

(continued)

(continued)

The relative viscosity of a liquid can be obtained by using a capillary viscometer and comparing data with a second liquid of known viscosity, provided the densities of the two liquids are known, as follows:

$$\eta' / \eta'_o = (\rho t)/(\rho_o t_o)$$

■ EXAMPLE 2

At 25°C, water has a density of 1 g/mL and a viscosity of 0.895 cP. The time of flow of water in a capillary viscometer is 15 seconds. A 50% aqueous solution of glycerin has a flow time of 750 seconds. The density of the glycerin solution is 1.216 g/mL. What is the viscosity of the glycerin solution?

$$\eta = \frac{(0.895)(750)(1.216)}{(1)(15)} = 54.4 \text{ cP}$$

■ EXAMPLE 3

The time of flow between marks on an Ostwald viscometer using water ($\rho = 1$) was 120 seconds at 20°C. The time for a liquid ($\rho = 1.05$) to flow through the same viscometer was 230 seconds. What is the absolute and relative viscosity of the liquid?

$$\eta = \frac{(0.01)(1.05)(230)}{(1.0)(120)}$$

$$\eta = 0.020 \text{ poise} = 2.0 \text{ cP}$$

Viscosity is related to temperature; thus,

$$\eta' = Ae^{Ev/RT}$$

where

A is a constant depending on the molecular weight and molar volume of the material,
Ev is the activation energy required to initiate flow between molecules,
R is the gas constant, and
T is the absolute temperature.

Viscosity is additive in ideal solutions, as follows:

$$\frac{1}{\eta} = \frac{1}{\eta}V_1 + \frac{1}{\eta}V_2$$

where

η is the viscosity of the solutions and
V_1 and V_2 are the volume fractions of the pure liquids.

■ EXAMPLE 4

What is the viscosity of the liquid resulting from mixing 300 mL of liquid A ($\eta = 1.0$ cP) and 200 mL of liquid B ($\eta = 3.4$ cP)?

$$\frac{1}{\eta} = \frac{1(0.6)}{1.0} + \frac{1(0.4)}{3.4}$$

$$\eta = 1.4 \text{ cP}$$

Nonnewtonian substances are those that fail to follow the Newton equation of flow. Example materials include colloidal solutions, emulsions, liquid suspensions, and ointments. There are three general types of nonnewtonian materials: plastic, pseudoplastic, and dilatant.

Substances that exhibit plastic flow are called *Bingham bodies*. Plastic flow does not begin until a shearing stress corresponding to a certain yield value is exceeded. The flow curve intersects the shearing stress axis and does not pass through the origin. The materials are elastic below the yield value.

(continued)

PHYSICAL PHARMACY CAPSULE **14.3** Rheology *(continued)*

Pseudoplastic substances begin flow when a shearing stress is applied; therefore, they exhibit no yield value. With increasing shearing stress, the rate of shear increases; consequently, these materials are also called shear-thinning systems. It is postulated that this occurs as the molecules, primarily polymers, align themselves along the long axis and slip or slide past each other.

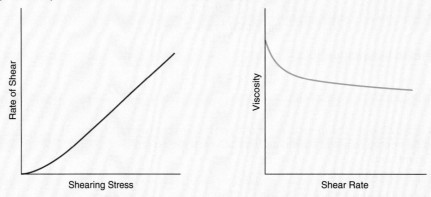

Dilatant materials are those that increase in volume when sheared, and the viscosity increases with increasing shear rate. These are also called shear-thickening systems. Dilatant systems are usually characterized by having a high percentage of solids in the formulation.

The viscosity of nonnewtonian materials is determined using a viscometer capable of producing differing shear rates, measuring the shear stress, and plotting the results. Other types of flow not detailed here include *thixotropic*, *antithixotropic*, and *rheopexic*. Thixotropic flow is used to advantage in some pharmaceutical formulations. It is a reversible gel–sol transformation. Upon setting, a network gel forms and provides a rigid matrix that will stabilize suspensions and gels. When stressed (by shaking), the matrix relaxes and forms a sol with the characteristics of a liquid dosage form for ease of use. All of these unique flow types can be characterized by studying their respective rheograms. ∎

FIGURE 14.4. Oral pediatric suspension package with calibrated dropper accompanying the medication container.

Support of the suspensoid by the dispersion medium may depend on several factors: the density of the suspensoid, whether it is flocculated, and the amount of material requiring support.

The solid content of a suspension intended for oral administration may vary considerably, depending on the dose of the drug to be administered, the volume of product to be administered, and the ability of the dispersion medium to support the concentration of drug while maintaining desirable features of viscosity and flow. Frequently, the usual adult oral suspension is designed to supply the dose of the particular drug in a convenient measure of 5 mL or one teaspoonful. Pediatric suspensions are formulated to deliver the appropriate dose of drug by administering a dose-calibrated number of drops or with the use of a teaspoon. Figure 14.4 shows an oral suspension administered as pediatric drops. Some pediatric drops are accompanied by a calibrated dropper, whereas other packages have the drop capability built into the container. On administration, the drops may be placed directly in the infant's mouth or mixed with a small portion of food. Because many of the suspensions of antibiotic drugs intended for pediatric use are prepared in a highly flavored, sweetened, colored base, they are frequently referred to by their manufacturers and also popularly as syrups, even though in fact they are suspensions.

Preparation of Suspensions

In the preparation of a suspension, the pharmacist must be acquainted with the characteristics of both the intended dispersed phase and the dispersion medium. In some instances, the dispersed phase has an affinity for the vehicle to be employed and is readily wetted by it. Other drugs are not penetrated easily by the vehicle and have a tendency to clump together or to float on the vehicle. In the latter case, the powder must first be wetted to make it

more penetrable by the dispersion medium. Alcohol, glycerin, propylene glycol, and other hygroscopic liquids are employed as wetting agents when an aqueous vehicle is to be used as the dispersion phase. They function by displacing the air in the crevices of the particles, dispersing the particles, and allowing penetration of dispersion medium into the powder. In large-scale preparation of suspensions, wetting agents are mixed with the particles by an apparatus such as a colloid mill; on a small scale in the pharmacy, they are mixed with a mortar and pestle. Once the powder is wetted, the dispersion medium (to which have been added all of the formulation's soluble components, such as colorants, flavorants, and preservatives) is added in portions to the powder, and the mixture is thoroughly blended before subsequent additions of vehicle. A portion of the vehicle is used to wash the mixing equipment free of suspensoid, and this portion is used to bring the suspension to final volume and ensure that the suspension contains the desired concentration of solid matter. The final product is then passed through a colloid mill or other blender or mixing device to ensure uniformity.

Whenever appropriate, suitable preservatives should be included in the formulation of suspensions to preserve against bacterial and mold contamination.

An example formula for an oral suspension follows (2). The suspensoid is the antacid aluminum hydroxide, the preservatives are methylparaben and propylparaben, and syrup and sorbitol solution provide the viscosity and sweetness.

Aluminum hydroxide compressed gel	326.8 g
Sorbitol solution	282.0 mL
Syrup	93.0 mL
Glycerin	25.0 mL
Methylparaben	0.9 g
Propylparaben	0.3 g
Flavor	qs
Purified water, to make	1,000.0 mL

The parabens are dissolved in a heated mixture of the sorbitol solution, glycerin, syrup, and a portion of the water. The mixture is then cooled and the aluminum hydroxide added with stirring. The flavor is added and purified water to the volume. The suspension is then homogenized, using a hand homogenizer, homomixer, or colloid mill. A high-speed industrial-size mixer used to prepare dispersions of various types, including suspensions and emulsions, is shown in Figure 14.5. A large storage holding tank with a liquid filling unit in the process of filling large-mouth suspension bottles is shown in Figure 14.6.

Sustained-Release Suspensions

The formulation of liquid oral suspensions having sustained-release capabilities has had only limited success because of the difficulty of maintaining the stability of sustained-release particles in liquid disperse systems (3).

FIGURE 14.5. An industrial mixer for the manufacture of disperse systems.

Product development research has centered on the same types of technologies used in preparing sustained-release tablets and capsules (e.g., coated beads, drug-impregnated wax matrix, microencapsulation, ion exchange resins). The use of a combination of ion exchange resin complex and particle coating *has* resulted in product success via the so-called Pennkinetic system. By this technique, ionic drugs are complexed with ion exchange resins, and the drug–resin complex particles coated with ethylcellulose (3). In liquid formulations (suspensions) of the coated particles, the drug remains adsorbed onto the resin

FIGURE 14.6. Liquid filling. Bottles being conveyed after cleaning for filling, valve insertion, and capping. (Courtesy of Shenzhen Penglai Industrial Corporation Ltd.)

but is slowly released by the ion exchange process in the gastrointestinal tract. An example of this product type is hydrocodone polistirex (Tussionex Pennkinetic Extended-Release Suspension, CellTech).

Extemporaneous Compounding of Suspensions

Not all medicines are available in a convenient, easy-to-take liquid dosage form. Consequently, patients who are not able to swallow solid medicines, such as infants and the elderly, may present a special need. Fortunately, pharmacists may use a solid dosage form of the drug and extemporaneously compound a liquid product. A difficulty that confronts the pharmacist is a lack of ready information on stability of a drug in a liquid vehicle. It is known that drugs in liquid form have faster decomposition rates than in solid form and some are affected by the pH of the medium. Leucovorin calcium when compounded from crushed tablets or the injectable form is most stable in milk or antacid and is unstable in acidic solutions.

To overcome this information gap, the pharmacist can attempt to contact the manufacturer of the solid dosage form to attain stability information. A number of extemporaneous formulations have appeared in the professional literature, such as for prednisone oral suspension (4) and ketoconazole suspension (5), and some manufacturers provide in the package insert a formula for preparation of an oral liquid form, such as Rifadin (rifampin, Aventis). A number of compilations of formulations based upon documented stability data and unpublished data compiled by manufacturers and practitioners are available for pharmacists to use, and hundreds of compounded liquid formulations are available through journals such as the *International Journal of Pharmaceutical Compounding*. The USP has recently focused on expanding the number of official monographs for compounded suspensions, especially for common pediatric formulations. USP monographs include a specific formulation, compounding instructions, and recommended beyond-use dates.

Typically, in formation of an extemporaneous suspension, the contents of a capsule are emptied into a mortar or tablets crushed in a mortar with a pestle. The selected vehicle is slowly added to and mixed with the powder to create a paste and then diluted to the desired volume. The selected vehicle can be a commercial product, such as the Ora family of preparations (Ora-Sweet, Ora-Sweet SF, Ora-Plus, Ora-Blend, Paddock Laboratories).

The extent of the formulation depends upon the patient. For example, a liquid suspension for a neonate should not include preservatives, colorings, flavorings, or alcohol because of the potential for each of these to cause either acute or long-term adverse effects. Because this liquid product will probably be administered through a tube threaded through the mouth into the stomach and because taste is usually underdeveloped in the neonate, a flavoring agent is not required.

In the neonate, alcohol can alter liver function, cause gastric irritation, and effect neurologic depression. So unless it is absolutely necessary, it should be omitted from an extemporaneous formulation. Pharmacists must be cautious because some vehicles, such as Aromatic Elixir, NF, contain a significant amount of alcohol, 21% to 23%, and are not suitable for use in these patients. The same problem holds for liquid formulations for the elderly or any patient who may be receiving another medication that depresses the central nervous system or would cause the patient to get violently ill, for example, metronidazole (Flagyl) and disulfiram (Antabuse).

Preservatives have been implicated in adverse effects in preterm infants. Benzyl alcohol should be omitted from neonate formulations because this agent can cause a gasping syndrome characterized by a deterioration of multiple organ systems and eventually death. Propylene glycol has also been implicated in problems such as seizures and stupor in some preterm infants. Thus, formulations for neonates should be kept simple and not compounded to supply more than a few days of medicine.

To minimize stability problems of the extemporaneous product, it should be placed in an airtight, light-resistant container by the pharmacist and stored in the refrigerator by the patient. Because it is a suspension, the patient should be instructed to shake it well prior to use and watch for any color change or consistency change that might indicate a stability problem.

Mixing Solids in Liquids

Pharmaceutical suspension mixing primarily involves the subdivision or deaggregation of one or more of the phases present, with subsequent dispersal throughout the vehicle or the rest of the material to be mixed. Liquid–solid mixing is usually done to suspend coarse free-flowing solids or to break up lumps of fine agglomerated solids. Two examples can be presented; one where the particles are lifted into suspension (and separated from one another) by bulk motion of the fluid; in the second, the mixer itself (or the high shear field near it) must destabilize the lumps and cause them to disintegrate.

Suspensions generally have increased viscosity to keep the suspended particles uniformly distributed. This is accomplished by introduction of a viscosity-increasing agent that also serves to enhance physical stability. A good thickening agent is one that has the required viscosity to keep the drug particles suspended separately from each other but would be sufficiently fluid to allow the preparation to be poured from the container. These agents can result in different types of rheological properties, including formation of newtonian and nonnewtonian liquids. This increased viscosity sometimes requires extended mixing times and/or a specific order of mixing.

Regarding rheological characteristics:

1. Shear-thinning (pseudoplastic) liquids get easier to mix after stress is applied.

2. Shear-thickening (dilatant) liquids become thicker and more difficult to mix after stress is applied.
3. Thixotropic liquids become easier to mix after stress is applied and they thin out, but increase in viscosity again after the shear stress is removed.
4. Generally, mixing nonnewtonian fluid requires heavier duty mixers.
5. Newtonian fluids tend to be more predictable with which to work.

Axial-flow impellers are preferred for solid suspensions, although radial-flow impellers can be used in a tank with baffles, which converts some of the rotational motion into vertical motion. When the solid is more dense than the liquid (and collects at the bottom of the container), the impeller is rotated so that the fluid is pushed downward; when the solid is less dense than the liquid (the floats on top), the impeller is rotated so that the fluid is pushed upward.

Very fine powders may agglomerate or form lumps during transportation and storage and are not easily mixed into liquids. Upon exposure to liquids, they tend to aggregate and wet on the outside but remain dry on the inside of the particle mass. In some ways, deagglomeration of solids is similar to the blending of immiscible liquids, except that coalescence is not usually a problem. Shear is often required to break the agglomerates up.

The mixing of finely divided solids with a liquid of low viscosity in the production of a suspension depends on the separation of aggregates into primary particles and the distribution of these particles throughout the fluid. These processes are often carried out in a single mixing operation, provided that shear forces of sufficient intensity to disrupt aggregates can be generated. High-speed turbines, frequently fitted with stators to produce increased shearing action, are often employed. When aggregation is not a problem, or when deaggregation is to be carried out following a general mixing step, the equipment used in mixing of suspensions is essentially the same as that previously discussed for liquids of comparable viscosity.

To prepare a suspension, one must first obtain uniform, small particles of the drug and any insoluble excipient. Then, the active pharmaceutical ingredient (API)-insoluble material should be thoroughly wetted before mixing with the vehicle. Hydrophilic materials are best wetted with water-miscible liquids (e.g., glycerin), whereas hydrophobic substances can be wetted with nonpolar liquids or with the use of a surfactant. Generally, one should use the minimal amount of wetting agent required to produce the desired product. Next, the vehicle is added geometrically with thorough mixing of each portion to obtain a uniform preparation.

Mixing suspensions is somewhat more complicated than mixing solutions or powders because many variables are involved, including agglomeration of particles and the viscosity of the vehicle to promote physical stability. However, when properly done, suspensions provide a necessary and efficacious dosage form for some patients.

Packaging and Storage of Suspensions

All suspensions should be packaged in wide-mouth containers having adequate airspace above the liquid to permit thorough mixing by shaking and ease of pouring. Most suspensions should be stored in tight containers protected from freezing, excessive heat, and light. It is important that suspensions be shaken before each use to ensure a uniform distribution of solid in the vehicle and thereby uniform and proper dosage. While it may seem obvious to a pharmacist, patients and caregivers should be shown how to shake the product to uniformity prior to measuring a dose. Insufficient or inconsistent shaking can lead to significant variability in the amount of active ingredient administered from dose to dose.

Examples of Oral Suspensions

Examples of official and commercial oral suspensions are presented in Table 14.1. Antacid and antibacterial suspensions are briefly discussed next as examples of this dosage form. In addition, kaolin mixture with pectin is widely used in the treatment of diarrhea.

Antacid Oral Suspensions

Antacids are intended to counteract the effects of gastric hyperacidity and, as such, are employed by persons, such as peptic ulcer patients, who must reduce the level of acidity in the stomach. They are also widely employed and sold over the counter (OTC) to patients with acid indigestion and heartburn. Many patients belch or otherwise reflux acid from the stomach to the esophagus and take antacids to counter the acid in the esophagus and throat.

Most antacid preparations are composed of water-insoluble materials that act within the gastrointestinal tract to counteract the acid and/or soothe the irritated or inflamed linings of the gastrointestinal tract. A few water-soluble agents are employed, including sodium bicarbonate, but for the most part, water-insoluble salts of aluminum, calcium, and magnesium are employed; these include aluminum hydroxide, aluminum phosphate, dihydroxyaluminum aminoacetate, calcium carbonate, calcium phosphate, magaldrate, magnesium carbonate, magnesium oxide, and magnesium hydroxide. The ability of each of these to neutralize gastric acid varies with the chemical agent. For instance, sodium bicarbonate, calcium carbonate, and magnesium hydroxide neutralize acid effectively, whereas magnesium trisilicate and

TABLE 14.1. Oral Suspensions by Category

Oral Suspension	Representative Commercial Products	Drug Concentration in Commercial Product	Comments
Antacids			
Alumina, magnesia, simethicone	Mylanta Liquid (Johnson & Johnson Merck)	Aluminum hydroxide, 200 mg; magnesium hydroxide, 200 mg; and simethicone, 20 mg/5 mL	Counteract gastric hyperacidity, relieve distress in the upper gastrointestinal tract
Magaldrate	Riopan Oral Suspension (Wyeth)	Hydroxymagnesium aluminate 540 mg aluminum (chemical entity of aluminum and magnesium hydroxides)	
Magnesia and alumina	Maalox Suspension (Novartis Consumer Health)	Aluminum hydroxide 225 mg; magnesium hydroxide 200 mg/5 mL	
Aluminum hydroxide, magnesium carbonate	Gaviscon Liquid Antacid (GlaxoSmithKline)	Aluminum hydroxide 95 mg; magnesium carbonate 358 mg/15 mL; sodium alginate	
Anthelmintics			
Pyrantel pamoate	Pin-X Oral Suspension (Effcon)	250 mg/5 mL	For worm infestations
Thiabendazole	Mintezol Oral Suspension (Merck)	500 mg/5 mL	
Antibacterials (Antibiotics)			
Ciprofloxacin	Cipro Oral Suspension (Schering-Plough)	50 and 100 mg/mL	Indicated in the treatment of specific susceptible microorganisms
Erythromycin estolate	Generic	125 and 250 mg/5 mL	Broad-spectrum macrolide antibiotic; bacteriostatic and bactericidal activity

(Continued)

TABLE 14.1. Oral Suspensions by Category *(Continued)*

Oral Suspension	Representative Commercial Products	Drug Concentration in Commercial Product	Comments
Antibacterials (Nonantibiotic Anti-infectives)			
Methenamine mandelate	Mandelamine Suspension Forte (various)	500 mg/5 mL	Oleaginous vehicle; chemical combination of approximately equal parts of methenamine and mandelic acid; destroys most pathogens commonly infecting urinary tract. Acid urine is essential for activity; maximum efficacy at pH 5.5. Methenamine in acid urine is hydrolyzed to ammonia and the bactericidal agent, formaldehyde. Mandelic acid exerts its antibacterial action, contributes to acidification of urine. Usual dose 1 g up to four times a day. Suspension form especially useful for children, adults who do not swallow a tablet (also official and commercially available)
Sulfamethoxazole and trimethoprim	Bactrim Suspension (Roche), Septra Suspension (Monarch)	Trimethoprim 40 mg, sulfamethoxazole 200 mg/5 mL	For acute middle ear infection (otitis media) in children, urinary tract infections because of susceptible microorganisms
Sulfamethoxazole	Gantanol Suspension (various)	500 mg/5 mL	Bacteriostatic sulfa drug suspensions useful for urinary tract infections. Sulfonamides competitively inhibit bacterial synthesis of folic acid and para-aminobenzoic acid
Sulfisoxazole acetyl oral suspension	Gantrisin Syrup and Gantrisin Pediatric Suspension (Roche)	500 mg/5 mL	
Antidiarrheal			
Bismuth subsalicylate	Pepto-Bismol Liquid (Procter & Gamble)	262 mg/15 mL	For indigestion without causing constipation, nausea, control of diarrhea. Unlabeled use for prevention and treatment of traveler's (enterotoxigenic *Escherichia coli*) diarrhea but not the first line of therapy for either
Antiflatulent			
Simethicone	Mylicon Drops (AstraZeneca)	40 mg/0.6 mL	Symptomatic treatment of gastrointestinal distress due to gas. Reduces surface tension of gas bubbles, enabling them to coalesce and be released through belching or flatus
Antifungals			
Nystatin	Nilstat (Wyeth)	100,000 U/mL	Antibiotic with antifungal activity. Suspension is held in mouth as long as possible before swallowing in treatment of mouth infections caused by *Candida* (*Monilia*) *albicans*, other *Candida* spp.
Antiprotozoal			
Atovaquone	Mepron Suspension (GlaxoSmithKline)	750 mg/5 mL	Indicated for the prevention of *Pneumocystis carinii* pneumonia
Antipsychotics, Sedatives, Antiemetics			
Hydroxyzine pamoate	Vistaril Oral Suspension (Pfizer)	25 mg/5 mL	Management of anxiety, tension, psychomotor agitation
Diuretic			
Chlorothiazide	Diuril Oral (Salix)	250 mg/5 mL	Interferes with renal tubular electrolyte reabsorption; increases sodium, chloride excretion
HIV Infections			
Nevirapine	Viramune Oral Suspension antiretroviral agents in treating HIV-1 (Boehringer Ingelheim)	50 mg/5 mL	Used in combination with other infections
Nonsteroidal Anti-inflammatory			
Indomethacin	Indocin Oral Suspension (Merck & Co.)	25 mg/5 mL	Active treatment of moderate to severe rheumatoid arthritis (including acute flares of chronic illness), moderate to severe osteoarthritis, acute painful shoulder (bursitis or tendinitis), acute gouty arthritis
Psychotropic			
Paroxetine HCl	Paxil Oral Suspension (Apotex)	10 mg/5 mL	Indicated for the treatment of major depressive disorder

aluminum hydroxide do so less effectively and much more slowly. In selecting an antacid, it is also important to consider the possible adverse effects of each agent in relation to the individual patient. Each agent has its own peculiar potential for adverse effects. For instance, sodium bicarbonate can produce sodium overload and systemic alkalosis, a hazard to patients on sodium-restricted diets. Magnesium preparations may lead to diarrhea and are dangerous to patients with diminished renal function because of those patients' inability to excrete all of the magnesium ion that may be absorbed; the gastric acid converts insoluble magnesium hydroxide to magnesium chloride, which is water soluble and is partially absorbed. Calcium carbonate carries the potential to induce hypercalcemia and stimulation of gastric secretion and acid production, the latter effect known as acid rebound. Excessive use of aluminum hydroxide may lead to constipation and phosphate depletion with consequent muscle weakness, bone resorption, and hypercalciuria.

The use to which an antacid is to be put is a major consideration in its selection. For instance, in the occasional treatment of heartburn or other infrequent episodes of gastric distress, a single dose of sodium bicarbonate or a magnesium hydroxide preparation may be desired. However, for treatment of acute peptic ulcer or duodenal ulcer in which the therapeutic regimen includes frequent administration of antacids, sodium bicarbonate provides too much sodium, and magnesium hydroxide induces diarrhea. Thus, in the treatment of ulcerative conditions, a combination of magnesium hydroxide and aluminum hydroxide is frequently used because the latter agent has some constipating effects that counter the diarrhea effects of the magnesium hydroxide.

When frequent dosage administration is required and when gastroesophageal reflux is being treated, liquid antacids generally are preferred to tablet forms. For one thing, the liquid suspensions assert more immediate action, because they do not require time to disintegrate. It is important that an antacid have a reasonably fast onset of action, because gastric emptying may not allow it much time in the stomach. Endoscopic studies have shown that very little antacid remains in the fasting stomach 1 hour after administration. Therefore, the U.S. Food and Drug Administration (FDA) requires that antacid tablets not intended to be chewed must disintegrate within 10 minutes in simulated gastric conditions. Generally, frequent food snacks prolong the time an antacid remains in the stomach and can prolong its action.

Because many antacids, especially aluminum- and calcium-containing products, interfere with absorption of other drugs, especially the fluoroquinolone and tetracycline antibiotics and iron salts, pharmacists must caution their patients against taking such drugs concomitantly.

In addition to the suspension forms of antacids, a number of official and commercial liquid antacid preparations of the magma and gel type will be mentioned later in this chapter. Generally, these liquid forms are pleasantly

flavored (usually with peppermint) to enhance their palatability and patient appeal. Because liquid antacid preparations characteristically contain a large amount of solid material, they must be shaken vigorously to redistribute the antacid prior to administration. Also, a large dose of antacid is frequently required. Thus, many patients prefer to swallow one or two tablespoonfuls of a liquid preparation than to swallow whole or chew the corresponding number of tablets (commonly three to six) for the equivalent dose of drug.

Antibacterial Oral Suspensions

The antibacterial oral suspensions include preparations of antibiotic substances (e.g., erythromycin derivatives and tetracycline and its derivatives), sulfonamides (e.g., sulfamethoxazole and sulfisoxazole acetyl), other anti-infective agents (e.g., methenamine mandelate and nitrofurantoin), or combinations of these (e.g., sulfamethoxazole-trimethoprim).

Many antibiotic materials are unstable when maintained in solution for an appreciable length of time, and therefore, from a stability standpoint, insoluble forms of the drug substances in aqueous suspension or as dry powder for reconstitution (discussed next) are attractive to manufacturers. The antibiotic oral suspensions, including those prepared by reconstitution, provide a convenient way to administer dosages to infants and children and to adult patients who prefer liquid preparations to solid ones. Many of the oral suspensions that are intended primarily for infants are packaged with a calibrated dropper to assist in the delivery of the prescribed dose. Some commercial pediatric antibiotic oral suspensions are pictured in Figure 14.4 and calibrated droppers in Figure 14.7.

The dispersing phase of antibiotic suspensions is aqueous and usually colored, sweetened, and flavored to render

FIGURE 14.7. Calibrated droppers used in the administration of pediatric medications.

the liquid more appealing and palatable. As noted previously, the palmitate form of chloramphenicol was selected for the suspension dosage form not only because of its water insolubility but also because it is flavorless, which eliminates the necessity to mask the otherwise bitter taste of the chloramphenicol base.

Rectal Suspensions

Barium Sulfate for Suspension, USP, may be employed orally or rectally for diagnostic visualization of the gastrointestinal tract. Mesalamine (5-aminosalicylic acid) suspension was introduced to the market in 1988 as Rowasa (Alaven) for treatment of Crohn disease, distal ulcerative colitis, proctosigmoiditis, and proctitis. It is no longer commercially available but is compounded by pharmacists. Colocort (Paddock Laboratories) is a hydrocortisone rectal suspension indicated as adjunctive therapy in the treatment of ulcerative colitis and is packaged in a convenient disposable single-dose enema designed for self-administration. It contains 100 mg of hydrocortisone in 60 mL of an aqueous solution also containing carbomer 934P, polysorbate 80, purified water, sodium hydroxide, and methylparaben.

Dry Powders for Oral Suspension

A number of official and commercial preparations consist of dry powder mixtures or granules that are intended to be suspended in distilled water or some other vehicle prior to oral administration. As indicated previously, these official preparations have "for Oral Suspension" in their official title to distinguish them from prepared suspensions.

Most drugs prepared as a dry mix for oral suspension are antibiotics. The dry products are prepared commercially to contain the antibiotic drug, colorants (FD&C dyes), flavorants, sweeteners (e.g., sucrose or sodium saccharin), stabilizing agents (e.g., citric acid, sodium citrate), suspending agents (e.g., guar gum, xanthan gum, methylcellulose), and preserving agents (e.g., methylparaben, sodium benzoate) that may be needed to enhance the stability of the dry powder or granule mixture or the liquid suspension. When called on to reconstitute and dispense one of these products, the pharmacist loosens the powder at the bottom of the container by lightly tapping it against a hard surface and then adds the label-designated amount of purified water, usually in portions, and shakes the slurry until all of the dry powder has been suspended (Fig. 14.2). It is important to add precisely the prescribed amount of purified water to the dry mixture if the proper drug concentration per dosage unit is to be achieved. Also, the use of purified water rather than tap water is needed to avoid the possibility of adding impurities that could adversely affect the stability of the resulting preparation. Generally, manufacturers provide the dry powder or granule mixture in a slightly oversized container to permit adequate shaking of the contents after the entire amount of purified water has been added. Pharmacists must realize that an oversized bottle is provided with each of these products,

and they must carefully measure out the required amount of purified water. They should not "eyeball" the amount of water to be added or fill up the bottle with purified water. There are devices available to aid in accurate reconstitution, including the Fillmaster and/or the Fillmaster Plus.

Water for reconstitution is frequently added in two portions. After adding the first portion, for example, 2/3 of the total water volume required, the bottle is capped tightly and inverted and tapped or shaken vigorously to incorporate all of the powder in the liquid. The second portion of water is then added and the mixture is shaken to achieve the final homogeneous suspension.

Among the official antibiotic drugs for oral suspension are the following:

Amoxicillin for Oral Suspension, USP (Amoxil for Oral Suspension, GlaxoSmithKline)

Ampicillin for Oral Suspension, USP (Principen for Oral Suspension, Geneva)

Cefaclor for Oral Suspension, USP (Ceclor for Oral Suspension, Lilly)

Cefixime for Oral Suspension, USP (Suprax Powder for Oral Suspension, Lupin Pharma)

Cephalexin for Oral Suspension, USP (Keflex for Oral Suspension, Victory Pharma)

Dicloxacillin Sodium for Oral Suspension, USP (Pathocil for Oral Suspension, Wyeth-Ayerst)

Doxycycline for Oral Suspension, USP (Vibramycin Monohydrate for Oral Suspension, Pfizer)

Erythromycin Ethylsuccinate for Oral Suspension, USP (E.E.S. Granules for Oral Suspension, Arbor Pharmaceuticals)

Several official antibiotics for oral suspension are also combined with other drugs. For example, erythromycin ethylsuccinate plus acetyl sulfisoxazole granules for oral suspension is indicated for the treatment of acute middle ear infection caused by susceptible strains of *Haemophilus influenzae*. Probenecid is combined with ampicillin for reconstitution and ultimate use for the treatment of uncomplicated infections (urethral, endocervical, or rectal) caused by *Neisseria gonorrhoeae* in adults.

Among the official drugs other than antibiotics prepared as dry powder mixtures for reconstitution to oral suspension are cholestyramine (Questran, Par), used in the management of hyperlipidemia, and barium sulfate (Barosperse, Mallinckrodt), used orally or rectally as a radiopaque contrast medium to visualize the gastrointestinal tract as an aid to diagnosis. Barium sulfate was introduced into medicine about 1910 as a contrast medium for roentgen ray examination of the gastrointestinal tract. It is practically insoluble in water, and thus, its administration even in the large doses required is safe because it is not absorbed from the gastrointestinal tract. The pharmacist must be careful not to confuse barium sulfate with other forms of barium, such as barium *sulfide* and barium *sulfite*, which are soluble salts and *are* poisonous. Barium sulfate is a fine, nongritty, odorless, and tasteless white powder. When prepared as a suspension and administered orally, it is used to diagnose conditions of the hypopharynx, esophagus, stomach, small intestine, and colon. The barium sulfate renders the gastrointestinal tract opaque to the x-ray so as to reveal any abnormality in the anatomic features of the tract. When administered rectally, barium sulfate allows visualization of the features of the rectum and colon.

Commercially, barium sulfate for diagnostic use is available as a bulk powder containing the required suspending agents for effective reconstitution to an oral suspension or enema. Enema units, which contain prepared suspension in a ready-to-use and disposable bag, are also available.

EMULSIONS

An emulsion is a dispersion in which the dispersed phase is composed of small globules of a liquid distributed throughout a vehicle in which it is immiscible (Fig. 14.8). In emulsion terminology, the dispersed phase is the *internal phase*, and the dispersion medium is the *external* or *continuous phase*. Emulsions with an oleaginous internal phase and an aqueous external phase are *oil-in-water* (o/w) emulsions. Conversely, emulsions having an aqueous internal phase and an oleaginous external phase are termed *water-in-oil* (w/o) emulsions. Because the external phase of an emulsion is continuous, an o/w emulsion may be diluted or extended with water or an aqueous preparation and a w/o emulsion, with an oleaginous or oil-miscible liquid. Generally, to prepare a stable emulsion, a third phase, an *emulsifying agent*, is necessary. Depending on their constituents, the viscosity of emulsions can vary greatly, and pharmaceutical emulsions may be prepared as liquids or semisolids. Based on the constituents and the intended application, liquid emulsions may be employed orally, topically, or parenterally and semisolid emulsions topically. Many pharmaceutical preparations that are actu-

ally emulsions are not classified as such because they fit some other pharmaceutical category more appropriately. For instance, emulsions include certain lotions, liniments, creams, ointments, and commercial vitamin drops that are discussed in this book under these various designations.

Purpose of Emulsions and of Emulsification

Emulsification enables the pharmacist to prepare relatively stable and homogeneous mixtures of two immiscible liquids. It permits administration of a liquid drug in the form of minute globules rather than in bulk. For orally administered emulsions, the o/w type permits palatable administration of an otherwise distasteful oil by dispersing it in a sweetened, flavored aqueous vehicle. The reduced particle size of the oil globules may render the oil more digestible and more readily absorbed or, if that is not the intent, more effective in its task, as for example, the increased efficacy of mineral oil as a cathartic when emulsified.

Emulsions to be applied to the skin may be o/w or w/o, depending on such factors as the nature of the therapeutic agents, the desirability for an emollient or tissue-softening effect, and the condition of the skin. Medicinal agents that irritate the skin generally are less irritating in the internal phase of an emulsified topical preparation than in the external phase, from which direct contact with the skin is more prevalent. Naturally, the miscibility or solubility in oil and in water of a medicinal agent dictates to a great extent the vehicle, and its nature in turn suggests the phase of the emulsion that the resulting solution should become. On the unbroken skin, a w/o emulsion can usually be applied more evenly because the skin is covered with a thin film of sebum, and this surface is more readily wetted by oil than by water. A w/o emulsion is also more softening to the skin because it resists drying and removal by contact with water. On the other hand, if it is desirable to have a preparation that is easily removed from the skin with water, an o/w emulsion is preferred. Also, absorption through the skin (percutaneous absorption) may be enhanced by the diminished particle size of the internal phase. Other aspects of topical preparations are discussed in Chapters 10 and 11.

Theories of Emulsification

Many theories have been advanced in an attempt to explain how emulsifying agents promote emulsification and maintain the stability of the emulsion. Although certain of these theories apply rather specifically to certain types of emulsifying agents and to certain conditions (e.g., the pH of the phases of the system and the nature and relative proportions of the internal and external phases), they may be viewed in a general way to describe the manner in which emulsions may be produced and stabilized. Among the most prevalent theories are the *surface tension theory*, the *oriented-wedge theory*, and the *plastic* or *interfacial film theory*.

All liquids have a tendency to assume a shape having the minimal surface area exposed. For a drop of a liquid, the shape with the lowest surface area is the sphere. Liquids

FIGURE 14.8. Mineral oil-in-water emulsion. (Courtesy of Viswas Sharad Purohit/Dreamstime.com.)

possess internal forces that tend to promote association of the molecules to resist distortion of the sphere. If two or more drops of the same liquid come into contact with one another, the tendency is for them to join or to *coalesce*, making one larger drop having a smaller surface area than the total surface area of the individual drops. The force that causes liquids to reduce their interfacial surface area may be measured quantitatively, and when the environment surrounding the liquid is air, it is referred to as the liquid's surface tension. When the liquid is in contact with a second liquid in which it is insoluble and immiscible, the force causing each liquid to resist breaking up into smaller particles is called interfacial tension. Substances that reduce interfacial tension encourage a liquid to break up into smaller drops or particles. These tension-lowering substances are called *surface-active* agents (surfactants) or *wetting agents*. According to the *surface tension theory* of emulsification, the use of these substances as emulsifiers and stabilizers lowers the interfacial tension of the two immiscible liquids, reducing the repellent force between the liquids and diminishing each liquid's attraction for its own molecules. Thus, the surface-active agents facilitate the breaking up of large globules into smaller ones, which then have a lesser tendency to reunite or coalesce.

The *oriented-wedge* theory assumes monomolecular layers of emulsifying agent curved around a droplet of the internal phase of the emulsion. The theory is based on the presumption that certain emulsifying agents orient themselves about and within a liquid in a manner reflective of their solubility in that particular liquid. In a system containing two immiscible liquids, presumably the emulsifying agent is preferentially soluble in one of the phases and is embedded more deeply and tenaciously in that phase than the other. Because many molecules of substances upon which this theory is based (e.g., soaps) have a hydrophilic or water-loving portion and a hydrophobic or water-hating portion (but usually lipophilic or oil loving), the molecules position or orient themselves into both phases. Depending on the shape and size of the molecules, their solubility characteristics, and thus their orientation, the wedge shape envisioned for the molecules causes either oil globules or water globules to be surrounded. Generally, an emulsifying agent having a greater hydrophilic than hydrophobic character will promote an o/w emulsion, and a w/o emulsion results from use of an emulsifying agent that is more hydrophobic than hydrophilic. Putting it another way, the phase in which the emulsifying agent is more soluble will become the continuous or external phase of the emulsion. Although this theory may not represent a totally accurate depiction of the molecular arrangement of the emulsifier molecules, the concept that water-soluble emulsifiers generally do form o/w emulsions is important and is frequently encountered in practice.

The *plastic* or *interfacial film theory* places the emulsifying agent at the interface between the oil and water, surrounding the droplets of the internal phase as a thin, but not necessarily monomolecular, layer of film adsorbed on the surface of the drops. The film prevents contact and coalescing of the dispersed phase; the tougher and more pliable the film, the greater the stability of the emulsion. Naturally, enough of the film-forming material must be available to coat the entire surface of each drop of the internal phase. Here again, the formation of an o/w or a w/o emulsion depends on the degree of solubility of the agent in the two phases, with water-soluble agents encouraging o/w emulsions and oil-soluble emulsifiers the reverse.

In actuality, it is unlikely that a single theory of emulsification can explain the means by which the many and varied emulsifiers promote emulsion formation and stability. It is more than likely that even within a given emulsion system, more than one of the aforementioned theories play a part. For instance, lowering of the interfacial tension is important in the initial formation of an emulsion, but the formation of a protective wedge of molecules or film of emulsifier is important for continued stability. No doubt certain emulsifiers are capable of both tasks. Physical Pharmacy Capsule 14.4 discusses Gibbs free energy and its application to the formulation of stable emulsions.

Preparation of Emulsions

Emulsifying Agents

The initial step in preparation of an emulsion is selection of the emulsifier. To be useful in a pharmaceutical preparation, the emulsifying agent must be compatible with the other formulative ingredients and must not interfere with the stability or efficacy of the therapeutic agent. It should be stable and not deteriorate in the preparation. The emulsifier should be nontoxic with respect to its intended use and the amount to be consumed by the patient. Also, it should possess little odor, taste, or color. Of prime importance is the capability of the emulsifying agent to promote emulsification and to maintain the stability of the emulsion for the intended shelf life of the product.

Various types of materials have been used in pharmacy as emulsifying agents, with hundreds, if not thousands, of individual agents tested for their emulsification capabilities. Although no attempt will be made here to discuss the merits of each of these agents in pharmaceutical emulsions, it would be well to point out the types of materials that are commonly used and their general application. Among the emulsifiers and stabilizers for pharmaceutical systems are the following:

1. Carbohydrate materials, such as the naturally occurring agents acacia, tragacanth, agar, chondrus, and pectin. These materials form hydrophilic colloids, which, when added to water, generally produce o/w emulsions. Acacia is frequently used in the preparation of extemporaneous emulsions. Tragacanth and agar are commonly employed as thickening agents in acacia-emulsified products. Microcrystalline cellulose is employed in a number of commercial suspensions and emulsions as a viscosity regulator to retard particle settling and provide dispersion stability.

2. Protein substances, such as gelatin, egg yolk, and casein. These substances produce o/w emulsions.

PHYSICAL PHARMACY CAPSULE **14.4** Gibbs Free Energy in an Emulsion

As previously discussed, pharmaceutical dispersions consist of two mutually insoluble phases or states of matter. In suspensions, settling and compaction of solid drug particles may occur as well as clumping or aggregation of particles (flocculation is aggregation that is reversible upon vigorous agitation or shaking). In emulsions, creaming (a reversible weak association of internal phase droplets) and cracking (an irreversible coalescence of internal phase droplets) may occur. The latter may result to minimize Gibbs free energy by minimizing the surface area of the internal phase.

Gibbs free energy states

$$\Delta G = \Delta A \gamma$$

where

Δ is the size of change in G and A,
ΔG naturally "seeks" to 0 or a minimum,
A is the total surface area of dispersed particles, and
γ is the interfacial tension, or interphase repulsion, that is,

liquid repels liquid in emulsions,
liquid repels solid in suspensions,
liquid repels gas, and
solid repels gas in inhalations.

A large "ΔG" forces "A" to a minimum unless "γ" is greatly reduced to compensate for a large "A."

Good emulsions and suspensions must have a very large "A" for dosing consistency; thus, they must also have a very small "γ."

The natural instability of dispersions is due to

A large "A" and a large "γ," which cause a large "G"
A large "G" and a large "γ," which cause emulsified droplets and suspended particles, or the internal phase, to aggregate to reduce "A" to reduce "G"

Stable emulsions and suspensions must have a large "A" and a small "G" concurrently for consistent and uniform dosing. This is done by decreasing "γ," which will decrease "G," which will decrease self-attraction of dispersed phase particles.

■ EXAMPLE

Area increase in o/w emulsion
Fifty milliliter of an oil in a graduated cylinder has a total A = 80 cm^2.
This 50 mL is processed to make 9.55×10^{13} droplets of 1×10^{-4} cm diameter each.
Each droplet has an A = 7.854×10^{-9} cm^2.
The total "A" of the 50 mL as 1-μm-diameter droplets is

$$\left(7.854 \times 10^{-9} \text{ cm}^2 / \text{droplet}\right) \times \left(9.55 \times 10^{13} \text{ droplets}\right) = 7.5 \times 10^5 \text{ cm}^2$$

$$\Delta A = \frac{7.5 \times 10^5 \text{cm}^2}{80 \text{ cm}^2} = 9.38 \times 10^3$$

For this emulsion to be stable, the "γ" must be decreased by nearly 9,400 times to minimize "G." ■

The disadvantage of gelatin as an emulsifier is that the emulsion frequently is too fluid and becomes more fluid upon standing, especially at higher temperatures.

3. High molecular weight alcohols, such as stearyl alcohol, cetyl alcohol, and glyceryl monostearate. These are employed primarily as thickening agents and

stabilizers for o/w emulsions of certain lotions and ointments used externally. Cholesterol and cholesterol derivatives may also be employed in externally used emulsions to promote w/o emulsions.

4. Wetting agents, which may be anionic, cationic, or nonionic. These agents contain both hydrophilic and lipophilic groups, with the lipophilic protein of the

molecule generally accounting for the surface activity of the molecule. In anionic agents, this lipophilic portion is negatively charged, but in the cationic agent, it is positively charged. Owing to their opposing ionic charges, anionic and cationic agents tend to neutralize each other and are thus considered incompatible. Nonionic emulsifiers show no inclination to ionize. Depending on their individual nature, certain members of these groups form o/w emulsions and others w/o emulsions. Anionic emulsifiers include various monovalent, polyvalent, and organic soaps, such as triethanolamine oleate, and sulfonates, such as sodium lauryl sulfate. Benzalkonium chloride, known primarily for its bactericidal properties, may be employed as a cationic emulsifier in products for external use. Agents of the nonionic type include the sorbitan esters and the polyoxyethylene derivatives, some of which appear in Table 14.2.

5. The ionic nature of a surfactant is a prime consideration. Nonionic surfactants are effective over pH range of 3 to 10, cationic surfactants are effective over pH range of 3 to 7, and anionic surfactants require a pH greater than 8 (6).

6. Finely divided solids such as colloidal clays, including bentonite, magnesium hydroxide, and aluminum hydroxide. Generally, these form o/w emulsions when the insoluble material is added to the aqueous phase if there is a greater volume of the aqueous phase than of the oleaginous phase. However, if the powdered solid is added to the oil and the oleaginous phase volume predominates, a substance such as bentonite is capable of forming a w/o emulsion. The relative volume of internal and external phases of an emulsion is important, regardless of the type of emulsifier used. As the internal concentration of an emulsion increases, so does the viscosity of the emulsion to a certain point, after which the viscosity decreases sharply. At this point, the emulsion has undergone *inversion*, that is, it has changed from an o/w emulsion to a w/o or vice versa. In practice, emulsions may be prepared without inversion with as much as about 75% of the volume of the product being internal phase.

The HLB System

Generally, each emulsifying agent has a hydrophilic portion and a lipophilic portion, with one or the other being more or less predominant and influencing in the manner already described the type of emulsion. A method has been devised (7,8) whereby emulsifying or surface-active agents may be categorized on the basis of their chemical makeup as to their hydrophilic–lipophilic balance, or HLB. By this method, each agent is assigned an HLB value or number indicating the substance's polarity. Although the numbers have been assigned up to about 40, the usual range is between 1 and 20. Materials that are highly polar or hydrophilic have been assigned higher numbers than

TABLE 14.2. HLB Values for Selected Emulsifiers

Agent	HLB
Ethylene glycol distearate	1.5
Sorbitan tristearate (Span 65[a])	2.1
Propylene glycol monostearate	3.4
Triton X-15[b]	3.6
Sorbitan monooleate (Span 80[a])	4.3
Sorbitan monostearate (Span 60[a])	4.7
Diethylene glycol monolaurate	6.1
Sorbitan monopalmitate (Span 40[a])	6.7
Sucrose dioleate	7.1
Acacia	8.0
Amerchol L-101[c]	8.0
Polyoxyethylene lauryl ether (Brij 30[a])	9.7
Gelatin	9.8
Triton X-45[b]	10.4
Methylcellulose	10.5
Polyoxyethylene monostearate (Myrj 45[a])	11.1
Triethanolamine oleate	12.0
Tragacanth	13.2
Triton X-100[b]	13.5
Polyoxyethylene sorbitan monostearate (Tween 60[a])	14.9
Polyoxyethylene sorbitan monooleate (Tween 80[a])	15.0
Polyoxyethylene sorbitan monolaurate (Tween 20[a])	16.7
Pluronic F-68[d]	17.0
Sodium oleate	18.0
Potassium oleate	20.0
Sodium lauryl sulfate	40.0

[a]ICI Americas; Wilmington, DE.
[b]Rohm and Haas; Philadelphia, PA.
[c]Amerchol Corporation; Edison, NJ.
[d]BASF-Wyandotte Chemical; Parsippany, NJ.

materials that are less polar and more lipophilic. Generally, surface-active agents having an assigned HLB value of 3 to 6 are greatly lipophilic and produce w/o emulsions, and agents with HLB values of about 8 to 18 produce o/w emulsions. Examples of assigned HLB values for some surfactants are shown in Table 14.2. The type of activity to be expected from surfactants of assigned HLB numbers is presented in Table 14.3.

TABLE 14.3. Activity and HLB Value of Surfactants

Activity	Assigned HLB
Antifoaming	1–3
Emulsifiers (w/o)	3–6
Wetting agents	7–9
Emulsifiers (o/w)	8–18
Solubilizers	15–20
Detergents	13–16

PHYSICAL PHARMACY CAPSULE **14.5** Blending of Surfactants

*W*etting agents are surfactants with HLB values of *7* to *9*. Wetting agents aid in attaining intimate contact between solid particles and liquids.

Emulsifying agents are surfactants with HLB values of *3* to *6* or *8* to *18*. Emulsifying agents reduce interfacial tension between oil and water, minimizing surface energy through the formation of globules.

Detergents are surfactants with HLB values of *13* to *16*. Detergents will reduce the surface tension and aid in wetting the surface and the dirt. The soil will be emulsified, and foaming generally occurs and a washing away of the dirt.

Solubilizing agents have HLB values of *15* to *20*.

HLB values are additive, and often, surfactants are blended. For example, if 20 mL of an HLB of 9.0 is required, two surfactants (with HLB values of 8.0 and 12.0) can be blended in a 3:1 ratio. The following quantities of each will be required:

$$0.75 \times 8.0 = 6.0$$
$$0.25 \times 12.0 = 3.0$$
$$\text{Total HLB} = 9.0 \blacksquare$$

In the HLB system, in addition to the emulsifying agents, values are assigned to oils and oil-like substances. One selects emulsifying agents having the same or nearly the same HLB value as the oleaginous phase of the intended emulsion. For example, mineral oil has an assigned HLB value of 4 if a w/o emulsion is desired and a value of 10.5 if an o/w emulsion is to be prepared. To prepare a stable emulsion, the emulsifying agent should have an HLB value similar to the one for mineral oil, depending on the type of emulsion desired. When needed, two or more emulsifiers may be combined to achieve the proper HLB value.

Physical Pharmacy Capsules 14.5 and 14.6 summarize the activities of surfactants and the calculations to determine the quantity of surfactant required for a stable emulsion.

PHYSICAL PHARMACY CAPSULE **14.6** Surface Area of Globules

*T*he following is a sample calculation for determining the quantity of surfactant required to prepare a stable o/w emulsion.

A surface-active agent will spread itself as a single layer when applied to the surface of still water. The dimensions of a molecule can be determined by their surface orientation. For example, if a micropipette is used to deliver 3 μL of a surfactant to the clean, quiet surface of water, the area over which it spreads, determined experimentally using a film balance, is 12,000 cm². The actual thickness of the film can be calculated by dividing the volume of surfactant applied by the surface area, as follows:

$$\frac{0.003 \text{ cm}^3}{12,000 \text{ cm}^2} = 2.5 \times 10^{-7} \text{ cm}$$

The surfactant has a density of 0.910 g/mL and a molecular weight of 325 g/mol. To calculate the cross-sectional area occupied by each molecule, divide the area of the monomolecular film by the number of molecules in the 3 mL of surfactant constituting the film, as follows:

1. Obtain the weight of the surfactant by multiplying the volume by the density (0.003 mL × 0.910 g/mL = 0.00273 g).
2. To calculate the number of moles present, divide the weight of the surfactant by its molecular weight (0.00273 g/325 g/mol = 8.4 × 10⁻⁶ mol).

(continued)

(continued)

3. The number of molecules present is the number of moles times Avogadro number ($8.4 \times 10^{-6} \times 6.02 \times 10^{23} = 5.0568 \times 10^{18}$ molecules).
4. The cross-sectional area can now be calculated by dividing the surface area by the number of molecules ($12,000$ cm^2/$5.0568 \times 10^{18} \times 2.373 \times 10^{-15}$ cm$^2 \times 23.73 \times 10^{-16}$ or approximately 24 square angstroms).

The quantity of surfactant required to emulsify a selected quantity of oil for the preparation of an oil-in-water emulsion can be calculated as follows:

■ EXAMPLE

To emulsify 50 mL of oil to an average globular diameter of 1 μg, the volume of each globule is

$$V_1 = \frac{4}{3}\pi r^3 = \frac{4}{3}\pi \left(0.5 \times 10^{-4}\right)^3 = 0.524 \times 10^{-12} \text{ mL}$$

To calculate the number of globules per milliliter, divide 1 mL by the volume of each globule:

$$\frac{1 \text{ mL}}{0.524 \times 10^{-12} \text{ mL/globule}} = 1.91 \times 10^{12} \text{ globules/mL}$$

The surface area (S) of each individual globule will be

$$S = 4\pi r^2 = 4\pi \left(0.5 \times 10^{-4}\right)^2 = 3.14 \times 10^{-8} \text{ cm}^2$$

and the surface area of all the globules in 1 mL of oil is

$$\left(1.91 \times 10^{12}\right) \times \left(3.14 \times 10^{-8}\right) = 6 \times 10^4 \text{ cm}^2$$

The number of surfactant molecules that will be adsorbed at the interface of the oil globules and the dispersion medium from 1 mL of oil is equal to the total surface area divided by the cross-sectional area of the surfactant:

$$\frac{6 \times 10^4 \text{ cm}^2}{2.373 \times 10^{-15} \text{ cm}^2/\text{molecule}} = 2.528 \times 10^{19} \text{ molecules}$$

The number of moles of surfactant required to emulsify 1 mL of oil is equal to the number of molecules adsorbed at the interface divided by Avogadro number:

$$\frac{2.528 \times 10^{19} \text{ molecules}}{6.02 \times 10^{23} \text{ molecules/mole}} = 4.199 \times 10^{-5} \text{ moles}$$

and the quantity required for 50 mL will be

$$50 \text{ mL} \times 4.199 \times 10^{-5} \text{ moles/mL} = 2.095 \times 10^{-3} \text{ moles}$$

$$2.095 \times 10^{-3} \text{ moles} \times 325 \text{ g/mole} = 0.681 \text{ g, or } 681 \text{ mg}$$

Therefore, 681 mg of surfactant will be required to emulsify 50 mL of the oil. ■

Methods of Emulsion Preparation

Emulsions may be prepared by several methods, depending upon the nature of the components and the equipment. On a small scale, as in the laboratory or pharmacy, emulsions may be prepared using a dry Wedgwood or porcelain mortar and pestle; a mechanical blender or mixer, such as a Waring blender or a milkshake mixer; a hand homogenizer (Fig. 14.9); a bench-type homogenizer (Fig. 14.10); or sometimes a simple prescription bottle. On a large scale, large mixing tanks (Fig. 14.5) may be used to form the emulsion through the action of a high-speed impeller. As desired, the product may be rendered finer by passage through a colloid mill, in which the particles are sheared between the small gap separating a high-speed rotor and the stator, or by passage through a large homogenizer, in which the liquid is forced under great pressure through a small valve opening.

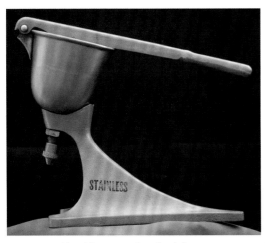

FIGURE 14.9. Hand homogenizer for laboratory preparation of emulsions.

FIGURE 14.10. Kinematica homogenizer model PT 3100 D with accessories. The equipment is used for homogenization, dispersion, and emulsification of solids or liquids. Volumes range from 0.5 mL to 25 L. (Courtesy of Kinematica, Inc.)

Industrial homogenizers have the capacity to handle as much as 100,000 L of product per hour.

In the small-scale extemporaneous preparation of emulsions, three methods may be used. They are the *continental* or *dry gum method*, the *English* or *wet gum method*, and the *bottle* or *Forbes bottle method*. In the dry gum method, the emulsifying agent (usually acacia) is mixed with the oil before the addition of water. In the wet gum method, the emulsifying agent is added to the water (in which it is soluble) to form a mucilage, and then the oil is slowly incorporated to form the emulsion. The bottle method is reserved for volatile oils or less viscous oils and is a variation of the dry gum method.

Continental or Dry Gum Method

The continental method is also referred to as the 4:2:1 method because for every four parts by volume of oil, two parts of water and one part of gum are added in preparing the initial or *primary emulsion*. For instance, if 40 mL of oil is to be emulsified, 20 mL of water and 10 g of gum would be employed in the primary emulsion, with any additional water or other formulation ingredients added afterward. In this method, the acacia or other o/w emulsifier is triturated with the oil in a perfectly dry Wedgwood or porcelain mortar until thoroughly mixed. A mortar with a rough rather than smooth inner surface must be used to ensure proper grinding action and reduction of the globule size. A glass mortar is too smooth to produce the proper reduction of the internal phase. After the oil and gum have been mixed, the two parts of water are added all at once, and the mixture is triturated immediately, rapidly, and continuously until the primary emulsion is creamy white and produces a crackling sound to the movement of the pestle. Generally, about 3 minutes of mixing is required to produce a primary emulsion. Other liquid formulative ingredients that are soluble in or miscible with the external phase may then be mixed into the primary emulsion. Solid substances such as preservatives, stabilizers, colorants, and any flavoring material are usually dissolved in a suitable volume of water (assuming water is the external phase) and added as a solution to the primary emulsion. Any substances that might interfere with the stability of the emulsion or the emulsifying agent are added as near last as is practical. For instance, alcohol has a precipitating action on gums such as acacia; thus, no alcohol or solution containing alcohol should be added directly to the primary emulsion, because the total alcoholic concentration of the mixture would be greater at that point than after other diluents were added. When all necessary agents have been added, the emulsion is transferred to a graduate and made to volume with water previously swirled about in the mortar to remove the last portion of emulsion.

Provided the dispersion of the acacia in the oil is adequate, the dry gum method can almost be guaranteed to produce an acceptable emulsion. Sometimes, however, the amount of acacia must be adjusted upward to ensure that an emulsion can be produced. For example, volatile oils, liquid petrolatum (mineral oil), and linseed oil usually require a 3:2:1 or 2:2:1 ratio for adequate preparation. Rather than using a mortar and pestle, the pharmacist can generally prepare an excellent emulsion using the dry gum method and an electric mixer or blender.

English or Wet Gum Method

By this method, the same proportions of oil, water, and gum are used as in the continental or dry gum method, but the order of mixing is different, and the proportion of ingredients may be varied during the preparation of the primary emulsion as is deemed necessary by the operator. Generally, a mucilage of the gum is prepared by triturating in a mortar granular acacia with twice its weight of water. The oil is then added slowly in portions, and the mixture is triturated to emulsify the oil. Should the mixture become too thick, additional water may be blended into the mixture before another portion of oil is added. After all of the oil has been added, the mixture is thoroughly mixed for several minutes to ensure uniformity. Then, as with the continental or dry gum method, the other formulative materials are added, and the emulsion is transferred to a graduate and brought to volume with water.

Bottle or Forbes Bottle Method

The bottle method is useful for the extemporaneous preparation of emulsions from volatile oils or oleaginous substances of low viscosities. Powdered acacia is placed in a dry bottle, two parts of oil are added, and the mixture is thoroughly shaken in the capped container. A volume of water approximately equal to that of the oil is then added in portions and the mixture thoroughly shaken after each addition. When all of the water has been added, the primary emulsion thus formed may be diluted to the proper volume with water or an aqueous solution of other formulative agents.

This method is not suited for viscous oils because they cannot be thoroughly agitated in the bottle when mixed with the emulsifying agent. When the intended dispersed phase is a mixture of fixed oil and volatile oil, the dry gum method is generally employed.

Auxiliary Methods

An emulsion prepared by either the wet gum or the dry gum method can generally be increased in quality by passing it through a hand homogenizer. In this apparatus, the pumping action of the handle forces the emulsion through a very small orifice that reduces the globules of the internal phase to about 5 μm and sometimes less. The hand homogenizer is less efficient in reducing the particle size of very thick emulsions, and it should not be employed for emulsions containing a high proportion of solid matter because of possible damage to the valve.

In Situ Soap Method

The two types of soaps developed by this method are calcium soaps and soft soaps. Calcium soaps are w/o emulsions that contain certain vegetable oils, such as oleic

acid, in combination with limewater (synonym: Calcium Hydroxide Solution, USP). They are prepared simply by mixing equal volumes of the oil and limewater. The emulsifying agent in this instance is the calcium salt of the free fatty acid formed from the combination of the two entities. In the case of olive oil, the free fatty acid is oleic acid, and the resultant emulsifying agent is calcium oleate. A difficulty that sometimes arises when preparing this self-emulsifying product is that the amount of free fatty acids in the oil may be insufficient on a 1:1 basis with calcium hydroxide. Typically, to make up for this deficiency, a little excess of the olive oil, or even a small amount of oleic acid, is needed to ensure a nice, homogeneous emulsion. Otherwise, tiny droplets of water form on the surface of the preparation. Because the oil phase is the external phase, this formulation is ideal where occlusion and skin softening are desired, such as for itchy, dry skin or sunburned skin. A typical example of this emulsion is calamine liniment:

Calamine	
Zinc oxide aa	80.0 g
Olive oil	
Calcium hydroxide solution aa qs ad	1,000.0 mL

Mixing Immiscible Liquids

The mixing of systems consisting of multiple immiscible liquid phases primarily involves the subdivision of the internal phase into the external phase with subsequent dispersal throughout the mass of material to be mixed. An example formulation is a mixture of oil and water, or an emulsion. An emulsion is a dispersion in which the dispersed phase is composed of small globules of a liquid distributed throughout a vehicle in which it is immiscible. Emulsification enables the pharmacist to prepare relatively stable and homogeneous mixtures of two immiscible liquids.

Most emulsified liquids for oral use are oils, which generally have lower density than the aqueous medium in which they are dispersed, so they tend to rise toward the top of the preparation. Complete and uniform redistribution of the dispersed phase is essential to the accurate administration of uniform doses. For a properly prepared dispersion, this should be accomplished by moderate agitation of the container prior to measuring a dose.

The mixing of two immiscible liquids requires the subdivision of one of the phases into globules, which are then distributed throughout the bulk of the fluid. The process usually occurs by stages during which the large globules are successively broken down into smaller ones. Two primary forces come into play here: (*a*) the interfacial tension of the globules in the surrounding liquid and (*b*) the forces of shear within the fluid mass. The former tends to resist the distortion of globule shape necessary for fragmentation into smaller globules, whereas the forces of shear act to distort and ultimately disrupt the globules. The relationship between these forces largely determines the final size distribution in the mixture. Multiphase mixing generally involves the use of high shear and low flow to create droplets of one liquid in another.

A variety of process functions like blending miscible liquids or dispersing immiscible liquids are carried out in agitated vessels by rotating impellers. The impellers are either axial or radial, depending on the angle that the impeller (also known as the agitator) blade makes with the plane of impeller rotation (described in previous newsletters).

On a large scale, large mixing tanks may be used to form the emulsion through the action of a high-speed impeller. As desired, the product may be rendered finer by passage through a colloid mill, in which the particles are sheared between the small gap separating a high-speed rotor and the stator, or by passage through a large homogenizer, in which the liquid is forced under great pressure through a small valve opening.

The quality of the final preparation/product is dependent upon complete and homogeneous mixing; this can be obtained only by understanding the various factors involved in "mixing" and the characteristics of the ingredients (solids, liquids, etc.) being mixed. Understanding which equipment to use, and when and how to use it, is also vital.

Microemulsions

Microemulsions are thermodynamically stable, optically transparent isotropic (or homogeneous) mixtures of a biphasic o/w system stabilized with surfactants. The diameter of droplets in a *micro*emulsion may be in the range of 100 Å (10 mμ) to 1,000 Å, whereas in a *macro*emulsion, the droplets may be 5,000 Å in diameter (6). Both o/w and w/o microemulsions may be formed spontaneously by agitating the oil and water phases with carefully selected surfactants. The type of emulsion produced depends on the properties of the oil and surfactants.

Hydrophilic surfactants may be used to produce transparent o/w emulsions of many oils, including flavor oils and vitamin oils such as A, D, and E. Surfactants in the HLB range of 15 to 18 have been used most extensively in the preparation of such emulsions. These emulsions are dispersions of oil, not true solutions; however, because of the appearance of the product, the surfactant is commonly said to solubilize the oil. Surfactants commonly used in the preparation of such oral liquid formulations are polysorbate 60 and polysorbate 80.

The advantages of microemulsions include the following:

- Increased physical stability.
- Increased solubilization.
- Improved bioavailability and efficacy.
- Provides aqueous dosage form for water-insoluble drugs.
- Can be used via various routes.
- Rapid and efficient penetration of the drug moiety.
- Helpful in taste masking.
- Protection from hydrolysis and oxidation when drug is in the oil phase, an o/w microemulsion.

- Liquid dosage form.
- Relatively ease in manufacturing/compounding.
- Generally, they appear as clear, transparent solutions.

The disadvantages of microemulsions include the following: (*a*) thermal stress can break them, (*b*) high surfactant levels are required, (*c*) higher cost, (*d*) higher risk of adverse events such as irritation and/or poor taste, (*e*) cosolvents may be costly and have unwanted toxicities, and (*f*) they are affected by the ionic strength of the gastrointestinal (GI) tract (6). Many microemulsions have very narrow ranges of oil, surfactant, and water phase composition where they are stable. Pharmacists should therefore not add anything to or dilute a microemulsion without first verifying they are compatible.

There can basically be three types of microemulsions:

1. Oil/water microemulsions where two emulsifiers required and the primary has a higher HLB. Common droplet diameters are between 20 and 50 nm.
2. Water/oil microemulsions where two emulsifiers are required and the primary has a lower HLB. Common droplet diameters are between 20 and 50 nm.
3. Bicontinuous phase microemulsions where there is a bicontinuous system consisting of microdomains of water and oil that are interdispersed within the system. There is no clearly defined internal or external phase in a bicontinuous system.

The general method of preparation for an oil-in-water emulsion with an oil-soluble drug is to (*a*) dissolve drug in the oil phase, (*b*) add surfactant and mix well, (*c*) add the cosurfactant and mix well, and (*d*) slowly add water with continued mixing. The actual method will vary depending upon the components used. An example compounded microemulsion is as follows:

Fluconazole 20 mg/mL Topical Microemulsion

Fluconazole		2 g
Lauryl alcohol		10 g
Labrasol:alcohol (1:1)		20 g
Purified water	qs	100 mL

1. Calculate the required quantity of each ingredient for the total amount to be prepared.
2. Accurately weigh and/or measure each ingredient.
3. Prepare the mixture of Labrasol and alcohol 95% (1:10 mixture).
4. Add the lauryl alcohol to the mixture and mix well.
5. Incorporate the fluconazole slowly and mix well with each addition of the powder.
6. Incorporate sufficient purified water slowly with continuous stirring to final volume and mix well.
7. Package and label.

There are a number of commercial products using microemulsions either are on the market or are being investigated and include the following:

- Cyclosporine (Neoral) is a self-emulsifying preconcentrate of cyclosporine, which is more rapidly and consistently absorbed than the original oil-based formulation of cyclosporine (SandImmune).
- w/o microemulsions incorporating medium chain glycerides have been used to deliver calcein intraduodenally and produce significantly higher plasma levels of the drug compared to an aqueous formulation.
- Microemulsions (w/o) have been prepared for fluorouracil, apomorphine HCl, diphenhydramine HCl, tetracaine HCl, and methotrexate.
- Microemulsions (o/w) have been prepared for estradiol, finasteride, ketoprofen, meloxicam, felodipine, and triptolide.
- Ophthalmic preparations studied include chloramphenicol microemulsions (Span 20, Tween 20, Isopropyl Myristate, Purified Water).
- Nasal delivery has been studied for diazepam for emergency treatment of status epilepticus. Dosing at 2 mg/kg reached a maximum drug plasma concentration within 2 to 3 minutes.
- Periodontal delivery using a microemulsion containing a thermoreversible gel containing poloxamers was studied as a local anesthetic for pain relief in conjunction with periodontal scaling and root planning.
- Ocular delivery using microemulsions containing pilocarpine formulated with lecithin, propylene glycol, and PEG 200 as cosurfactant and IPM as the oil phase have been studied.
- A dog shampoo "Allermyl" marketed by Virbac may be the first application of microemulsions for use as a therapeutic cleansing product.
- Solvium is a topical ibuprofen gel (Akzo) 5% as a transparent gel.

Microemulsions provide an innovative approach with numerous advantages and applicable to many different drugs. More on lipid and self-emulsifying drug delivery systems is discussed in Chapter 20 Novel Dosage Forms and Drug Delivery Technologies.

Stability of Emulsions

Generally speaking, an emulsion is considered to be physically unstable if (*a*) the internal or dispersed phase upon standing tends to form aggregates of globules, (*b*) large globules or aggregates of globules rise to the top or fall to the bottom of the emulsion to form a concentrated layer of the internal phase, and (*c*) if all or part of the liquid of the internal phase separates and forms a distinct layer on the top or bottom of the emulsion as a result of the coalescing of the globules of the internal phase. In addition, an emulsion may be adversely affected by microbial contamination and growth and by other chemical and physical alterations.

Aggregation and Coalescence

Aggregates of globules of the internal phase have a greater tendency than do individual particles to rise to the top of the emulsion or fall to the bottom. Such a preparation of the globules is termed the creaming of the emulsion, and provided coalescence is absent, it is a reversible process. The term is taken from the dairy industry and is analogous to creaming or rising to the top of cream in milk that is allowed to stand. The creamed portion of an emulsion may be redistributed rather homogeneously upon shaking, but if the aggregates are difficult to disassemble or if insufficient shaking is employed before each dose, improper dosage of the internal phase substance may result. Furthermore, a creamed emulsion is not esthetically acceptable to the pharmacist or appealing to the consumer. More important, it increases the risk that the globules will coalesce.

According to the Stokes equation (Physical Pharmacy Capsule 14.1), the rate of separation of the dispersed phase of an emulsion may be related to such factors as the particle size of the dispersed phase, the difference in density between the phases, and the viscosity of the external phase. It is important to recall that the rate of separation is increased by increased particle size of the internal phase, larger density difference between the two phases, and decreased viscosity of the external phase. Therefore, to increase the stability of an emulsion, the globule or particle size should be reduced as fine as is practically possible, the density difference between the internal and external phases should be minimal, and the viscosity of the external phase should be reasonably high. Thickeners such as tragacanth and microcrystalline cellulose are frequently added to emulsions to increase the viscosity of the external phase. Upward creaming takes place in unstable emulsions of the o/w or the w/o type in which the internal phase has a lesser density than the external phase. Downward creaming takes place in unstable emulsions in which the opposite is true.

More destructive to an emulsion than creaming is coalescence of the globules of the internal phase and subsequent separation of the emulsion into two distinct layers. Separation of the internal phase from the emulsion is called breaking, and the emulsion is described as being cracked or broken. This is irreversible, because the protective sheath about the globules of the internal phase no longer exists. Attempts to reestablish the emulsion by agitation of the two separate layers are generally unsuccessful. A broken emulsion indicates that it was incorrectly prepared, stored improperly, or was mixed or diluted with an incompatible additive. Additional emulsifying agent and reprocessing through appropriate machinery are usually necessary to reproduce an emulsion.

Generally, care must be taken to protect emulsions against extremes of cold and heat. Freezing and thawing coarsen an emulsion and sometimes break it. Excessive heat has the same effect. Because emulsion products may be transported to and used in locations with climates of extremely high or low temperature, manufacturers must know their emulsions' stability before they may be shipped. For most emulsions, the industry performs tests at 5°C, 40°C, and 50°C (41°F, 104°F, and 122°F) to determine the product's stability. Stability at both 5°C and 40°C for 3 months is considered minimal. Shorter exposure periods at 50°C may be used as an alternative test.

Because other environmental conditions, such as the presence of light, air, and contaminating microorganisms, can adversely affect the stability of an emulsion, appropriate formulative and packaging steps are usually taken to minimize such hazards to stability. For light-sensitive emulsions, light-resistant containers are used. For emulsions susceptible to oxidative decomposition, antioxidants may be included in the formulation and adequate label warning provided to ensure that the container is tightly closed to air after each use. Many molds, yeasts, and bacteria can decompose the emulsifying agent, disrupting the system. Even if the emulsifier is not affected by the microbes, the product can be rendered unsightly by their presence and growth and will of course not be efficacious from a pharmaceutical or therapeutic standpoint. Because fungi (molds and yeasts) are more likely to contaminate emulsions than are bacteria, fungistatic preservatives, commonly combinations of methylparaben and propylparaben, are generally included in the aqueous phase of an o/w emulsion. Alcohol in the amount of 12% to 15% based on the external phase volume is frequently added to oral o/w emulsions for preservation.

Examples of Oral Emulsions

Mineral Oil Emulsion

Mineral oil emulsion, or liquid petrolatum emulsion, is an o/w emulsion prepared from the following formula:

Mineral oil	500 mL
Acacia (finely powdered)	125 g
Syrup	100 mL
Vanillin	40 mg
Alcohol	60 mL
Purified water, to make	1,000 mL

It is prepared by the dry gum method (4:2:1), mixing the oil with the acacia and adding 250 mL of purified water all at once to make the primary emulsion. To this is slowly added with trituration the remainder of the ingredients, with the vanillin dissolved in the alcohol. A substitute flavorant for the vanillin, a substitute preservative for the alcohol, a substitute emulsifying agent for the acacia, and an alternative method of emulsification may be used as desired.

The emulsion is employed as a lubricating cathartic with a usual dose of 30 mL. The usual dose of plain (unemulsified) mineral oil for the same purpose is 15 mL. The emulsion is much more palatable than the unemulsified oil. Both are best taken an hour before bedtime. There are a number of commercial preparations of emulsified oil, with many containing additional cathartic agents such as phenolphthalein, milk of magnesia, agar, and others.

Castor Oil Emulsion

Castor oil emulsion is used as a laxative for isolated occurrences of constipation and in preparation of the colon for radiographic and endoscopic examination. The castor oil in the emulsion works directly on the small intestine to promote bowel movement. This and other laxatives should not be used regularly or excessively, as they can lead to dependence for bowel movement. Overuse of castor oil may cause excessive loss of water and body electrolytes, which can have a debilitating effect. Laxatives should not be used when nausea, vomiting, or abdominal pain is present, because these symptoms may indicate appendicitis, and use of a laxative in this instance could promote rupturing of the appendix.

The amount of castor oil in commercial emulsions varies from about 35% to 67%. The amount of oil influences the dose required. Generally, for an emulsion containing about two-thirds oil, the adult dose is 45 mL, about three tablespoonsful. For children 2 to 6 years of age, 15 mL is usually sufficient, and for children less than 2 years of age, 5 mL may be given. Castor oil is best taken on an empty stomach, followed with one full glass of water.

Simethicone Emulsion

Simethicone emulsion is a water-dispersible form of simethicone used as a defoaming agent for the relief of painful symptoms of excessive gas in the gastrointestinal tract. Simethicone emulsion works in the stomach and intestines by changing the surface tension of gas bubbles, enabling them to coalesce, freeing the gas for easier elimination. The emulsion in drop form is useful for relief of gas in infants due to colic, air swallowing, or lactose intolerance. The commercial product (Mylicon Drops, AstraZeneca) contains 40 mg of simethicone per 0.6 mL. Simethicone is also present in a number of antacid formulations (e.g., Mylanta, Johnson & Johnson Merck) as a therapeutic adjunct to relieve the discomfort of gas.

Examples of Topical Emulsions

Many of the hand and body lotions used to treat dry skin are o/w emulsions. A lotion is an emulsion liquid dosage form applied to the outer surface of the body. Historically, this term has also been applied to suspensions and solutions. A number of topical emulsions, or lotions, are used therapeutically to deliver a drug systemically. An example is Estrasorb (estradiol, Graceway), which contains estradiol for use in the treatment of hot flashes and night sweats accompanying menopause. It works by replacing the hormones lost during menopause. Corticosteroid-containing emulsions include Lotrimin AF (clotrimazole, Schering-Plough) and Diprolene (augmented betamethasone dipropionate, Schering-Plough).

A shampoo is a solution, emulsion, or suspension dosage form used to clean the hair and scalp. It may contain an API intended for topical application to the scalp.

GELS AND MAGMAS

Gels are defined as semisolid systems consisting of dispersions made up of either small inorganic particles or large organic molecules enclosing and interpenetrated by a liquid.

Gels are also defined as semirigid systems in which the movement of the dispersing medium is restricted by an interlacing three-dimensional network of particles or solvated macromolecules of the dispersed phase. A high degree of physical or chemical cross-linking may be involved. The increased viscosity caused by the interlacing and consequential internal friction is responsible for the semisolid state. A gel may consist of twisted matted strands often wound together by stronger types of van der Waals forces to form crystalline and amorphous regions throughout the system, such as tragacanth and CMC.

Some gel systems are as clear as water, and others are turbid because the ingredients may not be completely molecularly dispersed (soluble or insoluble), or they may form aggregates, which disperse light. The concentration of the gelling agents is mostly less than 10%, usually in 0.5% to 2.0% range, with some exceptions.

Gels in which the macromolecules are distributed so that no apparent boundaries exist between them and the liquids are called *single-phase gels*. When the gel mass consists of floccules of small, distinct particles, the gel is classified as a two-phase system and frequently called a *magma* or a *milk*. Gels and magmas are considered colloidal dispersions because they contain particles of colloidal dimension.

Colloidal Dispersions

Many of the various types of colloidal dispersions have been given appropriate names. For instance, *sol* is a general term to designate a dispersion of a solid substance in a liquid, solid, or gaseous medium. However, more often than not, it is used to describe the solid–liquid dispersion system. To be more descriptive, a prefix such as *hydro-* for water (*hydrosol*) or *alco-* for alcohol (*alcosol*) may be employed to indicate the dispersion medium. The term *aerosol* has similarly been developed to indicate a dispersion of a solid or a liquid in a gaseous phase.

Although there is no precise point at which the size of a particle in a dispersion can be considered to be colloidal, there is a generally accepted size range. A substance is said to be colloidal when its particles fall between 1 nm and 0.5 μm. Colloidal particles are usually larger than atoms, ions, or molecules and, generally, consist of aggregates of many molecules, although in certain proteins and organic polymers, single large molecules may be of colloidal dimension and form colloidal dispersions. One difference between colloidal dispersions and true solutions is the larger particle size of the disperse phase of the colloidal dispersion. Another difference is the optical properties of the two systems. True solutions do not scatter light and, therefore, appear clear, but colloidal dispersions contain opaque particles that do scatter light and thus appear turbid. This turbidity is easily seen, even with dilute preparations, when the dispersion is observed at right angles to a beam of light passed through the dispersion (Tyndall effect). Although reference is made here to dilute colloidal dispersions, most pharmaceutical preparations contain high concentrations of colloidal particles, and in these instances, there is no difficulty in observing turbidity. In fact, certain preparations are opaque, depending on the concentration of the disperse phase. Also, the particle size of the dispersed phase in some pharmaceutical preparations is not uniform, and a preparation may contain particles within and outside of the colloidal range, giving the preparation more of an opaque appearance than if all particles were uniformly colloidal.

Particle size is not the only important criterion for establishing the colloidal state. The nature of the dispersing phase with respect to the disperse phase is also of great importance. The attraction or lack of attraction between the disperse phase and the dispersion medium affects both ease of preparation and the character of the dispersion. Terminology has been developed to characterize the various degrees of attraction between the phases of a colloidal dispersion. If the disperse phase interacts appreciably with the dispersion medium, it is said to be *lyophilic*, meaning solvent loving. If the degree of attraction is small, the colloid is termed *lyophobic*, or solvent hating. These terms are more suitably used when reference is made to the specific dispersion medium, for a single substance may be lyophobic with respect to one dispersion medium and lyophilic with respect to another. For instance, starch is lyophilic in water but lyophobic in alcohol. Terms such as *hydrophilic* and *hydrophobic*, which are more descriptive of the nature of the colloidal property, have therefore been developed to refer to the attraction or lack of attraction of the substance specifically to water. Generally speaking, because of the attraction to the solvent of lyophilic substances, lyophilic colloidal systems are easier to prepare and have greater stability. Lyophobic colloids, on the other hand, are harder to prepare due to the lack of attraction between the phases. A third type of colloidal sol, termed an *association* or *amphiphilic colloid*, is formed by grouping or association of molecules that exhibit both lyophilic and lyophobic properties.

Lyophilic colloids are large organic molecules capable of being solvated or associated with the molecules of the dispersing phase. These substances disperse readily upon addition to the dispersion medium to form colloidal dispersions. As more molecules of the substance are added to the sol, the viscosity characteristically increases, and when the concentration of molecules is sufficiently high, the liquid sol may become a semisolid or solid dispersion, termed a *gel*. Gels owe their rigidity to an intertwining network of the disperse phase that entraps and holds the dispersion medium. A change in temperature can cause certain gels to resume the sol or liquid state. Also, some gels become fluid on agitation, only to resume their solid or semisolid state after remaining undisturbed for a period of time, a phenomenon known as *thixotropy*.

Lyophobic colloids are generally composed of inorganic particles. When these are added to the dispersing phase, there is little if any interaction between the two phases. Unlike lyophilic colloids, lyophobic materials do not spontaneously disperse but must be encouraged to do so by special individualized procedures. Their addition to the dispersion medium does not greatly affect the viscosity of the vehicle. Amphiphilic colloids form dispersions in both aqueous and nonaqueous media. Depending on their individual character and the nature of the dispersion medium, they may or may not become greatly solvated. However, they generally increase the viscosity of the dispersion medium with an increase in concentration.

For the most part, the colloidal sols and gels used in pharmacy are aqueous preparations. The various preparations composed of colloidal dispersions are prepared not according to any general method but according to the means best suited to the individual preparation. Some substances, such as acacia, are termed *natural colloids* because they are self-dispersing upon addition to the dispersing medium. Other materials that require special means for prompt dispersion are termed *artificial colloids*. They may require fine pulverization of coarse particles to colloidal size by a colloid mill or a micropulverizer, or colloidal size particles may be formed by chemical reaction under highly controlled conditions.

Terminology Related to Gels

A number of terms are commonly used in discussing some of the characteristics of gels, including imbibition, swelling, syneresis, thixotropy, and xerogel. *Imbibition* is the taking up of a certain amount of liquid without a measurable increase in volume. *Swelling* is the taking up of a liquid by a gel with an increase in volume. Only liquids that solvate a gel can cause swelling. The swelling of protein gels is influenced by pH and the presence of electrolytes. *Syneresis* occurs when the interaction between particles of the dispersed phase becomes so great that on standing, the dispersing medium is squeezed out in droplets and the gel shrinks. Syneresis is a form of instability in aqueous and nonaqueous gels. Separation of a solvent phase is thought to occur because of the elastic contraction of the polymeric molecules; in the swelling process during gel formation, the macromolecules become stretched, and the elastic forces increase as swelling proceeds. At equilibrium, the restoring force of the macromolecules is balanced by the swelling forces, determined by the osmotic pressure. If the osmotic pressure decreases, as on cooling, water may be squeezed out of the gel. The syneresis of an acidic gel from *Plantago albicans* seed gum may be decreased by the addition of electrolyte, glucose, and sucrose and by increasing the gum concentration. pH has a marked effect on the separation of water. At low pH, marked syneresis occurs, possibly as a result of suppression of ionization of the carboxylic acid groups, loss of hydrating water, and the formation of intramolecular hydrogen bonds. This would reduce the attraction of the solvent for the macromolecule. *Thixotropy* is a reversible gel–sol formation with no change in volume or temperature, a type of nonnewtonian flow. A *xerogel* is formed when the liquid is removed from a gel and only the framework remains. Examples include gelatin sheets, tragacanth ribbons, and acacia tears.

Classification and Types of Gels

Table 14.4 is a general classification of gels listing two classification schemes. The first scheme divides gels into inorganic and organic. Most *inorganic hydrogels* are two-phase systems, such as aluminum hydroxide gel and bentonite magma. Bentonite has also been used as an ointment base in about 10% to 25% concentrations. Most *organic gels* are single-phase systems and may include such gelling agents as carbomer and tragacanth and those that contain an organic liquid, such as *Plastibase*.

TABLE **14.4.** General Classification and Description of Gels		
Class	**Description**	**Examples**
Inorganic	Usually two-phase systems	Aluminum hydroxide gel
		Bentonite magma
Organic	Usually single-phase systems	Carbopol
		Tragacanth
Hydrogels	Organic hydrogels	Pectin paste, tragacanth jelly
	Natural and synthetic gums	Methylcellulose, sodium CMC, Pluronic
	Inorganic hydrogels	Bentonite gel (10%–25%), Veegum, silica
Organogels	Hydrocarbon type	Petrolatum, mineral oil/polyethylene gel (Plastibase)
	Animal, vegetable fats	Lard, cocoa butter
	Soap base greases	Aluminum stearate with heavy mineral oil gel
	Hydrophilic organogels	Carbowax bases (PEG ointment)
	Polar	
	Nonionic	

The second classification scheme divides gels into hydrogels and organogels with some additional subcategories. *Hydrogels* include ingredients that are dispersible as colloidals or soluble in water; they include organic hydrogels, natural and synthetic gums, and inorganic hydrogels. Examples include hydrophilic colloids such as silica, bentonite, tragacanth, pectin, sodium alginate, methylcellulose, sodium CMC, and alumina, which, in high concentration, form semisolid gels. Sodium alginate has been used to produce gels that can be employed as ointment bases. In concentrations greater than 2.5% and in the presence of soluble calcium salts, a firm gel, stable between pH 5 and 10, is formed. Methylcellulose, hydroxy ethylcellulose, and sodium CMC are among the commercial cellulose products used in ointments. They are available in various viscosity types, usually high, medium, and low. *Organogels* include the hydrocarbons, animal and vegetable fats, soap base greases, and the hydrophilic organogels. Included in the hydrocarbon type is *Jelene*, or *Plastibase*, a combination of mineral oils and heavy hydrocarbon waxes with a molecular weight of about 1,300. Petrolatum is a semisolid gel consisting of a liquid component together with a protosubstance and a crystalline waxy fraction. The crystalline fraction provides rigidity to the structure, while the protosubstance, or gel former, stabilizes the system and thickens the gel. The hydrophilic organogels, or polar organogels, include the polyethylene glycols of high molecular weight, the *Carbowax*. They are soluble to about 75% in water and are completely washable. The gels look and feel like petrolatum. They are nonionic and stable. *Jellies* are a class of gels in which the structural coherent matrix contains a high proportion of liquid, usually water. They usually are formed by adding a thickening agent such as tragacanth or carboxymethyl cellulose to an aqueous solution of a drug substance. The resultant product is usually clear and uniformly semisolid. Jellies are subject to bacterial contamination and growth, so most are preserved with antimicrobials. Jellies should be stored with tight closure because water may evaporate, drying out the product.

Some substances, such as acacia, are termed natural colloids because they are self-dispersing in a dispersing medium. Other materials that require special treatment for prompt dispersion are called artificial colloids. The special treatment may involve fine pulverization to colloidal size with a colloid mill or a micropulverizer.

Preparation of Magmas and Gels

Some magmas and gels (inorganic) are prepared by freshly precipitating the disperse phase to achieve a fine degree of subdivision of the particles and a gelatinous character to those particles. The desired gelatinous precipitate results when solutions of inorganic agents react to form an insoluble chemical having a high attraction for water. As the microcrystalline particles of the precipitate develop, they strongly attract water to yield gelatinous particles, which combine to form the desired gelatinous precipitate.

Other magmas and gels may be prepared by directly hydrating the inorganic chemical, which produces the disperse phase of the dispersion. In addition to the water vehicle, other agents such as propylene glycol, propyl gallate, and hydroxypropyl cellulose may be used to enhance gel formation.

Because of the high degree of attraction between the disperse phase and the aqueous medium in both magmas and gels, these preparations remain fairly uniform on standing, with little settling of the disperse phase. However, on long standing, a supernatant layer of the dispersion medium develops, but the uniformity of the preparation is easily reestablished by moderate shaking. To ensure uniform dosage, magmas and gels should be shaken before use, and a statement to that effect must be included on the label of such preparations. The medicinal magmas and gels are used orally for the value of the disperse phase.

Examples of Gelling Agents

Gelling agents include acacia, alginic acid, bentonite, carbomer, CMC sodium, cetostearyl alcohol, colloidal silicon dioxide, ethylcellulose, gelatin, guar gum, hydroxy ethylcellulose, hydroxypropyl cellulose, hydroxypropyl methylcellulose, magnesium aluminum silicate, maltodextrin, methylcellulose, polyvinyl alcohol (PVA), povidone, propylene carbonate, propylene glycol alginate, sodium alginate, sodium starch glycolate, starch, tragacanth, and xanthan gum. A few of the more common ones are discussed here.

Alginic acid is obtained from seaweed throughout the world, and the prepared product is a tasteless, practically odorless white to yellowish-white–colored fibrous powder. It is used in concentrations of 1% to 5% as a thickening agent in gels. It swells in water to about 200 to 300 times its own weight without dissolving. Cross-linking with increased viscosity occurs upon the addition of a calcium salt, such as calcium citrate. Alginic acid can be dispersed in water vigorously stirred for approximately 30 minutes. Premixing with another powder or with a water-miscible liquid aids dispersion.

Bentonite is discussed later, in the section on preparation of bentonite magma.

Carbomer (Carbopol) resins, first described in the literature in 1955, are ingredients in a variety of dosage systems, including controlled-release tablets, oral suspensions, and topical gels. Carbomer resins are high molecular weight allyl pentaerythritol–cross-linked acrylic acid–based polymers modified with C_{10} to C_{30} alkyl acrylates. They are fluffy white dry powders with large bulk density. The 0.5% and 1.0% aqueous dispersions are pH 2.7 to 3.5 and 2.5 to 3.0, respectively. There are many carbomer resins, with viscosity ranges from 0 to 80,000 cP.

Carbomer 934 is highly effective in thick formulations such as viscous gels. Carbomer 934P is similar to 934 but is intended for oral and mucosal contact applications and is the most widely used in the pharmaceutical industry.

In addition to thickening, suspending, and emulsifying in both oral and topical formulations, the 934 polymer is used in commercial products to provide sustained-release properties in the stomach and intestinal tract. Carbomer 940 forms sparkling clear water or hydroalcoholic gels. It is the most efficient of all the Carbopol resins and has very good nondrip properties.

The addition of alcohol to prepared carbomer gels may decrease their viscosity and clarity. An increase in the concentration of carbomer may be required to overcome the loss of viscosity. Also, gel viscosity depends on the presence of electrolytes and on the pH. Generally, a maximum of 3% electrolytes can be added before a rubbery mass forms. Too much neutralization also will result in decreased viscosity that cannot be reversed by the addition of acid. Maximum viscosity and clarity occur at pH 7, but acceptable viscosity and clarity begin at pH 4.5 to 5.0 and extend to a pH of 11.

Carbomer preparations are primarily used in aqueous systems, although other liquids can be used. In water, a single particle of carbomer will wet very rapidly, but like many other powders, carbomer polymers tend to form clumps of particles when haphazardly dispersed in polar solvents. As the surfaces of these clumps solvate, a layer forms and prevents rapid wetting of the interior of the clumps. When this occurs, the slow diffusion of solvent through this solvated layer determines the mixing or hydration time. To achieve fastest dispersion of the carbomer, it is wise to take advantage of the very small particle size of the carbomer powder by adding it very slowly into the vortex of the liquid while very rapidly stirring it. Almost any device, like a simple sieve, that can sprinkle the powder on the rapidly stirred liquid is useful. The goal is to prevent clumping by slowly sprinkling the very fine powder over the rapidly agitated water.

A neutralizer is added to thicken the gel after the carbomer is dispersed. Sodium hydroxide or potassium hydroxide can be used in carbomer dispersions containing less than 20% alcohol. Triethanolamine will neutralize carbomer resins containing up to 50% ethanol. Other neutralizer agents include sodium carbonate, ammonia, and borax.

Carboxymethylcellulose (CMC) in concentrations of 4% to 6% of medium viscosity can be used to produce gels; glycerin may be added to prevent drying. Precipitation can occur below pH 2; it is most stable at pH 2 to 10, and maximum stability is at pH 7 to 9. It is incompatible with ethanol.

CMC sodium is soluble in water at all temperatures. The sodium salt of CMC can be dispersed with high shear in cold water before the particles can hydrate and swell to sticky gel grains agglomerating into lumps. Once the powder is well dispersed, the solution is heated with moderate shear to about 60°C (140°F) for fastest dissolution. These dispersions are sensitive to pH changes because of the carboxylate group. The viscosity of the product falls markedly below pH 5 or above pH 10.

Colloidal silicon dioxide can be used with other ingredients of similar refractive index to prepare transparent gels. Colloidal silicon dioxide adsorbs large quantities of water without liquefying. The viscosity is largely independent of temperature. Changes in pH may affect the viscosity: It is most effective at pH values up to about 7.5. Colloidal silicon dioxide (fumed silica) will form a gel when combined with 1-dodecanol and *n*-dodecane. These are prepared by adding the silica to the vehicle and sonicating for about 1 minute to obtain a uniform dispersion and sealing and storing at about 40°C (140°F) overnight to complete gelation. This gel is more hydrophobic than the others.

Gelatin is dispersed in hot water and cooled to form gels. As an alternative, moisten the gelatin with about three to five parts of an organic liquid that will not swell the polymer, such as ethyl alcohol or propylene glycol, followed by the addition of the hot water and cooling.

Magnesium aluminum silicate, or *Veegum*, in concentrations of about 10% forms a firm thixotropic gel. The material is inert and has few incompatibilities but is best used above pH 3.5. It may bind to some drugs and limit their bioavailability.

Methylcellulose is a long-chain substituted cellulose that can be used to form gels in concentrations up to about 5%. Because methylcellulose hydrates slowly in hot water, the powder is dispersed with high shear in about one-third of the required amount of water at 80°C to 90°C (176°F to 194°F). Once the powder is finely dispersed, the rest of the water is added cold or as ice with moderate stirring to cause prompt dissolution. Anhydrous alcohol or propylene glycol may be used to prewet the powders. Maximum clarity, fullest hydration, and highest viscosity will be obtained if the gel is cooled to 0°C to 10°C (32°F to 50°F) for about an hour. A preservative should be added. A 2% solution of methylcellulose 4,000 has a gel point about 50°C (122°F). High concentrations of electrolytes will salt out the macromolecules and increase their viscosity, ultimately precipitating the polymer.

Plastibase, or *Jelene*, is a mixture of 5% low molecular weight polyethylene and 95% mineral oil. As a polymer, it is soluble in mineral oil above 90°C, close to its melting point. When cooled below 90°C, the polymer precipitates and causes gelation. The mineral oil is immobilized in the network of entangled and adhering insoluble polyethylene chains, which probably even associate into small crystalline regions. This gel can be heated to about 60°C (140°F) without substantial loss of consistency.

Poloxamer, or *Pluronic*, gels are made from selected forms of polyoxyethylene–polyoxypropylene copolymers in concentrations ranging from 15% to 50%. Poloxamers generally are waxy white free-flowing granules that are practically odorless and tasteless. Aqueous solutions of poloxamers are stable in the presence of acids, alkalis, and metal ions. Commonly used poloxamers include the 124 (L-44 grade), 188 (F-68 grade), 237 (F-87 grade), 338 (F-108 grade), and 407 (F-127 grade) types, which are freely soluble in water. The "F" designation refers to the flake form. The "L" designation refers to the liquid form. The trade name Pluronic is used in the United States by BASF for pharmaceutical and industrial-grade poloxamers. Pluronic F-127 has low toxicity and good solubilizing capacity and optical properties, and it is a good medium for topical drug delivery systems.

PVA is used at concentrations of about 2.5% in the preparation of various jellies that dry rapidly when applied to the skin. Borax is a good agent that will gel PVA solutions. For best results, disperse PVA in cold water, followed by hot water. It is less soluble in the cold water.

Povidone at the higher molecular weights can be used to prepare gels in concentrations up to about 10%. It has the advantage of being compatible in solution with a wide range of inorganic salts, natural and synthetic resins, and other chemicals. It has also been used to increase the solubility of a number of poorly soluble drugs.

Sodium alginate can be used to produce gels in concentrations up to 10%. Aqueous preparations are most stable at pH 4 to 10; below pH 3, alginic acid is precipitated. Sodium alginate gels for external use should be preserved, for example, with 0.1% chloroxylenol or the parabens. If the preparation is acidic, benzoic acid may be used. High concentrations will raise viscosity to the point of salting out the sodium alginate; this occurs at about 4% with sodium chloride.

Tragacanth gum has been used to prepare gels that are most stable at pH 4 to 8. These gels must be preserved with either 0.1% benzoic acid or sodium benzoate or a combination of 0.17% methylparaben and 0.03% propylparaben. These gels may be sterilized by autoclaving. Powdered tragacanth gum tends to form lumps when added to water. Thus, aqueous dispersions are prepared by adding the powder to vigorously stirred water. Also, the use of ethanol, glycerin, or propylene glycol to wet the tragacanth before mixing with water is very effective. If other powders are to be incorporated into the gel, they can be premixed with the tragacanth in the dry state.

Gel Formulation Considerations

In a gel preparation, the powdered polymers, when added to water, may form temporary gels that slow dissolution. As water diffuses into these loose clumps of powder, their exterior frequently turns into clumps of solvated particles encasing dry powder. The globs or clumps of gel dissolve very slowly because of their high viscosity and the low diffusion coefficient of the macromolecules.

As a hot colloidal dispersion of gelatin cools, the gelatin macromolecules lose kinetic energy. With reduced kinetic energy, or thermal agitation, the gelatin macromolecules are associated through dipole–dipole interaction into elongated or threadlike aggregates. The size of these association chains increases to the extent that the dispersing medium is held in the interstices among the interlacing network of gelatin macromolecules, and the viscosity increases to that of a semisolid. Gums, such as agar, Irish moss, algin, pectin, and tragacanth, form gels by the same mechanism as gelatin.

Polymer solutions tend to be cast as gels because the solute consists of long, flexible chains of molecules of such thickness that they tend to become entangled, attract each other by secondary valency forces, and even crystallize. Cross-linking of dissolved polymer molecules also causes these solutions to gel. The reactions produce permanent gels, held together by primary valence forces. Secondary valence forces are responsible for reversible gel formation. For example, gelatin will form a gel when lowered to about 30°C, the gel melting point, but aqueous methylcellulose solutions will gel when heated above about 50°C because the polymer, being less soluble in hot water, precipitates. Lower temperatures, higher concentrations, and higher molecular weights promote gelation and produce stronger gels. The reversible gelation of gelatin will occur at about 25°C for 10% solutions, 30°C for 20% solutions, and about 32°C for 30% solutions (77°F, 86°F, and 90°F, respectively). Gelation is rarely observed for gelatin above 34°C (93°F), and regardless of concentration, gelatin solutions do not gel at 37°C (98.6°F). The gelation temperature or gel point of gelatin is highest at the isoelectric point. Water-soluble polymers have the property of thermal gelation, that is, they gel on heating, whereas natural gums gel on cooling. The thermal gelation is reversed on cooling.

Inorganic salts will compete with the water in a gel and cause gelation at lower concentrations. This is usually reversible; upon addition of water, the gels will reform. Because alcohol is not a solvent or precipitant, it may cause precipitation or gelation, lowering the dielectric constant of the medium and tending to dehydrate the hydrophilic solute. Alcohol lowers the concentrations at which electrolytes salt out hydrophilic colloids. Phase separation by adding alcohol may cause coacervation.

Aqueous polymer solutions, especially of cellulose derivatives, are stored for approximately 48 hours after dissolution to promote full hydration and maximum viscosity and clarity. Any salts are added at this point rather than dissolving in water prior to adding polymer; otherwise, the solutions may not reach their full viscosity and clarity.

Examples of Magmas and Gels

One official magma, Bentonite Magma, NF, used as a suspending agent, finds application in the extemporaneous compounding of prescriptions. Sodium Fluoride and Phosphoric Acid Gel, USP, is applied topically to the teeth as a dental care prophylactic. Other official gels applied topically include Fluocinonide Gel, USP, an anti-inflammatory corticosteroid, and Tretinoin Gel, USP, an irritant that stimulates epidermal cell turnover, causes peeling, and is effective in the treatment of acne. Examples of such drugs and drug products are erythromycin and benzoyl peroxide topical gel (Benzamycin Topical Gel, Dermik Laboratories), clindamycin topical gel (Cleocin T Topical Gel, Pfizer), clindamycin and benzoyl peroxide topical gel (BenzaClin, Dermik), and benzoyl peroxide gel (Desquam-X 10 Gel, Westwood-Squibb) used in the control and treatment of acne vulgaris; hydroquinone gel

(Solaquin Forte Gel, ICN), a bleach for hyperpigmented skin; salicylic acid gel (Compound W Gel, Medtech), a keratolytic; and desoximetasone gel (Topicort Gel, Taro) and augmented betamethasone dipropionate topical gel (Diprolene, Schering-Plough), anti-inflammatory and antipruritic agents.

Other official magmas and gels are employed as antacids: Aluminum Phosphate Gel, USP; Aluminum Hydroxide Gel, USP; and Dihydroxyaluminum Aminoacetate Magma, USP. Some of these preparations are discussed briefly next.

Bentonite Magma, NF

Bentonite magma is a preparation of 5% bentonite, a native colloidal hydrated aluminum silicate, in purified water. It may be prepared mechanically in a blender with the bentonite added directly to the purified water while the machine is running, or it may be prepared by sprinkling the bentonite, in portions, upon hot purified water, allowing each portion to become thoroughly wetted without stirring before another portion is added. By the latter method, the mixture must be allowed to stand for 24 hours before it may be stirred. The standing period ensures complete hydration and swelling of the bentonite. Bentonite, which is insoluble in water, swells to approximately 12 times its volume upon addition to water. The NF monograph for bentonite contains a test for swelling power in which 2 g of a bentonite sample is added in portions to 100 mL water in a 100-mL glass-stoppered cylinder. At the end of a 2-hour period, the mass at the bottom of the cylinder is required to occupy an apparent volume of not less than 24 mL. Other required tests are for gel formation, fineness of powder, and pH, the latter being between 9.5 and 10.5. After bentonite magma has been allowed to stand undisturbed for some time, it sets to a gel. Upon agitation, the sol form returns. The process may be repeated indefinitely. As mentioned earlier, this phenomenon is termed *thixotropy*, and bentonite magma is a *thixotropic gel*. The thixotropy occurs only when the bentonite concentration is somewhat above 4%.

Bentonite magma is employed as a suspending agent. Its alkaline pH must be considered because it is undesirable for certain drugs. Furthermore, because the suspending capacity of the magma is drastically reduced if the pH is lowered to about pH 7, another suspending agent should be selected for drugs requiring a less alkaline medium rather than making bentonite magma more acidic.

Aluminum Hydroxide Gel, USP

Aluminum Hydroxide Gel, USP, is an aqueous suspension of a gelatinous precipitate composed of insoluble aluminum hydroxide and the hydrated aluminum oxide, equivalent to about 4% aluminum oxide. The disperse phase of the gel is generally prepared by a chemical reaction, using various reactants. Usually, the aluminum source of the reaction is aluminum chloride or aluminum alum, which yields the insoluble aluminum oxide and aluminum hydroxide precipitate. To the gel, the USP permits the addition of peppermint oil, glycerin, sorbitol, sucrose, saccharin, or other flavorants and sweeteners as well as suitable antimicrobial agents.

This antacid preparation is a white, viscous suspension. It is effective in neutralizing a portion of the gastric hydrochloric acid; coats the inflamed and perhaps ulcerated gastric surface by virtue of its gelatinous, viscous, and insoluble character; and is useful in the treatment of hyperacidity and peptic ulcers. The main disadvantage to its use is its constipating effects. The usual dose is 10 mL four or more times a day, that is, after meals and at bedtime. The analogous commercial product (Amphojel, Wyeth-Ayerst) at 10 mL has the capacity to neutralize about 13 mEq of acid. The preparation should be stored in a tight container, and freezing should be avoided.

Because it possesses a trivalent cation, aluminum hydroxide interferes with the bioavailability of tetracycline by chelating with the antibiotic in the gastrointestinal tract. Thus, when these two medicines are indicated for patient use, the doses should be staggered to ensure that the patient receives the benefit of both drugs. Aluminum hydroxide gel has also been implicated in decreasing the bioavailability of other drugs by adsorption onto the gel. This is usually illustrated by a decrease in the area under the concentration time curve (AUC) for the concomitantly administered drug. Suffice it to say that the clinical significance of the interaction may not be that great, but observation of the patient to ensure the proper therapeutic outcome is important. Thus, for example, if aluminum hydroxide gel is suspected of causing incomplete absorption of the second drug, an upward alteration in the dose of the second drug may be necessary provided the aluminum hydroxide gel administration remains the same.

Milk of Magnesia

Milk of magnesia is a preparation containing 7% to 8.5% magnesium hydroxide. It may be prepared by a reaction between sodium hydroxide and magnesium sulfate (1), diluted solutions being used to ensure a fine, flocculent, gelatinous precipitate of magnesium hydroxide. The precipitate so produced is washed with purified water to remove the sodium sulfate prior to its incorporation with additional purified water to prepare the required volume of product. Commercially, the product is more economically produced by the direct hydration of magnesium oxide:

$$2\,NaOH + MgSO_4 \rightarrow Mg(OH)_2 + Na_2SO_4$$
$$MgO + H_2O \rightarrow Mg(OH)_2$$

Irrespective of its method of preparation, milk of magnesia is an opaque white viscous preparation from which varying proportions of water separate on standing. For this reason, it should be shaken before use. The preparation has a pH of about 10, which may bring about a reaction between the magma and the glass container, imparting a bitter taste to the preparation. To minimize such an occurrence, 0.1% citric acid may be added. Also, flavoring oils at a concentration not exceeding 0.05% may be added to enhance the palatability of the preparation.

Milk of magnesia possesses reasonable acid-neutralizing ability, and a dose of 5 mL will neutralize about 10 mEq of stomach acid. However, to neutralize more acid, a higher dose, such as 15 mL, is usually necessary, and this may predispose the patient to the development of diarrhea, a common side effect of this drug. Thus, to circumvent the problem of diarrhea from magnesium hydroxide and the constipating effects of aluminum hydroxide, frequently these two drugs are combined in an antacid preparation. The combination results in a more palatable product with optimum buffering of stomach contents at a pH of 4 to 5 and less of a chance for either diarrhea or constipation to occur. When a laxative effect is desired, a bedtime dose of 30 to 60 mL of milk of magnesia will suffice very nicely by the next morning.

Milk of magnesia is best stored in a tight container, preferably at 0°C to 35°C. Freezing results in a coarsening of the disperse phase, and temperatures above 35°C decrease the gel structure.

Starch Glycerite

Starch	100 g
Benzoic acid	2 g
Purified water	200 g
Glycerin	700 g

The starch and benzoic acid are rubbed in the water to a smooth mixture. The glycerin is added and mixed. The mixture is heated to 140°C with constant gentle agitation until a translucent mass forms. The heat ruptures the starch grains and permits the water to reach and hydrate the linear and branched starch molecules, which trap the dispersion medium in the interstices to form a gel. Starch glycerite has been used as a topical vehicle and protectant.

Lubricating Jelly Formula

Methylcellulose, 4,000 cP	0.8%
Carbopol 934	0.24%
Propylene glycol	16.7%
Methylparaben	0.015%
Sodium hydroxide, qs ad	pH 7
Purified water, qs ad	100%

Disperse the methylcellulose in 40 mL of hot (80°C to 90°C) water. Chill overnight in a refrigerator to dissolve. Disperse the Carbopol 934 in 20 mL water. Adjust the pH of the dispersion to 7.0 by adding sufficient 1% sodium hydroxide solution (about 12 mL is required), and bring the volume to 40 mL with purified water. Dissolve the methylparaben in the propylene glycol. Mix the methylcellulose, Carbopol 934, and propylene glycol fractions, using caution to avoid incorporating air. Lubricating jellies are used to assist in medical procedures; to aid in insertion of various devices and drugs, including catheters and suppositories; and as vehicles for some drug products, especially in extemporaneous compounding.

Clear Aqueous Gel with Dimethicone

Water	59.8%
Carbomer 934	0.5%
Triethanolamine	1.2%
Glycerin	34.2%
Propylene glycol	2.0%
Dimethicone copolyol	2.3%

Prepare the carbomer gel, add the other ingredients, and mix well. Dimethicone copolyol is included to reduce the sticky feel associated with glycerin. These gels are commonly used as vehicles for drug products, especially for those that are extemporaneously compounded.

Poloxamer Gel Base

Pluronic F-127, NF	20–50 g
Purified water/buffer qs ad	100 mL

Poloxamer gel base is widely used as a vehicle for extemporaneous products. In a combination with isopropyl palmitate and lecithin, it is an absorption-enhancing topical vehicle.

▌ PROPER ADMINISTRATION AND USE OF DISPERSE SYSTEMS

Many dosage forms discussed thus far in this chapter are for oral use. As with the oral solutions discussed in the previous chapter, they can be measured by spoonful or administered dropwise, depending on the appropriate dosage. It is very important that the patient understands the proper quantity of product to use. For example, differences in dosage can occur between product categories, such as OTC antidiarrheal suspensions (tablespoonfuls) versus OTC antacid suspensions (teaspoonfuls). Differences in dosage can also occur within a category, most notably in antacid suspensions. Some are recommended in teaspoon doses because of higher concentration, whereas others are suggested in tablespoon quantities. It is important, therefore, that the pharmacist ensures that the patient knows how much to use and then use a calibrated device to make sure the right amount is taken. The dosing units in the instructions on the prescription label should match the units listed on the measuring device. If the graduated lines on a dropper have "mL" as the unit, then instructions on the label should state the dose in "mL," for example "give 0.5 mL by mouth every 12 hours." Patients or their caregivers are more likely to give an incorrect dose when the units on the label and on the device do not match.

Many reconstituted products, as mentioned earlier in the chapter, are suspensions. Several problems can emerge if the pharmacist is not careful to counsel the patient about them. Usually, the patient or guardian of the patient receives the product in an oversized bottle that allows for the proper shaking of the product prior to its use. To allay fears that the medicine may not all be in the bottle, the pharmacist must make the patient or the guardian aware of this and indicate that this feature enhances the ability to shake it up before administration. Furthermore, some patients do not make the connection that the medicine should be administered by mouth. Oral antibiotic suspensions intended to treat a middle ear infection have been mistakenly administered directly into the ear by some patients or guardians. Thus, the pharmacist should review with the patient the proper route of administration. Lastly, because these are reconstituted with purified water, stability problems with the drug usually dictate that it be stored in the refrigerator until it is consumed. The patient has to be informed of this. The consumer may overlook a tiny label directing refrigerator storage. Alternatively, not all suspensions need to be stored in the refrigerator, but because of prior experience with other liquid suspensions that necessitated refrigeration, a patient or guardian may assume that this is necessary.

Certain suspensions, such as aluminum hydroxide gel, cholestyramine, and kaolin, by virtue of their active ingredients interfere with absorption of other drugs. For example, cholestyramine has been shown to interfere with and decrease the bioavailability of warfarin, digoxin, and thyroid hormones. The pharmacist should be aware of this and make recommendations to help avoid this drug interaction whenever possible. The typical suggestion is to stagger the administration of the liquid cholestyramine away from other drug administration by several hours, and giving warfarin at least 6 hours after the cholestyramine reportedly avoids the impaired warfarin bioavailability (9). However, warfarin undergoes enterohepatic recycling in the body, and if cholestyramine is present in the intestine because of earlier administration, it can bind it and decrease warfarin's reabsorption. In this instance, use of one of the two drugs should be discontinued by the physician. However, if concurrent use is necessary, the pharmacist should monitor the patient more frequently for the possibility of an altered anticoagulant response. This is important because if adjustments in warfarin dosage are made on the basis of cholestyramine interference and then the cholestyramine is discontinued, the warfarin dosage also must be decreased according to the patient's prothrombin time.

AEROSOLS

Pharmaceutical aerosols are pressurized dosage forms that, upon actuation, emit a fine dispersion of liquid and/or solid materials containing one or more active ingredients in a gaseous medium (Physical Pharmacy Capsule 14.7).

PHYSICAL PHARMACY CAPSULE 14.7 Partial Pressure and Aerosol Formulation

Aerosols generally contain an active drug in a liquid gas propellant, in a mixture of solvents with a propellant, or in a mixture with other additives and a propellant. The gas propellants can be formulated to provide desired vapor pressures for enhancing the delivery of the medication through the valve and actuator in accordance with the purpose of the medication. Aerosols are used as space sprays, surface sprays, aerated foams, and for oral inhalation.

Various propellants have properties that may be important including molecular weight, boiling point, vapor pressure, liquid density, and flash point. An example of a calculation to determine the vapor pressure of a certain mixture of hydrocarbon propellants follows.

■ EXAMPLE

What is the vapor pressure of a 60:40 mixture of propane and isobutane? Information on the two propellants is as follows:

Property	Propane	Isobutane
Molecular formula	C_3H_8	C_4H_{10}
Molecular weight	44.1	58.1
Boiling point (°F)	−43.7	10.9
Vapor pressure (psig at 70°F)	110	30.4
Liquid density (g/mL at 70°F)	0.50	0.56
Flash point (°F)	−156	−117

(continued)

1. Assume an ideal solution:

$$n_{propane} = 60/44.1 = 1.36$$
$$n_{isobutane} = 40/58.1 = 0.69$$

2. From Raoult law, determine the number of moles of each propellant.
3. From Raoult law, the partial pressure exerted by the propane is

$$P_{propane} = \left[\left(n_{propane} \right) / \left(n_{propane} + n_{isobutane} \right) \right] P_{propane}$$
$$P_{propane} = \left[(1.36)/(1.36 + 0.69) \right] 110 = 72.98 \, \psi$$

4. The partial pressure exerted by the isobutane is

$$P_{isobutane} = [(0.69)/(1.36 + 0.69)] 30.4 = 10.23 \, \psi$$

5. The vapor pressure exerted by both gases, P_T, is

$$P_T = 72.98 + 10.23 = 83.21 \, \psi \text{ at } 70°F$$

The vapor pressure required for a specific application can be calculated in a similar manner, and different ratios of propellants may be used to obtain that pressure. ■

Pharmaceutical aerosols are similar to other dosage forms because they require the same types of considerations with respect to formulation, product stability, and therapeutic efficacy. However, they differ from most other dosage forms in their dependence upon the function of the container, its valve assembly, and an added component—the propellant—for the physical delivery of the medication in proper form.

The term *pressurized* package is commonly used when referring to the aerosol container or completed product. Pressure is applied to the aerosol system through the use of one or more liquefied or gaseous propellants. Upon activation of the valve assembly of the aerosol, the pressure exerted by the propellant forces the contents of the package out through the opening of the valve. The physical form in which the contents are emitted depends on the formulation of the product and the type of valve. Aerosol products may be designed to expel their contents as a fine mist; a coarse, wet, or dry spray; a steady stream; or a stable or a fast-breaking foam. The physical form selected for a given aerosol is based on intended use. For instance, an aerosol for inhalation therapy, as in the treatment of asthma or emphysema, must present particles in the form of a fine liquid mist or as finely divided solid particles. Particles less than 6 μm will reach the respiratory bronchioles, and those less than 2 μm will reach the alveolar ducts and alveoli (Fig. 14.11). By contrast, the particle size for a dermatologic spray intended for deposition on the skin is coarser and generally less critical to the therapeutic efficacy of the product. Some dermatologic aerosols present

the medication in the form of a powder, a wet spray, a stream of liquid (usually a local anesthetic), or an ointment-like product. Other pharmaceutical aerosols include vaginal and rectal foams.

Aerosols used to provide an airborne mist are termed *space sprays*. Room disinfectants, room deodorizers, and space insecticides characterize this group of aerosols. The particle size of the released product is generally quite small, usually below 50 μm, and must be carefully controlled so that the dispersed droplets or particles remain airborne for a long time. A 1-second burst from a typical aerosol space spray will produce 120 million particles, a substantial number of which will remain suspended in the air for an hour.

Aerosols intended to carry the active ingredient to a surface are termed *surface sprays* or *surface coatings*. The

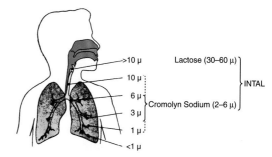

FIGURE 14.11. Relationship of INTAL (cromolyn sodium, Fisons) particle size to airway penetration. (Courtesy of Fisons Corporation.)

dermatologic aerosols can be placed in this group. Also included are a great many cosmetic and household aerosol products, including personal deodorant sprays, hair lacquers and sprays, perfumes and colognes, shaving lathers, toothpaste, surface pesticide sprays, paint sprays, spray starch, waxes, polishes, cleaners, and lubricants. A number of veterinary and pet products have been put into aerosol form, as have such food products as dessert toppings and food spreads. Some of these products are sprays; others, foams; and a few, pastes.

TYPES OF AEROSOLS

Inhalation aerosols, commonly known as metered-dose inhalers (MDIs), are intended to produce fine particles or droplets for inhalation through the mouth and deposition in the pulmonary tree. The design of the delivery system is intended to release measured quantities and of the appropriate quality of the active substance with each actuation.

Nasal aerosols, commonly known as nasal MDIs, produce fine particles or droplets for delivery through the nasal vestibule and deposition in the nasal cavity. Each actuation of the valve releases measured mass and appropriate quality of the active substance.

Lingual aerosols are intended to produce fine particles or droplets for deposition on the surface of the tongue. The design of the delivery system releases one dose with each actuation.

Topical aerosols produce fine particles or droplets for application to the skin. Topical aerosol drug products may be designed, as needed, to deliver a metered amount of formulation upon actuation of the designed valve or continuous release of formulation during depressed status of the valve.

Advantages of the Aerosol Dosage Form

Some features of pharmaceutical aerosols that may be considered advantages over other types of dosage forms are as follows:

1. A portion of medication may be easily withdrawn from the package without contamination or exposure to the remaining material.
2. By virtue of its hermetic character, the aerosol container protects medicinal agents adversely affected by atmospheric oxygen and moisture. Being opaque, the usual aerosol container also protects drugs adversely affected by light. This protection persists during the use and the shelf life of the product. If the product is packaged under aseptic conditions, sterility may also be maintained during the shelf life of the product.
3. Topical medication may be applied in a uniform thin layer to the skin without anything else touching the affected area. This method of application may reduce the irritation that sometimes accompanies mechanical (fingertip) application of topical preparations. The rapid volatilization of the propellant also provides a cooling, refreshing effect.

4. By proper formulation and valve control, the physical form and the particle size of the emitted product may be controlled, which may contribute to the efficacy of a drug, as with the fine controlled mist of an inhalant aerosol. Through the use of *metered valves*, dosage may be controlled.
5. Aerosol application is a clean process, requiring little or no washup by the user.

The Aerosol Principle

An aerosol formulation consists of two component parts: the *product concentrate* and the *propellant*. The product concentrate is the active ingredient of the aerosol combined with the required adjuncts, such as antioxidants, surface-active agents, and solvents, to prepare a stable and efficacious product. When the propellant is a liquefied gas or a mixture of liquefied gases, it frequently serves the dual role of propellant and solvent or vehicle for the product concentrate. In certain aerosol systems, compressed gases—carbon dioxide, nitrogen, and nitrous oxide—are employed as the propellant.

For many years, the liquefied gas propellants most used in aerosol products were the chlorofluorocarbons (CFCs). However, these propellants are being phased out and will be prohibited for nonessential use under federal regulations following recognition that they reduce the amount of ozone in the stratosphere, which results in an increase in the amount of ultraviolet radiation reaching the earth, an increase in the incidence of skin cancer, and other adverse environmental effects. Under the law, the FDA has the authority to exempt from the prohibition specific products under the agency's jurisdiction when there is sufficient evidence showing that (*a*) there are no technically feasible alternatives to the use of a CFC propellant in the product, (*b*) the product provides a substantial health or other public benefit unobtainable without the use of the CFC, and (*c*) the use does not involve a significant release of CFCs into the atmosphere, or, if it does, the release is warranted by the benefit conveyed. A number of metered-dose pharmaceutical products for oral inhalation have received such essential use exemptions. Among the CFCs used as propellants in pharmaceuticals were dichlorodifluoromethane, dichlorotetrafluoroethane, and trichloromonofluoromethane (Table 14.5).

Fluorinated hydrocarbons are gases at room temperature. They may be liquefied by cooling below their boiling point or by compression at room temperature. For example, dichlorodifluoromethane (Freon 12) will form a liquid when cooled to $-30°C$ ($-22°F$) or when compressed to 70 psig (pounds per square inch gauge) at $21°C$ ($70°F$). Both of these methods for liquefying gases are employed in aerosol packaging, as discussed later in this section.

When a liquefied gas propellant or propellant mixture is sealed within an aerosol container with the product concentrate, equilibrium is quickly established between the portion of propellant that remains liquefied and that which vaporizes and occupies the upper portion of the aerosol

TABLE 14.5. Physical Properties of Some Fluorinated Hydrocarbon Propellants

Chemical Name	Chemical Formula	Numeric Designation	Vapor Pressure[a] 70°F	Boiling Point (1 atm) °F	Liquid Density (g/mL) 70°F
Trichloromonofluoromethane	CCl_3F	11	13.4	74.7	1.485
Dichlorodifluoromethane	CCl_2F_2	12	13.4	74.1	1.485
Dichlorotetrafluoroethane	$CClF_2CClF_2$	114	21.6	38.4	1.468
Chloropentafluoroethane	$CClF_2CF_3$	115	17.5	−37.7	1.29
Monochlorodifluoromethane	CH_3CClF_2	142[b]	43.8	15.1	1.119
Difluoroethane	CH_3CHF_2	152[b]	76.4	−11.2	0.911
Octafluorocyclobutane	$CF_2CF_2CF_2CF_2$	C318	40.1	21.1	1.513

[a]Pounds per square inch absolute, equal to psig + 14.7.
[b]The numeric designations for fluorinated hydrocarbon propellants were designed in the refrigeration industry to simplify communications. The numeric designations are arrived at by the following method: (a) The digit at the extreme right refers to the number of fluorine atoms in the molecule. (b) The second digit from the right is one greater than the number of hydrogen atoms in the molecule. (c) The third digit from the right is one less than the number of carbon atoms in the molecule; if this number is zero, it is omitted and a two-digit number is used. (d) A capital C before a number indicates the cyclic nature of a compound. (e) The small letters following a number indicate decreasing symmetry of isomeric compounds, with "b" indicating less symmetry than "a," and so forth. The number of chlorine atoms in a molecule may be determined by subtracting the total number of hydrogen and fluorine atoms from the total number of atoms, which may be added to the carbon chain.

container (Fig. 14.12). The vapor phase exerts pressure in all directions—against the walls of the container, the valve assembly, and the surface of the liquid phase, which is composed of the liquefied gas and the product concentrate. It is this pressure that, upon actuation of the aerosol valve, forces the liquid phase up the dip tube and out of the orifice of the valve into the atmosphere. As the propellant meets the air, it expands and evaporates because of the drop in pressure, leaving the product concentrate as airborne liquid droplets or dry particles, depending upon the formulation. As the liquid phase is removed from the container, equilibrium between the propellant remaining

liquefied and that in the vapor state is reestablished. Thus, even during expulsion of the product from the aerosol package, the pressure within remains virtually constant, and the product may be continuously released at an even rate and with the same propulsion. However, when the liquid reservoir is depleted, the pressure may not be maintained, and the gas may be expelled from the container with diminishing pressure until it is exhausted.

Aerosol Systems

The pressure of an aerosol is critical to its performance. It can be controlled by (*a*) the type and amount of propellant

FIGURE 14.12. Cross-section sketches of contents and operation of a typical two-phase aerosol system. (Courtesy of Armstrong Laboratories, Division of Aerosol Techniques.)

and (b) the nature and amount of product concentrate. Thus, each formulation is unique unto itself, and a specific amount of propellant to be employed in aerosol products cannot be firmly stated, although some general statements may be made. Space sprays generally contain a greater proportion of propellant than do aerosols intended for surface coating; hence, they are released with greater pressure, and the resultant particles are projected more violently from the valve. Space aerosols usually operate at 30 to 40 psig at 21°C and may contain as much as 85% propellant. Surface aerosols commonly contain 30% to 70% propellant with pressures between 25 and 55 psig at 21°C. Foam aerosols usually operate between 35 and 55 psig at 21°C and may contain only 6% to 10% propellant.

Foam aerosols may be considered to be emulsions because the liquefied propellant is partially emulsified with the product concentrate rather than being dissolved in it. Because the fluorinated hydrocarbons are nonpolar organic solvents having no affinity for water, the liquefied propellant does not dissolve in the aqueous formulation. The use of surfactants or emulsifiers in the formulation encourages the mixing of the two components to enhance the emulsion. Shaking of the package prior to use further mixes the propellant throughout the product concentrate. When the aerosol valve is activated, the mixture is expelled to the atmosphere, where the propellant globules vaporize rapidly, leaving the active ingredient in the form of a foam.

Blends of the various liquefied gas propellants are generally used in pharmaceutical aerosols to achieve the desired vapor pressure and to provide the proper solvent features for a given product. Some propellants are eliminated from use in certain products because of their reactivity with other formulative materials or with the proposed container or valve components. For instance, trichloromonofluoromethane tends to form free hydrochloric acid when formulated with systems containing water or ethyl alcohol, the latter a commonly used cosolvent in aerosol systems. The free hydrochloric acid not only affects the efficacy of the product but also corrodes some container components.

The physiologic effect of the propellant must also be considered in formulating an aerosol to ensure safety of the product in its intended use. Even though an individual propellant or propellant blend and the active ingredient of a formulation are nontoxic when tested individually, the use of the combination in aerosol form may have undesirable features. For instance, when an active ingredient ordinarily used in a nasal or oral spray is placed in a fine aerosol mist, it may reach deeper into the respiratory tract than desired and result in irritation. With new dermatologic, vaginal, and rectal aerosol products, the influence of the aerosol form of the drug on the recipient tissue membranes must be evaluated for irritating effects and changes in the absorption of the drug from the site of application. The absorption pattern of a drug may change because of an increased rate of solubility of the fine particles usually produced in aerosol products.

Although the fluorinated hydrocarbons have a relatively low order of toxicity and are generally nonirritating, certain individuals who use an inhalation aerosol may be sensitive to the propellant agent and may exhibit cardiotoxic effects following rapid and repeated use (10).

Two-Phase Systems

As noted previously, the two-phase aerosol system consists of the liquid phase, containing the liquefied propellant and product concentrate, and the vapor phase.

Three-Phase Systems

The three-phase system consists of a layer of water-immiscible liquid propellant, a layer of highly aqueous product concentrate, and the vapor phase. Because the liquefied propellant usually has a greater density than the aqueous layer, it generally resides at the bottom of the container with the aqueous phase floating above it. As with the two-phase system, upon activation of the valve, the pressure of the vapor phase causes the liquid phase to rise in the dip tube and be expelled from the container. To avoid expulsion of the reservoir of liquefied propellant, the dip tube must extend only within the aqueous phase (product concentrate) and not down into the layer of liquefied propellant. The aqueous product is broken up into a spray by the mechanical action of the valve. If the container is shaken immediately prior to use, some liquefied propellant may be mixed with the aqueous phase and be expelled through the valve to facilitate the dispersion of the exited product or the production of foam. The vapor phase within the container is replenished from the liquid propellant phase.

Compressed Gas Systems

Compressed rather than liquefied gases may be used to prepare aerosols. The pressure of the compressed gas in the head space of the aerosol container forces the product concentrate up the dip tube and out of the valve. The use of gases that are insoluble in the product concentrate, as is nitrogen, will result in emission of a product in essentially the same form as it was placed in the container. An advantage of nitrogen as a propellant is its inert behavior toward other formulative components and its protective influence on products subject to oxidation. Also, nitrogen is an odorless and tasteless gas and thus does not contribute adversely to the smell or taste of a product.

Other gases, such as carbon dioxide and nitrous oxide, which are slightly soluble in the liquid phase of aerosol products, may be employed when their expulsion with the product concentrate is desired to achieve spraying or foaming.

Unlike aerosols prepared with liquefied gas propellants, compressed gas–filled aerosols have no reservoir of propellant. Thus, higher gas pressures are required in these systems, and the pressure in these aerosols diminishes as the product is used.

Aerosol Container and Valve Assembly

The effectiveness of a pharmaceutical aerosol depends on achieving the proper combination of formulation, container, and valve assembly. The formulation must not chemically interact with the container or valve components so as to interfere with the stability of the formulation or with the integrity and operation of the container and valve assembly. The container and valve must be capable of withstanding the pressure required by the product, it must resist corrosion, and the valve must contribute to the form of the product to be emitted.

Containers

Various materials have been used in the manufacture of aerosol containers, including (*a*) glass, uncoated or plastic coated; (*b*) metal, including tin-plated steel, aluminum, and stainless steel; and (*c*) plastics. The selection of the container for an aerosol product is based on its adaptability to production methods, compatibility with formulation components, ability to sustain the pressure intended for the product, the interest in design and aesthetic appeal on the part of the manufacturer, and cost.

Were it not for their brittleness and danger of breakage, glass containers would be preferred for most aerosols. Glass presents fewer problems with respect to chemical compatibility with the formula than do metal containers, and it is not subject to corrosion. Glass is also more adaptive to creativity in design. On the negative side, glass containers must be precisely engineered to provide the maximum in pressure safety and impact resistance. Plastic coatings are commonly applied to the outer surface of glass containers to render them more resistant to accidental breakage, and in the event of breaking, the plastic coating prevents the scattering of glass fragments. When the total pressure of an aerosol system is below 25 psig and no more than 50% propellant is used, glass containers are considered quite safe. When required, the inner surface of glass containers may be coated to render them more chemically resistant to formulation materials.

Tin-plated steel containers are the most widely used metal containers for aerosols. Because the starting material is in sheets, the completed aerosol cylinders are seamed and soldered to provide a sealed unit. When required, special protective coatings are employed within the container to prevent corrosion and interaction between the container and formulation. The containers must be carefully examined prior to filling to ensure that there are no flaws in the seam or in the protective coating that would render the container weak or subject to corrosion.

Most aluminum containers are manufactured by extrusion or by other methods that make them seamless. They have the advantage over the seam type of container of greater safety against leakage, incompatibility, and corrosion. Stainless steel is employed to produce containers for certain small-volume aerosols in which a great deal of chemical resistance is required. The main limitation of stainless steel containers is their high cost.

Plastic containers have met with varying success in the packaging of aerosols because of their inherent problem of being permeated by the vapor within the container. Also, certain drug–plastic interactions affect the release of drug from the container and reduce the efficacy of the product.

Valve Assembly

The function of the valve assembly is to permit expulsion of the contents of the can in the desired form, at the desired rate, and, in the case of metered valves, in the proper amount or dose. The materials used in the manufacture of valves must be inert to the formulations and must be approved by the FDA. Among the materials used in the manufacture of the various valve parts are plastic, rubber, aluminum, and stainless steel.

The usual aerosol valve assembly is composed of the following parts (Fig. 14.13):

1. *Actuator*: the button the user presses to activate the valve assembly for emission of the product. The actuator permits easy opening and closing of the valve. It is through the orifice in the actuator that the product is discharged. The design of the inner chamber and size of the emission orifice of the actuator contribute to the physical form (mist, coarse spray, solid stream, or foam) in which the product is discharged. The type and quantity of propellant used and the actuator design and dimensions control the particle size of the emitted product. Larger orifices (and less propellant) are used for products to be emitted as foams and solid streams than for those intended to be sprays or mists.

2. *Stem*: supports the actuator and delivers the formulation in the proper form to the chamber of the actuator.

3. *Gasket*: placed snugly with the stem and prevents leakage of the formulation when the valve is closed.

FIGURE 14.13. Valve assembly components.

4. *Spring*: holds the gasket in place and is the mechanism by which the actuator retracts when pressure is released, returning the valve to the closed position.
5. *Mounting cup*: attached to the aerosol can or container and holds the valve in place. Because the underside of the mounting cup is exposed to the formulation, it must receive the same consideration as the inner part of the container with respect to meeting criteria of compatibility. If necessary, it may be coated with an inert material (e.g., an epoxy resin or vinyl) to prevent an undesired interaction.
6. *Housing*: directly below the mounting cup, the housing links the dip tube and the stem and actuator. With the stem, its orifice helps to determine the delivery rate and the form in which the product is emitted.
7. *Dip tube*: extends from the housing down into the product; brings the formulation from the container to the valve. The viscosity of the product and its intended delivery rate dictate to a large extent the inner dimensions of the dip tube and housing for a particular product.

The actuator, stem, housing, and dip tube are generally made of plastic, the mounting cup and spring of metal, and the gasket of rubber or plastic resistant to the formulation.

Metered-Dose Inhalers

Metering valves are employed when the formulation is a potent medication, as in inhalation therapy (Fig. 14.14). In these metered valve systems, the amount of material

FIGURE 14.14. Metered-dose inhaler. Each metered dose is delivered through the mouthpiece upon actuation of the aerosol unit's valve. (Courtesy of Boehringer Ingelheim.)

discharged is regulated by an auxiliary valve chamber by virtue of its capacity or dimensions. A single depression of the actuator causes evacuation of this chamber and delivery of its contents. The integrity of the chamber is controlled by a dual-valve mechanism. When the actuator valve is closed, the chamber is sealed from the atmosphere. However, in this position, the chamber is permitted to fill with the contents of the container, to which it is open. Depression of the actuator causes a simultaneous reversal of positions; the chamber becomes open to the atmosphere, releasing its contents, at the same time becoming sealed from the contents of the container. Upon release of the actuator, the system is restored for the next dose. The USP contains a test to determine quantitatively the amount of medication from a metered valve.

As noted previously, the effectiveness of delivering medication to the lower reaches of the lungs for local or systemic effects depends in part on the particle size of the inhaled drug. Breathing patterns and the depth of respiration also play important roles in the deposition of inhaled aerosols to the lungs. Analysis of dose uniformity (11), particle size distribution patterns (12–14), and the respirable fractions of aerosol-delivered particles (15,16) are areas of research in developing aerosol products for optimal oral inhalation therapy.

A unique translingual aerosol formulation of nitroglycerin (Nitrolingual Spray, Rhône-Poulenc Rorer) permits a patient to spray droplets of nitroglycerin onto or under the tongue for acute relief of an attack or for prophylaxis of angina pectoris due to coronary artery disease. The product is not to be inhaled. At the onset of an attack, two metered spray emissions, each containing 0.4 mg of nitroglycerin, are administered. The product contains 200 doses of nitroglycerin in a propellant mixture of dichlorodifluoromethane and dichlorotetrafluoroethane.

Filling Operations

As explained earlier, fluorinated hydrocarbon gases may be liquefied by cooling below their boiling point or by compressing the gas at room temperature. These two features are used in the filling of aerosol containers with propellant.

Cold Filling

In the cold method, both the product concentrate and the propellant must be cooled to −34.5°C to −40°C (−30°F to 40°F). This temperature is necessary to liquefy the propellant gas. The cooling system may be a mixture of dry ice and acetone or a more elaborate refrigeration system. After the chilled product concentrate has been quantitatively metered into an equally cold aerosol container, the liquefied gas is added. The heavy vapors of the cold liquid propellant generally displace the air in the container. However, in the process, some of the propellant vapors are also lost. When sufficient propellant has been added, the valve assembly is inserted and crimped into place. Because of the low temperatures required, aqueous systems cannot be filled by this process, because the water turns to ice.

For nonaqueous systems, some moisture usually appears in the final product because of the condensation of atmospheric moisture within the cold containers.

Pressure Filling

By the pressure method, the product concentrate is quantitatively placed in the aerosol container, the valve assembly is inserted and crimped into place, and the liquefied gas, under pressure, is metered into the valve stem from a pressure burette (Fig. 14.15). The desired amount of propellant is allowed to enter the container under its own vapor pressure. When the pressure in the container equals that in the burette, the propellant stops flowing. Additional propellant may be added by increasing the pressure in the filling apparatus through the use of compressed air or nitrogen gas. The trapped air in the package may be ignored if it does not interfere with the quality or stability of the product, or it may be evacuated with a special apparatus. After the container is filled with sufficient propellant, the valve actuator is tested for proper function. This spray testing also rids the dip tube of pure propellant prior to consumer use.

Pressure filling is used for most pharmaceutical aerosols. It has two advantages over cold filling: There is less danger of moisture contamination of the product, and less propellant is lost in the process.

When compressed gases are employed as the propellant in aerosol systems, the gas is transferred from large steel cylinders into the aerosol containers. Prior to filling, the product concentrate is placed in the container, the valve assembly is crimped into place, and the air is evacuated from the container by a vacuum pump. The compressed gas is then passed into the container through a pressure-reducing valve attached to the gas cylinder; when the pressure within the aerosol container is equal to the predetermined and regulated delivery pressure, the gas flow stops, and the aerosol valve is restored to the closed position. For gases like carbon dioxide and nitrous oxide, which are slightly soluble in the product concentrate, the container is manually or mechanically shaken during the

FIGURE 14.15. Pressure filling of aerosol containers. (Courtesy of Umomos/Shutterstock.)

filling operation to achieve the desired pressure in the head space of the aerosol container.

Testing the Filled Containers

After filling by either method, the aerosol container is tested under various environmental conditions for leaks or weakness in the valve assembly or container.

Filled aerosol containers are also tested for proper function of the valve. The *valve discharge rate* is determined by discharging a portion of the contents of a previously weighed aerosol during a period and calculating, by the difference in weight, the grams of contents discharged per unit of time. As is deemed desirable, aerosols may be tested for their spray patterns, for particle size distribution of the spray, and for accuracy and reproducibility of dosage when using metered valves.

Packaging, Labeling, and Storage

A unique aspect of pharmaceutical aerosols compared to other dosage forms is that the product is actually packaged as part of the manufacturing process. With most other dosage forms, the product is completely manufactured and then placed in the appropriate container.

Most aerosol products have a protective cap or cover that fits snugly over the valve and mounting cup. This protects the valve against contamination with dust and dirt. The cap, which is generally made of plastic or metal, also serves a decorative function.

Medicinal aerosols that are to be dispensed only upon prescription usually are labeled by the manufacturer with plastic peel-away labels or easily removed paper labels so that the pharmacist may easily replace the manufacturer's label with his label containing the directions for use specified by the prescribing practitioner. Most other types of aerosols have the manufacturer's label printed directly on the container or on firmly affixed paper.

In addition to the usual labeling requirements for pharmaceutical products, aerosols have special requirements for use and storage. For example, for safety, labels must warn users not to puncture pressurized containers, not to use or store them near heat or an open flame, and not to incinerate them. Exposure to temperatures above 49°C (120°F) may burst an aerosol container. Most medications in aerosol containers are intended for use at ambient room temperatures. When the canisters are cold, less than the usual spray may result. This may be particularly important to users of metered-dose inhalation sprays. These products are generally recommended for storage between 15°C and 30°C (59°F and 86°F). Pharmaceutical aerosols are labeled with regard to shaking before use, holding at the proper angle and/or distance from the target; there are special detailed instructions for inhaler devices.

Aerosols should be maintained with the protective caps in place to prevent accidental activation of the valve assembly or contamination by dust and other foreign materials. Examples of pharmaceutical aerosols are shown in Figure 14.16 and presented in Table 14.6.

FIGURE 14.16. Pharmaceutical aerosols.

Proper Administration and Use of Pharmaceutical Aerosols

The pharmacist should make every attempt to educate the patient about aerosol dosage forms, particularly for oral or nasal administration, because these are only effective when properly used. To complement verbal instructions, the pharmacist should provide the patient with the written instructions in the product package and demonstrate the proper technique with a placebo inhaler if possible. It is difficult to predict what percentage of patients will read or understand the printed instruction. Thus, the pharmacist must verbally transmit instruction for proper use. Using the oral metered aerosols as a model, the pharmacist should demonstrate how the inhaler is assembled, stored, and cleaned. The patient should be told whether the inhaler requires shaking before use and how to hold it between the index finger and thumb so that the aerosol canister is upside down. The patient should understand that coordination must be achieved between inhalation (after exhaling as completely as possible) and pressing down the inhaler to release one dose. The patient should be instructed to hold the breath for several seconds or as long as possible to gain the maximum benefit from the medication, then remove the inhaler from the mouth, and exhale slowly through pursed lips.

Some patients cannot use MDIs properly. Thus, after a new prescription is dispensed, it is advisable for the pharmacist to follow up with the patient to make sure the patient can use the inhaler. If the patient cannot use the inhaler, it is advisable for the pharmacist to recommend to the patient or the patient's physician the use of an extender device with the inhaler. Extender devices, or spacers, were originally developed for patients who could not learn to coordinate release of the medication with inhalation. These are now considered an important therapeutic aid because they can effectively assist the delivery

TABLE 14.6. Examples of Inhalation Aerosols

Aerosol	Representative Commercial Products	Category and Comments
Albuterol	Proventil Inhalation Aerosol (Key), Ventolin Inhalation Aerosol (GlaxoSmithKline)	Beta-adrenergic agonist for prevention and relief of bronchospasm in patients with reversible obstructive airway disease and for relief of exercise-induced bronchospasm
Beclomethasone dipropionate	Beclovent Inhalation Aerosol (Glaxo Wellcome), Vanceril Inhaler (Schering)	Adrenocortical steroid; aerosol for oral inhalation to control bronchial asthma in patients requiring chronic treatment with corticosteroids plus other therapy, for example, xanthines, sympathomimetics
	Beconase Nasal Inhaler (GlaxoSmithKline), Vancenase Pockethaler Nasal Inhaler (Schering)	Adrenocortical steroid; aerosol for intranasal relief of seasonal or perennial rhinitis in cases poorly responsive to conventional treatment
Cromolyn sodium	Intal Inhaler (King)	Antiasthmatic, antiallergic, mast cell stabilizer; metered dose for oral use to prevent exercise-induced bronchospasm, acute bronchospasm induced by environmental pollutants and known allergens
Ipratropium bromide	Atrovent Inhalation Aerosol (Boehringer Ingelheim)	Anticholinergic (parasympatholytic) bronchodilator for bronchospasm
Metaproterenol sulfate	Alupent Inhalation Aerosol (Boehringer Ingelheim)	Sympathomimetic for bronchospasm in patients with reversible obstructive airway disease
Salmeterol xinafoate	Serevent Inhalation Aerosol (GlaxoSmithKline)	Beta-adrenergic agonist for long-term maintenance treatment of asthma, prevention of bronchospasm in patients with reversible obstructive airway disease
Terbutaline sulfate	Brethine (AAIPharma)	Beta-adrenergic agonist for relief of bronchospasm
Triamcinolone acetonide	Azmacort (Kos)	For patients who require chronic treatment with corticosteroids to control symptoms of bronchial asthma

of medication despite improper patient inhalation technique. By placing an extender device between the MDI's mouthpiece and the patient's mouth, the patient is permitted to separate activation of the aerosol from inhalation by up to 3 to 5 seconds (a valve in the spacer opens when the patient inhales). Another advantage of the extender is that aerosol velocity is reduced and droplet size is decreased because there is time for evaporation of the fluorohydrocarbon propellant. Thus, extender devices also cause less deposition of medication in the oropharynx. Extender devices can be used with most pressurized canisters, such as Brethancer Inhaler (Novartis) and InspirEase (Key).

It is wise for the pharmacist to share with the patient ways to assess how much medication is left in the canister. This is important to ensure continuity of therapy, especially for those who have respiratory illness and may need their medication on a moment's notice.

Examples of oral *inhalation aerosols* (solutions and powders) include Asmanex Twisthaler (mometasone furoate inhalation powder, Schering), Ventavis (iloprost inhalation solution, Cotherix), Pulmicort Flexhaler (budesonide inhalation powder, AstraZeneca), Atrovent HFA (ipratropium bromide HFA inhalation aerosol, Boehringer Ingelheim), and Brovana (arformoterol tartrate inhalation solution, Sepracor Inc.).

As presented in Table 14.6, a number of drug substances are administered through pressure-packaged inhalation aerosols like the type shown in Figure 14.14. For the inhaled drug substance or solution to reach the bronchial tree, the inhaled particles must be just a few microns in size.

Topical Aerosols

Convenient aerosol packages for use on the skin include the anti-infective agents povidone–iodine, tolnaftate, and thimerosal; the adrenocortical steroids betamethasone dipropionate and valerate, dexamethasone, and triamcinolone acetonide; and the local anesthetic dibucaine hydrochloride.

The use of topical aerosols provides the patient a means of applying the drug in a convenient manner. The preparation may be applied to the desired surface area without the use of the fingertips, making the procedure less messy than with most other types of topical preparations. Among the disadvantages to the use of topical aerosols are the difficulty in applying the medication to a small area and the greater expense associated with the aerosol package.

For topical administration of aerosol dosage forms, the patient should first clean the affected area gently and pat it dry. Holding the canister with the nozzle pointing toward the body area and about 6 to 8 inches away, the patient should press down the button to deliver enough medication to cover the area. The patient should allow the spray to dry and not cover the area with a bandage or dressing unless instructed to do so by the physician. The patient should avoid accidentally spraying the product into the eyes or mouth. If it is necessary to apply the product to a facial area, the patient should spray the product into the palm of the hand and apply it by this means.

Vaginal and Rectal Aerosols

Aerosol foams containing estrogenic substances and contraceptive agents are commercially available. The foams are used intravaginally in the same manner as for creams. The aerosol package contains an inserter that is filled with foam and the contents placed in the vagina through activation of the plunger. The foams are generally o/w emulsions resembling light creams. They are water miscible and nongreasy.

Some commercial rectal foams use inserters. One such product, Proctofoam (Alaven Pharmaceuticals), contains pramoxine hydrochloride to relieve inflammatory anorectal disorders (Fig. 14.17).

FIGURE 14.17. Foam for anal and perianal use. To fill the applicator, the foam container is shaken vigorously and held upright, and the applicator tip placed on the container opening. With the plunger of the applicator drawn out all the way, pressure is exerted on the container cap, and foam fills the applicator tube. (Courtesy of Reed & Carnrick.)

FOAMS

A foam is an emulsion dosage form containing dispersed gas bubbles. When dispensed, it has a fluffy, semisolid consistency. Medicated foams are emulsions containing a dispersed phase of gas bubbles in a liquid continuous phase containing the API. Medicated foams are packaged in pressurized containers or special dispensing devices and are intended for application to the skin or mucous membranes. The medicated foam is formed at the time of application. Surfactants are used to ensure the dispersion of the gas and the two phases. Medicated foams have a fluffy, semisolid consistency and can be formulated to break to a liquid quickly or to remain as foam to ensure prolonged contact. Medicated foams intended to treat severely injured skin or open wounds must be sterile.

PREPARATION OF FOAMS

A foam may contain one or more APIs, surfactants, aqueous or nonaqueous liquids, and propellants. If the propellant is in the internal, or discontinuous, phase, a stable foam is discharged. If the propellant is in the external, or continuous, phase, a spray or a quick-breaking foam is discharged. Quick-breaking foams formulated with alcohol create a cooling sensation when applied to the skin and may have disinfectant properties.

Foams containing flammable components should be appropriately labeled. Labeling indicates that a foam drug product must be shaken well to ensure uniformity prior to dispensing. The instructions for use must clearly note special precautions that are necessary to preserve sterility. In the absence of a metering valve, the delivered volume may be variable.

PATIENT COUNSELING

SUSPENSIONS

1. Discuss and demonstrate how to shake the suspension, shake vigorously or mix using a rolling action, and how to measure the required dose.
2. Describe and demonstrate the proper method for administering doses.
3. Instruct on the proper recapping and storage of the bottle, as well as the way to determine if the suspension has become physically unstable.

EMULSIONS

1. Discuss and demonstrate how to shake the emulsion and how to measure the required dose.
2. Instruct and demonstrate how to measure the required dose.
3. Instruct on the proper recapping and storage of the bottle.
4. Instruct on the way to determine if the emulsion has become physically unstable.

INHALERS AND NEBULIZERS, GENERAL INFORMATION

A patient or caregiver should be thoroughly instructed on how to administer oral inhalation solutions. If the solution does not include a preservative, the patient should be instructed to appropriately discard any remaining solution in the individual dosage vials and in the device used for aerosolization.

ADMINISTRATION USING METERED-DOSE INHALERS

1. Shake the inhaler and remove the mouthpiece cap.
2. Exhale fully and place the mouthpiece into the mouth. Some physicians may recommend either a spacer be used or to hold the inhaler 1 to 2 inches from the open mouth.

3. As a deep breath is being taken, squeeze the canister and mouthpiece together simultaneously.
4. Inhale the spray into the lungs with a slow, deep breath and hold the breath as long as is comfortable.
5. Exhale slowly. If a spacer or the space technique was not used, rinse the mouth before swallowing and expectorate to prevent swallowing the drug solution and reduce the incidence of side effects.
6. Wipe or rinse the mouthpiece and dry. Rinse the plastic actuator once weekly to prevent clogging. Remove the drug-filled canister and place the plastic actuator under warm running water and allow to air dry before reassembling.
7. Inhaled medications begin working generally within a minute. If more than one puff is prescribed, wait at least one minute between each administration.
8. If several different medicines from different inhalers are to be administered, it is best to give the bronchodilator before the others.

FOR CHILDREN 3 AND UNDER ADMINISTRATION USING SPACERS OR HOLDING CHAMBERS

1. Shake the inhaler and place the mouthpiece into the open end of the chamber ensuring a tight fit.
2. Place the facemask over the nose and mouth.
3. Actuate one dose into the chamber.
4. Allow the child to inhale and exhale normally into the chamber at least ten times.
5. Clean the face after the mask is taken off to remove any medication that may be deposited on the skin.

FOR CHILDREN OVER 3 ADMINISTRATION USING SPACERS OR HOLDING CHAMBERS

1. Shake the inhaler and place the mouthpiece into the open end of the chamber for a tight fit.
2. Have the child exhale completely.

3. Place the mouthpiece of the chamber into the mouth with lips sealed around it.

4. Actuate one dose into the chamber.

5. Have the child to inhale slowly through the mouthpiece.

6. Have the child hold their breath as long as possible.

ADMINISTRATION USING DRY POWDER INHALERS (DPI)

1. Prepare the dose and the mouthpiece of the inhaler for administration.

2. Keep the inhaler level, turn the head away from the DPI, and exhale completely to empty the lungs.

3. Begin the *inhalation* rapidly and forcefully through the mouthpiece.

4. Continue inhaling as long as reasonable.

5. Hold the breath for about 10 seconds.

6. If the inhaler contains a corticosteroid, rinse the mouth and expectorate.

7. Store the inhaler in a dry place at room temperature.

8. Wipe it out once weekly with a clean, dry cloth.

ADMINISTRATION USING OF A NEBULIZER

1. Assemble the nebulizer according to its instructions.

2. Fill the medicine cup or reservoir with the prescription medication according to the instructions.

3. Connect the nebulizer to the power source or compressor.

4. Place the mouthpiece in the mouth. Breathe through the mouth until all the medicine is used; this may take about 10 to 15 minutes. A nose clip may help to breathe only through the mouth.

5. Wash the medicine cup and mouthpiece with warm water and air dry until the next treatment.

6. After each use, rinse with distilled water; shake the excess moisture from the cup and let air dry on a clean towel.

7. Once or twice weekly follow the manufacturer's instructions on disinfection.

SUBLINGUAL AEROSOLS

1. Prime the metered dose several times prior to use, as applicable.

2. Hold the metered dose pump vertically with the dose chamber on top and the spray opening as close to the open mouth as possible.

3. Apply the spray under the tongue.

4. Do not inhale or swallow the spray as it should be absorbed under the tongue.

5. Avoid drinking or eating for several minutes until the drug has been absorbed.

FOAMS

1. Explain the proper storage, use, and disposal of foams.

2. Instruct on how to protect the preparation from heat and generally to avoid refrigeration.

3. Store at room temperature and out of direct sunlight.

4. For use, the area to be covered needs to be clean and dry.

5. Do not apply an excess of foam, but only what is needed to cover the area appropriately.

6. If the skin is intact, the foam can be rubbed in; if it is abraded, the foam should only be applied and not rubbed.

7. A protective cover can be added as directed.

8. Store the container away from the reach of children.

9. An empty container should be disposed of properly. If the container is not used and is no longer needed, the contents should be discarded appropriately and the container rinsed and then discarded in the trash.

PHARMACEUTICS CASE STUDY

SUBJECTIVE INFORMATION

Working for an innovative pharmaceutical company, you have received a request to develop an oral liquid formulation for a new organ rejection drug. The drug must be formulated so that a 5-mg dose can be reasonably easily administered either as the dosage form or immediately after mixing with water or juice. The formulation should be stable and easy to manipulate. The problem is that the drug is not water soluble but a solution dosage form is desired.

OBJECTIVE INFORMATION

The drug has a molecular weight of 1,015.2 and occurs as a white to off-white powder that is insoluble in water but freely soluble in benzyl alcohol, chloroform, acetone, and acetonitrile.

The drug may be prepared as an aqueous suspension or as a solution in a water-miscible liquid that can be diluted prior to administration. A reasonable dispersant liquid for the insoluble drug may include a blend of lecithin products that would form liposomes upon dilution in an aqueous vehicle. Some commercial blends occur as honey-colored fluids with a typical odor and nutty taste. These can be diluted with water and have densities of approximately 1 to 1.2 and viscosities in the range of 5,000 mPa.

It may be wise to add a dispersant such as polysorbate 80 to aid in mixing when this is added to water or juice. Polysorbate 80 (Tween 80, polyoxyethylene 20 sorbitan monooleate, $C_{64}H_{124}O_{26}$) has a molecular weight of 1,310 and occurs as a yellow oily liquid with a characteristic odor and a warm, somewhat

(continued)

(continued)

bitter taste. It has a specific gravity of 1.06 to 1.09, and its HLB is 15.0; it forms o/w emulsions. It is stable in the presence of electrolytes, weak acids, and weak bases. It should be stored in a well-closed, light-resistant container in a cool place (5).

ASSESSMENT

After viewing the options, you decide to select a solvent system for the drug and prepare it as a solution. The patient can obtain the dose and dilute it immediately prior to administration. This meets the criteria of stability and ease of administration.

You select a commercial dispersant liquid for oral use containing 50% phosphatidylcholine in propylene glycol, sunflower seed oil glycerides, soy acid, alcohol, and

ascorbyl palmitate. This product is used as a dispersant, emulsifier, penetrant, and solubilizer for pharmaceuticals, creams, lotions, emulsions, and liposome preparations for dermatology. It is suitable for oral use.

PLAN

You formulate the product as a 5-mg dose in 1 mL of the vehicle containing 0.5% polysorbate 80 in the described dispersant liquid. This will provide a stable, easy-to-use product.

For administration, the proper quantity of the oral liquid will be added to approximately 2 to 4 oz of water or juice. The preparation should be vigorously stirred and taken at once. Various juices can be used depending on the preference of the patient. ∎

CLINICAL CASE STUDY

HPI: M.H. is a 31-year-old WF who presents to the pharmacy with a prescription for metronidazole. Upon questioning, the patient reveals that she just returned from an appointment with her gynecologist. She has been having symptoms that she describes as "an unusual yellowish smelly discharge with itching and burning." The patient continues, "At first I thought it was just another yeast infection, but the discharge seemed a little different. I did not want to use another OTC product that might not work, so I went to see my doctor." Her gynecologist informed her that she had *trichomonal vaginitis*, a sexually transmitted disease (STD). When handing the prescription to the pharmacist, she complains that she "hates this medicine. I don't like taking pills even if they aren't big. And they leave an awful taste in my mouth." The pharmacist knows M.H. as a regular customer and decides to look up her profile to confirm that she had previously taken metronidazole. She also reviews M.H.'s past medical history.

PMH:	Asthma since childhood Vaginal yeast infections about once a year Bacterial vaginosis in 2001 Miscarriage in 1999
SH:	(+) EtOH: drinks cocktails on weekends, occasionally wine at dinner (−) Tobacco (−) Illicit drugs
FH:	Mother (+) for breast cancer Father (+) for hypertension and hypercholesterolemia Brother (+) for asthma

Allergies:	NKDA
Meds:	Advair 250/50 1 inhalation bid Albuterol MDI prn Gyne-Lotrimin 3 prn yeast infections

PHARMACEUTICAL CARE PLAN

S: Patient has vaginal symptoms, including itching, burning, and a yellowish, malodorous discharge. Patient complains about the size of the metronidazole tablets and its metallic taste.

O: The gynecologist has diagnosed *trichomonal vaginitis*. Previously, the patient has been prescribed metronidazole oral tablets for bacterial vaginosis.

A: M.H. is a 31-year-old WF diagnosed with *trichomonal vaginitis* that is to be treated with oral metronidazole tablets. Although she is in a monogamous relationship, unprotected sex increases the risk of transmitting STDs, such as *Trichomonas*. M.H.'s adherence to the metronidazole regimen is very important because untreated vaginitis may progress to urethritis and/or cystitis. Worried that the patient may not adhere to her regimen, the pharmacist considers compounding a metronidazole suspension so that the patient will not have to take the tablets and will have an easier dosage form.

(continued)

CLINICAL CASE STUDY (continued)

P:
1. The pharmacist offers the alternative of an extemporaneously prepared metronidazole suspension in lieu of the oral tablets. The patient agrees to try this option. So the pharmacist calls the patient's physician to seek permission to change the drug delivery system.

2. After securing permission to do so, the pharmacist decides to use metronidazole benzoate powder in lieu of metronidazole HCl, the active ingredient in the oral tablets. The benzoate form is relatively tasteless, which may also be a more suitable option for M.H. even though the metallic taste will occur from the therapy after administration.

3. The first step in preparation of the suspension is a mathematical calculation to determine the equivalent dose of metronidazole benzoate. The pharmacist confirms that 200 mg of the benzoate ester is equivalent to 125 mg of the HCl salt. The prescribed dose of metronidazole HCl tablets is 250 mg tid for 7 days. Thus, the pharmacist calculates the equivalent metronidazole benzoate dose that will be 400 mg tid for 7 days.

4. After weighing the required amount of metronidazole benzoate powder, the pharmacist triturates it in a mortar and selects Ora-Plus as the suspending agent and pestle to minimize the particle size. The pharmacist Ora-Sweet as the flavoring agent. The suspension will be compounded so that the final concentration (w/v) of metronidazole benzoate will be 400 mg/5 mL. With constant mixing, the pharmacist slowly adds Ora-Plus 50 mL to the metronidazole benzoate powder to create a slurry. The resultant suspension is transferred into a graduated cylinder and diluted with enough Ora-Sweet so that the total volume of the suspension is 105 mL. Before bringing the product to final volume, the pharmacist uses some Ora-Sweet to remove as much of the slurry from the mortar as possible.

   After stirring the suspension, the contents are transferred into an appropriate-sized plastic bottle, and the label with the appropriate information is affixed. The following auxiliary labels should also be affixed to the bottle: Keep refrigerated, shake well before using, finish the entire course of therapy, avoid alcoholic beverages, and take with food.

5. When dispensing the metronidazole suspension to the patient, the pharmacist counsels and instructs M.H. M.H. should take one teaspoonful by mouth three times daily for 7 consecutive days. The daily doses should be taken with food after each meal. The medication should be stored in the refrigerator when not being used and, because it is a suspension, shaken well before each dose. It is assumed that the suspension will be used up before the beyond-use date of 30 days. However, it is necessary for the pharmacist to label the product with the beyond-use date in the event that some is left over.

6. The pharmacist suggests that the medication be taken with food to help prevent stomach upset, nausea, and diarrhea. Although the benzoate form of metronidazole may help to lessen the bitter taste associated with its administration, the metallic taste may still occur after systemic absorption, and the patient should understand this. In addition, M.H. should be told about the interaction (disulfiram reaction) between metronidazole and alcohol. Alcohol must be avoided during therapy and for 72 hours after the last dose. This disulfiram reaction may result in severe flushing, headache, nausea, vomiting, or chest and abdominal pain. M.H. should also be aware that the medication may darken her urine.

7. Because *trichomonal vaginitis* is an STD, M.H. must be educated to take certain precautions to prevent transmission and reinfection of herself. During treatment, M.H. should refrain from sexual intercourse. The importance of practicing safe sex (e.g., condom use) should be emphasized to prevent contracting STDs and other serious infections (e.g., HIV, hepatitis). In addition, M.H.'s sexual partner should be treated with metronidazole. Although he may be asymptomatic, there is an elevated risk that he is carrying the *Trichomonas* organism and infecting M.H. during intercourse. Thus, with this prescription, her partner may or may not be treated. If the latter, it is important that the pharmacist tells M.H. not to share her medication with her sexual partner. She is to take a full course of therapy. If there is a primary treatment failure, it is likely that the male sexual partner will also be treated during the second course of therapy. Emphasis will be put on the importance of M.H. completing the full course of metronidazole therapy to prevent resistance, emergence, and recurrent infections. ■

APPLYING THE PRINCIPLES AND CONCEPTS

GROUP ACTIVITIES

1. Discuss specific patient circumstances and therapeutic circumstances where particular liquid disperse system dosage forms would be indicated or contraindicated for use.

2. Describe the three phases of a stable emulsion.

3. Identify and describe three methods for emulsion preparation.

4. Obtain representative extemporaneous prescriptions, which result in a suspension or emulsion dosage

form, and devise a procedure to compound each prescription.

5. Create a table of representative oral o/w products inclusive of active and inactive ingredients, indications and contraindications for their use, adverse effects associated with their use, dosage, and patient information.

6. Create a table of representative topical w/o and o/w products inclusive of active and inactive ingredients, indications and contraindications for their use, adverse effects associated with use, dosage, and patient information.

7. Create a table of topical gel products, which are also available as topical creams and ointments, and describe differences, which exist between the dosage forms.

8. Role-play proper counseling points a pharmacist should make when dispensing a liquid disperse system to a patient.

INDIVIDUAL ACTIVITIES

1. Identify three desired features in a suspension, and explain how these benefit patient administration.

2. Explain the role of suspending agents when added to a dispersion medium.

3. Compare and contrast the various suspending agents used in suspension dosage forms. Determine additional processes/techniques, which allow a drug to be more effectively penetrated by a given vehicle.

4. Differentiate the terms "for Oral Suspension" and "Oral Suspension," and create a table illustrating three product examples of each.

5. List advantages of emulsifying a liquid drug over pure liquid drug for oral administration.

6. Describe the chain of events that occur after aggregation or coalescence of an emulsion.

REFERENCES

1. Heyd A, Dhabhar D. Particle shape effect on caking of coarse granulated antacid suspensions. Drug Cosmet Ind 1979;125:42.
2. Oral Liquid Pharmaceuticals. Wilmington, DE: ICI Americas, 1975.
3. Chang RK. Formulation approaches for sustained-release oral suspensions. Pharm Technol 1992;16:134–136.
4. Allen LV Jr. Prednisone oral suspension. Int J Pharm Compd 2007;11(1):77.
5. Allen LV Jr. Ketoconazole oral suspension. Int J Pharm Compd 1997;1(6):414.
6. Allen LV Jr. Compounding microemulsions. Int J Pharm Compd 2018;22(2):137–143.
7. Griffin WC. Classification of surface-active agents by "HLB". J Soc Cosmet Chem 1949;1:311–326.
8. Griffin WC. Calculation of HLB values of non-ionic surfactants. J Soc Cosmet Chem 1954;5(1):249–256.
9. Baxter K, Preston CL, eds. Stockley's Drug Interactions. 10th Ed. London: Pharmaceutical Press, 2013.
10. Chiou WL. Aerosol propellants: Cardiac toxicity and long biological half-life. JAMA 1974;227:658.
11. Cyr TD, Graham SJ, Li KY, et al. Low first-spray drug content in albuterol metered-dose inhalers. Pharm Res 1991;8:658–660.
12. Miller NC, Marple VA, Schults RK, et al. Assessment of the twin impinger for size measurement of metered-dose inhaler sprays. Pharm Res 1992;9:1123–1127.
13. Ranucci JA, Chen FC. Phase Doppler anemometry: A technique for determining aerosol plume-particle size and velocity. Pharm Technol 1993;17:62–73.
14. Ranucci JA, Cooper D, Sethachutkul K. Effect of actuator design on metered-dose inhaler plume-particle size. Pharm Technol 1992;16:84–92.
15. Martonen TB, Katz IM. Deposition of aerosolized drugs within human lungs: Effects of ventilatory parameters. Pharm Res 1993;10:871–878.
16. Martonen TB, Katz I, Fults K, et al. Use of analytically defined estimates of aerosol respirable fraction to predict lung deposition patterns. Pharm Res 1992;9:1634–1639.

SECTION SEVEN

Sterile Dosage Forms and Delivery Systems

15 Parenterals

OBJECTIVES

After reading this chapter, the student will be able to:

List the advantages and disadvantages of parenteral administration

Define parenteral administration, and list the different parenteral methods of administration

Compare and contrast the risks and benefits of the various parenteral routes

Identify the challenges of using nonaqueous vehicles in parenteral products

Define osmolality and osmolarity, and explain their relationship with the tonicity of a substance

Compare and contrast a small-volume and a large-volume parenteral

Outline the different methods of sterilization for parenteral products

Differentiate between single- and multiple-dose packaging requirements

Identify the measures for proper handling and disposal of hazardous substances/chemotherapy

Compare and contrast total parenteral nutrition (TPN) preparations to total nutritional admixture (TNA) preparations

INTRODUCTION

Considered in this chapter are important pharmaceutical dosage forms with the common characteristic of sterility, that is, they are free from contaminating microorganisms. Among these sterile dosage forms are the various small- and large-volume injectable preparations, irrigation fluids intended to bathe body wounds or surgical openings, and dialysis solutions. Biologic preparations, including vaccines, toxoids, and antitoxins, also among this group are discussed in Chapter 16. Sterility in these preparations is essential because they are placed in direct contact with the internal body fluids or tissues, where infection can easily arise. Ophthalmic preparations, which are also prepared to be sterile, are discussed separately in Chapter 17.

INJECTIONS

Injections are sterile, pyrogen-free (endotoxin units [EU] limited) preparations intended to be administered parenterally. The term *parenteral* refers to the injectable routes of administration. It derives from the Greek words *para* (outside) and *enteron* (intestine) and denotes routes of administration other than the oral route. *Pyrogens*, or bacterial endotoxins, are organic metabolic products shed from Gram-negative bacteria, which can cause fever and hypotension in patients when they are in excessive amounts in intravenous (IV) injections. Pyrogens and the determination of their presence in parenteral preparations are discussed later in this chapter. In general, the parenteral routes are used when rapid drug action is desired, as in emergencies; when the patient is uncooperative, unconscious, or unable to accept or tolerate oral medication; or when the drug itself is ineffective by other routes. With the exception of insulin injections, which are commonly *self*-administered by diabetics, most injections are administered by the physician, physician's assistant, or nurse in the course of medical treatment. Thus, injections are employed mostly in the hospital, extended care facility, clinic, and, less frequently, at home. An exception is *home health care* programs, in which health professionals pay scheduled visits to patients at home, providing needed treatment, including IV medications. These programs enable patients who do not require or are unable to pay for more expensive hospitalization to remain at home while receiving appropriate medical care. The pharmacist supplies injectable preparations to the physician and nurse as required for use in the institutional setting, clinic, office, or home health care program.

Perhaps the earliest injectable drug to receive official recognition was the hypodermic morphine solution, which appeared first in the 1874 addendum to the 1867 *British Pharmacopeia* and, in 1888, in the first edition of the *National Formulary (NF) of the United States*. Today, literally hundreds of drugs and drug products are available for parenteral administration.

Parenteral Routes of Administration

Drugs may be injected into almost any organ or area of the body, including the joints (*intra-articular*), joint fluid area (*intrasynovial*), spinal column (*intraspinal*), spinal fluid (*intrathecal*), arteries (*intra-arterial*), and, in an emergency, even the heart (*intracardiac*). However, most injections go into a vein (*intravenous, IV*), into a muscle (*intramuscular, IM*), into the skin (*intradermal, ID; intracutaneous*), or under the skin (*subcutaneous, SC; sub-Q, SQ; hypodermic, hypo*) (Fig. 15.1).

Intravenous Route

IV injection of drugs had its scientific origin in 1656 in the experiments of Sir Christopher Wren, architect of St Paul's Cathedral and amateur physiologist. Using a bladder and quill for a syringe and needle, he injected wine, ale, opium, and other substances into the veins of dogs and studied their effects. IV medication was first given to humans by Johann Daniel Major of Kiel in 1662 but was abandoned for a period because of thrombosis and embolism in the patients so treated. The invention of the hypodermic syringe toward the middle of the 19th century created new interest in IV techniques, and toward the turn of the 20th century, IV administration of solutions of sodium chloride and glucose became popular. Today, IV administration of drugs is a routine occurrence in the hospital, although recognized dangers are still associated with the practice. Thrombus and embolus formation may be induced by IV needles and catheters, and the possibility of particulate matter in parenteral solutions poses a concern.

IV drugs provide rapid action compared with other routes of administration, and because drug absorption is not a factor, optimum blood levels may be achieved with accuracy and immediacy not possible by other routes. In emergencies, IV administration of a drug may be lifesaving because of the placement of the drug directly into the circulation and the prompt action that ensues. On the negative side, once a drug is administered intravenously, it cannot be retrieved. In the case of an adverse reaction to the drug, for instance, the drug cannot be easily removed from the circulation, as it could, for example, by induction of vomiting after oral administration of the same drug. Furthermore, the IV dose may differ greatly from the oral dose. Thus, great care must be taken to prevent overdosing or underdosing. The beta-blocker drug class, such as

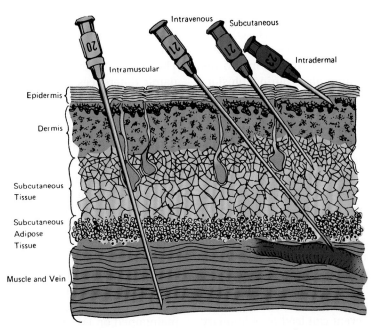

FIGURE 15.1. Routes of parenteral administration. Numbers on needles indicate gauge of the needles (outside diameter of shaft). (Reprinted from Turco S, King RE. Sterile Dosage Forms: Their Preparation and Clinical Applications. 3rd Ed. Philadelphia, PA: Lea & Febiger, 1987, with permission.)

metoprolol, is a perfect example of the vast differences between IV (three bolus injections of 5 mg each at about 2-minute intervals) and oral dosing (100 mg/d).

Although most superficial veins are suitable for venipuncture, the basilic and cephalic veins on the back of the hand and dorsal forearm are the best peripheral veins for IV therapy. The antecubital vein is not preferred for IV therapy because it is a point of great inflection with a high risk of extravasation. Most clinicians insert the needle with the bevel facing upward, at the most acute angle possible with the vein, to ensure that the direction of flow of the injectable is that of the flow of the blood. Strict aseptic precautions must be taken at all times to avoid the risk of infection. Not only are the injectable solutions sterile, the syringes and needles must also be sterilized, and the point of entrance must be disinfected to reduce the chance of carrying bacteria from the skin into the blood via the needle. Before injection, the health care worker must withdraw the plunger of the syringe or squeeze a special bulb found on most IV sets to ensure that the needle has been properly seated. A backflow of blood into the administration set or syringe indicates proper placement of the needle in the vein.

Both small and large volumes of drug solutions may be administered intravenously. The use of 1,000-mL containers of solutions for IV infusion is commonplace in the hospital. These solutions, containing such agents as nutrients, plasma volume expanders, electrolytes, amino acids, and other therapeutic agents, are administered through an indwelling needle or catheter by continuous infusion. The infusion or flow rate may be adjusted according to the needs of the patient. Generally, flow rates for IV fluids are expressed in milliliters per hour and range from 42 to 150 mL/h. Lower rates are used for keep open (KO, KVO) lines. For IV infusion, the needle or catheter is placed in a prominent vein of the forearm or leg and taped firmly to the patient so that it will not slip from place during infusion. The main hazard of IV infusion is thrombus formation induced by the catheter or needle touching the wall of the vein. Thrombi are most likely when the infusion solution is irritating to the biologic tissues. A *thrombus* is a blood clot formed within the blood vessel (or heart), usually because of slowing of the circulation or an alteration of the blood or vessel wall. Once such a clot circulates, it becomes an *embolus*, carried by the blood stream until it lodges in a blood vessel, obstructing it and resulting in a block or occlusion referred to as an *embolism*. Such an obstruction may be a critical hazard to the patient, depending on the site and severity of the obstruction.

IV drugs ordinarily must be in aqueous solution; they must mix with the circulating blood and not precipitate from solution. Such an event can lead to pulmonary microcapillary occlusion and blockage of blood flow. IV fat emulsions (e.g., Intralipid, 20% to 30%, Baxter; Liposyn II, 10% to 20%, Hospira; Liposyn III, 10% to 30%, Hospira) have gained acceptance for use as a source of calories and essential fatty acids for patients requiring parenteral nutrition for extended periods, usually more than 5 days. The product contains up to 30% soybean oil emulsified with egg yolk phospholipids in a vehicle of glycerin in water for injection. The emulsion is administered via a peripheral vein or by central venous infusion.

Naturally, the IV route is used for blood transfusions, and it also serves as the point of exit for removal of blood from patients for diagnostic work and for donation.

In the late 1980s, automated IV delivery systems for intermittent self-administration of analgesics became commercially available. Patient-controlled analgesia (PCA) has been used to control the pain associated with a variety of surgical procedures, labor, sickle cell crisis, and cancer. For patients with chronic malignant pain, PCA allows a greater degree of ambulation and independence (1).

The typical PCA device includes a syringe or chamber that contains the analgesic drug and a programmable electromechanical unit. The unit, which may be compact enough to be worn on a belt or carried in a pocket (e.g., WalkMed PCA, McKinley, Wheat Ridge, CO), controls the delivery of drug by advancing a piston when the patient presses a button. The drug can be loaded into the device by a health care professional or dispensed from preloaded cartridges available from the manufacturer. The devices deliver IV bolus injections to produce rapid analgesia, along with slower infusion to produce steady-state concentrations for sustained pain control.

The advantage of the PCA is its ability to provide constant and uniform analgesia. The typical injection of an opioid into a depot muscular site may result in variable absorption, leading to unpredictable blood concentrations. Furthermore, these injections are usually given when needed and are often inadequate to treat the pain. The PCA can prevent pharmacokinetic and pharmacodynamic differences between patients from interfering with the effectiveness of analgesia. Because opioid kinetics differ greatly among patients, the rates of infusion must be tailored (2).

The PCA also permits patients to medicate themselves for breakthrough pain. It eliminates the delay between the perception of pain and receiving the medication. Furthermore, it saves nursing time. Otherwise, the nurse must check the analgesic orders given by the physician; sign out the pain reliever from a controlled, locked location; and then administer the medication to the patient.

The PCA also provides better pain control with less side effects by minimizing the variations between suboptimal pain relief and overuse of opioids. When the side effect profile of PCA patients is compared to those of patients maintained on IM opioids, nausea, sedation, and respiratory depression occur less often in the PCA group. Finally, patients accept the PCA as a favorable mode of relief, perhaps because of the sense of being in control and taking an active part in their pain relief.

PCA devices can be used for IV, SC, or epidural administration. Usually, these devices are either *demand dosing* (a fixed dose of drug is injected intermittently) or *constant-rate infusion plus demand dosing* (2). Regardless of the type used, the physician or nurse establishes the loading dose, the rate of background infusion, dose per demand, lockout interval (minimum time between demand doses), and maximum dosage over a specified time. Figure 15.2 demonstrates the LifeCare PCA Infusion System. With this device, the patient pushes a button on a pendant to deliver a prescribed quantity of the analgesic.

Intramuscular Route

IM injections of drugs provide effects that are less rapid but generally longer lasting than those obtained from IV administration (3). Aqueous or oleaginous solutions or suspensions of drug substances may be administered intramuscularly. Depending on the type of preparation, absorption rates vary widely. Drugs in solution are more rapidly absorbed than those in suspension, and drugs in aqueous preparations are more rapidly absorbed than oleaginous preparations. The physical type of preparation is based on the properties of the drug itself and on the therapeutic goals.

IM injections are performed deep into the skeletal muscles. The point of injection should be as far as possible from major nerves and blood vessels. Injuries to patients from IM injection usually are related to the point at which the needle entered and where the medication was deposited. Such injuries include paralysis resulting from neural

damage, abscess, cyst, embolism, hematoma, sloughing of the skin, and scarring.

In adults, the upper outer quadrant of the gluteus maximus is the most frequently used site for IM injection. In infants, the gluteal area is small and composed primarily of fat, not muscle. The muscle is poorly developed. An injection in this area may come dangerously close to the sciatic nerve, especially if the child is resisting the injection and squirming or fighting. Thus, in infants and young children, the deltoid muscles of the upper arm or the mid-lateral muscles of the thigh are preferred. An injection in the upper or lower portion of the deltoid would be well away from the radial nerve. The deltoid may also be used in adults, but the pain is more noticeable here than in the gluteal area. If a series of injections are to be given, the injection site is usually varied. To be certain that a blood vessel has not been entered, the clinician may aspirate slightly on the syringe following insertion of the needle to observe any blood entering the syringe. The volume of medication that may be conveniently administered by the IM route is limited, generally to a maximum of 5 mL in the gluteal region and 2 mL in the deltoid of the arm.

The Z-track technique is useful for IM injections of medications that stain the upper tissue, such as iron dextran injection, and those that irritate the tissue, such as diazepam, by sealing these medications in the lower muscle. Because of its staining qualities, iron dextran must be injected only into the muscle mass of the upper outer quadrant of the buttock. The skin is displaced laterally prior to injection, then the needle is inserted and the syringe aspirated, and the injection performed slowly and smoothly. The needle is then withdrawn and the skin released. This creates a Z pattern that blocks infiltration of medication into the SC tissue. The injection is 2 to 3 inches deep, and a 20- to 22-gauge needle is used. To reduce any further staining of the upper tissue, usually one needle is used to withdraw the iron dextran from its ampul and replaced with another for the injection.

Subcutaneous Route

The SC route may be used for injection of small amounts of medication. Injection of a drug beneath the skin is usually made in the loose interstitial tissue of the outer upper arm, the anterior thigh, or the lower abdomen. The site of injection is usually rotated when injections are frequently given, as with daily insulin injections. Prior to injection, the skin at the injection site should be thoroughly cleansed. The maximum amount of medication that can be comfortably injected subcutaneously is about 1.3 mL, and amounts greater than 2 mL will most likely cause painful pressure. Syringes with up to 3-mL capacities and 24- to 26-gauge needles are used. These needles have cannula lengths of three-eighths of an inch to an inch. Most typically, SC insulin needles are 25 to 30 gauge with length of five-sixteenth to five-eighth of an inch. Upon insertion, if blood appears in the syringe, a new site should be selected.

FIGURE 15.2. LifeCare PCA Infusion System. (Courtesy of Hospira, Inc.)

Irritating drugs and those in thick suspension may produce induration, sloughing, or abscess and may be painful. Such preparations are not suitable for SC injection.

Intradermal Route

A number of substances may be effectively injected into the corium, the more vascular layer of the skin just beneath the epidermis. These substances include various agents for diagnostic determinations, desensitization, or immunization. The usual site for ID injection is the anterior forearm. A short (three-eighth of an inch) and narrow (23- to 26-gauge) needle is usually employed. The needle is inserted horizontally into the skin, with the bevel facing up. The injection is made with the bevel just disappearing into the corium. Usually, only about 0.1 mL may be administered in this manner.

Specialized Access

When it is necessary to administer repeated injections over time, it is prudent to employ devices that provide continued access and reduce pain associated with administration.

Several types of central venous catheters are used in institutions and on an outpatient basis for a variety of parenteral medications (e.g., cancer chemotherapy, long-term antibiotic therapy, TPN solutions). They can remain in place for a few days to several months. When not in use, they require heparinization to maintain patency of the catheter lumen.

The use of indwelling plastic catheters reduces the need for multiple punctures during IV therapy. Composed of polyvinyl chloride (PVC), Teflon, and polyethylene, these should be radiopaque to ensure that they are visible on radiographs. Usually, these must be removed within 48 hours after insertion. The choice of catheter depends on several factors, including length of time of the infusion, purpose of the infusion, and condition and availability of the veins. Three types of catheters are available: plain plastic, catheter over needle or catheter outside needle, and catheter inside needle.

The injection ports on Broviac and Hickman central vein catheters are not implanted subdermally. They are external usually at the abdomen after the catheter is tunneled under the abdomen and chest to access the superior vena cava. These do carry a risk of morbidity, including fracture of the catheters, entrance site infection, and catheter sepsis. Developed to overcome catheter complications, they are designed to provide repeated access to the infusion site. The delivery catheter can be placed in a vein, cavity, artery, or the central nervous system. A Huber point needle is used to inject through the skin into the rubber septum of a totally implanted central vein access device.

Official Types of Injections

According to the USP, injectable materials are separated into five general types. These may contain buffers, preservatives, and other added substances:

1. *Injection*: Liquid preparations that are drug substances or solutions thereof (e.g., Insulin Injection, USP)

2. *For injection*: Dry solids that, upon addition of suitable vehicles, yield solutions conforming in all respects to the requirements for injections (e.g., Cefuroxime for Injection, USP)

3. *Injectable emulsion*: Liquid preparation of drug substance dissolved or dispersed in a suitable emulsion medium (e.g., Propofol, USP)

4. *Injectable suspension*: Liquid preparation of solid suspended in a suitable liquid medium (e.g., Methylprednisolone Acetate Suspension, USP)

5. *For injectable suspension*: Dry solid that, upon addition of suitable vehicle, yields preparation conforming in all respects to the requirements for *injectable suspensions* (e.g., Imipenem and Cilastatin for Injectable Suspension, USP)

The form in which the manufacturer prepares a given drug for parenteral use depends on the nature of the drug itself with respect to its physical and chemical characteristics and on certain therapeutic considerations. Generally, if a drug is unstable in solution, it may be prepared as a dry powder intended for reconstitution with a proper solvent at the time of administration, or it may be prepared as a suspension. If the drug is unstable in water, that solvent may be replaced in part or totally by a solvent in which the drug is insoluble. If the drug is insoluble in water, an injection may be prepared as an aqueous suspension or as a solution in a suitable nonaqueous solvent, such as a vegetable oil. If an aqueous solution is desired, a water soluble salt form of the insoluble drug is frequently prepared. Aqueous or blood-miscible solutions may be injected directly into the bloodstream. Blood-immiscible liquids, such as oleaginous injections and suspensions, can interrupt the normal flow of blood, and their use is generally restricted to other than IV administration. The onset and duration of action of a drug may be somewhat controlled by its chemical form, the physical state of the injection (solution or suspension), and the vehicle. Drugs that are very much soluble in body fluids generally have the most rapid absorption and onset of action. Thus, drugs in aqueous solution have a more rapid onset of action than do drugs in oleaginous solution. Drugs in aqueous suspension are also more rapid acting than drugs in oleaginous suspension because of the greater miscibility of the aqueous preparation with the body fluids after injection and the more rapid contact of the drug particles with the body fluids. Oftentimes, long action is desired to reduce the frequency of injections. These long-acting injections are called repository or depot preparations.

The solutions and suspensions of drugs intended for injection are prepared in the same general manner as solutions (Chapter 13) and disperse systems (Chapter 14), with the following differences:

1. Solvents or vehicles must meet special purity and other standards ensuring their safety by injection.

2. The use of added substances, such as buffers, stabilizers, and antimicrobial preservatives, falls under

specific guidelines of use and is restricted in certain parenteral products. The use of coloring agents is strictly prohibited.

3. Parenteral products are always sterilized, must meet sterility standards, and must not exceed allowable endotoxin limits (ELs).

4. Parenteral solutions must meet compendial standards for particulate matter.

5. Parenteral products must be prepared in environmentally controlled areas, under strict sanitation standards, and by personnel specially trained and clothed to maintain the sanitation standards.

6. Parenteral products are packaged in special hermetic containers of specific and high quality. Special quality control procedures are used to ensure hermetic seal and sterile condition.

7. Each container of an injection is filled to a volume in slight excess of the labeled volume to be withdrawn. This overfilling permits ease of withdrawal and administration of the labeled volumes.

8. The volume of injection permitted in multiple-dose containers is restricted, as are the types of containers (single dose or multiple dose) that may be used for certain injections.

9. Specific labeling regulations apply to injections.

10. Sterile powders intended for solution or suspension immediately prior to injection are frequently packaged as lyophilized or freeze-dried powders to permit ease of solution or suspension upon the addition of the solvent or vehicle.

11. Extemporaneously prepared parenteral preparations must be compounded in a USP <797> compliant facility.

Solvents and Vehicles for Injections

The most frequently used solvent in the large-scale manufacturer of injections is *Water for Injection, USP*. This water is purified by distillation or by reverse osmosis and meets the same standards for the presence of total solids as does *Purified Water, USP*—that is, not more than 1 mg/100 mL Water for Injection, USP—and may not contain added substances. Although water for injection is not required to be sterile, it must be pyrogen-free. The water is intended to be used in the manufacture of injectable products to be sterilized after preparation. Water for injection should be stored in tight containers at temperatures below or above the range in which microbial growth occurs. Water for injection is intended to be used within 24 hours after collection. Naturally, the water should be collected in sterile and pyrogen-free containers. The containers are usually glass or glass lined.

Sterile Water for Injection, USP, is packaged in single-dose containers not larger than 1 L. As with water for injection, it must be pyrogen-free but does have an allowable endotoxin level, not more than 0.25 USP EU/mL. Also, it may not contain any antimicrobial agent or other added substance. This water may contain slightly more total solids than water for injection because of the leaching of solids from the glass-lined tanks during sterilization. This water is intended to be used as a solvent, vehicle, or diluent for already sterilized and packaged injectable medications. The 1-L bottles cannot be administered intravenously because they have no tonicity. Thus, they are used for reconstitution of multiple antibiotics. In use, the water is aseptically added to the vial of medication to prepare the desired injection. For instance, a suitable injection may be prepared from the dry powder Sterile Ampicillin Sodium, USP, by aseptic addition of sterile water for injection.

Bacteriostatic Water for Injection, USP, is sterile water for injection containing one or more suitable antimicrobial agents. It is packaged in prefilled syringes or in vials containing not more than 30 mL of the water. The container label must state the names and proportions of the antimicrobial agent or agents. The water is employed as a sterile vehicle in the preparation of small volumes of injectable preparations. Theoretically, presence of the bacteriostatic agent gives the flexibility for multiple-dose vials. If the first person to withdraw medication inadvertently contaminates the vial contents, the preservative will destroy the microorganism, although there has been debate on how much protection the antimicrobial agent can provide in a multiple-dose vial (4). Because of the presence of antimicrobial agents, the water must be used only in parenterals that are administered in small volumes. Its use in parenterals administered in large volume is restricted by the excessive and perhaps toxic amounts of the antimicrobial agents that would be injected along with the medication. Generally, if more than 5 mL of solvent is required, sterile water for injection rather than bacteriostatic water for injection is preferred. In using bacteriostatic water for injection, due regard must also be given to the chemical compatibility of the bacteriostatic agent or agents with the particular medicinal agent being dissolved or suspended.

USP labeling requirements demand that the label state NOT FOR USE IN NEONATES. This statement was the result of problems encountered with neonates and toxicity of the bacteriostat, that is, benzyl alcohol. This toxicity results from the high cumulative amounts (milligrams per kilogram) of benzyl alcohol and the limited detoxification capacity of the neonate liver. This solution has not been reported to cause problems in older infants, children, or adults.

Benzyl alcohol poisoning is recognized as gasping syndrome. In one study, 10 premature infants developed this clinical syndrome characterized by the development of multiorgan failure and eventually died (5). The typical clinical course included metabolic acidosis, respiratory distress requiring mechanical ventilation, central nervous system dysfunction, hyperactivity, hypotonia, depression of the sensorium, apnea, seizure, coma, intraventricular hemorrhage, hepatic and renal failure, and eventual cardiovascular collapse and death. In the study, the amount of benzyl alcohol received ranged from 99 to 234 mg/kg/d. Based on the concentration of 0.9% benzyl alcohol in the bacteriostatic water for injection and sodium chloride injection, death resulted from as little as 11 mL/kg/d.

Following toxicity reports and the deaths of infants in the early 1980s, the FDA issued a very strong recommendation to stop the use of fluids preserved with benzyl alcohol for use in neonates as a flush solution or to reconstitute medications.

Sodium Chloride Injection, USP, is a sterile isotonic solution of sodium chloride in water for injection. It contains no antimicrobial agents but has approximately 154 mEq each of sodium and chloride ions per liter. It may be used as a sterile vehicle in solutions or suspensions of drugs for parenteral administration.

Besides its use to reconstitute medications for injection, sodium chloride injection is frequently used as a catheter or IV line flush to maintain patency. Catheters or IV lines are constantly used to infuse fluids and IV medications and draw blood for laboratory analysis, among others. Usually, 2 mL is used to flush the line after each use or every 8 hours if the line is not used.

Bacteriostatic Sodium Chloride *Injection, USP*, is a sterile isotonic solution of sodium chloride in water for injection. It contains one or more suitable antimicrobial agents, which must be specified on the labeling. Sodium chloride 0.9% renders the solution isotonic. For the reasons noted for bacteriostatic water for injection, this solution may not be packaged in containers larger than 30 mL. When this solution is used as a vehicle, care must be exercised to ensure compatibility of the added medicinal agent with the preservative or preservatives and with the sodium chloride.

Bacteriostatic sodium chloride injection is also used to flush a catheter or IV line to maintain its patency. When used in only small quantities for flushing lines and reconstituting medications, the amount of benzyl alcohol is negligible and safe. But in neonates, especially premature infants with very low birth weights, accumulation of benzoic acid and unmetabolized benzyl alcohol may occur as a result of liver immaturity. Because of their low physical weight, their acute illness and consequent need for medications, and the frequent use of the umbilical catheter for various purposes, these patients may receive much more flush solution relative to their body weight than adults. Thus, bacteriostatic sodium chloride injection also carries the warning NOT FOR USE IN NEONATES.

Suffice it to say that benzyl alcohol may be present in other parenteral medications, and the pharmacist must be vigilant for its inappropriate use in neonates. Generally speaking, however, the amount of benzyl alcohol received through this means is negligible compared to the amount received from flush solutions. Preferably, the medication is available in a preservative-free formulation (i.e., single-use dose), and that should be used. However, if such a formulation is not available and there is no alternative, a medication preserved with benzyl alcohol may still be used if the physician's clinical judgment is that the risk-to-benefit ratio is appropriate.

Ringer Injection, USP, is a sterile solution of sodium chloride, potassium chloride, and calcium chloride in water for injection. The three agents are present in concentrations similar to those of physiologic fluids. Ringer's is employed as a vehicle for other drugs or alone as an electrolyte replenisher and plasma volume expander. *Lactated Ringer Injection, USP*, has different quantities of the three salts in Ringer injection, and it contains sodium lactate. This injection is a fluid and electrolyte replenisher and a systemic alkalizer.

Nonaqueous Vehicles

Although an aqueous vehicle is generally preferred for an injection, it may be precluded by the limited water solubility of a medicinal substance or its susceptibility to hydrolysis. When such physical or chemical factors limit the use of a wholly aqueous vehicle, the pharmaceutical formulator must turn to one or more nonaqueous vehicles.

The selected vehicle must be nonirritating, nontoxic in the amounts administered, and not sensitizing. Like water, it must not exert a pharmacologic activity of its own, nor may it adversely affect the activity of the medicinal agent. In addition, the physical and chemical properties of the solvent or vehicle must be considered, evaluated, and determined to be suitable for the task at hand. Among the many considerations are the solvent's physical and chemical stability at various pH levels, viscosity, which must be such as to allow ease of injection (suitable for use in syringes); fluidity, which must be maintained over a fairly wide temperature range; boiling point, which should be sufficiently high to permit heat sterilization; miscibility with body fluids; low vapor pressure to avoid problems during heat sterilization; and constant purity or ease of purification and standardization. No single solvent is free of limitations; hence, cross-consideration and assessment of each solvent's advantages and disadvantages help the formulator determine the most appropriate solvent for a given preparation. Among the nonaqueous solvents employed in parenteral products are fixed vegetable oils, glycerin, polyethylene glycols, propylene glycol, alcohol, and a number of less often used agents, including ethyl oleate, isopropyl myristate, and dimethylacetamide. These and other nonaqueous vehicles may be used provided they are safe in the amounts administered and do not interfere with the therapeutic efficacy of the preparation or with its response to prescribed assays and tests.

The USP specifies restrictions on the fixed vegetable oils in parenteral products. For one thing, they must remain clear when cooled to 10°C (50°F) to ensure the stability and clarity of the injectable product during refrigeration. The oils must not contain mineral oil or paraffin, as these materials are not absorbed by body tissues. The fluidity of a vegetable oil generally depends on the proportion of unsaturated fatty acids, such as oleic acid, to saturated acids, such as stearic acid. Oils to be employed in injections must meet officially stated requirements of iodine number and saponification number.

Although the toxicity of vegetable oils is generally considered to be relatively low, some patients exhibit allergic reactions to specific oils. Thus, when vegetable oils are employed in parenteral products, the label must state the specific oil. The most commonly used fixed oils in injections are corn oil, cottonseed oil, peanut oil, and sesame oil. Castor oil and olive oil have been used on occasion (Physical Pharmacy Capsule 15.1).

PHYSICAL PHARMACY CAPSULE **15.1** Colligative Properties of Drugs

Drug molecules have properties that are often divided into additive, constitutive, or colligative.
 Additive properties depend on the total contribution of the atoms in the molecule or on the sum of the properties of the constituents of the solution. An example is molecular weight.

 Constitutive properties depend on the arrangement and, to a lesser extent, the number and kind of atoms in a molecule. Examples are refraction of light, electrical properties, and surface and interfacial properties.

 Colligative properties depend primarily on the number of particles in solution. Example properties include changes in vapor pressure, boiling point, freezing point, and osmotic pressure. These values should be approximately equal for equimolar concentrations of drugs.

■ LOWERING OF VAPOR PRESSURE

A vapor in equilibrium with its pure liquid at a constant temperature will exert *vapor pressure*. When a solute is added to the pure liquid, it will alter the tendency of the molecules to escape the original liquid. In an ideal solution or one that is very dilute, the partial vapor pressure of one component (p_1) is proportional to the mole fraction of molecules (N_1) of that component in the mixture:

$$p_1 = N_1 p^\circ_1$$

where p°_1 is the vapor pressure of the pure component.

■ EXAMPLE 1

What is the partial vapor pressure of a solution containing 50 g dextrose in 1,000 mL of water? The vapor pressure of water is given as 23.76 mm Hg.

1. (50 g dextrose)/(MW of 180) = 0.28 mol of dextrose
2. (1,000 g water)/(MW of 18) = 55.56 mol of water
3. 0.28 + 55.56 = 55.84 total moles
4. (55.56)/(55.84) = 0.995 mole fraction of water
5. p_1 = (0.995)(23.76 mm Hg) = 23.64 mm Hg

The vapor pressure of the solution is 23.64 mm Hg. The decrease in vapor pressure by the addition of the 50 g dextrose is 23.76 − 23.64 = 0.12 mm Hg.

■ INCREASE IN BOILING POINT

The *boiling point* of a liquid is the temperature at which the vapor pressure of the liquid comes into equilibrium with the atmospheric pressure. The vapor pressure is reduced when a nonvolatile solute is added to a solvent, so that the solution must reach a higher temperature to reestablish the equilibrium, hence, an increase in the boiling point. This is described in the following equation:

$$\Delta T_b = k_b m$$

where

 ΔT_b is the change in boiling point,
 k_b is the molar elevation constant of water, and
 m is the molality of the solute.

■ EXAMPLE 2

What is the boiling point elevation of a solution containing 50 g dextrose in 1,000 mL of water? The molal elevation constant of water is 0.51.

1. (50 g dextrose)/(MW of 180) = 0.28 mol of dextrose in 1,000 mL of water or 0.28-molal solution
2. ΔT_b = (0.51) (0.28) = 0.143°C

(continued)

(continued)

■ DECREASE IN FREEZING POINT

The *freezing point* of a pure liquid is the temperature at which the solid and liquid phases are in equilibrium at 1 atm. The freezing point of a solution is the temperature at which the solid phase of pure solvent and the liquid phase of solution are in equilibrium at 1 atm pressure. When a solute is added to a solvent, the decrease in freezing point is proportional to the concentration of the solute. The relationship is described by the following equation:

$$\Delta T_f = k_f m$$

where

ΔT_f is the change in freezing point,
k_f is the molal freezing point depression constant of water, and
m is the molality of the solute.

■ EXAMPLE 3

What is the decrease in freezing point of a solution containing 50 g dextrose in 1,000 mL of water? The molal elevation constant of water is −1.86°C.

1. (50 g dextrose)/(MW of 180) = 0.28 mol of dextrose in 1,000 mL of water or 0.28-mol solution
2. ΔT_f = (−1.86) (0.28) = −0.52°C

■ OSMOTIC PRESSURE

The pressure that must be applied to a more concentrated solution to prevent the flow of pure solvent into the solution separated by a semipermeable membrane is called the *osmotic pressure*. This relationship can be expressed as follows:

$$PV = nRT$$

where

P is the pressure (atm),
V is the volume (L),
n is number of moles of solute,
R is the gas constant (0.082 L atm/mol deg), and
T is the absolute temperature (°C).

■ EXAMPLE 4

What is the osmotic pressure of 50 g dextrose in 1,000 mL of water at room temperature (25°C)?

1. (50 g dextrose)/(MW of 180) = 0.28 mol of dextrose.
2. 273°C + 25°C = 298°C.
3. Volume will be 1 L.
4. P = [(0.28)(0.082)(298)]/(1) = 6.84 atm.

Deviations from reality in these ideal examples of colligative properties are explained by the use of the van't Hoff term, which considers that electrolytes exert more pressure than nonelectrolytes and is related to the number of ionic species present. These deviations may be caused by ionic interaction, degree of dissociation of weak electrolytes, or associations of nonelectrolytes.

■ MILLIEQUIVALENTS

An *equivalent weight* is the atomic weight in grams of a material divided by its valence or charge. Milliequivalents are related to equivalents, which are also considered measures of combining power, chemical activity, or chemical reactivity. Equivalency, or milliequivalency, takes into consideration the total number of ionic charges in solution and the valence of the ions. Normally, plasma contains about 155 mEq of cations and anions in solution. The number of cations is always matched by the number of anions.

A *milliequivalent* is the quantity in milligrams of a solute equal to 1/1,000 of its gram equivalent weight. Consider the following example.

■ EXAMPLE 5

What is the milliequivalent weight of sodium?

1. The atomic weight of sodium is 23.
2. The valence of sodium is +1.

(continued)

3. The equivalent weight of sodium is (23 g)/(1) = 23 g.
4. The milliequivalent weight of sodium is (23 g)/1,000 = 0.023 g, or 23 mg.
5. Therefore, 1 mEq of sodium weighs 23 mg.

Milliequivalent calculations are commonly required in pharmacy practice today. The following are some examples.

■ EXAMPLE 6

How many milliequivalents of potassium chloride are in a solution containing 74.5 mg/mL?

1. The atomic weight of potassium is 39 and that of chloride is 35.5. The combined molecular weight is 74.5.
2. Because the valence is 1 for both potassium and chloride, the equivalent weight for potassium chloride is 74.5 g, and the milliequivalent weight is 74.5 mg.
3. The solution contains 74.5 mg/mL, and the milliequivalent weight is 74.5 mg; therefore, there is 1 mEq/mL of potassium chloride in the solution.

■ EXAMPLE 7

How many milliequivalents of calcium are in 10 mL of 10% calcium chloride ($CaCl_2 \cdot 2H_2O$) solution?

1. The formula weight for calcium chloride dihydrate is 147.
2. The equivalent weight is 147/2 = 73.5, because calcium is divalent (i.e., valence = +2).
3. Therefore, 1 mEq of calcium chloride weighs 73.5 mg.
4. (10 mL) (10%) = 1 g, or 1,000 mg, of calcium chloride dihydrate.
5. (1,000 mg)/(73.5 mg) = 13.6 mEq of calcium chloride dihydrate, which also is 13.6 mEq of calcium.

■ EXAMPLE 8

How many milliequivalents of sodium are contained in a 1-L bag of 0.9% sodium chloride?

1. (1,000 mL) (0.009) = 9 g, or 9,000 mg.
2. The formula weight for sodium chloride is 23 + 35.5 = 58.5.
3. The milliequivalent weight for sodium chloride is 58.5 mg.
4. (9,000)/(58.5) = 153.8 mEq or 154 mEq.

In these cases, because sodium chloride is monovalent, there is 154 mEq of sodium, 154 mEq of chloride, or 154 mEq of sodium chloride.

■ OSMOLALITY AND TONICITY

Biologic systems are compatible with solutions having similar osmotic pressures, that is, an equivalent number of dissolved species. For example, red blood cells, blood plasma, and 0.9% sodium chloride solution contain approximately the same number of solute particles per unit volume and are termed iso-osmotic and isotonic.

If solutions contain more (hypertonic) or fewer (hypotonic) dissolved species, it may be necessary to alter the composition of the solution to bring them into an acceptable range.

An osmol (Osm) is related to a mole (gram molecular weight) of the molecules or ions in solution. One mole of glucose (180 g) dissolved in 1,000 g of water has an osmolality of 1 Osm, or 1,000 mOsm/kg of water. One mole of sodium chloride (23 + 35.5 g = 58.5 g) dissolved in 1,000 g of water has an osmolality of almost 2,000 mOsm, because sodium chloride dissociates into almost two particles per molecule. In other words, a 1-molal solution of sodium chloride is equivalent to a 2-molal solution of dextrose.

Normal serum osmolality values are in the vicinity of 285 mOsm/kg (often expressed as 285 mOsm/L). Ranges may include values from about 275 to 300 mOsm/L. Pharmaceuticals should be close to this value to minimize discomfort on application to the eyes or nose or on injection.

Some solutions are iso-osmotic but not isotonic. This is because the physiology of the cell membranes must be considered. For example, the cell membrane of the red blood cell is not semipermeable to all drugs. It allows ammonium chloride, alcohol, boric acid, glycerin, propylene glycol, and urea to diffuse freely. In the eye, the cell membrane is semipermeable to boric acid, and a 1.9% solution of boric acid is an isotonic ophthalmic solution. But even though a 1.9% solution of boric acid is isotonic with the eye and is iso-osmotic, it is not isotonic with blood—because boric acid can freely diffuse through the red blood cells—and it may cause hemolysis.

Pharmacists are often called upon to calculate the quantity of solute that must be added to adjust a hypotonic solution of a drug to isotonic. This can be done using several methods, including L-value, sodium chloride equivalent, and cryoscopy.

(continued)

(continued)

One of the most frequently used methods for calculating the quantity of sodium chloride necessary to prepare an isotonic solution is the *sodium chloride equivalent method*. A sodium chloride equivalent is the amount of sodium chloride that is osmotically equivalent to 1 g of the drug. For example, the sodium chloride equivalent of ephedrine sulfate is 0.23, that is, 1 g of ephedrine sulfate is equivalent to 0.23 g of sodium chloride.

■ EXAMPLE 9

How much sodium chloride is required to make the following prescription isotonic?

Rx Ephedrine sulfate 2%
Sterile water, qs 30 mL
M. isoton with sodium chloride

1. (30 mL) (0.009) = 0.270 g sodium chloride is required if only sodium chloride is present in the 30 mL of solution.
2. (30 mL) (0.02) = 0.6 g ephedrine sulfate is to be present.
3. (0.6 g) (0.23) = 0.138 g is the quantity of sodium chloride represented by the ephedrine sulfate.
4. Because 0.270 g sodium chloride is required if only sodium chloride is used and the quantity of sodium chloride that is equivalent to 0.6 g of ephedrine sulfate is 0.138 g, then 0.270 g − 0.138 g = 0.132 g of sodium chloride required to render the solution isotonic.
5. Therefore, the solution requires ephedrine sulfate 0.6 g, sodium chloride 0.132 g, and sufficient sterile water to make 30 mL. ■

By selective employment of solvent or vehicle, a pharmacist can prepare injectable preparations as solutions or suspensions in either an aqueous or nonaqueous vehicle. For the most part, oleaginous injections are administered intramuscularly. They must not be administered intravenously, as the oil will occlude the pulmonary microcirculation. Some examples of official injections with oil as the vehicle are presented in Table 15.1.

Added Substances

The USP permits addition of suitable substances to official preparations intended for injection to increase stability or usefulness as long as the substances are not interdicted in the individual monographs, are harmless in the amounts administered, and do not interfere with the therapeutic efficacy of the preparation or with specified assays and tests. Many of these added substances are antibacterial preservatives, buffers, solubilizers, antioxidants, and other adjuncts. Agents employed solely for their coloring effect are strictly prohibited in parenteral products.

The USP requires that one or more suitable substances be added to parenteral products that are packaged in multiple-dose containers to prevent the growth of microorganisms regardless of the method of sterilization employed, unless otherwise directed in the individual monograph or unless the injection's active ingredients are themselves bacteriostatic. Such substances are used in concentrations that prevent the growth of or kill microorganisms. Because many of the usual preservative agents are toxic in large amounts or irritating when parenterally administered, special care must be exercised in the selection of the appropriate preservative agents. For the following preservatives, the indicated maximum limits prevail for use in a parenteral product unless otherwise directed: for agents containing mercury and the cationic surface-active compounds, 0.01%; for agents such as chlorobutanol, cresol, and phenol, 0.5%; and for sulfur dioxide as an antioxidant or for an equivalent amount of the sulfite, bisulfite, or metabisulfite of potassium or sodium, 0.2%.

In addition to the stabilizing effect of the additives, the air accompanying an injectable product is frequently replaced with an inert gas, such as nitrogen, to enhance the stability of the product by preventing a chemical reaction between oxygen and the drug.

Methods of Sterilization

The term *sterilization*, as applied to pharmaceutical preparations, means destruction of all living organisms and their spores or their complete removal from the preparation. Five general methods are used to sterilize pharmaceutical products:

1. Steam
2. Dry heat
3. Filtration
4. Gas
5. Ionizing radiation

The method is determined largely by the nature of the preparation and its ingredients. However, regardless of the method used, the resulting product must pass a test for sterility as proof of the effectiveness of the method and the performance of the equipment and personnel.

Steam Sterilization

Steam sterilization is conducted in an autoclave and employs steam under pressure. It is usually the method of choice if the product can withstand it (Fig. 15.3).

TABLE 15.1. Some Injections in Oil

Injection	Oil	Category
Dimercaprol	Peanut	Antidote to arsenic, gold, and mercury poisoning
Estradiol cypionate	Cottonseed	Estrogen
Estradiol valerate	Sesame or castor	Estrogen
Fluphenazine decanoate	Sesame	Antipsychotic
Fluphenazine enanthate	Sesame	Antipsychotic
Hydroxyprogesterone caproate	Castor	Progestin
Progesterone in oil	Sesame or peanut	Progestin
Testosterone cypionate	Cottonseed	Androgen
Testosterone cypionate and estradiol cypionate	Cottonseed	Androgen and estrogen
Testosterone enanthate	Sesame	Androgen
Testosterone enanthate and estradiol valerate	Sesame	Androgen and estrogen

Most pharmaceutical products are adversely affected by heat and cannot be heated safely to the temperature required for dry heat sterilization (about 150°C to 170°C or 302°F to 338°F). When moisture is present, bacteria are coagulated and destroyed at a considerably lower temperature than when moisture is absent. In fact, bacterial cells with a large percentage of water are generally killed rather easily. Spores, which contain a relatively low percentage of water, are comparatively difficult to destroy. The mechanism of microbial destruction in moist heat is thought to be by denaturation and coagulation of some of the organism's essential protein. It is the hot moisture in the microbial cell that permits destruction at relatively low temperature. Death by dry heat is thought to be by dehydration of the microbial cell followed by slow oxidation. Because it is not possible to raise the temperature of steam above 100°C (212°F) under atmospheric conditions, pressure is employed to achieve higher temperatures. It is the temperature, not the pressure, that destroys the microorganisms, and the application of pressure is solely to increase the temperature of the system. Time is another important factor in the destruction of microorganisms by heat. Most modern autoclaves have gauges to indicate to the operator the internal conditions of temperature and pressure and a timing device to permit the desired exposure time for the load. The usual steam pressures, the temperatures obtainable under these pressures, and the approximate length of time required for sterilization after the system reaches the indicated temperatures are as follows:

10-lb pressure (115.5°C or 240°F) for 30 minutes
15-lb pressure (121.5°C or 250°F) for 20 minutes
20-lb pressure (126.5°C or 260°F) for 15 minutes

As can be seen, the greater the pressure applied, the higher the temperature obtainable and the less the time required for sterilization.

Most autoclaves routinely operate at 121°C (250°F), as measured at the steam discharge line running from the autoclave. The temperature in the chamber of the autoclave must also be reached by the interior of the load being sterilized, and this temperature must be maintained for an adequate time. The penetration time of moist heat into the load varies with the nature of the load, and the exposure time must be adjusted to account for this latent period. For example, a solution packaged in a thin-walled 50-mL ampul may reach 121°C in 6 to 8 minutes after that temperature is registered in the steam discharge line, whereas 20 minutes or longer may be required to reach that temperature within a solution packaged in a completely filled, thick-walled 1,000-mL glass bottle. An estimate of these latent periods must be added to the total time to ensure adequate exposure times. This process depends on moisture and an elevated temperature, so air is removed from the chamber as sterilization begins, because a combination of air and steam yields a lower temperature than does steam alone under the same pressure. For instance, at 15-lb pressure, the temperature of saturated steam is 121.5°C, but a mixture of equal parts of air and steam will reach only about 112°C (234°F).

In general, steam sterilization is applicable to pharmaceutical preparations and materials that can withstand the required temperatures and are penetrated but not adversely affected by moisture. In aqueous solutions, the moisture is already present, and all that is required is elevation of the temperature of the solution for the pre-

FIGURE 15.3. Autoclaving of IV electrolyte solutions. (Courtesy of Hospira, Inc.)

scribed period. Thus, solutions in sealed containers, such as ampuls, are readily sterilized by this method. Sealed empty vials can be sterilized by autoclaving only if they contain a small quantity of water. Steam sterilization is also applicable to bulk solutions, glassware, surgical dressings, and instruments. It is not useful for oils, fats, oleaginous preparations, and other preparations not penetrated by moisture or for exposed powders that may be damaged by the condensed moisture.

Dry Heat Sterilization

Dry heat sterilization is usually carried out in ovens designed for this purpose. The ovens may be heated either by gas or by electricity and are generally thermostatically controlled.

Because dry heat is less effective in killing microorganisms than is moist heat, higher temperatures and longer periods of exposure are required. These must be determined for each product with consideration to the size and type of product and the container and its heat distribution characteristics. In general, individual units to be sterilized should be as small as possible, and the sterilizer should be loaded so as to permit free circulation of heated air throughout the chamber. Dry heat sterilization is usually conducted at 150°C to 170°C for not less than 2 hours. Higher temperatures permit shorter exposure for a given article; conversely, lower temperatures require longer exposure times. For example, if a particular chemical agent melts or decomposes at 170°C but is unaffected at 140°C (284°F), the lower temperature is used, and the exposure time is increased.

Dry heat sterilization is generally employed for substances that are not effectively sterilized by moist heat. Such substances include fixed oils; glycerin; various petroleum products, such as petrolatum, liquid petrolatum (mineral oil), and paraffin; and various heat-stable powders, such as zinc oxide. Dry heat is also an effective method for sterilizing glassware and surgical instruments. Dry heat is the method of choice when dry apparatus or dry containers are required, as in the handling of packaging of dry chemicals or nonaqueous solutions.

Sterilization by Filtration

Sterilization by filtration, which depends on the physical removal of microorganisms by adsorption on the filter medium or by a sieving mechanism, is used for heat-sensitive solutions. Medicinal preparations sterilized by this method must undergo extensive validation and monitoring because the effectiveness of the filtered product can be greatly influenced by the microbial load in the solution being filtered.

Commercially available filters are produced with a variety of pore size specifications. It would be well to mention briefly one type of modern filter, the Millipore filter (Fig. 15.4). The Millipore filter is a thin plastic membrane of cellulosic esters with millions of pores per square inch. The pores are made to be extremely uniform in size and

FIGURE 15.4. Membrane filters act as microporous screens that retain all particles and microorganisms larger than the rated pore size on their surface. (Courtesy of Millipore Corporation.)

occupy approximately 80% of the membrane's volume, the remaining 20% being the filter material. This high degree of porosity permits flow rates much in excess of those of other filters having the same particle retention capability. Millipore filters are made from a variety of polymers to be suitable for filtration of almost any liquid or gas system. Also, the filters have various pore sizes, 14 to 0.025 μm, to meet the specific requirements. For comparative purposes, the period that ended the last sentence is approximately 500 μm. The smallest particle visible to the naked eye is about 40 μm, a red blood cell is about 6.5 μm, the smallest bacterium is about 0.2 μm, and a poliovirus is about 0.025 μm.

Although the pore size of a bacterial filter is of prime importance in the removal of microorganisms from a liquid, other factors, such as the electrical charge on the filter and that of the microorganism, the pH of the solution, the temperature, and the pressure or vacuum applied to the system, are also important.

The major advantages of bacterial filtration include its speed in the filtration of small quantities of solution, its ability to sterilize thermolabile materials, the relatively inexpensive equipment required, the development and proliferation of membrane filter technology, and the complete removal of living and dead microorganisms and other particulate matter from the solution.

The class of filter medium lends itself to more effective standardization and quality control and also gives the user greater opportunity to confirm the properties of the filter assembly before and after use. The fact that membrane filters are thin polymeric films offers many advantages but also some disadvantages compared to depth filters, such as porcelain or sintered material. Because much of the membrane surface is a void or open space, the properly assembled and sterilized filter offers the advantage of a high flow rate.

One disadvantage is that because the membrane tends to be fragile, it is essential to determine that the assembly was properly made and that the membrane was not ruptured or flawed during assembly, sterilization, or use. The housing and filter assemblies should first be validated for

FIGURE 15.5. Luer-Lok syringes with syringe filters. (Courtesy of Olha Rohulya/Shutterstock.)

compatibility and integrity. This disadvantage is a circumstance not true of methods involving dry or moist heat sterilization, in which the procedures are just about guaranteed to give effective sterilization. Also, filtration of large volumes of liquids requires more time, particularly if the liquid is viscous, than, say, steam sterilization. In essence, bacterial filters are useful when heat cannot be used and also for small volumes of liquids.

Bacterial filters may be used conveniently and economically in the community pharmacy to filter extemporaneously prepared solutions (as ophthalmic solutions) that must be sterile (Figs. 15.5 and 15.6). Furthermore, the membrane filter is the method most commonly used in hospitals. Occasionally, in the past, hospitals used the autoclave (moist heat) to sterilize IV solutions, which were then unavailable commercially, for example, caffeine citrate, and many community pharmacies use autoclave sterilization for high-risk sterile compounding today.

To date, information about drug adsorption to membrane filters is limited. Several studies, however, have demonstrated that membrane filters can remove drug from solution (6–9). For example, 0.22-μm filters reduce the in vitro antimicrobial activity of amphotericin B (a colloidal suspension), whereas filtration of the amphotericin B through 0.85- and 0.45-μm filters did not. Butler et al. (10) demonstrated that the potency of drugs administered intravenously and in small doses could be significantly reduced during in-line filtration with a filter containing

a cellulose ester membrane. The literature indicates that drugs administered in low doses might present a problem of bonding to the filter. Many filters in clinical use are nitrate or acetate esters of cellulose. These compounds are polar and have residual hydroxyl groups that may adsorb drug. Hydrophobic interactions between hydrocarbon portions of drug molecules being filtered and linear cellulose molecules of filters are also thought to contribute to drug adsorption.

In general, current information suggests that little or no adsorption takes place with membrane filters. However, it is recommended that minute doses of drugs (<5 mg) should not be filtered until sufficient data demonstrate insignificant adsorption. With respect to amphotericin B, to ensure the passage of the antibiotic colloidal dispersion, the filter's mean pore diameter should be more than 1 μm.

Membrane filter media include cellulose acetate, cellulose nitrate, fluorocarbonate, acrylic polymers, polycarbonate, polyester, PVC, vinyl, nylon, polytef, and even metal membranes, and they may be reinforced or supported by an internal fabric.

Gas Sterilization

Some heat-sensitive and moisture-sensitive materials can be sterilized much better by exposure to ethylene oxide or propylene oxide gas than by other means. These gases are highly flammable when mixed with air but can be employed safely when properly diluted with an inert gas such as carbon dioxide or a suitable fluorinated hydrocarbon. Such mixtures are commercially available.

Sterilization by this process requires specialized equipment resembling an autoclave, and many combination steam autoclaves and ethylene oxide sterilizers are commercially available. Greater precautions are required for this method of sterilization than for some of the others, because the variables—for instance, time, temperature, gas concentration, and humidity—are not as firmly quantitated as those of dry heat and steam sterilization. In general, sterilization with gas is enhanced, and the exposure time required is reduced, by increasing the relative humidity of the system (to about 60%) and by increasing the exposure temperature to 50°C to 60°C. If the material being sterilized cannot tolerate either the moisture or the elevated temperature, exposure time must be increased. Generally, sterilization with ethylene oxide gas requires 4 to 16 hours of exposure. Ethylene oxide is thought to sterilize by interfering with the metabolism of the bacterial cell.

The great penetrating qualities of ethylene oxide gas make it a useful agent in certain special applications, such as sterilization of medical and surgical supplies and appliances such as catheters, needles, and plastic disposable syringes in their final plastic packaging just prior to shipment. The gas is also used to sterilize certain heat-labile enzyme preparations, certain antibiotics, and other drugs, after testing to ensure the absence of chemical reaction and other deleterious effects on the drug substance.

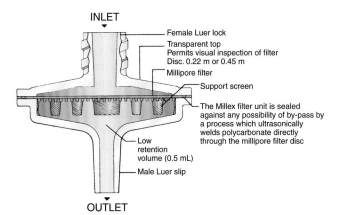

FIGURE 15.6. Cutaway showing composition of the Millex filter unit. (Courtesy of Millipore Corporation.)

Sterilization by Ionizing Radiation

Techniques are available for sterilization of some types of pharmaceuticals by gamma rays and by cathode rays, but application of such techniques is limited because of the highly specialized equipment required and the effects of irradiation on the products and their containers.

The exact mechanism by which irradiation sterilizes a drug or preparation is still subject to investigation. One of the proposed theories is alteration of the chemicals within or supporting the microorganism to form deleterious new chemicals capable of destroying the cell. Another theory proposes that vital structures of the cell, such as the chromosomal nucleoprotein, are disoriented or destroyed. It is probably a combination of irradiation effects that causes the cellular destruction, which is complete and irreversible.

Validation/Verification of Sterility

Regardless of the method, pharmaceutical preparations required to be sterile must undergo tests to confirm the absence of microorganisms. The USP contains monographs and standards for biologic indicators of sterilization. A *biologic indicator* is a characterized preparation of specific microorganisms resistant to a particular sterilization process. They may be used to monitor a sterilization cycle and/or periodically to revalidate the process. Biologic indicators are generally of two main forms. In one, spores are added to a carrier, such as a strip of filter paper, packaged to maintain physical integrity while allowing the sterilization effect. In the other, the spores are added to representative units of the product being sterilized, with assessment of sterilization based on these samples. In steam and ethylene oxide sterilization, spores of suitable strains of *Bacillus stearothermophilus* are commonly employed because of their resistance to these modes of sterilization. In dry heat, spores of *Bacillus subtilis* are commonly used. With ionizing radiation, spores of suitable strains of *Bacillus*, including *B. pumilus*, *B. stearothermophilus*, and *B. subtilis*, have been used.

The effectiveness of thermal sterilization has been quantified through the determination and calculation of *F value* to express the time of thermal death. *Thermal death time* is defined as the time required to kill a particular organism under specified conditions. The F_0 at a particular temperature other than 121°C is the time in minutes required to provide lethality equivalent to that provided at 121°C for a stated time.

Although heat distribution in an autoclave chamber is usually rapid, with 121°C obtained nearly instantaneously throughout the autoclave, the product being sterilized may not achieve identical conditions because of a variety of factors of heat transfer, including the thermal conductivity of the packaging components, the viscosity and density of the product, container proximity, passage of steam around containers, and other variables. F values may be computed from biologic data derived from the rate of destruction of known numbers of microorganisms, as shown in the following equation:

$$F_0 = D_{121}(\log A - \log B)$$

where

D_{121} is the time required for a one-log reduction in the microbial population exposed to a temperature of 121°C, A is the initial microbial population, and B is the number of microorganisms that survive after a defined heating time (11).

A one-log reduction is a 90% decrease in the number of microbes in the product. If there were 1,000 viable microbes in the starting product, a one-log reduction would decrease the number of viable microbes in the container to 100.

In compounding, verification is used that involves authoritatively signed assurance and documentation that a process, procedure, or piece of equipment is functioning properly and producing the expected results. Verification may require outside laboratory testing when in-house capabilities are not adequate.

Pyrogen and Endotoxin Testing

Endotoxins are a subset of pyrogens that come from Gram-negative bacteria. The terms endotoxin and lipopolysaccharide are often used interchangeably. However, to be more precise, endotoxins are the natural complex of lipopolysaccharides that occur in the outer layer of bilayered Gram-negative bacterial cells, whereas lipopolysaccharides are the purified form used as a standard for quality control and research purposes.

Inadvertent administration of endotoxins to humans may result in a number of events, ranging from fever, through a cascade of pathogenic responses, to death. Responses can include irreversible and fatal septic shock, hypotension, lymphopenia, neutrophilia, and elevated levels of cortisol and C-reactive protein.

Endotoxins are potent, toxic, and very stable and are present in many pharmaceutical ingredients and on surfaces that come into contact with preparations formulated for parenteral administration. They are water soluble, will pass through 0.2-μm filters, are not destroyed by autoclaving, and are insoluble in organic solvents. Endotoxins are very difficult to eliminate in a final preparation. Therefore, procedures are directed at eliminating endotoxins during the preparation process.

The body can tolerate a certain load of endotoxins (measured as endotoxin units, or EU) without adverse results. The generally accepted EL (Endotoxin Load) is defined as

$$EL = K / M$$

where K is the threshold human pyrogenic dose of endotoxin per kilogram of body weight per hour, which is 5.0 EU/kg for parenteral drugs (except those administered intrathecally) and 0.2 EU/kg for the intrathecal route of administration, and where M is maximum recommended human dose per kilogram of body weight that would be administered in a single 1-hour period.

The EL, then, is equal to the threshold pyrogenic response (K in EU/kg) divided by the dose in the units by which it is administered (milliliters, units, or milligrams) per 70-kg person per hour. The delivery method (multiple or bolus doses) and other factors must also be considered.

To use the EL = K/M formula, it is necessary to know the maximum endotoxin levels established for the drugs being prepared. Individual USP/NF monographs contain information regarding endotoxin level limits. The most recent edition of that compendium should be consulted to determine if the information has been updated.

See Physical Pharmacy Capsule 15.2 for example calculations.

PHYSICAL PHARMACY CAPSULE **15.2** Endotoxin Calculations

■ ALLOWABLE ENDOTOXIN LEVELS IN PARENTERAL PREPARATIONS

Pharmacists compounding high-risk sterile preparations from bulk substances must be proficient in calculating the endotoxin load for the compounded preparations. The endotoxin load in compounded sterile preparations (CSPs) can be calculated as follows:

1. Multiply the weight of the patient (in kilograms) times the allowable endotoxin units (EU) per kilogram (kg) [EU/kg] to obtain the endotoxin limit per hour for nonintrathecal or for intrathecal medication delivery.
   EU/kg × patient weight (kg) = EL per hour (nonintrathecal)
   or
   0.2 EU/kg × patient weight (kg) = EL per hour (intrathecal)
2. Obtain the required information for the calculations from *USP–NF* or a current EL table.
3. Determine the final volume of the preparation.
4. Input the information on the EL worksheet.
5. Determine the final endotoxin load.
6. Consider the route of administration, and determine if the calculated value exceeds the value in Step 1.
7. If the calculated value does not exceed the value in Step 1, the compound may be prepared.
8. If the calculated value exceeds the value in Step 1, check with the prescriber.
   The amount of endotoxin present in the sample must be less than the endotoxin release limit calculated for the given end preparation. If the endotoxin level is excessive and the parenteral has been dispensed, the patient's doctor should be notified, and the patient should be monitored for characteristic host reactions to pyrogens.

■ RESOURCES

1. Allen LV Jr. Quality-control analytical methods: Allowable endotoxin levels in sterile preparations. Int J Pharm Compd 2004;8(6):466–467.
2. Allen LV Jr. Quality-control analytical methods: Allowable endotoxin levels in sterile preparations. Int J Pharm Compd 2004;8(6):479–485.
3. Stockton S. Endotoxin calculations. Int J Pharm Compd 2004;8(6):468.

■ EXAMPLE

1. A 158-lb patient is to receive an intrathecal infusion of morphine sulfate at a rate of 0.3 mg/h. The solution will be prepared by diluting Infumorph 200 with 0.9% sodium chloride injection to produce an infusion rate of 2 mL/h.
   A. Infumorph 200 is preservative-free morphine sulfate 10 mg/mL in 20-mL ampuls. How much Infumorph 200 and 0.9% sodium chloride injection should be used to prepare a 24-hour infusion?
   • 0.3 mg/h × 24 hours = 7.2 mg morphine sulfate
   • 7.2 mg × 1 mL/10 mg = 0.72 mL Infumorph 200
   • 2 mL/h × 24 h = 48 mL total volume
   • 48 mL − 0.72 mL = 47.28 mL 0.9% sodium chloride injection

   B. What is the endotoxin load for this preparation?
   The USP specifies a limit of 14.29 USP EU/mg of morphine sulfate in solutions for intrathecal use and a limit of 0.5 EU/mL for solutions containing 0.5% to 0.9% sodium chloride:

(continued)

(continued)

- 7.2 mg × 14.29 EU/mg = 102.89 EU from morphine sulfate
- 47.28 mL × 0.5 EU/mL = 23.64 EU from 0.9% sodium chloride injection
- Endotoxin load = 102.89 EU + 23.64 EU = 126.53 EU
- 126.53 EU/24 h = 5.27 EU/h

C. Does this limit exceed the allowable EL for an intrathecal injection for this patient?
The maximum amount of endotoxin in a solution for intrathecal administration is 0.2 EU/kg/h.
Allowable limit: 0.2 EU/kg/h × 1 kg/2.2 lb × 158 lb = 14.36 EU/h
The endotoxin load in the preparation does not exceed the allowable limit.

2. Epinephrine is administered subcutaneously or intramuscularly as a 1:1,000 solution and is supplied in 1-mL ampuls.

A. What is the potential endotoxin load in a 1-mL ampul of epinephrine 1:1,000 solution?
- The USP specifies a limit of 357 USP EU/mL of epinephrine in solutions for injection.
- 1 mL × 1 g/1,000 mL × 1,000 mg/g × 357 EU/mg = 357 EU

B. What is the minimum weight (in pounds) of a patient that could receive this dose without exceeding the threshold pyrogenic dose of 5 EU/kg/h, assuming that the patient receives no more than one dose per hour?
- 357 EU × 1 kg/5 EU × 2.2 lb/kg = 157.08 lb

3. The following is an order for a parenteral nutrition solution to be administered to a patient weighing 184 lb at a rate of 70 mL/h:
Component Source
- Amino acids 4% 500 mL of 8.5% amino acids injection
- Dextrose 25% 500 mL of 70% dextrose injection
- Sodium acetate 20 mEq 50-mL vial of 32.8% solution
- Potassium chloride 15 mEq 25-mL vial of 14.9% solution
- Magnesium sulfate 10 mEq 10-mL vial of 12.5% magnesium sulfate heptahydrate solution
- Calcium gluconate 5 mEq 50-mL vial of 10% solution
- Potassium phosphate 15 mmol 10-mL vial of 3 mmol/mL solution
- Sterile water for injection 1,000 mL of sterile water for injection to make 1,000 mL

A. What is the endotoxin load for this solution?
- The ELs specified by the USP for each of the solutions are as follows:
- Amino acids: Endotoxin information is unavailable
- Dextrose: 10 EU/g of dextrose in solutions containing 5% to 70% dextrose
- Sodium acetate: 3.9 EU/mEq of sodium acetate
- Potassium chloride: 8.8 EU/mEq of potassium chloride
- Magnesium sulfate: 0.09 EU/mg of magnesium sulfate
- Calcium gluconate: 0.17 EU/mg of calcium gluconate
- Potassium phosphate: 1.1 EU/mg of potassium phosphates
- Sterile water for injection: 0.25 EU/mL of sterile water
- Dextrose: 25 g/100 mL × 1,000 mL = 250 g × 10 EU/g = 2,500 EU
- Sodium acetate: 20 mEq × 3.9 EU/mEq = 78 EU
- Potassium chloride: 15 mEq × 8.8 EU/mEq = 132 EU
- Magnesium sulfate (MgSO$_4$·7H$_2$O, MW = 246):
- 10 mEq × 246 mg/2 mEq = 1,230 mg × 0.09 EU/mg = 110.7 EU
- Calcium gluconate [Ca(C$_6$H$_{11}$O$_7$)$_2$, MW = 430]:
- 5 mEq × 430 mg/2 mEq = 1,075 mg × 0.17 EU/mg = 182.75 EU
- Potassium phosphate: 15 mmol × 1 mL/3 mmol = 5 mL
- Potassium phosphates injection contains 236 mg potassium phosphate, dibasic, and 224 mg potassium phosphate, monobasic per milliliter
- 5 mL × 236 mg K$_2$HPO$_4$/mL = 1,180 mg
- 5 mL × 224 mg KH$_2$PO$_4$/mL = 1,120 mg
- Total = 2,300 mg × 1.1 EU/mg = 2,530 EU
- In order to determine the amount of water to add, the volumes of each additive must be calculated:
- Amino acids: 4 g/100 mL × 1,000 mL = 40 g × 100 mL/8.5 g = 470.59 mL
- Dextrose: 25 g/100 mL × 1,000 mL = 250 g × 100 mL/70 g = 357.14 mL
- Sodium acetate (NaC$_2$H$_3$O$_2$, MW = 82):
- 20 mEq × 82 mg/mEq × 1 g/1,000 mg × 100 mL/32.8 g = 5 mL
- Potassium chloride (KCl, MW = 74.5):
- 15 mEq × 74.5 mg/mEq × 1 g/1,000 mg × 100 mL/14.9 g = 7.5 mL
- Magnesium sulfate: 1,230 mg × 1 g/1,000 mg × 100 mL/12.5 g = 9.84 mL

(continued)

- Calcium gluconate: 1,075 mg × 1 g/1,000 mg × 100 mL/10 g = 10.75 mL
- Potassium phosphate: 5 mL
- Total volume = 865.82 mL
- Amount of water to add:
- 1,000 mL − 865.82 mL = 134.18 mL × 0.25 EU/mL = 33.54 EU
- Total endotoxin load = 5,566.99 EU (without amino acids)

B. What is the maximum amount of endotoxin that this patient may receive per hour from the parenteral nutrition solution, and does this amount exceed the limit of 5 EU/kg/h?

5,566.99 EU/1,000 mL × 70 mL/h = 389.69 EU/h from parenteral nutrition solution
5 EU/kg/h × 184 lb × 1 kg/2.2 lb = 418.18 EU/h limit for patient

The nutrition solution does not exceed the EL for this particular patient; however, because the amino acid information is not available, there is potential for the solution to exceed the limit. ∎

USP injection monographs state a bacterial EU limit, USP EU. Thus, injections are not pyrogen- or endotoxin-free but are limited. The following are examples from the USP–NF (12):

Dextrose Injection: Contains not more than 0.5 USP EU/mL for injections containing less than 5% dextrose and not more than 10.0 USP EU/mL for injections containing between 5% and 70% dextrose.
Digoxin Injection: Contains not more than 200.0 USP EU/mg of digoxin.
Gentamicin Injection: Contains not more than 0.71 USP EU/mg of gentamicin.

Pyrogen Test Manufacturers of water for injection may employ any suitable method for removal of pyrogens from their product. Because pyrogens are organic, one of the more common means of removing them is by oxidizing them to easily eliminated gases or to nonvolatile solids, both of which are easily separated from water by fractional distillation. Potassium permanganate is usually employed as the oxidizing agent, with its efficiency increased by addition of a small amount of barium hydroxide to impart alkalinity to the solution and to make nonvolatile barium salts of any acidic compounds that may be present. These two reagents are added to water that has been distilled several times, and distillation is repeated, the chemical-free distillate being collected under strict aseptic conditions. When properly conducted, this method results in highly pure, sterile, and pyrogen-free water. However, in each instance, the official pyrogen test must be performed to ensure the absence of these fever-producing materials.

The USP pyrogen test uses healthy rabbits that have been properly maintained in terms of environment and diet before the test. Normal, or control, temperatures are taken for each animal to be used in the test. These temperatures are used as the base for the determination of any temperature increase resulting from injection of a test solution. A given test uses rabbits whose temperatures do not differ by more than 1°C from each other and whose body temperatures are considered not to be elevated. A synopsis of the procedure of the test is as follows.

Render the syringes, needles, and glassware free from pyrogens by heating at 250°C for not less than 30 minutes or by other suitable method. Warm the product to be tested to 37°C ± 2°C.

Inject into an ear vein of each of three rabbits 10 mL of the product per kilogram of body weight, completing each injection within 10 minutes of the start of administration. Record the temperature at 30-minute intervals 1 to 3 hours subsequent to the injection.

If no rabbit shows an individual rise in temperature of 0.5°C or more, the product meets the requirements for the absence of pyrogens. If any rabbit shows an individual temperature rise of 0.5°C or more, continue the test using five other rabbits. If not more than three of the eight rabbits show individual rises in temperature of 0.5°C or more and if the sum of the eight individual maximum temperature rises does not exceed 3.3°C, the material under examination meets the requirements for the absence of pyrogens.

Endotoxin Test An extract from the blood cells of the horseshoe crab (*Limulus polyphemus*) contains an enzyme and protein system that coagulates in the presence of low levels of lipopolysaccharides. This discovery led to the development of the *Limulus* amebocyte lysate (LAL) test for the presence of bacterial endotoxins. The Bacterial Endotoxins Test, USP, uses LAL and is considered generally more sensitive to endotoxin than the rabbit test. The FDA has endorsed it as a replacement for the rabbit test, and it is used for a number of parenteral products. The USP–NF has specific allowable endotoxin levels for various injections based on the dosage of the individual drugs to keep below a threshold level of administered endotoxins.

Some parenteral products, however, cannot be tested with LAL because the active ingredient interferes with the outcome. Such products include meperidine HCl and promethazine HCl, oxacillin sodium, sulfisoxazole, and vancomycin HCl, among others. These must be tested with the aforementioned Pyrogen Test, USP.

Because the LAL test is so sensitive for the presence of bacterial endotoxins, when the active ingredient of the small-volume parenteral can interfere with the test, a strategy to overcome this interference is to dilute the product more than twofold. Diphenhydramine HCl, ephedrine HCl, meperidine HCl, promethazine HCl, and thiamine HCl, among others, are tested in this manner.

The Industrial Preparation of Parenteral Products

Once the formulation for a particular parenteral product is determined, including selection of the proper solvents or vehicles and additives, the production pharmacist must follow rigid aseptic procedures in preparing the products. In most manufacturing plants, the area in which parenteral products are made is maintained bacteria-free by use of ultraviolet lights; a filtered air supply; sterile manufacturing equipment, such as flasks, connecting tubes, and filters; and sterilized work clothing (Fig. 15.7).

In the preparation of parenteral solutions, the required ingredients are dissolved according to good pharmaceutical practice in water for injection, in another solvent, or in a combination of solvents. The solutions are usually filtered through a membrane until sparkling clear. After filtration, the solution is transferred as rapidly as possible and with the least possible exposure into the final containers. The product is then sterilized, preferably by autoclaving, and samples of the finished product are tested for sterility and pyrogens. If sterilization by autoclaving is impractical because of the nature of the ingredients, the individual components of the preparation that are heat or moisture labile may be sterilized by other appropriate means and added aseptically to the sterilized solvent or solution of components that can be autoclaved.

Suspensions of drugs for parenteral use may be prepared by reducing the drug to a very fine powder with a ball mill, micronizer, colloid mill, or other appropriate equipment and then suspending the material in a liquid in which it is insoluble. It is frequently necessary to sterilize separately the individual components of a suspension before combining them, as frequently the integrity of a suspension is destroyed by autoclaving. Autoclaving of a parenteral suspension may alter the viscosity of the product,

affecting the suspending ability of the vehicle, or change the particle size of the suspended particles, altering both pharmaceutical and therapeutic characteristics. If a suspension remains unaltered by autoclaving, this method is generally employed to sterilize the final product. Because parenteral emulsions, which are dispersions or suspensions of a liquid throughout another liquid, are generally destroyed by autoclaving, an alternative method of sterilization must be employed for this type of injectable.

Some injections are packaged as dry solids rather than in conjunction with a solvent or vehicle because the therapeutic agent is unstable in the presence of the liquid component. These dry powders are packaged in the final container to be reconstituted, generally to a solution or less frequently a suspension. The method of sterilization of the powder may be dry heat or another appropriate method. These are examples of sterile drugs prepared and packaged *without* pharmaceutical additives such as buffers, preservatives, stabilizers, and tonicity agents:

Ampicillin sodium
Ceftizoxime sodium
Ceftazidime sodium
Cefuroxime sodium
Kanamycin sulfate
Nafcillin sodium
Penicillin G benzathine
Streptomycin sulfate
Tobramycin sulfate

Antibiotics are prepared industrially in large fermentation tanks.

Sterile drugs formulated *with* pharmaceutical additives and intended to be reconstituted prior to injection include the following:

Cyclophosphamide
Dactinomycin
Erythromycin lactobionate
Hydrocortisone sodium succinate
Mitomycin
Nafcillin sodium
Penicillin G potassium
Vinblastine sulfate

Sometimes, a liquid is packaged along with the dry powder for use at the time of reconstitution (Fig. 15.8). This liquid is sterile and may contain some of the desired pharmaceutical additives, such as the buffering agents. More frequently, the solvent or vehicle is not provided, but the label generally lists suitable solvents. Sodium chloride injection and sterile water for injection are perhaps most frequently employed to reconstitute dry-packaged injections. The dry powders are packaged in containers large enough to permit proper shaking with the liquid component when the latter is aseptically injected through the container's rubber closure during reconstitution. To facilitate dissolution, the dry powder is prevented from caking upon standing by the appropriate means, including lyoph-

FIGURE 15.7. Sterile filling of vials. (Courtesy of Wyeth Laboratories.)

FIGURE 15.10. ADD-Vantage system. (Courtesy of Hospira, Inc.)

FIGURE 15.8. The Mix-O-Vial contains dry ingredients in the bottom compartment and a liquid diluent in the top, separated by a specially formulated center seal. The bottom compartment can be filled either with a liquid that is frozen and dried to make a lyophilized product or with a powder. The diluent in the top contains a preservative and sometimes one or more active ingredients. To use the vial, the dust cover is removed (A and B) and pressure is applied (C) to the top plunger, which dislodges the center seal; and the vial is shaken well. The top of the plunger is then swabbed with a disinfectant; the syringe needle inserted through the target circle on the plunger; and the contents of the vial withdrawn into the syringe. The Mix-O-Vial offers stability of the product until it is activated, convenience, fast operation, and safety as regards the right drug with the proper diluent in the correct proportions.

ilization (Fig. 15.9). Powders so treated form a honeycomb lattice structure that is rapidly penetrated by the liquid, and solution is rapid because of the large surface area of powder exposed.

Pfizer manufactures the Mix-O-Vial, which incorporates the cover as part of the plunger. Once mixed, the small circle of plastic that covers the injection site is removed. This reduces the touch contamination potential.

The Hospira ADD-Vantage system is another example of a ready-to-mix sterile IV product designed for intermittent administration of potent drugs that do not have long-term stability in solution. With this system, antibiotics and other drugs do not have to be mixed until just prior

to administration. ADD-Vantage consists of two components (Fig. 15.10): a flexible plastic IV container partially filled with diluent and a glass vial of powdered or liquid drug. The vials containing the medication and the piggybacks (50 to 250 mL of dextrose 5% in water injection, 0.45% sodium chloride solution, or 0.9% sodium chloride injection) are specially designed to be used together. The vial locks into a chamber inside the plastic container, and the drug is released by removing the stopper on the vial, allowing the two components to mix. This simple process is performed by external manipulation of the container, preserving the closed, sterile system.

The ADD-Vantage unit may be assembled in a number of locations. Microbiologic tests and sterility tests have been conducted at various intervals following assembly of the units under a laminar flow hood, in a pharmacy on a countertop, and in a patient's hospital room. The final admixtures were sterile, demonstrating that the ADD-Vantage unit can be aseptically assembled under the conditions tested. The assembled but not activated ADD-Vantage system can be used within 30 days of removal of the diluent container from the outer wrapping. ADD-Vantage enables hospitals to reduce drug waste, often caused by canceled or changed prescriptions, and helps the pharmacy conserve labor and reduce material costs.

The BD UltraSafe Passive Needle Guard (Becton Dickinson Pharmaceutical Systems) is one example of an IV infusion system for use in preparing extemporaneous IV admixtures or for patient administration (Fig. 15.11).

FIGURE 15.9. Antibiotic lyophilizers. (Courtesy of Hospira, Inc.)

FIGURE 15.11. BD UltraSafe passive needle guard. (Courtesy of Becton Dickinson Pharmaceutical Systems.)

When compared to the two traditional methods of preparing small-volume infusions, that is, the transfer needle and vial (TFN) and syringe and vial (SYR) methods, the systems with needle guards performed quite favorably, saving time, using fewer materials, and costing less (13).

This system is an integrated drug transfer mechanism with a protective shield surrounding the attached transfer needle. Reconstitution and transfer of the drug into an infusion bag are accomplished safely, quickly, and with few materials. The needle is inserted into the port of the infusion bag, and the transfer set is pushed down toward the vial until it clicks. With the Monovial upright, the infusion bag is squeezed several times to transfer the fluid into the Monovial. The Monovial is shaken a few times to reconstitute the drug and inverted. Then the minibag is squeezed and released to transfer the drug back into the infusion bag. This process is repeated until the vial is empty.

Several manufacturers ship to the hospital pharmacy reconstituted IV antibiotic solutions, for example, cefazolin sodium, in the frozen state. When thawed, these nonpyrogenic solutions are stable for a finite period. Reconstituted cefazolin is stable for 48 hours at room temperature and for 10 days when refrigerated (5°C or 41°F). The product is packaged in a small plastic bag for piggyback use in IV administration.

Packaging, Labeling, and Storage of Injections

Containers for injections, including the closures, must not interact physically or chemically with the preparation so as to alter its strength or efficacy and are routinely tested for compatibility (Fig. 15.12). If the container is made of glass, it must be clear and colorless or light amber to permit inspection of its contents. The type of glass suitable for each parenteral preparation is usually stated in the individual monograph. Injections are placed either in single-dose containers or in multiple-dose containers (Figs. 15.13 to 15.15). By definition:

FIGURE 15.13. Packaging of injectable products.

Single-dose container: A hermetic container holding a quantity of sterile drug intended for parenteral administration as a single dose; when opened, it cannot be resealed with assurance that sterility has been maintained.

FIGURE 15.14. A typical vial for sterile injectable products, made from type I (borosilicate) glass. The rubber closure has been specially selected for compatibility with the product, desirable physical characteristics, and so on. The overseal holds the closure in place and provides ready access to the contents of the vial. (Courtesy of Hospira, Inc.)

FIGURE 15.12. Testing compatibility of rubber closures with a solution. (Courtesy of CMP PHAR.MA S.R.L.)

FIGURE 15.15. A 100-mL single-dose plastic bag for IV infusion. (Courtesy of AlteredR/Shutterstock.)

Multiple-dose container: A hermetic container that permits withdrawal of successive portions of the contents without changing the strength, quality, or purity of the remaining portion.

Single-dose containers may be ampuls or single-dose vials. Ampuls (Fig. 15.16) are sealed by fusion of the glass container under aseptic conditions (Fig. 15.17). The glass container is made so as to have a neck that may be easily separated from the body of the container without breaking the glass. After opening, the contents of the ampul should be withdrawn into a syringe with a 5-mm filter needle or straw apparatus. The filter needle is replaced with a regular needle. The filter needle is used to trap any glass particles that entered the sterile solution when the neck of the ampul was broken. If a filter needle is not available, withdrawal of glass can be minimized by holding the ampul upright, tilted slightly, when inserting the needle, and avoiding the outer surface of the neck of the ampul. The needle should not be lowered to the bottom of the ampul but held slightly above to avoid drawing glass into the syringe.

Once opened, the ampul cannot be resealed, and no unused portion may be retained and used later, as the contents would have lost sterility. Some injectable products are packaged in prefilled syringes, with or without special administration devices (Figs. 15.18 to 15.20). The types of glass for parenteral product containers are described in Chapter 5. Types I, II, and III are suitable for parenteral products, with type I being the most resistant to chemical deterioration. The type of glass to be used for a particular injection is indicated in the individual monograph for that preparation.

FIGURE 15.16. Ampul before filling and sealing.

One of the prime requisites of parenteral solutions is clarity. They should be sparkling clear and free of all particulate matter, that is, no mobile undissolved substances should be present. Such contaminants include dust, cloth fibers, glass fragments, material leached from the glass or plastic container or seal, and any other material that may find its way into the product during manufacture or administration or that develop during storage.

To keep unwanted particles out of parenteral products, a number of precautions must be taken during manufacture, storage, and use of the products. During manufacture, the parenteral solution is usually filtered just before it goes into the container. The containers are carefully

FIGURE 15.17. Ampul filling and sealing machine. (Courtesy of Alexander Tolstykh/Shutterstock.)

FIGURE 15.18. Disposable sterile cartridges compatible with the Carpuject holder. (Courtesy of Hospira, Inc.)

selected to be chemically resistant to the solution and of the highest available quality to minimize the chances of container components leaching into the solution. It has been recognized for some time that some particulate matter in parenteral products is leached material from the glass or plastic container. Once the container is selected, it must be carefully cleaned to be free of all extraneous matter (Fig. 15.21). During container filling, extreme care must be exercised to prevent the entrance of airborne dust, lint, or other contaminants. Filtered and directed airflow in production areas reduces the likelihood of contamination. Laminar flow hoods allow for draft-free flow of clean, filtered air over the work area. These hoods are commonly found in hospitals for both manufacture and incorporation of additives into parenteral and ophthalmic products (Fig. 15.22). The personnel who manufacture parenterals must be made acutely aware of the importance of cleanliness and aseptic techniques. They are provided with uniforms of monofilament fabrics that do not shed lint. They wear face hoods, caps, gloves, and disposable shoe covers to prevent contamination (Fig. 15.23).

After the containers are filled and hermetically sealed, they are visually (Fig. 15.24) or automatically (Fig. 15.25)

FIGURE 15.20. Inject-Ease automatically inserts the needle of an insulin syringe into the skin when activated. (Courtesy of AmbiMedInc.)

inspected for particulate matter. Usually, an inspector passes the filled container past a light source with a black background to observe for mobile particles. Particles of approximately 50 μm may be detected in this manner.

FIGURE 15.19. Carpuject, a prefilled unit dose injection system that includes a reusable, clear, plastic full-length holder. (Courtesy of Abbott Hospital products division.)

FIGURE 15.21. Filling and sealing of ampuls/vials (non–freeze-dried preparations). (Courtesy of Cozzoli Machine Company.)

FIGURE 15.22. Hyperalimentation being prepared in a horizontal laminar flow hood. (Courtesy of Allie Morrison, PharmD, RPh, MPH, https://www.pharmacytechshq.com/2019/04/21/certified-sterile-compounding-pharmacy-technicians/.)

Reflective particles, such as fragments of glass, may be visualized in smaller size, about 25 μm. Methods to detect smaller particulate matter include microscopic examination and use of sophisticated equipment such as the Coulter Counter, which electronically counts particles in samples. Having passed the inspection, the product may be labeled. However, the pharmacist should inspect each parenteral solution for evidence of particulate matter.

Although the total significance of injecting or infusing parenteral solutions containing particulate matter into a patient has not been ascertained, it is apparent that particulate matter has the potential to induce thrombi and vessel blockage, and depending on the chemical composition of the particles, it has the additional potential to introduce into the patient agents that are undesired and possibly toxic.

FIGURE 15.24. Semiautomatic inspection machine for parenteral products. (Courtesy of Syntegon Technology GmbH.)

In formulating a single-dose parenteral product, the pharmacist must consider not only the physicochemical aspects of the drug but also the intended therapeutic use of the product. Some single-dose preparations are to be administered rapidly in small volumes, but others infuse slowly into the circulatory system over hours. Most small-volume parenterals are formulated so that a convenient amount of solution, say 0.5 to 2 mL, contains the usual dose of the drug, although larger volumes of more diluted solutions are frequently administered intravenously and intramuscularly. Generally, several strengths of injections of a given drug are marketed to permit a wider dosage selection by the physician without waste, as would be the case if only part of a given single-dose parenteral solution was administered. The large-volume single-dose preparations generally are those used to expand the blood volume or to replenish nutrients or electrolytes and are given by slow IV infusion. However, in no instance may a single-dose parenteral container permit withdrawal and administration of more than 1,000 mL. In addition, preparations intended for intraspinal, intracisternal, or peridural administration must be packaged only in single-dose containers as a precaution against contamination.

In the hospital, physicians commonly order an additional agent to be placed in a large-volume parenteral solution for infusion. The person filling such an order must be certain that aseptic conditions are employed and that the additive is compatible with the original solution (14). Care must also be exercised not to introduce particulate

FIGURE 15.23. Pharmacist preparing a parenteral admixture in a laminar flow hood. (Courtesy of Richard Fincher/Shutterstock.)

FIGURE 15.25. Industrial automatic inspection machine, which detects particulate matter in injectables. (Courtesy of CMP PHAR.MA S.R.L.)

matter into the solution. Many pharmaceutical companies have developed special devices for aseptic transfer of pharmaceutical additives to large-volume parenterals. An ordinary sterile needle and syringe may be effectively employed to transfer solutions from one parenteral product to another by a pharmacist. However, a filtering device is employed when a transfer occurs from an ampul to a container (Fig. 15.26). Many hospital pharmacies have established well-controlled IV *additive* or *admixture* programs to ensure compatibility, safety, and efficacy of the additive and solution (14,15). An example of an inside view of a sterile compounding aseptic isolator is shown in Figure 15.26.

Multiple-dose containers are affixed with rubber closures to permit penetration of a hypodermic needle without removal or destruction of the closure. Upon withdrawing the needle from the container, the closure reseals and protects the contents from airborne contamination. The needle may be inserted to withdraw a portion of the prepared liquid injection, or it may be used to introduce a solvent or vehicle to a dry powder for injection. In either instance, the sterility of the injection may be maintained so long as the needle itself is sterile at the time of entry into the container. Unless otherwise indicated in the monograph, multiple-dose injectables are required to contain antibacterial preservatives. Also, unless otherwise specified, multiple-dose containers are not permitted to allow withdrawal of more than 30 mL to limit the number of penetrations into the closure and thus protect against loss of sterility. The limited volume also guards against an excessive amount of antibacterial preservative being inadvertently administered with the drug when unusually large doses of an injection are required, in which case a preservative-free single-dose preparation is advisable. The usual multiple-dose container contains about 10 usual doses of the injection, but the quantity may vary greatly with the individual preparation and manufacturer.

It is possible that rubber closures may contain latex, a problem for patients with latex allergies. Currently, nonla-tex closures are being developed, and manufacturers will provide a list of their latex-free products.

Because it is impossible in practice to transfer the entire volume of a single-dose container or the last dose in a multiple-dose container into a hypodermic syringe, a slight excess (or overfill) in volume of the contents of ampuls and vials over the labeled size or volume of the package is permitted. Table 15.2 presents the recommended overages permitted by the USP to allow withdrawal and administration of the labeled volumes.

For labeling purposes, revised injectable product nomenclature became official on January 1, 1995, and continues. The main points of the new process are as follows:

I. The term *sterile* was eliminated from the titles of injectable products except appropriate monograph titles for water intended for parenteral use, such as Sterile Water for Injection, USP.
II. For established names of injectable products, all of which are suitable and intended for parenteral administration, USP established the following criteria in determining the product's title:
A. Liquids
  1. *Injection*: Title for liquid preparations that are drug substances or solutions thereof
  2. *Injectable suspension*: Title for liquid preparations of solids suspended in a suitable liquid medium
  3. *Injectable emulsion*: Title for liquid preparations of drug substances dissolved or dispersed in a suitable emulsion medium
B. Solids
  1. *For injection*: Title for dry solids that, upon the addition of suitable vehicles, yield solutions conforming in all respects to the requirements for *injections*
  2. *For injectable suspension*: Title for dry solids that, upon the addition of suitable vehicles, yield preparations conforming in all respects to the requirements for *injectable suspensions*

FIGURE 15.26. Use of a filter syringe for aseptic addition of an ingredient to a large-volume parenteral solution during administration to a cancer patient. (Courtesy of Steven Tritton/Shutterstock.)

TABLE 15.2. Recommended Overages for Official Parenteral Products in Milliliters

Labeled Size	Excess Volume for Mobile Liquids	Excess Volume for Viscous Liquids
0.5	0.10	0.12
1.0	0.10	0.15
2.0	0.15	0.25
5.0	0.30	0.50
10.0	0.50	0.70
20.0	0.60	0.90
30.0	0.80	1.20
50.0 or more	2.00%	3.00%

Originally, to facilitate this transition to a new nomenclature, the Center for Drug Evaluation and Research encouraged parenteral drug manufacturers to place a flag, or reminder statement, on the labels of the product for 6 months, alerting practitioners to the changes. The intent was to help practitioners become familiar with the revised rules. An example of a flag is the following: FORMERLY STERILE [DRUG NAME].

In addition, the labels on containers of parenteral products must state the following:

- The name of the preparation
- For a liquid preparation, the percentage content of drug or the amount of drug in a specified volume
- For a dry preparation, the amount of active ingredient present and the volume of liquid to be added to prepare a solution or suspension
- The route of administration
- A statement of storage conditions and an expiration date
- The name of the manufacturer and distributor
- An identifying lot number capable of yielding the complete manufacturing history of the specific package, including all manufacturing, filling, sterilizing, and labeling operations

Injections for veterinary use are labeled so. Preparations intended to be used as dialysis, hemofiltration, or irrigation solutions should meet the requirements for injections except those relating to volume in the containers and should bear a statement indicating that the solution is not intended for use by IV infusion. Appropriately labeled containers allow a sufficient area of the container to remain free of label for its full length or circumference to permit inspection of the contents. Any injection that visual inspection reveals to contain particulate matter other than normally suspended material should be discarded.

Each individual monograph for the official injection states the type of container (single dose and/or multiple dose) permitted for the injection, the type of glass preferred for the container, exemptions if any to usual package size limitations, and any special storage instructions. Most injections prepared from chemically pure medicinal agents are stable at room temperature and may be stored without special concern or conditions. However, most biologic products—insulin injection and the various vaccines, toxoids, toxins, and related products—should be stored under refrigeration. Consult the individual monograph to find the proper storage temperature for a particular injection.

Environmental Issues

Major manufacturers, including Hospira, Inc., Baxter Healthcare, B. Braun, are shipping containers free from PVC and di-2-ethylhexylphthalate (DEHP). Some health care facilities are planning to phase out the use of PVC/DEHP products in future years. A concern, especially for male neonate patients, is that PVC bags can leach DEHP into the fluid of the container.

Another concern is the amount of plastic waste generated by PVC/DEHP containers. Hospitals for a Healthy Environment reported that hospitals produce approximately 6,600 tons of waste per day. Fifteen percent of the solid waste contains plastic. In response to the need for less plastic waste, Hospira, Inc., has launched its VISIV line of IV containers that are PVC/DEHP-free (Fig. 15.27). Also, these bags do not contain any overwrap, which reduces the amount of plastic needing discarding. Advances in material science allowed incorporation of the attributes of the overwrap into the original container. In addition, the VISIV container has a sterile port. Thus, in emergency situations, the pharmacist or health care provider does not have to sterilize the port prior to administration. In addition, this new system provides thermal stability, moisture barrier properties, and inertness required for IV medication administration while avoiding leaching associated with the presence of PVC. Baxter Healthcare has introduced its Aviva line of PVC/DEHP- and latex-free IV containers for large-volume parenteral administration.

FIGURE 15.27. VisIV container. (Courtesy of Hospira, Inc.)

In the past, the problems associated with PVC/DEHP resulted in IV admixtures still needing preparation in glass containers. Although glass containers are more expensive to prepare than PVC/DEHP containers, PVC/DEHP containers are more costly to manufacture than the non-PVC/DEHP plastic bags. In a cost-cutting environment, it is conceivable that eventually most hospitals will convert to the PVC/DEHP-free containers and not carry two types of large-volume containers.

Quality Assurance for Compounded Sterile Preparations

On June 1, 2008, the revised USP Chapter <797>, Pharmaceutical Compounding-Sterile Preparations, became official (12). Unlike guidelines published by groups starting with the National Coordinating Committee for Large-Volume Parenterals in the late 1970s and, more recently, the American Society of Health-System Pharmacists (ASHP), USP <797> is optionally enforceable by the state boards of pharmacy. Many state boards of pharmacy have incorporated USP <797> into their regulations by reference while others have written their own standards that are quite similar. USP <797> provides the minimum practice and quality standards for CSPs. The chapter is for those who compound sterile preparations including pharmacy staff, physicians, and nurses and all locations such as hospitals, clinics, and pharmacies where sterile preparations are compounded, stored, and transported. USP <797> does not relate to the clinical administration of the CSP via its prescribed route of administration. Practitioners who compound sterile preparations must be thoroughly familiar with the chapter.

Three risk levels of CSPs are described: low-risk level, medium-risk level, and high-risk level. Risk levels are based on the potential of contaminating a low-risk level or medium-risk level CSP or failure to sterilize a high-risk level CSP, which can cause harm to the patient, including death. With low-risk level and medium-risk level CSPs, sterile ingredients and devices are used, and sterility is maintained. High-risk level CSPs include nonsterile components; thus, they must be sterilized during the compounding process. Health care professionals are responsible for determining CSP risk levels; however, any CSP with a nonsterile component is always high-risk level.

Low-risk level CSPs include injecting sterile electrolyte solution into a large-volume IV fluid container or reconstituting a lyophilized antibiotic and then transferring the solution to a 100-mL fluid container. Compounding parenteral nutrition solutions via automated or manual methods would be considered medium-risk level as would pooling contents from multiple ampuls or vials of sterile products to provide a CSP to be administered once to multiple patients or to one patient multiple times. Sterilizing a solution made from a nonsterile bulk powder such as alum or glutamine qualifies as a high-risk level.

The immediate-use CSPs section is only for situations where there is an emergency or immediate need for the patient to receive an otherwise low-risk level CSP. This may occur in a respiratory or cardiac arrest, emergency room, operating room, and combat zone or with the preparation of a diagnostic agent. Hazardous drugs such as chemotherapy may not be compounded as immediate use or is batch preparation or compounding based on predicted needs of CSPs. The compounding process cannot exceed 1 hour. Immediate-use CSPs are exempt from low-risk level requirements only when all criteria noted in the chapter are met. Note that compounding under immediate-use conditions increases the likelihood of microbial contamination and potential patient harm.

Facilities for compounding CSPs are designed and environmentally controlled to minimize airborne contamination. Primary engineering controls (PECs) such as laminar airflow workbenches, compounding aseptic isolators, compounding aseptic containment isolators (CACI), and biological safety cabinets (BSC) are PECs or sources of ISO Class 5 air quality. After initial certification, PECs should be recertified by a qualified individual at least every 6 months or whenever the device or room is relocated or altered or a major service to the facility is performed.

Exposure to hazardous drugs presents a potential health risk to compounding personnel, USP <797>. Adverse events may range from skin rashes to effects on the reproductive system and possibly cancer (16). Hazardous drugs must be compounded under conditions that protect the health care professional and other workers who may come in contact with the agents, including personnel protective equipment. Preparation shall occur in an ISO Class 5 environment such as a BSC or CACI placed in an ISO Class 7 negative pressure area (net flow of air is into the area) physically separated from other preparation areas. Closed system transfer devices (CSTDs) that prevent venting or exposure of the hazardous drug to the environment shall be used within the ISO Class 5 environment. For institutions that compound a low number of hazardous drugs, a CSTD used within a BSC or CACI in a nonnegative pressure room is acceptable. Training for personnel who compound, stock, or distribute hazardous drugs shall encompass proper storage, handling, and disposal of the drugs. Verification of appropriate hazardous drug compounding techniques shall be done on an annual basis. Additional information can be obtained from EPA, OSHA, NIOSH, and in USP <800> Hazardous Drugs—Handling in the Healthcare Setting.

Proper hand hygiene and garbing practices, personnel aseptic technique, and the disinfection of compounding surfaces are key components in minimizing the risk to patients. Direct touch is the most likely source of contamination for CSPs prepared by compounding personnel. Sterile gloves must be used, as well as disinfectants such as sterile 70% isopropyl alcohol (IPA). Repeated disinfection of gloves with IPA during the compounding process has been shown to reduce the contamination rate of pharmacy CSPs (17). Recommended frequencies are defined for cleaning and disinfecting the compounding area.

Compounding personnel must be completely trained in the theoretical and practical aspects of aseptic manipulation using audiovisual materials, professional publications, and live demonstrations. They must pass written examinations and media-fill testing before being allowed to prepare CSPs for patients. Annual media-fill testing is required for low-risk level and medium-risk level compounding and semiannually for high-risk level compounding. Gloved fingertip sampling assesses competency in performing hand hygiene and garbing.

USP <797> also includes sections on establishing beyond-use dates, compounding radiopharmaceuticals and allergen extracts, characteristics of a quality assurance program, verification of compounding accuracy and sterility, finished preparation release checks and test, and elements of quality control. The appendices have useful information on required and recommended competencies, common disinfectants, and sample forms for assessing compounding personnel, cleaning, and disinfection practices.

Available Injections

Hundreds of injections of various medicinal agents are on the market. Tables 15.3 and 15.4 present some examples of those packaged in small-volume and large-volume containers, the latter for IV infusion.

TABLE 15.3. Some Injections Usually Packaged and Administered in Small Volume

Injection	Physical Form	Category and Comments
Botulinum toxin type A	Powder for injection	For temporary improvement in appearance of moderate to severe glabellar lines associated with corrugator or procerus muscle activity in adult patients 65 y or younger; administered IM
Butorphanol tartrate	Solution	Opioid agonist–antagonist analgesic; administered IM or IV for relief of moderate to severe pain, as preoperative or preanesthesia medication
Chlorpromazine HCl	Solution	Antipsychotic drug with antiemetic (antidopaminergic) effects; should not be administered SQ. Injection should be IM slowly, deep into upper outer quadrant of buttocks. Avoid injecting directly into vein. IV route used **only** for severe hiccoughs, surgery, and tetanus
Cimetidine HCl	Solution	Histamine H_2 antagonist; IM or IV for pathologic GI hypersecretory conditions or intractable ulcers
Dalteparin sodium	Solution	Sterile low molecular weight heparin for prophylaxis of deep vein thrombosis in patients at risk who are undergoing abdominal surgery. Available in a prefilled syringe; administered SQ
Dexamethasone sodium phosphate	Solution	Glucocorticoid; IM or IV for cerebral edema, unresponsive shock. Also intra-articular, intralesional, in soft tissue of joints, bursae, and ganglia
Digoxin	Solution	Cardiotonic given IM (not preferred) or IV with highly individualized and monitored dosage
Dihydroergotamine mesylate	Solution	Alpha-adrenergic blocking agent specific for migraine, IM or IV
Diphenhydramine HCl	Solution	Ethanolamine, nonselective antihistamine; IV or IM when PO impractical; indicated for type I (immediate) hypersensitivity reactions, active treatment of motion sickness
Furosemide	Solution	Loop diuretic; IM or IV slowly for edema or acute pulmonary edema
Granisetron HCl	Solution	5-HT$_3$ receptor antagonist for prevention of nausea and vomiting during cancer therapy, including high-dose cisplatin
Heparin sodium	Solution	Anticoagulant IV or SQ as indicated by activated partial prothrombin time or actuated coagulation time
Hydromorphone HCl	Solution	Opioid analgesic for relief of moderate to severe pain; SQ, IM, or slow IV
Ibutilide fumarate	Solution	Antiarrhythmic with predominantly class III (cardiac action potential prolongation) properties according to Vaughn Williams classification; infused IV undiluted or diluted in 50-mL diluent
Iron dextran	Solution	Hematinic agent; IV or IM for documented iron deficiency when oral administration is unsatisfactory or impossible
Isoproterenol HCl	Solution	Adrenergic (bronchodilator) given IM, SQ, or IV
Ketorolac tromethamine	Solution	NSAID for <5 d of moderately severe acute pain that requires analgesia at opioid level, usually postoperatively
Lidocaine HCl	Solution	Cardiac depressant given IV as antiarrhythmic; also local anesthetic epidurally, by infiltration, and in peripheral nerve block

(Continued)

TABLE 15.3. Some Injections Usually Packaged and Administered in Small Volume *(Continued)*

Injection	Physical Form	Category and Comments
Magnesium sulfate	Solution	Anticonvulsant/electrolyte; IM or direct IV injection, IV infusion, other IV administration for convulsive toxemia of pregnancy, parenteral nutrition therapy, mild magnesium deficiency, and severe hypomagnesemia
Meperidine HCl	Solution	Opioid analgesic given IM, SQ, or slow continuous IV infusion
Metoclopramide monohydrochloride	Solution	Gastrointestinal stimulant; administered IM, direct IV, or slow IV admixture to prevent chemotherapy emesis
Midazolam HCl	Solution	Short-acting benzodiazepine CNS depressant; IV or IM; for preoperative sedation, anxiolysis, amnesia
Morphine sulfate	Solution	Opioid analgesic. IM, IV, and PCA
Nalbuphine HCl	Solution	Opioid agonist–antagonist analgesic; administered SQ, IM, IV for moderate to severe pain, and preoperative analgesia
Naloxone HCl	Solution	Opioid antagonist; prevents or reverses effects of opioids, including respiratory depression, sedation, hypotension; IV, IM, and SQ
Oxytocin	Solution	Oxytocic, given IM (erratic) or IV obstetrically for therapeutic induction of labor
Phenytoin sodium	Solution	Anticonvulsant; IM (erratic absorption) prophylaxis for neurosurgery or slow IV for status epilepticus
Phytonadione	Dispersion	Vitamin K (prothrombogenic) for hemorrhage. Aqueous dispersion of phytonadione, a viscous liquid
Procaine penicillin G	Suspension	Anti-infective; IM for moderately severe infections of penicillin G–sensitive microorganisms
Prochlorperazine edisylate	Solution	Antidopaminergic; IM or IV for control of severe nausea and vomiting associated with adult surgery
Propranolol HCl	Solution	Beta-adrenergic receptor blocker for hypertension. Oral dosage (tablets) is usual; IV administration is reserved for life-threatening arrhythmias and those occurring under anesthesia
Sodium bicarbonate	Solution	Electrolyte; IV, undiluted or diluted for cardiac arrest, less urgent forms of metabolic acidosis
Sumatriptan succinate	Solution	Selective 5-hydroxytryptamine$_1$ receptor, subtype agonist, for acute migraine with or without aura. Self-administered SQ from unit-of-use syringe, *SELF-dose* unit
Verapamil HCl	Solution	Calcium channel blocker; slow IV over at least 2 min for supraventricular tachyarrhythmias

TABLE 15.4. Representative Marketed Frozen, Premixed Products Illustrating Stability Data When Frozen and After Thawing[a]

Drug[b]	Strength	Diluent	Expiration Dating		
			Frozen Stability	Refrigerated Stability	Room Temperature
Cefazolin sodium	1 g	Iso-osmotic in dextrose, 50 mL	24 mo	30 d	48 h
Ceftazidime sodium	1 g, 2 g	Iso-osmotic in dextrose, 50 mL	9 mo	7 d	24 h
Ceftriaxone sodium	1 g, 2 g	Iso-osmotic in dextrose, 50 mL	12 mo	21 d	48 h
Nafcillin sodium	1 g, 2 g	Iso-osmotic in dextrose, 50 mL, 100 mL	18 mo	21 d	72 h
Oxacillin sodium	1 g, 2 g	Iso-osmotic in dextrose, 50 mL	18 mo	21 d	48 h
Ticarcillin disodium and clavulanate potassium	3.1 g	Iso-osmotic in water, 100 mL	30 d	7 d	24 h
Vancomycin HCl	500 mg, 1 g	Iso-osmotic in dextrose, 100 mL	12 mo	30 d	72 h

[a]Stability information provided by Baxter Healthcare Corporation.

[b]Stability data based on packaging drug in a Galaxy container.

SMALL-VOLUME PARENTERALS

The USP designation small-volume injection applies to an injection packaged in containers labeled as containing 100 mL or less. Table 15.3 presents some commonly employed injections given in small volume. Some of these injections are solutions, and others are suspensions.

Premixed IV delivery systems have simplified delivery for small-volume parenterals in particular. A distinct advantage of these ready-to-use systems is that they require little or no manipulation to make them patient specific. Thus, they are a viable alternative to the traditional labor-intensive method of compounding parenteral medications from individual or multiple doses of IV medications and an appropriate parenteral solution. Since the introduction of the first ready-to-use systems in the late 1970s, the availability and variety of systems have increased (e.g., Baxter Healthcare Corporation, B. Braun Medical, Hospira) (Table 15.4).

The traditional method for preparing small-volume parenteral therapy from a partial-fill drug vial into a minibag can be labor intensive and costly in materials. The savings accrued through ready-to-use systems can be significant (18). Another key advantage of these systems is extended stability dating and reduced wastage. Doses can be put together (but not activated) in cycles, then activated just prior to use, and delivered to the nursing station by the pharmacy personnel (18).

The downside of these ready-to-use small parenteral products is that they do not offer flexibility in changing the volume or concentration of the product. This may pose a problem to the fluid-restricted patient (18). But the introduction of minibags in volumes of 100, 50, and 25 mL has helped this problem somewhat. Another disadvantage of the ready-to-use products is that some manufacturers' premixed products require thawing. Microwave use for quick thawing poses stability problems for some of these products (e.g., cefazolin). For example, before it was removed from the market, the high-energy microwave oven could cause a structural alteration of the cephalothin molecule. Another possibility was that a substance would leach from the rubber stopper when frozen ampuls of Neutral Keflin were thawed in the microwave, and oftentimes, thawing was not even, with the periphery thawed and the central portion still frozen.

General precautions (19) were once published for using a microwave to thaw frozen products. However, this practice is no longer suggested. Instead, many hospital pharmacies use the Saf-Thaw (MMI of Mississippi, Crystal Springs). This apparatus provides a layer of conditioned air continuously circulating around the frozen product. The thawing surface facilitates recirculating the conditioned air in the unit and thereby prevents collection of unconditioned air or moisture from the room where the Saf-Thaw is operating. The frozen product is placed on the thawing surface, which is approximately 37°C (99°F), warm to the touch when the unit is in operation. Several dozen frozen products can be placed on the thawing surface at one time, depending on their size.

In years past, some manufacturers recommended warming frozen premixed products in a water bath, with a warning not to submerge the product because there was a distinct possibility that water from the bath could enter and contaminate the product. Now, manufacturers recommend that the frozen container be thawed at room temperature or in a refrigerator (e.g., for 1 hour) and prohibit the use of a water bath or microwave. Thawed floor stock is usually available for emergency orders. Generally, these are kept in refrigerators and warm up quickly (e.g., 20 minutes) to room temperature.

The ready-to-use systems have not been used much in the pediatric and neonatal population. The unique dosing and fluid requirements of these patients make these systems inappropriate. In some institutions, the unique dosing and fluid requirements of pediatric and neonate patients are addressed by making dilutions of medications to standardized concentrations, filling and capping individual syringes, and administering these doses through a syringe pump.

INSULINS

Among the most used of the small-volume injections are the various insulin preparations. Insulin, the active principle of the pancreas gland, is primarily concerned with the metabolism of carbohydrates but also influences protein and fat metabolism. Insulin facilitates the cellular uptake of glucose and its metabolism in liver, muscle, and adipose tissue. It increases the uptake of amino acids and inhibits the breakdown of fats and the production of ketones. Insulin is administered to patients with abnormal or absent pancreatic *beta* cell function to restore glucose metabolism and maintain satisfactory carbohydrate, fat, and protein metabolism. It is used in the treatment of *diabetes mellitus* that cannot be controlled satisfactorily by dietary regulation alone or by oral antidiabetic drugs. Insulin may also be used to improve the appetite and increase the weight in selected cases of nondiabetic malnutrition and is frequently added to IV infusions.

Insulin is administered by needle, pen device, and pump (Figs. 15.28 to 15.30). A system for nasal administration of

FIGURE 15.28. InsuJet™, a jet injection device. The jet injection method uses pressure rather than a needle to provide subcutaneous distribution of medication. This device can be used with U-100 insulin or a combination of insulins and can deliver 2 to 100 units in half-unit increments. (Courtesy of European Pharma Group.)

FIGURE 15.29. Insulin syringes calibrated in units. (Courtesy of Alexvav/Shutterstock.)

insulin was introduced onto the market. However, it was withdrawn from the market because of the variability in drug delivery.

Originally, insulin was available as U-40 (i.e., 40 U/mL) and U-80 (i.e., 80 U/mL). However, confusion associated with dosing caused patient errors with injecting too much or too little of the required dosage. Ultimately, the U-100 (i.e., 100 U/mL) insulin was suggested as a replacement for the U-40 insulin, with the intention of making U-100 the

FIGURE 15.30. Packaging of disposable sterile insulin syringes and needles. (Courtesy of Becton, Dickinson and Company.)

single strength for in-home use by the patient. In December 1991, Eli Lilly announced that it would cease the production of U-40 insulins, and subsequently, other insulin manufacturers also decided to cease the production of this strength. Previously, the U-80 strength had been decertified. The basis for this decision was lack of demand (very low numbers of patients using this strength). Recognizing, however, that insulin under 100 U/mL might still be needed (i.e., for small children, veterinary use), Lilly markets a diluting fluid for Humalog, Humulin N, Humulin R, Humulin 70/30, Humulin 50/50, and Humulin R (U-500). This fluid can be used to prepare any strength of insulin below 100 U/mL. It is not commercially available, however, and can only be secured through a direct, special order request to Eli Lilly and Co.

The diluting solutions are identical to the diluent in the insulin in every way (e.g., preservative agent, buffer, pH) except for the presence of insulin. The recommended storage condition for opened and unopened diluting solutions is controlled room temperature, 25°C (77°F). Once the diluting solutions are opened, the material can be used for a month.

Age-associated sight difficulties and the vision deterioration associated with diabetes can interfere significantly with buying and using insulin products. Therefore, packaging of insulins must make allowances for visual deficits. To facilitate identification of the proper medication at the site of purchase, the arrangement and size of the package lettering must make it easy for the insulin-dependent patient to recognize the type and concentration of the product. For example, Humulin insulins, an international symbol also appears on the cartons and bottles of all formulations of Humulin insulins. These symbols help ensure that patients with diabetes secure the correct Humulin formulation anywhere in the world. Each manufacturer of insulin has its own distinct labeling for its insulin products.

The goal of insulin therapy is to achieve tight blood glucose control by mimicking insulin secretion by the normal pancreas. Normal insulin secretion consists of two components, basal and bolus insulins. These components are mimicked by the administration of two types of insulins. Basal insulins are intermediate-acting or long-acting insulins that mimic basal secretion of insulin. This is the small amount that the pancreas secretes continuously. These products help to suppress hepatic glucose production between meals and overnight. Basal insulins provide approximately 50% of a person's daily requirements. Bolus insulins are rapid-acting or short-acting insulins that mimic the extra insulin the pancreas secretes in response to the postprandial rise of blood glucose levels. Postprandial blood glucose values contribute significantly to hemoglobin A_{1C} values and consequently to the long-term complications of diabetes if these blood glucose values are not controlled. Thus, postprandial control of blood glucose is essential for optimal management. Bolus injections are estimated to provide 10% to 20% of a patient's total daily insulin requirement at each meal.

Regular Insulin

Regular insulin is a sterile aqueous solution of insulin. The solution was previously prepared from beef or pork pancreas or both. Currently, it is prepared exclusively through biosynthetic means (human insulin), discussed in the next section. The source must be stated on the labeling. In 1980, purified pork insulin (Iletin II, pork, Lilly) became available for individuals allergic to or otherwise adversely affected by the mixed pork and beef product. The first insulin developed for clinical use was amorphous. This type was then replaced by a purer zinc–insulin crystalline product that produced a clear aqueous solution. Originally, insulin injection (regular insulin) was produced at a pH of 2.8 to 3.5. This was necessary because particles formed in the vial when the pH was increased above the acid range. However, changes in manufacturing to produce insulin of greater purity have allowed for insulin injection with a neutral pH. The neutral product is more stable than the acidic product.

Regular insulin is prepared to contain 100 or 500 USP insulin units per milliliter. The labeling must state the potency in USP insulin units per milliliter and the expiration date, which must not be later than 24 months after the date of manufacture. As an added precaution against inadvertent use of the incorrect strength, the packages are color coded for strength. For instance, all insulins of the various types containing 100 U/mL have an orange code/label, and U-100 syringes have orange caps over the needles. The 500 U/mL preparation is labeled Humulin R U-500 in green type. The label is white with a bold blue-green border. It also carries a warning with white letters in a red box, "Warning—Highly Concentrated. Important: Use only with a U-500 syringe." Syringes for use with U-500 insulin have green caps over the needles and a bold "U-500" label at the bottom of the barrels. U-500 insulin is indicated for patients with a marked insulin requirement usually (more than 200 U/d) because a large dose may be administered subcutaneously in a small volume. Its effect lasts up to 24 hours, possibly because of delayed absorption of the concentration solution.

Regular insulin is a colorless to straw-colored solution, depending on its concentration; the 500 U/mL product is straw colored. It is substantially free from turbidity. A small amount of glycerin (1.4% to 1.8%) is added for stability, and 0.1% to 0.25% of either phenol or cresol is added for preservation. Insulin remains stable if stored in a cold place, preferably the refrigerator. However, because injection of cold insulin is uncomfortable, the patient may store the vial being used at room temperature (15°C to 30°C or 59°F to 86°F) for up to 28 days. Any insulin remaining in the vial after that time should be discarded. Freezing should be avoided, as this reduces potency.

The various insulin preparations differ as to their onset of action, peak of action, and duration of action (Table 15.5). Regular insulin, being a solution, is categorized as rapid acting. Insulin suspensions are slower acting. Only rapid and regular insulins may be administered intravenously; all others are normally given subcutaneously, usually 30 minutes to 2 hours before a meal so that physiologic effects will parallel absorption of glucose. The dosage is individually determined, with the usual range being 5 to 100 U. The pharmacist plays a vital role in the education of the diabetes patient, particularly in the proper use of insulin. The insulin dose should always be checked to ensure it is correct. Because it is a solution, regular insulin can be used in emergencies, such as ketoacidosis, to effect a rapid decrease in blood glucose levels. However, with the exception of diabetic ketoacidosis, it is rare for a patient to require a dose of regular insulin greater than 25 U. Previously, diabetes patients combined regular insulin with a modified insulin, such as NPH, to provide daily coverage in two injections (morning, late afternoon)

TABLE 15.5. Insulin Activity Profiles and Compatibility

Preparation	Onset (h)	Peak (h)	Duration (h)	Compatible with
Rapid Acting				
Insulin lispro	0.25	0.5–1.0	3	Ultralente; NPH
Insulin aspart	0.25	0.5–1.0	3	None
Short Acting				
Regular insulin	0.5	2–5	5–8	All
Intermediate Acting				
Isophane (NPH) insulin	1–2	6–10	16–20	Regular
Insulin–zinc (lente)	1–2	6–12	18–24	Regular, semilente
Long Acting				
Insulin–zinc extended (ultralente)	4–6	10–18	24–28	Regular, semilente
Insulin glargine	2	None	>24	None
Mixtures				
Isophane/regular insulin 70/30, 50/500.75	7–12	16–24	—	—
NPL/lispro mix 75/25	5 min	7–12	1–24	—

or use premixed preparations. So, it was important that the patient understood how much of each to use and in what order to mix them in the syringe. Regular insulin is drawn up first into the syringe. Now, however, a patient will inject a rapid-acting insulin before meals and a long-acting insulin one time per day.

Prior to use, the patient should be instructed to inspect the insulin carefully. Regular and rapid insulins, insulin glargine, and insulin detemir should appear clear, whereas the other insulins, which are suspensions, should appear uniformly cloudy. With the suspensions, the patient should be instructed how to prepare the insulin: the vial is rotated slowly and gently between the palms of the hands several times before the insulin is drawn into the syringe. This avoids frothing and bubble formation, which would result in an inaccurate dose. The patient should not shake the insulin vial as this may affect the insulin molecules rendering them somewhat ineffective and incorporate air in the solution/suspension resulting in an incorrect dose being measured.

Proper storage should also be encouraged. These preparations should be stored in a cool place or a refrigerator. The patient should be warned to avoid exposing the insulin to extremes of temperature, that is, freezing, such as overnight in the car in the winter and heat, as in the glove compartment of a car in summer or in direct sunlight. If this occurs, the patient should discard the insulin and get a new bottle (20). Any bottle of insulin that appears frosted or clumped should be returned to the pharmacy where it was purchased. Finally, the patient should use the insulin in a timely fashion, not beyond the expiration date indicated on the insulin vial.

Human Insulin

Biosynthetic human insulin was the first recombinant DNA drug product to receive approval from FDA. This product, Humulin (Lilly), became available in 1983. It is produced by using a special non–disease-forming laboratory strain of *Escherichia coli* and recombinant DNA technology. A recombined plasmid DNA coding for human insulin is introduced into the bacteria, and it is then cultured by fermentation to produce the A and B chains of human insulin. These A and B chains are freed and purified individually before they are linked by the specific disulfide bridges to form human insulin. The insulin produced is chemically, physically, and immunologically equivalent to insulin derived from the human pancreas. The biosynthetic insulin is free of contamination with *E. coli* peptides and is also free of the pancreatic peptides that are present as impurities in insulin preparations extracted from animal pancreas. These latter impurities include proinsulin and proinsulin intermediates, glucagon, somatostatin, pancreatic polypeptide, and vasoactive intestinal peptide.

Pharmacokinetic studies in some normal subjects and clinical observations in patients indicate that formulations of human insulin have a slightly faster onset of action and a slightly shorter duration of action than the original purified pork insulin counterparts. Two formulations of human insulin were initially marketed: neutral regular human insulin (Humulin R, Lilly) and NPH human insulin (Humulin N, Lilly). Neutral regular human insulin consists of zinc–insulin crystals in solution. It has a rapid onset of action and a relatively short duration of action at 6 to 8 hours. NPH human insulin is an intermediate-acting turbid preparation with a slower onset of action and longer duration of action (16 to 20 hours) than regular insulin.

Human insulins should be stored as other insulins, in a cold place, preferably a refrigerator. Freezing should be avoided.

Insulin Lispro

Insulin lispro solution consists of zinc–insulin lispro crystals dissolved in a clear aqueous fluid. It is created when the amino acids at positions 28 and 29 on the insulin B chain are reversed.

Insulin lispro solution is rapidly absorbed after SC administration and demonstrates no significant differences in absorption from abdominal, deltoid, and femoral sites of injection. Its bioavailability mimics that of regular insulin. However, peak serum levels of insulin lispro occur within 0.5 to 1.5 hours and are higher, and it is shorter acting than regular insulin with a duration of 3 to 4 hours. Peak hypoglycemic effects are more pronounced with lispro insulin solution. Thus, hypoglycemia is the primary complication associated with its use. Comparative studies have demonstrated, however, that hypoglycemic episodes have been less frequent with insulin lispro than with regular insulin. Insulin lispro solution should be stored in a refrigerator but not in the freezer. If accidentally frozen, it should not be used. It may be stored at room temperature for up to 28 days, but the storage temperature should be as cool as possible. Insulin lispro pens should be kept at room temperature once in use. The vial or cartridge should be kept away from direct light and heat. At the end of 28 days, any unused portion of the insulin lispro solution should be discarded.

Insulin Aspart

Insulin aspart is a recombinant, ultrashort-acting insulin using *Saccharomyces cerevisiae* (baker's yeast) as the production organism. It is homologous with regular human insulin except for a single substitution of the amino acid proline by aspartic acid in position B28. This insulin was developed to control postprandial glucose concentrations when administered 5 to 10 minutes before mealtime in a manner similar to that for insulin lispro. The dosage is individualized to the patient's needs.

Insulin aspart demonstrates pharmacokinetics very similar to those of insulin lispro solution in terms of onset of action (0.25 hours), peak effect (0.5 to 1 hour), and duration of action (3 hours). A few studies have demonstrated that patients treated with insulin aspart had better glucose control and fewer nocturnal hypoglycemic episodes than patients using insulin regular. These studies demonstrate that insulin aspart is a viable alternative therapy for patients who use insulin regularly.

Mixing insulin aspart with NPH human insulin immediately before injection may produce some attenuation in the peak concentration of the insulin aspart. However, the time to peak concentration and the total bioavailability of the insulin aspart should not be affected. When insulin aspart is mixed with NPH human insulin, the insulin aspart should be drawn up first. This combination should be injected immediately after mixing. Insulin aspart should not be mixed with crystalline zinc–insulin preparations because compatibility data are lacking.

Insulin Glulisine (Apidra)

Insulin glulisine is a recombinant rapid-acting insulin analog that differs from human insulin by the replacement of two amino acids on the *beta* chain at positions B3 (i.e., asparagine replaced by lysine) and B29 (i.e., lysine replaced by glutamic acid). This insulin is produced by recombinant DNA technology using a nonpathogenic strain of *E. coli* (K12). Apidra is equipotent to regular human insulin when administered intravenously. When given subcutaneously, insulin glulisine demonstrates a more rapid onset of action and shorter duration of action compared to regular insulin. It is a sterile, clear, aqueous, and colorless solution with a pH of approximately 7.3.

Insulin glulisine has the onset of action in 0.2 to 0.5 hours and reaches its peak effect in 1.6 to 1.8 hours. It has a duration of action of 3 to 4 hours. Apidra demonstrates distribution and elimination properties very similar to those of regular insulin with a volume of distribution of 13 L and a half-life of 13 minutes (IV) and 42 minutes (sub-Q).

Insulin glulisine can only be mixed with NPH insulin, and when mixed, it should be drawn into the syringe first. It is available in a concentration of 100 U/mL in 10-mL vials and 3-mL cartridges for use in the OptiClik insulin delivery device. Unopened vials of Apidra should be stored in the refrigerator (2°C to 8°C). It should not be stored in the freezer and should be discarded if frozen. Similarly, if inadvertently exposed to extremes in temperature (i.e., heat, freezing) in the glove compartment of an automobile, for example, it should be discarded. Open (in-use) vials can be stored in the refrigerator or at room temperature of not greater than 25°C. Open, in-use cartridges inserted into the OptiClik system should not be refrigerated but kept at room temperature. Any open vials or cartridges should be discarded after 28 days. The vial or the cartridges should be protected from direct light and heat. Infusion bags for IV use are stable at room temperature for 48 hours. Apidra is stable in the infusion sets for up to 48 hours and should be discarded if exposed to temperatures greater than 37°C.

Isophane Insulin Suspension (NPH Insulin)

Isophane insulin suspension is a sterile suspension in an aqueous vehicle buffered with dibasic sodium phosphate to pH 7.1 to 7.4. It is prepared from zinc–insulin crystals modified by the addition of protamine so that the solid phase of the suspension consists of crystals of insulin, zinc, and protamine. Protamine is prepared from the sperm or the mature testes of fish belonging to the genus *Oncorhynchus* and others. As mentioned in the discussion of the aqueous insulin solutions, suspensions of insulin with a pH on the alkaline side inherently have a longer duration of action than solutions. Insulin is least soluble at pH 7.2.

The rod-shaped crystals of isophane insulin suspension should be approximately 30 μm long and the suspension free of large aggregates of crystals following moderate agitation. This is necessary for it to pass freely through the needle and for absorption of the drug to be consistent from one batch to another. When a portion of the suspension is examined microscopically, the suspended matter is largely crystalline, with only traces of amorphous material. The official injection is required to contain glycerin and phenol for stability and preservation. The specified expiration date is 24 months after the immediate container was filled by the manufacturer. The suspension is packaged in multiple-dose containers having not less than 10 mL of injection. Each milliliter contains 100 U of insulin. The suspension is best stored in a refrigerator, but freezing must be avoided.

As indicated earlier, isophane insulin suspension is an intermediate-acting preparation administered as required mainly as hormonal replacement in diabetes mellitus. The usual dose range subcutaneously is 10 to 80 U. Its effects are comparable with those of a mixture of two to three parts of regular insulin and one part of protamine zinc–insulin.

The *NPH* used in some product names stands for neutral protamine Hagedorn because the preparation is neutral (pH about 7.2), contains protamine, and was developed by Hagedorn. The term *isophane* is based on the Greek words *iso* (equal) and *phane* (appearance) and refers to the equivalent balance between the protamine and insulin.

Isophane Insulin Suspension and Regular Insulin

In years past, patients needing a rapid onset of action and intermediate duration of activity, approximately 1 day, would routinely mix isophane insulin suspension, an intermediate-acting insulin, with regular insulin, a rapid-acting insulin. Unexpected responses, such as hypoglycemic episodes, were encountered. In addition, it was fairly common for the patient to contaminate one of the vials during mixing. Subsequently, a premixed formulation of isophane insulin suspension and regular insulin became available, and now, there are two formulations. The 70/30 combination consists of 70% isophane insulin suspension and 30% regular insulin, and the 50/50 combination consists of 50% isophane insulin suspension and 50% regular insulin. These combinations are stable and absorbed as if injected separately.

Humulin 50/50 achieves a higher insulin concentration (C_{max}) and maximum glucose infusion rates with more rapid elimination than Humulin 70/30. However, as expected, the cumulative amounts of insulin absorbed (area under the curve, or AUC) and the cumulative effects over 24 hours following injection are identical. Thus, the 70/30 combination provides an initial response tempered with a more prolonged release of insulin. The 50/50 mixture is useful when a greater initial response is required and for patients who have been using extemporaneously compounded insulin mixtures in a 50/50 ratio.

The Humulin 70/30 and 50/50 premixed insulins are cloudy suspensions with a zinc content of 0.01 to 0.04 mg/100 U. These insulins are neutral in pH and phosphate buffered. *m*-Cresol and phenol are the preservatives for both combinations. Protamine sulfate is the modifying protein salt.

Patients should not attempt to change the ratio of these products by adding NPH or regular insulin. If Humulin N and Humulin R mixtures are prescribed in a different proportion, the individual insulin products should be mixed in the amounts recommended by the physician.

Humalog Mix

Humalog Mix is a manufactured premixed insulin consisting of insulin lispro and neutral protamine lispro (NPL) in a fixed ratio. Humalog Mix 50/50 consists of 50% insulin NPL suspension and 50% insulin lispro injection. Humalog Mix 75/25 contains 75% insulin NPL suspension and 25% insulin lispro injection. It is estimated that these premixed combinations are used by more than 40% of diabetes patients who inject insulin twice daily.

These fixed combinations were developed to give better control for diabetes patients who use a combination of short- and long-acting insulins. In comparison to Humulin 70/30, Humalog Mix 75/25 demonstrated lower postprandial blood glucose levels and no difference between the afternoon and overnight glucose values. Furthermore, insulin NPL suspension was developed as an alternative to combinations employing NPH insulin. NPH insulin was unstable over weeks to months when mixed with lispro insulin.

Insulin Glargine

Insulin glargine is a long-acting (up to 24 hours) basal insulin preparation intended for once-daily SC administration at bedtime in the treatment of type 1 diabetes mellitus in adults and children. It can also be used by adults with type 2 diabetes who require long-acting insulin. It is created when the amino acids at position 21 of human insulin are replaced by glycine and two arginines are added to the C-terminus of the B chain.

Insulin glargine is a recombinant, human insulin analog. It is formulated as a clear solution at a pH of 4.0. However, once it is injected into SC tissue, it is neutralized to physiologic pH of approximately 7.4, which causes formation of microspheres. It is slowly absorbed and exhibits no distinct peak. Insulin glargine begins working in 2 hours and mimics basal insulin secretion more closely than other long-acting insulins for 24 hours. This allows for once-daily dosing. Because insulin glargine provides only basal coverage, it is often used in conjunction with other insulins or oral hypoglycemic drugs. However, because of the unique release characteristics of insulin glargine, it should not be mixed with any other insulin. Differences in pH can cause clumping. If it has to be used in combination with a rapid-acting insulin, the injections must be administered separately.

Insulin Detemir

Insulin detemir is an intermediate- to long-acting basal insulin, which is dosed subcutaneously either once or twice daily. It is supplied as a clear neutral (pH 7.4) solution and produced by recombinant DNA in *S. cerevisiae* (i.e., baker's yeast). It is similar in structure to human insulin with the exception of a deletion of the amino acid threonine in position B30 and a C14 fatty acid chain attached to the amino acid position B29.

Insulin detemir maintains its long-acting property through slow systemic absorption. The drug molecules have strong self-association and are highly albumin bound. Insulin detemir has an onset of action of 3 to 4 hours and a peak effect within 6 to 8 hours. The duration of action is dose dependent. At low dosages (i.e., 0.1 to 0.2 U/kg), its duration can range between 5.7 and 12.1 hours. This is the most variable dosage range. At a middle-range dosage (i.e., 0.6 U/kg), its duration of action approaches 20 hours, and at high dosages (i.e., >0.6 U/kg), its duration of action is the least variable between 22 and 23 hours. The administered dose of drug, therefore, determines if this insulin should be given once or twice daily.

Detemir should not be mixed with any other insulin. Short- or rapid-acting insulin given in a separate syringe is often used as a bolus, whereas insulin detemir is simultaneously used as the basal insulin. The conversion from NPH to insulin detemir is 1:1 with small adjustments as needed based on glucose monitoring. This insulin should never be frozen and should be stored in a refrigerator or a cool room out of direct light. Once the vial is in use, it can be kept for up to 42 days.

Insulin Pens

Advantages of the pen devices are that they improve the accuracy of insulin dose measurement and they are packaged five per box (21). These devices allow the dose of insulin to be dialed in, or some have audible dose selectors. This feature is particularly advantageous for administering low insulin dosages (22). These devices may be ideal for children, adolescents, and patients with visual and/or physical dexterity difficulties. Just as with the handling of a suspension form of insulin, for example, Novolin 70/30 PenFill (Novo Nordisk), the patients should be instructed to roll the cartridge in their hands gently before administering it.

Adherence to dosing schedules facilitates effective patient care and helps to decrease health care costs. This is particularly important with diabetes therapy. Getting patients to adhere to insulin dosages facilitates glycemic control and provides value to the payers of health care. Lee et al. (23) demonstrated that health care costs, for example, emergency room visits, decreased hospital length of stay, and physician visits, were reduced in patients studied who switched from insulin vials and syringes to a prefilled insulin analog pen device.

Insulin Infusion Pumps

Insulin infusion pumps allow an estimated 300,000 patients to achieve and maintain blood glucose at nearly normal levels on a *constant basis* through continuous SC insulin infusion (i.e., CSII) (24). CSII is achieved through the use of small and lightweight pumps and eliminates the need for the patient to adhere rigidly to a regimen of multiple daily injections of insulin. This provides convenience, better adherence, and control over the disease process. The main objective of pump therapy is strict control of the blood glucose level at 70 to 140 mg/dL to reduce blood glucose variations that increase the risk for micro- and macrovascular complications, for example, gangrene and diabetic retinopathy.

Today, an insulin pump is of the approximate size of 3.2 × 2.2 × 0.8 inch and weighs between 3 to 4 ounces with battery (i.e., AA, AAA) and full cartridge. It is a plastic-encased computer device that can be worn in a pocket or bra or on a belt. A computer chip in the pump allows the patient to program the amount of insulin for the pump to release. Inside the pump, depending upon the model, a syringe reservoir will hold up to 300 U of U-100 insulin. The reservoir delivers insulin through a plastic infusion set, available in 24- or 42-inch lengths. For optimal working efficiency, the patient should change the infusion site every 2 or 3 days or whenever blood glucose is above 240 mg/dL for two tests in a row. This may indicate that the infusion set is not working properly.

LARGE-VOLUME PARENTERALS

The USP designation large-volume IV solution applies to a single-dose injection intended for IV use and is packaged in containers labeled as containing more than 100 mL. Common examples of large-volume parenterals in use today are presented in Table 15.6 and are administered by IV infusion to replenish body fluids or electrolytes or to provide nutrition. They are usually administered in volumes of 100 mL to 1 L or more per day by slow IV infusion with or without a controlled-rate infusion system (Fig. 15.31). Because of the large volumes administered, these solutions must not contain bacteriostatic agents or other pharmaceutical additives. They are packaged in large single-dose containers (Figs. 15.32 and 15.33).

As indicated previously, electrolytes, vitamins, and antineoplastics are frequently incorporated into large-volume parenterals for coadministration to the patient. It is the responsibility of the pharmacist to understand the physical and chemical compatibilities of the additive in the solution or liquid in which it is placed. Obviously, a combination that results in formation of insoluble material or affects the efficacy or potency of the therapeutic agent of the vehicle is not acceptable. For example, deaths were associated with the administration of calcium and phosphate in total nutrient admixtures (TNAs) (25).

It is also important to be vigilant for incompatibilities associated with multiple infusions coadministered to a patient, as discussed later in this chapter. A typical nursing question may be, "Can the dopamine drip be run in with the heparin drip?" To answer these questions, the pharmacist must know about parenteral therapy and be aware of incompatibilities reported in the literature. Numerous references (e.g., *Handbook on Injectable Drugs (ASHP), King's Guide to Parenteral Admixtures* [King Guide Publications]) are available for sources listing and discussing parenteral incompatibilities. The pharmacist should use only the most current edition of these references. Popular

TABLE 15.6. Some IV Infusions That May Be Administered in Volumes of 1 L or More, Alone or with Other Drugs

Injection	Usual Contents	Category And Comments
Amino acid	3.5%, 5%, 5.5%, 7%, 8.5%, and 10% crystalline amino acid with or without varying concentrations of electrolytes or glycerin	Fluid and nutrient replenisher
Dextrose Injection, USP	2.5%, 5%, and 10% dextrose, other strengths	Fluid and nutrient replenisher
Dextrose and Sodium Chloride Injection, USP	Dextrose 2.5%–10%; NaCl 0.11%–0.9% (19–154 mEq sodium)	Fluid, nutrient, electrolyte replenisher
Mannitol Injection, USP	5%, 10%, 15%, 20%, and 25% mannitol	Diagnostic aid in renal function; diuretic; fluid and nutrient replenisher
Ringer Injection, USP	147 mEq sodium, 4 mEq potassium, 4.5 mEq calcium, and 156 mEq chloride per liter	Fluid and electrolyte replenisher
Lactated Ringer Injection, USP	2.7 mEq calcium, 4 mEq potassium, 130 mEq sodium, and 28 mEq lactate per liter	Systemic alkalinizer; fluid and electrolyte replenisher
Sodium Chloride Injection, USP	0.9% NaCl	Fluid and electrolyte replenisher; isotonic vehicle

FIGURE 15.31. Accurate delivery of IV fluids and medications by use of a controlled-rate infusion system. (Courtesy of Hospira, Inc.)

FIGURE 15.33. Peritoneal dialysis and irrigation fluids. (Courtesy of Manitoba Renal Program.)

drug information databases now incorporate these references for pharmacists to access on their smartphones.

Large-volume parenteral solutions are employed in *maintenance* therapy for the patient entering or recovering from surgery and for the patient who is unconscious and unable to take fluids, electrolytes, and nutrition orally. The solutions may also be used in *replacement therapy* for patients who have suffered a heavy loss of fluid and electrolytes.

Maintenance Therapy

When a patient is receiving parenteral fluids for only a few days, simple solutions providing adequate amounts of water, dextrose, and small amounts of sodium and potassium generally suffice. When patients are unable to take oral nutrition or fluids for slightly longer periods, say 3 to 6 days, solutions of higher caloric content may be used. If oral feeding must be deferred for periods of weeks or longer, TPN or TNAs must be implemented to provide all of the essential nutrients to minimize tissue breakdown and to maintain normalcy within the body. TNAs (three-in-one) include all substrates necessary for nutritional support—carbohydrates, protein, fat, electrolytes, and trace elements—mixed in a single plastic IV bag for convenient administration.

These admixtures are very useful for chemotherapy, gastrointestinal patients, and anorexic patients. The use of three-in-one admixtures in pediatrics, especially for neonates, is controversial. The concentrations of calcium, phosphorus, and necessary warm administration for pediatric TPN do not lend themselves to stable preparations. As a result, many pediatric institutions do not compound three-in-one admixtures for their patients but administer the fat emulsion separately.

When using TNA, the pharmacist must consider the order of substrate mixing, differentiate between various brands of substrate and their physicochemical properties, determine the type of plastic bag system that is most appropriate, determine how the product should be stored, and assess any potential complications. Per FDA ruling, TNAs must be filtered with a 1.2-μm filter. For example, the use of plastic bags with DEHP may result in plasticizer leaching into the solution.

In April 1994, the FDA issued a safety alert regarding the hazards of precipitation associated with parenteral nutrition (26). This was in response to two deaths

FIGURE 15.32. Accurate delivery of IV fluids and medications by use of a controlled-rate infusion system. (Courtesy of Patarapong Saraboon/Shutterstock.)

FIGURE 15.34. Nutrimix KS-240 Automated TPN Compounder System. (Courtesy of Kapsam Health Products.)

FIGURE 15.35. Parenteral nutrition automated mixing device accommodating multiple additives. (Courtesy of Phanie/Alamy Stock Photo.)

and at least two other cases of respiratory distress associated with the use of three-in-one admixtures. Autopsies revealed diffuse microvascular pulmonary emboli linked to a calcium phosphate precipitate in the admixture. Consequently, the FDA safety alert recommends that a filter be used when infusing either central or peripheral parenteral nutrition admixtures. A 0.22-µm filter containing both bacterial retentive and air-eliminating filters has been recommended for use with lipid-free (two-in-one) parenteral nutrient solutions.

Lipid emulsions and three-in-one parenteral nutrient solutions can be safely filtered at a pore size of at least 1.2 µm. A problem with the lipid emulsion in a three-in-one admixture is that it obscures any precipitate. Thus, if a lipid emulsion is needed, a preferable alternative is to employ a two-in-one admixture with a lipid infused separately via a Y-site. Driscoll et al. demonstrated that certain lipid injectable emulsions packaged in plastic containers have baseline abnormal globule size distributions (GSDs) compared with those packaged in glass containers. When used to compound TNAs, the abnormal GSD profile worsens and produces less stable TNAs than those compounded with lipid injectable emulsions packaged in glass (27).

Replacement Therapy

When the patient has undergone a heavy loss of water and electrolytes, as in severe diarrhea or vomiting, greater than usual amounts of these materials may be initially administered and then maintenance therapy provided. Patients with Crohn disease, AIDS, burns, or trauma are candidates for replacement therapy.

Water Requirement

In normal individuals, the daily water requirement is the amount needed to replace normal and expected losses. Water is lost daily in the urine and feces and from the skin and respiration. The normal daily requirement of water for adults is about 25 to 40 mL/kg of body weight or an average of about 2 L/m² of body surface area (28). Nomograms

for the determination of body surface area from height and weight are presented in Figure 2.10. Children and small adults need more water per pound of body weight than do larger adults; water requirements correlate more closely with body surface area than with weight, and a guideline to estimate normal daily requirement for water in these patients is as follows:

1. <10 kg: 100 mL/kg/d
2. 10 to 20 kg: 1,000 mL + 50 mL/kg/d for weight over 10 kg
3. 20 kg to maximum of 80 kg: 1,500 mL + 20 mL/kg/d for weight over 20 kg

However, in the newborn, the volume administered in the first week or two should be about half that calculated from body surface area.

In water replacement therapy for adults, 70 mL/kg/d may be required in addition to maintenance water requirements; a badly dehydrated infant may require an even greater proportion (28). Thus, a 50-kg patient may require 3,500 mL for replacement plus 2,400 mL for maintenance. To avoid fluid overload, especially in elderly patients and those with renal or cardiovascular disorders, monitoring of blood pressure is desirable.

Because water administered intravenously as such may cause osmotic hemolysis of red blood cells and because a patient who requires water generally requires nutrition and/or electrolytes, parenteral administration of water is generally as a solution with dextrose or electrolytes with sufficient tonicity (sodium chloride equivalency) to protect the red blood cells from hemolyzing.

Electrolyte Requirement

Potassium, the primary intracellular cation, is particularly important for normal cardiac and skeletal muscle function. The usual daily intake of potassium is about 100 mEq, and the usual daily loss is about 40 mEq. Thus, any replacement therapy should include a minimum of 40 mEq plus the amount needed to replace additional losses.

The most commonly used concentration of potassium chloride for continuous-infusion maintenance therapy is 20 to 40 mEq/L. With a peripheral line, that concentration may increase to 60 mEq/L, and with a central line, the maximum concentration can be up to 80 mEq/L.

Sodium, the principal extracellular cation, is vital to maintain normal extracellular fluids. Average daily intake of sodium is 135 to 170 mEq (8 to 10 g). The body is able to conserve sodium when this ion is lost or removed from the diet. When there is sodium loss or a deficit, the daily administration of 3 to 5 g of sodium chloride (51 to 85 mEq) should prevent a negative sodium balance. A low sodium level in the body may result from excessive sweating, use of certain diuretics, or diarrhea. Fatigue, muscle weakness, apprehension, and convulsions are among the symptoms of excessive sodium loss. Sodium concentrations can increase when a person does not drink enough water, especially in hot weather, or if kidney function is impaired. Dry, sticky mucous membranes, flushed skin, elevated body temperature, lack of tears, and thirst are among the symptoms of sodium excess. Sodium has been implicated as a causative factor in about 20% of cases of high blood pressure.

Chloride, the principal anion of the extracellular fluid, is usually paired with sodium. Chloride is also important for muscle contraction, balancing the fluid levels inside and outside the cells, and maintaining the acid–base balance of the extracellular fluid. An adequate supply of chloride is necessary to prevent bicarbonate, the second most prevalent anion, from tipping the acid–base balance to the alkaline side. In 1979, a lack of chloride in a brand of infant formula caused metabolic alkalosis in babies who had been exclusively fed that formula. As a result, the Congress passed the Infant Formula Act of 1980, which spells out the nutrients that must be in formulas and establishes quality control procedures for the manufacture of these infant foods. Although other electrolytes and minerals, including calcium, magnesium, and iron, are lost from the body, they generally are not required during short-term parenteral therapy.

Caloric Requirements

Generally, patients requiring parenteral fluids are given 5% dextrose to reduce the caloric deficit that usually occurs in patients undergoing maintenance or replacement therapy. The use of dextrose also minimizes ketosis and the breakdown of protein. Basic caloric requirements may be estimated by body weight; in the fasting state, the average daily loss of body protein is approximately 80 g per day for a 70-kg man. Daily ingestion of at least 100 g of glucose reduces this loss by half.

Parenteral Nutrition

Parenteral nutrition is infusion of enough basic nutrients to achieve active tissue synthesis and growth. It is characterized by the long-term IV feeding of protein solutions containing high concentrations of dextrose (~20%), electrolytes, vitamins, and, in some instances, insulin. Among the components used in parenteral nutrition solutions are the following, listed in quantities commonly provided per liter of fluid. The individual components and amounts vary with the patient's needs.

Electrolytes

Sodium	35 mEq
Potassium	30 mEq
Magnesium	5 mEq
Calcium	5 mEq
Chloride	40 mEq
Acetate	35 mEq
Phosphate	15 mM

Vitamins

Vitamin A	3,300 USP units
Vitamin D	200 USP units
Vitamin E	10 IU
Vitamin C	200 mg
Niacin	40 mg
Vitamin B_2	3.6 mg
Vitamin B_1	6 mg
Vitamin B_6	6 mg
Pantothenic acid	15 mg
Folic acid	600 mg
Vitamin B_{12}	5 mg
Biotin	60 mg
Vitamin K	150 µg

Essential Amino Acids

L-Isoleucine	590 mg
L-Leucine	770 mg
L-Lysine acetate	870 mg (free base 620 mg)
L-Methionine	450 mg
L-Phenylalanine	480 mg
L-Threonine	340 mg
L-Tryptophan	130 mg
L-Valine	560 mg

Nonessential Amino Acids

L-Alanine	600 mg
L-Arginine	810 mg
L-Histidine	240 mg
L-Proline	950 mg
L-Serine	500 mg
Aminoacetic acid	1.19 g

The large proportion of dextrose increases the caloric value of the solution while keeping the volume required to be administered to a minimum. The solution is administered slowly through a large vein, such as the superior vena cava. The superior vena cava is accessed through the subclavian vein immediately beneath the clavicle and near the heart. This permits rapid dilution of the concentrated hyperalimentation fluid and minimizes the risk of tissue or cellular damage because of the hypertonicity of the solution. Generally, final concentrations of dextrose (not >10%) can be given peripherally. Solutions containing more than 10% dextrose should be given via the superior vena cava.

Calcium, usually as calcium gluconate, and phosphate, usually as potassium or sodium phosphate, are frequently present in parenteral admixtures. A significant problem associated with their use is the formation of calcium phosphate, an insoluble precipitate. As mentioned earlier in this chapter, formation of calcium phosphate and deposition of its crystals in lung tissue led to the 1994 FDA safety alert (26).

Many factors have been implicated in the formation of the insoluble precipitate. Among these are the concentration of the individual ions, the salt form of the calcium, the concentration and type of amino acids, the concentration of the dextrose, the temperature and pH of the TPN, the presence of other additives (e.g., cysteine), and the order of mixing. The potential for calcium phosphate precipitation is especially challenging for compounding neonate and pediatric TPN admixtures because of the small volume they are able to tolerate and the need for aggressive replacement therapy. Thus, pharmacists must be alert to avoid this serious compatibility problem.

Figure 15.34 demonstrates a four-station Nutrimix Macro TPN Compounder. This device can pump four nutritional solutions (dextrose, water, amino acids, fat) simultaneously to compound nutritional admixtures by gravimetric means. The user programs the volume and specific gravity of the fluid to be pumped, and the device calculates the weight of the solution that has to be transferred from the source station to the bag. The fifth load cell serves as a confirmation of the weights programmed versus weights delivered. The picture demonstrates big flexible containers and the fat emulsion in glass. Figure 15.35 demonstrates a TPN Compounder. This automatically dispenses small-volume nutritional additives into flexible containers that already contain a base nutritional admixture. The figure depicts 10 stations of small vials. Typically, TPN Compounders are connected directly to a computer entry program, which automatically calculates the amount of each ingredient to be added and drives the compounder to deliver the required amount. These compounders, for example, Baxa Compounder, also have a bar code reader that "reads" each bottle hung on the machine, thereby reducing the chance of human error. They also deliver ingredients in a specific order to avoid incompatibilities, for example, calcium ion is delivered last, after a rinse to ensure all phosphates have been washed from the tubing.

With the increasing use of parenteral solutions in children, including nutritional solutions, pharmacists are frequently confronted with inquiries concerning the appropriate method of parenteral drug delivery (27). A dilemma with young patients is that they often have a limited fluid capacity caused by disease (e.g., congestive heart failure, renal insufficiency) and limited vascular access. As a consequence, pharmacists are asked whether a medication can be administered along with a parenteral nutrition solution. Although this practice is to be discouraged, it may be the only way to ensure that the patient is receiving adequate nutrition as well as appropriate drug therapy. Furthermore, administering the medication with the nutritive solution, rather than interrupting the feeding to administer medication, makes rebound hypoglycemia less likely. However, the practice of administering medication through a central venous line intended for parenteral nutrition solutions is not without risks. Catheter sepsis and occlusion can result.

Formerly, 1 L of TPN was prepared at a time. However, to conserve time, a 24-hour supply is much more efficient and now the norm. Indeed, if a patient encounters a problem necessitating remake of a bag, the cost difference between one or two 1,000-mL bags and a 2,000-mL bag is not that significant. Waste should not be a consideration because the attending physician should not use the TPN to adjust minutely for a patient's need. Typically, electrolyte requirements exceed the physical compatibilities of the TPN components (e.g., calcium–phosphate compatibilities in lipid-containing TPNs), and when this occurs, the pharmacist should encourage the physician to order a separate infusion to make up the deficiency.

The following abbreviations may be used in hospitals in describing the desired order for parenteral nutrition:

CVTPN (central vein TPN)
TPN (total parenteral nutrition)
PPN (peripheral parenteral nutrition)

Enteral Nutrition

As appropriate, hospitalized and home care patients may receive their nutritional needs through *enteral* rather than *parenteral* means. Enteral nutrition products may be administered orally, via nasogastric tube, via feeding gastrostomy, or via needle–catheter jejunostomy. These products are formulated to contain a variety of vitamins, minerals, carbohydrates, proteins, fats, and caloric requirements to meet the specific needs of patients. Although parenteral feeding is appropriate for short-term use in a hospital or long-term care facility or when the gastrointestinal tract is unable to absorb nutrients, enteral feeding is preferable whenever possible. It is just as effective as a source of nutrients, is less expensive than parenteral feeding, and has a low potential to cause serious complications.

The pharmacist can help select these products, because they do differ in the amounts of carbohydrate, fat, protein, and fiber. Furthermore, these products differ in taste and consumer acceptability criteria, such as mouthfeel and cost. Pharmacists may encounter consumers who wish to self-administer an enteral product. If the intent is to supplement calories or protein in an otherwise healthy individual who simply wishes to ensure a balanced dietary intake, a complete formula can be recommended. However, if it is intended to help a person regain weight lost unexpectedly, the individual should be instead referred to a doctor. Sudden weight loss may indicate a serious pathologic problem requiring medical attention.

Pharmacists can also help manage the cost of these products. Composition (oligomeric or polymeric) and form (ready to use vs. powder) influence cost. Generally, the polymeric products are less expensive than the oligomeric products. Although powder forms may be less expensive than ready-to-use formulations, there is an indirect cost of labor required in powder preparation.

Pharmacists are often requested to provide information on how to administer medication via enteral tubes (28,29). A first inclination is to use a liquid or crush a tablet. However, there are some important considerations to be made first. The type of tubing, for example, nasoenteric tubes, which clog easily, dictates a liquid medication. Location of the enteral tube is important too. For example, quinolones should not be administered via a jejunostomy tube because these are located beyond the duodenum, the primary site of absorption for quinolones.

Most immediate-release tablets can be crushed and mixed with water to create a slurry for administration down an enteral tube. However, sustained-release tablets, enteric-coated tablets, or those containing carcinogenic medicines cannot be crushed and administered as a slurry. Pellets from some microencapsulated products (e.g., Cardizem CD, Effexor XR, Micro-K) can be poured down a feeding tube provided they are not crushed.

The pharmacist must also be cognizant that enteral feedings can alter the absorption of certain drugs, for example, warfarin, levothyroxine, and quinolones. So the timing of administration is critical. For a patient maintained on phenytoin, enteral feedings can reduce absorption and subsequently plasma levels by as much as 75%. Thus, enteral tube feedings should be withheld for 2 hours prior to or after phenytoin administration.

Intravenous Infusion Devices

Since the early 1970s, the use of the IV route to administer drugs has become increasingly popular. In 1989, it was estimated that about 40% of drugs and fluid used in hospitals was administered intravenously (30). This increase has affected the development and use of mechanical infusion devices. Advances in infusion technology and computer technology have resulted in devices with extremely sophisticated drug delivery capabilities (e.g., multiple-rate programming, pumps) (31). As a result, these cost-efficient devices provide greater accuracy and reliability of drug delivery than the traditional gravity-flow infusion methods. They also help reduce the fluid volume attributable to the medication infusion and decrease the need for monitoring fluid input, saving nurses' time. Furthermore, multiple drug dosages can be administered, and incompatible drugs can be administered separately (30).

Originally, the disadvantages associated with these mechanical devices included the initial capital investment and extensive in-service education. Furthermore, the influence of infusion pump devices on the delivery of a drug was not fully recognized by clinicians. For example, intrinsic factors (e.g., operating mechanisms, flow accuracy, flow continuity, occlusion detection) and an extrinsic factor (back pressure) may have altered the rate of drug delivery and the therapeutic response of the patient.

Pumps were classified by their *mechanism of* operation (peristaltic, piston, diaphragm), *frequency or type of drug delivery* (continuous or intermittent, bolus dosing, single solution or multiple solution), or *therapeutic application* (PCA) (32). Current research focuses on the influence of drug delivery by these devices and the creation of new technologies (e.g., implantable pumps, pumps with chronobiologic applications, osmotic pressure devices, and open- or closed-loop systems) (32). Today, several features are to be considered in selecting an infusion pump system. Most important is patient safety, then convenience and versatility of the device, and cost efficiency. Table 15.7 lists several infusion devices used in parenteral nutrition support and features associated with each.

TABLE 15.7. Selected Infusion Devices Used in Large-Volume Infusions

Pump	Manufacturer	Features
Colleague CX	Baxter	Micro and macro rate range, basic delivery programming, and ability to piggyback secondary medications. Pump settings include patient weight limits, air detection sensitivity, rate limits, and medication parameters. The dose calculator may be used for up to nine delivery modes. Pump includes a label library of 64 drug and therapy labels. Guardian feature gives a warning when programmed doses are not within institutional limits. This feature also displays overrides, which are stored in the pump's history log for added security.[a]
Symbiq	Hospira	Simple to use and program. Allows hospitals to define soft and hard limits for up to 400 medications. Ability to track medication risk events and generate quality assurance reports. Rate accuracy of the Symbiq system is ±5% across the entire delivery range (0.1–1,000 mL/h) allowing hospitals to meet the needs of all care areas.[b]
Plum A +	Hospira	Easy-to-read display with programming options that include automated piggyback delivery, automated concurrent delivery, programmable standby settings, multistep delivery, loading dose automation, and programmable delayed starts. Can be upgraded with Hospira MedNet Software.[c]
Outlook safety infusion	B. Braun	Has DoseScan technology that allows the clinician to match the right drug to the right patient. This protects against the number one cause on IV medication errors. Outlook also has DoseGuard technology alerting the clinician when a dose limit is exceeded.[d]
Flo-Gard	Baxter	Flow check occlusion alarm (an in-line resistance display of incremental back pressure); flow rate calculation is automatic after volume and time are selected; slide clamp option offers an additional step to protect against inadvertent gravity free flow; front panel lockout protects against tampering; automatic restart once occlusion clears; automatic piggybacking of secondary medication; programmed delivery profile allows up to 10 steps; and individualizing control of infusion ramping and tapering.[e]

[a]http://www.baxter.com/products/medication_management/infusion_pumps/large_volume_infusion_pumps/colleague/index.html
[b]http://www.hospira.com/Products/Symbiqinfusionsystem.aspx
[c]http://www.hospira.com/Products/plumaplusinfusionsystem.aspx
[d]http://www.bbraunusa.com/index.cfm?uuid=598A9770D0B759A1E35DC94F1D834815
[e]http://www.baxter.com/products/medication_management/infusion_pumps/large_volume_infusion_pumps/flo_gard/index.html

FIGURE 15.36. A portable disposable system for infusion or irrigation therapy. (Courtesy of Hospira, Inc.)

The Symbiq Infusion System with Hospira MedNet Software (Fig. 15.36) requires users to select an entry from the drug library for all drug delivery programs. Human factors design was incorporated to provide intuitive ease of use, accelerate staff acceptance, and reduce the risk of programming errors. Hospitals can configure the device to focus on patient needs for each care area. Wireless communication enables customers to gather infusion data remotely. Hospitals can track medication risk events and generate quality assurance reports.

SPECIAL CONSIDERATIONS ASSOCIATED WITH PARENTERAL THERAPY

IV Admixtures

When parenteral dosage forms are combined for administration, admixtures are formed and may be either in-syringe, small volume or large volume. An in-syringe admixture example may be a combination of atropine and hydroxyzine in a syringe, a small volume example may include gentamicin in 25 mL sodium chloride injection and a large volume example may be a combination of vitamin B complex and vitamin C added to 1,000 mL of 5% dextrose in water injection. With the hundreds of drug products available, the preferences of physicians and other factors, there are literally tens of thousands of different combinations, doses, etc.

It is common practice to mix several parenterals in the same large-volume containers to minimize the number of injections a patient must tolerate. Individual components of an admixture have been specifically formulated for stability and administration individually and as separate units; when they are diluted with other vehicles or each other, the original stability and compatibility data no longer applies. Also, the same product may be manufactured by several companies using different formulations, further complicating the compatibility and stability issues. Despite the potential problems, pharmacists are routinely asked to combine single-entity and multiple-entity products into a single syringe, in small volume parenterals (SVPs) and large volume parenterals (LVPs) for patient convenience.

IV Admixture Incompatibilities

IV admixture incompatibilities may occur when parenteral drugs are combined. An incompatibility occurs when one drug is mixed with at least one other drug, solution or in a different container to produce, by physicochemical means, a product unsuitable for administration. A product may be unsuitable because it delivers a subtherapeutic quantity of the drug, or because an incompatibility results in toxic decomposition products, which are delivered to the patient. It has been estimated a number of years ago that 30% of common drug products are incompatible or unstable when added to common LVP vehicles. These incompatibilities may be therapeutic, physical, or chemical in nature (33).

Therapeutic Incompatibilities

Therapeutic incompatibilities, also called drug interactions, may arise when two or more drugs with antagonistic or synergistic pharmacological effects are concurrently administered. Checking for therapeutic incompatibilities should be routinely performed for each IV admixture.

Physical Incompatibilities

A physical incompatibility occurs when the combination of two or more drugs, or a drug and vehicle, results in a change in a solution's appearance, color, or clarity; the occurrence of turbidity; formation of a precipitate; or the evolution or a gas. In general, physical incompatibilities are the easiest to detect and are familiar to most pharmacists. In many cases, they can be predicted from the physicochemical characteristics of the drugs involved—when sodium salts of weak acids (e.g., phenytoin sodium or sodium pantoprazole) are added to intravenous fluids with an acidic pH, the free acids will often precipitate; calcium salts often precipitate in the presence of sodium bicarbonate; acid salts (e.g., dimenhydrinate) precipitate when added to an alkaline medium. Solubility considerations are important for drugs with low water solubility. For example, when a solution using a cosolvent system (e.g., diazepam injection) is diluted with water, the drug will often come out of solution.[2]

Chemical Incompatibilities

The term chemical incompatibility is generally applied when a drug in solution is more rapidly degraded by its combination with other drugs, although this is simplistic. Chemical incompatibilities are often the result of hydrolysis, oxidation, photolysis, reduction, or complexation and most often can only be detected using analytical methods (chromatography, spectroscopy, etc.).

Excipients

In compounding parenteral admixtures, one must be cognizant of excipients such as vehicles, cosolvents, buffers, preservatives, antioxidants, inert gases, surfactants, complexation agents, and chelating agents. In some cases, an additive may be the primary cause of an incompatibility and in other cases a contributing factor.

Factors Involved In Incompatibilities

1. pH. The most important factor responsible for incompatibilities is a change in the acid–base environment of the drug. The solubility and stability profile of a drug may be critically related to pH.
2. Solubility. Water is the most commonly used solvent in parenterals. When a compound is not soluble in water or is degraded by water, it may be dissolved in a nonaqueous solvent, which must be nontoxic, nonirritating, nonsensitizing, and pharmacologically inactive. Most of the solvents are low molecular weight alcohols, including ethanol, propylene glycol, glycerin, and some of the polymeric alcohols such as the polyethylene glycols. Combinations of water-miscible solvents are called cosolvents and are used to dissolve the drug and to enhance the stability of the active drug product. The effect of these cosolvent systems can be complicated and difficult to predict in working with admixtures. Changes resulting from these cosolvents include alteration in physicochemical parameters; for example, pKa, surface tension, viscosity, and reaction rate constants (including possibly new reaction pathways for degradation, etc.).
3. Also, fixed oils (e.g., corn oil, cottonseed oil, peanut oil, sesame oil) can be used as solvents for parenterals, and these vehicles should be considered. As these oils are insoluble in water, any preparation containing oils may be incompatible with the water-based parenterals.
4. Concentration. Some drug products are stable and compatible at some concentrations but not at others. For example, tetracycline hydrochloride in a small volume maintains its pH range over 24 hours; when diluted in a large volume, however, it degrades after 12 hours and becomes less therapeutically active.
5. Complexation. When tetracycline is in the presence of calcium ions, a complex is formed that reduces the activity of the tetracycline. Complexation can also occur and result in enhanced solubility of a drug, as occurs with caffeine and sodium benzoate.
6. Light. Some drugs are sensitive to light and therefore should be light protected. In the case of admixtures, these drugs are removed from their protective environment (amber container or light-resistant packaging) and mixed in a new medium, so they must be covered with aluminum foil, amber plastic, or some other light-resistant material to protect them during both storage and administration to prevent photodecomposition.
7. Temperature. Temperature is also an important factor in determining drug stability in admixtures and is primarily related to storage of the admixture after preparation and storage prior to administration.
8. Vehicle. There is a difference between the characteristics (e.g., pH) of 5% dextrose in water and 0.9% sodium chloride injections; dextrose has been found to have a catalytic effect on the degradation of sodium oxacillin where the sodium oxacillin degrades faster in dextrose solution than in sodium chloride solution.

Standardization of Intravenous Concentrations

Parenteral medications, including IV administration, account for twice as many errors as other methods of administration (i.e., 3% vs. 1.4%) (34). Consequently, stakeholders including representatives from the ASHP, Infusion Nurses Society, the Joint Commission, National Patient Safety Foundation, Institute for Safe Medication Practices, and the USP have recommended standardization in IV use, especially with regard to infusion concentrations and dosage units (35).

Different health care settings use different concentrations of IV medications, which foster errors because pharmacists and health care practitioners have to recalculate and re-compound medications for individual patients. Thus, this group called upon pharmaceutical manufacturers and the FDA to create products available in "ready-to-administer" or "ready-to-use" (RTU) form. That is, all IV medications should be available to the end user in the most readily available form, which does not have to be manipulated. Further, this group also recommended that medications, which cannot be provided in "ready-to-administer" dosage forms, be compounded exclusively in the pharmacy whenever possible.

Look-Alike Products

To prevent mix-ups in which one drug product is selected in error because of its similarity in appearance to another, storage shelves should be labeled to warn about this possibility. A recent example of a serious medication error occurred when Lupron Depot-Ped 11.25 mg (Leuprolide acetate-TAP), a 1-month gonadotropin-releasing analog used to treat central precocious puberty, was confused with Lupron Depot 3-Month. The latter is administered every 3 months to women with endometriosis or uterine leiomyomata (fibroids). The product releases its active ingredient over 3 months. Inadvertently, the second product was administered to children and caused them to receive therapy that was too low. It led attending physicians to believe that the drug therapy was a failure. One reason for the confusion was that the pharmacy staff inadvertently selected the wrong computer code during order entry, and this was repeated when, after referencing patients' drug profiles for monthly refills, the staff continued to select the 3-month dosage form instead of the monthly pediatric dosage form (36).

The manufacturer actually anticipated the problem and placed a picture of either an adult or a child to help discriminate the products. Unfortunately, price stickers were placed directly over the pictures and obscured the visual cues. To compound the problem, the products were taken to the pediatricians' offices, where the nurses administering the product also failed to note the mistake. The mistake might not have been detected except that a parent of one of the children questioned the pharmacy to ask about the increased prescription cost; Lupron Depot 3-Month costs more than Lupron Depot-Ped.

In the recent past, Heparin 10- and 10,000-U/mL vials from Baxter Laboratories were of the same size and both had blue labels, just differing in the degree of blue shading. A pharmacy technician inadvertently loaded an automated cabinet, that is, Pyxis, with the 10,000-U/mL vial instead of the 10-U/mL flush in the neonatal unit. Subsequently, the nurses pulled the drug and did not read the label. Then the catheters of several premature infants were flushed with doses 1,000 times greater than thought. The infants who received multiple doses developed bleeding and four ultimately died. The result was the 10,000-U/mL heparin product being removed from the hospital formulary and only one strength, that is, 10 U/mL is carried for a catheter flush (37). In addition, flush protocols have been rewritten to change the saline flush eliminating heparin altogether.

Adsorption of Drugs

Numerous studies have demonstrated that some drugs are adsorbed to the inner lining of IV containers and tubing or administration sets. Most often, these include proteins and peptides. Some of the drugs that have been implicated in this phenomenon include insulin and monoclonal antibodies, for example, laronidase (Aldurazyme). To obviate the adsorption phenomenon, human albumin is added. For laronidase, for example, the concentration of human albumin is 0.1% in 0.9% sodium chloride injection.

The adsorption of insulin onto glassware and tubing depends on several factors, including concentration of insulin, contact time of insulin with glass and tubing, flow rate of the infusion, and presence of negatively charged proteins (human serum albumin). Plastic IV infusion sets have reportedly removed up to 80% of a dose, but 20% to 30% is more common. The percent adsorbed is inversely proportional to the insulin concentration and will take place within 30 to 60 minutes. Because this phenomenon cannot be easily and accurately predicted, it is essential to monitor the patient.

Pharmacists must be cognizant of this phenomenon and take appropriate steps to prevent it. The significance of the loss is magnified with drugs that are used in small quantities because a small amount lost to adsorption results in a higher percentage loss of the drug delivered to the patient. One method to minimize this is to administer infusions through short lengths of small-diameter tubing made of inert plastics.

Absorption (Sorption) of Drugs

Plastic materials used for IV drug delivery may also facilitate drug absorption into the material itself. Absorption into a plastic material is most important to consider, as this phenomenon has been shown to occur in IV containers, delivery sets, syringes, filters, and other plastic apparatus, particularly associated with flexible PVC and can decrease the amount of drug delivered to the patient. This provides a hydrophobic environment for drug migration into the material. Most drug–plastic container interactions result from drug absorption by the DEHP in flexible PVC bags and tubing.

Examples of drugs lost from aqueous solutions during infusion through flexible PVC tubing include the following:

- Amiodarone HCl
- Chlorpromazine HCl
- Diazepam
- Lorazepam
- Nitroglycerin (NTG)
- Promazine HCl
- Promethazine HCl
- Thiopental sodium
- Thioridazine HCl
- Trifluoperazine HCl
- Warfarin sodium

NTG, for example, should always be prepared in glass and/or a plastic known to be compatible with it. It is adsorbed (40% to 80% of total dose) to PVC. Previously, some manufacturers packaged NTG for IV use with special non-PVC tubing to avoid loss (<5%) of the drug into the tubing during administration. However, many manufacturers have discontinued supplying NTG IV in the US market. Baxter Healthcare and Abbott Laboratories still manufacture NTG IV for injection, that is, 5 mg/mL. Baxter Healthcare, Hospira, and B. Braun market NTG premixed 100, 200, and 400 µg/mL in 250- and 500-mL glass bottles in 5% dextrose. However, the administration set, including tubing, is sold separately from the medication.

Special high-density polyethylene administration sets are recommended for NTG IV administration. Hard solid plastics, such as polyethylene and polypropylene, generally do not adsorb NTG. The amount of NTG adsorption depends on such factors as concentration, flow rate (e.g., a slow flow rate and long tubing increase the loss of NTG), surface area of the tubing, and contact time with the tubing.

IV NTG should be regulated by automatic infusion equipment (pumps, controllers) to enhance consistent dose administration. However, infusion pumps may fail to occlude the non-PVC infusion sets completely because the non-PVC tubing is stiffer than standard PVC tubing. Excessive flow at low infusion rate settings may occur, causing alarms or unregulated gravity flow when the infusion pump is stopped. This could lead to overinfusion of NTG.

Some practitioners have responded by using the PVC tubing with the NTG and working around the problem. This is justified by some in that even though a great amount of drug is lost, the amount of drug the patient receives is based on hemodynamic functions. But when the previous set is replaced, re-titration of the drug is necessary. To allay this problem, several manufacturers market non–PVC-containing pump administration sets.

In similar fashion to coping with the adsorption phenomenon of drugs to IV containers and/or administration sets, pharmacists must also be cognizant of the absorption phenomenon with flexible PVC materials and take appropriate steps to prevent it. The significance of the loss is magnified with drugs that are used in small quantities because a small amount lost to absorption results in a higher percentage loss of the drug delivered to the patient.

Handling and Disposal of Chemotherapeutic Agents for Cancer

In 1982, health care personnel became aware of environmental contamination from handling cytotoxic agents. Mutagenic and allergic case reports began to emerge in the literature, and in 1985, in response, the American Society of Hospital Pharmacists (now the ASHP) published its initial technical assistance bulletin on handling cytotoxic and hazardous drugs. This was revised in 1990. In 2006, ASHP issued their Guidelines on Handling Hazardous Drugs that replaced the technical assistance bulletin (38). These guidelines provide recommendations for the safe handling of hazardous drugs, environmental and ventilation controls, personal protective equipment, work practices, and hazardous waste containment and disposal. Practitioners should also be familiar with USP <800> Hazardous Drugs—Handling in Healthcare Settings, which can be enforced, if desired, by individual state boards of pharmacy and may be required by some certifying agencies. Practitioners must also be aware that the requirements of EPA, OSHA, and NIOSH must be met. Appendices include use of personal protective equipment, BSCs, and isolators, reducing exposure to hazardous drugs during administration, spill kits, and treatment of workers with direct skin or eye contact with hazardous drug.

Reconstituted Parenterals and Compatibility Resources

It should be noted that drugs that are prepared as "powders for reconstitution" generally have stability problems in solution. After reconstitution with the required diluent, these products generally have relatively short beyond-use dates that must be considered and observed.

Ready-to-use injections are the most stable at the pH at which they have been formulated. Any manipulation requiring a media of a different pH media may poses stability issues that must be considered.

Compatibility tables/charts and reference books are in wide use today. An entry in a reference that describes an admixture combination as physically compatible means that there are no observable changes in the solution. It does not rule out chemical changes involving drug degradation. The chemical compatibility information generally is presented as a beyond-use date that may be in hours, days, or weeks. These charts and books should be carefully evaluated during use to confirm the admixture or preparation being modified fits the data given in the reference source.

IRRIGATION AND DIALYSIS SOLUTIONS

Solutions for irrigation of body tissues and for dialysis are subject to the same stringent standards as parenteral preparations. The difference is in use. Irrigation and dialysis solutions are not injected into the vein but employed outside of the circulatory system. Because they are generally used in large volumes, they are packaged in large containers, generally of the screw cap type, which permits rapid pouring. Dialysis solutions generally appear similar to IV bags, and irrigation solutions are screw capped or bagged, so caution is necessary to avoid selecting the wrong product.

It is important to note that hemodialysis and peritoneal dialysis procedures have the capability to enhance the plasma clearance of a drug. In instances of clearance by 30% or more, supplemental dosing may be required or dosing after dialysis should be considered. Variations in duration of dialysis, flow rates, dialysis membrane type, and whether peritoneal dialysis is continuous or intermittent, all affect the extent of drug clearance. Drugs that have been shown to be cleared from plasma by hemodialysis, for example, include acetaminophen, captopril, cefaclor, imipenem, lithium, and metformin.

Irrigation Solutions

Irrigation solutions are intended to bathe or wash wounds, surgical incisions, or body tissues. Examples are presented in Table 15.8. Even though the actual contents of irrigation solutions are similar to parenteral solutions, their packaging and labeling is different and irrigation solutions must not be administered parenterally.

Dialysis Solutions

Dialysis is separation of substances from one another in solution by taking advantage of their differing diffusibility through membranes. *Peritoneal dialysis* solutions, allowed to flow into the peritoneal cavity, are used to remove toxic substances normally excreted by the kidney. In cases of poisoning or kidney failure, or in patients awaiting renal transplants, dialysis is an emergency lifesaving procedure. Solutions are commercially available containing dextrose as a major source of calories, vitamins, minerals, electrolytes, and amino acids or peptides as a source of nitrogen. The solutions are made to be hypertonic (with dextrose) to plasma to avoid absorption of water from the dialysis solution into the circulation.

TABLE 15.8. Examples of Irrigation Solutions

Solution	Description
Acetic Acid Irrigation, USP	0.25% solution applied topically to bladder for irrigation; pH 2.8–3.4, calculated osmolarity 42 mOsm/L; during urologic procedures, it washes away blood and surgical debris while maintaining suitable conditions for tissue and permitting unobstructed view
Neomycin and Polymyxin B Sulfates Solution for Irrigation, USP	Sterile urogenital solution contains 57 mg neomycin sulfate (40 mg neomycin) and polymyxin B sulfate 2,00,000 U/mL; topical antibacterial in continuous irrigation of bladder; pH 4.5–6; 1 mL added to 1 L 0.9% NaCl, administered via three-way catheter at 1 L/24 h (~40 mL/h)
Ringer Irrigation, USP	NaCl 8.6 g/L, potassium chloride 0.3 g/L, calcium chloride 0.33 g/L in purified water, in same proportions as in Ringer injection. Sterile and pyrogen-free; used topically to irrigate; must be labeled NOT FOR INJECTION; pH 5–7.5, calculated osmolarity 309 mOsm/L
Sodium Chloride Irrigation, USP	NaCl in water for injection; 77, 154 mEq/L of each sodium, chloride in 0.45% and 0.9% solutions, respectively; NaCl irrigation pH 5.3 approx.; 0.45%, 0.9% solutions calculated osmolarity 154, 308 mOsm/L, respectively. Employed topically to wash wounds and body cavities where absorption into blood not likely; also employed as enema; for simple evacuation, 150 mL; for colonic flush, 1,500 mL may be used
Sterile Water for Irrigation, USP	Sterilized and suitably packaged. Label designations FOR IRRIGATION ONLY, NOT FOR INJECTION must appear prominently. Must not contain any antimicrobial or other added agent

Peritoneal dialysis uses the principles of osmosis and diffusion across the semipermeable peritoneal membrane and includes osmotic and chemical equilibration of the fluid within the peritoneal cavity with that of the extracellular compartment. The semipermeable peritoneal membrane restricts the movement of formed elements (e.g., erythrocytes) and large molecules (e.g., protein) but allows the movement of smaller molecules (e.g., electrolytes, urea, water) in both directions across the membrane according to the concentration on each side of the membrane, with net movement occurring in the direction of the concentration gradient. Intraperitoneal instillation of dialysis solutions containing physiologic concentrations of electrolytes allows for movement of water, toxic substances, and/or metabolites across the membrane in the direction of the concentration gradient, removing these substances from the body following drainage of the solution from the peritoneal cavity (i.e., outflow).

Hemodialysis is employed to remove toxins from the blood. In this method, the arterial blood is shunted through a polyethylene catheter through an artificial dialyzing membrane bathed in an electrolyte solution. Following the dialysis, the blood is returned to the body circulation through a vein.

Various dialysis solutions are available commercially, and the pharmacist may be called upon to provide them or to make adjustments in their composition.

PHARMACEUTICS CASE STUDY

SUBJECTIVE INFORMATION

You have been asked to prepare progesterone injection 200 mg/mL in sesame oil for a physician's office. How will you formulate it?

OBJECTIVE INFORMATION

Progesterone is sparingly soluble in vegetable oils, and cosolvents must be used to obtain the 200 mg/mL concentration. Hormone injections in oil sometimes contain benzyl alcohol and/or benzyl benzoate. Benzyl alcohol, in addition to being a solvent, has preservative and anesthetic properties. Benzyl benzoate can be metabolized to benzyl alcohol and benzoic acid.

ASSESSMENT

It is apparent that a cosolvent system must be used, possibly consisting of sesame oil, benzyl alcohol, and benzyl benzoate, similar to other hormone injections. The product must be sterilized and suitably packaged.

PLAN

After reviewing the literature and the formulations for other hormone in oil injections, you determine that the formula will consist of benzyl alcohol 20%, benzyl benzoate 20%, and sesame oil 60%. The progesterone will be dissolved in the solvent system and be placed in a suitable container for dry heat sterilization. The dry heat sterilization will be validated but will start with 150°C for 1 hour. After sterilization, the injection will be aseptically packaged and labeled. ■

CLINICAL CASE STUDY

M.N. is an 18-year-old AA female diagnosed with type 1 diabetes mellitus 3 months ago. Today, she presents to the clinic for her regular checkup. Yesterday, she had her local pharmacist download her blood glucose (BG) levels for the past month from her home monitor. M.N. takes these to her physician for interpretation. M.N. tells her physician that she is "concerned about some of her BG levels, especially in the morning." She notes that her morning BG levels are usually around 160 mg/dL. She also states that she has been waking up from nightmares around 3 AM a few times every week. Three nights ago, after waking up, she checked her BG level at 3 AM, and her value was 192 mg/dL. She repeated the test to ensure that there was no error with her technique, and her reading was 188 mg/dL. Upon further questioning, the physician determines that M.N.'s knowledge of diabetes is increasing. However, the physician believes that M.N. would benefit from further education on diet and exercise. Because M.N. is newly diagnosed, the physician also wants her to review her insulin injection technique "from start to finish."

Meds: Humulin (NPH/Regular) 70/30 18 U before breakfast and 9 U before dinner.

Develop a pharmaceutical care plan addressing the following problems:
Hyperglycemia at 3:00 AM, 8:00 AM
Nutrition and exercise
Insulin injection technique

PHARMACEUTICAL CARE PLAN

S: M.N. is seen in the clinic for a regular checkup by her primary care physician. She is concerned with some BG levels that she has recorded over the past month. She says she has had nightmares a few times every week at that time. M.N. has been compliant with her insulin regimen and has requested additional education on insulin injection technique along with nutrition and exercise information.

O: Weight: 120 lb (54.5 kg)
See graph for average BG levels for April.
Current medications:
Humulin (NPH/Regular) 70/30 18 U before breakfast and 9 U before dinner.

A: 1. M.N.'s BG is uncontrolled with hyperglycemia at 3:00 AM and 8:00 AM. Hyperglycemia at these times is most likely because the patient is without appropriate insulin coverage throughout the night. M.N. checked her BG level at 3:00 AM after awakening from a nightmare, and the level was found to be elevated. The nightmares are an indication of high BG levels during sleep.
2. M.N. would like to review appropriate insulin injection preparation and administration technique with the pharmacist.
3. M.N. is a newly diagnosed patient and would like further information regarding diet and exercise.

P: 1. Because M.N.'s BG levels at 3:00 AM and 8:00 AM have been running high, it is appropriate to adjust the dinnertime dose of insulin. With a dinnertime dose of less than 10 U, the UKPDS suggests that the dose of insulin be increased by 1 U (if particular injection dose is more than 10 U, increase it by 2 U).
2. Therefore, M.N.'s Humulin 70/30 dose may be increased to 11 U at dinnertime to provide control during the night. M.N. should be instructed to monitor her 8:00 AM BG levels and three consecutive 3:00 AM BG levels and report these to her physician. If M.N. finds that her BG level after dinner is falling too low, she should increase her meal with one additional carbohydrate exchange.
3. The main points regarding insulin injection technique include in order:
Roll the vial of insulin in the palms to warm insulin and disperse it evenly.
Swipe the top of the vial once with an alcohol swab.
Swipe the body site for the injection with a different alcohol swab.
Pull air into the syringe. The amount of air pulled in should be equal to the amount of insulin that will be needed for the injection.
Insert the needle into the vial using the anticoring technique (demonstrated to the patient) and push the air into the vial.
While holding onto the vial and the syringe, invert both and remove the desired dose of insulin.
Remove the syringe from the vial.
At injection site, gather a fold of skin.
Insert the needle at a 90-degree angle to injection site.
Inject insulin.
Remove the needle from skin.
Discard the syringe in designated container for disposal.
Refer the patient to a registered dietitian for tailored meal planning. Some points M.N. should keep in mind:
Eat three scheduled meals per day. Skipping meals can cause BG to be uncontrolled.
Watch for serving sizes and control portion sizes.
Balance diet between carbohydrates, proteins, and fats.
It is important to monitor BG levels regularly.
Instruct the patient to make exercise a regular part of her day. Explain that exercise can help lower BG levels and any extra effort can be beneficial (e.g., parking further away from the store, taking the stairs instead of an elevator).
Caution: Start off slowly when beginning a new exercise program. For example, the patient may begin walking 3 days per week for 20 minutes and increase as tolerated. Instruct the patient to discuss the exercise regimen with a physician. ■

PATIENT COUNSELING

1. Instruct the patient on the proper storage and use of any parenteral preparation they use or for which they are responsible.
2. Explain the proper method of maintaining a sterile administration site and the proper handling of administration sets and equipment.
3. If applicable, demonstrate how to program ambulatory pumps and how to deal with emergencies.
4. Explain the importance of the expiration date or beyond-use date of the preparation.
5. Discuss the correct disposal of parenteral preparations, needles, syringes, and tubing so that patients are aware of the harm that can result from improper disposal.
6. Explain the importance of keeping the medication and the associated supplies (syringes, needles, etc.) out of the reach of children.

APPLYING THE PRINCIPLES AND CONCEPTS

GROUP ACTIVITIES

1. Prepare a chart outlining the differences in storage, administration, duration of activity, and compatibility of the different insulin products.
2. Develop an instruction sheet for health care professionals for proper use of an ampul (consider technique, reuse, Luer-Lok).
3. Review articles about parenteral and enteral nutrition and highlight the important advantages and disadvantages of each type.
4. Aseptic technique development:
   - Properly gown with personal protective equipment and gloves and assess hand hygiene by sampling the gloves with agar plate medium.
   - Perform media-fill testing using Soybean Casein Digest to develop and practice aseptic technique.
   - Practice aseptic volume transfers using a solution with the addition of methylene blue to demonstrate caution needed when preparing hazardous parenteral drugs.
5. Locate the standard operational procedure from your institution's IV room and compare it to the current USP <797> standards.
6. Discuss available references needed to determine:
   - If an oral dosage form can be crushed and added to an enteral feeding
   - The availability of alternative dosage forms for use in an enteral feeding
   - If it is acceptable to deliver a drug product through an enteral feeding tube

7. Discuss common technique mistakes when preparing compounded sterile products, and discuss how these technique mistakes can be overcome and corrected.

INDIVIDUAL ACTIVITIES

1. Summarize the five general types of injectable materials and identify which can be used directly/require reconstitution before administration: (*a*) injection, (*b*) for injection, (*c*) injectable emulsion, (*d*) injectable suspension, and (*e*) for injectable suspension.
2. Make a list of drugs that can cause electrolyte imbalance.
3. In a table, summarize the advantages and disadvantages of IV administration.
4. List examples of compounded sterile products from each risk category, that is, low, medium, and high.
5. Given simulated, daily blood glucose levels, follow a diabetes diet for 1 week, and calculate your insulin requirements at each meal.
6. Review the daily requirements of electrolytes, vitamins, and essential/nonessential amino acids, and then compare these values to your daily dietary intake and the contents found within a representative daily multivitamin product.
7. Perform a primary literature search that addresses the use of standardized versus individualized TPN orders, and compare/contrast the pros/cons of each.

REFERENCES

1. Rapp RP, Bivins BA, Littrell RA, et al. Patient-controlled analgesia: A review of effectiveness of therapy and an evaluation of currently available devices. DICP 1989;23:899–904.
2. Kwan JW. Use of infusion devices for epidural or intrathecal administration of spinal opioids. Am J Hosp Pharm 1990;47(Suppl 1):S18–S23.
3. Erstad BL, Meeks ML. Influence of injection site and route on medication absorption. Hosp Pharm 1993;28:853–856; 858–860; 863, 864; 867, 868; 871–874; 877, 878.
4. Highsmith AK, Greenhood GP, Allen JR. Growth of nosocomial pathogens in multiple-dose parenteral medication vials. J Clin Microbiol 1982;15:1024–1028.
5. Gershanik J, Boecler B, Ensley H, et al. The gasping syndrome and benzyl alcohol poisoning. N Engl J Med 1982;307:1384–1388.
6. Nema S, Avis KE. Loss of LDH activity during membrane filtration. J Parenter Sci Technol 1993;47:16–21.
7. Sarry C, Sucker H. Adsorption of proteins on microporous membrane filters: Part I. Pharm Technol 1992;16(Oct):72–82.

8. Sarry C, Sucker H. Adsorption of proteins on microporous membrane filters: Part II. Pharm Technol 1993;17:60–70.

9. McKinnon BT, Avis KE. Membrane filtration of pharmaceutical solutions. Am J Hosp Pharm 1993;50:1921–1936.

10. Butler LD, Munson JM, DeLuca PP. Effect of inline filtration on the potency of low-dose drugs. Am J Hosp Pharm 1980;37:935–941.

11. Akers MJ, Attia IA, Avis KE. Understanding and using F_0 values. Pharm Technol 1987;11:44–48.

12. USP-NF. Chapter <797> Pharmaceutical Compounding-Sterile Preparations, Current edition. Rockville, MD: U.S. Pharmacopeial Convention, Inc.

13. Wall DS, Noe LI, Abel SR, et al. A resource use comparison of monovial with traditional methods of preparing extemporaneous small-volume intravenous infusions. Hosp Pharm 1997;32:1647–1656.

14. Turco S, Miele WH, Barnoski D. Evaluation of an aseptic technique testing and challenge kit (Attack). Hosp Pharm 1993;28: 11–16.

15. Crawford SY, Narducci WA, Augustine SC. National survey of quality assurance activities for pharmacy-prepared sterile products in hospitals. Am J Hosp Pharm 1991;48:2398–2413.

16. NIOSH Publication 2004-165. Preventing Occupational Exposure to Anti-Neoplastic and Other Hazardous Drugs in Health Care Settings. Appendix A. http://www.cdc.gov/niosh/docs/2004-165/. (Accessed July 30, 2020)

17. Trissel LA, Gentempo JA, Saenz LM, et al. Effect of two work practice changes on the microbial contamination rates of pharmacy-compounded sterile preparations. Am J Health Syst Pharm 2007;64:837–841.

18. Maliekal J, Bertch KE, Witte KW. An update on ready-to-use intravenous delivery system. Hosp Pharm 1993;28:970–971; 975–977.

19. Turco S. Sterile Dosage Forms. 4th Ed. Philadelphia, PA: Lea & Febiger, 1994:263.

20. Chandler C, Gryniewicz CM, Pringle T, et al. Insulin temperature and stability under simulated transit conditions. Am J Health Syst Pharm 2008;65:953–963.

21. Meece J. Effects of insulin pen devices on the management of diabetes mellitus. Am J Health Syst Pharm 2008;65:1076–1082.

22. Keith K, Nicholason D, Rogers D. Accuracy and precision of low-dose insulin administration using syringes, pen injectors, and a pump. Clin Pediatr 2004;43:69–74.

23. Lee WC, Balu S, Cobden D, et al. Medication adherence and the associated health-economic impact among patients with type 2 diabetes mellitus converting to insulin pen therapy: An analysis of third-party managed care claims. Clin Ther 2006;28:1712–1725.

24. Potti LG, Haines ST. Continuous subcutaneous insulin infusion therapy: A primer on insulin pumps. Pharm Today 2009;15(1):54–67.

25. Lumpkin M. Safety alert: Hazards of precipitation associated with parenteral nutrition. Am J Hosp Pharm 1994;51:1427–1428.

26. McKinnon BT. FDA safety alert: Hazards of precipitation associated with parenteral nutrition. Nutr Clin Pract 1996;11:59–65.

27. Munzenberger PJ, Levin S. Home parenteral antibiotic therapy for patients with cystic fibrosis. Hosp Pharm 1993;28:20–28.

28. Shaver K, Woelfel JA. Pharmacist Letter, 2008;24(12):Document 241204.

29. Williams NT. Medication administration through enteral feeding tubes. Am J Health Syst Pharm 2008;65:2347–2357.

30. Kwan JW. High-technology IV infusion devices. Am J Hosp Pharm 1989;46:320–335.

31. KITS: Kit for Infusion Technology Self-Instruction. Proceedings from the Institute of Safe Medication Practices Summit on the use of Smart Infusion Pumps: Guidelines for Safe Implementation and Use. Abbott Park, IL: Abbott Laboratories. Available at: http://www.ismp.org/Tools/guidelines/smartpumps/comments/printer-Version.pdf. (Accessed July 30, 2020)

32. Keefner KR. Parenteral pumps and controlled-delivery devices. US Pharmacist 1992;17(8):H-3–H-16.

33. Allen Jr LV. Intravenous Admixture Preparation Considerations, Part 2: Incompatibilities and Factors Involved. Int J Pharm Compd. 24(1) Jan-Feb 2020, 44-50.

34. Thompson CA. ASHP evaluation of the USP MEDMARX data. 2002–2006. Surgical units have high potential for harmful medication errors, USP says. Am J Health Syst Pharm 2007;64(9):917,920. http://www.ashp.org/import/news/healthsystempharmacynews/newsarticle.aspx?id=2535. (Accessed April 13, 2016)

35. Egervary A. Industry groups call for IV concentration standards. Pharm Today 2009;15(1):HSE 8.

36. Institute for Safe Medication Practices. Look-alike products. Pharm Today 2003;9(5):20.

37. http://www.theindychannel.com/news/9884927/detail.html. (Accessed July 30, 2020)

38. American Society of Health-System Pharmacists. ASHP guidelines on handling hazardous drugs. Am J Health Syst Pharm 2006;63:1172–1193.

CHAPTER

16 Biologics

OBJECTIVES

After reading this chapter, the student will be able to:

1. Discuss the differences between biologics and biosimilars
2. Define, compare, and contrast the different types of immunity
3. List the standards and control requirements needed for the production of biologics
4. List various sources of valuable information for the proper use, storage, and administration of biologics
5. Compare and contrast the types of biologics for active immunity and their mechanism of action
6. List the sources of biologics for passive immunity
7. Describe the possible adverse drug reactions for biologics based on their mechanism of action, administration, and/or excipients
8. Describe the childhood and adult immunization schedules

▌ BIOLOGICS AND BIOSIMILARS

A biologic medicine is typically a large molecule derived from living cells and used in the treatment, diagnosis, or prevention of disease. Biologics include therapeutic proteins, DNA vaccines, monoclonal antibodies, and fusion proteins. Generally, they are from 200 to 1,000 times larger than the typical small molecule drug and are structurally far more complex. Biologics are also very sensitive to their manufacturing and handling conditions, making them very difficult to characterize and produce. Biologics are not made using a set of standard materials but are developed using unique biological systems and living cells; consequently, the active ingredient is impossible to duplicate and the specific cell lines from which the biologic originates are unique to each manufacturer. The manufacturing process involves dozens of steps involving hundreds of variables and is generally more complex than is the manufacturing process for small drug molecules. Biologics are generally given by the parenteral route.

Biosimilars are similar, but not identical, copies of the original biologic medicine. Biologics are so complex that it is impossible to reproduce them exactly. This is different from generic medicines of small molecule drugs where they must be the same. Biologics made by different manufacturers differ from the original product and from each other. Biosimilars are determined on the basis of analytical, nonclinical, and clinical data to be similar to an original biologic in terms of structural characteristics and safety and efficacy. Minor differences are expected and permitted as long as such differences are demonstrated to not be clinically significant. So, a biosimilar product is a biological product that is approved based on demonstrating that it is highly similar to an FDA-approved biological product and has no clinically meaningful differences in terms of safety and effectiveness from the reference product.

In 2015, the FDA approved the first biosimilar product for use in the United States; it was Sandoz Biopharmaceutical's Zarxio, which is a biosimilar version of Amgen Inc.'s Neupogen (filgrastim). It has been approved for the same indications. The approval results from the faster abbreviated regulatory approval pathway created by the Biologics Price Competition and Innovation Act of 2009, signed into law in March 2010. Biosimilars are neither a generic nor an original product. It is not a "biobetter" or a "stand-alone." Biosimilars are not "better," but they can be less expensive and may facilitate access to new treatments in many populations.

Although most states have passed legislation allowing pharmacists to substitute generics of small drug molecules without having to obtain prescriber approval, the same is not true for biosimilars; this is being handled on a state-by-state basis.

INTRODUCTION

The Food and Drug Administration (FDA) refers to immunizing agents as biologics. In an encompassing manner, a biologic is a substance produced by a living source; biologics include antibiotics, hormones, and vitamins, among others. The Advisory Committee on Immunization Practices (ACIP) refers to immunizing agents as *immunobiologics*.

According to the *Code of Federal Regulations*, a biologic product is any virus, therapeutic serum, toxin, antitoxin, or analogous product employed for prevention, treatment, or cure of diseases in humans. The purpose of these products is to help develop immunity in the person receiving them. Immunity is defined as natural or acquired resistance to disease.

Provision of immunity through the use of a biologic is immunization. *Vaccination* is the term more commonly used; it refers to the use of a biologic product (a vaccine) to develop active immunity in the patient.

The benefits of these products is apparent when one considers, for example, that the incidence of poliomyelitis fell dramatically after licensure of the inactivated polio vaccine in 1955 and the oral polio vaccine (OPV) in the 1960s. In the early 1950s, there were more than 20,000 cases of polio each year. By 1960, the number of polio cases had dropped to about 3,000, and by 1979, the last cases (about 10) of indigenously acquired polio in the United States were reported. Similarly, the largest annual number of cases of rubella, or German measles, an acute viral disease affecting people of all ages, occurred in the United States in 1969 (57,686 cases reported). Following rubella vaccine licensure in 1969, the incidence of this disease fell rapidly, and since 1992, the number of reported cases in the United States has been fewer than 500 per year.

TYPES OF IMMUNITY

Before discussing specific biologics, it is important to understand the different types of immunity. There are two main categories of immunity: natural and acquired.

Natural Immunity

Natural, innate, or native immunity depends on factors that are inborn and can be classified as species immunity, racial immunity, and individual immunity.

Species Immunity

In general, cold-blooded animals are not susceptible to diseases common to warm-blooded animals. Humans are not all susceptible to certain diseases of lower animals, such as chicken cholera. However, a number of infections that occur primarily in animals can be transmitted to humans. Among the most important are anthrax (in cattle, sheep, horses), plague (in rodents), and rabies (in cats, dogs, bats, and others). Correspondingly, many human diseases do not naturally occur in animals. Examples include gonorrhea, typhoid fever, influenza, measles, mumps, and poliomyelitis.

Racial Immunity

Human races differ in susceptibility to common infections (e.g., yellow fever, pneumonia, tuberculosis). Factors that determine racial immunity are elusive and not well known. Racial immunity should not be used synonymously or confused with environmental immunity. Environmental immunity may be the result of resistance to infection among individuals in a community resulting from the degree of acquired immunity and other factors (e.g., nutrition, genetic constitution, fatigue). For example, tuberculosis and smallpox wreaked havoc among the Eskimos and American Indians when these groups were first exposed to them. However, with the course of time, the disease tends to become less severe, and it may eventually reach the same level of incidence and severity as among other races with whom the disease has been endemic for a long time.

Individual Immunity

Apart from any specific immunity to a particular infectious agent, individuals vary in the ability to resist common microbiologic diseases. Some individuals have little capacity to resist skin disorders, the common cold, and other familiar diseases. The natural resistance of the same individual may vary from time to time.

General good health, demonstrated by healthy body tissues, skin, and mucous membranes; leukocytes in plentiful supply; and an active and positive lifestyle (i.e., little or no smoking, alcohol, social drug use), provides adequate barriers to bacterial infiltration. Resident bacteria in the gastrointestinal tract and upper respiratory tract, for example, provide resistance to infection. These play a vital role in resisting invasion by other species of microorganisms capable of producing infection. Also, stomach acid is to a degree capable of destroying ingested bacteria. Intestinal enzymes are also known to provide secondary defense mechanisms.

Acquired Immunity

Acquired immunity is a specific immunity that may be active or passive. *T lymphocytes* regulate cell-mediated immunity and are responsible for controlling certain bacterial and viral infections. These lymphocytes are responsible for mediating graft versus host disease, allograft rejection, and delayed hypersensitivity reactions.

T lymphocytes augment the activity of *B* lymphocytes, which are primarily involved with humoral immunity and antibody production. Once an antigen is introduced into the body, *B lymphocytes* differentiate into plasma cells that produce antibodies specific to the invading antigen. These antibodies, known synonymously as immunoglobulins, attach to the invading antigen and cause its destruction by phagocytes and the complement system.

Once exposed to an antigen, the *T* and *B lymphocytes* demonstrate memory that allows them to recognize and respond to a specific antigen when exposed again. The second response is far greater in magnitude to the first immunologic response. This memory of an antigen by the immune system allows sensitized individuals to resist infections on subsequent exposure.

Active Immunity

Active immunity develops in response to antigenic substances in the body. This may occur by natural means, as by infection, in which case it is termed *naturally acquired active immunity*, or it may develop in response to administration of a specific vaccine or toxoid, in which case it is *artificially acquired active immunity*. In either case, the body builds up its own defense in response to the antigen.

Vaccines are administered primarily for prophylactic action, to develop acquired active immunity. Vaccines may contain living attenuated (weakened) or killed microorganisms or fractions of these microorganisms. Toxoids are bacterial toxins modified and detoxified with moderate heat and chemical treatment so that the antigenic properties remain whereas the substance is rendered nontoxic. Although toxoids do not cause disease, exposure of immunocompetent persons may result in antibody production that will protect the person against disease caused by the natural toxin. A problem with toxoids is that they produce inadequate immunologic responses when administered alone. Therefore, they are often combined with adjuvants (e.g., alum, aluminum phosphate, aluminum hydroxide) that enhance their antigenicity. These agents do so through their insoluble nature, which acts to keep the immunogens in tissue for longer periods and, thus, prolongs the immune response.

A vaccine composed of killed whole bacteria or viruses or substructures of these is known as an inactivated vaccine. Vaccines that contain live but significantly weakened microorganisms are attenuated vaccines. Both types are capable of producing immunity. However, the attenuated vaccines typically have more antigenicity and so are more likely to confer permanent immunity. To maintain adequate antibody titers, inactivated vaccines must be administered again over time.

With live vaccines, caution must be exercised with immunocompromised patients. This group of patients includes those with HIV infection, thymic abnormalities, lymphoma, leukemia, generalized malignancy, or advanced debilitating diseases or who are receiving corticosteroids, alkylating agents, antimetabolites, or radiation chemotherapy. These patients are unable to mount immune responses against even weakened microorganisms. The result could be a disseminated bacterial or viral infection. Thus, inactivated vaccines should be employed for these patients.

Immunization during pregnancy is another concern. Live attenuated vaccines should be avoided for pregnant patients because of the danger of transmission of the microorganism to the fetus. For example, measles, mumps, and rubella (MMR) vaccine should not be administered during pregnancy, and pregnancy should be avoided for 1 month following vaccination with monovalent measles vaccine and 4 weeks following MMR or other rubella-containing vaccines.

Passive Immunity

Passive acquired immunity occurs by introduction of the immunoglobulins produced in another individual (human or animal) into the host, who is not involved in their production. In similar fashion to active acquired immunity, passive acquired immunity can be classified as natural or artificial.

Naturally acquired passive immunity occurs by placental transmission of immunoglobulin gamma (IgG) from the mother to the fetus. Because of the transfer of these immunoglobulins, the infant may have passive immunity to diphtheria, tetanus, measles, mumps, and other infections for the first 4 to 6 months of life.

Several biologic products containing immunoglobulins provide passive immunity. These are limited to provision of temporary prophylaxis to susceptible individuals, for example, during an epidemic, and to supplying immediate immunoglobulins for the treatment of infections and toxicities. Notable in this category are the antivenins for treatment of snakebite (e.g., North American coral snake antivenin) and spiders (e.g., black widow spider antivenin).

The acquired passive immunity provided by immunoglobulins is not long lasting, usually 1 to 2 weeks. Their important feature is that they offer the susceptible patient protection during a critical period of exposure (e.g., the patient exposed to diphtheria). Immunoglobulins do not last long because their function is to bind to the pathogen as needed. Immunoglobulin is metabolized by the body if not needed for immunologic purposes.

▌ PRODUCTION OF BIOLOGICS

Biologics are produced by manufacturers licensed to do so in accordance with the terms of the federal Public Health Service Act (58 Stat. 682) approved on July 1, 1944, and each product must meet specified standards as administered by the Center for Biologics Evaluation and Research of the FDA (1). Each lot of a licensed biologic is approved for distribution when it has been determined that the lot meets the specific control requirements for that product. Licensing includes approval of a specific series of production steps and in-process control tests as well as end product specifications that must be met lot by lot.

Generally, each lot of a biologic product must pass rigid control requirements before it may be distributed for general use. Provisions generally applicable to biologic products include tests for potency, general safety, sterility, purity, water (residual moisture), pyrogens, identity, and constituent materials. Constituent materials include preservatives, diluents, and adjuvants, which generally should meet compendial standards; extraneous protein in cell-cultured vaccines (which, if other than serum originating, is excluded); and antibiotics other than penicillin added to the production substrate of viral vaccines, for which compendial monographs on antibiotics and antibiotic substances are available. Additional safety tests on live vaccines and certain other items are also required.

Biologics to be administered by injection are packaged and labeled in the same manner as are other injections. In addition, the label of a biologic product must include the title or proper name (the name under which the product is licensed under the Public Health Service Act); the name, address, and license number of the manufacturer; the lot number; the expiration date; and the recommended individual dose for multiple-dose containers. The package label also includes the preservative and its amount; the number of containers if more than one; the amount of product in the container; the recommended storage temperature; a statement, if necessary, that freezing is to be avoided; and such other information as FDA regulations may require to ensure safe and effective use of the product.

With few exceptions, most biologics are stored in a refrigerator (2°C to 8°C, or 35°F to 46°F), and freezing is avoided. Besides the biologic substance that is harmed by freezing, the container may be broken because of the expansion of an aqueous vehicle resulting in loss of product. Diluents packaged with biologics should not be frozen. Some products are to be held at specified temperatures during shipment.

The expiration date for biologic products varies with the product and the storage temperatures. Most biologic products have an expiration date of a year or longer after the date of manufacture or issue. The stated date on each lot determines the dating period, which begins on the date of manufacture and beyond which the product cannot be expected to retain the required safety, purity, and potency. The dating period may be composed of an in-house storage period during which the lot is held under prescribed conditions followed by a period after issue. The individual monographs for biologics usually indicate both the after-issue time frame for use and (in parentheses) the permissible in-house storage period.

STORAGE, HANDLING, AND SHIPPING OF BIOLOGICS

Biologics are sensitive to extreme temperatures, and exposure to heat or freezing can decrease their potency and dramatically reduce their effectiveness. Poor storage, handling, and shipping conditions for these products not only waste the intrinsic value of the products but waste money as well. Biologics are expensive and can add significantly to one's inventory costs. An inventory of vaccines and other immunologic products can amount to tens of thousands of dollars or more.

A real danger is that if damaged products are administered, the person may get little or none of the intended benefit. The person may not be able to build up immunity and may result in an infection or inadequate protection from the disease.

The overriding theme for the pharmacist in storage, handling, and shipping of biologic products is to maintain the cold chain (2). This implies continuity from the manufacturer's refrigerator to one's pharmacy, clinic, or office to administration. If the cold chain is maintained, the pharmacist can be assured that the quality of the product will not be diminished.

In the pharmacy, there should be a clear understanding of primary and secondary individuals who are responsible for receiving, handling, and shipping these products. A key ingredient is good storage equipment. Whenever possible, separate commercial refrigerators and freezers should be used for these products. For small-volume biologics, a standard refrigerator-freezer should be used. Frost-free freezers are no longer recommended for storage of frozen products because periodic freeze–thaw cycling, inherent in the refrigerator's frost-free function, can significantly reduce the product stability.

Refrigerators and freezers cool by convection. Thus, cool air must have room to circulate around the product. Packing the refrigerator too tightly can lead to small incremental elevations in the temperature of the product.

A separate refrigerator dedicated to biologics is preferable to minimize the times the refrigerator door is opened. The World Health Organization recommends that the door not be opened more frequently than four times per day. Also, doors should be closed as quickly as possible after securing the product, and pharmacists should avoid using the inside of the refrigerator door to store products to avoid unacceptable temperature variations. The door shelving can be used to store diluents or bottles of water. This helps provide insulation and a thermal reserve (2).

If a vaccine must be kept outside of the refrigerator for a few minutes, it is advisable to put the product in an insulated container with coolant packs (thermal packs, blue ice packs, chemical packs) from the freezer. Coolant packs should be kept in the freezer and ready for use in shipping. An additional advantage of freezer packs is that they provide extra insulation and cooling power in the freezer in case of an interruption of electric power or outage.

Coolant packs that contain water have about as much cooling capacity as do ethylene glycol packs. An easy way to create a coolant pack is to fill a plastic bottle with water and freeze it. It is important, however, that the product not come in direct contact with these coolant packs because the vial contents may freeze and be damaged. A towel or sheet of cardboard may be used to separate the product from the coolant pack (2).

Periodically, it is advisable for the pharmacist to test the temperature of the refrigerator and freezer. The National Immunization Program (NIP) recommends twice daily temperature monitoring and recording. Furthermore, logs of these temperatures should be kept for 3 years. Some adult immunization programs recommend that refrigerator temperature be checked daily and recorded in a log. Refrigerator temperatures should range between 2°C and 8°C, and freezers should stay well below 0°C. Usually, an optimal temperature is −15°C (5°F).

With respect to personnel, pharmacists should educate and train every person who will handle biologics in good storage and handling procedures. These individuals should understand the importance of reporting any problems or interruptions associated with proper handling and storage guidelines. It is far more important to report a breach in handling and storage than to discount and overlook it intentionally. The use of a mishandled or poorly stored biologic could have devastating consequences on the person who receives it.

Store containers of the same vaccine together. To avoid selecting the wrong product or one having a similar sounding name or packaging, separate the products. A good example of this occurs with pediatric and adult dosage forms (e.g., tetanus–diphtheria toxoids), which could be confused. Keep them separate. Look-alike packaging as well as soundalike names can easily confuse any conscientious practitioner.

An online publication describing storage and handling requirements for currently recommended vaccines is available from the Centers for Disease Control and Prevention (CDC). Included in the publication are shipping and storage recommendations for specific vaccines, how to reconstitute them, information about vaccines' shelf life before and after reconstitution, and special handling instructions (3).

Biologics for Active Immunity

Bacterial Vaccines

A vaccine is a suspension of attenuated (live) or inactivated (killed) microorganisms or fractions thereof that are administered to induce immunity and prevent disease. Originally, the organism is grown in a suitable broth medium in a controlled environment of temperature, pH, and oxygen tension. To reduce the potential for hypersensitivity reactions to the finished product, the medium, whenever possible, should consist of chemically defined ingredients.

Following a suitable amount of time for bacterial growth, the culture is processed in two steps. If the vaccine is to be inactivated microorganisms, the organisms are treated with phenol or formaldehyde. Heat and phenol or heat and acetone are employed for the typhoid fever vaccine. Next, the organisms are separated from the medium through centrifugation and suspended in sterile water or 0.9% sodium chloride for injection. If necessary, the preparation may be further purified by several methods, including dialysis and/or additional centrifugation.

A live attenuated vaccine can also be produced by genetic alteration of the pathogenic organisms. This allows the organism to survive and multiply but not produce the disease. Usually, several base pairs of DNA in a key region of the gene structure are eliminated or altered. Thus, the organism is incapable of reverting to its more pathogenic form.

Another way to create a vaccine is to employ purified antigen subunits produced with use of recombinant DNA. With subunit vaccines, the genes that code for the desired antigen are introduced into the nonpathogenic organisms. There is no potential to harm the patient because there is no possibility that a pathogenic organism can be created from only a limited number of components of the original organism. Also, the subunit vaccine can be expected to have a lower incidence of side effects. As an example, the hepatitis B vaccine is produced through recombinant DNA technology by common baker's yeast, into which the gene for the hepatitis B surface antigen (HBsAg) has been inserted.

To date, subunit vaccines have had limited clinical utility because of inability to produce a sufficient, specific immune response. However, alternative biotechnologic strategies have been employed to produce subunit vaccine immunogens and adjuvant-active compounds that can be added to enhance the immune response.

The final vaccine may contain one single immunogen (monovalent), or it may contain multiple immunogens (polyvalent, trivalent) to promote immunity against the same disease state. The final product may also be a mixed vaccine. For example, MMR vaccine is a single product with three immunogens for three viral diseases. A mixed biologic may contain a vaccine and a toxoid in the same product, as with diphtheria, tetanus, and pertussis (DTP). Another example of a mixed biologic is the combination vaccine Pediarix (diphtheria and tetanus toxoids and acellular pertussis adsorbed, hepatitis B [recombinant], and inactivated poliovirus vaccine [IPV]) introduced in late 2002.

The strength of a vaccine may be expressed as total number of organisms, total protective units per milliliter or dose, or micrograms of immunogen in each milliliter or in each dose of vaccine.

A current list of vaccines licensed in the United States is posted at www.fda.gov/cber/.

Viral Vaccines

Viruses cannot be grown on inanimate media employed to grow bacteria and so are propagated on one of several types of animate media. Examples of animate media include embryonic egg, cell cultures of chick embryo, human diploid cell culture, monkey cell culture, skin of living calves, and intact mice.

In similar fashion to vaccine preparation, after growth of the culture, various techniques are employed to separate the virus from the host cell. Purification steps are taken to reduce the incidence of hypersensitivity reactions to animate media or host cells, most notably embryonic egg. The final viral product may contain a single immunogen (monovalent) or multiple immunogens (polyvalent) to elicit immunity against the same disease.

The vaccine may remain as the whole virion or be further chemically processed to split it into a subvirion vaccine, as is the case with the influenza virus vaccine. This virus is prepared yearly with three virus strains. Since 1977, influenza A (H1N1), influenza A (H3N2), and influenza B viruses have circulated globally. Each year's influenza vaccine contains a virus representing each of these three distinct influenza virus groups. The three viruses selected to be included for the 2008 to 2009 season vaccine were selected in February 2008 as the viruses that appeared most likely to be circulating during this influenza season (4). The 2008 to 2009 trivalent vaccine strains are A/Brisbane/59/2007-like (H1N1), A/Brisbane/10/2007-like (H3N2), and B/Florida/4/2006-like viruses. The degree of antigenic match between current influenza vaccine strains and the influenza viruses that are circulating this season will continue to be assessed as more viruses become available for analysis. To date, 91% of influenza A (H1N1) viruses sent to CDC for antigenic characterization were similar to A/Solomon Islands/3/2006, the influenza A (H1N1) component of the 2007 to 2008 influenza vaccine. Although the majority of influenza A (H3N2) and influenza B viruses are not optimally matched, vaccination with the trivalent influenza vaccine continues to be recommended because the vaccine can provide partial protection against related strains and reduce the risk for influenza-related complications and deaths. In addition, communities can experience outbreaks with more than one strain of influenza in a given year.

Strains are usually selected during the preceding February because of scheduling requirements for production, quality control, packaging, distribution, and vaccine administration before the onset of the next influenza season. Sometimes strains mutate and protection is not thorough as was the case for the 2007 to 2008 flu season. When there is a good match between the strains in the vaccine and those in the community, inactivated vaccine is 70% to 90% effective in preventing influenza in adults under 65 years of age.

To prolong stimulation of antibodies, the virion may be adsorbed onto aluminum phosphate, as is the case with rabies vaccine (adsorbed). Typically, viral vaccines are available as lyophilized (freeze-dried) products that require reconstitution prior to administration with the provided diluent. Some inactivated vaccines are available in suspensions for injection.

Belshe et al. (5) reported the effectiveness of a live attenuated, cold-adapted, trivalent influenza virus vaccine that was administered intranasally to more than 1,000 healthy school-aged children. This placebo-controlled trial demonstrated that children receiving the active vaccine had fewer febrile illnesses, including 30% fewer episodes of febrile otitis media, than did the placebo group. This was one significant outcome of the study, because otitis media is a recognized complication of influenza in children, and the influenza virus has been isolated from middle ear fluid in children with influenza and middle ear effusion. The incidence of otitis media increases in the 14-day period after influenza virus infection. Furthermore, administration of inactivated influenza virus vaccine has been shown to reduce outbreaks of otitis media in day care centers (6). Thus, if efforts are employed to immunize more day care children, this might ultimately result in lower incidence of otitis media and less need for prescribed antibiotics.

Historically, the influenza vaccine was strongly recommended annually for children aged 6 months or more with certain risk factors, including but not limited to asthma, cardiac disease, sickle cell disease, HIV, and diabetes. However, as of 2006, all children aged 6 to 59 months and their household contacts and out-of-home caregivers should be vaccinated against influenza.

In June 2003, the live intranasal influenza virus vaccine (FluMist, Wyeth; MedImmune) was approved for active immunization against influenza A and B viruses in healthy children aged 5 to 17 and adults 18 to 49 years of age. It is the first vaccine approved in the United States for administration as a nasal mist. The introduction of a nasal vaccine has much implication to help overcome barriers to immunization (fear of side effects, the need for yearly immunizations, perception of low vaccine effectiveness). Widespread use of the nasal vaccine in high-risk children may, therefore, be more easily achievable than use of injected vaccines. This would be a very effective way to reduce the incidence of influenza in this population. The only downside is its expense (ranging from $50 to $70 per patient) and that the cold chain, discussed earlier in this chapter, must be maintained to guarantee adequate stability.

The strength of viral vaccines can be provided in tissue culture infectious doses, the quantity of virus estimated to infect 50% of inoculated cultures. Also, micrograms of immunogen, international units, D-antigen units, and plaque-forming units for yellow fever vaccine are employed for these products.

Cancer Vaccines

For more than a century, the role of the immune system and its relationship to cancer has been researched. Recently, however, the immune response is being clinically explored as a mode to prevent and treat cancer. Cancer vaccines in development are intended to increase recognition of cancer cells by the immune system.

This approach to cancer treatment is exciting, as it offers another modality to complement surgery, radiation therapy, and chemotherapy. Another cause for guarded optimism is that the development of these vaccines may play a role in preventing cancer in patients at high risk because of familial diseases.

For the immune system to recognize and kill a tumor cell, immune cells must recognize antigens on the tumor cell as foreign to the body and receive costimulatory signals. Otherwise, tumor cells go undetected by the immune system and proliferate. Thus, a goal of cancer vaccine development is to increase antigen awareness of the immune cells or increase costimulatory signals that induce an immune response.

T cells, lymphokine-activated killer cells, and natural *killer cells* have antitumor activity. Thus, tumor vaccine development is to stimulate these immune cells instead of antibody-producing cells, the operational model used to protect one from an infection. Tumor-killing cells recognize tumor-associated antigens (TAAs) on the surface of the tumor cells. These antigens have peptide fragments that appear on the cell surface either by the cancer cell or taken up by a phagocytic cell.

TAAs fall into one of three categories. These are patient specific, tumor specific, and shared. Antigens unique to a specific patient are patient specific, such as an antigen expressed on the surface of a B-cell malignancy. A tumor-specific TAA is unique to a particular tumor. Most notable is prostate-specific antigen, found in prostate tumors. Shared TAAs are created by tumor cells with a common histology. A notable example of this is the carcinoembryonic antigen on adenocarcinoma cells found in colon, ovarian, and lung tumors.

Four types of cancer vaccines are under investigation, and a thorough explanation of each is beyond the scope of this book. Nonetheless, these types are important. They are autologous, allogeneic, anti-idiotypic, and gene therapy–derived vaccines.

Autologous tumor vaccines are developed from antigenic material procured from the tumor of the patient. Tumor cells are isolated from tissue procured during biopsy or surgery. These cells are killed or attenuated and reinfused into the patient. Typically, to enhance immunogenicity, they are combined with an adjuvant, such as bacille Calmette-Guérin (BCG) or *Corynebacterium parvum.* A major problem with this approach is the work and cost associated with the production of vaccine for the individual patient. Also, some tumors escape the immune system because their antigens are not expressed on the tumor surface.

Allogeneic tumor vaccines use the concept of shared or tumor-specific antigens. These vaccines are produced from cell lines that express tumor-specific or shared TAAs. To induce an immune response, either the fragment of the allogeneic tumor cell or the whole cell is injected. The beneficial aspect of this vaccine is that it can be used in a wide population of patients.

Anti-idiotypic vaccines are three-dimensional immunogenic regions on the antibody that binds antigen. Antibodies that bind TAAs are isolated and injected into mice. The resulting antibodies are harvested and used to vaccinate another mouse. The resulting antibodies have a three-dimensional binding site that mimics the original structure of the TAA. These antibodies are combined with an adjuvant and given as a vaccine. Because the anti-idiotypic antibody closely resembles the antigen, these can be used to induce immune responses (cellular, antibody–antigen) to a given antigen.

Gene therapy allows a DNA template to be placed within a cell, transcribed into messenger RNA, and expressed as a costimulatory protein. One can then induce a cell to synthesize this protein as part of its normal function. A gene that encodes for interleukins or other costimulatory proteins can be placed in cells expressing TAAs. This stimulates the immune response. In June 2006, the FDA approved the first quadrivalent human papillomavirus (HPV) (Types 6, 11, 16, 18) recombinant vaccine (Gardasil by Merck). Approximately 70% of cervical cancer is caused by infection with HPV types 16 and 18, and approximately 90% of genital warts are caused by HPV types 6 and 11. As this is a prophylactic measure, at present, this vaccine is only indicated for women 9 to 26 years of age. Subsequently, in September 2008, this vaccine was approved to prevent vulvar and vaginal cancers. To test the vaccine, 15,000 women from earlier cervical cancer studies were evaluated for a 2-year period. In the group that did not receive the vaccine, 10 women developed precancerous vulvar lesions and nine developed similar vaginal lesions. No women in the Gardasil-treated group developed such lesions.

Clinical trials are being undertaken for cancer vaccines for melanoma, colorectal cancer, renal cell carcinoma, breast and ovarian cancers, prostate cancer, and lung cancer.

Toxoids

In similar fashion to bacterial vaccines, bacteria are propagated, and after the required growth is achieved, the culture is filtered through a sterilizing membrane filter. The filtrate that contains the toxin (exotoxin) is then processed. Processing involves addition of a concentrated salt solution to precipitate the toxin from the filtrate. After the precipitated toxin is washed and dialyzed to purify it, the toxin is detoxified with formaldehyde.

The detoxified toxin (toxoid) may be plain or contain an adjuvant (e.g., alum, aluminum hydroxide, aluminum sulfate). The product may also contain single, multiple, or mixed immunogens (e.g., tetanus and diphtheria toxoids adsorbed for adult use, which contains two toxoids for active immunization against different toxins). A mixed biologic, such as diphtheria and tetanus toxoids and pertussis vaccine adsorbed for pediatric use, has two toxoids and a vaccine in a single-dosage form for active immunization against different toxicities and infection.

Their advantage is broad immunization coverage and minimum number of injections.

These mixtures or types of biologics differ from polyvalent products, which are used for different strains of the same toxicity or infection (e.g., influenza virus vaccine, pneumococcal vaccine polyvalent).

The strength of a toxoid is in flocculating (Lf) units (e.g., tetanus toxoid, 4 to 5 Lf U/0.5-mL dose). A flocculating unit is the smallest amount of toxin that flocculates most rapidly one unit of standard antitoxin in a series of mixtures containing fixed amounts of antitoxin and varying amounts of toxin.

Biologics for Passive Immunity

Human Immune Sera and Globulins (Homologous Sera)

Human immune sera, or homologous sera, include immunoglobulin and hyperimmune sera for specific diseases. These contain the specific antibodies obtained from the blood of humans and produced as a result of having had the specific disease or having been immunized against it with a specific biologic product. The source of homologous sera is the pooled plasma of adult donors, either from the general population (for immunoglobulin) or from hyperimmunized donors (for immunoglobulins for specific diseases). Thus, these products confer passive immunity.

The pooled plasma from adult donors must be free of hepatitis B antigen and antibodies to HIV. Processing steps include fractional precipitation (e.g., with cold ethanol), maintaining rigorous control of pH and ionic strength. Further purification takes place with a finished biologic product that contains not less than 15% and not more than 18% protein. There are of course exceptions (e.g., varicella–zoster immunoglobulins [VZIGs] contain not <10% protein).

These preparations are for intramuscular (IM) injection and should not be administered intravenously. However, immunoglobulin intravenous (3% to 12% protein) and cytomegalovirus immunoglobulin are administered intravenously.

Sera have the greatest value for the treatment of acute disease, although they are also useful in some instances to prevent illness when immediate protection is needed. Immunity resulting from the injection of an immune serum is brief (a few weeks) because the foreign serum and the antibodies it produces are eliminated from the body within a few weeks.

Animal Immune Sera (Heterologous Sera)

Most commonly employed immune sera are prepared by immunization of horses against the specific immunogen (e.g., toxin, venom). After the plasma is harvested, it is separated by fractional precipitation into two components: immunologically active (immunoglobulins) and immunologically inactive (albumins, clotting factors) ones. The immunologically active component is treated with pepsin to remove the complement-activating component of the molecules and render it less immunogenic.

Subsequently, the active component is recovered through dialysis and fractional precipitation or centrifugation.

This category of pharmaceuticals includes antitoxins and antivenins. Antitoxins are produced by inoculating horses with increasing doses of the toxoids and exotoxins. After several injections over weeks or months, the animal is bled with adequate safeguards to avoid contamination and the plasma harvested. Antivenins are produced similarly, by inoculating horses with the venom of selected species and harvesting the plasma.

Before using these products, precautions must be taken to ensure the safety of the patient, who may be sensitive to horse protein. Appropriate measures, including a sensitivity test with suitable controls, should be taken to detect any dangerous hypersensitivity.

Table 16.1 lists representative biologics by category. Although the scope of this book does not permit a thorough description of each according to its intended use, adverse effects, and so on, the list demonstrates the wide applicability of these products to produce active or passive immunity, provide prophylaxis, or serve as a diagnostic tool.

ADMINISTRATION AND TOXICITY ASSOCIATED WITH BIOLOGIC PRODUCTS

Table 16.1 lists examples of official biologics, and Table 16.2 lists the composition of some example biologic products.

Biologics must be dispensed in the original container to avoid contamination and deterioration. They are sterile when packaged and are injected by aseptic techniques. A few are administered by mouth.

Traditional vaccines, often constituted by inactivated whole cells, can cause unwanted side effects. Those developed from selected antigens have demonstrated fewer systemic side effects. Liposomal delivery has decreased side effects while enhancing the vaccine's effectiveness.

Itching, erythema, pain, and tenderness around the injection site occur with subcutaneous, IM, and intradermal administration. Vaccines that contain adjuvants (e.g., BCG) can cause these adverse effects in addition to induration and ulceration at the site. Low-grade fever, myalgia, and arthralgia have occurred in patients who received a BCG-containing biologic product.

These adverse effects are controlled with the use of over-the-counter analgesic agents. However, before these are used, the patient's drug history should be obtained to ensure that the use of an analgesic is permissible given a patient's health status and other drug therapy.

The foremost adverse effect of concern with immunization is hypersensitivity, most notably anaphylaxis, ranging from pruritus or urticaria to bronchospasm, respiratory distress, laryngeal edema, circulatory collapse, and death. Life-threatening anaphylaxis is a rarity but quite possible. The risk of an anaphylactic reaction is in the range of one for every 600,000 to 6.4 million doses of vaccine distributed (7).

TABLE **16.1.** Examples of Official Biologic Products

Biologic Product	Nature of Contents	Route[a]	Use
Vaccines and Vaccine Combinations			
Anthrax adsorbed	Toxigenic, nonencapsulated strain of *Bacillus anthracis* culture, protective antigens (proteins common to all harmful strains), and aluminum hydroxide as adjuvant to enhance antibody response	Subcutaneous	Active immunizing agent
BCG	Attenuated living culture of BCG strain of *Mycobacterium bovis*	Intradermal active immunizing agent from multidose vial	Active immunizing agent
Hepatitis B	Originally, biochemically, biophysically inactivated human HBsAg particles from chronic HBsAg carriers. Now, only recombinant vaccines produced in yeast cells are available in the United States.	IM	Active immunizing agent
Human papillomavirus	Recombinant vaccine from highly purified virus-like particles of capsid protein of HPV types 6, 11, 16, and 18	IM	Active immunizing agent
Influenza virus	Aqueous suspension of inactivated virus from allantoic fluid of infected chick embryo in phosphate-buffered isotonic NaCl injection	IM	Active immunizing agent
Influenza virus	Preservative-free, latex-free, egg-based aqueous solution. Each 0.5 mL contains ~$1 \times 10^{6.5-7.5}$ tissue culture infectious doses of virus. Egg base provides protein to increase reproducibility of virus.	Intranasal	Active immunizing agent
Measles virus, live	Live attenuated Enders line measles virus from attenuated Edmonston strain in chick embryo cell cultures	SQ	Active immunizing agent
Measles, mumps, rubella virus, live	Propagated in chick embryo (measles, mumps) and in human diploid cell cultures (rubella)	SQ	Active immunizing agent
Measles, mumps, rubella, varicella virus, live	Live, attenuated preparation propagated in chick embryo cell cultures (measles, mumps) and in human fibroblasts (rubella, varicella)	SQ	Active immunizing agent
Measles and rubella virus, live	Measles virus grown on chicken embryo tissue and rubella virus on duck embryo tissue	SQ	Active immunizing agent
Mumps virus, live	Live attenuated Jeryl Lynn (B level) strain of virus propagated in chick embryo tissue	SQ	Active immunizing agent
Pneumococcal, polyvalent	Sterile solution of antigenic capsular polysaccharides from *Streptococcus pneumoniae*. Contains 23 capsular polysaccharide types. Each 0.5-mL dose contains 25 μg of each type of capsule polysaccharide in 0.9% NaCl injection. Also contains phenol or thimerosal preservative	IM, SQ	Active immunizing agent
Pneumococcal 7-valent conjugate	Sterile 0.5-mL dose solution of saccharides of capsular antigens of *S. pneumoniae* serotypes 4, 6B, 9V, 14, 18C, 19F, and 23F individually conjugated to diphtheria CRM197 to form glycoconjugate	IM	Active immunizing agent
Rabies	Inactivated virus from HDCV or RDCV cultures	HDCV, IM, and ID; RDCV and IM only	Active immunizing agent
Rubella virus, live	Live rubella (German measles) virus propagated in human diploid (WI-38) cell culture	SQ	Active immunizing agent
Rubella and mumps, live	Rubella virus in human diploid cell culture and mumps virus on chicken embryo tissue	SQ	Active immunizing agent
Smallpox	Dried calf lymph live virus preparation of vaccinia virus	ID	Active immunizing agent
Typhoid	Parenteral form, solution of cell surface Vi polysaccharides extracted from *Salmonella typhi* Ty2 strain; oral form, enteric-coated capsules, lyophilized, live *S. typhi* of attenuated Ty21a strain	SQ or ID; oral	Active immunizing agent
Varicella virus, live	Varicella–zoster, Oka/Merck strain, attenuated by multiple passages through cultures of human embryonic lung cell, embryonic guinea pig cell, WI-38 strain of human diploid cell, MRC-5 strain of human diploid cell	SQ	Active immunizing agent
Yellow fever	Dried frozen attenuated strain of living yellow fever virus cultured in living chick embryo, prepared, processed, freeze-dried, and sealed in nitrogen	SQ	Active immunizing agent

(Continued)

TABLE 16.1. Examples of Official Biologic Products *(Continued)*

Biologic Product	Nature of Contents	Route[a]	Use
Zoster virus, live	Varicella–zoster, Oka/Merck strain, attenuated by multiple passages through cultures of human embryonic lung cell, embryonic guinea pig cell, WI-38 strain of human diploid cell, MRC-5 strain of human diploid cell	SQ	Active immunizing agent
Toxoids			
Diphtheria and tetanus, adsorbed	Suspension of purified diphtheria toxoid, tetanus toxoid alum precipitated or adsorbed onto aluminum phosphate	Deep IM	Active immunizing agent
Tetanus	Suspension of formaldehyde-treated tetanus *bacillus* (*C. tetani*)	IM, SQ	Active immunizing agent
Tetanus, adsorbed	Suspension of toxoid alum precipitated or adsorbed onto aluminum phosphate	Deep IM	Active immunizing agent
Tetanus, diphtheria adsorbed for adult use	Suspension of toxoids, alum precipitated or adsorbed onto aluminum phosphate	IM	Active immunizing agent
Antitoxins			
Botulism	Solution of refined, concentrated proteins, chiefly globulins, with antitoxin from blood serum or plasma of healthy horses immunized against toxins produced by type A, B, and E strains of *C. botulinum*	IM or IV	Passive immunizing agent
Tetanus	Solution of refined, concentrated proteins, chiefly globulins, with antitoxic antibodies from blood serum or plasma of a healthy animal, usually horse, immunized against tetanus toxoid or toxin. More commonly from pooled human plasma. Lyophilized concentrate, which contains IgG with minimum of 100 IU/mL of antitetanus antibodies. Only selected plasma is used (HIV and HB5 negative).	IM or SQ (prophylactic) or V (therapeutic)	Passive immunizing agent
Immune Sera			
Cytomegalovirus	IgG antibodies from large number of healthy persons who contributed to plasma pools	IV	Passive for kidney transplant recipients seronegative for CMV who receive kidney from CMV-seropositive donor
Immunoglobulin IM	Nonpyrogenic solution of globulins with many antibodies normally in adult human blood prepared by cold alcohol fractionation of pooled plasma from venous blood of at least 1,000 individuals	IM	Passive immunity to hepatitis A and B, measles, varicella–zoster, and primary immunodeficiency diseases
Immunoglobulin IV	Nonpyrogenic solution of globulins with many antibodies normally in adult human blood prepared by cold alcohol fractionation of pooled plasma from venous blood of at least 1,000 individuals	IV	Primary immunodeficiency diseases, HIV, ITP, bone marrow transplant, beta cell CLL
Rh_o (D) globulin	From plasma or serum of adults with high titer of anti-Rh_o antibody to red blood cell antigen Rh_o (D); contains 10%–18% protein; not <90% IgG. Commercial solutions contain glycine as a stabilizer and thimerosal as a preservative; pH is adjusted with sodium carbonate or NaCl.	IM	Passive immunizing agent
Tetanus immunoglobulin	Solution of globulins derived from blood plasma of adult human donors hyperimmunized with tetanus toxoid	IM	Passive immunizing agent
Miscellaneous Biologic Products			
Antivenin (Crotalidae) polyvalent	Dried frozen solution of specific venom-neutralizing globulins from serum of healthy horses immunized against venoms of four species of pit vipers, *Crotalus atrox*, *Crotalus adamanteus*, *Crotalus durissus terrificus*, and *Bothrops atrox*	IM or IV	Neutralizes venom of crotalids native to the Americas

TABLE 16.1. Examples of Official Biologic Products *(Continued)*

Biologic Product	Nature of Contents	Route[a]	Use
Candida albicans skin test antigen	From culture filtrate, cells of two strains of *C. albicans*	ID	Detects reduced cellular hypersensitivity and DTH; assesses diminished cellular immunity in HIV
Plasma Protein Fraction, USP	Blood plasma of adult human donors; contains ~5% protein, ~88% normal human albumin; 12% *alpha* and *beta* globulins	IV	Blood volume expansion
Tuberculin, USP	Solution of concentrated soluble products of MTB. Old tuberculin, soluble partially purified product of MTB in special liquid medium free of protein (purified protein derivative)	ID	Diagnostic aid (tuberculosis)

[a]The doses to be administered and the schedule of doses vary widely with the patient's age, exposure, previous record of immunizations, and so on.
BCG, bacille Calmette-Guérin; IM, intramuscular; SQ, subcutaneous; HBsAg, hepatitis B surface antigen; HDCV, human diploid cell vaccine; RDCV, rhesus diploid cell vaccine; ID, intradermal; ITP, idiopathic thrombocytopenic purpura; CLL, chronic lymphocytic leukemia; IgG, immunoglobulin gamma; DTH, delayed-type hypersensitivity; MTB, *Mycobacterium tuberculosis*.

TABLE 16.2. Composition of Some Example Biological Products

Product	Active	Vehicle	Tonicity Agent or Preservative	Other
Influenza				
Afluria	Influenza virus vaccine suspension, IM Single dose	Sterile water for injection	Sodium chloride	Monobasic sodium phosphate Dibasic sodium phosphate
	Multidose	Sterile water for injection	Sodium chloride Thimerosal	Monobasic potassium phosphate Potassium chloride Calcium chloride
Fluarix	Influenza virus vaccine	Sterile water for injection		Octoxynol-10 A-tocopheryl hydrogen succinate Polysorbate
Flulaval	Influenza virus vaccine		Thimerosal	Residual: Ovalbumin Formaldehyde Sodium deoxycholate
Tetanus Toxoid and Combinations				
Boostrix	Tetanus toxoid Reduced diphtheria toxoid Acellular pertussis vaccine suspension, IM	Sterile water for injection		Aluminum hydroxide Sodium dihydrogen phosphate dihydrate
Infanrix	Diphtheria and tetanus toxoids and acellular pertussis vaccine, adsorbed		Sodium chloride	Aluminum hydroxide Residual: Formaldehyde Polysorbate 80
Kinrix	Diphtheria and tetanus toxoids and acellular pertussis vaccine, adsorbed		Sodium chloride	Aluminum hydroxide Residual: Formaldehyde Polysorbate 80
Pediarix	Diphtheria and tetanus toxoids and acellular pertussis adsorbed hepatitis B and IPV		Sodium chloride	Aluminum salts Residual: Formaldehyde Polysorbate 80 Neomycin sulfate Polymyxin B
Human Papillomavirus				
Gardasil	HPV quadrivalent	Sterile water for injection	Sodium chloride	Aluminum hydroxyphosphate sulfate Yeast protein L-histidine Polysorbate 80 Sodium borate

(Continued)

TABLE 16.2. Composition of Some Example Biological Products *(Continued)*

Product	Active	Vehicle	Tonicity Agent or Preservative	Other
Hepatitis				
Havrix	Hepatitis A vaccine			Aluminum hydroxide Amino acids phosphate-buffered saline Polysorbate 20 residual: Formalin Neomycin sulfate
Vaqta	Hepatitis A vaccine, inactivated	0.9% Sodium chloride solution		Residual: Bovine albumin Formaldehyde Neomycin pH adjusted with sodium borate
Engerix	Hepatitis B vaccine		Sodium chloride	Aluminum hydroxide Disodium phosphate dehydrate Sodium dihydrogen phosphate dihydrate
Recombivax	Hepatitis B vaccine (recombinant)	Sterile water for injection		Aluminum hydroxyphosphate Residual: Formaldehyde
Twinrix	Hepatitis A and hepatitis B (recombinant vaccine)	Sterile water for injection	Sodium chloride	Aluminum phosphate Aluminum hydroxide Amino acids Phosphate buffer Polysorbate
Haemophilus B				
PedvaxHIB	Haemophilus B conjugate vaccine	0.9% Sodium chloride solution		Aluminum hydroxyphosphate sulfate
Rabies Vaccine				
RabAvert	Rabies vaccine			Polygeline Human serum albumin Potassium glutamate Sodium EDTA
Rotavirus				
Rotarix	Rotavirus vaccine, live, oral			Dextran Sorbitol Xanthan Dulbecco's Modified Eagle Medium
RotaTeq	Rotavirus vaccine, live, oral, pentavalent			Sucrose Sodium citrate Sodium phosphate monobasic monohydrate Sodium hydroxide Polysorbate 80 Fetal bovine serum
Meningococcal				
Menveo	Meningococcal oligosaccharide, diphtheria CRM conjugate vaccine	Sterile water for injection		Residual: Formaldehyde
Measles				
M-M-R II	Measles, mumps, and rubella virus vaccine live		Sodium chloride	Sorbitol Sodium phosphate Sucrose Hydrolyzed gelatin Recombinant human albumin Fetal bovine serum Neomycin

TABLE 16.2. Composition of Some Example Biological Products *(Continued)*

Product	Active	Vehicle	Tonicity Agent or Preservative	Other
ProQuad	Measles, mumps, rubella, and varicella virus vaccine		Sodium chloride	Sucrose Hydrolyzed gelatin Sorbitol Monosodium-L-glutamate Sodium phosphate dibasic Human albumin Sodium bicarbonate Potassium phosphate monobasic Potassium chloride Potassium phosphate dibasic Residual: Neomycin Bovine calf serum
Pneumococcal				
Pneumovax 23	Pneumococcal vaccine polyvalent	0.9% Sodium chloride solution	0.25% Phenol	
Varicella				
Varivax	Varicella virus vaccine live		Sodium chloride	Sucrose Hydrolyzed gelatin Monosodium-L-glutamate Sodium phosphate dibasic Potassium phosphate monobasic Potassium chloride Sodium phosphate monobasic EDTA Neomycin Fetal bovine serum
Zoster				
Zostavax	Zoster vaccine live		Sodium chloride	Sucrose Hydrolyzed porcine gelatin Monosodium-L-glutamate Sodium phosphate dibasic potassium phosphate monobasic Potassium chloride

The immunopathologic classification of allergic drug reactions places anaphylactic reactions in type I. In this situation, initial exposure to an antigen results in production of specific IgE antibodies. Upon reexposure, antigen reacts with antibodies bound to the surface of mast cells or basophils, causing the release of histamine and other mediators. Several weeks are required after initial exposure to antigen and sensitization before an anaphylactic reaction can occur. Once sensitized, however, the patient can demonstrate an attack within minutes of reexposure to small amounts of the drug administered by any route.

Because of the rare nature of anaphylactic reactions, it is difficult to determine whether the patient is allergic to the proteins that make up the active antigenic portion of the vaccine or to the excipients (e.g., neomycin, gelatin, aluminum gels). Several viruses that constitute vaccines are grown in animate media, including embryonic egg and cell cultures of chick embryo. Even though purification techniques decrease dramatically the amount of egg protein in the final product, even picograms or nanograms can elicit a response.

Before a vaccination is administered, it is important that a complete and thorough history of previous allergic reactions be taken. This includes the names of the offending agents and the type of reaction. Also, one should determine how long ago the reaction took place. One should inquire not only about drugs (e.g., neomycin, gelatin) but also about foods (e.g., severe allergy to egg products). It may be necessary for an allergist to perform skin testing to determine whether a patient may demonstrate an immediate type I hypersensitivity reaction to a vaccine.

Even though anaphylactic reactions to immunizations are rare, they can occur. Therefore, at the time of immunization, adequate safeguards, including proper emergency supplies and trained personnel, must be in place to handle such an emergency.

Thimerosal has been used in vaccines as a preservative since the 1930s. It is effective for killing bacteria in several vaccines and for preventing bacterial contamination, especially in opened multidose vials. Previously, several of the vaccines routinely recommended for children in the United States contained thimerosal. In high doses, both forms of organic mercury (methylmercury and ethyl mercury) formed from metabolism of thimerosal can cause neurotoxicity. Definitive information regarding the dose of thimerosal that produces developmental effects in infants is not available. Therefore, in September 1999, the American Academy of Pediatrics (AAP) Committee on Infectious Diseases and Committee on Environmental Health urged government agencies and the pharmaceutical industry to work rapidly toward reducing children's exposure to mercury from all sources, including vaccines. Specifically, these committees urged rapid elimination of thimerosal in vaccines. Since the end of 2001, all routine pediatric vaccinations contain either no thimerosal or only trace amounts, and it is estimated that the overall vaccine schedule for children now contains 98% less than it used to. The academy also issued guidelines to prevent exposure of women of childbearing age to amounts of mercury that might be toxic to the rapidly developing brain of the fetus, which is much more susceptible to toxicity than is the adult brain. It also stated that the specific window of highest susceptibility is not known, but exposure after birth should be associated with less toxicity than should in utero exposure.

When vaccines preserved with thimerosal have been administered in recommended doses, some hypersensitivity reactions have been reported, but no other harmful effects have been noted. However, massive overdoses with thimerosal-containing products have resulted in toxicity expressed in the central nervous system, kidneys, and immune system. Thus, as part of an ongoing review of biologic products in response to the FDA Modernization Act of 1997, the FDA determined that infants who would receive thimerosal-containing vaccines at several visits might be exposed to more mercury than recommended by federal guidelines.

Pichichero et al. (8) demonstrated that mercury does not accumulate in children who receive thimerosal-containing vaccines. After administration of such vaccines, mercury was measured in the urine, blood, and stool samples of 40 term infants less than 6 months old and in 21 control infants who received thimerosal-containing vaccines. The authors concluded from the data at 2 months and at 6 months of age that the amounts of mercury in the blood of infants receiving these vaccines are well below concentrations of mercury associated with toxicity. Thus, the conclusion was that thimerosal in these vaccines poses little risk to term infants but should not be administered at birth to very low birth weight premature infants.

The AAP also recommended that the benefits and risks of thimerosal-containing vaccines be discussed with parents. It emphasized that the larger risk of not vaccinating the child (e.g., more than 20% will develop pneumonia) far outweigh any known risk of exposure to a thimerosal-containing vaccine. Infants and children who have received vaccines preserved with thimerosal do not need to have blood, urine, or hair tested for mercury because the concentrations of mercury would be quite low and would not require treatment.

All infants need protection against debilitating and potentially harmful childhood diseases as well as consequences from the vaccinations. One concern has been the development of autism in some infants who were administered the MMR vaccination. In a study attempting to resolve the question, Madsen et al. (9) identified more than 537,000 children in Denmark from 1991 to 1998, 82% of whom had received the MMR vaccine. The scientists determined that the relative risk of autistic disorders among vaccinated children was 8% less than among unvaccinated children, not statistically significant. Furthermore, the risk of other autistic spectrum disorders was found to be 17% lower with vaccination, statistically equivalent to the risk of unvaccinated children. In addition, no relationship was identified between the infants' ages at the time of vaccination, time since vaccination, or date of vaccination and the development of the autistic disorder. This study on the possible link between autism and the MMR vaccine should have allayed the fears of parents, and pharmacists have been endeavoring to educate them on this matter as well as the thimerosal-containing vaccinations. However, concern persists even though two additional hypotheses have emerged recently concerning environmental exposure like vaccines might cause autism. In addition to the thimerosal hypothesis, putative association has centered on the MMR vaccine and the large number of vaccines administered. Gerber and Offit (10) discussed the genesis of each theory and reviewed relevant epidemiological evidence. Suffice it to say, 20 epidemiological studies reviewed demonstrated that neither thimerosal nor MMR vaccine causes autism. In addition, Tozzi et al. (11) compared the neuropsychological performance 10 years after vaccination in two groups of children exposed randomly to varying amounts of thimerosal through immunization. There was no conclusive evidence that thimerosal had an effect on the neuropsychological development of the children, and an association between thimerosal exposure through vaccination in infancy and eventual neuropsychological deficits was unlikely or clinically negligible.

Typically, IM injection is the preferred route of administration. The vastus lateralis muscle of the thigh is the preferred site for injection for infants up to 12 to 18 months of age. The deltoid muscle of the shoulder is preferred for children older than 18 months of age. Needle overpenetration of the IM injection into the bone or periosteum can cause pain and/or damage. Further, it can cause the needle to detach from the syringe. For vaccination into the thigh muscle, a 7/8-inch or longer needle is used for all children aged 6 years or younger. For vaccination into the shoulder, needle lengths ranging from ½ inch to ⅞ to 1 inch are recommended depending upon the weight of the child (12).

Given their ability to affect complex processes in the body, biological products including vaccines have a higher likelihood of adverse effects than do traditional or chemical agents. Nearly one-third of boxed warnings for biological pharmaceuticals approved by the FDA from January 1995 through 2007 have been added within 2 years of the product's availability on the market (13). Thus, it is important for pharmacists to participate in extensive adverse event monitoring of new products.

Influenza continues to be a major cause of morbidity and mortality in the United States. The U.S. Public Health Service has targeted elimination of HIB in children less than 5 years of age. It is characterized by an abrupt onset of fever, myalgia, headache, severe malaise, cough, sore throat, and rhinitis. Although it resolves within a few days, it can exacerbate chronic conditions (e.g., asthma, diabetes mellitus) and lead to secondary bacterial pneumonia. The ACIP makes recommendations on a yearly basis concerning the use and composition of the influenza virus vaccine to children aged 6 months through 18 years. But in spite of efforts to vaccinate persons at high risk, the annual rate of influenza remains high.

Influenza

Typically, the vaccine is administered parenterally, and it causes concern among parents over the threat of adverse reactions. As mentioned earlier, in June 2003, the first intranasal live attenuated influenza virus (LAIV) vaccine, FluMist, was approved for clinical use in the United States. However, its use was originally restricted to healthy children aged 5 to 17 and adults aged 18 to 49. For healthy individuals aged 5 to 49, LAIV is an acceptable alternative to the IM trivalent inactivated influenza vaccine (TIV). At that time, the FDA's Vaccines and Related Biological Products Advisory Committee determined that the vaccine was not safe for patients under age 5 because of concerns over increased rates of asthma within 6 weeks of vaccination. In a randomized clinical trial, FluMist and TIV were compared among children aged 6 to 59 months (14). Excluded children were those with medically diagnosed or treated wheezing within 42 days before enrollment or a history of severe asthma. FluMist demonstrated a 55% greater efficacy compared with TIV in preventing culture-confirmed influenza illness.

Subsequently, on October 24, 2007, the ACIP recommended that either the LAIV or TIV can be used to vaccinate healthy nonpregnant persons aged 2 to 49 years. Healthy persons were defined as those who do not have an underlying medical condition that predisposes them to influenza complications. For patients 50 years of age and older, the safe and effective use of FluMist has not been established. Hence, it is restricted from use in this patient population. When considering the use of the LAIV in children aged 2 to 4 years, health care providers should consult the medical record, when available, to identify children in this age group with recurrent wheezing that might indicate

asthma. Parents should also be asked, "In the past 12 months, has a health care provider ever told you that your child had wheezing or asthma?" Children whose parents respond "yes" to the question or demonstrate an asthmatic or wheezing episode noted in the medical record within the last 12 months should not receive FluMist, and the injective TIV should be administered instead.

FluMist must be used cautiously and never administered parenterally. Patients with a history of anaphylactic reactions to eggs should not generally receive this vaccine. Children and adolescents receiving chronic aspirin therapy, because of the risk of Reye syndrome, and patients with a history of Guillain-Barré syndrome should not receive FluMist. Pregnant women should not receive FluMist. Whenever the nasal vaccine is administered, epinephrine injection should be available in case of an anaphylactic reaction. The most common adverse effects encountered with FluMist are nasal congestion, runny nose (45%), sore throat (28%), cough (14%), and chills (9%). Serious adverse events occurred at similar rates in healthy children aged 60 to 71 months receiving FluMist and those receiving the placebo dosage form. It is important that suspected adverse events be reported by telephone to the VAERS (1-800-822-7967). Three other changes in the use of FluMist and its 2007 to 2008 formulation should be noted: the amount of vaccine administered, the temperature at which FluMist is shipped and stored after delivery to the end user, and the minimum interval between doses have changed compared with the 2006 to 2007 influenza-season formulation. FluMist is now supplied in a prefilled, single-use sprayer containing 0.2 mL of vaccine instead of the previous 0.5-mL dose. Those administering the FluMist should spray 0.1 mL (i.e., one-half of the total sprayer contents) into the first nostril while the recipient is in the upright position. The attached dose-divider clip should then be removed from the sprayer and the second half of the dose administered into the second nostril (Fig. 16.1).

Note: Active inhalation (i.e., sniffing) is not required by the patient during FluMist administration

FIGURE 16.1. Instructions for intranasal administration of FluMist, live attenuated influenza vaccine. (Courtesy of MedImmune, LLC.)

Previously, FluMist was shipped and stored frozen. It is now approved to be shipped to end users at 35°F to 46°F (2°C to 8°C). The product should be stored within this temperature range upon receipt and up to the time the expiration date is reached. Lastly, the recommended interval from the first to the second dose in children requiring two doses has changed from a minimum of 6 weeks to a minimum of 4 weeks, the same interval recommended between doses for TIV.

Because FluMist is a live vaccine, IM inactivated vaccine is preferred for health care workers and for family members and other close contacts of immunosuppressed patients. The package insert advises FluMist recipients to avoid close contact (e.g., within the same household) with any immunocompromised patients for at least 21 days.

A new catch-up immunization schedule for children and adolescents who start vaccinations late or who are more than 1 month behind has been published by the CDC (15). Minimum ages and minimum intervals between dosages are provided for each of the routinely recommended childhood and adolescent vaccines. The schedules are divided into two distinct age groupings, ages 4 months to 6 years and ages 7 to 18 years.

Toxins

Botulinum toxin type A (i.e., Botox) is indicated to treat axillary hyperhidrosis; cervical dystonia (CD), that is, to decrease the severity of abnormal head position and neck pain associated with CD; and strabismus and blepharospasm associated with dystonia. Botulinum toxin type A (i.e., Botox Cosmetic) is only indicated for the temporary improvement in the appearance of moderate to severe glabellar lines associated with corrugators and/or procerus muscle activity, that is, facial frown lines, in adult patients ≤65 years of age (16).

Botulinum toxin type A is available as a powder for injection in a single-use vial. Unopened vials are to be stored in a refrigerator (2°C to 8°C) for up to 24 months. It is to be administered within 4 hours of reconstitution and, during this time period, must be stored in a refrigerator. The reconstituted injection should appear clear, colorless, and without particulate matter. Prior to injection, the vacuum-dried botulinum toxin type A is reconstituted with sterile normal saline without a preservative; 0.9% w/v sodium chloride injection is the recommended diluent.

As an example, for glabellar line injection, using Botox Cosmetic, a 21-gauge needle and an appropriately sized syringe are used to draw up a total of 2.5 mL of 0.9% sterile saline solution without preservative. The needle is inserted at a 45-degree angle, and the diluent is slowly injected into the botulinum toxin A (cosmetic) vial. The vial is discarded if a vacuum does not pull the diluent into the vial. The vial is gently rotated, and the date and time of the reconstitution are recorded on the label space. Then, at least 0.5 mL of the properly reconstituted toxin is drawn up into the sterile syringe, preferably a tuberculin syringe,

expelling air bubbles in the syringe barrel. The needle used for reconstitution is removed, and a 30-gauge needle is attached, and the concentration will be 4 U/0.1 mL and a total dose of 20 U in 0.5 mL. The duration of activity of botulinum toxin type A cosmetic for glabellar lines is approximately 3 to 4 months.

The safe and effective use of botulinum toxin type A depends upon the proper product storage, selection of the correct dose, proper reconstitution, and proper administration. Physicians administering botulinum toxin type A must have a clear understanding of the relevant neuromuscular or orbital anatomy of the area involved and any alterations to the anatomy caused by prior surgical procedures.

Botulinum toxin type A must not be confused with botulinum toxin type B. Botulinum toxin type B is a preservative-free injectable solution, that is, 5,000 U/mL. Type B is also indicated for cervical dystonia and chronic sialorrhea in adults. The clinical doses of botulinum toxin are not interchangeable between products.

▌ RESPONDING TO BIOTERRORISM

In the wake of the events of September 11, 2001 (9/11), awareness of the necessity for vigilance to illness patterns and diagnostic clues that might indicate an unusual infectious disease outbreak heightened. Pharmacists and allied health professionals were asked to report any indication of suspicious symptoms to local and state health departments. Evidence of intentional release of biologic agents includes infection in these groups: (*a*) people in the same location with symptoms that suggest an infectious disease outbreak (e.g., unexplained febrile illness associated with sepsis, pneumonia, respiratory failure, rash, or botulism-like syndrome with flaccid muscle paralysis), (*b*) age groups not normally associated with the disease in question, and (*c*) numerous cases of acute flaccid paralysis with prominent bulbar palsies that suggest the release of botulinum toxin.

Pharmacists are also encouraged to participate in their community's disaster preparedness efforts (17). The pharmacist can bring an important and unique perspective to determining and preparing for health care needs during times of natural disasters or man-made crises. The American Pharmacists Association has attempted to assist involved pharmacists by creating a National Pharmacists Response Team. The 10 teams will assist communities with chemoprophylaxis or vaccinations during times of need. Interested pharmacists can apply for the team online at www.aphanet.org/pharmcare/NPRTform.pdf.

After 9/11, the news media concentrated on the threat of an anthrax outbreak without realizing there were other more prominent diseases with greater potential harm to the public. Those listed by the CDC as the biggest biologic threats in addition to anthrax included smallpox and pneumonic plague. Other agents of concern include *Clostridium botulinum* toxin (botulism), *Francisella tularensis* (i.e., tularemia), and hemorrhagic fevers.

Smallpox, caused by variola virus, has initial symptoms that include high fever, fatigue, headache, and backaches. These symptoms are followed by a rash. Although most patients recover, up to 30% of cases result in death. This disease is spread by face-to-face contact. Routine vaccination against smallpox ended in 1972, so the level of immunity among persons vaccinated up until this time is unknown. Therefore, all individuals are considered susceptible. In 2002, after evaluating the risk of a bioterrorist attack and the adverse effects of the smallpox vaccine (e.g., lymph node swelling, rash, fever, scarring, severe skin reactions, encephalitis), the ACIP concluded that the risks outweighed the benefits and recommended that the general public not be inoculated against smallpox. It recommended that vaccinations be offered to a total of about 15,000 health care workers around the country who would be designated to investigate smallpox cases and provide direct care at designated hospitals (18).

Botulism is a muscle-paralyzing disease caused by the toxin produced by *C. botulinum*. Food-borne botulism is a public health emergency because the contaminated food may still be available to other people. This form of botulism occurs when the preformed toxin is ingested in contaminated food and causes illness within 6 hours to 2 weeks. Symptoms include double vision, blurred vision, drooping eyelids, slurred speech, difficulty swallowing, dry mouth, and muscle weakness that leads to paralysis of the breathing muscles. Botulism is not communicable from one person to the next.

Pneumonic plague occurs when *Yersinia pestis* infects the lung. The initial symptoms of this illness include fever, headache, weakness, and cough with a bloody or watery sputum. This disease progresses over 2 to 4 days and may cause septic shock. If treatment is not initiated, the result is death. This disease is communicable with face-to-face contact with the infected person. Early treatment with antibiotics (e.g., tetracycline, streptomycin, chloramphenicol) is imperative. There is no vaccine against this disease.

Anthrax has three forms: cutaneous (skin surface is exposed to anthrax particles and skin lesions develop), gastrointestinal (particles are ingested), and inhalation (often fatal). Cutaneous anthrax demonstrates typically on the arms or hands as a swelling of the skin that develops into a central area of ulceration or a depression, and then a dark, blackish-brown scab forms over the area. This manifestation of anthrax can be painless, and a fever may be present. Gastrointestinal anthrax is characterized by an acute inflammation of the intestines, loss of appetite, vomiting, and pain. This is followed by a bout of abdominal pain, vomiting of blood, and severe diarrhea. Initial symptoms of inhalation anthrax resemble those of the common cold and, within a few days, progress to severe respiratory problems and shock.

Anthrax cannot be transmitted from one person to another. Treatment is with antibiotics (e.g., penicillin, doxycycline, fluoroquinolones), but only those exposed to this disease should be treated. Initially, with the anthrax scare after 9/11, prescriptions for Cipro, a fluoroquinolone, increased as concerned individuals were stockpiling to protect themselves and their families from the threat of anthrax. This was not a good practice because the drug should be used only by patients exposed to the disease and because storage conditions and validation of expiration dates cannot be ensured.

■ DIAGNOSTIC SKIN ANTIGENS

It may be necessary to use antigens in vivo as diagnostic tools. Typically, these are injected intradermally and the site inspected for development of a hypersensitivity reaction. A positive reaction is determined by the extent of induration (in millimeters) and degree of reaction, from slight induration to vesiculation and necrosis. These signs demonstrate sensitivity to the antigen and the presence of antibodies due to present or past infection with the particular organism.

The number of diagnostic skin biologics is relatively small. In the late 1970s, many were removed from the market as a result of the recommendations of the FDA panel on Review of Skin Antigens (19). Specifically, the panel questioned the reliability of skin test antigens for trichinosis, lymphogranuloma venereum, and mumps and recommended that these be withdrawn from the market and not licensed.

Some diagnostic skin antigens are featured in Table 16.1. One of the more recent in vivo diagnostic biologics, *Candida albicans* skin test antigen, is useful in the assessment of diminished cellular immunity in persons infected with HIV. Because HIV infection can modify the delayed-type hypersensitivity (DTH) response to tuberculin, it is advisable to skin test HIV-infected patients at high risk for tuberculosis with antigens in addition to tuberculin, to assess their competency to react to tuberculin. Responses to DTH antigens also have prognostic value in patients with cancer.

The Multiple Skin Test Antigens (Multitest CMI, Merieux) is a skin test for multiple antigens consisting of a disposable applicator with eight sterile heads preloaded with seven delayed hypersensitivity skin test antigens and a glycerin negative control for percutaneous administration. The seven antigens are tetanus toxoid antigen, diphtheria toxoid antigen, *streptococcus* antigen, old tuberculin, *Candida* antigen, *Trichophyton* antigen, and *Proteus* antigen. The intent of this multiple test is to detect anergy (lack of response to antigens) through delayed hypersensitivity skin testing.

PHARMACEUTICS CASE STUDY

SUBJECTIVE INFORMATION

You are in charge of providing a vaccine for a statewide program to vaccinate a select population of patients at 10 sites throughout the state. The vaccine will go to about 10,000 patients. What will you recommend to the organizing committee to ensure that the vaccine arrives intact, stable, and active?

OBJECTIVE INFORMATION

The vaccine is a lyophilized vaccine that must be stored in a freezer until it is reconstituted with sterile water for injection and administered. After reconstitution, it is stable for only 1 hour. Prior to reconstitution, it must remain frozen, and if allowed to reach room temperature prior to reconstitution, it must be discarded after 3 hours.

ASSESSMENT

Of the 10 sites for administration, 2 are within 50 miles, 2 more within 100 miles, 3 more within 150 miles, and 3 within approximately 225 miles of your facility.

PLAN

The vaccine will be ordered to arrive at your facility, shipped overnight from the manufacturer with sufficient dry ice to keep it frozen, the week before it is to be shipped to the vaccination sites. On Monday of the week of the vaccinations, the vaccines will be packaged in sufficient dry ice and shipped overnight to arrive at each of the 10 sites the next morning (Tuesday). Upon arrival, the vaccine will be placed in freezers until used. The vaccinations can be scheduled for Wednesday through Friday of that week; this will minimize storage and potential handling problems of the vaccine. ∎

CLINICAL CASE STUDY

PHARMACEUTICS CLINICAL CASE STUDY

Vaccines are antigenic substances administered for prophylactic purposes to achieve active immunity. The body's response helps to build up its own immune defenses. Vaccines may be living, attenuated, or killed microorganisms or fractions of microorganisms. They may also be a toxoid, a bacterial toxin that is modified and detoxified by use of moderate heat and chemical treatment. The end result of the processing is considered nontoxic, although the antigenic properties remain. Children and adults are vaccinated, and immunization schedules have been developed for both groups. For example, the pediatric immunization schedule includes 20 immunizations that are administered before the person is 2 years of age.

PHARMACEUTICAL CARE PLAN

S: J.C. is an 8-week-old female. Her mother brought J.C. to the emergency department at 3:00 PM. J.C. had been restless and crying inconsolably for the past 4 hours. J.C. was given her 2-month immunization of Pediarix yesterday by her pediatrician. Her mother took a rectal temperature today at 2:00 PM and found it to be elevated. J.C. has also had one seizure while in the emergency department.

O: Age: 8 weeks

Temperature (rectal) at 2:00 PM: 101°F per mother

Currently, 105°F in ER

A: The patient is reacting to the immunization Pediarix, a combination of diphtheria and tetanus toxoids and acellular pertussis adsorbed hepatitis B (recombinant) and IPV.

J.C. needs these immunizations to protect against many disease states. Diphtheria is an acute toxin-mediated infectious disease caused by toxigenic strains of *Corynebacterium diphtheriae*. Tetanus is a condition of neuromuscular dysfunction as a result of a potent exotoxin released from *Clostridium tetani*. Pertussis, or whooping cough, is a respiratory tract condition caused by *Bordetella pertussis*. Hepatitis B is a condition that affects the liver. Poliomyelitis is a highly contagious disease that can cause paralysis.

J.C. is most likely reacting to the acellular pertussis adsorbed component of Pediarix based on her presenting symptoms of fever above 105°F within 48 hours of Pediarix administration, inconsolable crying for longer than 3 hours within 48 hours of Pediarix administration, and seizure (with or without fever) within 3 days of Pediarix administration.

P: Because J.C. has had a reaction to the pertussis component, she may no longer be a candidate for immunization with Pediarix. Subsequent pertussis vaccinations must be withheld. Her 4- and 6-month immunizations will have to be individual injections of diphtheria and tetanus toxoid, hepatitis B vaccine, and IPV. ∎

APPLYING THE PRINCIPLES AND CONCEPTS

GROUP ACTIVITIES

1. Differentiate between currently available monovalent and polyvalent biological products.
2. Role-play a scenario between a health care professional and a parent in communicating the benefits versus risks of a child receiving a thimerosal-containing vaccine.
3. Compare and contrast the different methods for creating each type of biological product.
4. Create a flowchart for a patient to navigate a mass immunization event utilizing the information provided for immunizations from the Centers for Disease Control's Web site (www.cdc.gov).

INDIVIDUAL ACTIVITIES

1. List vaccination resources health care providers can refer patients and caregivers to regarding scheduled vaccines for adults and children.

2. Define and explain the term "cold chain" as it relates to the storage, handling, and shipping of biologics.
3. Describe the different methods of inducing immunity via bacterial vaccines.
4. List the required components of maintaining permanent vaccination records.
5. Compare and contrast the different types of oncological vaccinations.
6. List the organisms that are considered the most likely to be used in bioterrorism. Identify those that have approved vaccines.

List the various populations who should receive an influenza vaccination and the timing of the vaccination. List those patient types in whom this vaccine is contraindicated.

REFERENCES

1. Vaccines, Blood & Biologics. Available at: http://www.fda.gov/Cber/vaccines.htm. (Accessed May 2, 2016)
2. Grabenstein JD, Kendal AP, Snyder RH. Storing, handling, and shipping immunologic drugs. Hosp Pharm 1996;31:936–948.
3. Selected Vaccine Storage & Handling Resources. Available at: http://www.cdc.gov/vaccines/pubs/pinkbook/downloads/appendices/C/storage-handling-resources.pdf. (Accessed May 2, 2016)
4. Tanzi M. Flu vaccine revamped for 2008–2009 season. Pharm Today Immun Suppl 2008;14(8):15.
5. Belshe RB, Mendelman PM, Treanor J, et al. The efficacy of live attenuated, cold-adapted, trivalent, intranasal influenza virus vaccine in children. N Engl J Med 1998;338(20):1405–1412.
6. Clements DA, Langdon L, Bland C, et al. Influenza A vaccine decreases the incidence of otitis media in 6- to 30-month old children in day care. Arch Pediatr Adolesc Med 1995;149:1113–1117.
7. Grabenstein JD. Clinical management of hypersensitivities to vaccine components. Hosp Pharm 1997;32(1):77–84.
8. Pichichero ME, Cernichiari E, Lopreiato JD, et al. Mercury concentrations and metabolism in infants receiving vaccines containing thimerosal: A descriptive study. Lancet 2000;360:1737–1741.
9. Madsen KM, Hvid A, Vestergaard M, et al. A population-based study of measles, mumps, and rubella vaccination and autism. N Engl J Med 2002;347:1477–1482.
10. Gerber JS, Offit PA. Vaccines and autism: A tale of shifting hypothesis. Clin Infect Dis 2009;48:456–461.

11. Tozzi AE, Bisiacchi P, Tarantino V, et al. Neuropsychological performance 10 years after immunization in infancy with thimerosal-containing vaccines. Pediatrics 2009;123:475–482.
12. Barclay L. Needle-length guidelines for thigh and shoulder vaccinations may need revision. Medscape Med News. Available at: http://www.medscape.com/view article/579120. (Accessed May 2, 2016)
13. Giezen TJ, Mantel-Teeuwise AK, Straus SMJM, et al. Safety-related regulatory actions for biologicals approved in the United States and the European Union. JAMA 2008;300(16):1887–1896.
14. Belshe RB. Live attenuated versus inactivated influenza vaccines in infants and young children. N Engl J Med 2007;356:685–696.
15. Immunization Schedules. Available at: http://www.cdc.gov/vaccines/schedules/index.html. (Accessed May 2, 2016)
16. Trinza Z. Dermatologic Use of Botulinum Toxin. Available at: http://emedicine.medscape.com/article/1126453-overview#a0101. (Accessed May 2, 2016)
17. Hoeben BJ, Dennis MS, Bachman RL, et al. Role of the pharmacist in childhood immunizations. J Am Pharm Assoc (Wash) 1997;37(5):557–562.
18. Frey SE, Couch RB, Tacket CO, et al. Clinical responses to undiluted and diluted smallpox vaccine. N Engl J Med 2002;346:1265–1274.
19. Biological Products; Bacterial Vaccines and Related Biological Products; Implementation of Efficacy Review; Proposed Order. Available at: https://www.federalregister.gov/articles/2000/05/15/00-12116/biological-products-bacterial-vaccines-and-related-biological-products-implementation-of-efficacy. (Accessed May 2, 2016)

CHAPTER AT A GLANCE Ophthalmic Drug Delivery • Pharmacologic Categories of Ophthalmic Drugs • Pharmaceutical Requirements • Packaging Ophthalmic Solutions and Suspensions • Proper Administration of Ophthalmic Solutions and Suspensions • Nasal Preparations • Otic Preparations • Patient Counseling

OBJECTIVES

After reading this chapter, the student will be able to:

Describe ophthalmic, nasal, otic, and inhalation drug delivery

List drugs that are typically administered by each of these drug delivery methods

Explain the advantages/disadvantages of using one of these drug delivery methods over oral administration

Describe the use of the various pharmaceutical adjuvants, which are employed in the formulation of these dosage forms

Explain the proper administration of each of these drug delivery systems

Explain how patients can misuse/abuse these products intentionally or unintentionally

■ INTRODUCTION

Pharmaceutical dosage forms and drug delivery systems applied topically to the eye, nose, or ear can include solutions, suspensions, gels, ointments, and drug-impregnated inserts. This chapter builds on the general considerations of solutions and suspensions presented in Chapters 13 and 14 by describing additional requirements of these dosage forms when designed specifically for ophthalmic, nasal, or otic use.

■ OPHTHALMIC DRUG DELIVERY

Pharmaceutical preparations are applied topically to the eye to treat surface or intraocular conditions, including bacterial, fungal, and viral infections of the eye or eyelids; allergic or infectious conjunctivitis or inflammation; elevated intraocular pressure and glaucoma; and dry eye due to inadequate production of fluids bathing the eye. In treating certain ophthalmic conditions, such as glaucoma, both systemic drug use and topical treatments may be employed.

The normal volume of tear fluid in the cul-de-sac of the human eye is about 7 to 8 µL (1–4). An eye that does not blink can accommodate a maximum of about 30 µL of fluid, but, when blinked, can retain only about 10 µL (2). Because the capacity of the eye to retain liquid and semisolid preparations is limited, topical applications are administered in small amounts, liquids dropwise, and ointments as a thin ribbon applied to the margin of the eyelid. Larger volumes of liquid preparations may be used to flush or bathe the eye.

Excessive liquids, both normally produced and externally delivered, rapidly drain from the eye. A single drop of an ophthalmic solution or suspension measures about 50 µL (based on 20 drops/mL), so much of an administered drop may be lost almost immediately. The optimal volume to administer, based on eye capacity, is 5 to 10 µL (1). Microliter-dosing medication droppers are not generally available for personal use; consequently, loss of instilled medication using standard eye droppers is a common occurrence. The average dropper delivers about 25 to 50 µL/drop.

Because of the dynamics of the lacrimal system, the retention time of an ophthalmic solution on the eye surface is short, and the amount of drug absorbed is usually only a small fraction of the quantity administered. For example, following administration of pilocarpine ophthalmic solution, the solution is flushed from the precorneal area within 1 to 2 minutes, resulting in the ocular absorption of less than 1% of the administered dose (5,6). This necessitates repeated administration of the solution. Decreased frequency of dosing, increased ocular retention time, and greater bioavailability are achieved by formulations that extend corneal contact time, such as gel systems, liposomes, polymeric drug carriers, and ophthalmic suspensions and ointments (7,8). Systemic absorption of the active ingredient(s) that may result from drainage of the drug through the nasolacrimal duct and then swallowing can be minimized by applying gentle pressure to the lacrimal sac for 3 to 5 minutes after administration.

PHARMACOLOGIC CATEGORIES OF OPHTHALMIC DRUGS

The major categories of drugs applied topically to the eye are as follows:

- *Anesthetics*: Topical anesthetics, such as tetracaine, cocaine, and proparacaine, are employed to provide pain relief preoperatively, postoperatively, for ophthalmic trauma, and during ophthalmic examination.
- *Antibiotic and antimicrobial agents*: Used systemically and locally to combat ophthalmic infection. Among the agents used topically are azithromycin, gentamicin sulfate, sodium sulfacetamide, ciprofloxacin hydrochloride, ofloxacin, polymyxin B–bacitracin, and tobramycin.
- *Antifungal agents*: Among the agents used topically against fungal endophthalmitis and fungal keratitis are amphotericin B, natamycin, and flucytosine.
- *Anti-inflammatory agents*: Used to treat inflammation of the eye, as allergic conjunctivitis. Among the topical anti-inflammatory steroidal agents are fluorometholone, prednisolone, and dexamethasone salts. Nonsteroidal anti-inflammatory agents include diclofenac, flurbiprofen, ketorolac, and suprofen.
- *Antiviral agents*: Used against viral infections, as that caused by herpes simplex virus. Among the antiviral agents used topically are trifluridine, ganciclovir, and vidarabine.
- *Astringents*: Used in the treatment of conjunctivitis. Zinc sulfate is a commonly used astringent in ophthalmic solutions.
- *Beta-adrenergic blocking agents*: Agents such as betaxolol hydrochloride, levobunolol hydrochloride, metipranolol hydrochloride, and timolol maleate are used topically in the treatment of intraocular pressure and chronic open-angle glaucoma.
- *Miotics and other glaucoma agents*: Miotics are used in the treatment of glaucoma, accommodative esotropia, and convergent strabismus and for local treatment of myasthenia gravis. Among the miotics are pilocarpine, echothiophate iodide, and demecarium bromide. Several other types of agents are used in the treatment of glaucoma, including carbonic anhydrase inhibitors, such as acetazolamide (oral); beta-blockers, such as timolol; *alpha*-adrenergic agents, such as apraclonidine hydrochloride; sympathomimetics, such as dipivefrin hydrochloride; and an ester prodrug analog of prostaglandin F2a (e.g., bimatoprost, latanoprost, travoprost).
- *Mydriatics and cycloplegics*: Mydriatics allow examination of the fundus by dilating the pupil. Mydriatics having a long duration of action are termed *cycloplegics*. Among the mydriatics and cycloplegics are atropine, scopolamine, homatropine, cyclopentolate, phenylephrine, hydroxyamphetamine, and tropicamide.
- *Protectants and artificial tears*: Solutions employed as artificial tears or as contact lens fluids to lubricate the eye contain agents such as carboxymethyl cellulose, methylcellulose, hydroxypropyl methylcellulose, and polyvinyl alcohol.
- *Vasoconstrictors and ocular decongestants*: Vasoconstrictors applied topically to the mucous membranes of the eye cause transient constriction of the conjunctival blood vessels. They are intended to soothe, refresh, and remove redness due to minor eye irritation. Among the vasoconstrictors used topically are naphazoline, oxymetazoline, and tetrahydrozoline hydrochlorides. Antihistamines, such as emedastine difumarate, ketotifen fumarate, and olopatadine hydrochloride, are included in some products to provide relief of itching due to pollen, ragweed, and animal dander.

PHARMACEUTICAL REQUIREMENTS

The preparation of solutions and suspensions for ophthalmic use requires special consideration with regard to sterility, preservation, isotonicity, buffering, viscosity, ocular bioavailability, and packaging.

Sterility and Preservation

Ophthalmic solutions and suspensions must be sterilized for safe use. Although it is preferable to sterilize ophthalmics in their final containers by autoclaving at 121°C (250°F) for 15 minutes, this method sometimes is precluded by thermal instability of the formulation. As an alternative, bacterial filters may be used. Although bacterial filters work with a high degree of efficiency, they are not as reliable as the autoclave. However, because final product testing is used to validate the absence of microbes, sterility may be ensured by either method. One advantage of filtration is the retention of *all* particulate matter (microbial, dust, fiber), the removal of which has substantial importance in the manufacture and use of ophthalmic solutions. Figures 17.1 and 17.2 show bacterial filtration equipment that may be used in the extemporaneous preparation of ophthalmic solutions.

FIGURE 17.1. Sterilization by filtration. (Reproduced with permission from Merck KGaA, Darmstadt, Germany and/or its affiliates.)

To maintain sterility during use, antimicrobial preservatives generally are included in ophthalmic formulations; an exception is for preparations to be used during surgery or in the treatment of traumatized eyes because some preservatives irritate the eye. These preservative-free preparations are packaged in single-use containers.

During preformulation studies, antimicrobial preservatives must demonstrate stability, chemical and physical compatibility with other formulation and packaging components, and effectiveness at the concentration employed. Among the antimicrobial preservatives used in ophthalmic solutions and suspensions and their effective concentrations are benzalkonium chloride, 0.004% to 0.01%; benzethonium chloride, 0.01%; chlorobutanol, 0.5%; phenylmercuric acetate, 0.004%; phenylmercuric nitrite, 0.004%; and thimerosal, 0.005% to 0.01%. Certain preservatives have limitations; for example, chlorobutanol cannot be autoclaved because it decomposes to hydrochloric acid even in moderate heat. This degradation renders a

FIGURE 17.2. Examples of sterilizing filters. (Courtesy of Elkay Laboratory Products.)

product susceptible to microbial growth and could alter its pH and thereby affect the stability and/or physiologic activity of the therapeutic ingredient.

Pseudomonas aeruginosa can invade an abraded cornea and cause ulceration or even blindness. In concentrations tolerated by the eye, all of the aforementioned preservative agents are *in*effective against some strains of *P. aeruginosa*. However, preservative mixtures of benzalkonium chloride (0.01%) and either polymyxin B sulfate (1,000 USP U/mL) or disodium ethylenediaminetetraacetate (0.01% to 0.1%) *are* effective against most strains of *Pseudomonas*. The latter agent, which is commonly employed as a chelating agent for metals, renders strains of *P. aeruginosa* more sensitive to benzalkonium chloride.

Isotonicity Value

If a solution is placed behind a membrane that is permeable only to solvent molecules and not to solute molecules (a *semipermeable membrane*), *osmosis* occurs as the molecules of solvent traverse the membrane. If a solution-filled membrane is placed in a solution of a higher solute concentration than its own, the solvent, which has free passage in either direction, passes into the more concentrated solution until equilibrium is established on both sides of the membrane and an equal concentration of solute exists on the two sides. The pressure responsible for this movement is termed *osmotic pressure*.

The concentration of a solution with respect to osmotic pressure is concerned with the number of particles of solute in solution. That is, if the solute is not an electrolyte (as with sucrose), the concentration of the solution will depend solely on the number of molecules present. However, if the solute is an electrolyte (as with sodium chloride), the number of particles that it contributes to the solution will depend not only on the concentration of the molecules present but also on their degree of ionization. A chemical that is highly ionized will contribute a greater number of particles to the solution than will be the same amount of a poorly ionized substance. The effect is that a solution with a greater number of particles, whether they are molecules or ions, has higher osmotic pressure than does a solution having fewer particles.

Body fluids, including blood and tears, have an osmotic pressure corresponding to that of a 0.9% solution of sodium chloride. Thus, a 0.9% sodium chloride solution is said to be *iso-osmotic*, or having an osmotic pressure equal to that of physiologic fluids. The term *isotonic*, meaning equal tone, is commonly used interchangeably with iso-osmotic, although it is correctly used only with reference to a specific body fluid, whereas *iso-osmotic* is a physicochemical term comparing the osmotic pressure of two liquids that may or may not be physiologic fluids. Solutions with a lower osmotic pressure than body fluids or a 0.9% sodium chloride solution are commonly called *hypotonic*, whereas solutions having a greater osmotic pressure are termed *hypertonic*.

Theoretically, a hypertonic solution added to the body's system will have a tendency to draw water from the body tissues toward the solution in an effort to dilute and establish a concentration equilibrium. In the bloodstream, a hypertonic injection can cause *crenation* (shrinking) of blood cells; in the eye, the solution can draw water toward the site of the topical application. Conversely, a hypotonic solution may induce hemolysis of red blood cells or passage of water from the site of an ophthalmic application through the tissues of the eye.

In practice, the isotonicity limits of an ophthalmic solution in terms of sodium chloride or its osmotic equivalent may range from 0.6% to 2% without marked discomfort to the eye. Sodium chloride itself does not have to be used to establish a solution's osmotic pressure. Boric acid in a concentration of 1.9% produces the same osmotic pressure as does 0.9% sodium chloride. All of an ophthalmic solution's solutes, including the active and inactive ingredients, contribute to the osmotic pressure of a solution.

The calculations necessary to prepare iso-osmotic solutions may be made in terms of data relating to the colligative properties of solutions (9). Like osmotic pressure, the other colligative properties of solutions, namely, vapor pressure, boiling point, and freezing point, depend on the number of particles in solution. These properties, therefore, are related, and a change in any one of them will be accompanied by corresponding changes in the others. Although any one of these properties may be used to determine iso-osmoticity, a comparison of freezing points between the solutions in question is most used.

When 1 mole of a nonelectrolyte, such as boric acid, is dissolved in 1,000 g of water, the freezing point of the solution is about 1.86°C below the freezing point of pure water. By simple proportion, therefore, the weight may be calculated for any nonelectrolyte to be dissolved in each 1,000 g of water to prepare a solution iso-osmotic with lachrymal fluid and blood serum, which have freezing points of −0.52°C.

Boric acid, for example, has a molecular weight of 61.8, so 61.8 g in 1,000 g of water should produce a freezing point of −1.86°C. Therefore,

$$\frac{1.86\,(°C)}{0.52\,(°C)} = \frac{61.8\,(g)}{x\,(g)}$$
$$x = 17.3\,(g)$$

Hence, 17.3 g of boric acid in 1,000 g of water theoretically should produce a solution iso-osmotic with tears and blood.

The calculation employed to prepare a solution iso-osmotic with tears or blood when using electrolytes is different from the calculation for a nonelectrolyte. Because osmotic pressure depends on the number of particles, substances that dissociate have an effect that increases with the degree of dissociation; the greater the dissociation, the smaller the quantity required to produce a given osmotic pressure. If we assume that sodium chloride in weak solutions is about 80% dissociated, each 100 molecules yield 180 particles, or 1.8 times as many particles as are yielded by 100 molecules of a nonelectrolyte. This dissociation factor, commonly symbolized by the letter i, must be included in the proportion when we seek to determine the strength of an iso-osmotic solution of sodium chloride (molecular weight, 58.5):

$$\frac{1.86\,(°C) \times 1.8}{0.52\,(°C)} = \frac{58.5\,(g)}{x\,(g)}$$
$$x = 9.09\,g$$

Therefore, 9.09 g of sodium chloride in 1,000 g of water should make a solution iso-osmotic with blood or lacrimal fluid. As indicated previously, a 0.9% (w/v) sodium chloride solution is taken to be iso-osmotic (and isotonic) with the body fluids.

Simple iso-osmotic solutions, then, may be calculated by this general formula:

$$\frac{0.52 \times \text{molecular weight}}{1.86 \times \text{dissociation (i)}} = \text{g of solute per 1,000 g of water}$$

Although the i value has not been determined for every medicinal agent that might be named, the following values may be generally used:

Nonelectrolytes and substances of slight dissociation	1.0
Substances that dissociate into 2 ions	1.8
Substances that dissociate into 3 ions	2.6
Substances that dissociate into 4 ions	3.4
Substances that dissociate into 5 ions	4.2

Because 0.9% sodium chloride is considered to be iso-osmotic and isotonic with tears, other medicinal substances are compared with regard to their "sodium chloride equivalency." An often-used rule states (9):

Quantities of two substances that are tonicic equivalents are proportional to the molecular weights of each multiplied by the i value of the other.

Using the drug atropine sulfate as an example,

Molecular weight of sodium chloride = 58.5;

    i = 1.8

Molecular weight of atropine sulfate = 695;

    i = 2.6

$$\frac{695 \times 1.8}{58.5 \times 2.6} = \frac{1\,(g)}{x\,(g)}$$

x = 0.12 g of sodium chloride represented by 1 g of atropine sulfate.

Thus, the *sodium chloride* equivalent for atropine sulfate is 0.12 g. To put it one way, 1 g of atropine sulfate equals the tonic effect of 0.12 g of sodium chloride. To put it another way, atropine sulfate is 12% as effective as an equal weight of sodium chloride in contributing to tonicity. When a combination of drugs is used in a prescription or formulation to be rendered isotonic, each agent's contribution to tonicity must be taken into consideration. For instance, consider the following prescription:

Atropine sulfate:	1%
Sodium chloride:	qs to isotonicity
Sterile purified water, ad:	30 mL

To make the 30 mL isotonic with sodium chloride, 30 mL × 0.9% = 0.27 g or 270 mg of sodium chloride would be required. However, because 300 mg of atropine sulfate is to be present, its contribution to tonicity must be taken into consideration. The sodium chloride equivalent of atropine sulfate is 0.12. Thus, its contribution is calculated as follows:

$$0.12 \times 300 \text{ mg} = 36 \text{ mg}$$

Thus, 270 − 36 mg = 234 mg of sodium chloride required.

Table 17.1 presents a short list of sodium chloride equivalents. A more complete list may be found in pharmaceutical calculations or physical pharmacy textbooks.

As a convenience, some earlier pharmacy reference books list amounts of some common ophthalmic drugs that may be used to prepare isotonic solutions. Some of the drugs and the related values are presented in Table 17.2. The data are used in the following manner. Of each of the drugs listed, 1 g added to purified water will prepare the corresponding volume of an isotonic solution. For instance, 1 g of atropine sulfate will prepare 14.3 mL of isotonic solution. This solution may be diluted with an isotonic vehicle to maintain the isotonicity while changing the strength of the

active constituent in the solution to any desired level. For instance, if a 1% isotonic solution of atropine sulfate is desired, 14.3 mL of isotonic solution containing 1 g of atropine sulfate should be diluted to 100 mL (1 g atropine sulfate in 100 mL = 1% w/v solution) with an isotonic vehicle. By using sterile drug, sterile purified water, a sterile isotonic vehicle, and aseptic techniques, a sterile product may be prepared. In addition to being sterile and isotonic, the diluting vehicles generally used are buffered and contain suitable preservative to maintain the stability and sterility of the product.

Buffering

The pH of an ophthalmic preparation may be adjusted and buffered for one or more of the following purposes (10): (*a*) for greater comfort to the eye, (*b*) to render the formulation more stable, (*c*) to enhance the aqueous solubility of the drug, (*d*) to enhance the drug's bioavailability (i.e., by favoring unionized molecular species), and (*e*) to maximize preservative efficacy.

The pH of normal tears is considered to be about 7.4, but it varies; for example, it is more acidic in contact lens wearers (9). Tears have some buffer capacity. The introduction of a medicated solution into the eye stimulates the flow of tears, which attempts to neutralize any excess hydrogen or hydroxyl ions introduced with the solution. Most drugs used ophthalmically are weakly acidic and have only weak buffer capacity. Normally, the buffering action of the tears neutralizes the ophthalmic solution and thereby prevents marked discomfort. The eye apparently can tolerate a greater deviation from physiologic pH toward alkalinity (and less discomfort) than toward acidic range (10). For maximum comfort, an ophthalmic solution should have the same pH as the tears. However,

TABLE 17.1. Some Sodium Chloride Equivalents

Substance	Molecular Weight	Ions	I	Sodium Chloride Equivalent
Atropine sulfate·H_2O	695.0	3	2.6	0.12
Benzalkonium chloride	360.0	2	1.8	0.16
Benzyl alcohol	108.0	1	1.0	0.30
Boric acid	61.8	1	1.0	0.52
Chlorobutanol	177.0	1	1.0	0.18
Cocaine hydrochloride	340.0	2	1.8	0.17
Ephedrine sulfate	429.0	3	2.6	0.20
Epinephrine bitartrate	333.0	2	1.8	0.18
Ethylmorphine hydrochloride·$2H_2O$	386.0	2	1.8	0.15
Naphazoline hydrochloride	247.0	2	1.8	0.27
Physostigmine salicylate	413.0	2	1.8	0.14
Pilocarpine hydrochloride	245.0	2	1.8	0.24
Procaine hydrochloride	273.0	2	1.8	0.21
Scopolamine hydrobromide·$3H_2O$	438.0	2	1.8	0.13
Tetracycline hydrochloride	481.0	2	1.8	0.12
Zinc sulfate·$7H_2O$	288.0	2	1.4	0.16

TABLE 17.2. Isotonic Solutions Prepared from Common Ophthalmic Drugs

Drug (1 g)	Volume of Isotonic Solution (mL)
Atropine sulfate	14.3
Boric acid	55.7
Chlorobutanol (hydrous)	26.7
Cocaine hydrochloride	17.7
Colistimethate sodium	16.7
Dibucaine hydrochloride	14.3
Ephedrine sulfate	25.7
Epinephrine bitartrate	20.0
Eucatropine hydrochloride	20.0
Fluorescein sodium	34.3
Homatropine hydrobromide	19.0
Neomycin sulfate	12.3
Penicillin G potassium	20.0
Phenylephrine hydrochloride	35.7
Physostigmine salicylate	17.7
Physostigmine sulfate	14.3
Pilocarpine hydrochloride	26.7
Pilocarpine nitrate	25.7
Polymyxin B sulfate	10.0
Procaine hydrochloride	23.3
Proparacaine hydrochloride	16.7
Scopolamine hydrobromide	13.3
Silver nitrate	36.7
Sodium bicarbonate	72.3
Sodium biphosphate	44.3
Sodium borate	46.7
Sodium phosphate (dibasic, heptahydrate)	32.3
Streptomycin sulfate	7.7
Sulfacetamide sodium	25.7
Sulfadiazine sodium	26.7
Tetracaine hydrochloride	20.0
Tetracycline hydrochloride	15.7
Zinc sulfate	16.7

this is not pharmaceutically possible, because at pH 7.4 many drugs are insoluble in water. A few drugs—notably pilocarpine hydrochloride and epinephrine bitartrate—are quite acid and overtax the buffer capacity of the tears.

Most drugs, including many used in ophthalmic solutions, are most active therapeutically at pH levels that favor the undissociated molecule (Physical Pharmacy Capsule 17.1). However, the pH that permits greatest activity may also be the pH at which the drug is least stable. For this reason, a compromise pH is generally selected for a solution and maintained by buffers to permit the greatest activity while maintaining stability.

An isotonic phosphate vehicle prepared at the desired pH (Table 17.3) and adjusted for tonicity may be employed in the extemporaneous compounding of solutions. The desired solution is prepared with two stock solutions, one containing 8 g of monobasic sodium phosphate (NaH_2PO_4) per liter and the other containing 9.47 g of dibasic sodium phosphate (Na_2HPO_4) per liter, the weights being on an anhydrous basis.

The vehicles listed in Table 17.3 are satisfactory for many ophthalmic drugs, excepting pilocarpine, eucatropine, scopolamine, and homatropine salts, which show instability in the vehicle. The vehicle is used effectively as the diluent for ophthalmic drugs already in isotonic solution, such as those prepared according to the method presented in Table 17.2. When drug substances are added directly to the isotonic phosphate vehicle, the solution becomes slightly hypertonic. Generally, this provides no discomfort to the patient. However, if such a solution is not desired, the appropriate adjustment can be made through calculated dilution of the vehicle with purified water.

Viscosity and Thickening Agents

Viscosity is a property of liquids related to the resistance to flow. The reciprocal of viscosity is *fluidity*. Viscosity is defined in terms of the force required to move one plane surface past another under specified conditions when the space between is filled by the liquid in question. More simply, it can be considered as a relative property, with water as the reference material and all viscosities expressed in terms of the viscosity of pure water at 20°C (68°F). The viscosity of water is given as 1 centipoise (actually 1.0087 cP). A liquid material 10 times as viscous as water at the same temperature has a viscosity of 10 cP. The centipoise is a more convenient term than the basic unit, the poise; 1 poise is equal to 100 cP.

Specifying the temperature is important because viscosity changes with temperature; generally, the viscosity of a liquid decreases with increasing temperature. The determination of viscosity in terms of poise or centipoise results in the calculation of *absolute* viscosity. It is sometimes more convenient to use the kinematic scale, in which the units of viscosity are *stokes* and *centistokes* (1 stoke equals 100 centistokes). The kinematic viscosity is obtained from the absolute viscosity by dividing the latter by the density of the liquid at the same temperature:

$$\text{kinematic viscosity} = \frac{\text{absolute viscosity}}{\text{density}}$$

Using water as the standard, these are examples of some viscosities at 20°C:

Ethyl alcohol:	1.19 cP
Olive oil:	100.00 cP
Glycerin:	400.00 cP
Castor oil:	1,000.00 cP

PHYSICAL PHARMACY CAPSULE **17.1** pH and Solubility

pH is one of the most important factors in formulation. The effects of pH on solubility and stability are critically important. The effect of pH on solubility is critical in the formulation of liquid dosage forms, from oral and topical solutions to intravenous solutions and admixtures.

The solubility of a weak acid or base is often pH dependent. The total quantity of a monoprotic weak acid (HA) in solution at a specific pH is the sum of the concentrations of both the free acid and salt (A^-) forms. If excess drug is present, the quantity of free acid in solution is maximized and constant because of its saturation solubility. As the pH of the solution is increased, the quantity of drug in solution increases because the water-soluble ionizable salt is formed. The expression is

$$HA \overset{K_a}{\leftrightarrow} H^+ + A^-$$

where K_a is the dissociation constant.

At a certain pH level, the total solubility (S_T) of the drug solution is saturated with respect to both the salt and acid forms of the drug, that is, the pH_{max}. The solution can be saturated with respect to the salt at pH values higher than this but not with respect to the acid. Also, at pH values less than this, the solution can be saturated with respect to the acid but not to the salt. This is illustrated in the accompanying figure.

To calculate the total quantity of drug that can be maintained in solution at a selected pH, either of two equations can be used, depending upon whether the product is to be above or below the pH_{max} (figure). The following equation is used when below the pH_{max}:

$$S_T = S_a \left(1 + \frac{K_a}{[H^+]} \right) \qquad \textbf{Equation 17.1}$$

The next equation is used above the pH_{max}:

$$S_T = S'_a \left(1 + \frac{[H^+]}{K_a} \right) \qquad \textbf{Equation 17.2}$$

where

S_a is the saturation solubility of the free acid and
S'_a is the saturation solubility of the salt form.

■ EXAMPLE

A pharmacist prepares a 3% solution of an antibiotic as an ophthalmic solution and dispenses it to a patient. A few days later, the patient returns the eye drops to the pharmacist because the product contains a precipitate. The pharmacist, checking the pH of the solution and finding it to be 6.0, reasons that the problem may be pH related. The physicochemical information of interest on the antibiotic includes the following:

Molecular weight:	285 (salt) 263 (free acid)
3% Solution of the drug:	0.1053 M solution
Acid form solubility (S_a):	3.1 mg/mL (0.0118 M)
K_a:	5.86×10^{-6}

Using Equation (17.1), the pharmacist calculates the quantity of the antibiotic in solution at pH 6.0 (pH 6.0 = $[H^+]$ 1×10^{-6}):

$$S_T = 0.0118 \left(1 + \frac{5.86 \times 10^{-6}}{1 \times 10^{-6}} \right) = 0.0809 \; M$$

(continued)

(continued)

From this, the pharmacist knows that at pH 6.0, a 0.0809-M solution can be prepared. However, the concentration that was to be prepared was 0.1053 M; consequently, the drug is not in solution at that pH. The pH may have been all right initially but shifted lower over time, resulting in precipitation of the drug. At what pH (hydrogen ion concentration) will the drug remain in solution? This can be calculated using the same equation and the available information. The S_T value is 0.1053 M:

$$0.1053 = 0.0118 \left(1 + \frac{5.86 \times 10^{-6}}{[H^+]} \right)$$

$$[H^+] = 7.333 \times 10^{-7}, \text{ or a pH of } 6.135$$

The pharmacist prepares a solution of the antibiotic, adjusting the pH above about 6.2 using a suitable buffer system and dispenses the solution to the patient—with positive results.

An interesting phenomenon concerns the close relationship of pH to solubility. At pH 6.0, only a 0.0809-M solution could be prepared, but at pH 6.13, a 0.1053-M solution could be prepared. In other words, a difference of 0.13 pH units resulted in the following:

$$\frac{0.1053 - 0.0809}{0.0809} = 30.1\% \text{ more drug in solution at the higher pH}$$

In other words, a very small change in pH resulted in about 30% more drug going into solution. According to the figure, the slope of the curve would be very steep for this example drug, and a small change in pH (X-axis) results in a large change in solubility (Y-axis). From this, it can be reasoned that if one observes the pH–solubility profile of a drug, it is possible to predict the magnitude of the pH change on its solubility.

In recent years, more and more physicochemical information on drugs is being made available to pharmacists in routinely used reference books. This type of information is important for pharmacists in many types of practice, especially those who do compounding and pharmacokinetic monitoring. ■

Viscosity can be determined by any method that will measure the resistance to shear offered by the liquid. For ordinary newtonian liquids, it is customary to determine the time required for a given sample of the liquid to flow at a regulated temperature through a small vertical capillary tube and to compare this time with that required to perform the same task by the reference liquid. Many capillary tube viscosimeters have been devised, and nearly all are modifications of the Ostwald type. With an apparatus such as this, the viscosity of a liquid may be determined by the following equation:

$$\frac{\eta_1}{\eta_2} = \frac{\rho_1 t_1}{\rho_2 t_2}$$

TABLE 17.3. Isotonic Phosphate Vehicle

Monobasic Sodium Phosphate Solution (mL)	Dibasic Sodium Phosphate Solution (mL)	Resulting Buffer Solution (pH)	Sodium Chloride Required for Isotonicity (g/100 mL)
90	10	5.9	0.52
80	20	6.2	0.51
70	30	6.5	0.50
60	40	6.6	0.49
50	50	6.8	0.48
40	60	7.0	0.46
30	70	7.2	0.45
20	80	7.4	0.44
10	90	7.7	0.43
5	95	8.0	0.42

where

η_1 is the unknown viscosity of the liquid

η_2 is the viscosity of the standard

ρ_1 and ρ_2 are the respective densities of the liquids, and

t_1 and t_2 are the respective flow times in seconds.

In the preparation of ophthalmic solutions, a suitable grade of methylcellulose or other thickening agent is frequently added to increase the viscosity and thereby aid in maintaining the drug in contact with the tissues to enhance therapeutic effectiveness. Generally, methylcellulose of 4,000 cP is used in concentrations of 0.25% and the 25-cP type at 1% concentration. Hydroxypropyl methylcellulose and polyvinyl alcohol are also used as thickeners in ophthalmic solutions. Occasionally, a 1% solution of methylcellulose without medication is used as a tear replacement. Viscosity for ophthalmic solutions is considered optimal in the range of 15 to 25 cP.

Ocular Bioavailability

Ocular bioavailability is an important factor in the effectiveness of an applied medication. Physiologic factors that can affect a drug's ocular bioavailability include protein binding, drug metabolism, and lacrimal drainage. Protein-bound drugs are incapable of penetrating the corneal epithelium because of the size of the protein–drug complex (1). Because of the brief time an ophthalmic solution may remain in the eye, the protein binding of a drug substance can quickly negate its therapeutic value by rendering it unavailable for absorption. Normally, tears contain 0.6% to 2% of protein, including albumin and globulins, but disease states (e.g., uveitis) can raise these protein levels (1). Although ocular protein binding is reversible, tear turnover results in the loss of both bound and unbound drug (2).

As in the case with other biologic fluids, tears contain enzymes (e.g., lysozyme) capable of metabolic degradation of drug substances. However, only a limited amount of research has been conducted on the ocular metabolism of pharmacologic agents, so the full extent to which drug metabolism occurs and affects therapeutic effectiveness is undetermined (11).

In addition to physiologic factors affecting ocular bioavailability, other factors, such as the physicochemical characteristics of the drug substance and product formulation, are important. Because the cornea is a membrane barrier containing both lipophilic and hydrophilic layers, it is permeated most effectively by drug substances having both lipophilic and hydrophilic characteristics (1).

As discussed previously, ophthalmic suspensions, gels, and ointments mix with lacrimal fluids less readily than do low-viscosity solutions and so remain longer in the cul-de-sac, enhancing drug activity.

Additional Considerations

Ophthalmic solutions must be sparkling clear and free of all particulate matter for comfort and safety. The formulation

of an ophthalmic suspension may be undertaken when it is desired to prepare a product with extended corneal contact time, or it may be necessary when the medicinal agent is insoluble or unstable in an aqueous vehicle.

Drug particles in an ophthalmic suspension must be finely subdivided, usually micronized, to minimize eye irritation and/or scratching of the cornea. The suspended particles must not associate into larger particles upon storage and must be easily and uniformly redistributed by gentle shaking of the container prior to use.

PACKAGING OPHTHALMIC SOLUTIONS AND SUSPENSIONS

Although a few commercial ophthalmic solutions and suspensions are packaged in small glass bottles with separate glass or plastic droppers, most are packaged in soft plastic containers with a fixed built-in dropper (Figs. 17.3 and 17.4). This type of packaging is preferred both to facilitate administration and to protect the product from external contamination. Ophthalmic solutions and suspensions are commonly packaged in containers holding 2, 2.5, 5, 10, 15, and 30 mL of product.

Patients must be careful to protect an ophthalmic solution or suspension from external contamination. Obviously, the fixed-dropper containers are less likely to

FIGURE 17.3. Commercial ophthalmic solution in a plastic container with built-in dropper device. (Courtesy of Alcon.)

FIGURE 17.4. Ophthalmic product packaging. Liquids are in 5- and 15-mL Drop-Tainer dispensers, and ointments are in tubes containing 3.5 g of product. (Courtesy of Alcon.)

acquire airborne contaminants than are screw-type bottles, which are fully opened when in use. However, each type is subject to contamination during use by airborne contaminants and by the inadvertent touching of the tip of the dropper to the eye, eyelids, or other surface.

Ophthalmic solutions used as eyewashes are generally packaged with an eye cup, which should be cleaned and dried thoroughly before and after each use.

PROPER ADMINISTRATION OF OPHTHALMIC SOLUTIONS AND SUSPENSIONS

Prior to the administration of an ophthalmic solution or suspension, the patient or caregiver should be advised to wash the hands thoroughly. If the ophthalmic drops are supplied with a separate dropper, the person should inspect the dropper to make sure it has no chips or cracks. Ophthalmic solutions should be inspected for color and clarity. Out-of-date or darkened solutions should be discarded. Ophthalmic suspensions should be shaken thoroughly prior to administration to distribute the suspensoid evenly.

The cap of an eye drop container should be removed immediately prior to use and returned immediately after use. The combined dropper with container as shown in Figure 17.3 is used by holding it between the thumb and middle finger with the index finger on the bottom of the container. One or more drops are delivered by gently squeezing the container. A product packaged with a separate dropper is used by holding the dropper between the thumb and forefinger, then drawing up and discharging the medication dropwise in the usual and familiar manner.

To instill eye drops, the person should tilt the head back and, with the index finger of the free hand, gently pull downward the lower eyelid of the affected eye to form a pocket or cup. While looking up, and without touching the dropper to the eye, the prescribed number of drops should be instilled into the formed pocket. The lower eyelid should be released and the eye closed to allow the medication to spread over the eye. The eye should be held closed, preferably for a full minute, without blinking, rubbing, or wiping. While the eye is closed, gentle pressure should be applied just under the inner corner of the eye by the nose to compress the nasolacrimal duct to prevent drainage and enhance corneal contact time. Then, any excess liquid may be wiped away with a tissue. When multiple drops are prescribed for the same eye, the patient should wait about 5 minutes before instilling the second drop. Otherwise, the second drop will drain too quickly and have little effect in the eye.

During handling and administration, care must be taken not to touch the dropper to the eye, eyelid, or any other surface. If a separate dropper is used, it should be returned to the container and capped tightly. The dropper should not be rinsed or wiped off. If a combined dropper and container unit is used, the container cap should be returned and tightly closed.

In every case, the patient should be advised about the correct number of drops to instill, the frequency of application, the duration of treatment, proper storage of the medication, and usual side effects specific to the product. Among the side effects encountered with the use of ophthalmic medication are transient stinging or burning, foreign body sensation, itching, tearing, decreased vision, margin crusting, and occasionally a bad (drug) taste.

Examples of some commercially available ophthalmic solutions and suspensions are presented in Table 17.4.

An example ophthalmic formulation with the purpose of each ingredient is given as follows:

Ophthalmic Decongestant Solution

Phenylephrine hydrochloride	0.125%	Active
Polyvinyl alcohol	1.4%	Viscosity
Disodium edetate	0.05%	Chelator
Sodium acetate	0.1%	Buffer
Monobasic sodium phosphate	0.1%	Buffer
Dibasic sodium phosphate	0.05%	Buffer
Sodium thiosulfate	0.1%	Antioxidant
Sterile water for injection	qs 100%	Vehicle

NASAL PREPARATIONS

Most preparations intended for intranasal use contain adrenergic agents and are employed for their decongestant activity on the nasal mucosa. Most of these preparations are in solution form and are administered as nose drops or sprays; however, a few are available as jellies. Examples of products for intranasal use are shown in Figure 17.5 and in Table 17.5.

TABLE 17.4. Some Ophthalmic Agents by Category

Agent	Commercial Product	Active Ingredient (%)	Comments
Decongestant			
Naphazoline HCl	Naphcon-A Ophthalmic Solution (Alcon)	0.025	Topical ocular vasoconstrictor
Antiallergic			
Cromolyn sodium	Opticrom Ophthalmic Solution (Fisons)	4	For allergic ocular disorders, for example, vernal conjunctivitis
Antibacterial			
Ciprofloxacin hydrochloride	Ciloxan Sterile Ophthalmic Solution (Alcon)	0.35	For superficial eye infections due to susceptible microorganisms
Gentamicin sulfate		0.3	
Tobramycin	Tobrex Ophthalmic Solution (Alcon)	0.3	
Sulfacetamide sodium	Sodium Sulamyd Ophthalmic Solution (Schering-Plough)	10, 30	
Sulfacetamide sodium and prednisolone acetate	Blephamide Ophthalmic Suspension (Allergan)	10%/0.2%	For steroid-responsive anti-inflammatory conditions
Antiviral			
Trifluridine	Viroptic Ophthalmic Solution (Monarch)	1	For herpes simplex keratitis
Artificial Tears			
Dextran 70, hydroxypropyl methylcellulose	Tears Naturale II (Alcon)		For relief of dry eyes
Astringent			
Zinc sulfate	Zincfrin Ophthalmic Solution (Alcon)	0.25	Relief of discomfort, congestion of minor irritations to eyes, such as dust, fatigue, allergies
Anti-inflammatory			
Dexamethasone sodium phosphate		0.1	Combats inflammation of mechanical, chemical, immunologic causes
Antibacterial–Anti-inflammatory Combinations			
Tobramycin and dexamethasone	TobraDex Sterile Ophthalmic Suspension (Alcon)	0.3 tobramycin, 0.1 dexamethasone	
Beta-adrenergic Blocking Agents			
Betaxolol HCl	Betoptic-S Sterile Ophthalmic Solution (Alcon)	0.5	For ocular hypertension, chronic open-angle glaucoma
Timolol maleate	Timoptic Sterile Ophthalmic Solution (Aton Pharma)	0.25, 0.5	For chronic open-angle glaucoma, aphakic patients with glaucoma
Cholinergic			
Pilocarpine HCL	Isopto Carpine Ophthalmic Solution (Alcon)	0.25–10	Miotic for glaucoma, especially open-angle; neutralizes mydriasis following ophthalmoscopy or surgery
Cholinesterase Inhibitor			
Demecarium bromide	Humorsol Sterile Ophthalmic Solution (Merck & Co.)	0.125, 0.25	Intense miosis, ciliary muscle contractions by inhibiting cholinesterase. Used in open-angle glaucoma when shorter-acting miotics inadequate
Prostaglandin Analog			
Travoprost	Travatan Z Ophthalmic Solution	0.004%	Treatment of elevated intraocular pressure

Nasal Decongestant Solutions

Most nasal decongestant solutions are aqueous, rendered isotonic to nasal fluids (approximately equivalent to 0.9% sodium chloride), buffered to maintain drug stability while approximating the normal pH range of the nasal fluids (pH 5.5 to 6.5), and stabilized and preserved as required. The antimicrobial preservatives are the same as those used in ophthalmic solutions. The concentration of adrenergic

FIGURE 17.5. Commercial packages of nasal solutions, showing drop and spray containers and a nasal inhaler.

agent in most nasal decongestant solutions is quite low, ranging from about 0.05% to 1%. Certain commercial solutions are available in adult and pediatric strengths, the pediatric strength being approximately half of the adult strength.

Nasal decongestant solutions are employed in the treatment of rhinitis of the common cold, for vasomotor and allergic rhinitis including hay fever, and for sinusitis. Frequent or prolonged use may lead to chronic edema of the nasal mucosa, that is, rhinitis medicamentosa, aggravating the symptom that they are intended to relieve. Thus, they

are best used for short periods (no longer than 3 to 5 days), and the patient should be advised not to exceed the recommended dosage and frequency of use.

The easiest but least comfortable approach to treat rebound congestion is complete withdrawal of the topical vasoconstrictor. Unfortunately, this approach will promptly result in bilateral vasodilation with almost total nasal obstruction. A more acceptable method is to withdraw application of drug in only one nostril, with the patient continuing to use the medication in the other nostril. Once the rebound congestion subsides in the drug-free nostril, after about 1 to 2 weeks, a total withdrawal is instituted. Another approach is substitution of a topical saline solution or spray for the topical vasoconstrictor. This keeps the nasal mucosa moist and provides psychological assistance to patients who are dependent on placing medication into their nostrils.

Most of the adrenergic drugs used in nasal decongestant solutions are synthetic compounds similar in chemical structure, pharmacologic activity, and side effects to the parent compound, naturally occurring epinephrine. Epinephrine as a pure chemical substance was first isolated from suprarenal (adrenal) gland in 1901 and was called both suprarenin and adrenaline. Synthetic epinephrine was prepared just a few years later.

TABLE 17.5. Some Commercial Nasal Preparations

Product	Manufacturer	Active Ingredient	Use/Indications
Afrin nasal spray, Afrin nose drops	Schering-Plough	Oxymetazoline HCl 0.05%	Adrenergic, decongestant
Beconase AQ nasal spray	GlaxoSmithKline	Beclomethasone dipropionate 0.042%	Synthetic corticosteroid for relief of seasonal, perennial allergic, vasomotor rhinitis
Diapid nasal spray	Sandoz	Lypressin 0.185 mg/mL	Antidiuretic; control, prevention of diabetes insipidus of deficiency of endogenous posterior pituitary antidiuretic hormone
Imitrex nasal spray	GlaxoSmithKline	Sumatriptan 5 or 20 mg/ 100 µL	Acute treatment of migraines
Nasalcrom nasal spray	Pharmacia	Cromolyn sodium 4%	Prevention and treatment of symptoms of allergic rhinitis
Nasalide nasal solution	Dura	Flunisolide 0.025%	Symptoms of seasonal or perennial rhinitis
Neosynephrine nose drops, spray	Bayer Consumer Care	Phenylephrine HCl 0.125%–1.0%	Adrenergic, decongestant
Neosynephrine maximum strength 12 h	Bayer Consumer Care	Oxymetazoline HCl 0.05%	Adrenergic, decongestant
Ocean mist	Wonder Labs	Sodium chloride 0.65%	Restore moisture; relieve dry, crusted, inflamed nasal membranes
Privine HCl nasal solution	Insight	Naphazoline HCl 0.05%	Adrenergic, decongestant
Rhinocort aqua	AstraZeneca	Budesonide 32 µg/spray	Anti-inflammatory corticosteroid
Syntocinon nasal spray	Sandoz	Oxytocin 40 U/mL	Synthetic oxytocin for initial milk letdown preparatory to breast-feeding
Tyzine pediatric nose drops	Kenwood	Tetrahydrozoline HCl (0.05%)	Adrenergic, decongestant
Veramyst nasal spray	GlaxoSmithKline	Fluticasone furoate 27.5 µg/ l50 µL spray	Treatment of allergic rhinitis

Most solutions for nasal use are packaged in dropper bottles or in plastic spray bottles, usually containing 15 to 30 mL of medication. The products should be determined to be stable in the container and the package tightly closed while not in use. The patient should be advised to discard the solution if it becomes discolored and/or contains precipitated matter.

The patient should also understand that there is a difference in the duration of the effect of topical decongestants. For example, phenylephrine should be used every 3 to 4 hours, whereas oxymetazoline, which is longer acting, should only be used every 12 hours. Patients should be advised to read and adhere to the directions for use to avoid misuse/overuse.

Inhalation Solutions and Inhalants

Background

One of the earliest forms of inhaling drug products was by the burning of materials and the inhalation of the smoke. A natural vegetable product was dried and broken up and burned, or an oil was burned, or other material burned and the vapors inhaled. Until recent years, an asthma "cigarette" (Asthmador) was available containing the drug that was "smoked" and inhaled delivering the bronchodilator to the lungs. This principle is still used by recreational drug users for substances such as marijuana and opium. Some recreational drugs are simply inhaled as the powder form, resulting in a very rapid onset of action. There is no question about the effectiveness of this route of administration for drugs.

Formerly, inhalations were simple solutions of volatile medications, usually volatile oils, in alcohol or an alcoholic preparation. Often Compound Benzoin Tincture was used. An example formula is as follows:

Pine oil	5 mL
Eucalyptus oil	5 mL
Compound benzoin tincture	30 mL

Sig: Inhale the vapor of one teaspoonful when added to one pint of hot water.

Other inhalations designed for addition to hot water were aqueous preparations containing a volatile oil, water, and light magnesium carbonate. The purpose of the light magnesium carbonate was as a distributive or dispersing agent. The volatile material was distributed on the light magnesium carbonate, which was then mixed with the water. This ensured uniform dispersion of the oil upon shaking as the oil was distributed throughout the mixture, rather than remaining as a globule or being dispersed as large globules. The presence of the light magnesium carbonate did not interfere with the free volatilization of the oil when the product was added to hot water. If the oil would emulsify, this would actually retard volatilization. An approximate ratio of 100 mg of light magnesium

carbonate to 0.2 mL of oil was used. An example formula is as follows:

Menthol		325 mg
Eucalyptus oil		3.7 mL
Light magnesium carbonate		2 g
Purified water	qs	30 mL

Sig: Add one teaspoonful to a pint of hot water (not boiling). Inhale the vapor. Shake the bottle before using.

Introduction and Definitions

Inhalations are sterile drugs or sterile solutions of drugs administered by the nasal or oral respiratory route. The drugs may be administered for local action on the bronchial tree or for systemic effects through absorption from the lungs. Certain gases, such as oxygen and ether, are administered by inhalation, as are finely powdered drug substances and solutions of drugs administered as fine mists. Sterile Water for Inhalation, USP, and Sodium Chloride Inhalation, USP, may be used as vehicles for inhalation solutions.

As discussed in Chapter 14, a number of drug substances are administered through pressure-packaged inhalation aerosols. For the inhaled drug substance or solution to reach the bronchial tree, the inhaled particles must be just a few microns in size.

There are numerous advantages of oral inhalation products, including a rapid onset of action, bypassing the first-pass effect, avoiding drug degradation in the gastrointestinal tract, low dosages to minimize adverse reactions, dose titration capability, good for prn dosing, alternate route when other drugs may chemically or physically interact with concurrent drugs, and an alternate route for drugs with erratic oral or parenteral administration pharmacokinetics. The ultimate deposition of inhalation aerosols is dependent upon (*a*) the products formulation, (*b*) the design of components/packaging/container, (*c*) administration skills and techniques of the product user, and (*d*) the anatomical and physiological status of the respiratory system.

Numerous terms are used to describe the various dosage forms and methods of drug administration by inhalation, including aerosols, atomizers, inhalations, insufflations, metered-dose inhalers, nebulizers, and vaporizers.

By definition, an *aerosol* is a colloidal dispersion of a liquid or a solid in a gas. Oral inhalation and nasopharyngeal medications can both be administered in the form of an aerosol. These products are commonly produced by manual sprays or from pressurized packages. Aerosols have become so widespread in use that the term has come to mean a self-contained product that is sprayed and the propelling force is supplied by either a liquefied or a compressed gas. In pharmacy, these pressure-packaged products consist of the active drug dissolved in, suspended in, or emulsified in a propellant or a mixture of a solvent and a propellant. These aerosols are generally designed for either topical administration or for inhalation into the nasopharyngeal region or bronchopulmonary system. For pulmonary delivery, particles greater than 60 µm are usually deposited in the trachea and those greater than 20 µm between the trachea and the bronchioles but not into the bronchioles. Particles about 1 µm often remain airborne and are exhaled. Consequently, particles between about 5 to 20 µm would be desired to reach the bronchioles. Inhalation aerosols are the largest group of oral aerosol products formulated as either solutions or suspensions. Factors influencing the deposition of inhalation aerosols include the formulation, device, administrative technique of the user, and the anatomical and physiological status of the respiratory system.

An *atomizer* is an instrument used to disperse a liquid in a fine spray. Many of the older pressure-type atomizers used the Bernoulli principle. When a stream of air moves at a high velocity over the tip of a dip tube, the pressure is lowered resulting in the liquid being drawn into the airflow. The liquid is broken up into a spray as it is taken up into the air stream. To produce smaller droplets, a baffle, bead, or other device may be put in the flow to break the droplets into smaller droplets as they collide with the stationary device. These smaller droplets are then carried by the airflow into the inhaled stream of air. Many different configurations are available using the Bernoulli principle. A finer spray can be obtained using a pressure type atomizer. Today's plastic spray bottles are similar to the pressure atomizers. When the plastic bottle is squeezed, the air inside is compressed forcing the liquid up a dip tube into the tip. The liquid stream is mixed with air as it is emitted from the nozzle producing a spray.

Inhalations are preparations designed to deliver the drug into the respiratory tree of the patient for local or systemic effect. Rapid relief is obtained when the vapors or the mist/droplets reach the affected area. The USP-NF definitions of inhalations states "inhalations are drugs or solutions or suspensions of one or more drug substances administered by the nasal or oral respiratory route for local or systemic effect." The drugs may be nebulized to produce droplets sufficiently fine and uniform in size to reach the bronchioles. The mist may be breathed directly from the nebulizer of a face mask, tent, or intermittent positive pressure breathing (IPPB) machine; the IPPB machine may be used to produce a contained environment to maximize the quantity of drug available in the breathing environment to be delivered into the lungs.

Inhalants are drugs that are characterized by a high vapor pressure and can be carried by an air current into the nasal passage where they generally exert their effect. The devices or the container from which the inhalant is generally administered is called an "inhaler." An inhalant consists of cylindrical rolls of a fibrous material that has been impregnated with the drug, usually containing an aromatic substance in addition to an active substance.

These devices are often cylindrical in nature with a cap in place to retard the loss of the medication. To use, the cap is removed and the inhaler inserted into a nostril. Upon inhaling, the air passes through the inhaler and carries the vapor of the medication into the nasal passage. An actual "drug vapor" is being delivered to the patient. For example, menthol, camphor, amyl nitrite, propylhexedrine, and tuaminoheptane inhalants are of this type. Another type, the amyl nitrite inhalant, is packaged with the drug contained in a thin glass ampule encased in a gauze netting. When the product is squeezed and the glass ampule broken, the amyl nitrite is released and is absorbed on the gauze netting and inhaled by the patient. There are currently 25 inhalation products and 2 inhalants listed in the USP-NF.

Insufflations are powders administered using a powder blower (puffer) or *insufflator*. These may consist of a rubber bulb connected to a container and a delivery pipe. As the bulb is squeezed, air is blown into the container causing turbulence resulting in the powder flying around. As the air leaves the container, some of the fine particles are carried out with the air through the delivery tube and are ready for inhalation. Another device (puffer) consists of a plastic accordion-shaped container with a spout on one end. The powder is placed in the "puffer" and as the puffer is sharply squeezed, a portion of the powder is ejected from the spout into the air available for inhalation or application. Contemporary delivery systems include powders that may be delivered by various mechanical devices designed for the patient to breathe deeply to inhale the powder particles. The inspiration step provides energy to spin a propeller that serves to break up and distribute the particles as they are inhaled.

Metered-Dose Inhalants (MDIs) are propellant-driven drug products, either as solutions or as suspensions, containing the drug, a liquefied gas propellant with or without a cosolvent, and are designed to deliver a metered dose of the drug. These devices commonly deliver from 25 to 100 µL volumes of liquid drug for inhalation.

Nebulae, or spray solutions were intended for spraying into the throat and nose. Generally, these were simple solutions. Sprays in plastic spray bottles work similar to the pressure atomizers. When the flexible plastic container is squeezed, the air is compressed forcing the liquid in the container up through a dip tube into the tip where it mixes with a stream of air. Droplets are formed depending upon the geometry of the device and the pressure of the individual squeezing the bottle.

A *nebulizer* was formerly described as a small, vacuum type of atomizer inside a chamber. Large droplets would strike the walls of the chamber, fall back, and be reprocessed. The smaller particles are carried in the air stream out of the unit. For use, the nebulizer is placed in the mouth and the patient inhales while simultaneously squeezing the bulb. The Latin term for mist is nebula. Nebulizers must produce droplets sufficiently fine and uniform in size (optimally 0.5 to 7 µm) such that the mist reaches the bronchioles, in order for nebulizers to be suitable for the administration of inhalation solutions. An advantage to the newer pressurized aerosols is the fine mist they produce and more uniform doses as compared to the older manual nebulizers.

A *vaporizer* is an electrical device producing moist steam, either with or without medication, for inhalation. It is often used to soothe upper respiratory irritations but is relatively ineffective in providing medications to the deeper areas of the respiratory tract.

Formulation Considerations

Solution aerosols can be formulated reasonably easily if the active drug is soluble in the propellant system. If not, a suspension or emulsion aerosol can be prepared. For oral inhalation, either solution or suspension aerosols are used. Example ingredients in an oral inhalation or nasal aerosol solution are shown in Example 1 below.

Suspension aerosols have been used to formulate antiasthmatic aerosols, steroids, antibiotics, and others. Precautions to be considered include caking, agglomeration, particle size growth, and clogging of the valve systems. Example ingredients in a nasal aerosol solution or suspension are shown in Example 2 below.

Example 1: General formula components for oral, inhalation, and nasal aerosol solutions

Component	Example
Active ingredient	Soluble in vehicle
Solvents	Ethyl alcohol, propylene glycol, purified water
Surfactants	Polysorbate
Antioxidants	Ascorbic acid
Flavor	Aromatic oils
Propellants	As needed

Example 2: General formula components for nasal aerosol solutions or suspensions

Component	Example
Active ingredient	Solubilized or suspended
Antioxidants	Ascorbic acid, bisulfites
Preservatives	Benzalkonium chloride
Buffers	Phosphate buffer
Tonicity adjustment	Sodium chloride
Surfactants	Sorbitan esters
Vehicle	Purified water

Variables to Consider

When compounding, or formulating, products for oral inhalation, the variables to consider include particle size, solubility, vehicles, tonicity, pH, sterility, preservatives, viscosity, buffers, surfactants, and moisture content.

Particle size Generally, the particle size should lie within the range of about 0.5 to 10 μm, more preferably between about 3 to 6 μm, for a drug that, when inhaled, is intended to penetrate to the small bronchioles and the lung alveoli and to provide a rapid effect. This size range of particles will deposit in the lung by gravitational sedimentation, by inertial impaction, and by diffusion into terminal alveoli via Brownian motion. For inhalation aerosols, particles 5 to 10 μm are common, whereas for topical sprays, 50 to 100 μm are common.

Solubility Active drugs soluble in the matrix and in the pulmonary fluids will have a rapid onset of action and ordinarily a shorter duration of action, compared to drugs that are somewhat less soluble in the matrix and in the pulmonary fluids. Drugs that are poorly soluble in the pulmonary fluids may cause problems by irritating the lung tissue. For suspensions, it is best to select a vehicle in which the drug is not very soluble to minimize the phenomenon of particle size growth, resulting from the drug in solution crystallizing out onto the crystals that are present. Polymorphic forms of crystalline drugs should not be used for suspension aerosols. To enhance the stability of a suspension aerosol, the selection of a liquid phase with a density similar to that of the suspensoid, the tendency to settle will be minimized.

Vehicle Sterile Water for Inhalation and 0.9% Sodium Chloride Inhalation Solution are commonly used vehicles to carry the drugs in inhalations. Some inhalations are simple solutions of nonvolatile or volatile medications in water or cosolvent mixtures. Small quantities of alcohol or glycerin may be used to solubilize ingredients.

Tonicity Generally, it is best to have inhalation solutions that are isotonic with physiological fluids, that is, equivalent to 0.9% sodium chloride, or an osmolality of about 290 mOsm. To enhance movement of the fluid and drug through the alveoli, it may be best to have the solution slightly hypotonic. If it was hypertonic, the tendency would be to move fluids from the alveoli into the pulmonary space to reach an isotonic equilibrium. If hypotonic, the administered drug solution may have a greater tendency to move into the tissue for more rapid absorption and therapeutic effect.

pH A pH in the neutral range, similar to body fluids, would be desired to minimize any cough reflex that might occur if the pH was too low. Consideration must be made, however, for the solubility and stability characteristics of the drug.

Sterility A new requirement for inhalation solutions is sterility. This requirement is due to contamination problems with different inhalation solution products and adverse experience reports of commercially available products. To ensure patients get the best products available, extemporaneously compounded oral inhalation solutions should be sterilized. This can be easily accomplished using

0.2-μm filtration systems designed for extemporaneous compounding.

Preservative Any preparation that is not in unit dose containers should contain a preservative, especially with the latest requirement of sterility for this class of dosage forms. The minimum amount of preservative that is still effective should be used. If too high a concentration is used, it may initiate a cough reflex in the patient. Also, too high a concentration of preservatives that are also surfactants may result in foaming that may interfere with the delivery of the complete dose.

Viscosity The viscosity of the external phase for most aerosol products is very low; consequently, they are very sensitive systems. Evaporation, sedimentation, and increase in the particle size are processes that may occur and change rapidly.

Buffer A buffer, if used, should be at low buffer strength to maintain the desired pH and not induce pH changes in a microenvironment in the pulmonary cavity.

Surfactants Surfactants can be used as dispersing agents for suspensions, as solubilizing agents to enhance solubility of the drug, and as spreading agents when the drug is deposited in the lungs. The sorbitan esters, especially sorbitan trioleate, are used as well as lecithin derivatives, oleyl alcohol, and others. One should be cautious and keep the surfactant concentration as low as possible to minimize foaming that might interfere with proper administration.

Moisture content For inhalation dispersion aerosols, generally, the moisture content should be kept extremely low for all active and inactive ingredients. The ingredients should be anhydrous to minimize caking.

Example Formulas

Some example formulas illustrated here are for preservative-free formulations. These should be packaged as single-use or unit-dose products. Formulations are provided for 100 mL quantities for ease of calculations. The formulas should be reduced or expanded based upon the total quantity to be compounded. These solutions can be preserved by the addition of 4 mg benzalkonium chloride per 100 mL of solution (This would be 3 mL of a Benzalkonium Chloride 1:750 Solution.)

General Method of Preparation:

1. Calculate the quantity of the individual ingredients required for the total amount to be prepared.
2. Accurately weigh/measure each of the ingredients.
3. Dissolve the solids in about two-thirds of the volume of vehicle for the preparation.
4. Add the liquid ingredients and mix well.
5. Add sufficient vehicle to volume and mix well.
6. Filter through a 0.2-μm filter system into sterile containers.
7. Package and label.

Rx	Albuterol Sulfate 0.5% Inhalant Solution (Preservative Free)		
	Albuterol sulfate		500 mg
	Citric acid, anhydrous		100 mg
	Sodium chloride		800 mg
	Sterile water for inhalation	qs	100 mL
Rx	Beclomethasone Dipropionate 0.042% Nasal Solution (Preservative Free)		
	Beclomethasone dipropionate, monohydrate		43 mg
	Dextrose		5.4 g
	Polysorbate 80		1 mL
	Hydrochloric acid (3% to 5%)		Adjust to pH 7
	Ethanol, 95%		13 mL
	0.9% Sodium chloride solution	qs	100 mL
Rx	Ipratropium Bromide 0.02% Solution (Preservative Free)		
	Ipratropium bromide		20 mg
	Citric acid, anhydrous		50 mg
	0.9% Sodium chloride solution	qs	100 mL
Rx	Metaproterenol Sulfate 0.3% Solution (Preservative Free)		
	Metaproterenol sulfate		300 mg
	Citric acid, anhydrous		250 mg
	0.9% Sodium chloride solution	qs	100 mL

Administration

A widely used instrument capable of producing fine particles for inhalation therapy is the nebulizer. This apparatus, shown in Figure 17.6, contains an atomizing unit in a bulbous glass chamber. A rubber bulb at the end of the apparatus is depressed, and the medicated solution is drawn up a narrow glass tube and broken into fine particles by the passing airstream. The particles produced range between 0.5 and 5 μm. The larger, heavier droplets of the mist do not exit the apparatus but fall back into the reservoir of medicated liquid. The lighter particles do escape with the airstream and are inhaled by the patient, who operates the nebulizer with the exit orifice in the mouth, inhaling while depressing the rubber bulb.

The pharmacist should advise the patient on the proper technique to use the nebulizer and provide additional instructions, such as not to exceed physician's instructions and to use the smallest amount of product necessary to afford relief. The pharmacist may also advise on how to cope with any dryness of the mouth and should emphasize the need to clean the nebulizer after use and explain how to do it.

The common household vaporizer, like the one depicted in Figure 17.7, produces a fine mist of steam that may be used to humidify a room. When a volatile medication is added to the water in the chamber or to a medication cup, the medication volatilizes and is also inhaled by the patient. Humidifiers, as shown in Figure 17.8, are used to provide a cool mist to the air in a room. Moisture in

A

B

FIGURE 17.6. A: A handheld manual nebulizing device. B: An electronic nebulizing device. (Courtesy of DeVilbiss Co.)

the air is important to prevent mucous membranes of the nose and throat from becoming dry and irritated. Vaporizers and humidifiers are commonly used in the adjunctive treatment of colds, coughs, and chest congestion.

The pharmacist can help a patient select a vaporizer or humidifier according to personal needs. Both devices have advantages and disadvantages. Manufacturing guidelines and legal regulations, such as lock tops, have made vaporizers safer today than in years past, so the possibility of

FIGURE 17.7. A commercial vaporizer. (Photo provided by Kaz, Inc. Vicks is a registered trademark of The Procter & Gamble Co. Manufactured by Kaz, Inc. under license from The Procter & Gamble Company, Cincinnati, OH.)

FIGURE 17.8. A commercial humidifier. (Photo provided by Kaz, Inc., maker of Honeywell Portable Humidifiers. The Honeywell trademark is used by Kaz, Inc. under license from Honeywell Intellectual Properties, Inc.)

scalding because of an overturned vaporizer is less with newer models. Furthermore, the heat generated in a vaporizer kills any mold and bacteria in the water tank. Humidifiers are more costly but use less electricity than do vaporizers. In addition, humidifiers are noisier, can deposit minerals on woodwork and furniture, and can cool down a room by 1°F to 3°F (a problem with young children). The patient should learn about these subtle differences from the pharmacist and/or caregiver.

Ultrasonic humidifiers are effective and operate at an almost noiseless level, but they apparently pose a health problem. While they are highly efficient at nebulizing water into fine droplets, they are also efficient at nebulizing up to 90% of water contaminants. These contaminants include mold, bacteria, lead, and dissolved organic gases, which could ultimately cause acute respiratory irritation or chronic lung problems in unsuspecting patients. Thus, patients should either be advised to run water through a high-grade demineralization filter before filling their ultrasonic humidifier or buy a humidifier with a built-in filter that works.

Examples of Medicated Inhalation Solutions

A number of inhalations pressure packaged as inhalation aerosols are discussed in Chapter 14. Several other inhalations used in medicine are solutions intended to be administered by nebulizer or other apparatus. Among these are isoetharine inhalation solution (Bronkosol, Sanofi) and isoproterenol inhalation solution (Isuprel Solution, Sanofi), both used to relieve bronchial spasms of bronchial asthma and related conditions.

Inhalants

Inhalants are drugs or combinations of drugs that by virtue of their high vapor pressure can be carried by an air current into the nasal passage, where they exert their effect. The device that holds the drug or drugs and from which they are administered is an inhaler.

Aromatherapy is another contemporary term used to describe one of the age-old methods of drug administration. Today, however, the term aromatherapy is used primarily to refer to the use of volatile/aromatic oils that are used as room sprays, massage products, and room fresheners and even as inhalants when placed in hot water.

Certain nasal decongestants are in the form of inhalants. For instance, propylhexedrine is a liquid that volatilizes slowly at room temperature. This quality makes it effective as an inhalant.

Amyl Nitrite Inhalant

Amyl nitrite is a clear yellowish volatile liquid that acts as a vasodilator when inhaled. It is prepared in sealed glass vials that are covered with a protective gauze cloth. Upon use, the glass vial is broken in the fingertips, and the cloth soaks up the liquid from which the vapors are inhaled. The vials generally contain 0.3 mL of the drug substance. The effects of the drug are rapid and are used in the treatment of anginal pain.

Propylhexedrine Inhalant

Propylhexedrine (Benzedrex, B.F. Ascher & Company) is a liquid adrenergic (vasoconstrictor) agent that volatilizes slowly at room temperature. This quality enables it to be effectively used as an inhalant. The official inhalant consists of cylindrical rolls of suitable fibrous material impregnated with propylhexedrine, usually aromatized to mask its amine-like odor and contained in a suitable inhaler. The vapor of the drug is inhaled into the nostrils when needed to relieve nasal congestion because of colds and hay fever. It may also be employed to relieve ear block and pressure pain in air travelers.

Each plastic tube of the commercial product contains 250 mg of propylhexedrine with aromatics. The containers should be tightly closed after each opening to prevent loss of the drug vapors. The counterpart commercial product is Benzedrex Inhaler (Menley & James Laboratories).

Proper Administration and Use of Nasal Drops and Sprays

To minimize the possibility of contamination, the pharmacist should point out to the patient that the nasal product should be used by one person only and kept out of the reach of children. If the nasal product is intended for a child, the directions for use should be clear to the child if old enough to understand, the parent, or the caregiver. If an over-the-counter product is used, the parent should note the directions on the label.

Before using the drops, the patient should be advised to blow the nose gently and wash the hands thoroughly with soap and water. For maximum penetration with drops, a patient should lie down on a flat surface, such as a bed,

hanging the head over the edge and tilting the head back as far as comfortable. The prescribed number of drops is then gently placed in the nostrils, and to allow the medication to spread in the nose, the patient should remain in this position for a few minutes. After this, the dropper should be replaced in the bottle and tightened.

Before using the spray, the patient should gently blow the nose to clear the nostrils and wash the hands thoroughly with soap and water. The patient should be told not to shake the plastic squeeze bottle but to be sure to remove the plastic cap. While holding the head upright, the patient should insert the nose piece into the nostril, pointing it slightly backward, and close the other nostril with one finger. The patient should then spray the prescribed or recommended amount, squeezing the bottle sharply and firmly while sniffing. Remove the bottle tip from the nose while maintaining pressure on the bottle sides so as not to aspirate any nasal material into the bottle. Wipe the tip with alcohol or some other appropriate agent, release the pressure on the sides, and repeat the application as necessary. Sprays should always be administered with the patient upright. Spraying medicine into the nostrils should not be performed with the head over the edge of a bed (the preferred procedure for administration of nasal drops) because it could result in systemic absorption of the drug rather than a local effect.

The patient should be advised not to overuse the product. Some decongestant medicines, such as oxymetazoline and xylometazoline, can predispose the patient to rebound congestion if used for more than 3 to 5 consecutive days. The patient should also understand the normal time frame in which to see results and be advised to consult the physician after a certain number of days if relief is not achieved. Finally, patients should not share their medicated spray with another person to prevent the possibility of cross-contamination between individuals. Certain nasal medications, such as beclomethasone dipropionate (Vancenase, Schering), are available for administration through aerosol inhalers.

Nasal Route for Systemic Effects

The nasal route for drug delivery is of interest because of the need to develop a route that is neither oral nor parenteral for newly developed synthetic, biologically active peptides and polypeptides (12–18). Polypeptides, such as insulin, that are subject to destruction by the gastrointestinal fluids are administered by injection. However, the nasal mucosa has been shown to be amenable to the systemic absorption of certain peptides as well as to nonpeptide drug molecules including scopolamine, hydralazine, progesterone, and propranolol (16,17). The nasal route is advantageous for nonpeptide drugs that are poorly absorbed orally.

The adult nasal cavity has about a 20-mL capacity, with a large surface area (about 180 cm^2) for drug absorption afforded by the microvilli along the pseudostratified columnar epithelial cells of the nasal mucosa (14,16). The nasal tissue is highly vascularized, providing an attractive site for rapid and efficient systemic absorption. One great advantage to nasal absorption is that it avoids first-pass metabolism by the liver. However, identification of metabolizing enzymes in the nasal mucosa of certain animal species suggests the same possibility in humans and the potential for some intranasal drug metabolism (14). Some drugs can be transported directly to the brain after nasal administration (15).

For some peptides and small molecular compounds, intranasal bioavailability has been comparable to that of injections. However, bioavailability decreases as the molecular weight of a compound increases, and for proteins composed of more than 27 amino acids, bioavailability may be low (13). Various pharmaceutical techniques and formulation adjuncts, such as surface-active agents, have been shown to enhance nasal absorption of large molecules (13,17).

Pharmaceuticals on the market or in various stages of clinical investigation for nasal delivery include oxytocin (Syntocinon, Sandoz), desmopressin (DDAVP, Sanofi-Aventis), vitamin B_{12} (Ener-B Gel, Nature's Bounty), progesterone, insulin, calcitonin (Miacalcin, Novartis), propranolol, and butorphanol (Stadol, Bristol-Myers Squibb) (12,13).

OTIC PREPARATIONS

Otic preparations are sometimes referred to as ear or aural preparations. Solutions are most frequently used in the ear, with suspensions and ointments also finding some application. Ear preparations are usually placed in the ear canal by drops in small amounts for removal of excessive cerumen (earwax) or for treatment of ear infections, inflammation, or pain. Because the outer ear is a skin-covered structure and susceptible to the same dermatologic conditions as other parts of the body's surface, skin conditions are treated using the variety of topical dermatologic preparations discussed in Chapter 10.

Cerumen-Removing Solutions

Cerumen is a combination of the secretions of the sweat and sebaceous glands of the external auditory canal. The secretions, if allowed to dry, form a sticky semisolid that holds shed epithelial cells, fallen hair, dust, and other foreign bodies that make their way into the ear canal. Excessive accumulation of cerumen in the ear may cause itching, pain, and impaired hearing, and it impedes otologic examination. If not removed periodically, the cerumen may become impacted and its removal made more difficult and painful.

Through the years, light mineral oil, vegetable oils, and hydrogen peroxide have been commonly used agents to soften impacted cerumen for its removal. Recently, solutions of synthetic surfactants have been developed for their ability to remove earwax. One commercial product uses carbamide peroxide in glycerin and propylene glycol (Debrox drops, GSK). On contact with the cerumen, the carbamide peroxide releases oxygen, which disrupts the integrity of the impacted wax, allowing its easy removal.

Cerumen removal usually involves placing the otic solution in the ear canal with the patient's head tilted at a 45-degree angle, inserting a cotton plug to retain the medication in the ear for 15 to 30 minutes, and followed by gentle flushing of the ear canal with lukewarm water using a soft rubber ear syringe.

Anti-infective, Anti-inflammatory, and Analgesic Ear Preparations

Drugs used topically in the ear for their anti-infective activity include such agents as ciprofloxacin, colistin sulfate, neomycin, ofloxacin, polymyxin B sulfate, and nystatin, the latter agent used to combat fungal infections. These agents are formulated into eardrops (solutions or suspensions) in a vehicle of anhydrous glycerin or propylene glycol. These viscous vehicles permit maximum contact time between the medication and the tissues of the ear. In addition, their hygroscopicity causes them to draw moisture from the tissues, reducing inflammation and diminishing the moisture available for the life process of the microorganisms. To assist in relieving the pain that frequently accompanies ear infections, a number of anti-infective otic preparations also contain analgesic agents, such as antipyrine, and local anesthetics, such as pramoxine hydrochloride and benzocaine.

Topical treatment of ear infections is frequently considered adjunctive, with concomitant systemic treatment with orally administered antibiotics.

Liquid ear preparations of the anti-inflammatory agents hydrocortisone and dexamethasone sodium phosphate are prescribed for their effects against the swelling and inflammation that frequently accompany allergic and irritative manifestations of the ear and for the inflammation and pruritus that sometimes follow treatment of ear infections. In the latter instance, some physicians prefer the use of corticosteroids in ointment form, packaged in ophthalmic tubes. These packages allow placement of small amounts of ointment in the ear canal with a minimum of waste. Many commercial products used in this manner are labeled EYE AND EAR to indicate their dual use.

Aside from the antibiotic–steroid combinations that are used to treat otitis externa, or swimmer's ear, acetic acid 2% in aluminum acetate solution and boric acid 2.75% in isopropyl alcohol are used. These drugs help to reacidify the ear canal, and the vehicles help dry the ear canal. Drying the ear canal keeps in check growth of the offending microorganisms, usually *P. aeruginosa*. Pharmacists may also be called on for extemporaneous preparation of a solution of acetic acid 2% to 2.5% in rubbing alcohol (70% isopropyl alcohol or ethanol), propylene glycol, or anhydrous glycerin. The source of the acetic acid can be Glacial

Acetic Acid, USP, which contains at least 99.5% acetic acid by weight or Acetic Acid, NF, which contains approximately 36.5% acetic acid by weight. Boric acid 2% to 5% dissolved in either ethanol or propylene glycol has also been recommended for use in the ear. This substance, however, may be absorbed from broken skin and be toxic. Thus, it should not be used in children with burst eardrums.

Pain in the ear frequently accompanies ear infection or inflamed or swollen ear tissue. Frequently, the pain is far out of proportion to the actual condition. Because the ear canal is so narrow, even a slight inflammation can cause intense pain and discomfort. Topical analgesic agents generally are employed together with internally administered analgesics, such as aspirin, and other agents, such as anti-infectives, to combat the cause of the problem.

Most topical analgesics for the ear are solutions, and many contain the analgesic antipyrine and the local anesthetic benzocaine in a vehicle of propylene glycol or anhydrous glycerin (antipyrine 54 mg, benzocaine 14 mg, dehydrated glycerin qs 10 mL). Again, these hygroscopic vehicles reduce the swelling of tissues (and thus some pain) and the growth of microorganisms by drawing moisture from the swollen tissues into the vehicle. These preparations are commonly employed to relieve the symptoms of acute otitis media. Examples of some commercial otic preparations are presented in Table 17.6.

As determined on an individual product basis, some liquid otic preparations require preservation against microbial growth. When preservation is required, such agents as chlorobutanol 0.5%, thimerosal 0.01%, and combinations of the parabens are commonly used. Antioxidants, such as sodium bisulfite, and other stabilizers are also included in otic formulations as required. Ear preparations are usually packaged in 5- to 15-mL glass or plastic containers with a dropper.

Otic Suspensions

Subtle differences in the formulation of otic suspensions may be bothersome to the patient. This is so especially as it relates to differences in inactive or inert ingredients that are considered equivalent on the basis of active

ingredients and strength. For example, several suspension combinations of polymyxin B sulfate, neomycin sulfate, and hydrocortisone have been shown to be more acidic at pH 3 to 3.5 than the standard product, Cortisporin-TC Otic (Monarch), whose pH is 4.8 to 5.1. Consequently, there is a risk that when drops are legally substituted, a burning and stinging sensation can occur when the drops are introduced into the ear of young children, especially those with tympanostomies. It has also been demonstrated that with time, the pH of these formulations, including Cortisporin, becomes more acidic, possibly pH 3. Thus, if it is stored over time, the acidity may irritate the ear canal on later use. For this reason, this antibiotic–hydrocortisone combination has been formulated into a new suspension product, PediOtic (Glaxo Wellcome), with a minimum pH of 4.1.

Proper Administration and Use of Otic Drops

When eardrops are prescribed, it is important for the pharmacist to determine how the drops are to be used. For example, earwax removal drops should be instilled and then removed with an ear syringe. Drops intended to treat external otitis infection are intended to be instilled and left in the ear.

The pharmacist should make sure the child, parent, or caregiver understands that administration is intended for the ear and the frequency of application. To facilitate acceptance, the pharmacist should point out that the bottle or container of medication should first be warmed in the hands and, if the product is a suspension, shaken prior to withdrawal into the dropper. The pharmacist should also explain the need to store the medication in a safe place out of the reach of children and away from extremes of temperature.

When instilled into the ear, to allow the drops to run in deeper, the earlobe should be held up and back. For a child, the earlobe should be held gently down and back. For convenience, it is probably easier to have someone other than the patient to administer the drops.

Some eardrops by virtue of their low pH may cause stinging upon administration. Parents and children should

TABLE **17.6.** Some Commercial Otic Preparations

Product	Manufacturer	Active Ingredient	Vehicle	Use/Indications
Americaine otic	Insight Pharmaceuticals	Benzocaine	Glycerin, polyethylene glycol 300	Local anesthetic for ear pain, pruritus in otitis media, swimmer's ear, similar conditions
Cerumenex eardrops	Purdue Frederick	Triethanolamine polypeptide oleate condensate	Propylene glycol	Removes impacted earwax
Chloromycetin otic	Parke-Davis	Chloramphenicol	Propylene glycol	Anti-infective
Cortisporin otic solution	Glaxo Wellcome	Polymyxin B sulfate, neomycin sulfate, hydrocortisone	Glycerin, propylene glycol, water for injection	Superficial bacterial infections
Debrox drops	GlaxoSmithKline	Carbamide peroxide	Anhydrous glycerin	Earwax removal
PediOtic suspension	Glaxo Wellcome	Polymyxin B sulfate, neomycin sulfate, hydrocortisone	Mineral oil, propylene glycol, water for injection	Superficial bacterial infections

be forewarned, especially if a child has tympanostomy tubes in the ear. The patient or parent should also understand how long to use the product. For antibiotic eardrops, it is not necessary to finish the entire bottle, because therapy could last 20 to 30 days, depending upon the dosage regimen. Therefore, patients should be instructed to continue using the drops for 3 days after symptoms disappear. Products for otitis externa may take up to 7 to 10 days to demonstrate efficacy.

If a child is prone to develop ear infections as a result of swimming or showering, it might be advisable to recommend that the parents consult a physician for prophylactic medication to use during swimming season and consider using ear plugs that fit snugly in the ear when swimming or showering. After the child emerges from the water or shower, the parents can be advised to use a blow dryer on a low setting to dry the ear quickly without trauma. The dryer should not be held too close to the child's ear.

PATIENT COUNSELING

If applicable, explain that the dropper or spray container has been calibrated to deliver a consistent and uniform dose and must use the dosage device properly. Patient counseling on products and preparations for inhalation are discussed in Chapter 14 Disperse Systems.

ADMINISTERING SOLUTIONS, SUSPENSIONS, OINTMENTS, AND GEL-FORMING SOLUTIONS TO THE EYE

1. Before starting, wash and dry hands.
2. Instruct and demonstrate how to administer drops or ointments to the eye.
3. If drops or an ointment tube are used, do not to allow the tip to touch any part of the eye.
4. Tilt the head back and make a pouch by pulling out the lower eye lid. One can lie down if needed if having difficulty making a pouch.
5. If drops are used, allow the drug to fall freely into the eye/pouch and not to allow the drug to touch the eye and then be drawn back into the bottle.
6. Immediately after instilling a drop into the eye, place pressure on the lacrimal sac for a minute or two to help decrease systemic absorption of the drug that occurs when the drug is removed by the nasolacrimal duct and swallowed, thereby entering the gastrointestinal tract.
7. Since the normal volume of tear fluid in the eye is about 10 μL and the volume of an average drop is 25 to 50 μL, only 1 drop should be administered to the eye at one time.
8. If more than 1 drop or more than one drug is to be administered, wait at least 5 minutes between doses to allow the drug to be distributed and absorbed.
9. Explain that ophthalmic suspensions dissolve slowly and remain in the cul-de-sac longer.
10. Explain that ophthalmic ointments provide maximum contact between the drug and the eye because they are cleared quite slowly (0.5% per minute) from the eye.
11. Explain that the size of a drop delivered can vary with the angle of the dropper and the size of the dropper orifice and be consistent in the application process.

12. Close the eye to spread the medicine across the surface and prevent drainage due to blinking.
13. Do not touch the dropper with the fingers or to the eye or any other surface.
14. Eye drops should be used 30 minutes before putting on contact lenses, if worn.
15. Contact lenses should be removed before administering eye drops.
16. If using antibiotic drops, do not wear contact lenses.
17. The onset of most drug effects is within 30 to 60 minutes after administration to the eye.
18. Some ophthalmic products require refrigeration.
19. If a suspension, shake it well prior to administration.
20. Do not reuse unit-dose eye drops once opened.
21. Discard preserved eye drops after 60 days (after opening) or manufacturer's recommendation.

ADMINISTRATION OF NASAL LIQUIDS (DROPS AND SPRAYS)

1. Nose drops should be used in the lying-head-back position or the lateral-head-low position.
2. Nose sprays can be delivered with the head in the upright position (some spray bottles will deliver a constant stream of liquid if not held upright) or tilted as appropriate.
3. Deposit the nasal medication in the area of the nose just behind the anterior turbinate region where it can be spread across the respiratory mucosa by the cilia.
4. Nose drops that are administered into the nasal cavity as a small bolus of medication may flow out either the front or the back of the nose without contacting much surface area unless the patient is careful about the placement and movement of the head.
5. Generally nasal sprays are preferred over drops as they spread over the nasal cavity better.

ADMINISTRATION OF OTIC LIQUIDS

1. Explain and demonstrate how to apply drops to the ear from dropper bottles by tilting the head or lying down.
2. After application, a cotton or gauze pad can be placed in the ear to keep the liquid from escaping.

PHARMACEUTICS CASE STUDY

SUBJECTIVE INFORMATION

Working as a pharmacist in a local hospital, you receive a prescription for 5 mL of fluorouracil 10 mg/mL ophthalmic solution for topical use in the eye. What is a reasonable technique to compound the preparation so the patient can begin treatment within a couple of hours?

OBJECTIVE INFORMATION

Fluorouracil is an antineoplastic agent that is used as ancillary treatment of glaucoma, pterygium, retinal detachment, and premalignant eye lesions. The 10 mg/mL is often used in the treatment of premalignant lesions of the cornea, conjunctiva, and eyelids.

Fluorouracil occurs as a white to practically white, practically odorless crystalline powder that is sparingly soluble in water and slightly soluble in alcohol. Fluorouracil is commercially available as a solution for injection at a concentration of 50 mg/mL in 10, 20, and 100 mL vials and a 10-mL ampule. The injection has a pH adjusted to approximately 8.6 to 9.4 with sodium hydroxide and hydrochloric acid as needed. It is also available as Fluorouracil Powder, USP, that can be used to compound the preparation.

ASSESSMENT

Fluorouracil is water soluble and can be prepared as a sterile, isotonic ophthalmic solution. Two options are available. First, the commercial injection dosage forms can be diluted with sterile sodium chloride injection to the proper concentration. Second, it can be prepared from the fluorouracil powder in sterile water for injection, adjusted to isotonicity with sodium chloride, and sterile-filtered into a sterile container.

PLAN

The physician would like to have this preparation soon, so you select the first option. You obtain a 10-mL vial of fluorouracil 50 mg/mL injection. Using aseptic technique, cytotoxic handling procedures, and an appropriate aseptic clean air environment, you remove 1 mL of the injection, add sufficient sterile 0.9% sodium chloride injection to make 5 mL, and mix well. You package the preparation and add an appropriate label, and then dispose of the used materials appropriately for chemotherapy handling and disposal. ∎

CLINICAL CASE STUDY

HPI: K.P. is a 22-year-old WM who presents to the pharmacy with a prescription for olopatadine hydrochloride (Patanol) for allergic conjunctivitis. K.P. explains to the pharmacist, "My allergies have been so bad this spring that they have been bothering my eyes too. I tried to use Visine, but that just helped with the redness." The patient continues to explain that his eyes are excessively watery, itchy, and burning, and at times, he can barely see because the tears make his vision so blurry. He further complains that he has not been able to wear his contacts for almost a week because of his eye problems. K.P. is a college student who just moved to campus and is new to the pharmacy. Before preparing his prescription, the pharmacist takes his medical history.

PMH:	Seasonal allergic rhinitis since high school
	Seasonal allergic conjunctivitis
SH:	(+) EtOH: Drinks 3–4 beers/night on the weekends
	(–) Tobacco
	(–) Illicit drugs
FH:	Mother (+) for allergic rhinitis

	Father (+) for hypertension
	Sister (+) for asthma
Allergies:	PCN (rash, hives)
Meds:	Loratadine 10 mg po qd
	Visine prn red eyes
	Tylenol 1,000 mg po prn headaches
	Centrum 1 tab po qd

PHARMACEUTICAL CARE PLAN

S:	Patient has itching, burning, watery red eyes. Excessive tearing is causing blurred vision.
O:	Redness relieved by Visine.
A:	K.P. is a 22-year-old WM with uncontrolled allergic conjunctivitis. The patient is at high risk for seasonal allergic conjunctivitis because of his history of seasonal allergic rhinitis. K.P. also has a family history significant for allergic rhinitis. Although patient's allergic rhinitis symptoms are controlled by his use of loratadine 10 mg po qd, his ocular symptoms persist even though he uses Visine.

(continued)

(continued)

P: Based on patient's symptoms and medical and medication histories, olopatadine hydrochloride is an appropriate option for treatment of his allergic conjunctivitis. Thus, after verifying that K.P.'s prescription is complete, the pharmacist dispenses the medication.

The pharmacist should counsel K.P. on his medication. The prescribed dosage is one drop in each affected eye two times daily at an interval of at least 6–8 hours (e.g., morning and late afternoon or early evening). To administer the eye drops, the patient should follow these instructions:

Wash hands thoroughly before using the product.

With the index finger of the free hand, gently pull the lower outer eyelid down and away from the eye to create a pouch.

While tilting the head back, place the dropper over the eye without the tip of the dropper touching the eye.

Just prior to instilling a drop into the eye, look up toward the dropper.

As soon as the drop is instilled into the eye, release the eyelid slowly. Keep the eye closed for a full minute afterward.

While the eye is closed, use a finger to apply gentle pressure over the opening of the tear duct on the innermost (closest to the nose) portion of the eye. This serves to keep the medication in contact with the eye longer.

Excess solution may be gently wiped away with a tissue.

Replace the cap onto the ophthalmic product and keep it tightly closed when not in use.

Advise K.P. against wearing his contact lenses until his eye redness has resolved. Because the preservative in olopatadine hydrochloride may be absorbed by soft contact lenses, K.P. should follow necessary precautions if he decides to resume wearing his contact lenses. K.P. should wait at least 10 minutes after instilling the drops before inserting his contact lenses.

Explain to K.P. the common side effects associated with olopatadine hydrochloride use (e.g., burning or stinging, dry eyes, headache, sinusitis, blurred vision). In addition, K.P. should be instructed to discontinue using Visine while using his prescription.

Remind K.P. to store the eye drops at room temperature in an upright position with the cap tightly secured. He should follow the expiration date on the bottle. In addition, he should know not to rinse or tamper with the dropper. ∎

APPLYING THE PRINCIPLES AND CONCEPTS

GROUP ACTIVITIES

1. Select one ophthalmic, one nasal, and one inhalation product. In groups of three, one student serves as the pharmacist, the second the patient, and the third the observer. The pharmacist will counsel the patient on the specific product. After the session, the observer and patient provide constructive criticism on the session. The roles then should be rotated utilizing a different product until the three students have participated in each of the three roles.

2. Brainstorm how each one of these three dosage forms (ophthalmic, nasal, and inhalation) can be misused/abused by a patient and/or caregiver. Determine how a hard contact lens cleaning solution differs from a wetting solution, a wetting/soaking solution, and a rewetting/lubricating solution.

3. Go to the American Optometric Association Web site, that is, www.aoa.org, and complete activity sheets no. 2 and 3, which are created for parents and educators (lower left corner).

4. Interview a fellow student who uses contact lenses. Determine the type of lens used, review use and care procedures, and identify any problems associated with the use of the lenses and care products.

5. Organize and execute a health care booth at a local high school event, for example, swimming meet. Provide information and education materials to parents and participants on common ear ailments, including otitis externa, *syn.* swimmer's ear.

INDIVIDUAL ACTIVITIES

1. List eye care resources that health care providers can refer patients and caregivers to regarding proper use of contact lens products.

2. Go to the American Optometric Association Web site, that is, www.aoa.org, and perform the classroom exercises, which are created for parents and educators (lower left corner).

3. Describe the procedure for the chemical disinfection of an RGP or soft contact lens.

4. List precautions associated with contact lens use, and write out how you would counsel a patient to avoid adverse effects associated with misuse.

5. Isotonicity Calculation Exercise:
   a. How many milligrams of sodium chloride should be used to compound the following prescription? Given: Ephedrine sulfate SCE = 0.20
   b. How many grams of anhydrous dextrose (SCE = 0.18) should be used to prepare 1 L of a 0.5% isotonic ephedrine sulfate nasal spray?

6. List the antibiotic drugs that are currently available as ophthalmic drops.

7. List the antibiotic drugs that are currently available as otic drops.
8. Which ophthalmic drops can be used in the ear when there is no comparable otic product?
9. Select a special solution/suspension product and develop step-by-step instructions (with illustrations) demonstrating its appropriate use. The student then instructs his/her fellow students on the selected product. Because each student's selection should differ from fellow classmates' instructions, these can be collected at the end of the exercise, duplicated, and handed out as a packet to the class as a whole.

R_x:	Ephedrine sulfate	0.3
	Sodium chloride	qs
	Purified water qsad	30
Sig:	Use as directed	

REFERENCES

1. Mitra AK, ed. Ophthalmic Drug Delivery Systems. 2nd Ed. New York, NY: Marcel Dekker, 2003.
2. Reddy IK, Ganesan MG. Ocular therapeutics and drug delivery: An overview. In: Reddy IK, ed. Ocular Therapeutics and Drug Delivery. Lancaster, PA: Technomic publishing company, 1996:3–29.
3. Reddy IK, Azia W, Sause RB. Artificial tear formulations, irrigating solutions and contact lens products. In: Reddy IK, ed. Ocular Therapeutics and Drug Delivery. Lancaster, PA: Technomic publishing company, 1996:171–211.
4. Edman P. Biopharmaceutics of Ocular Drug Delivery. Ann Arbor, MI: CRC Press, 1993.
5. Lee VHL, Robinson JR. Mechanistic and quantitative evaluation of precorneal pilocarpine distribution in albino rabbits. J Pharm Sci 1979;68:673–684.
6. Shell JW. Pharmacokinetics of topically applied ophthalmic drugs. Surv Ophthalmol 1982;26:207–218.
7. Xiao Q, Hu Y, Chen F, et al. A comparative assessment of the efficacy of carbomer gel and carboxymethyl cellulose containing artificial tears in dry eyes. Med Sci 2008;28(5):592–595.
8. Del Amo EM, Urtti A. Current and future ophthalmic drug delivery systems. A shift to the posterior segment. Drug Discov Today 2008;13(3–4):135–143.
9. Ansel HC, Stockton SJ. Pharmaceutical Calculations. 15th Ed. Baltimore, MD: Williams & Wilkins, 2017.
10. Gangrade NK, Gaddipati NB, Ganesan MG, et al. Topical ophthalmic formulations: Basic considerations. In: Reddy IK, ed. Ocular Therapeutics and Drug Delivery. Lancaster, PA: Technomic publishing company, 1996:377–403.
11. Kumar GN. Drug metabolizing enzyme systems in the eye. In: Reddy IK, ed. Ocular Therapeutics and Drug Delivery. Lancaster, PA: Technomic publishing company, 1996:149–167.
12. Kaye RS, Purewal TS, Alpar OH. Development and testing of particulate formulations for the nasal delivery of antibodies. J Control Release 2009;135(2):127–135.
13. Csaba N, Garcia-Fuentes M, Alonso MJ. Nanoparticles for nasal vaccination. Adv Drug Deliv Rev 2009;61(2):140–157.
14. Boyaka PN, McGhee JR. Cytokines as adjuvants for the induction of mucosal immunity. Adv Drug Deliv Rev 2001;51(1–3):71–79.
15. Dhuria SV, Hanson LR, Frey WH II. Intranasal delivery to the central nervous system: mechanisms and experimental considerations. J Pharm Sci 2010;99(4):1654–73. doi: 10.1002/jps.21924
16. Liang MT, Davies NM, Blanchfield JT, et al. Particulate systems as adjuvants and carriers for peptide and protein antigens. Curr Drug Deliv 2006;3(4):379–388.
17. Kim HJ, Kim JK, Seo SB, et al. Intranasal vaccination with peptides and cholera toxin subunit B as adjuvant to enhance mucosal and systemic immunity to respiratory syncytial virus. Arch Pharm Res 2007;39(3):366–371.
18. Castaman G. Desmopressin for the treatment of haemophilia. Haemophilia 2008;14(Suppl 1):15–20.

SECTION EIGHT

Novel and Advanced Dosage Forms, Delivery Systems, and Devices

18 Radiopharmaceuticals

CHAPTER AT A GLANCE Background Information • Diagnostic Imaging • Therapeutic Use of Radiopharmaceuticals • Radiopharmaceuticals • Positron Emission Tomography • Drug Antidote for Radiation Exposure • Nonradioactive Pharmaceutical Use in Nuclear Medicine • Practice of Nuclear Pharmacy • Regulatory Process

OBJECTIVES

After reading this chapter, the student will be able to:

Compare and contrast the three principal types of radioactive decay (i.e., alpha, beta, gamma)

Compare and contrast the use of radiopharmaceuticals in diagnostics and therapeutics

Identify the diagnostic and/or therapeutic role(s) and delivery method(s) for the following radiopharmaceuticals: ^{99m}Tc, ^{89}Sr, ^{90}Y, ^{201}Tl, ^{67}Ga, ^{111}In, ^{123}I/^{131}I, and ^{153}Sm

Describe the concept and therapeutic utility of positron emission tomography (PET)

Identify indications for the following nonradioactive pharmaceuticals in nuclear medicine: Prussian blue, acetazolamide, captopril, dipyridamole, adenosine, and furosemide

Describe the organization of a nuclear pharmacy in a community and hospital setting

Define the role of the nuclear pharmacist (e.g., radiopharmaceutical preparation, quality assurance, dispensing, safety, consultation)

■ INTRODUCTION

By definition, a radiopharmaceutical is a radioactive pharmaceutical agent that is used for diagnostic or therapeutic procedures (1). For a product to be classified as a radiopharmaceutical agent safe for human use, the preparer must satisfy a state agency, the State Board of Pharmacy, and two branches of the federal government whose responsibilities in this category have overlapping jurisdictions. They are the Food and Drug Administration (FDA) and the Nuclear Regulatory Commission (NRC). The extent of oversight by the board of pharmacy differs between states. Because of the stringent regulations of the NRC, some state boards defer and do not have specific rules for nuclear pharmacies. Other state boards have rules within their pharmacy practice acts that relate to the practice of nuclear pharmacy.

Over the past four decades, the discipline of nuclear pharmacy, or radiopharmacy, has become highly

specialized and contributed positively to the practice of nuclear medicine. Nuclear pharmacy, the first specialty in pharmacy recognized (in 1978) by the Board of Pharmaceutical Specialties, focuses on the safe and effective use of radioactive drugs or radiopharmaceuticals.

The application of radiopharmaceuticals is divided into two major areas, diagnostic and therapeutic. The diagnostic side is well established, whereas the therapeutic side of nuclear medicine is evolving. For example, more than 100 radiopharmaceutical products are available, with the largest proportion of these having application in cardiology (e.g., myocardial perfusion), oncology (e.g., tumor imaging and localization), and neurology (e.g., cerebral perfusion). Diagnostically, they are also used for infection imaging and in nephrology. Historically, nuclear medicine has been well established as a therapeutic modality for thyroid cancer, Graves disease, hyperthyroidism, and bone pain palliation associated with skeletal metastasis. However, recent radiopharmaceuticals (e.g., ^{131}I- or ^{123}I-labeled

MIBG [*m*-iodobenzylguanidine]) are being used to treat pheochromocytoma and neuroblastoma, and radiolabeled somatostatin analogs are used for the treatment of neuroendocrine tumors (e.g., neuroblastoma) (2). Ongoing investigative studies involving radiopharmaceuticals are being conducted for numerous other diseases (e.g., primary bone cancers, ovarian cancer) using innovative means (e.g., targeting agents) to deliver the drug to the tumor. It is anticipated that many of these radiopharmaceuticals will become available for amelioration of diseases.

A radiopharmaceutical consists of a drug component and a radioactive component. Substances that have different numbers of protons and neutrons as compared to stable elements are called *radionuclides*. Nuclides may be stable or unstable; those that are unstable are radioactive because their nuclei undergo rearrangement while changing to a stable state, and energy is released. Most radionuclides emit gamma radiation.

An important distinction between radiopharmaceuticals and traditional drugs is lack of pharmacologic activity on the part of radiopharmaceuticals. For intensive purposes, radiopharmaceuticals have been used as tracers of physiologic processes. Their huge advantage is that their radioactivity allows noninvasive external monitoring or targeted therapeutic irradiation with very little effect on the biologic processes in the body. Indeed, radiopharmaceuticals have an excellent safety record, and their incidence of adverse effects is extremely low (3). However, in the past two decades, there has been committed interest to developing unsealed radionuclides for treatment of cancers arising from the diversity of newer molecular carriers (e.g., immune-derived molecules, receptor-avid tracers). Technologic advances in molecular pharmacology, combinatorial chemistry, and peptide biochemistry are providing innovative means (e.g., targeting vectors) to enhance radionuclide specificity and targeting cancerous cells in vivo.

Systemic administration of radiopharmaceuticals for site-specific use allows the physician to treat widely disseminated diseases. Optimally, therapeutic radiopharmaceuticals are designed for site specificity and based solely upon physiological function of the target organ even if the actual location of the cancerous tumor is unknown. The mechanism of localization of the radiopharmaceutical in a particular target organ depends upon processes as varied as antigen–antibody reactions, physical trapping of particles, receptor site binding, and transport of a chemical species across a cell membrane, among others. Ideally, the radiopharmaceutical will cause minimal or tolerable damage to healthy, adjacent tissue. However, a variety of factors related directly to the physical and chemical characteristics of the radiopharmaceutical make this goal difficult to achieve. Research will continue to address problems related to efficient radiopharmaceutical delivery to the target site. For example, the residence time of radioactivity at the target site, the in vivo catabolism and metabolism of the drug, and the optimization of relative rates of radiolabeled drug or drug metabolite clearance from the target site are factors to be determined.

Development of an effective radiopharmaceutical for therapeutic use is a complex, difficult undertaking.

BACKGROUND INFORMATION

Not all of the atoms of an unstable radionuclide completely rearrange at the same instant. The time required for a radionuclide to decay to 50% of its original activity is termed its radioactive half-life. Radionuclides range widely in their half-life; for ^{14}C, it is 5,730 years, whereas for ^{24}Na, it is 15 hours, and for ^{81}Kr, it is 13 seconds.

The activity of radioactive material may be calculated by a decay equation that allows the clinician to predict the activity at any time, earlier, or later than the specific assay. The specific decay equation:

$$A_e = A_0 e^{-\lambda t}$$

where

A_e is the specific activity at time t,
A_0 is the initial activity, and
λ is the decay constant calculated as ln 2/half-life, and
   t is time.

Decay tables have been formulated for various radionuclides by calculating the last portion of the decay equation ($e^{-\lambda t}$). Thus,

$$A_e = A_0 \left(\text{decay factor} \right)$$

The activity of a radioactive material is expressed as the number of nuclear transformations per unit of time. Because of decay, all radioactivity decreases with time because fewer atoms remain as the atoms decay. The fraction of nuclei disintegrating with time is always constant, and fewer and fewer atoms are left. The larger the decay constant, the faster the decay and the shorter the half-life. Thus, as demonstrated by the following, the half-life is inversely proportional to the decay constant:

$$t_{1/2} = \frac{0.69315}{\lambda}$$

where λ is the transformation or decay constant, which has a characteristic value for each radionuclide.

The fundamental unit of radioactivity is the *curie* (Ci), defined as 3.700×10^{10} nuclear transformations per second or disintegrations per second (dps). Multiplying this unit by 60 allows the definition to be expressed as disintegrations per minute. Multiples and submultiples (e.g., *millicurie* [mCi], *microcurie* [μCi], and *nanocurie* [nCi]) of the curie can be expressed also:

$$1 \text{ mCi} = 10^{-3} \text{ Ci}$$
$$1 \text{ μCi} = 10^{-6} \text{ Ci}$$
$$1 \text{ nCi} = 10^{-9} \text{ Ci}$$

In July 1974, at the meeting of the International Commission of Radiation Units and Measurements, a recommendation was made that within no less than 10 years, the curie would be replaced with a new SI (Système International d'Unites) unit, the reciprocal second (sec^{-1}) (4). The intent was that this new unit be used to express the unit of activity as a function of the rate of spontaneous nuclear transformations of radionuclides, as one per second (dps). It was further recommended that this new unit of activity be given the name *becquerel* and bear the symbol *Bq*. The intent was that the becquerel would be equivalent to 1 dps or approximately 2.703×10^{-11} Ci. For example, a 15-mCi dose of ^{99m}Tc would be referred to as a 555-megabecquerel (MBq) dose. To date, the conversion to SI units in the United States has been slow.

The amount of radiation absorbed by body tissue in which a radioactive substance resides is called the radiation dose. Traditionally, this is measured in rad (*radiation absorbed dose*); 1 rad = 100 ergs of energy absorbed by 1 g of tissue. The gray (Gy) is the international unit of absorbed dose, equal to 1 J of energy absorbed in 1 kg of tissue, that is, 1 Gy = 100 rad.

Radiopharmaceutical doses are dispensed to patients in units of activity, typically mCi or µCi. Traditional therapeutic agents are dispensed according to weight-based calculations to determine appropriate activity. The pharmacist remains responsible to ensure that the proper prescribed dose is prepared and dispensed. Because of the nature of radiopharmaceuticals, the amount of radioactivity in the unit dose at the time of preparation must be greater than the prescribed dose to allow for decay of radioactivity before the product is administered.

The three main types of radiation decay are alpha particles, beta particles, and gamma photons (or gamma rays). Of the three types, alpha particles have the largest mass and charge of radiation, consisting of two protons and two neutrons and a charge of +2, identical with the helium nucleus. Alpha particles carry a large amount of kinetic energy from being ejected from the nucleus. As an alpha particle loses energy, its velocity decreases. It then attracts electrons and becomes a helium atom. Most alpha particles are unable to pierce the outer layers of skin or penetrate a thin piece of paper. However, because the charge is large, it does cause a great deal of damage to cells in the immediate area by breaking down DNA. Beta particles may be either electrons with negative charge, *negatrons*, or positive electrons, *positrons*. These two particles, β$^-$ and β$^+$, have a range of more than 100 feet in air and up to about 1 mm in tissue. Beta particles are not as destructive as alpha particles, but they can be used therapeutically. The beta particle possesses a lot of kinetic energy, thousands to millions of electron volts. Nuclear medicine depends mostly on radiopharmaceuticals that decay by gamma emission. Gamma rays are electromagnetic vibrations comparable with light but with much shorter wavelength and much higher energy. Because of their short wavelength and high energy, they penetrate easily through soft tissue.

Auger electrons originate from the orbital electrons rather than from the nucleus. Whenever there is a vacancy in a lower orbital, an electron from a higher orbital falls down into that lower orbital, and the difference in energy between the two orbitals is emitted in the form of an x-ray with characteristic energy. Most of the time, the characteristic x-ray leaves the atom. But sometimes, the characteristic x-ray hits a higher orbital electron of the same atom. Then, the transfer of energy from the x-ray to the electron is enough to free it from the atom. This free electron, known as an auger electron, is similar to a beta particle except that it has much less energy, typically only tens to hundreds of electron volts. In materials with large atomic numbers, there are several higher electron orbitals, so several different auger electrons may be produced, each with a different kinetic energy. Thus, the term auger cascade is sometimes used to indicate the production of multiple different auger electrons.

The optimum dose of a radiopharmaceutical is that which allows acquisition of the desired information with the least amount of radiation dose or exposure to the patient. Consequently, the clinical utility of a radiopharmaceutical is determined mainly by the radionuclide's physical properties (e.g., radiation, energy, half-life). Therefore, the best diagnostic images at the lowest radiation dose are attained if the radionuclide has a short half-life and emits only gamma radiation. ^{99m}Tc is a prime example of a radionuclide with these properties. Its half-life is 6 hours, and gamma emission is in the order of 140 keV, efficiently detected by the gamma camera. It is commonly known as the "ideal" radionuclide for diagnostic imaging. For therapeutic use, however, radionuclides should emit particulate radiation (beta particles), which deposits the radiation within the target organ. ^{131}I is a prime example, used for hyperthyroidism and eradication of metastatic disease of the thyroid gland. Because ^{131}I emits both beta and gamma radiation, it can be used diagnostically (gamma rays) and therapeutically (beta particles).

Most radiopharmaceuticals are produced by nuclear activation in a nuclear reactor. In a reactor, stable atoms are bombarded with excess neutrons. The resulting neutron additions to the stable atoms produce unstable atoms and radionuclides. The facilities for the production, use, and storage of radioactive pharmaceuticals are subject to licensing by the NRC or, in certain instances, to appropriate state agencies. Many states, known as agreement states, have taken over licensing for the NRC. They agree to follow all NRC regulations and, in some instances, may be more stringent. As for all pharmaceuticals, the FDA enforces good manufacturing practice and proper labeling and use of the products. The Federal Department of Transportation regulates shipment of radiopharmaceuticals, as do state and local agencies.

Radiopharmaceuticals are used to diagnose disease or evaluate the progression of disease following specific therapy intervention. They can also be used to evaluate drug-induced toxicity and to an increasing extent are being used to treat diseased tissue.

The distribution pattern of radiopharmaceuticals can be used for imaging purposes to attain diagnostic information about organs or various body systems (5). Imaging procedures are classified as either *dynamic* or *static*. The dynamic study provides useful information through the rate of accumulation and removal of the radiopharmaceutical from a specific organ. A static study merely provides perfusion and morphologic information, such as assessing adequacy of blood flow; organ size, shape, and position; and any space-occupying lesions.

DIAGNOSTIC IMAGING

Some radiopharmaceuticals are formulated to accumulate within a target organ. ^{131}I is taken up actively by thyroid cells following absorption into the bloodstream after oral administration of a capsule or solution. The extent of uptake of the dose by the gland helps assess thyroid function, or an image of the gland can be obtained after administration. Alternatively, when ^{131}I was labeled with orthoiodohippuric acid (^{131}I-orthoiodohippurate, or OIH) and intravenously injected, kidney tubules would actively secrete this agent into urine. Measuring the time course of activity over the kidney with a gamma camera and plotting the rate of radioactivity accumulation and removal versus time yield a measure of kidney function. This dynamic study, termed a *renogram*, is particularly useful to assess renal function in patients with transplanted kidneys. The visualization of the entire kidney anatomically is known as a pyelogram (Fig. 18.1).

There are, however, limitations to the use of ^{131}I-orthoiodohippurate. Because of the risk of toxicity to normal tissues from its beta emissions, the dose must be no higher than 200 to 400 µCi. With this required lower dose, its relatively low energy gamma photons produce a

poorer image than ^{99m}Tc-Mag-3, which has pure gamma emissions of 140 keV, allowing for a higher dose and enhanced image quality without increasing the total body radiation burden. ^{99m}Tc-Mag-3 undergoes tubular secretion and glomerular filtration in the kidney and provides excellent renograms.

The most common diagnostic imaging procedure is myocardial perfusion imaging (MPI). For many years, this procedure was performed using ^{201}Tl-thallous chloride. However, in recent years, ^{201}Tl has been replaced as the "gold standard" in MPI by the ^{99m}Tc-based radiopharmaceuticals (e.g., ^{99m}Tc sestamibi, ^{99m}Tc tetrafosmin) (6).

Radiopharmaceuticals are useful to evaluate a patient's response to drug therapy and surgery. These agents can detect early changes in physiologic function that come before morphologic or biochemical end points. An example is perfusion lung imaging using ^{99m}Tc macroaggregated albumin particles to detect pulmonary embolism. Once the embolism is confirmed and thrombolytic and/or anticoagulant therapy initiated, this lung-perfusing agent can be administered again to evaluate its resolution with drug therapy. Cardiac radionuclide ventriculograms using ^{99m}Tc-labeled red blood cells are performed to assess left ventricular function (e.g., ejection fraction, regional wall motion) to evaluate the effect of surgery (e.g., coronary artery bypass graft, valve repair) or the response to drug therapy. Also, a ^{99m}Tc ejection fraction study can be performed to assess the benefits of heart medications, such as digoxin.

Radiopharmaceuticals also find utility to help monitor drug therapy, including toxicity. For example, the ability of doxorubicin to cause irreversible heart failure is well known, and the cumulative dose of this drug should not exceed 550 mg/m². Because there is much variation in the individual response to this drug, serial determinations of left ventricular ejection fraction using ^{99m}Tc are useful to determine the risk of developing doxorubicin-induced heart failure on an individual basis.

THERAPEUTIC USE OF RADIOPHARMACEUTICALS

Therapeutic radiopharmaceuticals are radiolabeled molecules designed to deliver therapeutic doses of cytotoxic ionizing radiation to specific disease sites, such as cancerous tumors, with high specificity in the body. The design of each radiotherapeutic agent requires optimizing the balance between specific targeting of the disease, such as a cancerous tumor, and the clearance of radioactivity from nontarget radiosensitive tissues; it is also necessary to consider the physical radioactive decay properties of the radionuclide. As mentioned earlier, difficulties in the design and development of a highly selective radiolabeled drug carrier include drug delivery, maximizing the residence time of radioactivity at target sites, in vivo catabolism and metabolism of the drug, and optimization of

FIGURE 18.1. Intravenous pyelogram in a patient. (Courtesy of Science Photo Library.)

relative rates of the radiolabeled drug or metabolite clearance from nontarget sites, among others.

Unsealed source radiolabeled agents have been used for treatment of cancers for more than five decades. Thyroid disease has been treated with sodium iodide, ^{131}I; polycythemia vera can be treated with sodium phosphate, ^{32}P; peritoneal effusions can be treated with chromic phosphate, ^{32}P; and ^{89}Sr-chloride, ^{153}Sm-EDTMP, and ^{186}Re-HEDP are used for pain relief associated with metastatic bone lesions. The intent is to use beta radiation to destroy diseased tissue selectively. Thus, a minimum sufficient dosage must be administered although this dose can be much larger than doses for diagnostics. In the case of ^{131}I, the therapeutic dose is 5 to 10,000 times the dose used to assess organ function. The major indications for radioiodine therapy include hyperthyroidism (diffuse toxic goiter or Graves disease and toxic multinodular goiter) and eradication of metastatic disease (thyroid cancer).

A major focus of current research is to enhance drug targeting to internal target sites (e.g., solid tumors, specific organs). The objective is to enhance the drug by concentrating it at the target site and minimize its effect in healthy sites. This approach is being investigated for cancer chemotherapy and radioimmunotherapy (RIT). RIT uses antigen-specific monoclonal antibodies (MABs) or their derived reagents to deliver therapeutic radionuclides to tumorous tissue (2). Improved bioengineered delivery vehicles (e.g., humanized and chimeric whole antibodies, Fv fragments, and hypervariable domain region peptides) have reinvigorated RIT, and more and more pretargeting protocols are becoming available (2).

Most chemotherapeutic drugs and radiotherapeutic peptides are small molecules. Consequently, low concentration of drug is obtainable at the target site, largely because of rapid excretion and metabolism by the kidneys and liver. This limits the amount of drug available for localization in the target site from the bloodstream. Increasing the dosage of drug is not an option because of the toxicologic implications for one or more body organ systems. Covalent conjugates of MABs were the first generation of drug-targeting agents that were employed to attain the concentrating effect in tumors (7).

In 1996, the FDA granted licenses to three manufacturers to market four radiolabeled antibodies for diagnostic imaging. CEA-Scan was a murine MAB fragment linked to ^{99m}Tc. It was reactive with carcinoembryonic antigen, a tumor marker for cancer of the colon and rectum and indicated with other standard diagnostic modalities for the detection of recurrent and/or metastatic colorectal cancer. Cytogen Corporation developed a linker payload system with the attachment of diagnostic (OncoScint colorectal/ovarian) or therapeutic substances (cancer cell–killing yttrium in OncoRad ovarian and OncoRad prostate systems) on the carbohydrate region of MABs. After injection, the MABs bind to the targeted tumor antigen to facilitate diagnosis or treatment. Although tumor targeting was somewhat successful with the large, long-circulating radiolabeled MABs, normal organ activity (e.g., blood, kidneys, liver, bone marrow) became problematic. Consequently, both CEA-Scan and OncoScint colorectal/ovarian are now off the market.

In the past two decades, extensive research for radionuclide therapy has attempted to use ions (molecular weight or MW, 10^2), low molecular weight drugs (MW 10^{2-3}), peptides (MW 10^3), radiolabeled antibody fragments and various proteins (MW 10^4), intact antibodies (MW 10^5), chase molecules, metabolizable linkers, local delivery, antibody-directed enzyme prodrugs, and liposomes for targeting purposes (MW 10^6) (8). The extensive size range demonstrated for a few of these molecules illustrates the several orders of magnitude that these substances cover with respect to molecular weight range (8). Thus, there is much potential for research involving an enormous number of agents with various properties.

One strategy to increase the concentration of a dose-limited, rapidly cleared radionuclide in a tumor was to couple it covalently to a large molecule (e.g., MAB directed against a tumor marker on the surface of the tumor) (9). Because of their large size, these radionuclide conjugates are not rapidly excreted by the kidneys; they are slowly removed from the systemic circulation over several days by the reticuloendothelial system (RES). Still, however, data demonstrate that while the radionuclide has high systemic circulation, very little is localized in the tumor. Thus, getting high tumor uptake with large antibody conjugates has posed a significant challenge. The most popular MAB pretargeting techniques employ either biotin and avidin or the hapten–antibody system and prodrug–enzyme systems or ligand–receptor systems (2). All of these methods employ a long-circulating targeting conjugate to get high tumor uptake with a diffusible, rapidly excreted effector molecule. The result is higher ratios of target to normal tissue and consequently less toxicity.

Molecular weight, lipophilicity, and charge of the targeting agents are important properties that influence hepatic and renal excretion. Small water-soluble peptides demonstrate effective excretion, which is beneficial in ridding the body of excess circulating radionuclide-labeled compounds. However, if excretion is too rapid, effective levels of the agent reaching the tumor are never achieved.

Creating a targeting agent with a very high molecular weight is thought to reduce the ability of the agent to diffuse through the capillary walls and thereby hinder the ability to target disseminated tumor cells in normally vascularized tissues. Thus, this may only allow tumor targeting in areas of pathologic tumor vasculature of the primary tumor or metastases. The limited passage through the capillary walls may also prolong systemic circulation and cause undesired exposure of normal tissue to radiation. Alternatively, enhanced circulation times may result in higher tumor uptake.

To avoid trapping and degradation of the agents by the RES (liver, spleen, and lymphoid tissue), therapeutic entities must be designed not to be recognized by the RES (9).

Pretherapeutic administration of nonradioactive antibodies (preload) can be used to saturate the RES and modify the distribution of the radiolabeled antibody. Pegylation and other preventive modifications have demonstrated some reduction in the RES's ability to uptake macromolecular agents.

In the spring of 2002, the FDA approved a new treatment regimen for low-grade B-cell non-Hodgkin lymphoma. It was the first regimen that combined a MAB with radionuclides. Rituximab is administered in a therapeutic regimen with ibritumomab tiuxetan (Zevalin). This therapy is recommended for patients who have not responded to standard chemotherapeutic treatments or to the prior use of rituximab (Rituxan). Rituximab and ibritumomab tiuxetan target the CD20 antigen on the surface of mature white blood cells (B cells) and B-cell lymphocytes occurring in non-Hodgkin lymphoma. This is discussed further later in the chapter.

Peptides have been investigated to succeed antibodies as delivery vehicles for linked diagnostic or therapeutic agents. Peptides have the advantage over MABs of being more rapidly cleared from the body, potentially with a lower level of toxicity (7). Further, they provide physiologic evidence of the nature of the disease process or progress of treatment. Radiolabeled peptides are a new class of radiotracers that target a cell or tissue and deliver a diagnostic signal or therapeutic agent to the site of the disease. Peptides are naturally occurring or synthetic compounds that contain one or more amino acid sequences or groups. On their plasma membranes, cells express receptor proteins with high affinity for regulatory peptides, such as somatostatin. Changes in the density of these receptors during disease, such as the overexpression found in many tumors, provide the basis for new imaging and therapeutic applications (10). The first peptide analogs successfully applied for visualization of receptor-positive tumors were radiolabeled somatostatin analogs. The next step was to label these analogs with therapeutic radionuclides for peptide receptor radionuclide therapy (PRRT). Results from preclinical and clinical multicenter studies have already shown an effective therapeutic response to radiolabeled somatostatin analogs to treat receptor-positive tumors. Infusion of positively charged amino acids reduces kidney uptake, enlarging the therapeutic window. For PRRT of CCK-B receptor–positive tumors, such as medullary thyroid carcinoma, radiolabeled minigastrin analogs are being successfully applied (7).

An example of this new class of radiopharmaceuticals is octreotide, a synthetic analog of the aforementioned peptide hormone, somatostatin, with the ^{111}In-labeled analog pentetreotide. The resulting product, OctreoScan, became the first radiolabeled peptide approved by the FDA. This agent has made possible the detection of small (0.5 to 1.0 cm) primary and metastatic tumors, including those of several brain tumor types, pancreatic islet tumors, neuroblastomas, carcinoids, thymomas, and melanomas, among others.

Small antimicrobial peptides are also thought to be candidates to be new antimicrobial agents. Lupetti et al. (11) have developed a scintigraphic approach to studying these pharmacokinetically in animals. These peptides, radiolabeled with ^{99m}Tc, demonstrated rapid accumulation at sites of infection but not at sites of sterile inflammation. This outcome indicated that these radiolabeled antimicrobial peptides could be used in infection detection and allows the effectiveness of antibacterial therapy in animals to be monitored. Another outcome of this research was that the process allowed reliable real-time whole-body imaging and quantitative biodistribution studies without the need to kill animals at each time interval.

RADIOPHARMACEUTICALS

The USP/NF (10) lists more than 75 official radioactive pharmaceuticals (12). Examples are presented in Table 18.1. The following describes some of the radiopharmaceuticals frequently used in daily practice. Several of these radiopharmaceuticals are being used for the delivery of MABs, biotechnologic drugs. For a deeper understanding of these biotechnologic drugs, including terminology, see Chapter 19.

Technetium-99M (^{99m}Tc)

Technetium-99m (^{99m}Tc) possesses a relatively short half-life of 6 hours, which allows administration of higher amounts of activity for faster and clearer images while exposing the patient to a low radiation dose. It offers an abundance of gamma photons for imaging without the hazardous effects of beta particles. Also, its chemistry profile is flexible, which allows it to be used as a binding agent for several pharmaceuticals used for imaging. Kits are available for preparation of various technetium ^{99m}Tc compounds that assist in hepatobiliary imaging (mebrofenin) and ischemic heart disease (sestamibi, tetrofosmin).

[99m]Tc has also been used as a radiolabel for MABs because of its wide availability in nuclear pharmacies and because it is relatively inexpensive and easy to obtain. It provides low radiation dosimetry and highly efficient detection of photons by planar scintigraphy. Unfortunately, widespread use of this radionuclide in immunoscintigraphy has been hindered by the lack of a simple, efficient, and stable method for attaching the ^{99m}Tc to the antibody molecule.

[99m]Tc sulfur colloid is used for imaging areas of functioning reticuloendothelial (RE) cells in the liver, spleen, and bone marrow (13). Phagocytosis, that is, physical entrapment, of the colloidal particles by the Kupffer cells in the RE system localizes the radiopharmaceutical to the specific target organ. In addition, it has also been used for other diagnosing purposes, for example, imaging of lymphatic vessels and nodes draining a particular organ or disease site. The subcutaneous, intradermal, and interstitial administration of this preparation causes pain and

TABLE 18.1. Representative Radiopharmaceutical Drugs and Primary Uses

Drug	Trade Name	Primary Uses
^{111}In oxyquinoline	Indium-111 Oxine	Radiolabel autologous leukocytes and platelets
^{111}In chloride	—	Used for radiolabeling Zevalin
^{111}In pentetreotide	OctreoScan	Imaging of neuroendocrine tumors
^{123}I sodium iodide	—	Thyroid imaging and uptake
^{131}I sodium iodide	—	Thyroid imaging, uptake, therapy
^{131}I tositumomab	Bexxar	Treatment of non-Hodgkin lymphoma
^{131}I-MIBG	—	Treatment of neuroendocrine tumors
^{99m}Tc exametazime	Ceretec	Cerebral perfusion, radiolabeling autologous leukocytes
^{99m}Tc macroaggregated	Pulmonite	Pulmonary perfusion albumin
^{99m}Tc mebrofenin	Choletec	Hepatobiliary imaging
^{99m}Tc medronate (MDP)	—	Bone imaging
^{99m}Tc mertiatide	TechneScan MAG3	Renal imaging
^{99m}Tc oxidronate (HDP)	OctreoScan HDP	Bone imaging
^{99m}Tc pentetate (DTPA)	Techneplex, TechneScan DTPA	Renal imaging and function studies; radioaerosol ventilation imaging
^{99m}Tc pertechnetate	—	Imaging of thyroid, salivary glands, ectopic gastric mucosa, parathyroid glands, dacryocystography, cystography
^{99m}Tc red blood cells	Ultratag	Imaging of gastrointestinal bleeding, cardiac chambers, cardiac first pass, gated equilibrium imaging
^{99m}Tc sestamibi	Cardiolite, Miraluma	Imaging of myocardial perfusion, breast tumor
^{99m}Tc sulfur colloid		Imaging of RES, bone marrow, gastric emptying, gastrointestinal bleeding, lymphoscintigraphy, arthrograms
^{99m}Tc tetrofosmin	Myoview	Myocardial perfusion imaging
^{201}Tl	—	Myocardial perfusion imaging; parathyroid and tumor imaging
^{133}Xe	DuPont Xenon, Mallinckrodt Xenon, GE Healthcare Xenon	Pulmonary ventilation imaging
^{90}Y microspheres	TheraSphere	Therapy for biopsy-proven, unresectable hepatocellular carcinoma
^{90}Y ibritumomab tiuxetan	Zevalin	Non-Hodgkin lymphoma
^{153}Sm-lexidronam (EDTMP)	Quadramet	Palliation of bone pain of skeletal metastases

discomfort at the site of injection, and consequently, lidocaine HCl is used simultaneously in a separate injection prior to administration of the ^{99m}Tc sulfur colloid. Dura and Hinkle evaluated the stability of a mixture of the colloid mixture with lidocaine HCl 1% and determined that adding 0.2 mL of lidocaine HCl 1% to the colloidal mixture and storing the syringes up to 8 hours did not affect the radiochemical purity of the mixture or alter the pH of the mixture substantially (13).

Because of availability, cost, radiation dose, and image quality, ^{99m}Tc-DPTA (diethylenetriaminepentaacetic acids; pentetate) is preferred for use of cerebrospinal fluid procedures that require shorter imaging times via intrathecal injection. However, unlike indium-111 chloride (^{111}In)-DPTA, ^{99m}Tc-DPTA is not FDA approved for intrathecal injection (14).

Strontium-89 Chloride (^{89}Sr)

Strontium-89 chloride (^{89}Sr) (Metastron) is a sterile, nonpyrogenic aqueous solution for intravenous use and contains no preservative. It decays by beta emission, with a physical half-life of 51 days. ^{89}Sr is retained much longer and accumulates in significantly greater concentration in metastatic bone lesions than in normal bone. Its beta emission is very harmful to skeletal tissue, and thus, its clinical use is reserved for bone pain palliation associated with primary bone tumors and metastatic involvement (blastic lesions).

Following intravenous administration, strontium compounds demonstrate similar characteristics to calcium analogs. They clear rapidly from the bloodstream and selectively localize in bone mineral. The uptake of ^{89}Sr by bone occurs preferentially in sites of osteogenesis imperfecta, a condition characterized by the formation of brittle bones prone to fractures. Thus, as mentioned, it finds utility with primary bone tumors and metastatic bone lesions.

Prior to administration of ^{89}Sr, a risk-to-benefit ratio must be determined because of its bone marrow toxicity. It should be used with caution in patients with platelet counts below 60,000 and white cell counts below 2,400. After administration of ^{89}Sr, weekly blood tests should be performed and the patient's status monitored. Because the average hematologic recovery time is 6 months of treatment, at least 90 days is required prior to retreatment.

A small percentage of patients receiving ^{89}Sr report a transient increase in bone pain 36 to 72 hours after injection. This is usually mild, self-limiting, and controllable with analgesic therapy. Pain relief from the administration of ^{89}Sr typically manifests 7 to 20 days postinjection, and a key benefit of its use is a decreased dependence on opioids.

Yttrium-90 (^{90}Y)

Yttrium-90 (^{90}Y), a trivalent radioactive metal, is a pure beta-emitting radionuclide. It possesses a physical half-life of 64.2 hours (2.68 days) and is frequently used in human studies, in part because of its routine availability from commercial vendors as a sterile, pyrogen-free product with high specific activity (15). Its principal therapeutic application is in RIT of solid large tumors and lymphomas. In addition, it is employed in pain palliation involving soft tissue.

TheraSphere is a therapeutic device approved for use in patients with liver cancer (Fig. 18.2). It is being used for patients with biopsy-proven unresectable hepatocellular carcinoma. It is administered to a conscious patient via a catheter inserted into the femoral artery and is delivered directly into the hepatic artery in an interventional vascular radiology suite to go to the left or right lobe of the liver. Usually, patients receive two treatments to each liver lobe.

Patented in 1988, it consists of microspheres having a mean diameter of 20 to 30 mm (the approximate size of two red blood cells) that are bonded chemically to a radioactive pure beta emitter (^{90}Y). After injection, the product produces radiation to tissue with an average range of 2.5 mm and a maximum range of less than 1 cm. These lodge in end arterioles and capillaries in tumors, which minimizes or prevents delivery of the injected radionuclide to other body organs and tissues.

The sterile, pyrogen-free glass spheres are preformed by incorporating [89]Y oxide into the glass matrix. Subsequently, neutron bombardment is used to convert the [89]Y in the glass to [90]Y. Because the ^{90}Y is embedded in the spheres, it is not leached from the glass or metabolized. This prevents in vivo mobilization to distant body tissues and organs (15).

The ^{90}Y decays to stable zirconium-90. Each treatment delivers approximately 150 Gy or 15,000 rad to the liver lobe. Typically, 135 to 540 mCi of [90]Y (5 to 10 GBq) is delivered in 10 mL of saline that contains 2 million to 8 million microspheres. This is injected over a few minutes into the right or left hepatic artery. Patients are evaluated every month thereafter. Regular blood work that analyzes blood counts and liver function is performed, as is computed tomography (CT) or magnetic resonance imaging (MRI) of the liver.

Thallous-201 Chloride (^{201}Tl)

Thallous-201 chloride (^{201}Tl) is available as a sterile, isotonic nonpyrogenic solution for intravenous administration (Fig. 18.3). It demonstrates a physical half-life of

FIGURE 18.2. TheraSphere™. (Image provided courtesy of Boston Scientific. © 2021 Boston Scientific Corporation or its affiliates. All rights reserved.)

FIGURE 18.3. Product package of thallous chloride [201]Tl. (Courtesy of Curium, copyright © 2021 Curium US LLC.)

73.1 hours and decays by electron capture to mercury, ^{201}Hg. ^{201}Tl is a potassium analog that undergoes rapid active transport into the myocardium. Thus, it is an advantageous agent in MPI for the diagnosis and localization of myocardial infarction. It may also have prognostic value regarding survival. When administered to a clinically stable patient following the onset of myocardial infarct symptoms, it helps to assess the site and size of the perfusion defect. ^{201}Tl may also be used as an adjunct to the diagnosis of ischemic heart disease, that is, atherosclerotic coronary artery disease, when used in conjunction with exercise stress testing. Identified ischemia on ^{201}Tl scanning has been demonstrated to be a strong predictor of long-term mortality in coronary artery disease (16). However, long-term survival after major vascular surgery is improved significantly if patients with moderate to severe ischemia on preoperative ^{201}Tl scanning undergo selective coronary revascularization (16).

When used in conjunction with exercise stress testing to help differentiate between ischemic and infarcted tissue, ^{201}Tl should be administered at the inception of a period of maximum stress sustained for 30 seconds after injection of the agent. Imaging commences within 10 minutes after administration to obtain maximum target-to-background ratios. If the patient is unable to undergo a treadmill stress exercise because of physical limitation, pharmaceutical agents such as adenosine (Adenocard) or dipyridamole (Persantine) may be used to induce cardiac stress.

^{201}Tl undergoes fast redistribution in normal myocardium. Because of decreased blood flow, the uptake and washout of ^{201}Tl are slower in ischemic cardiac tissue. If the image demonstrates no uptake, the tissue is classified as infarcted.

Gallium-67 Citrate (^{67}Ga)

Gallium-67 citrate (^{67}Ga) is available as a sterile, pyrogen-free aqueous solution. Chemically, this drug behaves similarly to ferric ion (Fe^{+3}) and demonstrates a half-life of 78 hours.

^{67}Ga can localize in certain viable primary and metastatic tumors and in focal sites of infection. Investigational studies demonstrate that perhaps ^{67}Ga accumulates in lysosomes and is bound to a soluble intracellular protein. ^{67}Ga may be useful in demonstrating the presence and extent of malignancies associated with Hodgkin disease, lymphomas, and bronchogenic carcinoma. It can also be useful for localization of focal inflammatory lesions (e.g., sarcoidosis, abscesses, pyelonephritis). Its most important use is in the diagnosis and monitoring of *Pneumocystis carinii* pneumonia of AIDS and can be used as a diagnostic screen in cases of prolonged fever when physical examination, laboratory tests, and other imaging studies have not disclosed the source of the fever (fever of undetermined origin) (17). This is because 2-[^{18}F], fluoro-2-deoxy-D-glucose (FDG) has replaced the other uses of ^{67}Ga.

Concurrent use of ferric ion can increase ^{67}Ga renal excretion from the body. Although the exact mechanism is not clear, it is thought that elevated serum iron levels may displace ^{67}Ga from plasma protein–binding sites and hasten its excretion, resulting in decreased tumor and abscess localization.

The optimal target-to-background concentration ratios are often obtained 48 hours postinjection, and delayed imaging is necessary to allow for the ideal target-to-background ratio. However, considerable biologic variation can occur in individuals, and acceptable imaging may be performed 6 to 120 hours after injection. The optimal target-to-background ratios also depend on the area of interest. For example, a lower abdominal scan can be hindered by ^{67}Ga fecal excretion. Thus, the use of laxatives facilitates faster scanning of the patient. Both ^{201}Tl and ^{67}Ga injections contain benzyl alcohol as their preservatives. This could be problematic for those patients who demonstrate hypersensitivity to this preservative.

Indium-111 Chloride (^{111}In)

Indium-111 chloride (^{111}In) has become a popular radionuclide as a label for MABs (Fig. 18.4). The advantage of using ^{111}In for immunoscintigraphy is its long half-life, which allows multiple images to be taken up to 10 to 14 days after administration. In addition, its dual photon peaks provide superior planar (2-dimensional) and tomographic (3-dimensional) images. Because it lacks beta emission, it can be administered in rather high doses. Lastly, unlike radioiodine complexes, ^{111}In–MAB complexes are relatively stable in the body.

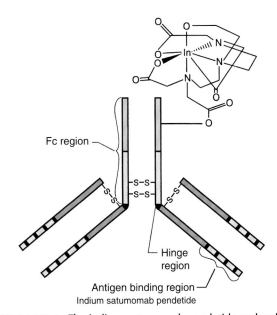

Indium satumomab pendetide

FIGURE 18.4. The indium satumomab pendetide molecule demonstrating attachment to the MAB. The antigen-binding region is also depicted. (Reprinted from Hunter TB, Walsh TK, Hall JN. Agents for diagnostic imaging. In: Block JH, Beale JM Jr, eds. Wilson and Gisvold's Textbook of Organic Medicinal and Pharmaceutical Chemistry. 11th Ed. Baltimore, MD: Lippincott Williams & Wilkins, 2004:470, with permission.)

FIGURE 18.5. Product package of Zevalin. (Courtesy of Acrotech Biopharma.)

Capromab pendetide (ProstaScint) is a MAB imaging agent linked to ^{111}In. This drug seeks out and attaches itself to prostate cancer and its metastases. ProstaScint images can aid management by helping identify when the cancer has metastasized from the prostate bed to regional lymph nodes or to distant soft tissues. It is also used as a diagnostic imaging agent in postprostatectomy patients with a rising prostate-specific antigen level and a negative or equivocal standard metastatic evaluation in whom there is a high clinical suspicion of occult metastatic disease. This product was approved for use by the FDA in late 1996.

Ibritumomab tiuxetan (Zevalin), approved for use in 2002, is a MAB that is separately labeled with ^{111}In and ^{90}Y in a two-phase regimen for the treatment of refractory low-grade follicular or transformed B-cell non-Hodgkin lymphoma, including patients with rituximab-refractory follicular non-Hodgkin lymphoma (Fig. 18.5). ^{111}In is used for the biodistributive study and administered 1 week prior to the final ibritumomab tiuxetan and ^{90}Y administration. This procedure ensures adequate biodistribution of the test dose. If the biodistribution is deemed unacceptable, the second step of the process is not implemented. This product works like a smart bomb. It is an antibody with a radionuclide attached that seeks and binds to cells with the CD20 receptor. Rituximab is administered prior to Zevalin (an unbound antibody) for both steps to clear most normal B cells and thus reduce the toxicity of the Zevalin.

The therapeutic regimen consists of two steps, as follows:

1. Initially, rituximab is infused in an amount equal to 250 mg/m^2 at 50 mg/h. The dose is increased by 50 mg/h every 30 minutes up to a maximum of 400 mg/h. During the infusion, the patient should be monitored for any hypersensitivity reaction and the infusion stopped if hypersensitivity occurs. If hypersensitivity does occur and is treated, the infusion is resumed at half the previous rate when symptoms improve. After rituximab infusion has been administered, within 4 hours, the diagnostic biodistribution dose of 5 mCi of ^{111}In-labeled ibritumomab tiuxetan is injected over 10 minutes with use of a syringe shield to reduce exposure during administration. The biodistribution of the drug is assessed by imaging within 2 to 24 hours and again 48 hours postinjection. If the biodistribution is acceptable, the second step is administered after 7 days of initial therapy. Alternatively, if the biodistribution is not acceptable, the therapy does not proceed to the second step.

2. Initiated within 7 to 9 days after step one, the patient receives another rituximab infusion of 250 mg/m^2 at an initial rate of 100 mg/h. The dosage is increased by 100 mg/h every 30 minutes to a maximum of 400 mg/h as tolerated. The therapeutic dose is then administered according to the patient's platelet count. Because the most commonly reported adverse effect of this therapy is thrombocytopenia and neutropenia, after the rituximab infusion, if the patient's platelet count is above 150,000 cells/mm^3, a 0.4-mCi/kg dose of ^{90}Y-labeled ibritumomab tiuxetan is administered. If the patient's platelet count is between 100,000 and 150,000 cells/mm^3, a reduced dose of 0.3 mCi/kg of ^{90}Y-labeled ibritumomab tiuxetan is administered over 10 minutes. In any case, the total administered dose may not exceed 32 mCi. If the patient's platelet count is below 100,000 cells/mm^3, the drug is not administered.

The regimen is supplied in two distinct kits (Fig. 18.5) that contain all of the nonradioactive ingredients necessary to create the single doses of ibritumomab tiuxetan labeled with ^{111}In and ^{90}Y. Because ^{90}Y is a pure beta particle–emitting radionuclide, extreme precaution must be taken to protect the caregivers and the patient to keep radiation exposure levels to a minimum. Although control of contamination is important in the handling of any radiopharmaceutical, it is paramount when handling a pure *beta* emitter, for example, ^{90}Y. A primary concern of handling a *gamma* emitter such as ^{99m}Tc is the shielding of its penetrating radiation, which is inversely proportional to the square of the distance from it. Radiation from pure *beta* emitters extends only a few millimeters from the source and may be shielded with acrylic shields, but skin contamination from these agents will result in a large tissue dose to caregivers.

Sodium Iodide-123 (^{123}I)

Sodium iodide-123 (^{123}I) is available as an oral capsule and is generally preferable to ^{131}I because it delivers lower radiation doses and has better imaging properties. It is used diagnostically to evaluate thyroid function and morphology. ^{123}I emits only gamma rays. In the euthyroid patient, 5% to 30% of the administered dose is concentrated in the thyroid gland at 24 hours and has an effective half-life of 13 hours. The remaining administered activity is distributed within the extracellular fluid and has an effective half-life of 8 hours. Although it is more expensive than ^{99m}Tc, ^{123}I produces a superior image because of its higher target-to-background ratio. Also, it gives a lower radiation dose.

Pharmacists must be aware that concurrently administered drugs can decrease the thyroid uptake of ^{123}I for a variety of reasons. Thus, it is recommended that these medications be withheld for a period prior to the administration of ^{123}I. For example, corticosteroids should be withheld 1 week prior to ^{123}I administration. Benzodiazepines should be withheld up to 4 weeks prior to ^{123}I administration. Vitamins, expectorants, antitussives, and topical medications containing iodine (e.g., clioquinol, Betadine) should be withheld for 2 to 4 weeks prior to the administration of ^{123}I.

Sodium Iodide-131 (^{131}I)

Sodium iodide-131 (^{131}I) is available as a volatile solution that can be purchased from a manufacturer or compounded by the nuclear pharmacist into an oral capsule or solution. In small amounts, it is used for thyroid function studies or thyroid uptake tests by determining the fraction of administered radioiodine activity taken up by the thyroid gland. The thyroid uptake test is used in the diagnosis of hyperthyroidism and in calculating the activity to be administered for radioactive iodine therapy.

Typically, the diagnostic dose of ^{131}I is 2 to 5 mCi. The therapeutic dose is higher, usually 5 to 200 mCi. The upper limit can be calculated to determine just how much radiation a particular patient can withstand. However, more than 200 mCi is usually not given.

^{131}I is also indicated for the evaluation of size, thyroid nodules, carcinoma, and masses in the lingual region, neck, and mediastinum and in the localization of functioning metastatic thyroid tumors. It finds utility in the preoperative and postoperative evaluation of patients with thyroid carcinoma and can be used to assess therapeutic effects in these patients.

The beta emissions from the ^{131}I destroy thyroid tissue and, in small amounts, can be used for diagnostic thyroid imaging. It is not recommended for this use because of its relatively long half-life (8 days), its beta emission, and its poor resolution on gamma camera images. However, if cost is a consideration, ^{131}I is used *in lieu* of ^{123}I. It is also used when availability of ^{123}I is a concern.

The time to radioactivity visualization is generally 18 to 24 hours. However, imaging of functional thyroid metastases is generally performed at 24 to 96 hours to allow maximal uptake and minimal blood pool retention.

Tositumomab with ^{131}I (Bexxar) is a MAB product that has a radioactive substance, ^{131}I, attached to it. The MAB seeks and binds to a protein receptor (CD20) on the surface of normal and malignant cells. It is indicated for treatment of patients with CD20-positive follicular non-Hodgkin lymphoma, with and without transformation, whose disease is refractory to rituximab, and who have relapsed following chemotherapy. Once it is bound to target cells, the product delivers radiation, which enhances the killing effect of the antibody. Normal B cells recover in about 9 months because the parent B cells do not possess the CD20 receptor.

Neuroendocrine tumors, such as neuroblastoma and pheochromocytoma, in adults are treated with ^{131}I-MIBG (11). Metaiodobenzylguanidine (i.e., MIBG, iobenguane) is a structural analog of guanethidine that has structural similarities to norepinephrine. This drug is selectively taken up by adrenergic neurons, the adrenal medulla, and some neuroendocrine cancer cells by an active uptake mechanism at the cell membrane. It is a good example of how targeted radionuclide therapy can be used for alternative treatment of neuroendocrine tumors, such as neuroblastoma, a heterogeneous pediatric cancer with clinical behavior related to the biologic features of the tumor. It is estimated that 50% of these patients have high-risk disease features, with overall survival rates less than 40%. Most of these children have significant tumor-related pain at the end of life. Often, too, the pain is difficult to treat. In targeted radiotherapy with submyeloablative doses, ^{131}I-MIBG has demonstrated effective palliation in highly refractory neuroblastoma. Most patients showed subjective improvement in pain and/or performance status (18). A retrospective review by Bomanji et al. (19) demonstrated that ^{131}I-MIBG also provides a good therapeutic response in adult patients with metastatic neuroendocrine tumors.

Samarium-153 (^{153}Sm)

Samarium-153 (^{153}Sm) has a short half-life, 46.3 hours (1.9 days), which can be advantageous for administering repeated doses; the difficulty is manufacturing and delivery. It is a low-energy beta emitter, which is advantageous for treating small clusters of tumorous cells. The range of its beta emissions is short and provides a good bone-to-marrow ratio. Myelotoxicity has been manageable at its approved dose schedule (1 mCi, or 37 MBq, per kilogram) (2).

^{153}Sm is chelated with ethylenediamine tetramethylene phosphonate (^{153}Sm-EDTMP, Quadramet) for the relief of pain in patients with confirmed osteoblastic metastatic bone lesions that enhance on radionuclide bone scan (2). The recommended dose is 1.0 mCi (37 MBq)/kg administered intravenously over 1 minute through a secure indwelling catheter and followed with a saline flush. Excretion of this radiolabeled chelate occurs almost exclusively via the kidneys into urine. Within the first 15 minutes of administration of the complex, localization in the kidneys and the skeleton is high to all other organs and tissues. By 30 minutes postadministration, most of the non–bone-associated radioactivity is in the urine. The patient should be advised to urinate often after administration of the product to minimize radiation exposure to the bladder.

Several clinical trials have demonstrated significant pain relief in approximately 70% to 80% of patients studied at the standard intravenous dosage of 1 mCi/kg. Toxicity is limited to bone marrow suppression manifested by decreased leukocyte counts and thrombocytopenia. The nadir for this is 4 weeks postadministration with recovery to normal levels in 6 weeks.

[153]Sm-labeled MABs are being used in animal research to study angiogenesis, the development of new blood vessels from preexisting ones. Central to this process is the activator vascular endothelial growth factor, and research is being performed in laboratory animals using radiolabeled ([153]Sm and ^{99m}Tc) antiendothelial MABs that localize in new cancerous vasculature (20).

Lutetium-177 (^{177}Lu)

Lutetium-177 (^{177}Lu) is being investigated in more than 30 clinical applications, including treatment of colon cancer, metastatic bone cancer, non-Hodgkin lymphoma, ovarian cancer, and lung cancer. It is estimated that more than 500,000 new cases of these cancers occur each year in the United States and nearly 2 million cases worldwide. [177]Lu is a rare earth metal with a physical half-life of 6.75 days and beta emissions (E = 149 keV) that penetrate 0.2 to 0.3 mm in soft tissues. In comparison to ^{90}Y, a higher percentage of ^{177}Lu radiation energy will be absorbed in very small tumors and micrometastases (6).

[177]Lu also emits two relatively low-abundance, low-energy gamma rays (113 and 208 keV) that allow imaging with a gamma camera but pose less radiation risk hazard to health care personnel than [131]I. Its most common side effects were delayed transient arthralgia and marrow suppression.

[177]Lu-dotatate (Lutathera) is approved for treatment of somatostatin receptor–positive neuroendocrine tumors. It is given as a series of 4 doses, each containing 200 mCi of [177]Lu. A continuous infusion of amino acid solution, containing specified amounts of L-lysine and L-arginine, must be administered with Lutathera. The infusion should begin 30 minutes before and continue at least 3 hours after the Lutathera dose is given. The purpose of the amino acids is to protect the kidney from excess radiation damage.

Lutathera administration is rather unique: the drug is not diluted directly in the solution for infusion. Rather, Lutathera is left in the original vial and normal saline is pumped through the vial and into the patient (Fig. 18.6). The normal saline is pumped at 50 to 100 mL/h for the first 5 to 10 minutes, then increased to 200 to 300 mL/h for 25 to 30 minutes more.

Rhenium-186 ([186]Re) and Rhenium-188 ([188]Re)

Rhenium-186 ([186]Re) and Rhenium-188 ([188]Re) are important radionuclides with therapeutic potential. The availability of [186]Re and [188]Re provides flexibility in design of radiolabeled agents that are compatible with their in vivo applications and pharmacokinetic properties. [188]Re has a higher beta particle energy and shorter half-life than [186]Re. Thus, it is generally more appropriate for larger tumor targeting and possesses a reasonably fast clearance from

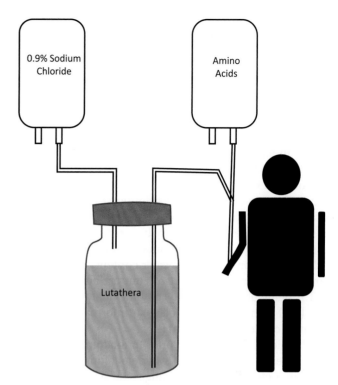

FIGURE 18.6. Dilution of Lutathera during administration.

the blood and other nontarget tissues. Alternatively, [186]Re is a medium-energy beta particle emitter with a 3.7-day half-life, which makes it more appropriate for use with biomolecules that are not cleared from the bloodstream very rapidly. Its lack of availability as a high specific activity product limits [186]Re use to applications in which high specific activity formulations are not mandatory.

POSITRON EMISSION TOMOGRAPHY

Since the early 1970s, positron emission tomography (PET) has been employed to study cerebral physiology (21). Since that time, it is a rapidly growing noninvasive modality for the diagnosis and management of cancer. PET yields high-quality images that characterize substrate metabolism, cellular proliferation, receptor density, and other parameters used to identify cancer and evaluate its response to treatment (22). Radiolabeled tracers injected in nonpharmacologic doses are used to construct three-dimensional images to demonstrate the location and concentration of the tracer of interest (23). PET allows the physician to secure an image showing the regional concentration of a positron-emitting nuclide inside the body (24). It is a method for quantitative imaging of regional function and chemical reactions within various organs of the human body. Imaging applications of PET have shown great use, for instance, in mapping regional blood flow, oxygen metabolism, regional blood volume, rates of use of metabolic substrates, receptor-specific tracer binding, bone remodeling, tumor receptor density, and reporter gene expression (23).

The tracers used in PET imaging are natural biochemicals labeled with radionuclides of carbon, nitrogen, oxygen, and fluorine. This allows analysis in terms of physiology and biochemistry at a level of sophistication beyond that encountered in traditional nuclear medicine. No other technology can image body chemistry with such sensitivity, so that the moment-to-moment change in concentration of a tracer in the blood or tissue can be determined in absolute units. Other imaging modalities, such as CT and MRI, provide predominantly anatomic information, and this is thought to be the future of imaging. CT is based on portrayal of the distribution of attenuation of x-rays passing through the body. MRI exploits the variation in regional concentrations of hydrogen and nuclear relaxation parameters to generate image contrast and to provide information about free water content, relative blood flow, and the concentration of contrast agents. Clinical PET is being used with CT to combine anatomic information (CT) with functional molecular information (PET) to advance cancer management (23).

Chemical changes occur prior to anatomic changes in most disease states, and PET can detect functional abnormalities before anatomic changes have occurred. PET evolved with its main focus on studies of the brain and heart. However, it has emerged as a valued diagnostic tool for diagnosis and therapy monitoring of patients with lymphoma, as a means to assess estrogen receptors in primary and metastatic breast cancers and to identify resectable colorectal tumor recurrence. In epilepsy, PET and surface electroencephalography are used in concert with clinical assessment of symptoms and signs to try to localize areas of the brain that are the foci of epileptic seizures when surgical intervention is the only remaining method to prevent the seizures.

Tumors have more intermediary metabolism than normal tissue, and PET use is advantageous because it can qualitatively and quantitatively study metabolism. Several processes, including glycolysis, increased membrane glucose transfer capability, and RNA, DNA, and protein synthesis are demonstrated and/or accelerated in tumors. In the 1930s, Warburg demonstrated that glucose was used more in tumorous tissue than in normal tissue, and this remains today as a foundation for PET imaging in oncology (25). The radiopharmaceutical most widely used for evaluating tumors with PET imaging is [^{18}F]-fluorodeoxyglucose because it has been demonstrated useful for tracing glucose metabolism, for detecting malignant tissue, and for quantifying changes in tumor glycolysis during and after treatment. Thus, it is useful for diagnosis, staging, and monitoring various cancers, including lung, colorectal, melanoma, lymphoma, and head and neck, among others. [^{18}F]-FDG has a 110-minute half-life, which is much easier to work with than a 2-minute half-life. PET scanning has also been demonstrated to predict accurately a patient's clinical and pathological response and survival in patients who undergo preoperative chemotherapy on the treatment strategy for esophageal carcinoma (26).

When a radionuclide within the body decays by emission of a positron, that particle travels a very short distance (1 to 4 mm) in body tissues or water before expending its kinetic energy and combining with an electron. This interaction, one positron annihilation, results in simultaneous emission of two photons, each having a specific energy (511 keV) and emitted exactly 180 degrees from each other. Therefore, two scintillation detectors are placed, one on either side of the tissue that contains the radionuclide. Detectors are connected to a coincident circuit that provides an output only when a certain level of gamma ray radiation can be simultaneously detected by both. The result is a low-background detector, highly specific for the particular radionuclide and providing excellent resolution.

Radionuclides that undergo positron decay generally have very short half-lives (e.g., ^{15}O; $t_{1/2}$ = 2.04 minutes), which permit administration of large doses of activity without subjecting the patient to excessive radiation exposure. The resulting high count rates facilitate collection of statistically significant images in a very short time and a dynamic study of physiologic processes that produces a quick fluctuation in tissue concentrations of the tracer. The short half-lives also allow repeat image studies within a brief time with no confounding background activity from the prior injection.

It is optimal to label radiopharmaceuticals using radionuclides with the shortest half-life that is compatible with the time scale of the physiologic process to be studied. However, a practical consequence of using short-lived ($t_{1/2} < 1$ hour) radionuclides in diagnostic medicine is the necessity for the radionuclide production and radiotracer synthesis to occur in the hospital where the imaging procedure will be conducted. Originally, the major production of radionuclides for PET imaging (^{11}C, ^{13}N, ^{15}O, ^{18}F) was generally with in-house biomedical cyclotrons. Today, however, there are numerous commercial cyclotrons nationwide.

For tracers that have demonstrated great utility in PET imaging studies, robotic technique and automated systems have been created for routine radiopharmaceutical synthesis. These systems cannot reduce the personnel needed to supply PET radiopharmaceuticals, but the automated systems encourage frequent syntheses using large amounts of activity to be performed without exposing the personnel to unnecessary or excessive radiation exposure.

PET was once conducted primarily in large medical centers. A prime consideration was that PET radionuclides had short half-lives, often 2 to 20 minutes, which made it difficult to get them from commercial sources. However, commercial dispensing is now possible in certain markets where a PET cyclotron is adjacent to the pharmacy. In other markets, out of necessity, the production facility must be on-site, and after rapid synthesis, the pharmaceutical must be purified. Thus, research continues to focus upon sources of PET radionuclides other than cyclotrons, such as radionuclide generators, that would allow PET technology in community-based nuclear medicine and pharmacy environments.

Parent–daughter generator systems are now being investigated as a possible mode to produce PET radionuclides.

Potentially, it would free PET imaging from its dependence on cyclotron generation within a hospital. Also, this could make PET a viable clinical diagnosis tool away from the hospital or large medical center. To date, very few positron emitters can be created by these systems, and only two radionuclides, ^{82}Rb and ^{68}Ga, have been extensively reported in the nuclear medicine literature. In late 2003, Ion Beam Applications was granted FDA approval of a generator (CardioGen-82) to make ^{82}Rb a PET agent for the evaluation of coronary artery disease. It is capable of distinguishing normal from abnormal myocardium in patients with suspected myocardial infarction, and it helps identify patients most likely to benefit from further intervention while reducing the risks of unnecessary medical, radiologic, and/or surgical procedures. The use of this infusion system is growing and is especially useful in obese/diabetic patients who have more adipose tissue, which causes attenuation artifacts. A real perfusion defect may be exaggerated in size and severity using single-photon emission CT. Alternatively, a real perfusion defect can be hidden within an area of apparent attenuation. PET imaging, utilizing a transmission scan in addition to an emission scan, corrects this problem. It gives a truer picture of cardiac perfusion and viability during stress. Only pharmaceutical stressing agents can be used with this system.

The ^{82}Rb generator is very expensive and has a 30-day useful life. Typically, this generator was cost prohibitive unless the facility had a significant patient volume. Commercial nuclear pharmacies have developed a service that allows various departments to share a generator. They deliver and pick up generators on a daily basis.

Future studies of new drug entities will include pharmacokinetic determination using PET technology. Further, PET will allow the manufacturer to quantify how much of the drug reaches a specific drug receptor. Thus, comparative PET studies will shed light on which drug, for example, within a therapeutic category can attain the best distribution and concentration at the intended receptor site. It is also conceivable that PET technology will open new vistas for interpretation of drug interactions, particularly where there is competition by two drugs for one receptor site. PET imaging is also being investigated as a mechanism for the early diagnosis of infection and the capacity to distinguish between bacterial and sterile inflammation. Investigations have included radiolabeled antibiotics such as ^{18}F-ciprofloxacin and ^{18}F-fleroxacin (27). Attempts are being made to understand the mechanisms of binding and accumulation of radiopharmaceuticals to bacteria. The goal is to discover a specific, reliable method to image infection that can be used to replace or complement scintigraphy with radiolabeled autologous leukocytes or radiolabeled MABs to granulocyte antigens (27).

Longer-lived PET radionuclides, such as ^{89}Zr ($t_{\frac{1}{2}}$, 78.1 hours), ^{76}Br ($t_{\frac{1}{2}}$, 61.1 hours), ^{124}I ($t_{\frac{1}{2}}$, 4.15 days), and ^{64}Cu ($t_{\frac{1}{2}}$, 12.8 hours), are being investigated as radiolabels for MAB-based PET imaging. Early clinical research has demonstrated that these may be useful for detecting metastases smaller than 1.5 cm. About 2% to 4% of cancer patients have an initial diagnosis of cancer of unknown primary origin (28). In addition to cancer diagnosis, radiolabeled MABs have been used to evaluate cardiovascular disorders. Clinical uses of ^{111}In antimyosin include detection of acute myocardial infarct, perioperative myocardial damage assessment, detection of acute myocarditis, diagnosis of rejection and management of patients after heart transplantation, and diagnosis of active rheumatic carditis, among others. The European Council of Nuclear Cardiology published its position paper that summarized the current and future potential of PET as a clinical cardiovascular diagnostic imaging tool (29). Included in the statement was evidence demonstrating the superior diagnostic accuracy of PET and its value to guide clinical decision-making.

Table 18.2 lists PET radiopharmaceuticals used in common imaging procedures, and the following section highlights a few of the more frequently used PET radiopharmaceuticals.

TABLE 18.2. Positron-Emitting Radiopharmaceuticals Used in Common PET Imaging Procedures

Radiopharmaceutical	Application	Typical Dose (mCi), Procedure[a]
[^{15}O]-oxygen	Cerebral oxygen extraction, metabolism	50–100
[^{15}O]-carbon monoxide	Cerebral blood volume	50–100
	Myocardial blood volume	50–100
[^{15}O]-water	Cerebral blood flow	80
	Myocardial blood flow	150
[^{13}N]-ammonia	Myocardial blood flow	15–25
[^{11}C]-acetate	Myocardial metabolism	30
[^{11}C]-*N*-methyl spiperone	Dopamine receptor binding	20
[^{18}F]-fluorodeoxyglucose	Cerebral glucose metabolism	5–20
	Myocardial glucose metabolism	
	Tumor glucose metabolism	
[^{82}Rb]-Rb$^+$	Myocardial blood flow	10–40

[a]Many PET studies combine imaging procedures (e.g., measurements of both blood flow and metabolism); the doses given here are typical of those actually used in each procedure of the study. For a single imaging procedure, an allowable dose (a dose that does not lead to excessive radiation exposure) may be significantly higher than these values.

Carbon-11 Radiopharmaceuticals

[11]C has been incorporated into a number of organic molecules (e.g., carboxylic acids, alcohols, glucose) for use in diagnostic imaging despite its relatively long half-life (20 minutes). To date, palmitic acid is the carboxylic acid used most in PET imaging. As a tracer, it has found utility in the study of myocardial metabolism.

Glucose randomly labeled with ^{11}C has been produced photosynthetically for use in studies of cerebral glucose metabolism. The use of ^{11}C glucose for cerebral glucose metabolism requires imaging less than 5 minutes after injection.

Nitrogen-13 Radiopharmaceuticals

[13]N ammonia has been used as a tracer for cerebral and myocardial blood flow and demonstrates a half-life of 10 minutes. It undergoes a relatively long extraction into these organs and exhibits prolonged retention, as a major fraction of extractor tracer is metabolically incorporated into amino acids. For study of pulmonary ventilation, ^{13}N gas is superior to the radioactive noble gases because of its lower solubility in blood.

Oxygen-15 Radiopharmaceuticals

[15]O is the radionuclide of oxygen with the longest half-life, 2.04 minutes. Because very little time is available for tracer synthesis, PET imaging studies employing [15]O are restricted to use of a few relatively simple molecules.

Four [15]O radiopharmaceuticals are available for clinical use. These are [15]O oxygen gas ([15]OO), [15]O carbon monoxide (C[15]O), [15]O carbon dioxide (CO[15]O), and [15]O water (H_2[15]O) having been used in hemodynamic studies that take advantage of their short half-life to allow administration of large doses of activity (up to 100 mCi) in imaging studies that can be repeated within 8 to 10 minutes with no carryover effect.

Labeled oxygen gas, that is, [15]OO, can be used directly in studies of oxygen metabolism or can be converted to carbon monoxide, carbon dioxide, or water. C[15]O can be safely administered via inhalation and serves as a tracer for red blood cell volume upon binding of the C[15]O to hemoglobin.

H_2[15]O can be used in equilibrium studies of tissue water content and finds its greatest use as a tracer for regional blood flow. Commonly used as a tracer in PET evaluation of cerebral and myocardial perfusion, its 2-minute half-life outweighs its limitation of ability to diffuse freely across the blood–brain barrier at high flow rates.

Fluorine-18 Radiopharmaceuticals

[18]F has a relatively long half-life among positron emitters, 110 minutes. Compared to radiopharmaceuticals with a shorter half-life, this presents several distinct advantages for synthesis and allows delivery of the radionuclide to imaging centers at a distance from the generating cyclotron.

[18]F also demonstrates specific activity that makes it attractive for use as a receptor-specific tracer binding. It is taken up by cells, is phosphorylated by hexokinase whose mitochondrial form is greatly elevated in rapidly growing malignant tumors, and is retained by tissues that demonstrate high metabolic activity, for example, malignant tumors. As a result, its major use has expanded beyond the imaging of cerebral, myocardial, and tumor metabolism with 2-[^{18}F]-FDG to include colorectal cancer, breast cancer, melanoma, and lung cancer (30). In brain imaging procedures, FDG maps normal brain metabolic activity and highlights glucose consumption patterns within the hippocampus and identifies specific images associated with normal brain function, mild cognitive impairment, and different types of dementia, including Alzheimer disease (31). In cardiac studies, it identifies ischemic regions in which glucose metabolism increases as a consequence of decreased fatty acid metabolism. As mentioned earlier, glucose metabolism increases in tumor tissue, and FDG localization in that tissue is extremely helpful in the imaging study (32).

Gallium-68 Radiopharmaceuticals

[68]Ga is rapidly bound by the iron-binding sites of transferrin following intravenous injection of ^{68}Ga citrate and is very useful in studies of regional plasma volume. When combined with a C[15]O measurement of regional blood cell volume, the ^{68}Ga-transferrin PET study allows calculation of the regional hematocrit. ^{68}Ga-transferrin has also been employed in pulmonary studies of vascular permeability.

DRUG ANTIDOTE FOR RADIATION EXPOSURE

In October 2003, the FDA approved Prussian blue (ferric hexacyanoferrate, Radiogardase) to treat patients from the harmful levels of ^{137}Cs or thallium radiation exposure and contamination (Fig. 18.7). These are radioactive agents

FIGURE 18.7. Radiogardase capsules. (Courtesy Heyl Chemisch-pharmazeutische Fabrik GmbH & Co.)

that terrorists might conceivably use to release from a dirty bomb that would be inhaled or ingested by victims. The two radioactive substances can cause serious illness and death when they gain entry, as the organs absorb high doses of radiation. At lower doses, these agents can cause cancer. Conventionally, ^{137}Cs is used in a wide range of devices to treat certain cancers. Nonradioactive thallium is used industrially and as a rat poison. In small quantities, radioactive thallium is used for medical imaging.

Prussian blue was first manufactured in 1704 as a dye for Prussian military uniforms. To treat cesium and/or thallium radiation exposure, Prussian blue is administered orally in a dose of 3 g three times daily in adults and adolescents. In children aged 2 to 12 years, the dosage is 1 g/d. It works by trapping cesium and thallium ions in the gastrointestinal tract and interrupts their reabsorption back into the systemic circulation. Prussian blue is not absorbed from the gastrointestinal tract to a significant degree. Studies have demonstrated that 99% of the oral dose is excreted in the stool. The duration of treatment depends on the extent of exposure. Preferably, it should be administered as soon as possible after exposure and is continued for 30 days. After this treatment period, the patient should be reassessed.

Counseling a patient prescribed Prussian blue is very important. Food has been demonstrated to increase its effectiveness by stimulating bile secretion. If it is more convenient, as for patients (e.g., young children, geriatric patients) who cannot swallow solid doses, the capsules may be opened and mixed with liquid or bland food. Patients should be forewarned that constipation may occur, and if so, they should increase their dietary fiber. In addition, because the drug is a dye, it may discolor the stool blue, and if it is administered as a liquid or with bland food, it may discolor the lining of the mouth.

It is important that pharmacists help the patient identify the source of the radiation and take appropriate safety measures to minimize exposure to others. Also, men should urinate in a stool rather than a urinal and flush the toilet several times after relieving themselves. Prussian blue is available as an artist's dye, so patients should be forewarned and dissuaded from using that source as a means to treat themselves, as it is not prepared in accordance with pharmaceutical safety procedures.

NONRADIOACTIVE PHARMACEUTICAL USE IN NUCLEAR MEDICINE

The advantage of radiopharmaceutical imaging is that it is a noninvasive modality in the diagnosis and workup of a disease. Generally, radiopharmaceuticals used diagnostically help to monitor a physiologic process without altering it. Sometimes, however, the information gained from the procedure is inadequate to address the clinical questions. To overcome this deficiency, interventional pharmaceutical drugs are used to complement the radiopharmaceutical (33).

These interventional pharmaceutical drugs alter the physiologic process being studied with radiopharmaceuticals. When the interventional drug is used in conjunction with nuclear medicine, the amount of information gained is greatly improved. This intervention improves the information about the process under study and may increase the specificity and sensitivity of the procedure or decrease the time necessary for imaging.

Acetazolamide (Diamox)

Acetazolamide (Diamox), an agent used to treat glaucoma by diuretic action, has been shown to increase cerebral blood flow following intravenous administration. On average, it can increase cerebral blood flow 23% ± 8% in normal vessels. Its use in cerebral perfusion studies is to enhance the differentiation between normal vessels and diseased vessels, which cannot easily dilate. It is indicated for use in patients with transient ischemic attack, carotid artery disease, or a cerebrovascular accident to help identify areas of the brain that are at risk for an infarct. The drug also is used in other neurologic conditions (e.g., Alzheimer disease, multi-infarct dementia) with which cerebral perfusion is far from optimal.

Captopril (Capoten)

Captopril (Capoten) is used to help diagnose renovascular hypertension in hypertensive patients with abdominal bruits, declining renal function, and poorly controlled hypertension with drug therapy. As an angiotensin-converting enzyme inhibitor, this drug blocks conversion of angiotensin I to angiotensin II and prevents vasoconstriction of the efferent arterioles of the kidney. This decreases glomerular filtration pressure in the affected kidney.

Cimetidine

Among children, Meckel diverticulum, a congenital anomaly of the gastrointestinal tract, presents itself in about a quarter of the cases as rectal bleeding and abdominal pain. This diverticulum, an abnormal remnant of the developing gastrointestinal tract, contains gastric mucosa that bleeds abnormally. This gastric mucosa concentrates ^{99m}Tc pertechnetate as normal mucosa, and cimetidine (i.e., Tagamet) demonstrates usefulness in Meckel diverticulum imaging by virtue of its action as a histamine H_2 receptor antagonist. Cimetidine reduces the volume and concentration of stomach acid, and following its administration in a Meckel's study, the cells of the gastric mucosa continue to accumulate ^{99m}Tc pertechnetate, but secretion of acid into the gastric lumen is reduced or prevented. This allows for continual ^{99m}Tc pertechnetate accumulation in the gastric mucosa with little transit through the intestinal tract. This results in an enhanced ability to visualize the small area of ectopic gastric mucosa.

Dipyridamole (Persantine) and Adenosine (Adenocard)

Dipyridamole (Persantine) is used as an alternative to a treadmill stress test prior to cardiac imaging. Typically, patients who are candidates to receive pharmaceutical stress as part of the imaging procedure rather than perform the stress test are those with cardiac, respiratory, and/or orthopedic problems; those maintained on beta-blocker or calcium channel blocker medications; and those with poor motivation. Dipyridamole blocks adenosine deaminase, the enzyme responsible for the degradation of adenosine, a potent coronary vasodilator. Adenosine can increase coronary blood flow up to four to five times the resting values. Blood flow through stenosed arteries is less than normal.

Adenosine (Adenocard) is an ideal agent in combination with MPI agents. It possesses an ultra short half-life, less than 10 seconds, and is a potent coronary vasodilator. This drug can increase coronary blood flow four to five times that of rest and can be beneficial as a pharmaceutical stress agent to help diagnose and identify stenosed arteries.

Dipyridamole and adenosine are available from commercial nuclear pharmacies in patient-specific unit dosage forms. In preparation for the use of adenosine or dipyridamole, theophylline- and caffeine-containing drugs, beverages, and foods must be discontinued, and the patient must take nothing by mouth overnight. An advantage of adenosine use over dipyridamole is that adverse effects caused by adenosine (e.g., chest pain; pain in the throat, jaw, or arm; headache; flushing; and dyspnea) generally disappear within 1 to 2 minutes after discontinuation of the infusion. Dipyridamole has a longer half-life (15 to 30 minutes) with a peak effect 2 to 3 minutes after infusion. When this agent is used, chest pain, headache, and dizziness occur most often.

To reverse the effects of adenosine and dipyridamole, aminophylline can be given intravenously if necessary. Nitroglycerin can be given to relieve the chest pain that follows dipyridamole administration.

Furosemide (Lasix)

Furosemide (Lasix), a loop diuretic, is administered to help confirm or rule out mechanical renal obstruction during renal scintigraphy when significant retention of radioactivity is noted in the renal pelvis. It inhibits the reabsorption of electrolytes, most notably sodium, in the ascending limb of the loop of Henle and in the proximal and distal tubules. In an obstructed kidney, furosemide diuresis will have little effect on clearance of the radioactivity retained in the kidney. An unobstructed kidney will rapidly clear the radioactivity into the bladder following furosemide administration, and the renograms will show rapid emptying with a steeply declining radioactivity curve.

Vitamin B$_{12}$

Schilling test determines a patient's capability to absorb radioactive vitamin B$_{12}$ from the intestine. Normally, vitamin B$_{12}$ is released from food sources (e.g., meat, eggs, milk) and bound to intrinsic factor in the stomach. Ultimately, this intrinsic factor–vitamin B$_{12}$ complex is absorbed in the ileum and stored in the liver. Once the liver's storage capacity for this complex is exceeded, vitamin B$_{12}$ is excreted in urine. In cases of vitamin B$_{12}$ deficiency, it is crucial to determine the cause of the deficiency, either lack of a proper diet or inadequate absorption. For the procedure, 1 mg of nonradioactive vitamin B$_{12}$ is given intramuscularly 2 hours before the ^{57}Co-labeled vitamin B$_{12}$ is administered orally. This large dose is intended to saturate the storage sites and helps flush absorbed radiolabeled B$_{12}$ into the urine. Thus, the excreted radioactivity demonstrates the amount absorbed. Excretion of 5% or less is diagnostic of B$_{12}$ malabsorption. Typical urinary excretion of B$_{12}$ ranges from 15% to 40%.

▌PRACTICE OF NUCLEAR PHARMACY

As nuclear medicine has evolved from a research tool into a mainstream clinical, diagnostic, and therapeutic tool, so has the practice of pharmacy evolved within nuclear medicine. The skills of pharmacists play an important role in the safe and efficient operation of nuclear pharmacies and modern PET facilities. In particular, the role of the pharmacist in PET increases as the use of PET radiopharmaceuticals grows from research to clinical to commercial environments.

Internal dose models and methods in use for many years are well established in nuclear medicine. These allow calculation of radiation doses to stylized models representing reference individuals. In the future, kinetic analyses will have to be carefully planned, and dose conversion factors that are most similar to the subject in question should be chosen to increase patient specificity. The important point is that the pharmacist uses his or her expertise to become a part of this and use patient image data to construct individualized models for more detailed and patient-specific dose calculations (34).

The Nuclear Pharmacy Practice Guidelines were created by the American Pharmacists Association Academy of Pharmacy Practice and Management Section of Nuclear Pharmacy. They were adopted in 1994, and the Specialty Council on Nuclear Pharmacy of the Board of Pharmaceutical Specialties validated them in 1995. The Specialty Council surveyed all board-certified nuclear pharmacists about the importance and frequency of each domain, task, and knowledge statement in the guidelines. This validation served as the underpinning for creation of the board examination in nuclear pharmacy. It established the proportion allotted to each of the nine identified domains on the nuclear pharmacy specialty examination (35).

Nuclear pharmacy is a patient-oriented service that embodies the scientific knowledge and professional judgment required to improve and promote health through safe and efficacious use of radioactive drugs for diagnosis and therapy. The pharmacist is expected to understand nuclear medicine procedures and their advantages and disadvantages for diagnostic or therapeutic purposes (36).

Typically, nuclear pharmacy practice occurs primarily in two settings: a large teaching hospital or a centralized commercial operation. Approximately, 95% of radiopharmaceuticals are produced in the commercial setting. With practice site differences, activities may not be all-inclusive at each site. The nine general activities encompassing nuclear pharmacy practice are procurement, compounding, quality assurance, dispensing, distribution, health and safety, provision of drug information and consultation, monitoring patient outcomes, and research and development.

Procurement and Storage

Nuclear pharmacists are responsible for securing radiopharmaceuticals, other appropriate drugs, supplies, and materials necessary to effect appropriate outcomes. The effectiveness of some diagnostic radiopharmaceuticals is enhanced or toxicity lessened by coadministration of other drugs. For example, some patients (e.g., elderly, obese, those with orthopedic problems) may not be capable of undergoing an exercise stress test prior to administration of a radiopharmaceutical intended to visualize cardiac perfusion. Thus, as mentioned earlier in this chapter, dipyridamole, a vasodilator, can be used as a substitute for the exercise stress test.

The short half-life of radiopharmaceuticals poses a special problem to the pharmacist in that the traditional pathways (e.g., drug wholesaler) to secure the drug may take longer than the lifetime of the drug. Typically, in the past, the nuclear pharmacist would order the drug directly from the manufacturer, primarily by overnight delivery. Therefore, knowledge of calibration time, shipping and delivery schedules, and radioactive decay associated with the ordered radiopharmaceutical weigh heavily in ordering. Limited quantities also played a vital role in the attempt to obtain products. All of this has led to the rise of centralized radiopharmacies.

Commercial radiopharmacies set up two distinct areas. The first includes general office workspace (e.g., storage, break rooms, restrooms). The second area is dedicated as a laboratory or pharmacy area. The latter area having restricted access, thus, is called the "restricted area." Within the "restricted area," there are separate areas for radioactive material storage, compounding and dispensing, quality control testing, and packaging and distribution. Dose calibration (i.e., counting) is performed in the compounding and dispensing area. Typically, this is an area that consists of laminar flow hoods and counter space. Each laminar flow hood contains a dose calibrator so that each unit dose can be "counted" by the dispensing

pharmacist or nuclear pharmacy technician. There is no patient treatment area. Imaging clinics (e.g., cardiology, oncology, general nuclear), typically, purchase unit dose radiopharmaceuticals from a commercial nuclear pharmacy.

Typically, hospital nuclear pharmacies are separate from the hospital pharmacy and are adjacent to the nuclear medicine or radiology departments. Usually, doses are prepared in the hospital nuclear pharmacy area and transported to the nuclear medicine department for administration by a nurse or certified nuclear medicine technologist in a treatment/administration room or private patient area. The patient is then brought to the "camera room" for imaging.

Preparation of the Radiopharmaceutical

Compounding of the radiopharmaceutical can be a simple (e.g., reconstituting reagent kits with ^{99m}Tc sodium pertechnetate) to very complex task (e.g., operating a cyclotron). Aside from the typical compounding procedures with a normal prescription (e.g., receipt of order, validation, safety of dose, supplies, and equipment to prepare), the preparation of a radiopharmaceutical is confounded by issues of radioactivity and chemical reactions.

Compounding of a radiopharmaceutical involves chemical reactions to label a molecule with a radionuclide. For most ^{99m}Tc-labeled compounds, stannous chloride is used to reduce Tc(VII) pertechnetate to a lower oxidation state. This then is followed by chelation of the technetium atoms by multidentate ligands. For other radiopharmaceuticals, covalent bonding, transchelation, and coordination complexation reactions are used.

Manufacturers produce ready-to-use radiopharmaceuticals (e.g., ^{201}Tl-thallous chloride) and radionuclides used in compounding radiopharmaceuticals at the nuclear pharmacy. Expense, limited availability, and shipping schedules, however, dictate that some radiopharmaceuticals be created on-site at a central radiopharmacy using a cyclotron, particularly for PET, because of their very short half-lives. Because of this necessary path of preparation, these are usually more expensive than those purchased directly from the manufacturer. A significant number of radiopharmaceuticals use ^{99m}Tc in the form of sodium pertechnetate plus sodium chloride for isotonicity. ^{99m}Tc is formed by decay of ^{99}Mo, a radioactive radionuclide of molybdenum obtained by neutron bombardment of ^{98}Mo. Commonly, a generator or "cow" containing ^{99}Mo (half-life, 67 hours) produces the ^{99m}Tc sodium pertechnetate at a rate that permits daily elutions of the generator (Fig. 18.8). "Milking the cow" is slang for eluting the generator to obtain the sodium pertechnetate. Other cyclotron-produced radiopharmaceuticals (e.g., ^{111}In, ^{123}I, ^{201}Tl) may be ordered for the next day. Many cyclotrons are operated as manufacturers and follow cGMP guidelines although this has not been mandated as yet by the FDA. It is anticipated that a mandate will be forthcoming and compliance will be expected in 2 years thereafter. At this

FIGURE 18.8. Cross section of a radionuclide generator for production of ^{99m}Tc by sterile 0.9% sodium chloride elution of a sterile alumina (Al$_2$O$_3$) column that has ^{99}Mo adsorbed onto it. (Reprinted with permission from Hunter TB, Walsh TK, Hall JN. Agents for diagnostic imaging. In: Block JH, Beale JM Jr, eds. Wilson and Gisvold's Textbook of Organic Medicinal and Pharmaceutical Chemistry. 11th Ed. Baltimore, MD: Lippincott Williams & Wilkins, 2004:462. Courtesy of Dupont-Pharma, Billerica, MA.)

writing, the publishing of the final rule is anticipated soon. As a result, many independent nuclear pharmacy owners have expanded and installed cyclotrons. The elution or the process of elution is related to the act of obtaining a radiopharmaceutical from a solid column generator or "cow." The eluate can then be used as is or added to another "cold" pharmaceutical to compound a radiopharmaceutical. The elution process usually uses a liquid, that is, 0.9% sodium chloride solution (NSS), but there have been generators that use gas, for example, air and oxygen. This process is similar, for example, to ion-exchange chromatography.

A significant majority of radiopharmaceuticals are produced for parenteral administration. Aseptic technique and methods must be maintained during preparation of the radiopharmaceutical and when radiolabeling biologic products (e.g., MABs, peptides). For example, to compound a vial of ^{99m}Tc radiopharmaceutical, the pharmacist takes an elution and removes the required amount of eluent and injects it aseptically into a vial and then adds a sufficient amount of normal saline to bring it to its proper concentration. Further, strict adherence to universal precautions and appropriate infection control handling are a necessity when radiolabeling patient blood cells.

There are no differences between commercially available products and pharmacy-compounded products other than the fact that the compounded products are dispensed in syringes. With solid, commercially available oral dosage forms such as capsules, there might be different colors of capsules or sizes, but other than physical appearance of the dosage form, they look alike and work the same.

Hung et al. (37) identified potential deficiencies in manufacturers' product package insert instructions for the preparation of radiopharmaceutical products. Five categories were identified as follows: (*a*) absent or incomplete instructions, particularly with respect to quality assurance procedures; (*b*) restrictive directions, such as specific instructions for chromatography solvents, counting devices, and reconstitution processes; (*c*) inconsistent instructions, such as different reconstituted volumes for the same final drug product, and unworkable expiration dates; (*d*) impractical directions, such as unrealistically low reconstituted activity limits and dangerously high numbers of radiolabeled particulate matter; and (*e*) vague instructions, such as use of "should," "may," and "recommend." The authors concluded that the manufacturers' instructions for the preparation of these products should be viewed as standard guidance rather than as requirements. They also advocated that nuclear pharmacists be allowed to use alternative validated methods to prepare radiopharmaceutical products as long as they do not conflict with normal pharmacy practice.

Quality Assurance

To ensure the safe use of radiopharmaceuticals in patients, the pharmacist must carry out appropriate tests (e.g., chemical, physical, biologic). USP monographs dictate that radiopharmaceuticals meet delineated specifications, including radionuclidic purity, radiochemical purity, chemical purity, pH, particle size, sterility, pyrogenicity (or bacterial endotoxin), and specific activity. When the pharmacist uses an already prepared radionuclide (e.g., ^{201}Tl, ^{123}I, ^{131}I), these qualities are assured by the manufacturer.

Radionuclidic purity is the proportion of activity present as the stated nuclide. It can be measured by gamma ray spectroscopy, half-life measurement, and/or other physical measurements that help to detect the presence of extraneous nuclides. Examples of the lack of radionuclidic purity are ^{198}Au contaminated with ^{199}Au and ^{99m}Tc contaminated with ^{99}Mo.

Radiochemical purity is the fraction of the stated radionuclide in the stated chemical form. If there are nonradioactive contaminants, the radioactive drug may be radiochemically pure but not chemically pure. Similarly, if there are small amounts of radioactive contaminants, the material may be chemically pure but not radiochemically pure. Column or thin-layer chromatography is useful for purity determination.

Dispensing of a Radiopharmaceutical

A distinct difference between radiopharmaceutical dispensing and the traditional mode by which ordinary prescriptions are dispensed is that radiopharmaceuticals never go directly to the patient; they are provided to trained health care professionals at the hospital or clinic and then administered to the patient. Also, because of the nature of the product, radiopharmaceuticals typically are dispensed in unit doses and, typically, as injectables.

When the radiopharmaceutical is ordered, the dispensing pharmacist must ensure that the ordered dose is safe for the patient. Thus, the pharmacist must weigh and consider patient factors such as age, weight, surface area, and gamma camera sensitivity with each order. Usually, prescriptions are ordered and shipped. Therefore, radioactive decay must be considered to accommodate the time from manufacture to administration. Because the product is a radiopharmaceutical, it is subject to special labeling requirements (e.g., standard radiation symbol, CAUTION—RADIOACTIVE MATERIAL).

Radiopharmaceuticals compounded from sterile components in closed sterile containers and with a volume of 100 mL or less for a single-dose injection or not more than 30 mL taken from a multiple-dose container are designated as and conform to the USP <797> standards for Low-Risk Compounded Sterile Products (CSPs) (12). Radiopharmaceuticals are to be compounded using appropriately shielded vials and syringes in a properly functioning and certified ISO class 5, primary engineering control room located in an ISO class 8 or cleaner air environment to permit compliance with special handling, shielding, and negative air flow requirements.

Radiopharmaceutical vials designed for multiuse, compounded with ^{99m}Tc, exposed to ISO class 5 environment, and punctured by needles with no direct contact contamination may be used up to the time indicated by the manufacturer's recommendations. Storage and transport of properly shielded vials or radiopharmaceutical CSPs may occur in a limited access ambient environment without a specific ISO class designation.

^{99m}Tc/^{99}Mo generator systems are to be stored and eluted under conditions recommended by the manufacturer and applicable state and federal regulations. Such generator systems are to be eluted in an ISO class 8 or cleaner air environment to permit special handling, shielding, and air flow requirements. To limit acute and chronic radiation exposure of inspecting personnel to a level that is as low as reasonably achievable (i.e., ALARA), direct visual inspection of radiopharmaceutical CSPs containing high concentrations of radioactivity doses shall be conducted in accordance with ALARA.

Radiopharmaceuticals prepared as low-risk level CSPs with 12-hour or less beyond-use date are to be prepared in a segregated compounding area. A line of demarcation defining the segregated compounding area shall be established. Materials and garb exposed in a patient care and treatment area shall not cross a line of demarcation into the segregated compounding area.

Radiopharmaceuticals for PET compounding conform to the USP <823> standards (12). This section of the USP provides the requirements for the control of components, materials, and supplies of the PET radiopharmaceuticals. In addition, compounding procedure verification and stability testing and expiration dating are provided. USP <823> also delineates PET radiopharmaceutical compounding for human use. In this section, quality control procedures are to be established by a designated, qualified, and trained individual who is responsible to ensure that the activities are conducted and properly completed by qualified and trained personnel.

Quality control tests to be performed on individual batches of PET radiopharmaceuticals, the analytical procedures, and the corresponding acceptance criteria are to be established in writing. The procedures are for PET radiopharmaceuticals labeled with a nuclide having a $t_{1/2}$ greater than 20 minutes and PET radiopharmaceuticals labeled with a nuclide having a $t_{1/2}$ less than 20 minutes. For each batch of PET radiopharmaceutical intended for parenteral administration, a membrane filter integrity test must be performed immediately after completion of product filtration. In addition, an in-process 20-minute endotoxin "limit test" and a standard 60-minute bacterial endotoxin test on each batch or quality control subbatch of the radiopharmaceutical must be performed prior to release for human use.

Written procedures for the performance of quality control tests must be established on batches of PET radiopharmaceuticals intended for human use. Verification testing of equipment and procedures used for quality control testing of PET radiopharmaceuticals must be conducted. For example, using internal or external standards, the correct operation of analytical equipment, for example, gas chromatography, must be confirmed upon initial installation or upon major repair. After the performance of quality control tests on PET batches of radiopharmaceuticals, the results must be initialed. Acceptance or rejection of individual batches of PET radiopharmaceuticals must be based on conformity of quality control test results with established acceptance criteria. Each batch that is acceptable must be signed and the date approved indicated. Unacceptable quality control test results must be investigated and the outcome documented.

USP <823> also delineates procedures for PET radiopharmaceutical sterilization and sterility assurance. This includes compounding equipment and components, environmental controls, and microbiological testing of the prepared products.

Distribution of Radiopharmaceuticals

Institutional procedures and policies dictate how a radiopharmaceutical is distributed within a health care facility. Generally, a lead-lined syringe container shipped in Department of Transportation–approved and tested cases are used with appropriate identifying information. Some nuclear pharmacies are converting from lead to tungsten containers. Tungsten is lighter, which results in less weight per shipment, and is less hazardous than lead. Local, state (e.g., State Board of Pharmacy), and federal (e.g., Department of Transportation, NRC) regulations are relevant when a radiopharmaceutical is distributed from a central nuclear pharmacy to another institution. Generally, these requirements relate to packaging, labeling, shipping papers, record keeping, shipper and carrier licensing, and personnel training.

Health and Safety

The NRC establishes and enforces radiation safety standards (e.g., limits for radiation doses, levels of radiation in an area, concentrations of radioactivity in air and waste water, waste disposal, precautionary procedures) for the compounding facility. Beyond the radiopharmaceuticals, related aspects of health and safety are a necessity. Hazardous chemicals (e.g., chromatography solvents) must be stored appropriately, handled safely, and disposed of properly. Attention must also be paid to the use of personal protective devices, containers, and the physical environment in which the radiopharmaceuticals are prepared. Personal monitoring devices are used to monitor and track annual radiation exposure (e.g., whole-body exposure [film badges or optically stimulated luminescence badges] and extremity exposure [ring badges]). Both are evaluated weekly or monthly, and the information is used to refine handling processes continually to manage occupational radiation exposure in accordance with the ALARA concept, that is, to keep occupational radiation exposures as low as is reasonably achievable.

Provision of Drug Information and Consultation

It is very important that the nuclear pharmacist possess oral and written communication skills. His or her knowledge and expertise are useful only when they can be conveyed to an allied health professional, the patient, and the patient's caregiver, among others. The nuclear pharmacist must be able to answer inquiries and know where to find requested information.

The type of information can include, among others, the following:

- Biologic effects of radiation
- Radiation physics and protection
- Radiopharmaceutical chemistry, compounding, quality assurance, and products
- Diagnostic and therapeutic applications of radiopharmaceuticals
- Ancillary medications used to enhance radiopharmaceutical procedures
- Drug interactions associated with radiopharmaceuticals (Tables 18.3 to 18.6)
- Precautions associated with the use of radiopharmaceuticals
- Regulatory requirements affecting the use of radiopharmaceuticals
- This information can be used for educational purposes (e.g., allied health professionals, consumer groups), for setting policies and procedures, and for diagnostic or therapeutic value in the care of patients

Monitoring Patient Outcomes

Patient safety and optimal outcomes are the goal of the nuclear pharmacist and a central tenet of pharmaceutical care. In that regard, the nuclear pharmacist can be instrumental in providing quality patient care. The nuclear pharmacist can, among other things,

- Develop institutional standards for the rationale and appropriate use of radiopharmaceuticals.
- Prospectively screen and review patient data to ensure appropriate use of radiopharmaceuticals and ancillary medicines.
- Ensure that patients are selected appropriately for radionuclide therapy and monitored after therapy to prevent complications and/or provide necessary therapy.

TABLE 18.3. Concurrent Administered Drugs Known to Interfere with Tumor and Abscess Localization Scintigraphy

Interfering Drug	Effect on Image
Phenytoin	Localization of RP in mediastinum, pulmonary hilar structures (patients without clinical evidence of lymphadenopathy)
Amiodarone, bleomycin, busulfan, nitrofurantoin, bacille Calmette-Guérin, chemotherapy, lymphangiographic contrast media, addictive drugs of abuse	Diffuse pulmonary localization (sometimes local pulmonary uptake)
Metoclopramide, reserpine, phenothiazines, oral contraceptives, diethylstilbestrol	Localization of RP in breast
Methotrexate, cisplatin, gallium nitrate, mechlorethamine HCl, vincristine, various chemotherapeutic agents, iron	Increased skeletal uptake Increased renal elimination Decreased hepatic accumulation Decreased tumor or abscess uptake
Clindamycin	Localization of RP in bowel
Calcium gluconate, IM injections	Soft tissue accumulation of RP
Ampicillin, sulfonamides, sulfinpyrazone, ibuprofen, cephalosporins, hydrochlorothiazide, methicillin, erythromycin, rifampin, pentamidine, phenylbutazone, gold salts, allopurinol, furosemide, phenazone, phenobarbital, phenytoin, phenindione	Increased accumulation of RP in the kidneys
Chemotherapeutic agents, antibiotics	Localization of RP in the thymus

RP, radiopharmaceutical.

- Evaluate the safety and effectiveness of radiopharmaceuticals and ancillary medications.
- Ensure proper preparation of patients prior to administration of the radiopharmaceutical and ancillary medications.
- Prevent, minimize, and/or rectify clinical problems associated with the use of radiopharmaceuticals and ancillary medications.
- Monitor patients for potential adverse effects following administration of a radiopharmaceutical or interventional medication.
- Discontinue incompatible medications before the nuclear medicine study, restart them after the study, and appropriately manage the patient during discontinuation.
- Ensure that patients with special needs, problems, or conditions (e.g., pregnancy, nursing mothers, dialysis patients, children, and the elderly) are given appropriate consideration before, during, and after radiopharmaceutical administration.

- Ensure that information gained from the nuclear medicine procedure is considered during development of the patient's therapeutic plan.
- Perform and enhance the effectiveness of nuclear pharmacy procedures, including administration of therapeutic or diagnostic radiopharmaceuticals and ancillary medications to the patient.

An example of a nuclear pharmacist intervention is use of radiopharmaceuticals in a breast-feeding woman. Specifically, recommendations are made for interruption of breast-feeding in patients who are undergoing a nuclear medicine diagnostic procedure. The nuclear pharmacist should review the patient's data, especially if the woman is of childbearing age. These recommendations include the following:

- Breast-feeding should be noted in the patient history from the attending physician.
- A member of the interdisciplinary team should inquire about the patient's breast-feeding status and notify the nuclear physician when a patient is breast-feeding.

TABLE 18.4. Drugs Known to Interfere with Brain Imaging

Interfering Drug	Effect on Image
Cancer chemotherapeutic agents	Patchy increased uptake of RP as a result of chemoneurotoxicity
Corticosteroids	Decreased uptake into brain lesions
Psychotropic drugs	Rapid accumulation of RP in nasopharyngeal area during arterial or capillary phase (cerebral radionuclide angiography)

RP, radiopharmaceutical.

TABLE 18.5. Concurrent Administered Drugs Known to Interfere with Myocardial Perfusion Scintigraphy

Interfering Drug	Effect on Image
Beta-blockers, nitrates, calcium channel blockers	Decreases number and size of exercise-induced ^{201}Tl perfusion defects
Vasopressin	Appearance of myocardial defects in patients without coronary artery disease
Propranolol, cardiac glycosides, procainamide, lidocaine, phenytoin, doxorubicin	Decreased myocardial localization, increased liver localization

TABLE 18.6. Drugs Known to Interfere with Renal Imaging

Interfering Drug	Effect on Image
Iodinated contrast agents, aminoglycosides	Decrease in effective plasma flow values; decreased glomerular filtration rate
Cyclosporine, cisplatin	Decreased urinary excretion; decreased tubular function
Furosemide	Misleading renogram and flow curves resulting in false-positive/false-negative studies
Probenecid	Decreased renal accumulation and accumulation

- Breast-feeding should be interrupted for the period during which radioactivity is known to appear in the breast milk.
- Close contact with an infant should be restricted to 5 hours within 24 hours of the procedure for ^{99m}Tc MIBI, ^{99m}Tc-labeled red blood cells, and ^{131}I (>3 mCi) whether or not the mother is breast-feeding (38).

Indirectly, the nuclear pharmacist can provide clinical services that include consultation with other caregivers (e.g., explain a nuclear medicine study), prepare institutional guidelines for the use of radiopharmaceuticals and ancillary medications, provide information and literature reviews related to specific questions or studies, formulate special drugs and/or dosage forms, and conduct drug use evaluation studies or drug use reviews.

REGULATORY PROCESS

Pharmacist expertise and experience in the drug regulatory process are very important in nuclear pharmacy practice, and the role of the pharmacist in nuclear medicine is complementary to all health professions practicing within it. The role of the pharmacist will become even more important in the future, with more players entering the marketplace, particularly in the domain of PET. Already there is a variety of corporate and institutional facility partnerships, and with the continual evolution of PET, this should exponentially increase the clinical demand for these agents and increase the role of nuclear pharmacy even further.

PHARMACEUTICS CASE STUDY

SUBJECTIVE INFORMATION

You are a pharmaceutical researcher assigned to work on a new drug, Radhot-1. Your project is to determine where Radhot-1 localizes in the body and the rate at which its two major metabolites are eliminated from the body.

OBJECTIVE INFORMATION

Radhot-1 contains carbon, hydrogen, sulfur, iodine, and nitrogen; it has been determined that these can be labeled appropriately for the study.

ASSESSMENT

To determine its location in the body, you use a gamma-emitting radionuclide. To follow the elimination of the two major metabolites, you label the two different parts of the molecule with two different beta-emitting radionuclides that can be counted separately.

PLAN

Radhot-1 will be prepared with a gamma-emitting iodine, beta-emitting carbon in one part of the molecule, and a beta-emitting hydrogen in a second part of the molecule, the two parts for beta counting being on the two separate parts of the molecule that split when metabolized. External body counting will be used to determine the source of the iodine localization. Urine samples will be collected and analyzed for the two different beta-emitting isotopes and the data plotted. ∎

CLINICAL CASE STUDY

M.G. is a 56-year-old woman who presents to her family physician with blood pressure of 210/120. Following thyroid function tests, ultrasound, a nuclear medicine scan, and fine-needle biopsy, she was diagnosed with Hashimoto thyroiditis and papillary carcinoma of the thyroid gland.

The patient underwent a total thyroidectomy 4 weeks ago and is scheduled today for a 100-mCi radioactive ^{131}I ablation of any residual thyroid tissue. Upon questioning, the patient states that she is allergic to iodine, having had a severe rash following the administration of iodinated contrast medium in the past. The nuclear medicine technologist calls the nuclear pharmacist for advice on how to handle the situation.

(continued)

(continued)

SUBJECTIVE INFORMATION

Patient with history of allergy to iodine scheduled to receive ^{131}I ablation.

PMH:	HTN 20 years
	Anxiety disorders × 10 years
	Autoimmune thyroid disorder × 1 year
	Thyroidectomy × 4 weeks
Meds:	Calcium carbonate (TUMS) 500 mg po qid
	KCl 10 mEq po bid
	Diovan 160/12.5 mg po qd
	Levoxyl 0.175 mg po qd
	Meprobamate 400 mg po tid prn
	Calcitriol 0.5 mg po qd
	Diltiazem 240 mg po qd
Family history:	Father HTN × 20 years
Social history:	(−) Smoking
	(−) Alcohol
	(−) Illicit drugs
Insurance:	IPDA
Allergies:	Penicillin, iodine

OBJECTIVE INFORMATION

BP: 134/72 **Ca:** 8.6 (8.7 to 10.5 mg/dL)

Wt: 195 **Ca, ionized:** 4.5 (4.7 to 5.2 mg/dL)

Pulse: 67

TSH: 75 (normal 0.35 to 5.5 uIU/mL) (TSH was 0.275 prior to thyroidectomy)

PHARMACEUTICAL CARE PLAN

1. Potential allergic reaction to ^{131}I. The recommended daily allowance is 0.15 mg of dietary iodine per day. The total therapeutic dose given in this situation would be 0.0008 mg of iodine. This amount would not likely cause an allergic reaction to iodine even in the most iodine-allergic patient.
2. Potential pregnancy teratogenicity. The patient is postmenopausal, and no pregnancy test was ordered.
3. Patient education on radioactive ablation therapy. Patient was educated on procedure and precautions to be taken regarding close contact with other people, particularly children and pregnant women, after radionuclide therapy. Patient was also educated about radioactive ablation therapy and had her questions answered, and written, informed consent was secured.
4. In 4 months, will follow-up with endocrinologist who will order a Thyrogen-stimulating thyroglobulin test.
5. Reference: Radiopharmaceuticals in Nuclear Medicine Practice, Kowalski and Perry, 1987. ■

APPLYING THE PRINCIPLES AND CONCEPTS

GROUP ACTIVITIES

1. Create a comparative table of radiopharmaceuticals for diagnostic use inclusive of indication(s), dosage regimen, adverse drug reactions, precautions, and route of administration.
2. Create a comparative table of radiopharmaceuticals for therapeutic use inclusive of dosage regimen, adverse drug reactions, precautions, and route of administration.
3. Interview a nuclear pharmacist, and determine how practice in a nuclear pharmacy differs from that of community and hospital pharmacy practice.
4. Identify a new radiopharmaceutical through the primary literature, and prepare a group PowerPoint presentation to educate the remainder of the recitation session students.

INDIVIDUAL ACTIVITIES

1. Secure an article from the primary literature, which features a radiopharmaceutical for either diagnostic or therapeutic use. Critique it, and prepare and deliver a journal club presentation.
2. List typical adverse drug reactions encountered by radiopharmaceuticals, and describe the treatment/antidote for each.
3. Describe patient circumstances, for example, age, gender, pharmacogenetic background, and organ function, which contraindicate the use of certain radiopharmaceutical drugs, and determine an alternative mode to pursue to take care of the patient.
4. Search an electronic database, and be able to discover within 5 minutes all significant drug interactions between the drugs and the radiopharmaceutical, and be capable to explain the interaction.
5. Compare three different ^{99m}Tc radiopharmaceuticals and explain the physiologic processes responsible for the different radioactivity localization patterns expected for the products.

REFERENCES

1. Nickel RA. Radiopharmaceuticals. In: Early PJ, Sodee DB, eds. Principles and Practice of Nuclear Medicine. 2nd Ed. St. Louis, MO: Mosby, 1995:94–117.
2. Srivastava S, Dadachova E. Recent advances in radionuclide therapy. Semin Nucl Med 2001;31:330–341.
3. Silberstein EB, Ryan J. Prevalence of adverse reactions in nuclear medicine. J Nucl Med 1996;37(1):185–192.
4. Early PJ. Methods of radioactive decay. In: Early PJ, Sodee DB, eds. Principles and Practice of Nuclear Medicine. 2nd Ed. St. Louis, MO: Mosby, 1995:23–49.
5. Shaw SM. Diagnostic imaging and pharmaceutical care. Am J Pharm Educ 1994;58:190–193.
6. Leslie WD, Tully SA, Yogendran MS, et al. Prognostic value of lung sestamibi uptake in myocardial perfusion imaging of patients with known or suspected coronary artery disease. J Am Coll Cardiol 2005;45:1676–1682.
7. de Jong M, Kwekkeboom D, Valkema R, et al. Radiolabeled peptides for tumour therapy: Current status and future directions. Plenary Lecture at the EANM 2002. Eur J Nucl Med Mol Imaging 2003;30:463–469.
8. Carlsson J, Aronsson EF, Hietala S-O, et al. Tumour therapy with radionuclides: Assessment of progress and problems. Radiother Oncol 2003;66:107–117.
9. Goodwin DA, Meares CF. Advances in pretargeting biotechnology. Biotechnol Adv 2001;19:435–450.
10. Krennin EP, Kwekkeboom DJ, Valkema R, et al. Peptide receptor radionuclide therapy. Ann N Y Acad Sci 2004;1014:234–245.
11. Lupetti A, Nibbering PH, Welling MM. Radiopharmaceuticals: New antimicrobial agents. Trends Biotechnol 2003;21:70–73.
12. U.S. Pharmacopeia–National Formulary. Current edition. Rockville, MD: U.S. Pharmacopeial Convention.
13. Dura JV, Hinkle GH. Stability of a mixture of technetium Tc-99m sulfur colloid and lidocaine hydrochloride. Am J Health Syst Pharm 2007;64:2477–2479.
14. Ponto JA. Special safety considerations in preparation of technetium Tc-99m DTPA for cerebrospinal fluid-related imaging procedures. J Am Pharm Assoc (2003) 2008;48(3):413–416.
15. Volkert WA, Hoffman TJ. Therapeutic radiopharmaceuticals. Chem Rev 1999;99:2269–2292.
16. Landesberg G, Mosseri M, Wolf YG, et al. Preoperative thallium scanning, selective coronary revascularization, and long-term survival after major vascular surgery. Circulation 2003;108:177–183.
17. http://www.emedicine.com/Radio/topic534.htm. (Accessed April 18, 2016)
18. Kang TI, Brohpy P, Hickeson M, et al. Targeted radiotherapy with submyeloablative doses of ^{131}I-MIBG is effective for disease palliation in highly refractory neuroblastoma. J Pediatr Hematol Oncol 2003;25:769–773.
19. Bomanji JB, Wong W, Gaze MN, et al. Treatment of neuroendocrine tumors in adults with ^{131}I-MIBG therapy. Clin Oncol 2003;15:193–198.
20. Bouziotis P, Fani M, Archimandritis SC, et al. Samarium-153 and technetium-99m-labeled monoclonal antibodies in angiogenesis for tumor visualization and inhibition. Anticancer Res 2003;23:2167–2171.
21. Hoffman JM, Hanson MW, Coleman RE. Clinical positron emission tomography imaging. Radiol Clin North Am 1993;31:935–959.
22. Coleman RE, Bednarczyk EM, Chilton H. Positron emission tomography: From production and distribution to drug research and clinical applications. J Am Pharm Assoc (Wash) 2000;40(5 Suppl 1):S66–S67.
23. Gambhir SS. Molecular imaging of cancer with positron emission tomography. Nat Rev Cancer 2002;2:683–693.
24. Green MA, Welch MJ. Radiopharmaceuticals for positron emission tomography (PET). In: Early PJ, Sodee DB, eds. Principles and Practice of Nuclear Medicine. 2nd Ed. St. Louis, MO: Mosby, 1995:739–751.
25. Warburg O. The Metabolism of Tumors. London: A. Constable, 1930:75–327.
26. Port JL, Lee PC, Korst RJ, et al. Positron emission tomographic scanning predicts survival after induction chemotherapy for esophageal carcinoma. Ann Thorac Surg 2007;84:393–400.
27. Signore A, D'Alessandria C, Lazzeri E, et al. Can we produce an image of bacteria with radiopharmaceuticals? Eur J Nucl Med Mol Imaging 2008;35(6):1051–1055.
28. Jerusalem G, Hustinx R, Geguin Y, et al. PET scan imaging in oncology. Eur J Cancer 2003;39:1525–1534.
29. LeGuludex D, Lautamaki R, Knuuti J, et al. Present and future of clinical cardiovascular PET imaging in Europe—A position statement by the European Council of Nuclear Cardiology (ECNC). Eur J Nucl Med Mol Imaging 2008;35(9):1709–1724.
30. Port ER, Yeung H, Gonen M, et al. ^{18}F-2-fluor-2-deoxy-d-glucose positron emission tomography scanning effects surgical management in selected patients with high-risk, operable breast carcinoma. Ann Surg Oncol 2006;13:677–684.
31. Mosconi L. Multicenter standardized ^{18}F-FDG PET diagnosis of mild cognitive impairment, Alzheimer's disease, and other dementias. J Nucl Med 2008;49:390–398.
32. Romer W, Schwaiger M. Positron emission tomography in diagnosis and therapy monitoring of patients with lymphoma. Clin Positron Imaging 1998;1:101–110.
33. Park HM, Duncan K. Nonradioactive pharmaceuticals in nuclear medicine. J Nucl Med Technol 1994;22:240–248.
34. Stabin MG. Developments in the internal dosimetry of radiopharmaceuticals. Radiat Prot Dosimetry 2003;105:575–580.
35. Talbert RL, Bertin RJ. Specialization in pharmacy practice. In: Hendrickson R, ed. Remington: The Science and Practice of Pharmacy. 21st Ed. Philadelphia, PA: Lippincott, Williams and Wilkins, 2006:2155–2162.
36. Rhodes BA, Hladik WB III, Norenberg JP. Clinical radiopharmacy: Principles and practices. Semin Nucl Med 1996;26(2):77–84.
37. Hung JC, Ponto JA, Gadient KR, et al. Deficiencies of product labeling directions for the preparation of radiopharmaceuticals. J Am Pharm Assoc (2003) 2004;44:30–35.
38. Harding LK, Bossuyt A, Pellet S, et al. Recommendations for nuclear pharmacy physicians regarding breast-feeding mothers. Eur J Nucl Med 1995;22:BP17.

CHAPTER

19 Products of Biotechnology

CHAPTER AT A GLANCE Techniques Used to Produce Biotechnologic Products • Products of Biotechnology • Tissue Plasminogen Activators • The Future of Biotechnology Products • The FDA Office of Biotechnology Products • Patient Information from the Pharmacist • Pharmacist Self-Help with Biotechnology Drugs

OBJECTIVES

After reading this chapter, the student will be able to:

1. Differentiate between the various techniques using living organisms in the production or modification of biotechnology drugs

2. Describe the classification of products of biotechnology used in clinical practice

3. Provide examples of biotechnology drugs for each classification of biotechnology drug type

4. Summarize important concepts associated with biotechnology product handling, storage, and administration

5. Describe the mission of the Food and Drug Administration (FDA) Office of Biotechnology Products and its structure

6. Discuss the general composition of biotechnology products

INTRODUCTION

The term *biotechnology* encompasses any technique that uses living organisms (e.g., microorganisms) in the production or modification of products. The classic example of biotechnologic drugs was proteins obtained from recombinant DNA (rDNA) technology. However, biotechnology now encompasses the use of tissue culture, living cells, or cell enzymes to make a defined product. rDNA and monoclonal antibody (MAb) technologies have provided exciting opportunities for the development of more pharmaceuticals and approaches to the diagnosis, treatment, and prevention of disease.

The biotechnology pharmaceutical market in the United States is forecast to grow at a compound annual growth rate of 11.9% and exceed $625 billion in value in 2026. Some factors driving this growth include the following:

1. Increased demand for new therapies with biotechnology drugs
2. Revised regulations and standards in encouraging more companies to invest in the field
3. Increased aging population and incidence of chronic illnesses (1)

Biotechnologic products will continue to have a marked impact upon the practice of pharmacy. Research will continue to generate potent new medications that require the pharmacist's unique expertise in custom dosing for individual patients and use of sophisticated drug delivery systems.

Pharmacogenomics is the application of genomic technology to genetic variation in response to pharmaceutical compounds. It is an emerging discipline and an outgrowth of pharmacogenetics that seeks to describe the genetic basis for interindividual differences in drug effectiveness and toxicity, using genome-wide approaches to identify genes that govern an individual's response to specific medications. The initial draft of the human genome has demonstrated that the human genome has more than 1.4 million single nucleotide polymorphisms, with more than 60,000 of these residing in the coding regions of human genes. Some of these have already been associated with significant differences in metabolism or effects with commonly used medications. Some genetic polymorphisms (e.g., thiopurine *S*-methyltransferase, CYP2D6) have a marked effect on drug pharmacokinetics, such that appropriate dosages of drugs for patients with these genotypes are significantly higher or lower than the normal dosages. The ultimate goal of pharmacogenomics is to define the contributions of inherited differences in drug disposition and/or targets to drug response and thereby improve safety and effectiveness of medications through genetically guided individualized treatments.

Biotechnology drugs that have become known synonymously as specialty pharmaceuticals hold great promise for people living with an increasing number of chronic diseases (2). Coupled with advances in genetic-based diagnostic techniques, specialty drugs could conceivably redefine the way illnesses will be treated in the future. As the use of novel technologies is incorporated into routine clinical practice, opportunities exist to make pharmaceutical care even more personalized. The goal is to create oral products to supplant injection or infusion administration. Accompanying this will be increased costs (3). Because of their uniqueness, these agents often require special handling, administration, patient education, and clinical support, all of which add to cost. Specialty products are conveniently placed into one of the three categories: (*a*) self-administered therapies (e.g., rheumatoid arthritis, multiple sclerosis, psoriasis); (*b*) products injected or infused in an office or clinic setting (e.g., vaccines, asthma, immune disorders); and (*c*) office or clinic-administered chemotherapeutic agents (e.g., cancer, neutropenia, anemia).

As a result of the increased risk of clinically important adverse effects, these agents dictate increased safety surveillance. The U.S. Food and Drug Administration (FDA) has mandated the implementation of a risk minimization action plan (i.e., RiskMAP) for those products with high risk. The plan is a strategic risk assessment plan designed to minimize product risk while preserving its benefits to the patient (4). Given their ability to affect complex processes in the body, biological products including vaccines have a higher likelihood of adverse effects than traditional or chemical agents. Nearly one-third of boxed warnings for biological pharmaceuticals between January 1995 and 2007 were added within 2 years after the products' approval by the FDA. Thus, it is important for pharmacists to participate in extensive adverse event monitoring of new products because a significant number of serious adverse reactions are not identified until the products are marketed for clinical use.

It is important to indicate that specialty products are not constituted solely with biotechnology products, which typically implies peptide products developed with recombinant technology. There are some nonpeptide injectables, for example, treprostinil sodium, and some oral specialty products, for example, bosentan and imatinib, for rare diseases that fall under this umbrella definition. Thus, the definition of specialty products will continue to evolve.

The first novel *biotechnologic* pharmaceuticals were proteins, but eventually, an increasing number will be smaller molecules, discovered through biotechnology-based methods that will determine just how proteins work. Clearly, biotechnology has established itself as a mainstay

in pharmaceutical research and development, and new products will continue to enter the market at an increasing pace in the future. Biotechnologic products are produced through highly complex processes from genetically engineered cell cultures, rather than synthesized chemically like small-molecule pharmaceuticals (5).

Biosimilars, also known as follow-on biologics, are biologic products that are "highly similar to and have [sic] no clinically meaningful differences from an existing FDA-approved biologic product." Biosimilars are produced by a different manufacturer following patent and exclusivity expiration on the original innovator product. For example, adalimumab was originally marketed as Humira®. Since the market exclusivity period for Humira® expired, the FDA has approved adalimumab biosimilar products from four different manufacturers.

Biologics differ from the more common small-molecule drugs as they generally exhibit high molecular complexity and may be quite sensitive to changes in manufacturing processes. The manufacturers of biosimilars do not have access to the originator's molecular clone and original cell bank, to the exact fermentation and purification process, or to the active drug substance. However, they do have access to the commercialized innovator product. Because differences in impurities and/or breakdown products can potentially have serious health implications, there is a concern that copies of biologics might perform differently than the original branded version of the product. Health insurers tend to view these as potentially cost-saving equivalents.

A vast number of biotechnology-derived medications have been approved and made available since human insulin became the first therapeutic recombinant protein drug in 1982. The commercial success of biotechnology spurred the entry of many additional products into the development pipelines since that time. This abundant activity grew out of entrepreneurism among many small venture-funded, narrowly focused groups. Several of these small companies have by now prospered to the point of becoming fully integrated pharmaceutical companies. It was anticipated then that patients with hemophilia, serious sepsis, skin ulcers, rheumatoid arthritis, and a number of cancers would benefit in future years as drugs in clinical trials secured market approval, and this has come to fruition. As some of those biotechnologic products are now on the market (e.g., ReFacto for hemophilia, Fuzeon for HIV therapy, Kineret for mild to moderate rheumatoid arthritis in patients who have failed one or more disease-modifying antirheumatic drugs [DMARDs], Xigris for severe sepsis), it is anticipated that this trend will continue.

As of 2020, there were more than 500 biologic and specialty products approved by the FDA (5,6). The growth of this grouping of pharmaceuticals is fueled with higher costs for existing specialty products (e.g., $10,000 treatment regimen cost per month), the introduction of new drugs to treat conditions where few drug alternatives exist, new indications for existing drugs, and an increasing degree of off-label use.

TECHNIQUES USED TO PRODUCE BIOTECHNOLOGIC PRODUCTS

Numerous techniques are used to create biotechnologic products. These include rDNA technology, MAb technology, polymerase chain reaction, gene therapy, nucleotide blockade or antisense nucleic acids, and peptide technology. The following section describes each of these techniques.

Recombinant DNA

DNA, deoxyribonucleic acid, has been called the substance of life. It is DNA that constitutes genes, allowing cells to reproduce and maintain life. Of more than 1 million kinds of plants and animals known today, no two are exactly alike; however, the similarity within families is the result of genetic information stored in cells, duplicated, and passed from cell to cell and from generation to generation. It is DNA that provides this continuity.

DNA was first isolated in 1869. Its chemical composition was determined in the early 1900s, and by the 1940s, it had been proved that the genes within cell chromosomes are made of DNA. It was not until the 1950s when James D. Watson and Francis H.C. Crick postulated the structure of DNA that biologists began to comprehend the molecular mechanisms of heredity and cell regulation. Watson and Crick described their model of DNA as a double helix, two strands of DNA coiled about themselves like a spiral staircase. It is now known that the two strands of DNA are connected by the bases adenine, guanine, cytosine, and thymine (A, G, C, and T). The order of arrangement of these bases with the two strands of DNA comprises a specific gene for a specific trait. A typical gene has hundreds of bases that are always arranged in pairs. When A occurs on one strand, T occurs opposite it on the other; G pairs with C. A gene is a segment of DNA that has a specific sequence of these chemical base pairs. The pattern constitutes the DNA message for maintaining cells and organisms and building the next generation. To create a new cell or a whole new organism, DNA must be able to duplicate (clone) itself. This is done by unwinding and separating the two strands and attaching new bases to each from within the cell according to the A-T/C-G rule. The result is two new double strands of DNA, each of the same structure and conformation.

DNA also plays an essential role in the production of proteins for cellular maintenance and function. DNA is translated to messenger RNA (mRNA), which specifies the amino acid sequence of a protein. Amino acids can be arranged in a vast number of combinations to produce hundreds of thousands of proteins. In essence, a cell is a miniature assembly plant for production of thousands of proteins. A single *Escherichia coli* bacterium is capable of making about 2,000 proteins.

The ability to selectively hydrolyze a population of DNA molecules with a number of endonucleases enabled a technique for joining two different DNA molecules: recombinant DNA, or *rDNA*. This technique uses nucleic acid replication, separation, and identification methods that permit production of large quantities of purified DNA fragments. These combined techniques, referred to as *rDNA technology*, allow the selection and removal of a specific desired piece of DNA out of a larger, more complex molecule. Consequently, rDNAs have been prepared with DNA fragments from bacteria combined with fragments from humans, viruses with viruses, and so forth. The ability to join two different pieces of DNA at specific sites within the molecules is achieved with two enzymes: a restriction endonuclease and a DNA ligase.

With rDNA technology, scientists can use nonhuman cells (e.g., a special strain of *E. coli*) to manufacture proteins identical to those produced in human cells. This process has enabled scientists to produce much larger quantities of human biomolecules than was previously available from human sources. For example, approximately 50 cadaver pituitary glands were required to treat a single growth hormone–deficient child for 1 year until rDNA-produced growth hormone became available. Further, the biosynthetic product does not have the viral contamination that was associated with the cadaver source. Human growth hormone (hGH) and insulin were the first rDNA products to become available for patients' use.

DNA probe technology is being used to diagnose disease. It uses small pieces of DNA to search a cell for viral infection or for genetic defects. DNA probes have application in testing for infectious disease, cancer, genetic defects, and susceptibility to disease. Using DNA probes, scientists can locate a disease-causing gene, which in turn can lead to the development of replacement therapies. In producing a DNA probe, the initial step is synthesis of the specific DNA sequence that is complementary to the gene being investigated. For instance, to test for a particular virus, a DNA sequence complementary to a viral gene is developed. The second step is to tag the synthetic gene with a dye or radioactive isotope. When introduced into a specimen, the synthetic strand of DNA acts as a probe, searching for a matching or complementary strand. When one is found, the two hybridize or join together via A–T and G–C base pairing. When the probe is bound to the virus, the dye or radioactive tag reveals the location of the viral gene through specialized imaging techniques.

Monoclonal Antibodies (MAbs)

When a foreign protein or antigen molecule enters the body, an immune response begins. Each antigen molecule may contain several different epitopes or antigenic sites, and lines of B lymphocytes will proliferate, each secreting an immunoglobulin (antibody) molecule that fits a single epitope. The mixture of several antibodies against the same antigen is called a polyclonal antibody.

By contrast, MAbs are produced by perpetuating the expression of a single B lymphocyte. Consequently, all of the antibody molecules secreted by a series of daughter cells derived from a single dividing parent B lymphocyte are genetically identical. Through the development of hybridoma technology emanating from Kohler and Milstein's research (7), it became possible to produce identical monospecific antibodies in almost unlimited quantities. These are constructed by the fusion of B lymphocytes, stimulated with a specific antigen, with immortal myeloma cells (8). The resultant hybridomas can be maintained in cultures and produce large amounts of antibodies.

Most MAbs now in use belong to the immunoglobulin G (IgG) subclass. The IgG molecule has a molecular weight between 150 and 180 kDa and consists of two heavy and two light polypeptide chains connected by disulfide bonds (Fig. 19.1). The heavy and the light chains can be divided into a variable and a constant domain. The constant domain amino acid sequence is relatively conserved among immunoglobulins of a specific class (e.g., IgG, IgM). The variable domains of an antibody population are highly heterogeneous. It is the variable domain that gives the antibody its binding specificity and affinity. Thus, the antibody engineer must be cautious to maintain the tertiary structure and orientation of the complementary determining region.

MAbs were originally derived from mouse B lymphocytes, and patients exposed to them have developed human antimouse antibody (HAMA) responses, which limited the utility of these MAb products. Presence of HAMA tended to cause a typical allergic reaction (chills, urticaria, wheezing) and decrease drug activity when the patient received subsequent doses of the MAb.

Failed efforts with murine MAbs led to the development of MAbs with human components and evolution of a new class of antibody-like molecules, or *man-made antibodies* (9). Consequently, chimeric and humanized antibodies have been constructed to overcome the lack of intrinsic antitumor activity and the immunogenicity of many murine MAbs. These MAbs retain the binding specificity of the original rodent antibody determined by the variable region but have the potential to activate the human immune system through their human constant region (10). They are also less likely to generate production of HAMA.

As an example, smaller fragments that contain intact immunoglobulin-binding sites, such as F[ab']$_2$ and Fab', do not contain the lower binding domain of the molecule (Fig. 19.2). A smaller molecule will tend to be less immunogenic when administered systemically and is more likely to have a greater tumor penetration than a larger structure (9). Also, in diagnostic imaging applications, smaller fragments have demonstrated greater renal, biliary, and colonic uptake at 24 hours than the whole IgG, because of filtering by the kidneys and excretion via the biliary system of small protein compounds. All three smaller antibody forms have had success at detecting smaller (<2 cm) lesions not seen on computed tomography (CT) and are superior to the IgC anticarcinoembryonic antigen antibody.

Another example is the smaller Sfv molecule, which contains the heavy and light chains of the binding sites joined by the shorter link (Fig. 19.2). These molecules also have been engineered to attach toxins, cytokines, radiolabeled elements, or genes, thus broadening their ability as delivery vehicles for cancer therapy.

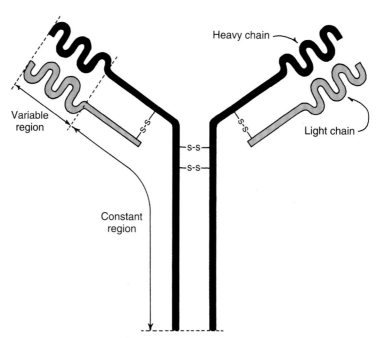

FIGURE 19.1. Basic shape of an immunoglobulin molecule akin to the class IgG, a heterogeneous population of molecules sharing a y-shaped structure composed of a heavy and light molecular chain linked by disulfide bonds. (Illustration by Alan J. Slade.)

IgG molecule   F[ab']₂   Fab'   Sfv

FIGURE 19.2. An IgG molecule and its fragments. (Illustration by Alan J. Slade.)

Today, fully human MAbs are produced in the mouse whose murine genes are inactivated and replaced by human sequences. The immunogenicity of fully human MAbs is low because they are 100% human and contain no mouse protein. At present, there are four types of MAbs. The suffix used in the name of the MAb indicates the source. The suffix *-omab* indicates murine, the earliest type of MAb derived entirely from mice, that is, mouse protein. The suffix *-ximab* indicates chimeric, which has a human constant region and a murine variable region. This was the second-generation MAb and emerged because of the high incidence of HAMA reactions with murine MAbs. The immune response and incidence of HAMA reactions were much lower for chimeric MAbs than with murine MAbs. Further, there was now a broader range of antigenic specificities, enhanced therapeutic activity, and more optimal pharmacodynamics (i.e., increased affinity for the antigen) and pharmacokinetic changes (e.g., longer $t_{½}$). The third generation of MAbs was the humanized MAbs that are 90% human, containing only 10% mouse protein in the variable region. The suffix *-zumab* indicates a humanized MAb. Eventually, the fourth-generation MAb was created and fully human. The suffix is *-umab*, and these MAbs are created in mice whose murine genes are inactivated and replaced with human sequences. As would be expected, the immunogenicity of fully human MAbs is low because there is no mouse protein. In addition, the fourth-generation MAbs are cleared at a slower rate from plasma because of the lack of the mouse component.

Polymerase Chain Reaction

Polymerase chain reaction is a biotechnologic process whereby there is substantial amplification (more than 100,000-fold) of a target nucleic acid sequence (a gene). This enzymatic reaction occurs in repeated cycles of a three-step process. First, DNA is denatured to separate the two strands. Next, a nucleic acid primer is hybridized to each DNA strand at a specific location within the nucleic acid sequence. Finally, a DNA polymerase enzyme is added for extension of the primer along the DNA strand to copy the target nucleic acid sequence.

Each cycle doubles the number of DNA molecules. This cycle is repeated until sufficient DNA sequence material is copied. For example, 20 cycles with a 90% success rate will yield 375,000, that is, 1.9^{20}, copies of each DNA strand in the starting solution.

Gene Therapy

Gene therapy is a process in which exogenous genetic material is transferred into somatic cells to correct an inherited or acquired gene defect. Also, it is intended to introduce a new function or property into cells. These common and life-threatening diseases include cystic fibrosis, hemophilia, sickle cell anemia, and diabetes.

Scientific technology has developed safe and efficient means to transfer genes into cells. Consequently, genetic and molecular delineation of the underlying pathophysiology of many of the primary immunodeficiency disorders has occurred, and gene-based therapy is now a viable option as long as the transferred genetic material can be delivered to the appropriate target cell or tissue.

Controversial ethical considerations over genetic intervention of germ line cells have fostered bioengineering to focus on gene therapy of somatic cells. Because somatic cells are end-stage differentiated cells, research has examined the use of a self-renewing stem cell population for therapeutic transfer of genetic material. Stem cells can renew themselves, and the inserted gene will remain in place through subsequent generations of differentiated cells or tissue populations.

As an example, a patient's cells (e.g., T lymphocytes) are harvested and grown in the laboratory. The cells receive the gene from a viral carrier (e.g., Moloney murine leukemia virus) and start to produce the missing protein necessary to correct the deficiency. These cells with the extra functional gene are then returned to the patient, and the normal protein is produced and released, alleviating the disease.

The genetic cause of numerous primary immunodeficiency disorders has been discovered and described. As a result, gene therapy can now be used as an alternative therapy, particularly in patients for whom bone marrow transplantation may not be suitable (e.g., a bone marrow donor cannot be identified, or preparation for transplantation carries substantial risk to the patient). The first primary immunodeficiency disease to be defined was adenosine deaminase (ADA) deficiency. The gene encoding for ADA is found on chromosome 20. Gene deletions and point mutations result in a loss or severe reduction in ADA enzymatic activity, leading to a clinical presentation of severe combined immunodeficiency disease (SCID) and often causing death in childhood or adolescence.

The first human protocol for gene therapy was performed in ADA patients in 1990 at the National Institutes of Health. Since that time, the genetic defects of several other primary immunodeficiency disorders have been defined, and the defects have been at least partially corrected by gene therapy using hemopoietic stem cells in vitro. For SCID and other diseases, gene therapy is lifesaving (11). As of July 2020, there were more than 100 phase 3 clinical trials of gene therapies registered with clinicaltrials.gov.

Nucleotide Blockade/Antisense

Nucleotide blockade and antisense technology focuses on the study of function of specific proteins and intracellular expression. The sequence of a nucleotide chain that contains the information for protein synthesis is called the sense sequence. The nucleotide chain that is complementary to the sense sequence is called the antisense sequence. Antisense drugs recognize and bind to the nucleotide sense sequence of specific mRNA molecules, preventing synthesis of unwanted proteins and actually destroying the sense molecules in the process.

The introduction of antisense nucleic acids into cells has provided new ideas to explore how proteins, whose expression has been selectively repressed in a cell, function within that cell. Another goal is to arrest the expression of dysfunctional mRNA or DNA and control disease processes. Antisense technology is part of a new approach termed *reverse genetics.*

Antisense RNA, for example, can be introduced into the cell by cloning. The specific gene of interest is cloned in an expression vector in the wrong orientation so that complementary mRNA is created to match abnormal mRNA. Then when the two mRNA strands complex together, translation of the mRNA to form disease-producing proteins is prevented. Anti-DNA strands also can be created to complex with DNA to form a triple helix. Oligonucleotides, or short single strands of nucleic acids, instead of the full mRNA, also can be employed to block RNA expression. This form of biotechnology is being used for viral disease (e.g., herpes simplex, HIV) and cancer (oncogenes).

Peptide Technology

Peptide technology entails screening for polypeptide molecules that can mimic larger proteins. This is intended to afford relatively simple products that can be stable and easy to produce. These peptides can serve as either protein receptor agonists or antagonists.

Formulation Composition

Most of the biotechnology products are proteins, but some may soon be smaller peptide-like molecules. Proteins are inherently unstable molecules, and their degradation profiles can be quite complex. Biotechnology products differ from conventional small-molecule drug products in their method of preparation and in the potential problems presented in their formulation. Pharmacists involved in compounding with biologically active proteins will be interested in their stabilization, formulation, and delivery.

In working with biotechnologically derived drugs, one must be cognizant of both the active drug constituent and the total drug delivery system, or carrier. Protein drugs are extremely potent and are generally used in quite low concentrations. The bulk of most compounded preparations may be the excipients. In addition to the vehicle, buffers, and the like, stabilizers are often incorporated in these products. A number of different stabilizers can be used, including surfactants, amino acids, polyhydric alcohols, fatty acids, proteins, antioxidants, reducing agents, and metal ions. Table 19.1 describes agents used as stabilizers.

pH is one of the key factors in developing a stable product. The optimal pH range for a specific product can be achieved through the selection of appropriate physiologic buffers. Usually, buffer concentrations are in the range of 0.01 to 0.1 M. In general, an increase in the buffer concentration means an increase in pain on injection.

Chelating agents can be incorporated to bind trace metals such as copper, iron, calcium, and manganese. Ethylenediaminetetraacetic acid (EDTA) is commonly used at a concentration of about 0.01% to 0.05%.

Antioxidants are often incorporated because oxidation is one of the major factors in protein degradation. Ascorbic acid, sodium disulfide, monothioglycerol, and α-tocopherol are frequently used at a concentration of about 0.05% to 0.1%.

Preservatives may be necessary; these could include phenol (0.3% to 0.5%), chlorobutanol (0.3% to 0.5%), and benzyl alcohol (1.0% to 3.0%).

Polyols are good stabilizers and are commonly used in concentrations from 1% to 10%.

Tonicity-adjusting agents include sodium chloride and dextrose in concentrations necessary to achieve isotonicity with 0.9% sodium chloride solution, or approximately 290 mOsm/L.

Preparation

A general rule for working with biotechnology formulations is to keep procedures as simple as possible. Sterility must be maintained in any preparation of parenteral products, because most do not contain a preservative. It is recommended that only one dose be prepared from each vial or container to minimize contamination. Many times this is not practical, however, as specific manipulations are needed to meet patient needs. Facilities should be clean, and proper techniques should be used.

TABLE 19.1. Stabilizing Agents for Biotechnology Preparations

Class	Agent	Action
Amino acids	Alanine Arginine Aspartic acid Glycine Glutamic acid Leucine	Serves as a solubilizer Serves as a buffer Inhibits isomerism Serves as a stabilizer Serves as a thermostabilizer Inhibits aggregation
Antioxidants	Ascorbic acid, cysteine hydrochloride, glutathione, thioglycerol, thioglycolic acid, thiosorbitol	Help stabilize protein conformation
Chelating agents	EDTA salts	Inhibit oxidation by removing metal ions, glutamic acid, and aspartic acid
Fatty acids	Phosphatidyl choline, ethanolamine	Serve as stabilizers
Proteins	Human serum albumin	Prevents surface adsorption; stabilizes protein conformation; serves as a complexing agent and cryoprotectant
Metal ions	Ca^{2+}, Ni^{2+}, Mg^{2+}, Mn^{2+}	Help stabilize protein conformation
Polyhydric alcohols	Ethylene glycol Glucose Lactose Mannitol Propylene glycol Sorbitol Sucrose Trehalose	Serves as a stabilizer Strengthens conformation Serves as a stabilizer Serves as a cryoprotectant Prevents aggregation Prevents denaturation and aggregation Serves as a stabilizer Serves as a stabilizer
Polymers	PEG, povidone	Prevent aggregation
Surfactants	Poloxamer 407 Polysorbate 20 and polysorbate 80	Prevents denaturation and stabilizes cloudiness Retard aggregation

Source: Bontempo JA. Development of Biopharmaceutical Parenteral Dosage Forms. New York, NY: Marcel Dekker, 1997:112–113.

A kit for testing aseptic technique in preparing formulations is available from equipment suppliers. At a minimum, a laminar-airflow hood should be used and appropriate attire worn. All equipment must be sterile. Any additive used in compounding parenteral drug products must be free of pyrogens; if a preparation becomes contaminated with pyrogens, it should be discarded. Two special considerations in working with biotechnologically derived preparations—the use of filters and the sorption of these drugs to containers—are discussed in the following sections.

The use of filters in manipulating biotechnology products can result in some loss of the drug available to the patient. For example, muromonab-CD3 (Orthoclone OKT3) injection should be filtered with a low–protein-binding filter of 0.2 to 0.22 μm. Many biotechnology products should not be filtered at all. If a filtration device is part of the IV administration apparatus, biotechnology drugs should generally be administered distal to the site of the filter. Filters that have been shown to minimize protein adsorption are those made from polyvinylidene difluoride, polycarbonate, polysulfone, and regenerated cellulose. As a precaution, low–protein-binding filters should be used.

Sorption of proteins to containers can result in drug loss. This loss can be minimized either by the use of albumin or by siliconization. Adding about 0.1% albumin to the product can decrease the sorption of proteins to containers. If glass mixing vessels are used, the albumin solution should be added before the drug. If siliconization is used, the compounding pharmacist should prepare a silicon solution or emulsion and soak or rinse the glass vials in it. The drained vials should then be placed in an oven at about 250°C for 5 to 6 hours. This procedure will minimize protein adsorption to glass; it can be used for both the preparation equipment and the packaging containers.

Physicochemical Considerations

To retain a drug's biologic activity up to the time of administration to the patient, some factors associated with handling proteins must be considered: selecting an appropriate vehicle for drug delivery, individualizing dosages, administering drugs through novel drug delivery systems, preparing drugs for delivery through these systems, monitoring their efficacy, and counseling patients on their use.

Some issues specific to protein pharmaceuticals are as follows:

- Their high molecular weight and potential for aggregation (i.e., a small change in structure can result in a change in activity)
- Their immunogenic potential, because some are produced by a fermentation-type process and proteins can copurify with proteins

- The assignment of potency to the reference standards (when traditional pharmaceuticals are about 98% pure, these materials may be only 0.1% to 1% active, with their activity assigned by potentially variable assays)
- The use of micropipettes, which can require frequent calibration
- Concern that constituted products can be less stable than lyophilized products
- The effect of agitation on a product's stability
- Possible interaction of the product with the inner wall of the glass vial and with the elastomeric closure
- The effectiveness of the preservative if a multidose product is mixed with other products

Physicochemical factors to be considered in compounding protein drug products include the structure of the protein drug, isoelectric point, molecular weight, solubility and factors affecting solubility (e.g., surfactants, salts, metal ions, pH), stability and factors affecting stability (e.g., pH, temperature, light, oxygen, metal ions, freeze–thaw cycles, mechanical stress), polymorphism, stereoisomers, filtration media compatibility, shear, and surface denaturation.

Solubility depends on a number of factors, including chemical structure, pH, and temperature. Proteins are generally more soluble in their native environment or medium or in a matrix that mimics their native environment, such as sodium chloride, trace elements, lipids, and other proteins in an aqueous medium. Before compounding these products, pharmacists must consider the ingredients' effects on the solubility of the active drug, especially because most of the products are currently administered parenterally. This task is critical because the actual drug is present in a small quantity and can go unnoticed if it precipitates. Sterile water for injection and 0.9% sodium chloride solution usually are good vehicles for use in a formulation.

The pH of the compound should be maintained close to the pH of the originally approved, manufactured product; changes in pH can affect proteins in numerous ways. Chemical degradation rate constants are pH related, and hydrogen ion concentration can affect the actual structure of proteins (i.e., quaternary structure). Buffer systems may be needed in compounding; they should be prepared at the minimum buffer strength required to produce the most stable drug product.

Chemical instability of proteins is the modification of protein structures by bond formation or cleavage to yield a new compound. *Physical instability* generally involves changes in structure, conformation, or behavior in a particular environment. Stability, both chemical and physical, depends on pH, temperature, and agitation, as well as on the overall environment in which the drug is contained.

Sorption is a problem with colony-stimulating factors (CSFs) and with aldesleukin (Proleukin) at low concentrations. To minimize "sticking" of the protein to the glass, it may be helpful to add about 0.1% albumin to the product to occupy the potential binding sites in the container. Pharmacists must consider this problem before making any changes in packaging.

Agitation, which is frothing created by the physical decomposition of the protein, can adversely affect the product in two ways. First, frothing can cause difficulties in using a syringe to withdraw the required amount of drug from a vial. To avoid this problem, the formulator should mix the product by rolling the vial in the hands or gently swirling it. Second, excessive agitation can cause changes in a protein's quaternary structure that often reduce or eliminate a drug's therapeutic activity. Some products, such as filgrastim (Neupogen) and sargramostim (Leukine), are reconstituted by directing a soft stream of diluent against the inside of the container wall. Others, such as recombinant tissue plasminogen activator (tPA; alteplase), are reconstituted by directing a stream of diluent directly into the product at the bottom of the vial.

Quality Control

The compounding pharmacist should follow standard quality control procedures. The compounded preparations can be tested for pH, final volume, sterility, and pyrogenicity and physically observed for clarity, presence of gas bubbles and particulate matter, and change in color.

■ PRODUCTS OF BIOTECHNOLOGY

Biotechnologic drugs fall into major classes, such as antisense, clotting factors, hematopoietic factors, hormones, interferons, interleukins (ILs), MAbs, tissue growth factors, and vaccines. Biotechnologic drugs are distinguished by whether they are physiologic or nonphysiologic peptides or new biotechnology products.

Physiologic peptides can be further subdivided by intended use. For example, those for substitution include clotting factors, insulin, hGH, and erythropoietin. Biotechnologic products intended for therapeutic purposes in nonphysiologic concentrations include interferons, cytokines, tPA, and urokinase. Nonphysiologic peptides include mutants of physiologic peptides, vaccines, thrombolytic agents, and antithrombics.

The following sections describe by classification products of biotechnology that have been approved by the FDA or are being developed for submission for approval (Table 19.2). The section describing indication also lists in brackets for some biotechnology drugs and products proposed uses under the Orphan Drug Act. (The FDA Office of Orphan Products Development provides an information packet that includes an overview of the FDA's orphan drug program, a brief description of the orphan products grant program, and a current list on designated orphan products.)

TABLE 19.2. Representative Biotechnology Products in Use in the United States

Generic Name	Trade Name (Manufacturer)	Indications [Proposed Use][a]
Aldesleukin	Proleukin (Prometheus)	Metastatic renal cell carcinoma, melanoma; primary immunodeficiency disease of T-cell defects
Alteplase	Activase (Genentech)	Ischemic stroke
Conjugate vaccine	PedvaxHIB (Merck & Co.)	Routine immunization of children aged 2–71 mo
Efavirenz	Sustiva (Bristol-Myers Squibb)	Treatment of HIV-1 in combination with 2, 3, or 4 other anti-HIV drugs
Epoetin alfa	Epogen (Ortho Biotech, Procrit)	Certain anemias; chronic renal disease; AIDS; cancer chemotherapy [anemia associated with end-stage renal disease or HIV infection or treatment; myelodysplastic syndrome; anemia of prematurity in preterm infants]
Filgrastim G-CSF	Neupogen (Amgen)	Decrease incidence of infection (febrile neutropenia) in nonmyeloid malignancies treated with myelosuppressive drugs. Reduce duration of neutropenia, neutropenia-related sequelae in nonmyeloid malignancies treated with myeloablative chemotherapy followed by bone marrow transplant [severe chronic neutropenia (absolute neutrophil count <500/mm^3); neutropenia of bone marrow transplant; CMV retinitis of AIDS treated with ganciclovir; mobilization of peripheral blood progenitor cells for collection prior to myeloablative or myelosuppressive chemotherapy; reduce duration of neutropenia, fever, antibiotic use, hospitalization following induction, consolidation for acute myeloid leukemia.]
Haemophilus B conjugate vaccine	ActHIB (Aventis Pasteur)	Routine immunization of children against invasive diseases of HIB
Hepatitis B vaccine	Engerix-B (GlaxoSmithKline), Recombivax HB (Merck)	Hepatitis B prophylaxis
Human growth hormone	Protropin (Genentech), Humatrope (Lilly)	hGH deficiency in children
Human insulin	Humulin (Lilly), Rapid, Velosulin (Novo Nordisk)	Insulin-dependent diabetes mellitus
Imciromab pentetate	Myoscint (Centocor)	[Detection of early necrosis as indication of rejection of orthotopic cardiac transplant]
Infliximab	Remicade (Centocor)	Active and fistulizing Crohn disease
Interferon alfa-2b	Intron A (Schering)	Hairy cell leukemia; AIDS-related Kaposi sarcoma; chronic hepatitis B and C (non-A, non-B); condylomata acuminate
Interferon alfa-n3	Alferon N (Hemispherx Biopharma)	Condylomata acuminata
Interferon beta-1b	Betaseron (Bayer)	Multiple sclerosis
Interferon gamma-1b	Actimmune (Intermune)	Chronic granulomatous disease
Muromonab-CD3	Orthoclone (Ortho Biotech), OKT 3 (Biotech)	Acute allograft rejection in renal transplant patients
Recombinant factor VIII	Kogenate (Bayer), Recombinate (Baxter)	Hemophilia A
Rituximab	Rituxan (Biogen, IDEC/Genentech)	Relapsed or refractory low-grade or follicular CD20-positive beta-cell NHL
Sargramostim (GM-CSF)	Leukine (Genzyme)	Myeloid reconstitution after bone marrow transplantation [Leukine: neutropenia of bone marrow transplant, graft failure, delay of engraftment, promotion of early engraftment; reduce neutropenia, leukopenia; decrease incidence of death from infection in AML]
Somatropin	Genotropin (Pfizer), Humatrope (Lilly), Norditropin (Novo Nordisk)	[Long-term treatment of children with growth failure of inadequate endogenous growth hormone; growth failure in children with inadequate growth hormone; idiopathic or organic growth hormone deficiency in children with growth failure; enhancement of nitrogen retention in hospitalized patients with severe burns; short stature in Turner syndrome; adults with growth hormone deficiency]

(Continued)

TABLE 19.2. Representative Biotechnology Products in Use in the United States *(Continued)*

Generic Name	Trade Name (Manufacturer)	Indications [Proposed Use][a]
Somatropin for injection	Humatrope (Lilly), Nutropin (Genentech)	Long-term treatment for growth failure in children who lack endogenous growth hormone secretion. [Long-term treatment of children with growth failure of inadequate secretion of normal endogenous growth hormone; short stature in Turner syndrome; growth retardation in CRF; catabolism/weight loss in AIDS; children with AIDS-associated failure to thrive, including wasting; replacement therapy for growth hormone deficiency in adults with epiphyseal closure]
tPA (alteplase)	Activase (Genentech)	Management of AMI in adults to improve ventricular function and reduce incidence of CHF and mortality of AMI. Management of acute ischemic stroke in adults to improve neurologic recovery and reduce disability. Management of acute massive PE, lysis of acute PE, defined by obstruction of blood flow to a lobe or multiple segments of the lungs, and for lysis of PE with unstable hemodynamics
Reteplase	Retavase (Centocor)	Management of AMI in adults to improve ventricular function following AMI, reduce incidence of CHF, reduce mortality of AMI
Trastuzumab	Herceptin (Genentech)	Treatment of metastatic HER2-positive breast cancer or cancer spread beyond breast and lymph nodes under arm. Used alone in patients with primary failure with other chemotherapies or as a first-line treatment of metastatic disease in combination with paclitaxel. Approved as part of an adjuvant treatment including chemotherapy for early-stage HER2-positive breast cancer that may or may not have spread to the lymph nodes. If the cancer has not spread into the lymph nodes (node-negative), the cancer needs to be estrogen receptor/progesterone receptor negative or have one high-risk fact

[a]Listing includes proposed uses for orphaned drugs in [brackets]. The Orphan Drug Act defines an orphan drug as a drug or biologic product for the diagnosis, treatment, or prevention of a rare disease or condition. A rare disease is one that affects fewer than 200,000 persons in the United States or more than 200,000 persons but without reasonable expectation that the cost of developing and marketing the drug will be recovered from sales in the United States.

Antisense Drugs

Golodirsen (Vyondys 53)

Golodirsen injection is an antisense drug approved for treatment of Duchenne muscular dystrophy patients with a specific mutation in the *DMD* gene. Golodirsen binds to exon 53 of the *DMD* gene and prevents its expression. This causes the patient's skeletal muscles to produce greater amounts of dystrophin, which is deficient in muscular dystrophy. Golodirsen is primarily excreted in the urine, so it is advisable to determine the patient's renal function before initiating therapy. Golodirsen is supplied as a sterile solution in single dose vials of 100 mg in 2 mL. The solution contains sodium chloride as an osmotic agent and is buffered with potassium phosphate monobasic and sodium phosphate dibasic. It should be stored in the refrigerator at 2°C to 8°C and protected from light. It should not be frozen. To prepare the solution for infusion, the vials are allowed to warm to room temperature and the appropriate volume of drug solution is diluted in normal saline to a total volume between 100 and 150 mL. The diluted product must be inspected of particulates prior to administration to the patient. The infusion is administered over 35 to 60 minutes and should not be mixed with any other drugs.

Efavirenz (Sustiva)

Efavirenz is a nonnucleoside reverse transcriptase inhibitor and the first anti-HIV drug to be approved by the FDA for once-daily dosing in combination with other anti-HIV drugs.

Clinical trials demonstrated that efavirenz reduces plasma viral RNA to below quantifiable levels in a majority of HIV-1–infected naive and treatment-experienced individuals in two-, three-, and four-drug combinations.

Efavirenz is available as an oral capsule and can be taken once a day on an empty stomach, preferably at bedtime to improve any nervous system symptoms. However, if taken with food, it is advised that it should not be administered with high-fat meals, because this interaction may increase the drug's systemic absorption.

Clotting Factors

Hemophiliacs bleed internally because of a lack of clotting protein factors. Historically, treatment has been infusions of protein derived from human blood. Now, genetic engineering can create, without donor blood, factors that produce more nearly contaminant-free products and therefore expose the patient to fewer contaminants.

Systemic Antihemophilic Factors (Kogenate FS, Recombinate)

Recombinant antihemophilic factor (AHF) is indicated for the treatment of classical hemophilia A, in which there is a demonstrated deficiency of activity of plasma clotting factor (factor VIII). Human recombinant AHF (rAHF) is a sterile, nonpyrogenic concentrate with biologic and pharmacokinetic activity comparable to that of plasma-derived AHF. Additional clinical trials are being conducted to determine whether antibodies to rAHF form more often than with plasma-derived products (11).

rAHF contains albumin as a stabilizer and trace amounts of mouse, hamster, and bovine proteins. These products are made by modifying hamster cells so that they produce a highly purified version of AHF factor VIII.

Each vial of AHF is labeled with the AHF activity expressed in international units (IU). The assignment of potency is referenced to the WHO International Standard. One IU of factor VIII activity, approximately equal to the AHF activity of 1 mL of fresh plasma, increases the plasma concentration of factor VIII by 2%. The specific factor VIII activity ranges from 2 to 200 AHF IU per milligram of total protein.

The dose–response relation is linear, with an approximate yield of a 2% rise in factor VIII activity for each unit of factor VIII per kilogram transfused. The following formulas provide a guide for dosing calculations:

$$\text{Expected factor VIII increase (\%normal)}$$
$$= \frac{\text{dose AFH/IU administered} \times 2}{\text{body weight (kg)}}$$

$$\text{AFH/IU required}$$
$$= \text{body weight (kg)}$$
$$\times \text{desired factor VIII increase}$$
$$(\%\text{normal}) \times 0.5$$

Kogenate FS is available in strengths of 250 IU, 500 IU, and 1,000 IU with 2.5 mL sterile water for injection provided as diluent, and 2,000 IU and 3,000 IU with 5 mL sterile water for injection provided as diluent. Each strength contains 2 to 3 mmol/L of calcium chloride, 26 to 36 mEq/L of sodium, and 31 to 40 mEq/L of chloride. The product is stabilized with sucrose, glycine, and histidine. Kogenate is supplied in a single-dose vial along with the diluent, a sterile filter needle, and a sterile administration set.

Recombinate is available in strengths of 250, 500, and 1,000 IU, 1,500 IU, and 2,000 IU each with 10 mL sterile water for injection provided as diluent. Each strength contains 12.5 mg/mL of human albumin, 180 mEq/L of sodium, 200 mEq/L of calcium, and a small quantity of foreign protein.

Dry concentrates of rAHF should be stored at 2°C to 8°C (35°F to 46°F) and the diluent protected from freezing. Kogenate may be stored at room temperatures not exceeding 25°C for 3 months. After reconstitution, the solution should not be refrigerated.

The diluent and dry concentrate should be brought to room temperature (~25°C) prior to reconstitution. These may be allowed to warm to room temperature or, in an emergency, warmed via water bath to a range of 30°C to 37°C (86°F to 98.6°F). Once reconstituted, the solution should not be shaken, because shaking could make it foam. The solution should be administered within 3 hours of reconstitution and any partially used vial discarded. This preparation should be administered alone through a separate line, without mixing with other intravenous fluids or medications.

Recombinant Factor VIII (ReFacto)

Approved for clinical use in March 2000, recombinant factor VIII is indicated for control and prevention of bleeding episodes and surgical prophylaxis to reduce the frequency of spontaneous bleeding episodes (Fig. 19.3). This product is the only factor VIII product indicated for short-term routine prophylaxis.

Hemophilia A is the most common form of hemophilia, an inherited blood disorder. Approximately, 17,000 American patients have hemophilia A. This form of the disease is the result of deficiency in blood clotting factor VIII.

Recombinant technology allows preparation of clotting factors without human blood or plasma products. This eliminates the risk of blood-borne viral contamination associated with nonrecombinant factor VIII products prepared from pooled human blood. Also, ReFacto does not contain human serum albumin, whereas previously approved recombinant products (e.g., Kogenate, Bayer) add albumin during the cell culture phase and during the final product formulation. This procedure theoretically increases the possibility of viral contamination in the final product.

Colony-Stimulating Factors

CSFs are four glycoprotein regulators that bind to specific surface receptors and control the proliferation and differentiation of marrow cells into macrophages, neutrophils, basophils, eosinophils, platelets, or erythrocytes (12,13). These recombinant human CSFs have demonstrated use in oncology (e.g., chemotherapy-induced leukopenia, cancer patients having marrow transplants), inherited disorders (e.g., congenital neutropenia), and infectious disease (e.g., AIDS) (14). Patients with low amounts of endogenous

FIGURE 19.3. The product package of ReFacto. (Courtesy of Genetics Institute.)

CSFs are prone to secondary infections because of diminished resistance associated with some forms of cancer or more commonly suppressed marrow function after the use of myelotoxic chemotherapy.

Granulocyte Colony-Stimulating Factor (Filgrastim)

Produced by rDNA technology, this drug stimulates the production of neutrophils in the bone marrow. It is approved for chemotherapy-related neutropenia and is indicated (to decrease the incidence of infection, as manifested by febrile neutropenia) in patients with nonmyeloid malignancies who are receiving myelosuppressive anticancer drugs and exhibiting severe neutropenia with fever. This drug can also be used as an adjunct to myelosuppressive cancer chemotherapy to help speed the recovery of neutrophils after treatment and to reduce serious infection risk.

Filgrastim injection contains no preservative and should be stored at 2°C to 8°C. It is not to be frozen. Before use, the injection may be allowed to reach room temperature for a maximum of 24 hours, after which time it should be discarded. A clear, colorless solution, it should be inspected visually prior to injection. This product is supplied as a 1- or 1.6-mL single-dose vial (Fig. 19.4). Filgrastim is also available as a 0.5- or 0.8-mL Singleject prefilled syringe with a concentration of 300 µg/0.5 mL with no preservatives. Each syringe is protected with an Ultrasafe needle guard.

Filgrastim is supplied in boxes containing 10 glass vials, which are packaged in a gel–ice insulating container with a temperature indicator to detect freezing. For convenience and to minimize the risk of breakage, filgrastim should be dispensed to the patient in its original packaging and the patient instructed to refrigerate the product promptly after arriving home.

FIGURE 19.4. The product package of filgrastim. (Used with permission of Amgen Inc.)

If the patient has to travel a considerable distance or the outside temperature is high, it may be necessary to place the medication in a small cooler with a gel refrigerant (e.g., blue ice) for transport. It is suggested that the vials be wrapped in a towel to avoid direct contact between them and the blue ice. The drug must be physically separated from the refrigerant to prevent freezing. Dry ice should not be used because of the possibility of freezing the product through inadvertent contact.

It is conceivable that when it is used as an adjunct to cancer chemotherapy, prescriptions for this product will be written for 7 to 10 vials. Indeed, patients may have extra vials of this product at home from previous courses of cancer chemotherapy. The pharmacist should question such patients about having any unexpired, properly stored unused vials from the previous course of therapy. Filgrastim injection repackaged in 1-mL plastic tuberculin syringes stored at 2°C to 8°C remains sterile for 7 days.

Because granulocyte CSF (G-CSF) is a protein, it can be denatured if severely agitated. If the vial is shaken vigorously, the solution may foam or appear frothy, making withdrawal difficult. Thus, the pharmacist should instruct the patient or caregiver to avoid shaking the vial before use. If it is shaken, the vial should be allowed to stand until the froth diminishes.

If it is necessary to dilute filgrastim, use 5% dextrose injection. When filgrastim is diluted to concentrations ranging between 5 and 15 mg/mL, it should be protected from inadvertent adsorption to plastic materials by the addition of albumin (human) to a final concentration of 2 mg/mL. When diluted in 5% dextrose injection or 5% dextrose plus albumin, filgrastim is compatible with glass bottles, polyvinyl chloride and polyolefin intravenous bags, and polypropylene syringes. Filgrastim should never be diluted with saline at any time, as the product may precipitate.

The manufacturer of filgrastim has developed a step-by-step guide to subcutaneous self-injection. However, the pharmacist should always emphasize the use of proper aseptic technique when preparing and administering the drug, to avoid product contamination and possible infection.

Granulocyte Colony-Stimulating Factor and Monomethoxypolyethylene Glycol (Pegfilgrastim)

Pegfilgrastim was approved in late January 2002 by the FDA for use in conjunction with myelosuppressive anticancer drugs to decrease the incidence of infection and neutropenic fever in patients with nonmyeloid malignancies. It is marketed under the trade name Neulasta (Fig. 19.5). It is derived by adding a 20-kDa monomethoxypolyethylene glycol (PEG) molecule to the N-terminal methionine residue of filgrastim. The covalent conjugation of the recombinant human G-CSF filgrastim and PEG alters the pharmacokinetic properties of filgrastim. The pegylation of filgrastim significantly prolongs the drug's half-life ($t_{1/2}$, 15 to 80 hours) over that of filgrastim ($t_{1/2}$, 3 to 4 hours)

FIGURE 19.5. The product package of pegfilgrastim. (Used with permission of Amgen Inc.)

by altered clearance. As a result, it is administered as a single fixed dose of 6 mg injected per chemotherapy cycle. This is in comparison to 10 to 14 injections normally needed for filgrastim during a chemotherapy cycle. The significantly lower number of injections required with pegfilgrastim is anticipated to increase adherence to the regimen and decrease the demands on medical personnel. Furthermore, early experience suggests that pegfilgrastim may be slightly more effective in reducing febrile neutropenia in breast cancer patients receiving docetaxel and doxorubicin.

Granulocyte–Macrophage Colony-Stimulating Factor (Sargramostim)

Sargramostim is a recombinant human granulocyte–macrophage CSF (GM-CSF) produced by rDNA technology in a yeast (*Saccharomyces cerevisiae*) expression system. GM-CSF is a growth factor that stimulates proliferation and differentiation of hematopoietic progenitor (precursor) cells into neutrophils and monocytes. It is a glycoprotein composed of 127 amino acids. The sequence of rGM-CSF differs from the natural human GM-CSF at position 23, where leucine is substituted.

This drug is indicated for acceleration of myeloid (marrow) recovery in patients with non-Hodgkin lymphoma (NHL), acute lymphoblastic leukemia (ALL), and Hodgkin disease undergoing autologous bone marrow transplantation (a procedure in which the patient's bone marrow is removed, treated to destroy malignant cells, and reinfused into the patient). It is also indicated in failure of bone marrow transplantation or engraftment delay (it takes 3 to 4 weeks for the new marrow to begin to produce new white blood cells).

Sargramostim is available in a multidose solution vial of 500 mg/mL and a preservative-free single-dose vial of 250 mg powder for reconstitution. It is reconstituted with 1 mL Sterile Water for Injection, USP (without preserva-

tive). The reconstituted solution should appear clear and colorless, and will be isotonic, with a pH of 7.4 ± 0.3. During reconstitution, the Sterile Water for Injection, USP, should be directed at the side of the vial and the contents gently swirled to avoid foaming during dissolution. The product must not be shaken or vigorously agitated. It can also be diluted for intravenous infusion in 0.9% Sodium Chloride Injection, USP. If the final concentration of GM-CSF is below 10 mg/mL, human albumin (0.1%) should be added to the saline before adding GM-CSF. This prevents adsorption of the drug to the components of the drug delivery system. To create a 0.1% albumin solution, the pharmacist should add 1 mg albumin (human) per milliliter of 0.9% sodium chloride injection.

An inline membrane filter for intravenous administration of this drug should not be used. In the absence of compatibility and stability information, other medications should not be admixed to infusion solutions containing sargramostim. Only 0.9% sodium chloride injection should be used to prepare the drug for intravenous infusion.

Because this product is preservative-free, it should be administered as soon as possible and within 6 hours following reconstitution or dilution for intravenous infusion.

Erythropoietins

Erythropoietin is a sialic acid–containing glycoprotein that enhances erythropoiesis by stimulating the formation of proerythroblasts and the release of reticulocytes from bone marrow. It is secreted by the kidney in response to hypoxia and transported to the bone marrow in the plasma. It resembles an endocrine hormone more than any other cytokines (15).

Anemia (a deficiency of red blood cell production) is a frequent complication of chronic renal failure (CRF), cancer, and cancer therapy. Although it is easily corrected with blood transfusions, erythropoietins are available to treat only the severest forms of anemia and not to maintain the red blood cell mass required for normal activity and well-being. As anemic patients with solid tumors often have lower serum levels of erythropoietin, correction of the erythropoietin deficiency through erythropoietin therapy may be as beneficial for these cancer patients as it has been for uremic patients (15).

Kidney disease also impairs the body's ability to produce this substance and thus results in anemia. In the past, patients received blood transfusions. However, a problem with transfusions was possible exposure to infectious agents (hepatitis, HIV). Now, genetically engineered drugs, such as epoetin alfa and darbepoetin, are available to stimulate erythropoiesis. Although expensive, these drugs may prove beneficial for patients who require extensive transfusions because of the high cost of transfusions, the risk of infectious disease, and the consequent additional health care costs.

Epoetin Alfa (Epogen, Procrit)

Epoetin alfa, a glycoprotein produced by rDNA technology, contains 165 amino acids in an identical sequence to that of endogenous human erythropoietin. Erythropoietin also affects the release of reticulocytes from the bone marrow into the bloodstream, where these mature into erythrocytes. It is approved for anemia related to cancer chemotherapy, chronic dialysis, and zidovudine (AZT) therapy.

Epoetin alfa stimulates erythropoiesis in anemic patients, dialyzed or not. The first evidence of a response to this drug is an increase within 10 days of the reticulocyte count. Coupled with this are subsequent increases in the red blood cell count, hemoglobin, and hematocrit, usually within 2 to 6 weeks. Once the hematocrit reaches the suggested target range, 30% to 36%, that level can be sustained in the absence of iron deficiency and concurrent illnesses by epoetin alfa therapy.

Epoetin alfa is available in 1-mL preservative-free single-dose vials (Fig. 19.6) in strengths of 2,000, 3,000, 4,000, 10,000, 20,000, and 40,000 U/mL. Each vial contains human albumin of 2.5 mg to prevent adsorptive losses. The product should be refrigerated at 2°C to 8°C and protected from freezing. The vial of epoetin alfa, recombinant injection, should not be shaken because this may denature the glycoprotein and render it biologically inactive. Each vial should be used to administer a single dose only, and any unused portion of the solution must be discarded.

The 10,000 U/mL is available in a 2-mL multidose vial. The 20,000 U/mL injection is available in a 1-mL multidose vial. These are preserved with 1% benzyl alcohol and contain 2.5 mg albumin (human) per milliliter. These vials should be stored at 2°C to 8°C after initial entry and between doses and discarded 21 days after initial entry.

Epoetin alfa should not be administered in conjunction with other solutions. However, just before subcutaneous administration, the solution can be admixed in a syringe

FIGURE 19.6. The product package of Epogen. (Used with permission of Amgen Inc.)

at a ratio of 1:1 with bacteriostatic 0.9% sodium chloride injection with benzyl alcohol 0.9%. The benzyl alcohol, a local anesthetic, may ameliorate pain associated with subcutaneous injection.

In early 2003, a counterfeit version of epoetin alfa (Procrit) was discovered. It posed a serious health threat because it contained a concentration of the active ingredient one-twentieth of the expected and was contaminated with two types of bacteria. The FDA identified three batches of the fake drug product. Ortho Biotech Products, the manufacturer of the legitimate drug, advised consumers to check for differences on the packaging and vials. For example, the aluminum seal on a vial of real Procrit is smooth, not dented. Also, the closure seals on the outer carton of the real Procrit have writing on the underside and leave a residue when peeled away. In years past, counterfeit drugs were a problem in developing countries. Now, however, these drugs are becoming problematic in the United States, with the FDA investigating more than a half dozen counterfeit drug cases in 2002.

Darbepoetin Alfa (Aranesp)

Darbepoetin alfa, a recombinant erythropoietic protein, was first approved for the treatment of anemia associated with chronic kidney disease or CRF. It is now approved for the treatment of chemotherapy-induced anemia in patients with nonmyeloid malignancies (Fig. 19.7).

Darbepoetin alfa is available as a solution for injection. The injection is preservative-free in 1-mL single-dose

FIGURE 19.7. The product package of Aranesp. (Used with permission of Amgen Inc.)

FIGURE 19.8. The product package of Fuzeon. (Courtesy of Genentech, Inc.)

vials. The polysorbate injection contains polysorbate 80, sodium phosphate monobasic monohydrate, sodium phosphate dibasic anhydrous, and sodium chloride. The albumin solution contains human albumin, sodium phosphate monobasic monohydrate, sodium phosphate dibasic anhydrous, and sodium chloride.

Prior to administration, the vial should be visually inspected for particulate matter and any discoloration. Vials demonstrating particulate matter and/or discoloration should not be used. The vial should not be shaken, as this will denature the darbepoetin and render it inactive. It should not be diluted or administered with other drug solutions. If there is any unused portion, it should be discarded and not pooled with other unused portions. The product should be stored in a refrigerator (2°C to 8°C), not frozen, and protected from light.

Darbepoetin alfa is available in strengths ranging from 25 mg/0.42 mL to 500 mg/mL. All solutions for injection are preservative-free in polysorbate or albumin solutions in single-dose prefilled, Singleject syringes and single-dose, prefilled SureClick autoinjectors. Several strengths are available in less than 1 mL solutions. Thus, the pharmacist has to be careful not to miscalculate the dosage required from the latter by assuming that the solution contains the drug in 1 mL.

Fusion Inhibitors: Enfuvirtide (Fuzeon)

Fusion inhibitors act through a unique mechanism. Enfuvirtide is a 36-amino acid synthetic peptide that corresponds to the C-terminal heptad repeat region (HR2) of the transmembrane subunit of the HIV-1 envelope surface glycoprotein gp41. Enfuvirtide binds to gp41 on the surface of the HIV and prevents the HIV from binding with T cells. Thus, it prevents the virus from infecting healthy cells. Once bound, it inhibits the conformational change in HIV-1 transmembrane glycoprotein gp41 that is required for fusion between HIV-1 and target cell membranes, blocking cell fusion and viral entry into the CD4 cell.

Approved in March 2003, enfuvirtide (known as T-20) is indicated only for patients who have used other anti-HIV medications and have ongoing evidence of viral replication despite ongoing antiretroviral therapy (Fig. 19.8). It is unknown if enfuvirtide is safe and effective for use in children under 6 years of age. Because enfuvirtide is a protein, it must be injected under the skin, making it the first injectable HIV drug. Adherence to the dosage regimen is extremely important, as studies on antiretroviral therapy have demonstrated increased resistance unless nearly every dose is properly administered and on time. The goal is 100% compliance because rates of compliance less than 95% can lead to further resistance (17). If a patient misses a dose, it should be administered as soon as possible, but not if it is almost time for the next dose. In this instance, the patient should know to administer only one dose.

Patient education including proper injection technique is crucial. For convenience, patients may mix both daily doses at the same time, but the second dose must be refrigerated until shortly before it is to be injected. As with insulin, it should be warmed to room temperature prior to injection. The patient should realize the importance of inspecting the injectable, and if particles are observed floating in the vial after mixing, it should not be used. Other injectable medications should not be mixed with enfuvirtide.

This drug is prescribed for patients with drug-resistant HIV infection, so the patient should understand to take precautions, discarding the syringes and needles into a sharps container. They are not to be discarded into the household garbage.

Growth Factor: Becaplermin (Regranex)

Endogenous platelet-derived growth factor increases the proliferation of cells that repair wounds and form granulation tissue. This factor promotes the chemotactic recruitment and proliferation of cells that participate in wound repair and enhances the formation of granulation tissue.

Becaplermin is a recombinant human platelet-derived growth factor for topical adjunctive treatment of diabetes ulcers, a form of pressure ulcer, of the lower extremities that extend into subcutaneous tissue or beyond, having a sufficient blood supply. It is reasonable to assume that it may find utility as an adjunct to good pressure ulcer care.

A measured quantity of the 0.01% gel formulation is spread evenly over the ulcerated area to yield a thin, continuous 1/16 inch thickness over the ulcerated area. The prescribed calculated length of the gel is placed on a clean, firm, nonabsorbent surface (e.g., waxed paper). A clean cotton swab, tongue depressor, or similar aid applicator is used to spread the gel over the surface of the ulcer to obtain an even layer, and the ulcer is covered with a saline-moistened gauze dressing.

After approximately 12 hours, the ulcer should be gently rinsed with saline or water to remove the residual gel and covered with a saline-moistened gauze dressing without the gel for the remainder of the day. The process is repeated daily until the ulcer has healed. The ulcer should demonstrate size reduction (about 30%) within 10 weeks. If complete healing has not occurred within 20 weeks, the therapy should be reassessed. To facilitate acceptance and convenience, bedtime application can be considered.

Becaplermin gel must be refrigerated for stability but need not be allowed to come to room temperature before it is applied. However, the cold gel may cause discomfort when it is applied. The gel itself has an expiration date of 9 months from the manufacture date, but because one tube lasts for about 2 to 4 weeks, pharmacists can dispense the gel up to a month prior to its expiration date.

Human Growth Hormone

The pituitary gland secretes hGH, which stimulates growth. It is estimated that approximately 15,000 American children are deficient in hGH and consequently will not achieve normal height as an adult.

In the late 1950s, cadaver pituitaries were harvested to produce hGH and treat these children. Besides the enormous expense, this method exposed the children to the risk of infection from viral contamination of the hormone (18). Genetic engineering now produces highly purified hGH.

Somatropin, recombinant, for injection, is administered subcutaneously at 0.16 to 0.24 mg/kg body weight per week divided into six or seven subcutaneous injections. This drug is available in various strengths ranging from 1.5 mg (~4 IU/mL) to 10 mg (~30 IU/vial). As Genotropin, for example, the 5.8-mg Intra-Mix two-chamber cartridge (with preservative) is preassembled in a reconstitution device and packaged with a pressure release needle. The front chamber contains 1.5 mg of recombinant somatropin (~4.5 IU), glycine, sodium dihydrogen phosphate anhydrous, and disodium phosphate anhydrous. The rear chamber contains 1.13 mL of water for injection. Depressing the stopper allows the two components to mix. If the diluent and somatropin are in separate vials, aseptic technique must be used to add the desired amount of diluent (1.5 to 5 mL) provided by the manufacturer or sterile water for injection to a 5-mg vial. Like Somatrem, somatropin is stable when refrigerated for up to 14 days following reconstitution with the diluent containing a preservative provided by the manufacturer. When sterile water for injection is used to reconstitute this product, each vial should be refrigerated and used within 24 hours because there is no preservative.

Interferons

In 1957, two British scientists, Alick Isaacs and Jean Lindenmann, found that infected chick embryo cells released a naturally produced glycoprotein that allowed uninfected cells to resist viral infection. They named this factor *interferon* because it appeared "to interfere with the transmission of infection." Later, these researchers demonstrated that interferon does not activate viruses directly but rendered the host cells resistant to viral multiplication. Interferons exert virus-nonspecific but host-specific antiviral activity. By the mid-1970s, it appeared that interferon might also curtail the spread of certain types of cancer (e.g., small cell lung cancer, renal cell carcinoma, basal cell carcinoma).

As a class, interferons are a part of the large immune regulatory network within the body that includes lymphokines, monokines, growth factors, and peptide hormones. Interferons are classified into two types: type I, alpha and beta, which share the same molecular receptor, and type II, gamma or immune, which have a different receptor (19).

Interferon Beta-1b (Betaseron)

Interferon beta-1b (IFNB-1b) is a type I interferon made in *E. coli* using recombinant technology; it differs from natural IFNB-1b only by the substitution of a serine residue for a cysteine at position 17. This manipulation enhances the stability of the drug while retaining the specific activity of natural IFNB-1b.

IFNB-1b is effective in the treatment of relapsing and remitting types of multiple sclerosis, an inflammatory demyelinating disease of the central nervous system (20). This form of disease is characterized by recurrent attacks followed by complete or incomplete recovery.

The effectiveness of lower doses has not been documented, and there is no evidence of efficacy when this drug is used longer than 2 years.

Lyophilized IFNB-1b (Fig. 19.9) 0.3 mg (9.6 mIU) is reconstituted using a sterile syringe and needle to inject 1.2 mL of supplied diluent (sodium chloride 0.54%) into the vial. The diluent should be added down the side of the vial and the vial then gently swirled, but not shaken, to dissolve the drug completely. After reconstitution with the accompanying diluent, the solution has a strength of 0.25 mg/mL. This product also contains dextrose and

FIGURE 19.9. The product package of Betaseron. (Courtesy of Bayer AG.)

albumin (often used in recombinant protein products to prevent sorption of the product to the glass vial, plastic tubing, or syringe). Reconstituted solution 1 mL is withdrawn from the vial into a sterile syringe fitted with a 27-gauge needle, and the drug is injected subcutaneously. For purposes of self-injection, the sites may include the arms, abdomen, hips, and thighs.

Because the product has no preservative, the vial is suitable for single use only. Before and after reconstitution, the product should be refrigerated. No more than 3 hours should elapse between reconstitution and use.

Interferon Beta-1a (Avonex, Rebif)

IFNB-1a was approved for use in multiple sclerosis therapy in 1996, 3 years after IFNB-1b was approved. It is indicated for the treatment of relapsing forms of multiple sclerosis to slow the progression of physical disability and decrease the frequency of clinical exacerbations.

The lyophilized powder for injection, that is, Avonex, is reconstituted by using a sterile syringe and Micro Pin to inject 1.1 mL of the supplied diluent and swirled gently to dissolve the active ingredient. One milliliter is withdrawn from the vial into the sterile syringe. A sterile 23-gauge, 1.25-inch needle is used to inject IM. The prepared product should be used as soon as possible but no later than 6 hours after reconstitution, if stored at 2°C to 8°C. Avonex is also available in a prefilled, single-use syringe, 30 mg/0.5 mL.

Rebif, available in prefilled syringes, is administered subcutaneously with a targeted dosage of 22 and 44 mg, three times weekly. If possible, administration should be consistent, preferably in the late afternoon or evening, on the same 3 days, for example, Monday, Wednesday, and Friday, at least 48 hours apart. Initial therapy should be 20% of the targeted dose three times per week and scaled upward over a 4-week period to the targeted dosage. Thus, the 8.8 mg/0.2 mL prefilled syringe is used for this purpose.

Vials of IFNB-1a must be refrigerated (2°C to 8°C), and if refrigeration is not available, the product can be stored at 25°C (77°F) for up to 30 days. A recent pharmacoeconomic study demonstrated Avonex to be cost-effective relative to other interferon therapies for multiple sclerosis (21).

Interleukins

Originally, ILs were thought to oversee interactions among white blood cells, key components of the immune system. Now, however, it is known that these substances affect a wider variety of cell types. Most clinical interest centers on IL-1, secreted primarily by the monocyte–macrophage that activates T cells and B cells, and IL-2, secreted by the T cell that supports growth and differentiation of T cells and B cells. There are 14 known ILs.

IL-1 was discovered in 1972, and within 7 years, its structure and function were delineated. It was first manufactured by rDNA technology in 1984. This substance is a key immune system regulator. It sets into motion a chain reaction that intensifies the immune response. IL-1 responds to the initial presence of an antigen. It activates T cells to mature, proliferate, and produce other *cytokines* (a generic term for soluble substances produced by cells that communicate with other cells to trigger or suppress cellular activity after interaction with an antigen).

IL-1 also intensifies the production of collagenase, prostaglandins, and antibodies. Because of this activity, excessive IL-1 is suspected to be behind many inflammatory disorders (collagenase breaks down connective tissue; prostaglandins are associated with inflammation). Patients with rheumatoid arthritis have an imbalance in which nine times as much IL-1 as IL-1a is present in the synovium. This imbalance favors agonist-derived inflammation and destruction. The cytokine may also be responsible for the fever, headache, fatigue, and weakness of influenza.

IL-2, like other cytokines, was initially greeted with much enthusiasm. Since that time, it has been found to be an essential component in the development of antigen-specific and antigen-nonspecific immune responses but has found few applications (21). Discovered in 1976, it became available through rDNA technology in 1984. When applied to white blood cells removed from patients and then reinfused as "lymphokine-activated killer cells" along with a booster injection of IL-2, spectacular remissions occurred in some patients with devastating conditions such as advanced malignant melanoma. Unfortunately, highly toxic side effects occurred because appropriate dosing was unknown. A combination of lower doses and physician experience managing its side effects will make IL-2 safer to use in the future.

Other ILs are in the research pipeline. IL-11 is being investigated in vitro and in mice to stimulate platelet function. If successful, this substance could help counter the platelet-depleting effects of chemotherapeutic agents. IL-6 (also known as beta-2 interferon) may also be a stimulator of platelet growth, and it is being investigated as an antiproliferative treatment for breast, colon, and skin cancer.

Aldesleukin (Proleukin)

Aldesleukin is synthetically produced by an rDNA process involving genetically engineered *E. coli* containing an analog of the human IL-2 gene. An expression clone that encodes a modified human IL-2 results from genetic engineering used to modify the human IL-2 gene. Aldesleukin differs from naturally occurring IL-2 in that it is not glycosylated because it is derived from *E. coli*, the molecule has no N-terminal alanine, and the molecule has serine substituted for cysteine at amino acid position 125.

Designated as an orphan drug, aldesleukin is approved for the treatment of metastatic renal carcinoma (about 10,000 cases diagnosed annually) in adults (over 18 years), melanomas, and primary immunodeficiency disease associated with T-cell defects. Aldesleukin is being investigated in phase II clinical trials for efficacy with zidovudine for HIV.

Because of its life-threatening toxicities (drug-related mortality rate is 4%), the physician should consider the benefit-to-risk ratio for the patient. The dosage of IL-2 is usually expressed in units of activity in promoting proliferation in a responsive cell line. Conversion to units from milligrams of protein varies with the source of IL-2. The strength and dosage of commercially available aldesleukin are expressed in IUs; 18 million IU equals 1.1 mg protein.

The manufacturer of aldesleukin recommends that plastic bags be used as the dilution containers instead of glass bottles for more consistent drug delivery. Inline filters are not recommended because of the risk of adsorption of aldesleukin to the filter.

Each single-use vial contains 22 million IU (1.3 mg of drug) reconstituted for intravenous or subcutaneous injection by addition of 1.2 mL of sterile water for injection.

The diluent should be directed to the side of the vial and the contents swirled gently to avoid foaming. The resultant solution should be clear and colorless to slightly yellow. It contains 18 million IU (1.1 mg) per milliliter. The vial should not be shaken. The appropriate dose is withdrawn, diluted in 50 mL of 5% dextrose injection, and infused over 15 minutes. Neither bacteriostatic water for injection nor 0.9% sodium chloride injection should be used to reconstitute this product because of the increased aggregation of the product.

Because the vial has no preservative, the reconstituted and diluted solutions should be refrigerated. However, it should be brought back to room temperature prior to administration. Reconstituted solutions should be used within 48 hours.

Anakinra (Kineret)

Approved in November 2001, anakinra is a recombinant IL-1 receptor antagonist. It competitively binds to the IL-1 receptor, thereby blocking the biologic action of IL-1. Anakinra is an unglycosylated form of human IL-1ra, which occurs naturally but in insufficient amounts to compete for higher levels of IL-1 in the synovium.

Anakinra is indicated for use in adult patients who have been treated unsuccessfully with at least one DMARD. It can be used as the sole agent or combined with other DMARDs except the tumor necrosis factor (TNF)-α–blocking agents, specifically because of the increased risk of infection. The recommended dosage of anakinra is 100 mg/d subcutaneously. Clinical trials demonstrated a mild pain sensation at the site of injection and some inflammation, redness, and/or bruising. Anakinra is packaged in single-use prefilled syringes (Fig. 19.10). These contain no preservatives and should be stored in the refrigerator and protected from light. Patients and caregivers should

FIGURE 19.10. The product package of Kineret. (Copyright © Sobi, Inc. 2018.)

be educated on the importance of proper disposal and caution against the reuse of needles, syringes, and drug product. The patient should have a puncture-resistant container available for the disposal of used syringes.

Monoclonal Antibodies

Historically, MAbs have found use in laboratory diagnostics, site-directed therapies, immunology, and home test kits (e.g., pregnancy, ovulation prediction). In the 1980s, monoclonals were expected to provide a tremendous potential for tumor therapy and immunomodulation. By coupling tracers and toxins to antibodies, tissue-selective or cell-specific targets can be attained. However, initial clinical trials demonstrated less than expected results because of (a) insufficient characterization of the product and its performance in vitro; (b) inadequate preclinical testing; (c) unrealistic expectations of clinical performance, for example, short circulating half-lives (patients frequently developed antibodies to the mouse-derived proteins); and (d) inadequately designed clinical trials.

Advances in genetic engineering provided more ways to design MAbs, and from 1980 to 2005, a total of 206 unique therapeutic MAbs were studied in clinical trials for a variety of cancer indications (22). By 2004, 13 intact, unconjugated, MAb antibodies; three intact immunoconjugates; and one Fab fragment were approved in the United States for therapeutic use in organ transplantation, rheumatoid arthritis, Crohn disease, breast cancer, and colorectal cancer, among others (23). MAbs are purified antibodies produced by a single source or clone of cells. These substances are engineered to recognize and bind to a single specific antigen. Thus, a MAb will target a particular protein or cell having the specific matching antigenic feature. When coupled with a drug molecule, radioactive isotope, or toxin, a MAb theoretically can target the desired cells or tissues with great precision. Specificity for the target antigen is the primary characteristic for the MAb and reflects affinity and strength of binding for the target antigen and cross-reactivity with normal cells. The ideal target organ antigen, hopefully, serves a vital biological function necessary for tumor cell survival because the tumor cell growth can continue unaffected if a target organ is not vital or can be circumvented. In addition, there must be sufficient antigen quantity to mediate a disease-relevant response. Also, the target organ antigen should not be shed or secreted because such antigens bind to, neutralize, and clear MAbs without causing an antitumor effect.

Diagnostically, the specificity of MAbs helps to detect the presence of endogenous hormones (e.g., luteinizing hormone [LH], human chorionic gonadotropin) in the urine to establish the test results (24). They are also used to detect allergies, anemia, and heart disease, and commercial MAb diagnostic kits are available for drug assays, tissue and blood typing, and infectious diseases including hepatitis, AIDS-related CMV, streptococcal infections, gonorrhea, syphilis, herpes, and chlamydia. When covalently linked with radioisotopes, contrast agents, or

FIGURE 19.11. The product package of Humira. (Courtesy of AbbVie, Inc.)

anticancer drugs, MAbs can be used to diagnose and treat malignant tumors (8).

Adalimumab (Humira)

Adalimumab was approved by the FDA in early 2003 for reducing signs and symptoms in rheumatoid arthritis patients who have not responded to previous treatments with methotrexate and other DMARDs (Fig. 19.11). Administered subcutaneously every 2 weeks, this drug now offers an attractive alternative for patients who require TNF-α blocker therapy (25). TNF-α is responsible for much of the pain and inflammation associated with rheumatoid arthritis. Adalimumab is also indicated for psoriatic arthritis, ankylosing spondylitis, and Crohn disease.

Adalimumab was approved for monotherapy or combination treatment with methotrexate or other DMARDs. Compared with other biologic response–modifying rheumatoid arthritis medications, it offers an easier, that is, subcutaneous, and less frequent dosing regimen chronically, that is, every other week. Enbrel, another TNF-α blocker, requires twice weekly injections, and natalizumab, that is, Remicade, another TNF-α blocker, requires an infusion for administration in the physician's office.

Adalimumab is administered subcutaneously as an easy-to-use, single-use, prefilled syringe or disposable, single-use pens for subcutaneous injection (40 mg/0.8 mL). The injections should be kept refrigerated but not frozen. The injectables should be removed from the refrigerator 15 to 20 minutes prior to injection and the patient should select an injection site on his/her thigh or stomach that is at least 1 inch from the previous site of injection (i.e., rotating the injection sites) and 2 inches from the navel. The drug should not be injected into skin that is inflamed, tender to the touch, bruised, or hard. The medication should also be protected from light and stored in its original carton until it is to be administered.

Basiliximab (Simulect)

Basiliximab is an IL-2 receptor antagonist. It is an example of a chimeric (murine–human) MAb (IgG_{1K}) produced by rDNA technology. It functions as an immunosuppressive agent, specifically binding to and blocking the IL-2 receptor alpha chain (IL-2Ra, also known as the CD25 antigen), which is selectively expressed on the surface of activated T lymphocytes. This high-affinity binding specificity of the drug to IL-2Ra competitively inhibits IL-2–mediated activation of lymphocytes, a critical pathway in the cellular immune response of allograft rejection.

Like daclizumab, basiliximab is indicated for the prophylaxis of acute organ rejection in patients receiving renal transplants. It is used as part of an immunosuppressive regimen that includes cyclosporine and corticosteroids.

Basiliximab demonstrates an adverse effect profile similar to that of daclizumab. Administration of this drug is by central or peripheral intravenous infusion only. The dilute reconstituted basiliximab (20 mg/5 mL) is brought to a 50-mL volume with 0.9% sodium chloride injection or 5% dextrose injection and administered as an intravenous infusion over 20 to 30 minutes.

Bevacizumab (Avastin)

Approved by the FDA in 2004, bevacizumab is used in combination with IV 5-fluorouracil–based chemotherapy for first- or second-line treatment of patients with metastatic carcinoma of the colon or rectum. It is a recombinant humanized IgG MAb that binds with vascular endothelial growth factor A (VEGF-A), a target antigen that binds to VEGF tyrosine kinase receptors on the surfaces of endothelial cells, signaling intracellular tyrosine kinases resulting in angiogenesis (26). Angiogenesis is a term used to describe the growth of new blood vessels and plays a crucial role in the development and maturation of tissues. It also plays a central feature in a number of diseases. In cancer, this process supplies the increased demand for oxygen and nutrients that facilitate tumor growth and metastasis. Thus, inhibition of angiogenesis is a possible treatment for some cancers.

This drug is available for injection, 25 mg/mL in single-use 4- and 16-mL vials. It is diluted for infusion using aseptic technique and the necessary amount withdrawn and diluted in a total volume of 100 mL 0.9% sodium chloride injection. The initial dosage is delivered over 90 minutes as an IV infusion following chemotherapy. If the first infusion is well tolerated, the second infusion may be administered over a 60-minute period. If the second, 60-minute infusion is well tolerated, subsequent infusions can be administered over a 30-minute period.

The vials for injection must be refrigerated at 2°C to 8°C and protected from light. Freezing must be avoided and the vials not shaken. Diluted bevacizumab solutions for infusion may be stored at 2°C to 8°C for up to 8 hours.

Gemtuzumab Ozogamicin (Mylotarg)

Gemtuzumab ozogamicin targets myeloid leukemic cells, leaving precursor pluripotent stem cells relatively unscathed and is less toxic than daunorubicin and cytarabine. It was the first drug specifically approved for treating relapsed AML. It is a MAb linked to a highly potent chemotherapeutic agent, calicheamicin. The antibody targets CD33, a glycoprotein on the surface of most AML cells.

Thus, it is now also indicated for patients who are older than 60 years and who demonstrate CD33-positive AML and not considered candidates for conventional therapy.

The product is light sensitive and must be protected from direct and indirect sunlight and unshielded fluorescent light during the preparation and administration of the infusion. In a shielded fluorescent-lighted hood, the contents of each vial should be reconstituted with 5-mL sterile water for injection using sterile syringes. The vial is gently swirled and inspected to assure complete dissolution of contents. The final concentration of the prepared solution should be 1 mg/mL.

Ibritumomab Tiuxetan (Zevalin)

Approved by the FDA in February 2002, ibritumomab tiuxetan is the first commercially available radiolabeled antibody for cancer therapy. When infused into the patient, the antibody binds to the surface of the specific cells and delivers radiation directly to the cancer cells. It is indicated for the treatment of relapsed or refractory low-grade follicular or transformed B-cell NHL.

Infliximab (Remicade)

Infliximab is the only approved drug therapy specifically indicated for the treatment of fistulizing Crohn disease, an inflammation of the intestine.

Approved in 1998, infliximab was originally indicated for short-term treatment. In 2002, this indication was expanded to reduction of the signs and symptoms of and induction and maintenance of clinical remission in patients with moderate to severely active Crohn disease who demonstrated an inadequate response to conventional therapies. In addition, in 1999, infliximab was approved for the treatment of rheumatoid arthritis, an indication that was expanded in 2002 to include improvement of physical function in patients without an adequate response to methotrexate therapy.

This MAb binds and neutralizes TNF-α, one of the primary cytokines that propagate the inflammatory response in patients with Crohn disease and rheumatoid arthritis. Thus, infliximab reduces the intestinal inflammation indicative of this disease process. Administration of single induction doses of infliximab when patients with Crohn disease are not receiving immunosuppressive drugs can lead to the development of antibodies to the chronic MAb itself. When antibodies to infliximab are present in high concentrations, patients demonstrate shortened duration of benefit, complete loss of response, and/or infusion reactions to the drug itself.

Infliximab is supplied in single-use 20-mL vials containing 100 mg of the drug. It has been associated with hypersensitivity reactions, including urticaria, dyspnea, and hypotension, and should be discontinued in case of a severe reaction. Additionally, anti-TNF therapy may result in the formation of autoimmune antibodies and rarely in the development of a lupus-like syndrome. If a patient develops symptoms suggestive of a lupus-like syndrome

FIGURE 19.12. The product package of Xolair. (Courtesy of Genentech, Inc.)

and is positive for antibodies against double-stranded DNA, infliximab therapy should be discontinued.

Omalizumab (Xolair)

Omalizumab is the first humanized therapeutic antibody for the treatment of asthma and the first approved therapy designed to target immunoglobulin E (IgE) in the management of asthma. It was approved by the FDA in 2003 for subcutaneous treatment of moderate to severe persistent asthma in patients more than 12 years of age who demonstrate a positive skin test or in vitro reaction to a perennial aeroallergen (Fig. 19.12). Another requisite for its use is that the patient is inadequately controlled with inhaled corticosteroids.

Palivizumab (Synagis)

Palivizumab is a humanized MAb (IgG_{1K}) produced by rDNA technology, directed to the epitope in the A antigenic site of the F protein of respiratory syncytial virus (RSV). It is a composite of human (95%) and murine (5%) antibody sequences.

Palivizumab demonstrates neutralizing and fusion-inhibitory activity against RSV and is used to prevent serious lower respiratory tract disease caused by RSV in children. The safety and efficacy of this drug were established in infants with bronchopulmonary dysplasia (BPD) and infants with a history of prematurity ($\leq$35 gestational weeks).

Palivizumab is for intramuscular use only, and the single-use vials of the drug do not contain a preservative. The injection must be administered within 6 hours after reconstitution.

Rituximab (Rituxan)

In November 1997, rituximab was the first MAb approved to treat cancer. It is a chimeric human–murine MAb directed against the CD20 antigen found on the surface of normal and malignant beta lymphocytes. The Fab domain of rituximab binds to the CD20 antigen on beta lymphocytes, and the Fc domain recruits immune effector functions to mediate beta-cell lysis in vitro.

Rituximab is used to treat patients with relapsed or refractory low-grade or follicular CD20-positive beta-cell

NHL. The recommended dosage is 375 mg/m^2 given as an intravenous infusion weekly for four doses (days 1, 8, 15, and 22). It may be administered in an outpatient setting.

Premedication with acetaminophen and diphenhydramine may attenuate infusion-related events. Because hypotension may occur during infusion, it is suggested that one consider withholding any antihypertensive medication 12 hours prior to rituximab infusion.

Rituximab (as Rituxan) is available in 10- and 50-mL single-unit vials (10 mg/mL). The required amount of drug is withdrawn and diluted to a final concentration of 1 to 4 mg/mL into an infusion bag containing either 0.9% sodium chloride or 5% dextrose injection. The bag is gently inverted to mix the solution. Any unused portion is discarded.

Satumomab Pendetide (OncoScint CR/OV Kit)

OncoScint CR/OV-In (^{111}In-satumomab pendetide) is a diagnostic imaging agent that is indicated for determining the extent and location of extrahepatic malignant disease in patients with known ovarian carcinoma.

Satumomab pendetide is a conjugate produced from the murine MAb CYT-099 (MAb B72.3). MAb B72.3 is a murine MAb of the IgG_{1K} subclass, which is directed to, localizes, and binds with a high molecular weight tumor–associated glycoprotein (TAG-72) that is expressed differentially by adenocarcinomas. (Adenocarcinoma is a technical name for a malignant tumor derived from a gland or glandular tissue or a tumor whose gland-derived cells form glandlike structures.) In vitro immunohistologic studies have reported MAb B72.3 to be reactive with about 83% of colorectal adenocarcinomas, 97% of common epithelial ovarian carcinomas, and most breast, non–small cell lung, pancreatic, gastric, and esophageal cancers evaluated.

OncoScint CR/OV is prepared by site-specific conjugation of the linker–chelator, glycyl tyrosyl-(N,e-diethylenetriamine pentaacetic acid)-lysine hydrochloride, to the oxidized oligosaccharide component of MAb B72.3. Each kit contains all of the nonradioactive ingredients necessary to produce a single-unit dose of OncoScint CR/OV-In for use as an intravenous injection. Each kit contains two vials. A single-dose vial of OncoScint CR/OV, formulated with sterile water for injection, contains 1 mg of satumomab pendetide in 2 mL of sodium phosphate–buffered saline solution adjusted to pH 6 with hydrochloric acid. OncoScint CR/OV is sterile, pyrogen-free, clear, and colorless, and it may contain some translucent particles. A vial of sodium acetate buffer contains 136 mg of sodium acetate trihydrate in 2 mL of water for injection adjusted to pH 6 with glacial acetic acid. It is sterile, pyrogen-free, clear, and colorless. Neither solution contains a preservative. Each kit also contains one sterile 0.22-mm Millex GV filter, prescribing information, and two identification labels. The kit should be stored upright in a refrigerator (2°C to 8°C) but not frozen.

Proper aseptic technique and precautions for handling radioactive materials should be employed. Waterproof gloves should be worn during radiolabeling. Consistent with the instructions provided, the sodium acetate buffer solution must be added to the ^{111}In chloride solution to buffer it prior to radiolabeling satumomab pendetide. After radiolabeling with ^{111}In, the immunoscintigraphic agent, OncoScint CR/OV-In (^{111}In-satumomab pendetide), is formed. The injection should be administered within 8 hours after radiolabeling.

Tocilizumab (Actemra)

IL-6, a proinflammatory cytokine, plays a primary role in causing local and systemic manifestations of rheumatoid arthritis. Tocilizumab is the first IL-6 receptor inhibiting MAb for the treatment of rheumatoid arthritis. It competitively inhibits the binding of IL-6 to its receptor, thereby preventing IL-6 signal transduction to inflammatory mediators to summon B and T cells.

Tocilizumab is a fusion of murine and human components. The drug was engineered by grafting the antigen-binding regions of the murine antihuman IL-6R antibody to the human IgG1 framework, which is associated with complement fixation. The resulting antibody has a longer half-life, that is, 240 hours, achieved after the third dose of 8 mg/kg in humans. The drug is administered as an IV infusion every 4 weeks for 3 months. The final assessment is performed 4 weeks after the third infusion. Because the drug is a humanized antibody, infusion-related adverse effects, that is, hypersensitivity reactions, might be expected.

Trastuzumab (Herceptin)

In September 1998, trastuzumab became the second MAb approved to treat cancer. It is indicated for the treatment of metastatic HER2-positive breast cancer or cancer that has spread beyond the breast and lymph nodes under the arm. The drug is approved for monotherapy in certain patients who have attempted chemotherapy with little success or as a first-line treatment of metastatic disease in combination with paclitaxel (Taxol) in patients whose tumors overexpress the HER2 protein. In 2006 and 2008, it was approved as part of an adjuvant treatment including chemotherapy for early-stage HER2-positive breast cancer that may or may not have spread to the lymph nodes. If the cancer has not spread into the lymph nodes (node-negative), the cancer needs to be estrogen receptor/progesterone receptor negative or have one high-risk fact.

Specifically, trastuzumab is a chimeric human–murine MAb that binds to the HER2 (or c-erbB2) protooncogene found on the surface of normal cells and plays a role in regulating cell growth. In the case of metastatic breast cancer cells, approximately 15% to 20% of tumors overexpress excess amounts of HER2. Thus, only patients who have tumors with this characteristic have shown benefit from trastuzumab. It should be used to treat only tumors that

FIGURE 19.13. The product package of Herceptin. (Courtesy of Genentech, Inc.)

have HER2 protein overexpression. Trastuzumab may be given weekly or every 3 weeks with different chemotherapy regimens (Fig. 19.13).

TISSUE PLASMINOGEN ACTIVATORS

tPAs are substances produced in small quantity by the inner lining of blood vessels and by the muscular wall of the uterus. They prevent abnormal blood clotting by converting plasminogen, a component of blood, to the enzyme plasmin, which breaks down fibrin, the main constituent of a blood clot.

Genetic engineering has prepared these substances artificially, and they are used as *thrombolytic agents* (agents that dissolve blood clots). They are used for conditions such as heart attack, angina, and occluded arteries. Unlike other anticoagulant drugs, tPA acts only on the site of the clot.

Recombinant Alteplase (Activase)

Alteplase, a tPA produced by rDNA, is used in the management of acute massive pulmonary embolism (PE). It is a sterile, purified glycoprotein of 527 amino acids. It is synthesized using the complementary DNA for natural

FIGURE 19.14. The product package of Activase (alteplase). (Courtesy of Genentech, Inc.)

human tissue-type plasminogen activator obtained from a human melanoma cell line.

The biologic activity of alteplase is determined by an in vitro clot lysis assay. The activity is expressed in IUs as tested against the WHO standard. Its specific activity is 580,000 IU/mg. Alteplase is an enzyme (serine protease) that has the property of fibrin-enhanced conversion of plasminogen to plasmin. It produces limited conversion of plasminogen in the absence of fibrin. When administered, alteplase binds to fibrin in a thrombus and converts the trapped plasminogen to plasmin. This initiates local fibrinolysis with limited systemic proteolysis.

In the 50-mg and 100-mg vials, an appropriate volume of the accompanying sterile water for injection (without preservatives) is added to the vial containing the lyophilized powder (50 or 100 mg) (Fig. 19.14). Reconstitution for the 50-mg vial should be with a large-bore (e.g., 18 gauge) needle and the stream of sterile water for injection directed into the lyophilized cake; for the 100-mg vial, reconstitution is done using the supplied transfer device. A slight foaminess can be expected; when allowed to stand undisturbed, it should dissipate within several minutes. The resultant solution appears as a colorless to pale yellow transparent solution having a pH of approximately 7.3 and containing 1 mg/mL. The 2 mg vial is not copackaged with sterile water for injection.

There are no antibacterial preservatives in the product, so it should be prepared just before use and must be administered parenterally, usually intravenously. The solution may be used for direct intravenous administration within 8 hours of reconstitution when stored at 2°C to 30°C (36°F to 86°F). Before diluting or administering the product, it is necessary to inspect it visually for particulate matter and discoloration whenever the solution and container permit.

This product may be administered as reconstituted at 1 mg/mL, or the reconstituted solution may be diluted further immediately preceding administration with an equal volume of 0.9% sodium chloride injection or 5% dextrose injection. Alteplase is stable for up to 8 hours in these solutions at room temperature, and either polyvinyl chloride

bags or glass bottles are acceptable. Light exposure has no influence upon stability.

Recombinant Reteplase (Retavase)

Reteplase is a nonglycosylated deletion mutein of tPA containing 355 of the 527 amino acids of native tPA. It is produced by rDNA in *E. coli*. Its mechanism of action is the same as that of alteplase.

Reteplase is indicated for management of AMI in adults, improvement of ventricular function following an AMI, reduction of the incidence of CHF, and reduction in mortality associated with an AMI.

Reteplase is for intravenous administration only. It is administered as a 10 + 10 U double-bolus injection. Each 10-mL bolus is administered intravenously over 2 minutes. The second bolus is given 30 minutes after initiation of the first bolus injection. An important requirement is that the bolus injection be given via a line in which no other medication is being injected or infused. If reteplase must be injected through an intravenous line containing heparin, the health professional should flush the line with 0.9% sodium chloride injection or 5% dextrose injection before and after reteplase administration.

The lyophilized powder for injection of reteplase should be reconstituted only with sterile water for injection (without preservatives) immediately before use. A colorless solution should be created containing 1 U/mL. A slight foaminess at this point is fairly common, and allowing the solution to stand undisturbed for a few minutes will allow dissipation of any large bubbles.

Reteplase (as Retavase) is available in kits. Each kit contains a two single-use reteplase vials of 10.8 U (18.8 mg), two single-use diluent vials for reconstitution (10-mL sterile water for injection), two sterile 10-mL syringes with 20-gauge needle attached, two sterile dispensing pins, two sterile 20-gauge needles for dosage administration, and two alcohol swabs.

Recombinant Tenecteplase (TNKase)

This thrombolytic agent is marketed with a needleless administration set that can be used to deliver the medication with just one dose in only 5 seconds. It is packaged in a 10-mL syringe, a dual-cannula device, and a 10-mL vial of sterile water for injection. Doses are calculated on the basis of body weight. After reconstitution of the lyophilized powder, patients will receive 6 to 10 mL. The agent is administered via an intravenous line with saline, as dextrose may cause precipitation. This product contains no bacteriostatic agent and so must be prepared immediately before administration. However, if it is not used immediately, it can be refrigerated for use within 8 hours.

Produced in Chinese hamster ovary cells using rDNA technology, it demonstrated comparable effectiveness (demonstrated mortality rates) and safety (intracranial hemorrhage, major bleeding episodes) as an accelerated infusion of recombinant alteplase in the ASSENT-2

(ASsessment of the Safety and Efficacy of a New Thrombolytic agent) trial. The tenecteplase protein is a modified form of natural tPA. The three letters in the name derive from amino acid substitutions at three regions of the tPA protein. These substitutions have provided a prolonged half-life that enables single-bolus dosing, an enhanced specificity for fibrin (which reduces the agent's disruption of other parts of the coagulation system), and an increased level of resistance to plasminogen activator inhibitor, which can otherwise interfere with the drug's therapeutic action. To be effective, tenecteplase, like the other clot busters, must be used within the first hours of a heart attack.

Tyrosine Kinase Inhibitor

The Philadelphia (Ph) chromosome, a truncated chromosome 22, was the first consistent chromosomal abnormality identified in human malignancy (27). Improved chromosome banding techniques demonstrated that this chromosome was the result of a reciprocal translocation between the long arms of chromosomes 9 and 22. The molecular consequences cause the fusion of the c-Abl oncogene (chromosome 9) and the Bcr sequence (chromosome 22) into the Bcr-Abl gene. This fusion catalyzes the phosphorylation of tyrosine residues from adenosine triphosphate (ATP). Ultimately, this activates several other multiple signaling pathways that affect cell growth, adhesion, and proliferation.

The size of the protein generated by this fusion gene depends on the breakpoint in the Bcr region. For example, 95% of patients with chronic myelogenous leukemia (CML) and up to approximately 20% of adult patients with ALL will demonstrate a 210-kDa fusion protein. Alternatively, a 185-kDa fusion protein is observed in 10% of adult patients with ALL and is the predominant Bcr-Abl fusion protein in Ph chromosome–positive children with ALL. The product of this fusion gene is a constitutively active tyrosine kinase with markedly enzymatic activity when compared to the Abl kinase. Because all of these events (cell growth, adhesion, proliferation) depend on the increased tyrosine kinase activity of the fusion protein, it is apparent that inhibition of the enzymatic activity of Bcr-Abl would be an effective treatment of CML. Bcr-Abl is present in most patients with CML, and the causative abnormality of the disease and its kinase activity are central for transformation.

Imatinib Mesylate (Gleevec)

Imatinib mesylate demonstrates potent and selective inhibitory activity in vivo against Abl tyrosine kinases, such as Bcr-Abl, through competitive inhibition at the ATP-binding site (28) (Fig. 19.15). It does so having minimal effect on normal cells by inhibiting cellular events that are mediated by activation of certain receptor kinases. Phase I clinical trials of the drug (as ST1571) conducted in June 1998 demonstrated significant activity against CML

FIGURE 19.15. The product package of Gleevec. (Copyright © 2021 Novartis AG. SAMPLE. FOR EDUCATIONAL USE ONLY.)

even in patients who were interferon refractory. A significant finding was that the drug is most advantageous when used early in the disease, in the chronic phase. Thus, some experts have proposed a treatment algorithm that calls for all CML patients to receive imatinib, whereas stem cell transplantation (SCT) is being evaluated. In patients whose condition responded to imatinib and for whom the risk of death from SCT is higher (all except the youngest patients with sibling donors), the procedure could be withheld or deferred.

Nilotinib (Tasigna)

Nilotinib, a Bcr-Abl tyrosine kinase inhibitor, was approved in late 2007 for the treatment of chronic and accelerated-phase CML in adults resistant or intolerant to prior therapies, including imatinib. The capsule dosage form should be swallowed whole at least 2 hours after a meal. The patient should then refrain from eating for 1 hour. Grapefruit juice should not be consumed while taking this drug.

Nilotinib is metabolized by the CYP3A4 liver enzymes, and therefore, patients should consult their health care provider prior to initiating any other drug therapy. Similarly, patients receiving concurrent therapy with CYP3A4 inhibitors or inducers should be monitored closely and dosage adjustments made accordingly. Nilotinib can cause QT prolongation, and patients are educated to be aware of possible symptoms, for example, irregular heartbeat and fainting.

Vaccines

Genetically engineered vaccines use a synthetic copy of the protein coat of a virus to fool the body's immune system into mounting a protective response. This avenue avoids the use of live viruses and minimizes the risk of causing the disease the vaccine was intended to prevent. Further, these vaccines will all but eliminate concern about the natural vaccine, which could be derived from blood donor carriers who may harbor the AIDS virus.

The first genetically engineered vaccine for use in the United States was approved by the FDA in 1986 for hepatitis B, a widespread liver infection. This vaccine has now replaced the plasma-derived vaccine.

Hepatitis B Vaccine Recombinant (Engerix-B, Recombivax HB)

The plasma-derived hepatitis B vaccine is no longer being produced in the United States, and its use is limited to hemodialysis patients, other immunocompromised patients, and persons with known allergies to yeast. Recombinant hepatitis B vaccine has demonstrated an ability to induce antibody to hepatitis B surface antigen (anti-HBs) that is biochemically and immunologically comparable to antibody induced by the plasma-derived hepatitis B vaccine. Studies demonstrate that the two are interchangeable in use.

Hepatitis B recombinant vaccine is indicated for immunization of persons of all ages against infection caused by all types of hepatitis B virus. A dialysis formulation (Recombivax HB Dialysis Formulation) is indicated for immunization of adult predialysis and dialysis patients. The vaccine should be administered by intramuscular injection into the deltoid muscle (outer aspect of the upper arm) for immunization of adults and older children. The anterolateral thigh is recommended for infants and younger children. For patients with a risk of hemorrhage following intramuscular injection, the vaccine may be administered subcutaneously, although the subsequent antibody titer may be lower and there may be an increased risk of a local reaction.

Haemophilus B Conjugate Vaccine (HibTITER, Liquid PedvaxHIB, ActHIB)

Prior to the introduction of *Haemophilus B* conjugate vaccines, *Haemophilus influenzae* type B (HIB) was the most frequent cause of bacterial meningitis and leading cause of serious systemic bacterial disease among children worldwide. HIB disease occurred primarily in children less than 5 years of age in the United States prior to the initiation of a vaccine program and was estimated to account for nearly 20,000 cases of invasive infections annually, about 12,000 of which were meningitis. The mortality rate from HIB meningitis is about 5%. Among children, the most prevalent cause of *H. influenzae* meningitis is by the capsular strains of type B. In addition to meningitis, *Haemophilus B* is responsible for numerous other invasive disease processes (e.g., epiglottitis, sepsis, septic arthritis, osteomyelitis, pericarditis).

HIB conjugate vaccines use a new technology, covalent bonding of the capsular polysaccharide of HIB to diphtheria toxoid, diphtheria CRM_{197} protein, or an outer membrane protein complex (OMPC) of *Neisseria meningitidis*, to produce an antigen that is postulated to convert the T-independent antigen to a T-dependent antigen. The protein carries both its own antigenic determinants and those of the covalently bound polysaccharide. Thus, the polysaccharide is theorized to be presented as a T-dependent antigen, resulting in both an enhanced antibody response and an immunologic memory.

Liquid PedvaxHIB is available as an injection of 7.5 mg *Haemophilus B* PRP, 125 mg *N. meningitidis* OMPC, and 225 mg aluminum (as aluminum hydroxide) per 0.5 mL in a single-dose vial. HibTITER is also available as an injection of 10 mg purified *Haemophilus B* saccharide capsular oligosaccharide and about 25 mg diphtheria CRM_{197} protein/5 mL in 1- and 10-mL dose vials. ActHIB is available as a lyophilized powder for injection containing 10 mg purified *Haemophilus B* capsular polysaccharide and 24 mg tetanus toxoid/5 mL. This is available in single-dose vials with 7.5-mL vials of diphtheria and tetanus toxoids and pertussis vaccine as diluents or with 0.6-mL vial containing 0.4% sodium chloride diluent.

Others

Rasburicase (Elitek)

Rasburicase is a recombinant urate oxidase enzyme produced by a genetically modified *S. cerevisiae* strain. In humans, uric acid is the final step in the catabolic pathway of purines. Rasburicase catalyzes enzymatic oxidation of uric acid into an inactive and soluble metabolite, allantoin. Rasburicase is active only at the end of the purine catabolic pathway.

Rasburicase is indicated for initial management of elevated plasma uric acid levels in children with leukemia, lymphoma, and solid tumor malignancies who are receiving oncologic therapy expected to result in tumor lysis.

Recombinant Human DNase I (Pulmozyme)

In 1989, the cystic fibrosis gene was discovered, and it has helped to lay the groundwork for new therapies to treat this disease, which is the most common inherited fatal disease affecting whites. Cystic fibrosis transmembrane conductance regulator, the protein product of the cystic fibrosis gene, is defective in its ability to facilitate ion transport across the airway epithelial cells in the lung. This defective regulator allows excessive absorption of sodium and adequate amounts of chloride across the cell membrane. Consequently, water from the mucus of the lung gets absorbed into the cell, and the mucus dries out, resulting in thick, tenacious mucus that accumulates in the small airways of the lung. This leads to a domino effect of chronic infection and inflammation, followed by chronic lung disease, pulmonary hypertension, and heart failure.

DNase (recombinant human deoxyribonuclease I), or dornase alfa, is a DNA enzyme indicated in conjunction with standard therapies for the management of cystic fibrosis to improve pulmonary function. This enzyme

FIGURE 19.16. The product package of Pulmozyme. (Courtesy of Genentech.)

specifically cleaves extracellular DNA, such as that found in the thick, sticky, mucous secretions of cystic fibrosis patients. As a result, airflow in the lung improves, and the risk of bacterial infection may decrease. This drug offers hope for breaking the cycle of chronic lung infection and inflammation associated with cystic fibrosis disease, and it demonstrates no effect upon the DNA of intact cells.

DNase is indicated to treat cystic fibrosis and is available in 2.5-mL single-use polyethylene ampuls for use with compressed air nebulizers (Fig. 19.16). Six nebulizer systems are recommended, and the safety and efficacy of the administration of DNase with other nebulizer systems have not been demonstrated. Clinical trials have been performed with and support the use of DNase with the following nebulizers:

- Marquest Acorn II nebulizer with Pulmo-Aide compressor
- Hudson T Updraft II nebulizer with Pulmo-Aide compressor
- Pari LC Jet plus nebulizer with the Pari Proneb compressor
- Pari Baby nebulizer with Pari Proneb compressor
- Durable Sidestream nebulizer with Mobilaire compressor
- Durable Sidestream nebulizer with Porta-Neb compressor

Patients who are unable to inhale or exhale orally throughout the entire nebulization period may use the Pari Baby nebulizer.

Portable jet models and ultrasonic nebulizers should not be used to administer DNase. The ultrasonic nebulizers may heat the protein enough to alter its structure. The portable jet nebulizers simply may not be capable of generating enough force or appropriate particle size to ensure optimal delivery of the drug into the lung.

To make administration efficient, it may be tempting to coadminister other compounds (e.g., albuterol, tobramycin) with DNase. However, no other medication should be mixed in the nebulizer system with this drug because of the possibility that a pH change could alter the DNase protein structure. Bronchodilator and antimicrobial agents that are delivered via nebulizer should be administered to patients sequentially, not mixed together. To date, no literature suggests the optimal sequence for all of these drugs to be administered.

The ampuls have an 18-month expiration date when stored in the refrigerator at 2°C to 8°C and should be protected from strong light. The product cannot be exposed to room temperatures for more than 24 hours. The patient or caregiver should discard the solution if it is cloudy or discolored and should be told to make sure that the product is within the expiration date on the ampul. Unused ampuls should be stored in their protective foil pouch under refrigerated.

THE FUTURE OF BIOTECHNOLOGY PRODUCTS

The future will continue to demonstrate the development of more protein-based pharmaceuticals as a result of modern biotechnologic strategies. These protein-based drugs present unique challenges because of intrinsic instability, multifaceted metabolic properties, and limited gastrointestinal absorption. Their problems include variable tissue penetration (because of the size of the molecules) and toxicity related to the stimulation of an immune or allergic reaction.

A distinct advantage of these biotechnologic proteins over proteins from natural sources is enhanced purity. Hepatitis B virus and the HIV are capable of contaminating proteins and enzymes from human plasma. If their presence is known, they can be isolated or neutralized. However, sometimes, their presence has been confirmed only after disastrous results. Products derived from recombinant technology will not have coextracted contaminants.

Research is also directed toward the discovery of new methods of delivery for these agents. Delivery systems being explored include transdermal and nasal routes, other forms of injectables, and oral tablets for smaller proteins. Few protein biopharmaceutical products can be administered orally because of their instability in the strong acid environment of the stomach and the low systemic absorption through gastrointestinal mucosa. A challenge is to deliver regulatory proteins (e.g., insulin, growth hormone) to distant organs or tissue without biotransformation. One strategy that is bearing fruit is nanotechnology defined as the study, manipulation, and manufacture of ultrasmall structures made of as few as one molecule.

The past two decades has resulted in nanoparticle-based diagnostic and therapeutic drugs developed for the treatment of cancer, diabetes, pain relief, asthma, and allergy, among others (29). Nanotechnology involves the control of matter in the 1- to 100-nm dimension range. Nanomaterials demonstrate unique physicochemical properties, for example, ultrasmall size, large surface area-to-mass ratio, and high reactivity, which differ from bulk materials of the same composition.

To date, nanoparticle-based drug delivery has demonstrated distinct advantages. For example, the solubility of poorly water-soluble drugs is improved; by reducing immunogenicity, a prolongation of a drug's systemic circulation is shown; the release of the drug is sustained; and consequently, administration frequency is reduced. Further, drugs are delivered in a target manner that is advantageous to minimize systemic effects. This technology can also deliver two or more drugs at the same time to effect combination therapy, thereby generating a synergistic effect and allaying drug resistance (29).

Among the nanoparticle-based products, the primary products are liposomal drugs and polymer–drug conjugates. Liposomes encapsulate the protein-based compound in a lipid complex and, typically, are composed of some combination of phosphatidylcholine, cholesterol, phosphatidylglycerol, other glycolipids, and/or phospholipids (30,31). These are water-filled vesicular structures composed of several phospholipid layers surrounding an aqueous core, with the outer shell capable of providing direction to specific target cells (e.g., tumors). Usually, liposomes concentrate the drug in cells of the reticuloendothelial system of the liver and spleen and reduce drug intake in the heart, kidney, and gastrointestinal tract. Liposomes are popular among particulate carriers because of their relatively low toxicity and the versatility of their release characteristics and disposition in vivo, which can be altered by changing preparation techniques and bilayer constituents. Depending on their size, charge, and bilayer rigidity, among other characteristics, liposomes circulate only for a short time (minutes) in the circulation before degradation and uptake by macrophages of the mononuclear phagocyte system. Sometimes, their residence in the systemic circulation can be for hours and even days if they are stable and not recognized as foreign bodies by the mononuclear phagocyte system.

For example, use of liposome-associated doxorubicin reduces cardiotoxicity, and liposome-associated amphotericin B reduces nephrotoxicity and other adverse effects. Doxil is doxorubicin produced within microscopic pegylated lipid spheres that are grafted to the liposome surface. The pegylated drug delivery platform is an example of a polymer–drug conjugate. The pegylated liposomal shell protects the inner compartment. A single lipid bilayer membrane composed of hydrogenated soy phosphatidylcholine and cholesterol separates this internal aqueous compartment from the external medium. In essence, the drug, doxorubicin, is encapsulated within this internal compartment by the pegylated polymer layer, which protects the drug from rapid capture and clearance from the blood stream by the liver, spleen, and bone marrow (32). It is theorized that the long residence times and stability of pegylated doxorubicin in plasma are related to a steric stabilization effect provided by the PEG coating (32). This provides a protective layer and suppresses recognition by opsonins. An opsonin is any molecule that acts as a binding enhancer for the process of phagocytosis. The previously mentioned pegylated doxorubicin and pegfilgrastim are prime examples of this strategy. The polyethylene glycol coating reduces mononuclear phagocyte system uptake and provides long plasma residence times and plasma stability.

Insoluble polymers composed of PEG are now used to form a protective sheath around a drug, inhibiting its degradation (32). PEG is a highly hydrated flexible polymer chain. It reduces plasma protein adsorption and biofouling, that is, the accumulation of undesired substances onto the membrane of nanoparticles that decrease renal clearance of the relatively small drug molecules, thus effecting a prolonged half-life. Other advantages of PEG include it being nontoxic and nonimmunogenic. Other hydrophilic polymers that are grafted to liposomes and demonstrate increased circulation times include poly(acryloylmorpholine), polyvinylpyrrolidone, and poly(2-oxazoline).

Studies have shown that liposome size is critical to the effective delivery of encapsulated drugs when the desired outcome requires deposition of liposomes outside of the capillary bed (32). Most solid tumors exhibit unique features (e.g., extensive angiogenesis, hyperpermeable and defective vasculature, impaired lymphatic drainage, increased production of mediators that enhance vascular permeability). Liposomes extravasate in solid tumors through gaps in the normally continuous vascular endothelium. The gaps in these solid tumors have been found to be no larger than 380 to 780 nm (32). If the liposome is too big, it will not be able to extravasate through defects in the capillary endothelium. However, if it is too small, the liposome may have an inadequate amount of drug encapsulated to be effective.

Additional nanoscale systems for drug delivery include phospholipid micelles, pluronic micelles, poly(L-amino acid) micelles, polyester micelles, nanoemulsions, drug nanoparticles, solid nanoparticles, lipid-based nanoparticles, ceramic-based nanoparticles, albumin nanoparticles, nanogels, and dendrimer nanocomposites for drug deliver. As research continues forward in nanomedicine, research moving toward developing smaller and smaller agents will require larger, multidisciplinary teams from numerous disciplines including medicine, pharmacy, engineering, materials science, information technology, and physics (32).

It is entirely feasible that in the future, engineered protein complexes will combine a transporting protein with one that encodes the gene sequence to produce a therapeutic protein in the target tissue. In this instance, the gene will become functional only in certain tissue, decreasing delivery to an unintended site. There is also a growing knowledge base and research about signaling transduction pathways. This has led to the creation of antibodies that target receptors, enzymes, or other growth-regulating molecules.

The future should also see the creation of more diagnostic products for in-home testing. MAb-based diagnostic tests that are now restricted to physician use are under development for home testing. These include products for infectious disease processes (e.g., AIDS, Chlamydia trachomatis, streptococcal throat infections). In addition, it is anticipated that MAb-based tests will also be available to assay blood or plasma concentrations of a number of drugs (e.g., digoxin, phenytoin, theophylline).

THE FDA OFFICE OF BIOTECHNOLOGY PRODUCTS

In 1989, the FDA Office of Biotechnology was created. The office did not evaluate submissions to the FDA for approval of clinical investigations or for product marketing approvals; these functions were executed by the appropriate FDA centers. Nor was this office intended to perform laboratory research or mandate research priorities to the FDA centers. Instead, it was created to serve a central coordinating, problem-solving, and advisory role within the Office of the Commissioner. It was to become an effective point of contact with the FDA for those outside of the agency on issues related to new biotechnology.

Originally, the FDA Office of Biotechnology had the following responsibilities:

1. It was to advise and assist the commissioner and other central officials about scientific issues related to biotechnology policy, direction, and long-range goals.
2. It represented the FDA on biotechnologic issues to other governmental agencies and intergovernmental groups, state and local governments, industry, consumer organizations, congress, national and international organizations, and the scientific community.
3. It provided leadership and direction on scientific and regulatory issues related to biotechnology through an agency-wide coordinating group, the Biotechnology Coordinating Committee, to promote communication and consistency on biotechnology matters across organizational lines.
4. It provided a problem-solving function for individuals, companies, associations, and organizations with concerns, questions, or complaints about biotechnology policies or procedures or about product jurisdiction and other aspects of product regulation.
5. It coordinated and facilitated guidance on cross-cutting or controversial biotechnology program policies.

Subsequently, the Office of Biotechnology has given way to the Office of Biotechnology Products. The mission of the Office of Biotechnology Products is to protect the public health by assuring the quality, safety, efficacy, availability, and security of recombinant therapeutic protein and MAb products. The Office of Biotechnology Products has two divisions: the Division of Therapeutic Proteins and the Division of Monoclonal Antibodies. The Office is also supported by a Biological Products Facility Staff in the Center for Drug Evaluation and Research Office of Compliance. The Division of Monoclonal Antibodies (http://www.fda.gov/cder/biologics/research/dma.htm) ensures that safe, efficacious, and high-quality MAb products are available to the American people to diagnose, prevent, and treat the illnesses that afflict them. Its main activities include application review (Chemistry, Manufacturing, and Controls: CMC), facility inspection (Prior Approval Inspections and biannual Good Manufacturing Practices), research supporting biotechnology policy, policy and guidance document development, as well as training (internal and external).

PATIENT INFORMATION FROM THE PHARMACIST

For products that can be parenterally self-administered, the pharmacist should instruct patients in the use of aseptic technique. Appropriate verbal instruction that reinforces the printed information sheet should also be provided when the product requires reconstitution. It is desirable to perform the first injection under the supervision of an appropriately qualified health care professional to ensure that the patient understands the technique and can perform the injection. Some products (e.g., Betaseron) come with a training video that demonstrates reconstitution and self-administration techniques.

Patients who self-administer these products must be taught how to prepare (Fig. 19.17) and give the injection and how to rotate injection sites (Fig. 19.18). Some products provide a schematic illustration of this on the patient information sheet. Patients should understand that changing sites each time helps avoid injection reactions and gives the site opportunity to bounce back from the previous injection. It is important that the patient understands not to administer an injection into the same area as the prior injection or in areas that are tender, red, or hard. The pharmacist should provide a method for the patient to record where previous injections were made. One simple way is to suggest that the patient note the injection site on a calendar.

Patients should be advised about the proper disposal of needles and syringes. In this day of the cost-conscious consumer, patients must be advised against reusing needles and syringes. It is advantageous to provide the patient with a puncture-resistant container for disposal of used needles and syringes along with instruction for the safe disposal of full containers.

The patient should understand that periodic injection site reactions may occur. These may be transient (as in the case of IFNB-1b) and not require discontinuation of the therapy. It is advisable, however, periodically to reevaluate the patient's understanding and use of aseptic self-administration technique and procedures.

Patients should be educated about the proper storage, for example, 2°C to 8°C, and, when necessary, the need to protect these products from light (Table 19.2). In addition, some products must be accompanied by an FDA-approved medication guide. Some products are also classified as Institute for Safe Medication Practices (ISMP) High-Alert Medications requiring special handling.

Reconstituting Betaseron

1. Remove the Betaseron vial from the well and take the cap off the vial.
2. Place the vial back into the vial holder. Use an alcohol prep pad to clean the top of the vial. Move the prep pad in one direction. Leave the alcohol prep pad on top of the vial until step 4.
3. Peel the label off the blister pack with the vial adapter in it, but do not remove vial adapter. The vial adapter is sterile; avoid touching the vial adapter.
4. Remove the alcohol prep pad from the top of the Betaseron vial. Keeping the vial adapter in the blister pack, place the adapter on top of the Betaseron vial and push down on the adapter until it pierces the rubber top of the Betaseron vial and snaps in place (**Figure 1**). Remove the blister packaging from the vial adapter.

5. Remove the rubber cap from the diluent syringe using a twist and pull motion. Discard the rubber cap.
6. Remove the vial with the vial adapter attached from the tray. Be careful not to pull the vial adapter off the top of the vial.
7. Connect the syringe with the yellow label to the vial adapter by turning clockwise and tighten carefully. This will form the syringe assembly (**Figure 2**).

8. Slowly push the plunger of the diluent syringe all the way in. This will transfer all of the diluent in the syringe to the Betaseron vial (**Figure 3**). Continue to hold the plunger in during the mixing process; otherwise the plunger may return to its original position after you release it.

9. Gently swirl the vial to completely dissolve the white cake of Betaseron. Do not shake. Shaking can cause Betaseron to foam; even gently mixing the solution can cause foaming. If there is foam, allow the vial to sit undisturbed until the foam settles.

10. After the cake is dissolved, look closely at the solution to make sure the solution is clear and colorless and does not contain particles. If the mixture contains particles, or is discolored, do not use. Repeat the steps to prepare your dose using a new tray of Betaseron, prefilled syringe, vial adapter and alcohol prep pads. Contact Bayer HealthCare Pharmaceuticals Inc. at 1-800-788-1467 to obtain replacement product.

Preparing the Injection

You have completed the steps to reconstitute your Betaseron and are ready for the injection. The injection should be given immediately after mixing and allowing any foam in the solution to settle. If you must delay giving yourself the injection, you may refrigerate the solution and use within three hours of reconstitution. Do not freeze.

1. With your thumb still pushing the plunger, turn the syringe assembly so that the vial is on top. (The syringe is horizontal.)

2. Slowly pull the plunger back to withdraw the entire contents of the Betaseron vial into the syringe (**Figure 4**).

NOTE: The syringe barrel is marked with numbers from 0.25 to 1.0 mL. If the solution in the vial cannot be drawn up to the 1.0 mL mark, discard the vial and syringe and start over with a new tray containing a Betaseron vial, prefilled diluent syringe, vial adapter and alcohol prep pads.

3. Turn the syringe assembly so that the needle end is pointing up. Remove any air bubbles by tapping the outer wall of the syringe with your fingers. Slowly push the plunger to the 1.0 mL mark on the syringe (or to the amount prescribed by your doctor).

NOTE: If too much solution is pushed into the vial, repeat steps 1, 2, and 3.

4. Turn the syringe assembly so that the vial is at the bottom. Remove the vial adapter and the vial from the syringe by twisting the vial adapter as shown in Figure 5. This will remove the vial adapter and the vial from the syringe, but will leave the needle on the syringe (**Figure 5**).

FIGURE 19.17. Preparing Betaseron for injection. (Courtesy of Bayer Health Care Pharmaceuticals, Inc.)

As with traditional "sound-alike–look-alike" products, biotechnology product names can be confused, and pharmacists have to be very careful to avoid medication errors as well.

It is very important for the patient to understand that these products should not be agitated or shaken. Otherwise, there is the possibility of product (protein) denaturation and resultant ineffectiveness. Much like the suspension forms of insulin, which should be rolled (or rotated) in the palms of the hands, these products should be gently swirled to dissolve their contents.

Whenever possible, pharmacists must emphasize the need for compliance with dosage regimens. Betaseron, for example, is administered every other day. A calendar reminder system may be helpful for a patient using this medication.

FIGURE 19.18. Rotation of injection sites. (Courtesy of Bayer Health Care Pharmaceuticals, Inc.)

PHARMACIST SELF-HELP WITH BIOTECHNOLOGY DRUGS

The advent of biotechnology drugs poses a real dilemma to some pharmacists. They may be reluctant to stock these medications because of their high cost and special storage and handling requirements and because of poor understanding of the drug's therapeutics (including side effects and counseling information required) and/or the difficult issue of reimbursement. These products also are far more expensive than ordinary pharmaceuticals. Table 19.3 demonstrates some representative biotechnology products illustrating storage conditions, handling and storage precautions, possible sound-alike/look-alike precautions, and other considerations.

Most biotechnologic drugs must be administered parenterally, which poses a threat to some pharmacists, who are wary of this administration route and cognizant of their limitations in counseling the patients in appropriate technique. Suffice it to say that the pharmacist should assume the professional responsibility to secure educational materials (videotapes, print) from the manufacturer. Self-injection products contain instruction sheets that offer a step-by-step guide for preparing and administering the injection at home.

Aside from being knowledgeable about such things as therapeutic use, side effects, precautions, and drug interactions, the pharmacist must also be able to identify monitoring parameters to ensure safety and efficacy. For physiologic peptide molecules used for substitution therapy (e.g., insulin, clotting factors, erythropoietin), therapeutic drug monitoring (measurement of serum drug concentrations) is not indicated because alternative methods are routinely available to assess the efficacy and toxicity of these compounds. As an example, in insulin-dependent diabetes mellitus patients, insulin is routinely monitored through the use of blood glucose measurements and glycosylated hemoglobin measurements. For clotting factors, efficacy is assessed by measuring the specific factor being monitored or prothrombin time or partial thromboplastin time.

TABLE 19.3. Representative Biotechnology Products Featuring Storage and Handling Requirements, Sound-Alike/Look-Alike Comparisons, and Special Considerations

Drug	Storage	Freeze	Shake	Protect from Light	Sound-Alike/Look-Alike Issues*	Other
Aranesp (darbepoetin alfa)	2°C–8°C	No	No	Yes	Darbepoetin alfa may be confused with epoetin alfa.	Do not dilute with other drug solutions
Avastin (bevacizumab)	2°C–8°C	No	No	Yes	Bevacizumab may be confused with cetuximab.	ISMP High-Alert Medication; do not mix with dextrose containing solutions
Avonex, Rebif (interferon beta-1a)	2°C–8°C	No	No	Yes	Avonex may be confused with Avelox.	Allow to warm to room temperature prior to use; FDA-approved medication guide must be given to the patient; some formulations contain albumin.
Betaseron (interferon beta-1b)	15°C–30°C, refrigerate if not used immediately after reconstitution	No	No	No	N/A	FDA-approved medication guide must be given to the patient, contains albumin
Combivir (zidovudine and lamivudine)	2°C–30°C	No	N/A	No	Combivir may be confused with Combivent or Epivir; AZT is an error-prone abbreviation (mistaken as azathioprine, aztreonam).	None
Copaxone (glatiramer acetate)	2°C–8°C; excursions to room temperature for up to 1 wk do not have a negative impact on potency	No	No	No	Copaxone may be confused with Compazine.	Antigenic, not for IV administration
Enbrel (etanercept)	2°C–8°C	No	No	Yes	N/A	Reconstituted vials should be administered immediately (if not, Enbrel may be stored at 2°C–8°C for up to 14 d); do not filter reconstituted solution during preparation
Epogen, Procrit (epoetin alfa)	2°C–8°C	No	No	No	Epoetin alfa may be confused with darbepoetin alfa.	None
Epzicom (abacavir and lamivudine)	15°C–30°C	No	N/A	No	N/A	FDA-approved medication guide and warning card must be given to the patient
Erbitux (cetuximab)	2°C–8°C	No	No	No	Cetuximab may be confused with bevacizumab.	Do not dilute
Evista (raloxifene)	15°C–30°C	No	N/A	No	Evista may be confused with Avinza.	Pregnancy Category X

(Continued)

TABLE 19.3. Representative Biotechnology Products Featuring Storage and Handling Requirements, Sound-Alike/Look-Alike Comparisons, and Special Considerations *(Continued)*

Drug	Storage	Freeze	Shake	Protect from Light	Sound-Alike/Look-Alike Issues*	Other
Fluvirin (influenza virus vaccine)	2°C–8°C	No	N/A	Yes	Influenza virus vaccine (human strain) may be confused with the avian strain (H5N1) of influenza virus vaccine.	Influenza virus vaccine may be confused with tetanus toxoid and tuberculin products. Medication errors have occurred when tuberculin skin tests (PPD) have been inadvertently administered instead of tetanus toxoid products and influenza virus vaccine. These products are refrigerated and often stored in close proximity to each other. Some formulations are manufactured with chicken/egg protein or gentamicin. Some products may contain thimerosal or latex
Forteo (teriparatide)	2°C–8°C	No	No	Yes	N/A	None
Gamunex (IVIG)	2°C–8°C for 36 mo or ≤25°C for up to 6 mo anytime during the 36-mo shelf life	No	No	No	N/A	Product of human plasma; may contain maltose or sucrose
Genotropin (somatropin)	2°C–8°C	No	No	Yes	Somatropin may be confused with somatrem or sumatriptan.	None
Gleevec (imatinib)	15°C–30°C	No	N/A	No	N/A	ISMP High-Alert Medication. **Special handling required: hazardous agent;** protect from moisture
Herceptin (trastuzumab)	2°C–8°C	No	No	No	N/A	ISMP High-Alert Medication. **Special handling required: hazardous agent;** do not prepare with D5W; do not mix or dilute with other drugs
Humira (adalimumab)	2°C–8°C	No	N/A	Yes	Humira may be confused with Humulin.	Packaging (needle cover) contains latex; store in original container
Integrilin (eptifibatide)	2°C–8°C, can be kept at room temperature for 2 mo	No	N/A	Yes (until administration)	N/A	Discard unused portion left in vial
Neulasta (pegfilgrastim)	2°C–8°C; allow to reach room temperature prior to injection (may be kept at room temperature for 48 h)	No	No	Yes	Neulasta may be confused with Neumega or Lunesta.	Packaging (needle cover) contains latex

Drug	Storage Temperature				May be confused with	Comments
Neupogen (filgrastim)	2°C–8°C	Protect from freezing/temperatures >30°C—if inadvertently frozen, thaw in a refrigerator and use within 24 h.	No	Yes	Neupogen may be confused with Epogen, Neumega, Neupro, or Nutramigen.	Packaging of some dosage forms contain latex
Pegasys (peginterferon alfa-2a)	2°C–8°C	No	No	Yes	N/A	FDA-approved medication guide must be given to the patient; Pregnancy Category X when given with ribavirin; discard unused solution
Remicade (infliximab)	2°C–8°C	No	No	No	Remicade may be confused with Renacidin or Rituxan; infliximab may be confused with rituximab.	FDA-approved medication guide must be given to the patient
Rituxan (rituximab)	2°C–8°C	No	No	Yes	Rituxan may be confused with Remicade; rituximab may be confused with infliximab.	ISMP* High-Alert Medication; rituximab dose is NOT based on BSA; FDA-approved medication guide must be given to the patient
Sustiva (efavirenz)	15°C–30°C	No	N/A	No	N/A	None
Synagis (palivizumab)	2°C–8°C	No	No	No	Synagis may be confused with Synalgos-DC or Synvisc	Do not dilute; store in original container
Tarceva (erlotinib)	15°C–30°C	No	N/A	No	Erlotinib may be confused with gefitinib.	ISMP High-Alert Medication. **Special handling required: hazardous agent**
Trizivir (abacavir, lamivudine, and zidovudine)	15°C–30°C	No	N/A	No	N/A	FDA-approved medication guide must be given to the patient
Truvada (emtricitabine and tenofovir)	15°C–30°C	No	N/A	No	N/A	None
Varivax (varicella virus vaccine)	−15°C, may be stored at 2°C–8°C for 72 h prior to reconstitution	Yes (do NOT freeze reconstituted vaccine)	No	Yes (before reconstitution)	N/A	Store diluent separately at room temperature or in the refrigerator; discard if reconstituted vaccine is not administered within 30 min
Viread (tenofovir)	15°C–30°C	No	N/A	No	N/A	None
Xolair (omalizumab)	2°C–8°C, may be shipped at room temperature	No	No	Yes (following reconstitution)	N/A	FDA-approved medication guide must be given to the patient

*Institute for Safe Medication Practices

Approved Biotechnology Drugs. http://www.bio.org/speeches/pubs/er/approveddrugs.asp#P. (Accessed May 4, 2016). Lamb E. Top 200 prescription drugs of 2006. Pharma Times 2007;May:34–37.

Lexi-Comp/Lexi-Drugs Online. (Accessed May 4, 2016).

Prepared by Nicole Costa Purdue University Doctor of Pharmacy Class of 2008.

PHARMACEUTICS CASE STUDY

SUBJECTIVE INFORMATION

Working for an up-and-coming biotechnology company, you have been assigned to formulate a new GM-CSF product called CSF-110.

OBJECTIVE INFORMATION

CSF-110 is a glycoprotein consisting of 143 amino acids and a dose of 100 to 200 mg. It is stable for only 24 hours in aqueous solution at a pH in the range of 6.5 to 7.5 and less stable outside of this pH range. It is adsorbed to the interior of glass vials in aqueous solution. A reasonable shelf life is required, so the drug can be commercially marketed.

ASSESSMENT

This product will be marketed as a dry powder for reconstitution; the powder may be simply preblended or lyophilized. Because of the difficulty of maintaining uniform blends during packaging of a product containing particles of different densities, it may be best to prepare the solutions and lyophilize them in the vials in which they are dispensed. This may also be supported by the coating action of human serum albumin on the interior of the vials in solution form to minimize sorption of the drug to the vial after reconstitution.

PLAN

A lyophilized product that can be reconstituted with sterile water for injection prior to use may be feasible. The product could include the drug, a 0.05-M phosphate buffer system at pH 7.0, 0.1% human albumin to minimize sorption, and sodium chloride for tonicity adjustment. The solution will be prepared, poured into vials, lyophilized, labeled, and packaged. ∎

CLINICAL CASE STUDY

SUBJECTIVE INFORMATION

CC:	J.S. is a 31-year-old WF who arrives at the clinic with her husband. He explains that J.S. has been feeling depressed ever since she started her new drug therapy a year ago. He is extremely concerned because she does not have any interest in the activities that she normally enjoyed to do.
HPI:	J.S. was diagnosed with multiple sclerosis a year ago, when she had complaints of blurred vision, fatigue, and tingling sensations in her right leg. She received intravenous corticosteroid therapy for her acute exacerbation. Since then, J.S. has been receiving interferon therapy (Betaseron).
PMH:	MS diagnosed 1 year ago DM type I since age 5 Pneumonia 2 months ago, treated and resolved Upper neck injury and concussion from a rugby game at age 22 Automobile accident at age 17 (concussion and shattered left)

Meds:	Regular 30 U SQ q12h for DM, started at age 5 IFNB-1b (Betaseron) 0.25 mg QOD (powdered vial) for MS, started 1 year ago
OTC:	Patient denies taking herbal, homeopathic medications, or other supplements
PSH:	Left elbow replacement surgery at age 17
FH:	Father: H/o DM (type unknown), died of stroke at age 57 Mother: HTN since age 55 Brother: DM type I
SH:	(+) Tobacco: smoked for 5 years, quit 6 years ago (−) ETOH (−) Caffeine (−) Illicit drugs
Exercise/daily activities:	Used to run and lift weights two to three times per week, hiking and mountain biking during summers
Diet:	Eats fast food and snacks of chips and candy; meal timing varies

(continued)

(continued)

The patient used to play professional rugby in Europe. Now she is a sales manager for Nike.

The patient lives with husband, married for 5 years.

ALL:	NKA
MS:	The patient reports that blurred vision, fatigue, and tingling sensations have subsided after Betaseron therapy. No allergic reactions or injection site reactions have been reported. The patient has been very compliant with therapy. The patient complains of difficulty in reconstituting the Betaseron.
DM:	The patient reports no sings/symptoms (s/s) of hyperglycemia or hypoglycemia. The patient is not aware of the recommended American Diabetic Association (ADA) diet. The patient also reports compliance with insulin shots but denies any glucose monitoring at home. The patient made an effort to exercise three times per week, but after interferon therapy, the patient does no exercise anymore.

OBJECTIVE INFORMATION NONE

A 31-year-old WF

Ht:	5'8" Wt: 63.6 kg
BP:	121/78 P: 72 T: 98° RR: 19
Pain:	None 137\104\13/112 4.3/25/0.8\ 6.3\13.1/269\ /40\
HgbA1c:	6.5
LFT:	wnl

ASSESSMENT

Betaseron therapy is effective in reducing recurrence of symptoms and exacerbations, but the patient has depression induced by Betaseron therapy. Studies indicate that interferon in Betaseron is responsible for the depression by suppressing circulating tryptophan and therefore serotonin synthesis. According to the patient's husband, the depression is interfering with the patient's quality of life.

Based on the patient's blood glucose and HgbA1c levels, the patient's diabetes is controlled.

PLAN

Recommend cessation of Betaseron therapy and substitute with glatiramer acetate (Copaxone). Although there are reports that using serotonin-specific reuptake inhibitors (SSRIs) (citalopram, paroxetine) may treat depression associated with interferon therapy, J.S. states having trouble reconstituting vials, and Copaxone comes as a prefilled syringe and is not associated with depression. In addition, follow-up on depression may be time consuming and cost money, and the side effect associated with SSRIs is another reason not to continue patient on Betaseron. Evaluate therapy at each clinic visit by monitoring side effects and s/s of disease progression, and magnetic resonance imaging should be done at least once a year to assess the reduction of neuronal lesions. Check complete blood count, perform a neurologic examination, and monitor the patient's compliance at each clinic visit. Monitor resolution of depression at next visit and encourage the patient to exercise regularly and to begin hobbies and activities (avoid activities that put the patient at high risk for trauma).

Continue insulin therapy. Recommend J.S. to obtain a glucose monitor and monitor blood glucose daily at home. Also recommend keeping a glucose diary (goal fasting blood glucose [FBG], 60 to 110 mg/dL; goal HgbA1c, 4% to 6%). Educate the patient on the importance of eating a healthy diet and following a consistent daily meal schedule. Recommend J.S. to start a 1,800-cal ADA diet. Also recommend the patient to check foot and skin daily and teeth and gums every 6 months and to get an annual eye and foot examination. Monitor for s/s of hypoglycemia and hyperglycemia at each clinic visit and perform urinary analysis (U/A) every 6 months. Recommend the patient to obtain a medical bracelet in case of emergency. Encourage J.S. to slowly begin exercising again. ∎

APPLYING THE PRINCIPLES AND CONCEPTS

GROUP ACTIVITIES

1. Describe the various technologies used in producing biotechnology drugs.
2. Select five biotechnology drugs featured in this chapter and determine the average patient cost of each for a 1-year period.
3. Select a high-risk biotechnology product and investigate the implementation of a risk minimization action plan (i.e., RiskMAP) for the specific product.
4. Make a listing of "biosimilars" instituted by the United States.
5. Identify three examples of biotechnology drugs that are classified by the ISMP as "High-Alert Medications" and explain the reasoning for the classification.
6. Create a table of disease states treated with biotechnological drug products and classify their treatment in which the drug products are self-administered, administered in a clinic/office, or as clinic/office administered chemotherapy.
7. Make a checklist for diluting biologic drugs for infusion.

INDIVIDUAL ACTIVITIES

1. Create a table of biotechnology products within a specific product classification and include indication(s), contraindication(s), adverse effect profile, dosage, and storage and administration. Note which products are especially susceptible to damage by foaming.

2. Select a biotechnology product that is available for patient or caregiver administration, and develop a counseling information sheet to facilitate its appropriate use by the patient or his/her caregiver.

3. Create a listing of pharmacist precautions needed when handling, storing, and dispensing biotechnology products.

4. Create a patient advisory brochure to facilitate patient or caregiver administration of an injectable biotechnology drug product.

5. Create a list of factors that might make a patient apprehensive about using a biotechnological product and describe how each factor can be overcome to allay patient apprehension.

6. List marketed examples of each type of Mab drug: -omab, -ximab, -zumab, and -umab.

REFERENCES

1. https://www.reportsanddata.com/report-detail/biologics-market#utm_source=globenewswire&utm_medium=referral&utm_campaign=shuv10oct2019&utm_content=DP. (Accessed May 21, 2020)
2. Sullivan SD. The promise of specialty pharmaceuticals: Are they worth the price? J Manag Care Pharm 2008;14(4):S3–S6.
3. http://www.fda.gov/downloads/RegulatoryInformation/Guidances/UCM126830.pdf. (Accessed May 4, 2016)
4. Gottlieb S. Biosimilars: Policy, clinical, and regulatory considerations. Am J Health Syst Pharm 2008;65(Suppl 6):S2–S8.
5. https://purplebooksearch.fda.gov/downloads. (Accessed July 21, 2020)
6. Kohler G, Milstein C. Continuous culture of fused cells secreting antibody of predefined specificity. Nature 1975;256:495–497.
7. Vermeij P, Blok D. New peptide and protein drugs. Pharm World Sci 1996;18(3):87–93.
8. Peterson NC. Recombinant antibodies: Alternative strategies for developing and manipulating murine-derived monoclonal antibodies. Lab Anim Sci 1996;46(1):8–14.
9. Goodin S. Development of monoclonal antibodies for the treatment of colorectal cancer. Am J Health Syst Pharm 2008;65(Suppl 4):S3–S7.
10. Jurcic JG, Scheinberg DA, Houghton AN. Monoclonal antibody therapy for cancer. In: Pinedo HM, Longo DL, Chabner BA, eds. Cancer Chemotherapy and Biological Response Modifiers Annual 17. Edinburgh, UK: Elsevier Science BV, 1997:195–216.
11. Sahai J, Louis SG. Overview of the immune and hematopoietic systems. Am J Hosp Pharm 1993;50(Suppl 3):S4–S18.
12. Metcalf D. The colony stimulating factors. Cancer 1990;65:2185–2195.
13. Blackwell S, Crawford J. Colony-stimulating factors: Clinical applications. Pharmacotherapy 1992;12(2, Part 2):20S–31S.
14. Oettgen HF. Cytokines in clinical cancer therapy. Curr Opin Immunol 1991;3:699–705.
15. Erickson A. Drotrecogin alfa (activated) has potential to save thousands of sepsis patients annually. Pharm Today 2002;8(1):1, 7.
16. Posey LM. FDA approves first fusion inhibitor for HIV. Pharm Today 2003;9(4):8.
17. Bagley JL. Biotech. Am Drug 1986;195(7):57–63.
18. Wordell CJ. Use of beta interferon in multiple sclerosis. Hosp Pharm 1993;28:802–807.
19. http://www.medicalnewtoday.com/articles/68108.php. (Accessed May 4, 2016)
20. Giedlin MA, Zimmerman RJ. The use of recombinant human interleukin-2 in treating infectious diseases. Curr Opin Biotechnol 1993;4:722–726.
21. Reichert JM, Valge-Archer VE. Development trends for monoclonal antibody cancer therapeutics. Nat Rev Drug Discov 2007;6:349–356.
22. Roskos LR, Davis CG, Schwabg GM. The clinical pharmacology of therapeutic monoclonal antibodies. Drug Dev Res 2004;6(3):108–120.
23. Newton GD. Monoclonal antibody-based self-testing products. Am Pharm 1993;NS33(9):22–23.
24. Weinblatt ME, Keystone EC, Furst DE, et al. Adalimumab, a fully human anti-tumor necrosis factor alpha monoclonal antibody, for the treatment of rheumatoid arthritis in patients taking concomitant methotrexate: The ARMADA trial. Arthritis Rheum 2003;48:35–45.
25. Yang JC, Haworth L, Sherry RM, et al. A randomized trial of bevacizumab, an anti-vascular endothelial growth factor antibody, for metastatic renal cancer. N Engl J Med 2003;349:427–434.
26. Nowell PC, Hungerford DA. A minute chromosome in human chorionic granulocytic leukemia. Science 1960;132:1497–1501.
27. Buchdunger E, O'Reilly T, Wood J. Pharmacology of imatinib (ST1571). Eur J Cancer 2002;38(Suppl 5):S28–S36.
28. Zhang L, Gu FX, Chan JM, et al. Nanoparticles in medicine: Therapeutic applications and developments. Clin Pharmacol Ther 2008;83(5):761–769.
29. Brannon-Peppas L, Blanchette JO. Nanoparticle and targeted systems for cancer therapy. Adv Drug Deliv Rev 2004;56:1649–1659.
30. Kawasaki ES, Player A. Nanotechnology, nanomedicine, and development of new, effective therapies for cancer. Nanomedicine 2005;1:101–109.
31. Martin FJ, Huang T. STEALTH liposomal technology: Current therapies and future directions. Drug Deliv Technol 2003;3(5):66–73.
32. Koo OM, Rubinstein I, Onyuksel H. Role of nanotechnology in targeted drug delivery and imaging: A concise review. Nanomedicine 2005;1:193–212.

Novel Dosage Forms and Drug Delivery Technologies

CHAPTER AT A GLANCE Composition • Topical Administration • Oral Administration • Vaginal Administration • Ophthalmics • Parenteral Administration • Self-Emulsifying Drug Delivery Systems • Hot Melt Extrusion • Pegylated Dosage Forms • Fusion Protein: Special Handling • Implants • Other Novel Delivery Systems • 3D Printing • Patient Counseling

OBJECTIVES

After reading this chapter, the student will be able to:

1. Describe the benefits of new, innovative drug delivery systems
2. Describe the mechanisms utilized to develop new, novel dosage forms
3. List novel drug delivery systems for each topical, oral, vaginal, ophthalmic, and parenteral route
4. List drugs that are typically administered by each of these drug delivery systems
5. Explain the advantages each novel delivery system may or may not have over traditional oral administration
6. Describe the principles of iontophoresis and phonophoresis and their benefits in advancing topical drug administration
7. Differentiate between liposomes for parenteral administration and standard parenteral solutions; describe a situation where liposomes for parenteral administration would be the preferred therapeutic dosage form over standard parenteral solutions
8. Describe self-emulsifying drug delivery systems and their application to enhance bioavailability
9. Identify the appropriate indication for two implantable medications and describe the mechanism of drug release for each
10. Describe the basic mechanism of 3D printing and their applications to personalized medicine

▌ INTRODUCTION

This chapter discusses novel drug delivery systems that are modifications of those previously presented, are relatively new on the market, or do not fit into the categories in the previous chapters. They may be relatively new, use new or relatively new delivery systems, or use unique delivery systems or unique devices before, during, or after administration. Dramatic changes have been introduced, with new technology and new devices now on the market. In some cases, traditional capsules and ointments have been replaced by osmotic pumps, wearable ambulatory pumps, electrically assisted drug delivery, and a host of other delivery methods based on various polymer technologies. Feedback mechanisms are now feasible: Actual drug delivery may be a response to a sensor detecting variations in certain body chemicals and prompting infusion of a drug to correct the imbalance.

Changes are coming about as new technologies are developed and reduce the limitations of existing therapies. In some cases, the new drugs require new delivery systems because the traditional systems are inefficient or ineffective; this may be true especially of some of the recombinant DNA and gene therapies of the future. We may soon be manipulating genes as active drugs and as drug delivery systems and even work in nanotechnology (nanopharmacy) in the future. Some therapies may become very site specific and require very high concentrations of drugs in selected sites of the body, as more controlled drug delivery systems will be available in the very near future. Traditional oral medications may not be as effective in some of these cases.

New drug delivery system development is largely based on promoting the therapeutic effects of a drug and minimizing its toxic effects by increasing the amount and persistence of a drug in the vicinity of a target cell and reducing the drug exposure of nontarget cells. This is still largely based on Paul Ehrlich's magic bullet concept.

New drug delivery systems can provide improved or unique clinical benefits, such as (*a*) improvement of the patient's compliance, (*b*) improved outcomes, (*c*) reduction of adverse effects, (*d*) improvement of the patient's acceptance of the treatment, (*e*) avoidance of costly interventions such as laboratory services, (*f*) allowing the patients to receive medication as outpatients, and possibly (*g*) a reduction in the overall use of medicinal resources.

Novel drug delivery systems can include those based on physical mechanisms and those based on biochemical mechanisms. Physical mechanisms, also referred to as controlled drug delivery systems, include osmosis, diffusion, erosion, dissolution, and electrotransport. Biochemical mechanisms include monoclonal antibodies, gene therapy and vector systems, polymer drug abducts, and liposomes.

Therapeutic benefits of some of the new drug delivery systems include optimization of the duration of action of the drug, decreasing dosage frequency, controlling the site of release, and maintaining constant drug levels. Safety benefits include reducing adverse effects, decreasing the number of concomitant medications a patient must take, decreasing the need for interventions, and reducing the number of emergency department visits. Economic benefits of novel drug delivery systems include simplifying administration regimens, enhancing the patient's compliance, and an overall reduction of health care costs.

COMPOSITION

Associated with the various mechanisms that are characteristic of or the basis of the newer drug delivery systems, their composition can be quite variable—ranging from naturally derived substances, such as gelatin and sugars, to the more complex polymers. New drug delivery systems also incorporate mechanical, electronic, and computer components.

The therapeutic efficacy of selected products can be enhanced, and in some cases, the toxicity can be decreased by incorporating novel polymer technology. For example, degradable bonds can be used to attach an active drug to a synthetic or naturally occurring polymer. Upon delivery to the target site and in the presence of certain enzymes or through hydrolysis or a comparable mechanism, the product can be cleaved, releasing the active drug at a specific site of action. Oral, topical, parenteral, and implantable drugs have the potential to be used with this approach.

A number of release profiles using polymers are possible, as are actual penetration into specific tissues and selection of specific target sites. Potential problems of polymers include the following: (*a*) Their high molecular weight may cause them to be very slowly excreted from the body. (*b*) Because of their size, permeability through various membranes may be slow. (*c*) Immunologic or toxic reactions may occur. (*d*) Because they are complex, they may be labor intensive and expensive to develop. Novel drug delivery systems will be discussed in the general categories of topical, oral, vaginal, implanted, ophthalmic, and parenteral preparations.

TOPICAL ADMINISTRATION

The basis for the development of transdermal drug delivery systems (patches) involves percutaneous absorption. See Chapters 10 and 11 for background information on transdermal systems and penetration enhancers. Novel topical systems also include iontophoresis (IP) and phonophoresis.

Iontophoresis

IP is an electrochemical method that enhances the transport of some solute molecules by creating a potential gradient through the skin with an applied electrical current or voltage. It induces increased migration of ionic drugs into the skin by electrostatic repulsion at the active electrode: Negative ions are delivered by the cathode and positive ions by the anode. A typical IP device consists of a battery, microprocessor controller, drug reservoir, and electrodes.

Advantages of IP include (*a*) control of the delivery rates by variations of current density, pulsed voltage, drug concentration, and ionic strength; (*b*) eliminating gastrointestinal incompatibility, erratic absorption, and first-pass metabolism; (*c*) reducing side effects and variation among patients; (*d*) avoiding the risks of infection, inflammation, and fibrosis associated with continuous injection or infusion; and (*e*) enhancing compliance with a convenient and noninvasive therapeutic regimen.

The main disadvantage of IP is skin irritation at high current densities; this can be eliminated or minimized by reducing the current.

IP is gaining increasing acceptance in the pharmaceutical industry with small, efficient iontophoretic patches projected to be on the market within the next few years. Miniaturization is now possible with smaller, more powerful batteries and electronics. The next generation of IP patch may also include an electronic record of the date, time, and quantity of each dose delivered, providing information for determining patient compliance. Also, units may soon be capable of reverse IP that serves to collect a sample noninvasively and determine the analyte levels in the body with feedback mechanisms for dosing. Currently, however, most IP involves the use of an iontophoretic device attached to electrodes containing a solution of the drug.

As previously mentioned, IP involves the use of small amounts of physiologically acceptable electric current to move charged, or ionized, drugs through the skin. Placing an ionized solution of the drug in an electrode of the same charge and applying a current repel the drug from the electrode into the skin. This method of drug delivery has been around for at least 100 years. Since the 1930s, IP of pilocarpine has been used to induce sweating in the diagnosis of cystic fibrosis. More recently, IP has been used in the topical delivery of fluoride to the teeth, dexamethasone as an anti-inflammatory into joints, and lidocaine as a topical anesthetic. Drugs such as corticosteroids, nonsteroidal anti-inflammatory agents, and anesthetics are commonly delivered via IP. Other drugs under study include a number of analgesics, nicotine, anti-AIDS drugs, cancer drugs, insulin, and proteins. IP is also useful in veterinary medicine.

In the IP process, the current, beginning at the device, is transferred from the electrode through the ionized drug solution as ionic flow. The drug ions move to the skin, where the repulsion continues, moving the drug through whatever pathways are available, namely, pores, and possibly through a disrupted stratum corneum. The drug-containing electrode is termed the active electrode, and the other electrode, the passive electrode, is placed elsewhere on the body. Current densities up to 0.5 mA/cm^2 can be tolerated with little or no discomfort. The larger the electrode surface, the greater the current the device must supply to provide a current density for moving the drug.

The delivery of a drug iontophoretically is quite complex, depending on the interactions between the drug and the vehicle electrolyte or buffer, partitioning of the drug between the vehicle and the skin, and then diffusion through a highly heterogeneous membrane under the influence of both chemical and electrical potential gradients.

The movement of ions across the skin is described by the relationship known as the Nernst-Planck equation:

$$J_i = -D_i \frac{dC_i}{dX} - Z_i\, mFC_i \frac{dE}{dX}$$

where
  J_i is flux;
  D_i is diffusivity;
  dC_i/dx is concentration gradient;
  z_i is valence of the species I;
  m is mobility;
  F is Faraday constant;
  C_i is concentration; and
  dE/dx is electrostatic potential gradient.

Variables affecting IP include aspects of the current, the physicochemical properties of the drug, formulation factors, biologic factors, and electroendosmotic flow.

The *current* can be direct, alternate, or pulsed and can have various waveforms, including square, sinusoidal, triangular, and trapezoidal. There may not be much advantage to the more complex forms, as direct current is most commonly used at this time.

Physicochemical variables include the charge, size, structure, and lipophilicity of the drug. The drug should be water soluble, low dose, and ionizable with a high charge density. Smaller molecules are more mobile, but large molecules are also usable.

Formulation factors include drug concentration, pH, ionic strength, and viscosity. Increasing drug concentration usually results in greater drug delivery to a certain degree. Buffer ions in a formula will compete with the drug for the delivery current, decreasing the quantity of drug delivered, especially because buffer ions are generally smaller and more mobile than the larger active drug. The pH of solutions can be adjusted and maintained by larger molecules, such as ethanolamine: ethanolamine HCl rather than the smaller hydrochloric acid and sodium hydroxide. An increase in ionic strength of the system will also increase the competition for the available current, especially because the active drugs are generally potent and present in a small concentration as compared to these extraneous ions.

Biologic factors pertain to the skin to which the electrodes are applied, its thickness, permeability, presence of pores, and so on.

Electroendosmotic flow results when a voltage difference is applied across a charged porous membrane, resulting in a bulk fluid flow in the same direction as the flow of counter ions. This fluid flow can actually carry a drug with it into the skin, especially positively charged, cationic, drugs. Neutral drugs can also be carried via electroendosmotic flow.

Iontophoretic devices have changed remarkably over the years, ranging from the galvanometers of the past to the small, specially designed units of today. Example IP units and electrodes are shown in Figures 20.1 to 20.3.

Iontophoretic units are now sized similarly to today's transdermal patches. They may be slightly thicker to accommodate the power source and small microprocessor controllers. The future may include IP patches capable of sampling and testing (e.g., glucose levels) and adjusting the delivery rate of a drug (e.g., insulin), all in the same IP system. Reverse IP can be used to extract chemicals or drugs from the body for testing. Many types of patches with electrodes may require pharmacists to add the drug prior to dispensing, as is done today in filling reservoirs for parenteral administration. Drugs currently administered using IP are listed in Tables 20.1 (human) and 20.2 (veterinary). Because most solutions designed specifically for IP are not commercially available, they must be compounded. It is best to have only the drug and water present to minimize competition for the active ions.

An IP system called Numby Stuff (IOMED) is used to achieve local anesthesia of the skin and is promoted as a painless, needleless system.

FIGURE 20.1. The DuPel iontophoresis system showing the connections to which a passive and an active (drug-containing) electrode will be attached.

FIGURE 20.3. Sample electrodes used in IP. The active electrode will generally receive up to 3 mL of a solution containing the drug to be delivered.

FIGURE 20.2. The Phoresor II iontophoresis system with example electrodes attached.

TABLE 20.1. Drugs Used in IP

Drug Solution	Concentration (%)	Use/Indication	Polarity
Acetic acid	2–5	Calcium deposits, calcified tendonitis	Negative
Atropine sulfate	0.001–0.01	Hyperhidrosis	Positive
Calcium chloride	2	Myopathy, myospasm, immobile joints	Positive
Sodium chloride	2	Sclerolytic, scar tissue, adhesions, keloids	Negative
Copper sulfate	2	Astringent, fungus infection	Positive
Dexamethasone sodium phosphate	0.4	Tendonitis, bursitis, arthritis, tenosynovitis, Peyronie disease	Negative
Estriol	0.3	Acne scars	Positive
Fentanyl citrate		Analgesic	Positive
Fluoride sodium	2	Desensitize teeth	Positive
Gentamicin sulfate	0.8	Ear chondritis	Positive
Glycopyrronium bromide	0.05	Hyperhidrosis	Positive
Hyaluronidase	150 U/mL solution	Absorption enhancement, edema, scleroderma, lymphedema	Positive
Idoxuridine	0.1	Herpes simplex	Negative
Iodine ointment	4.7	Sclerolytic, antimicrobial, fibrosis, adhesions, scar tissue, trigger finger	Negative
Iron/titanium oxide		Skin pigmentation	Positive
Lidocaine hydrochloride	4 (with or without epinephrine 1:50,000–1:100,000)	Skin anesthesia, trigeminal neuralgia	Positive
Lithium chloride	2	Gouty arthritis	Positive
Magnesium sulfate	2	Muscle relaxant, vasodilator, myalgias, neuritis, deltoid bursitis, low back spasm	Positive
Mecholyl chloride	0.25	Vasodilator, muscle relaxant, radiculitis, varicose ulcers	Positive
Meladinine sodium	1	Vitiligo	Negative
Methylphenidate hydrochloride		Attention deficit disorder	Positive
Morphine sulfate	0.2–0.4	Analgesic	Positive
Pilocarpine hydrochloride		Sweat test for cystic fibrosis	Positive
Poldine methylsulfate	0.05–0.5	Hyperhidrosis	Negative
Potassium iodide	10	Scar tissue	Negative
Sodium salicylate	2	Analgesic, sclerolytic, plantar warts, scar tissue, myalgias	Negative
Tretinoin		Acne scars	Positive
Water	100	Palmar, plantar, axillary hyperhidrosis	Both
Zinc oxide suspension	20	Antiseptic, ulcers, dermatitis, wound healing	Positive

Iontophoretic administration is also used in veterinary pharmacy, using drugs such as those listed in Table 20.2. Because of the difference in the size and anatomy of the animal patient, different electrodes may be required. IP has been studied to enhance drug penetration into the nails for the treatment of fungal infections. IP does moderately increase penetration as compared to passive diffusion (1).

Phonophoresis

Phonophoresis (syn, ultrasound, sonophoresis, ultrasonophoresis, ultraphonophoresis) is the transport of drugs through the skin using ultrasound; it is a combination of ultrasound therapy with topical drug therapy to achieve therapeutic drug concentrations at selected sites in the skin. It is widely used by physiotherapists. In this technique, the drug is generally mixed with a coupling agent, usually a gel, but sometimes a cream or ointment, that transfers ultrasonic energy from the phonophoresis device to the skin. The ultrasonic unit has a sound transducer head emitting energy at 1 MHz at 0.5 to 1 W/cm². Although the exact mechanism is not known, it may involve a disruption of the stratum corneum lipids, allowing the drug to pass through the skin.

Originally, the drug-containing coupling agent was applied to the skin and immediately followed by the

TABLE 20.2. Drugs Used in Veterinary IP

Drug Solution	Commercial Concentration (mg/mL)	Total/6 mL Electrode (mg)	Polarity
NSAIDs			
Phenylbutazone	200	1,200	Negative
Flunixin meglumine	50	300	Negative
Ketoprofen	100	600	Negative
Corticosteroids, anti-inflammatory agents			
Dexamethasone sodium phosphate	2 or 4	12 or 24	Negative
Betamethasone	4	24	Negative
Prednisolone sodium succinate	10 or 50	60 or 300	Negative
Antibiotics			
Gentamicin sulfate	50 or 100	300 or 600	Positive
Amikacin sulfate	50	300	Positive
Ceftiofur sodium	50	300	Negative
Local anesthetic			
Lidocaine hydrochloride	20	120	Positive

ultrasound unit. Today, the product is applied to the skin, and some time is allowed for the drug to begin absorption into the skin; then the ultrasound unit is applied. The ultrasound emitted from the unit is actually sound waves outside the normal human hearing range. As ultrasound waves, they can be reflected, refracted, and absorbed by the medium, just as regular sound waves can. Consequently, these are factors that must be considered as affecting phonophoresis efficiency.

Three effects of ultrasound are cavitation, microstreaming, and heat generation. Cavitation is formation and collapse of very small air bubbles in a liquid in contact with ultrasound waves. Microstreaming, closely associated with cavitation, results in efficient mixing by inducing eddies in small-volume elements of a liquid; this may enhance dissolution of suspended drug particles, resulting in a higher concentration of drug near the skin, for absorption. Heat results from the conversion of ultrasound energy to heat energy and can occur at the surface of the skin as well as in deeper layers of the skin.

The vehicle containing the drug must be formulated to provide good conduction of the ultrasonic energy to the skin. The product must be smooth and not gritty, as it will be rubbed into the skin by the head of the transducer. The product should have relatively low viscosity for ease of application and ease of movement of the transducer head. Gels work very well as a medium. Emulsions have been used, but the oil–water interfaces in emulsions can disperse the ultrasonic waves, reducing the intensity of the energy reaching the skin. It may also cause some local heat. Air should not be incorporated into the product, as air bubbles may disperse the ultrasound waves, resulting in heat at the liquid–air interface.

Hydrocortisone is the drug most often administered, in concentrations ranging from 1% to 10% in a phonophoresis gel.

ORAL ADMINISTRATION

The oral cavity consists of the lips, cheek (buccal), tongue, hard palate, soft palate, and floor of the mouth. The "oral mucosa" refers to the lining of the oral cavity and includes the buccal, sublingual, gingival, palatal, and labial mucosae. The buccal and sublingual tissues are the primary areas for drug delivery via the oral mucosa as they are more permeable than the other regions of the mouth.

Numerous drugs, including nitroglycerin, captopril, midazolam, triazolam, scopolamine, prochlorperazine, testosterone, estrogen, and others have been studied for transmucosal administration and some are on the market today. Dosage forms include sublingual tablets (nitroglycerin), lozenges (fentanyl), buccal tablets (prochlorperazine), chewing gums (nicotine), patches, sublingual drops and others.

Films

A film is a rapidly dissolving dosage form for oral use in the form of a thin flexible sheet. Films are prepared by mixing the polymer with the drug, sweetener, and flavor and casting, forming, drying, and packaging. Commercial films include the following as shown in Table 20.3.

Typical components of a film are as follows:

Ingredients	Amounts (w/w)	Purpose
Active pharmaceutical ingredient (API)	5%–30%	API
Water-soluble polymer	45%	Vehicle
Plasticizer	0%–20%	Pliability
Saliva stimulation	2%–6%	Dissolution increaser
Surfactant	qs	Wettability enhancer
Sweetener	3%–6%	Taste masker
Flavors, colors, fillers	qs	Compliance enhancer

TABLE 20.3. Commercial Oral Thin Films

Brand Name	Formulation Type	Application
Gas-X Thin Strips	Simethicone SL Film	Bloating and gas
KP106	D-amphetamine ODF	ADHD
Onsolis	Fentanyl buccal soluble film	Breakthrough pain (Cancer)
Pedia-Lax Quick Dissolve Strip	Sennosides ODF	Constipation
RapidFilm	Ondansetron and donepezil ODF	Nausea, psychosis
Setofilm	Ondansetron ODF	Nausea
Suboxone	Buprenorphine and naloxone SL Film	Opioid dependence
Sudafed PE quick dissolve strips	Phenylephrine ODF	Cough and cold
Triaminic Thin Strips	Phenylephrine and diphenhydramine ODF	Cough and cold
Zolmitriptan RapidFilm	Zolmitriptan oral disintegrating film (ODF)	Migraine

Shanmugam S. Oral thin films-misconceptions, advantages & limitations about an emerging drug delivery system. Drug Develop Deliv 2020;20(3):40–44.

An example of a drug-containing fast dissolving film and the method of preparation is as follows:

Rx	Montelukast 5 mg Fast Dissolving Film	
	For 10 Films	
	Montelukast sodium	52.79 mg
	Hypromellose	400 mg
	Crospovidone	400 mg
	Sucrose	400 mg
	Citric acid	400 mg
	Glycerin	3 mL (3.75 g)
	Flavor	qs
	Purified water	10 mL

Method of Preparation

1. Calculate the required quantity of each ingredient for the total amount to be prepared.
2. Accurately weigh/measure each ingredient.
3. Levigate the hypromellose and crospovidone with the glycerin.
4. Incorporate the montelukast sodium and mix well.
5. Add the sucrose, citric acid, and flavor to about 4 mL of purified water.
6. Combine the two mixtures and mix well.
7. Add sufficient purified water to final volume and mix well.
8. Cast onto a glass plate with boundaries situated to prevent the film from overflowing.
9. Allow to dry in a hot air oven at 40°C for 24 hours.
10. Cut or punch out the required size of film calculated to provide the desired dose.
11. Note: Weigh the dried films and divide by 10 to get the required weight of each film. It may vary somewhat based on the residual water content.
12. Package and label.

Mucoadhesive System

The Striant mucoadhesive testosterone buccal system is designed to adhere to the gum or inner cheek to provide a controlled and sustained release of testosterone through the buccal mucosa (2). Using a Striant system twice daily, morning and evening, provides continuous systemic delivery of testosterone to the patient. Each Striant buccal system contains 30 mg of testosterone, along with the inactive ingredients such as anhydrous lactose, Carbomer 934P, hypromellose, magnesium stearate, lactose monohydrate, polycarbophil, colloidal silicon dioxide, starch, and talc. When used as directed in hypogonadal males, the circulating testosterone levels should approximate the physiologic levels in healthy men at 300 to 1,050 ng/dL.

When applied, Striant begins hydrating, and testosterone is absorbed through the gum and cheek surfaces that are in contact with it. Venous drainage from the mouth into the superior vena cava circumvents first-pass (hepatic) metabolism. Following initial application, the serum testosterone concentration rises to a maximum within 10 to 12 hours; steady-state levels are usually obtained after the first two Striant systems are used. When removed and not reapplied, the serum testosterone levels fall below the normal range within 2 to 4 hours.

What is the effect of food when using Striant? No specific studies were reported in the package literature. The effects of toothbrushing, mouthwashing, chewing gum, and drinking alcoholic beverages on the use and absorption of testosterone from the Striant system were not specifically studied but were allowed in the phase 3 clinical studies, and no significant effect was attributed to these activities.

Medicated Gums

A medicated gum is a semisolid confection that is designed to be chewed rather than swallowed. Medicated gums release their active ingredient(s) into the saliva and can deliver therapeutic agents for both local action and systemic absorption. Most medicated gums are manufactured using the conventional melting process of the confectionary industry, or, alternatively, they may be directly compressed from gum powder. They are formulated from insoluble synthetic gum bases, such as polyisoprene, polyisobutylene, isobutylene–isoprene copolymer, styrene butadiene rubber, polyvinyl acetate, polyethylene, or poly-terpenes.

Softening agents, or plasticizers such as propylene glycol, glycerin, oleic acid, or vegetable oils, are added to maintain pliability and aid in the incorporation of the active and inactive ingredients, including sweeteners and flavoring agents. Sugars and artificial sweeteners and fla-vorings are added to improve taste. Some medicated gums are coated with magnesium stearate to reduce tackiness and improve handling during packaging; sometimes a pre-servative may be added.

Preparation by melting includes melting the gum base to about 115°C until it achieves the viscosity of a thick syrup, at which point it is filtered through a fine-mesh screen. Then sweeteners, plasticizers, and active drugs are added with mixing. Colorings, flavorings, and preserva-tives are added and mixed while the melted gum is cool-ing. It is then shaped by extrusion or rolling and cutting. Any additional coating is applied to improve taste and aid in bulk packaging.

Preparation by direct compression involves using the gum base in a free-flowing granular powder. It is dry blended with sweeteners, flavors, the active drug, and a lubricant. It is then processed using a conventional tab-let press into the desired shape and size. The tablets can be further coated with sugar or sugar-free excipients and packaged in blister or bottles as desired.

VAGINAL ADMINISTRATION

Intravaginal Drug Delivery System

Vaginal administration of drugs, especially hormones, has several advantages, including self-insertion and removal, continuous drug administration at an effective dose level, and good patient compliance. The continuous release and local absorption of drug minimize systemic toxicity that may result from the peak-and-valley blood level profile associated with oral drug administration.

In a polymeric vaginal drug delivery system, such as a resilient medicated vaginal ring, shown in Figure 20.4 or a copper-containing intrauterine contraceptive device, the drug may be uniformly distributed throughout the polymeric matrix. Upon administration and when in con-tact with vaginal fluids, the drug will slowly dissolve and migrate out of the device. Drug inside the device will dif-fuse toward the surface along a concentration gradient, resulting in a long-acting drug delivery system. Mirena (levonorgestrel-releasing intrauterine system) consists of a T-shaped polyethylene frame with a steroid reservoir (hormone elastomer core) around the vertical stem. It is designed to prevent pregnancy for up to 5 years (3).

Intrauterine Progesterone Drug Delivery System

The Progestasert system shown in Figure 20.5 slowly releases an average of 60 mg of progesterone per day for

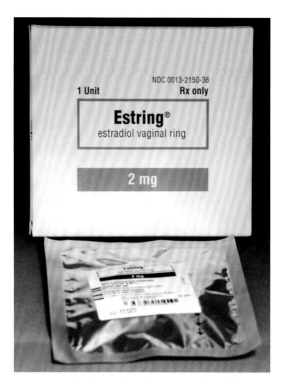

FIGURE 20.4. Estring polymeric vaginal drug delivery system.

1 year after insertion. The continuous release of progester-one into the uterine cavity provides local rather than sys-temic action. Two hypotheses for the contraceptive action have been offered: progesterone-induced inhibition of sperm capacity for survival and alteration of the uterine milieu to prevent nidation (implantation of a fertilized ovum). The intrauterine device contains 38 mg of proges-terone, a much smaller amount than would be taken by other routes of administration over the same period for the same purpose. The intrauterine device is replaced annu-ally for the maintenance of contraception (4).

The Progestasert provides contraception without the need for daily self-medication and has the advantages

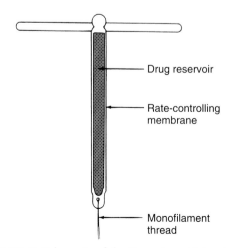

FIGURE 20.5. Schematic of the Progestasert intrauterine drug delivery system.

of (*a*) using a natural hormone; (*b*) containing no estrogens; (*c*) using a T-shaped delivery device to ensure comfort, safety, and retention, which minimizes mechanically induced irritation; and (*d*) confining the hormonal action to the uterus.

The device contains the progesterone suspended in silicone oil; barium sulfate is added to make it radiopaque. The ethylene vinyl acetate (EVA) membrane surrounding the drug core controls the rate of drug release. Titanium dioxide is added to the EVA for a white color. At the end of a year, the device will contain approximately 14 mg of progesterone, the excess being required to maintain the thermodynamic activity of the drug reservoir and consistent sustained drug release rate.

Dinoprostone Vaginal Insert

Dinoprostone (Cervidil, Forest Pharmaceuticals) is a thick, flat, rectangular polymeric slab enclosed in a pouch of a knitted polyester retrieval system. The buff-colored semitransparent polymeric hydrogel slab contains 10 mg of dinoprostone. The retrieval system is in the shape of a long knitted tape used to retrieve, or remove, the unit after the dosing interval is complete. The product is designed to release dinoprostone in vivo at a rate of about 0.3 mg/h. The unit contains 10 mg of dinoprostone in 236 mg of a cross-linked polyethylene oxide–urethane polymer slab that measures 29 mm by 9.5 mm and is 0.8 mm thick. When placed in a moist environment, the unit absorbs water, swells, and releases dinoprostone.

It is indicated for initiation and/or continuation of cervical ripening in patients at or near term when there is medical or obstetrical indication for labor induction.

The product is dosed at 10 mg of dinoprostone (1 U) inserted vaginally and removed upon onset of active labor or 12 hours after insertion. After administration, the patient should remain supine for 2 hours but may be ambulatory after that time.

This product should be stored in a freezer at −20°C to −10°C (−4°F to 14°F); it is packaged in foil and is stable in the freezer for 3 years. After opening and upon exposure to humidity, it is hygroscopic, and the release characteristics of the dinoprostone may be altered if it is improperly stored (5). An example is shown in Figure 20.6.

Estring

A unique method of administering estradiol is through the use of the estradiol vaginal ring (Estring, Pharmacia Corp., A Division of Pfizer) shown in Figure 20.4. The core of the ring contains a reservoir of estradiol, which is released immediately and then at a continuous rate of 75 mg per 24 hours over 90 days. The ring, composed of silicone polymers and barium sulfate, has an outer diameter of 55 mm and a core diameter of 2 mm. The ring is inserted into the upper third of the vaginal vault and is worn continuously for the treatment of urogenital symptoms associated with postmenopausal atrophy of the vagina.

FIGURE 20.6. Cervidil (dinoprostone) vaginal insert. (Courtesy Ferring Pharmaceuticals, Inc.)

Crinone Gel

Another type of vaginal product with extended action is the bioadhesive vaginal gel Crinone Gel (Wyeth-Ayerst), which contains micronized progesterone and the polymer polycarbophil in an oil-in-water emulsion system. The polymer, which is insoluble in water, swells within the vagina and forms a bioadhesive gel coating on the walls of the vagina. This allows the absorption of progesterone through the vaginal tissue over 25 to 50 hours. The product is used to assist in reproduction and is shown in Figure 20.7.

OPHTHALMICS

One of the problems associated with the use of ophthalmic solutions is the rapid loss of administered drug because of the blinking of the eye and the flushing effect of lacrimal fluids. Up to 80% of an administered dose may be lost through tears and the action of nasolacrimal drainage

FIGURE 20.7. Crinone (progesterone 8% gel). Commercial package contains six single-use, individually wrapped prefilled applicators.

within 5 minutes of installation. Extended periods of therapy may be achieved by formulations that increase the contact time between the medication and the corneal surface. This may be accomplished by the use of agents that increase the viscosity of solutions, by ophthalmic suspensions in which the drug particles slowly dissolve, by slowly dissipating ophthalmic ointments, or by the use of ophthalmic inserts.

Gels Extended Release

Although ophthalmic dosage forms are discussed at length in Chapter 17, it is useful to note here certain preparations designed to extend drug action. The following are but two examples of proprietary products that use viscosity-increasing agents to increase corneal contact time. Pilocarpine (Pilopine HS Gel, Alcon) employs Carbopol 940, a synthetic high molecular weight cross-linked polymer of acrylic acid. Timolol maleate (Timoptic-XE, Merck) employs gellan gum (Gelrite), which forms a gel upon contact with the precorneal tear film.

Ophthalmic Inserts

Lacrisert

Lacrisert (Merck) is a rod-shaped water-soluble form of hydroxypropyl cellulose. The insert is placed in the inferior cul-de-sac of the eye once or twice daily for the treatment of dry eyes. The inserts soften and slowly dissolve, thickening the precorneal tear film and prolonging the tear film breakup.

Pilocarpine Insert

Pilocarpine is available in a membrane-controlled reservoir system that is used in the treatment of glaucoma. Pilocarpine is sandwiched between two EVA membranes. It also contains alginic acid, a seaweed carbohydrate, which serves as a carrier for pilocarpine. The small, clear device has a white annular border made of EVA copolymer impregnated with titanium dioxide (pigment) that makes it easier for the patient to see. The insert is placed in the cul-de-sac, where it will float with the tears. The pilocarpine will diffuse from the device and exert its pharmacologic effect (Figs. 20.8 and 20.9).

The tear fluid penetrates the microporous membrane, dissolving the pilocarpine. The release rate of pilocarpine is in the range of 20 or 40 mg/h for 4 to 7 days. One advantage of this system is enhanced compliance, as the patient does not have to remember to instill the drops and has no blurred vision or slight discomfort that occurs when applying drops to the eyes.

The release rate of pilocarpine from the EVA system is shown in the following equation:

$$\frac{dm}{dt} = \frac{ADK\Delta C}{h}$$

Where dm/dt is the release rate; D is the diffusion coefficient of the drug in the membrane; K is the partition

FIGURE 20.8. Ocusert ocular therapeutic systems are thin, flexible wafers placed under the eyelid to provide a week's dose of pilocarpine in the treatment of glaucoma. Ocusert systems cause less blurring of vision than do conventional pilocarpine eye drops, which must be administered four times daily.

coefficient, that is, the ratio of drug concentration at equilibrium inside the membrane to that outside the membrane; ΔC is the difference of the drug concentration between the inside and the outside walls of the membrane; and A and h are the area and thickness of the system, respectively. Under routine conditions, the concentration of the drug in the tears is negligible (2 to 3 mg/mL) compared to that inside the membrane, which is essentially the solubility of the drug, so the equation can be rewritten

$$\frac{dm}{dt} = \frac{ADKS}{h}$$

The systems are designed to release at 20 or 40 mg/h for 1 week. Over a week's time, the total drug released by the system is 3.4 or 6.7 mg, for the 20 or 40 mg/h units, respectively.

FIGURE 20.9. Construction of the Ocusert ocular therapeutic system containing pilocarpine between transparent rate-controlling membranes.

The units contain either 5 or 11 mg of drug initially and are designed to retain about 40% of the initial quantity of drug to provide for a constant delivery rate and a safety margin of an extra day's delivery of drug.

PARENTERAL ADMINISTRATION

Long-Acting Parenteral Systems

Extended durations of drug action following injection may be achieved in a number of ways, including the use of crystal or amorphous drug forms having prolonged dissolution characteristics, slowly dissolving chemical complexes of the drug entity, solutions, or suspensions of drug in slowly absorbed carriers or vehicles (e.g., oleaginous vehicle), large particles of drug in suspension, or injection of slowly eroding microspheres of drug (6). The duration of action of the various forms of insulin, for example, is based in part on its physical form (amorphous or crystalline), complex formation with added agents, and dosage form (solution or suspension) (7).

Matrix carrier systems based on biodegradable materials for parenteral application have been examined as a potential means of delivering peptides and proteins (see "Gliadel Wafer Implant"). In such systems, a material such as purified insoluble collagen is used as a matrix that releases the drug contents through controlled diffusion and enzymatic matrix degradation.

In addition to these means of achieving extended drug action, the rate and duration of drug delivery may be controlled mechanically using controlled-rate drug infusion pumps.

Examples of proprietary parenteral products having long-acting features are presented in Table 20.4. Conventional parenteral products and methods of administration are discussed in Chapter 15.

Liposomes

Liposomes are composed of small vesicles of a bilayer of phospholipid encapsulating an aqueous space ranging from about 0.03 to 10 µm in diameter. They are composed of one or many lipid membranes enclosing discrete aqueous compartments. The enclosed vesicles can encapsulate water-soluble drugs in the aqueous spaces, and lipid-soluble drugs can be incorporated into the membranes. Liposomes can be administered parenterally, topically, by inhalation, and possibly by other routes of administration. Current products are administered parenterally.

The following is an oversimplification but will serve to illustrate the preparation of liposomes. Prepare a solution of a lipid (lecithin) in an organic solvent (acetone, chloroform) in a beaker. Allow the solvent to evaporate, leaving a thin film of the lipid on the walls of the container. Add an aqueous solution of the drug to the beaker and place it in an ultrasonic bath. As the lipid is displaced from the beaker walls, it forms spheres or cylinders, trapping the aqueous solution inside. The liposomes can be collected, sized, and used.

Numerous configurations are possible for liposomes, including spheres and cylinders. Spherical liposomes can be unilamellar (only one layer) or multilamellar (many layers). They are often designated LUV (large unilamellar vesicle), SUV (small unilamellar vesicle), and MLV (multilamellar vesicle). The smaller vesicles, or liposomes, generally range in size from 0.02 to 0.2 µm and the large vesicles from about 0.2 mm to more than 10 mm. The MLVs may have an onionskin structure of several layers.

The phospholipids composing liposomes are amphipathic, possessing both a hydrophilic or polar head and a hydrophobic or nonpolar tail. This is similar to the hydrophilic–lipophilic balance (HLB) and wedge orientation theories of emulsification. The hydrophobic tail is composed of fatty acids containing generally 10 to 24 carbon atoms, and the polar end may contain phosphoric acid bound to a water-soluble portion; the composition may vary considerably. Lecithin (phosphatidylcholine) is a backbone structure that has been studied extensively. When these phospholipids are exposed to water and line up, they do so in a manner that the fatty acid tails associate together as the lipophilic phase and the polar head groups

TABLE 20.4. Examples of Proprietary Extended Action Parenteral Products

Product	Contents and Comments
Bicillin C-R Injection (Monarch)	Contains penicillin G benzathine and penicillin G procaine, which have low solubility and are slowly released from IM injection sites. Hydrolyze to penicillin G. Hydrolysis plus slow absorption results in prolonged blood serum levels. Usual dose interval, 2–3 days
Decadron-LA Sterile Suspension (Merck)	Contains dexamethasone acetate, very insoluble ester of dexamethasone. Repository IM injection may be repeated as needed at 1–3 weeks
Depo-Provera Contraceptive Injection (Pharmacia)	Medroxyprogesterone acetate, water insoluble, in aqueous suspension. Single IM dose is repeated q3mo
Abelcet Amphotericin B Lipid Complex Injection (Enzon)	Suspension of amphotericin B complexed with two phospholipids administered by IV infusion qd
Lupron Depot for Suspension (TAP Pharmaceuticals)	Sterile lyophilized microspheres; mixed with diluent, form IM injection suspension q3–4 mo

IM, intramuscular; IV, intravenous.

associate toward the bulk water phase. Depending on the lipid composition and the water solubility of the drug, the drug may be in the aqueous compartments (if water soluble) or in the lipophilic bilayers (if oil soluble).

Some liposomes are unique because they can be selectively absorbed by tissues rich in reticuloendothelial cells, such as the liver, spleen, and bone marrow. This can serve as a targeting mechanism, but it also removes liposomes from the circulation rather rapidly. To extend the half-life of liposomes in the body, "stealth liposomes" have been developed by coating the liposomes with materials, such as the polymer polyethylene glycol (PEG), enabling liposomes to evade detection through the components of the body's immune system. This extends their half-life and may also alter their biodistribution.

Advantages of liposomes include the following: (*a*) Liposome-encapsulated drugs are delivered intact to various tissues and cells and can be released when the liposome is destroyed, enabling site-specific and targeted drug delivery. (*b*) Liposomes can be used for both hydrophilic and lipophilic drugs without chemical modification. (*c*) Other tissues and cells of the body are protected from the drug until it is released by the liposomes, decreasing the drug's toxicity. (*d*) The size, charge, and other characteristics can be altered depending on the drug and the intended use of the product.

Disadvantages of liposomes include their tendency to be taken up by cells of the reticuloendothelial system (RES) and the slow release of the drug when the liposomes are taken up by phagocytes through endocytosis, fusion, surface adsorption, or lipid exchange.

Many advances in liposome preparation, including composition, sizing, classification, and enhancing stability, have been made. Stability has been a problem, but stable liposomes can now be prepared. Liposomes have been investigated for a number of years as potential drug delivery systems and now are on the market.

One product is Abelcet Injection (Enzon). It is a sterile, pyrogen-free suspension for intravenous infusion consisting of amphotericin B complexed with two phospholipids in a 1:1 drug-to-lipid molar ratio. The two phospholipids, L-alpha-dimyristoyl phosphatidylcholine (DMPC) and L-alpha-dimyristoyl phosphatidylglycerol (DMPG), are present in a 7:3 molar ratio. The product is yellow and opaque with a pH in the range of 5 to 7. The formulation per milliliter is provided as the following (8):

Amphotericin B, USP	5 mg
DMPC	3.4 mg
DMPG	1.5 mg
Sodium Chloride, USP	9 mg
Water for Injection, USP qs	1 mL

The product contains the following bolded note, indicating that Abelcet is not interchangeable with the other available lipid-based amphotericin B products:

NOTE: Liposomal encapsulation or incorporation in a lipid complex can substantially affect a drug's functional properties relative to those of the unencapsulated or non–lipid-associated drug. In addition, different liposomal or lipid-complexed products with a common active ingredient may vary from one another in the chemical composition and physical form of the lipid component. Such differences may affect functional properties of these drug products.

AmBisome is amphotericin B liposome for injection. It is a sterile, nonpyrogenic lyophilized product for intravenous infusion; each vial contains 50 mg amphotericin B intercalated into a liposomal membrane consisting of approximately 213 mg of hydrogenated soy phosphatidylcholine, 52 mg of cholesterol, 84 mg of distearoyl phosphatidylglycerol, 0.64 mg of alpha-tocopherol, 900 mg of sucrose, and 27 mg of disodium succinate hexahydrate as a buffer. When reconstituted with sterile water for injection, the pH of the solution is between 5.0 and 6.0. AmBisome is a true, single bilayer liposomal drug delivery system. When the powder is reconstituted, multiple concentric bilayer membranes are formed; these are changed by microemulsification into single bilayer liposomes using a homogenizer. AmBisome contains liposomes that are less than 100 nm in diameter. Amphotericin B is a macrocyclic polyene antifungal antibiotic that is produced from a strain of *Streptomyces nodosus.*

Amphotec (amphotericin B cholesteryl sulfate, Sequus Pharmaceuticals) is a sterile, pyrogen-free lyophilized powder for reconstitution and intravenous administration. It is a 1:1 molar ratio complex of amphotericin B and cholesteryl sulfate that upon reconstitution forms a colloidal dispersion of microscopic disk-shaped particles. Each 50-mg single-dose vial contains amphotericin B 50 mg, sodium cholesteryl sulfate 26.4 mg, tromethamine 5.64 mg, disodium edetate dihydrate 0.372 mg, lactose monohydrate 950 mg, and hydrochloric acid qs. The 100-mg single-dose vial contains amphotericin B, 100 mg; sodium cholesteryl sulfate, 52.8 mg; tromethamine, 11.28 mg; disodium edetate dihydrate, 0.744 mg; lactose monohydrate, 1,900 mg; and hydrochloric acid, qs.

Amphotec is indicated for the treatment of invasive aspergillosis in patients when renal impairment or unacceptable toxicity precludes the use of amphotericin B deoxycholate in effective doses and in patients with aspergillosis when prior amphotericin B deoxycholate therapy has failed.

The drug is reconstituted with sterile water for injection by rapidly adding the water to the vial; it is shaken gently by hand, rotating the vial until all the solids have dissolved. The fluid may be opalescent or clear. It is further diluted in 5% dextrose injection for infusion. The product should not be reconstituted with any fluid other than sterile water for injection; do not reconstitute with dextrose or sodium chloride solutions. Also, for further dilution, it should not be admixed with sodium chloride or electrolytes. Solutions containing benzyl alcohol or any other bacteriostatic agent should not be used, as they may cause precipitation. An inline filter should not be used, and the infusion admixture should not be mixed with other drugs. If infused using a Y-injection site or similar device, flush the line with 5% dextrose injection before and after infusion of Amphotec.

After reconstitution, the drug should be refrigerated and used within 24 hours; do not freeze. If further diluted with 5% dextrose injection, it should be refrigerated and used within 24 hours (9).

Daunorubicin citrate liposome injection (DaunoXome, Gilead Sciences) is an aqueous solution of daunorubicin citrate encapsulated with liposomes composed of distearoyl phosphatidylcholine and cholesterol (2:1 molar ratio), with a mean diameter of about 45 nm (range 35 to 65 nm). The weight ratio of lipid to drug is 18.7:1 (total lipid–daunorubicin base), equivalent to a 10:5:1 molar ratio of distearoyl phosphatidylcholine, cholesterol, and daunorubicin, respectively.

DaunoXome is formulated to maximize the selectivity of daunorubicin for solid tumors in situ. The liposomal formulation helps to protect the daunorubicin from chemical and enzymatic degradation, minimizes protein binding, and generally decreases uptake by normal tissues.

The product should be diluted 1:1 with 5% dextrose injection prior to administration. Each vial contains the equivalent of 50 mg daunorubicin base at a concentration of 2 mg/mL after preparation; it is recommended to be diluted to 1 mg/mL for administration. The only fluid recommended for preparation is 5% dextrose injection; it must not be mixed with a solution containing sodium chloride or benzyl alcohol or with any other solution. An inline filter should not be used for the intravenous infusion of DaunoXome. The final product appears as a red translucent dispersion of liposomes that does scatter light, but it should not be used if it appears opaque or has precipitate or foreign matter in it. It should be stored in a refrigerator (2°C to 8°C; 36°F to 46°F); do not freeze and protect from light (10).

Stealth Liposomes

Liposome research has resulted in liposomes that avoid detection by the body's immune system, specifically the cells of the RES. These liposomes are known as "stealth liposomes" and are prepared with PEG on the outside of the membrane. The PEG coating, which is inert in the body, allows for longer circulatory life for the drug delivery mechanism. In addition to the PEG coating, most stealth liposomes also have some type of biological species attached as a ligand to the liposome in order to enable binding via a specific expression on the targeted drug delivery site. These targeting ligands could be monoclonal antibodies (making an immunoliposome), vitamins, or specific antigens. Targeted liposomes can target nearly any cell type in the body and deliver drugs that would naturally be systemically delivered. Naturally toxic drugs can be much less toxic if delivered only to diseased tissues. In case of tumor development, certain anticancer drugs like doxorubicin (Doxil) and daunorubicin are provided through liposomes.

Doxorubicin hydrochloride (Doxil) liposome injection consists of the drug encapsulated in stealth liposomes for intravenous administration. Doxorubicin is a cytotoxic anthracycline antibiotic that is isolated from *Streptomyces peucetius* var. *caesius*. The product is available as a sterile translucent red liposomal dispersion containing in each 10-mL single-use glass vial 20 mg doxorubicin HCl at a pH of 6.5. The stealth liposomes consist of 3.19 mg/mL of N-(carbonyl-methoxypolyethylene glycol 2000)-1,2-distearoyl-sn-glycero-3-phosphoethanolamine sodium salt, 9.58 mg/mL of fully hydrogenated soy phosphatidylcholine, and 3.19 mg/mL of cholesterol; also, each milliliter contains approximately 2 mg ammonium sulfate along with histidine as a buffer, sucrose for tonicity, and hydrochloric acid and/or sodium hydroxide for adjustment of pH. The doxorubicin is at least 90% encapsulated in the stealth liposomes. These stealth liposomes are protected from detection by the mononuclear phagocyte system by the coating with surface-bound methoxy PEG; this increases blood circulation time. These liposomes have a half-life of approximately 55 hours in humans (11).

SELF-EMULSIFYING DRUG DELIVERY SYSTEMS

Oral administration of drugs is preferred; however, more than 40% of new chemical entities (APIs) exhibit poor aqueous solubility; this results in poor oral drug delivery/bioavailability. Low aqueous solubility and low bioavailability is a major concern for developing oral formulations. One approach to this problem involves the use of self-emulsifying lipid formulations (SELFs), also called self-emulsifying oil formulations (SEOFs).

The main types of SELF systems include the following:

- Self-emulsifying drug delivery systems (SEDDSs)
- Self-micro-emulsifying drug delivery systems (SMEDDSs)
- Self-nano-emulsifying drug delivery systems (SNEDDS)

SEDDS are increasing in popularity for improving the solubility of lipophilic drugs. SEDDS are generally defined as isotropic mixtures of drug, oil, surfactant and/or cosurfactant, and sometimes cosolvents. Upon administration, the formulations rapidly disperse in the gastrointestinal (GI) fluids and the GI tract itself provides the necessary agitation for self-emulsification. The micro- or nano-emulsified drug is now exposed to a large interfacial surface area for absorption. This "in situ solubilization of drug" can be absorbed via lymphatic pathways, bypassing the hepatic first-pass effect.

SEDDS can be orally administered in soft or hard gelatin capsules and form fine, relatively stable oil-in-water emulsions upon aqueous dilution. When compared with standard emulsions, which are sensitive and metastable dispersed forms, SEDDSs are physically stable formulations that are easily prepared. These systems may offer an improvement in the rate and extent of absorption and result in more reproducible blood-time profiles for problematic drugs with poor solubility and bioavailability.

The droplet sizes of SEDDS formulations are generally in the 200 nm to 5 µm range, and the dispersion may have a turbid appearance. SMEDDSs have a smaller lipid droplet size (<200 nm), and the dispersion is generally optically clear to a translucent appearance. Both of these systems generate a large surface area of dispersions that provide optimum conditions for the increased absorption of poorly soluble drugs. A formulator's choice of whether to develop a SEDDS or a SMEDDS is usually dependent on the relationship between the characteristics of the API, its solubility, dissolution profile, and data obtained during in vitro screening with a number of excipients.

SELFs are usually liquid or semisolid formulations and are appropriate for soft or hard capsule filling. Currently, SEDDS drugs are developed in soft or hard gelatin capsules since, until recently, getting a SELF into tablet form was a challenge. There are actually more than 150 patents published on SEDDS (12,13). Table 20.5 is a list of commercial products incorporating SELFs (12,13).

The advantages of SEDDS include the following:

- High drug solubilization capacity
- Good thermodynamic stability
- Improvement in oral bioavailability with reduction in dose
- High drug payloads
- Reduce the intrasubject and intersubject variability and food effects
- Useful for drug targeting toward specific absorption window
- Control of delivery profile
- More consistent drug absorption rate profiles
- Protection of drug(s) from the hostile environment in gut
- Protection of sensitive drug substances
- Suitability for liquid or solid dosage forms

Some disadvantages of SEDDS include the following:

- A lack of an in vitro model for assessment of the formulations.
- Potential chemical instabilities of drugs and high surfactant concentrations.
- Volatile cosolvents in the conventional self-emulsifying formulations are known to migrate into the shells of soft or hard gelatin capsule, resulting in the precipitation of the lipophilic drugs.
- Formulations are potentially dependent on dissolution prior to release the drug.

Dosage forms utilizing SELFs and SEDDS are shown in Table 20.5 Commercial Products Using Lipid-Based Formulations include the following:

- Dry emulsions
- Self-emulsifying capsules
- Self-emulsifying sustained/controlled-release tablets
- Self-emulsifying sustained/controlled-release pellets
- Self-emulsifying solid dispersions
- Self-emulsifying suppositories

TABLE 20.5. Commercial Products Using Lipid-Based Formulations

Amlodipine SE Dry emulsion	—	—
Amprenavir	Agenerase	Capsule, Solution
Astaxanthin SE Capsules	—	—
Calcitriol	Rocaltrol	Solution
Carmustine Implants	—	—
Cyclosporine	Neoral	Capsule, Solution
Cyclosporine	Sandimmune	Capsule, Solution
Cyclosporine A	Gengraf	Capsule
Diclofenac SE tablets	—	—
Dutasteride	Avodart	Capsule
Halofantrine SEF powder	—	—
Indomethacin Suppositories	—	—
Isotretinoin	Accutane	Capsule
Lopinavir + Ritonavir	Kaletra	Tablet, Solution
Loratadine SEF (Beads)	—	—
Nitrendipine Pellets	—	—
Paclitaxel SE nanoparticles	—	—
Phenacetin Solid Dispersion	—	—
Progesterone	Prometrium	Capsule
Ritonavir	Norvir	Capsule
Saquinavir	Fortavase	Capsule
Bexarotene	Targretin	Capsule
Tipranavir	Aptivus	Capsule, Solution
Tretinoin	Vesanoid	Capsule
Valproic acid	Depakene	Capsule

- Self-emulsifying implants
- Melt granulations
- Self-emulsifying powders

The commonly used approach to formulating SEDDS is to incorporate the active lipophilic component into a lipid vehicle, surfactant dispersions, self-emulsifying formulations, emulsions, or liposomes. Every formulation technique has its advantages and limitations. The formulation of SEDDS is dependent on the following:

- The nature of the oil–surfactant pair
- The surfactant concentration
- The temperature at which self-emulsification occurs

There is a large variety of liquid or waxy excipients available ranging from oils to biological lipids, hydrophobic and hydrophilic surfactants, as well as water-soluble cosurfactant/cosolvents. There is a multitude of different combinations that could be formulated for encapsulation in hard or soft gelatin or mixtures which disperse to give fine colloidal emulsions. Examples of oils, surfactants, cosurfactants, and cosolvents used in SELFs are listed in Table 20.6 and popular emulsifiers employed in SEDDS formulations with their HLB Values are listed in Table 20.7.

TABLE 20.6. Examples of Oils, Surfactants, Cosurfactant, and Cosolvents Used in SELFs

Oils	Surfactants	Cosurfactants/Cosolvent
Cotton seed oil	Polysorbate 20 (Tween 20)	Span 20
Soybean oil	Polysorbate 80 (Tween 80)	Span 80
Corn oil	D-alpha Tocopheryl polyethylene glycol 1000 succinate (TPGS)	Capryol 90
Sunflower oil	Polyoxyl-35-castor oil (Cremophor EL)	Lauroglycol
Castor oil	Polyoxyl-40-hydrogenated castor oil (Cremophor RH40)	Transcutol
Sesame oil	Labrasol	Capmul
Peanut oil		Ethanol
Labrafac		Propylene glycol
Labrafil		Polyethylene glycol

Prior to formulating a SELF, the following should be considered, including

- The solubility of the drug indifferent oils, surfactants and cosurfactant/ co-solvents
- The selection of oil, surfactant and cosolvent based on the solubility of the drug and the preparation of an appropriate phase diagram
- The methods and procedure for preparation of the SEDDS formulation by dissolving the drug in a mixture of oil, surfactant, and cosurfactant/cosolvents

Preparing SELFs/SEDDs Formulations

Numerous methods can be used for preparing SELFs, including

- Capsule filling with liquid and semisolid self-emulsifying formulations
- Adsorption to solid carriers and encapsulating/tableting
- Spray drying
- Melt granulation
- Melt extrusion/extrusion spheronization

TABLE 20.7. Popular Emulsifiers Employed in SEDDS Formulations with Their HLB Values

Chemical Name	HLB	Commercial Name
Ethoxylated castor oil	12–15	Emulphor El-620
Glyceryl monooleate	3–4	Peceol
Methyl-oxirane polymer with oxirane	12–18	Pluronic L-64
L-α-Phosphatidylcholine	4–9	Lecithin
PEG-20 sorbitan monooleate	15	Tween 80
PEG-20 sorbitan trioleate	11	Tween 85
PEG-4 lauryl ether	9.7	Brij-30
PEG-6 corn oil	4	Labrafil M 2125 CS
PEG-6 apricot kernel oil	4	Labrafil M1944CS
PEG-8 caprylic/capric glycerides	14	Labrasol
PEG-8 caprylic/capric glycerides	>10	Labrafac CM 10
PEG-8 corn oil	6–7	Labrafil WL 2609 BS
PEG-20 sorbitan monolaurate	17	Tween 20
PEG-20 sorbitan tristearate	11	Tween 65
PEG-25 trioleate	11	Tagat TO
PEG-35 castor oil	12–14	Cremophor-EL Cremophor-ELP
PEG-35 hydrogenated castor oil	13	Cremophor EL
PEG-40 hydrogenated castor oil	13	Cremophor RH40
Polyoxyethylene hydrogenated castor oil 40	13	HCO-40
Polyoxyethylene–polyoxypropylene copolymers	18–23	Pluronic F 127
Sorbitan monooleate	4.3	Span 80

Examples of SEDDS Formulas

Ceftriaxone Rectal SEDDS

Ceftriaxone	40%
Capryol 90	15%
Kolliphor EL	22.5%
Kolliphor PS20	22.5%

Coenzyme Q10 Oral SEDDS

Coenzyme Q10	x mg
Myvacet 9-45	40%
Labrasol	50%
Lauroglycol	10%

Ibuprofen Oral SEDDS

Ibuprofen	x mg
Labrafac PG	20%
Tween 80	25%
Polyethylene glycol 200	55%

HOT MELT EXTRUSION

Various extrusion processes have been used in pharmacy for many years. In earlier times, suppositories were made using a cold-extrusion process both at the manufacturing and compounding levels. Cold or room-temperature extrusion is used in some instances today for mixing and in preformulation steps. Hot melt extrusion has been around for a long time but has become more popular in recent decades by large scale manufacturers. It simply involves comingling two or more substances together (typically polymer and drug), heating them beyond their glass transition (T_g) temperature and sometimes above their melting temperature (T_m) to bind them on a molecular level, achieving a homogenous amorphous solid (14).

The potential advantages of this process include taste masking, targeted drug delivery, implants, controlled-release dosage forms, and it is a component of 3D printing (discussed later).

PEGYLATED DOSAGE FORMS

Neulasta (pegfilgrastim) is a covalent conjugate of recombinant methionyl human granulocyte colony-stimulating factor (G-CSF) (filgrastim) and monomethoxy PEG. Filgrastim is a water-soluble 175-amino acid protein obtained from bacterial fermentation of a strain of *Escherichia coli*; it has a molecular weight of approximately 19 kDa. Pegfilgrastim is produced by covalently bonding a 20-kDa PEG molecule to the N-terminal methionyl residue of filgrastim, resulting in an average molecular weight of pegfilgrastim of approximately 39 kDa. Neulasta is available in 0.6-mL prefilled syringes for subcutaneous injection. The syringe contains 6 mg of pegfilgrastim (based on protein weight) in a clear, colorless, sterile, preservative-free solution containing 0.35 mg acetate, 30 mg sorbitol, 0.02 mg polysorbate 20, and 0.02 mg sodium in water for injection; the pH of the injection is 4.0. Depending on the therapeutic indication, Neulasta is administered either as a single injection or as two injections a week apart, while filgrastim is administered daily for the entire treatment cycle.

Pegasys (peginterferon *alfa*-2a), used in the treatment of hepatitis C virus, is a covalent conjugate of recombinant *alfa*-2a interferon (molecular weight ~20 kDa) with a single-branched bis-PEG chain of approximately 40-kDa molecular weight. The PEG moiety is linked at a single site to the interferon *alfa* moiety via a stable amide bond to lysine; the final product has an approximate molecular weight of 60 kDa.

Each vial of Pegasys contains approximately 1.2 mL of solution to deliver 1 mL of drug for subcutaneous administration. The 1-mL volume delivers 180 mg of drug product (expressed as the amount of interferon *alfa*-2a), 8 mg sodium chloride, 0.05 mg polysorbate 80, 10 mg benzyl alcohol, 2.62 mg sodium acetate trihydrate, and 0.05 mg acetic acid; the solution has a pH of 6.0 ± 0.01 and is colorless to light yellow.

Pegasys produces maximal serum concentrations at 72 to 96 hours after dosing that are sustained for up to 168 hours. In comparison to Roferon-A (non-PEGylated interferon *alfa*-2A), the mean systemic clearance for Pegasys was 94 mL/h, which is approximately one-hundredth of that for Roferon. The mean terminal half-life after subcutaneous dosing in patients with chronic hepatitis C was 80 hours (range 50 to 140 hours) compared to 5.1 hours (range 3.7 to 8.5 hours) for Roferon-A (15).

PEG-Intron (peginterferon alfa-2b Powder for Injection) is a covalent conjugate of recombinant *alfa* interferon with PEG; approximate molecular weight of the PEG portion is 12 kDa, and the approximate molecular weight of the PEG-Intron molecule is 31 kDa. The product is a white to off-white lyophilized powder supplied in 2-mL vials for subcutaneous use. Each vial contains 74, 118.4, 177.6, or 222 mg of PEG-Intron and 1.11 mg dibasic sodium phosphate anhydrous, 1.11 mg monobasic sodium phosphate dihydrate, 59.2 mg sucrose, and 0.074 mg polysorbate 80. After reconstitution with 0.7 mL of the supplied diluent, which is sterile water for injection, each vial contains PEG-Intron in strength of 100, 160, 240, or 300 mg/mL.

Compared to interferon *alfa*-2b, PEG-Intron has one-seventh the mean apparent clearance and a fivefold greater mean half-life, permitting a reduced dosing frequency. At effective therapeutic doses, PEG-Intron has approximately a tenfold greater maximum concentration (C_{max}) and a 50-fold greater area under the curve than interferon *alfa*-2b (16).

FUSION PROTEIN: SPECIAL HANDLING

Ontak

Denileukin diftitox (Ontak) is included in this chapter because of its unusual nature and handling. Ontak is a fusion protein designed to direct the cytocidal action of diphtheria toxin to cells that express the interleukin-2 (IL-2) receptor. Ontak is a recombinant DNA–derived cytotoxic protein composed of the amino acid sequences for diphtheria toxin fragments A and B (Met_1-Thr_{387})-His followed by the sequences for IL-2 (Ala_1-Thr_{133}); it is produced in an *E. coli* expression system. Ontak has a molecular weight of 58 kDa. The single-use vials (2 mL) contain 300 mg of recombinant denileukin diftitox in a sterile solution of 20 mM citric acid, 0.05 mM ethylenediaminetetraacetic acid (EDTA), and less than 1% polysorbate 20 in water for injection; the pH of the solution is between 6.9 and 7.2.

The drug is indicated in the treatment of patients with persistent or recurrent cutaneous T-cell lymphoma whose malignant cells express the CD25 component of the IL-2 receptor. It should be used only by physicians experienced in the use of antineoplastic therapy and management of patients with cancer. Use of this drug should be in patients managed in a facility equipped and staffed for cardiopulmonary resuscitation and where the patients can be closely monitored for an appropriate period based on their health status.

Ontak requires special handling as follows: (*a*) It must be brought to room temperature before preparing the dose. The vials may be thawed in the refrigerator for not more than 24 hours or at room temperature for 1 to 2 hours. (*b*) The solution in the vial may be mixed by gentle swirling: *Do not vigorously shake Ontak solution.* (*c*) After thawing, a haze may be visible. This haze should clear when the solution is at room temperature. (*d*) Ontak solution must not be used unless the solution is clear, colorless, and without visible particulate matter. (*e*) *Ontak must not be refrozen.* The following are a few administration items of interest: (*a*) Diluted Ontak solution should be prepared and held in plastic syringes or soft plastic intravenous bags. *Do not use a glass container* because adsorption to glass may occur in a dilute state. (*b*) The concentration of Ontak must be at least 15 mg/mL in all steps in the preparation of the solution for intravenous infusion. This is best accomplished by withdrawing the calculated dose from the vial or vials and injecting it into an empty infusion bag. Then, for each 1 mL of Ontak, no more than 9 mL of sterile saline without preservative should be added to the intravenous bag. (*c*) Ontak solution should not be physically mixed with any other drugs. (*d*) Do not administer Ontak solution through an inline filter. (*e*) Prepared solutions of Ontak should be administered within 6 hours, using a syringe pump or intravenous infusion bag. (*f*) Unused portions of Ontak should be discarded immediately.

Prior to handling this drug, pharmacists, nurses, and physicians should carefully read and understand all of the precautions explained in the package labeling (17).

IMPLANTS

Implants are long-acting dosage forms that provide continuous release of the drug, often for periods of months to years. They are administered by the parenteral route; for systemic delivery, they may be placed subcutaneously, or for local delivery, they can be placed in a specific region in the body. They can be made by compression, melting, or sintering. They generally consist of the drug and rate-controlling excipients. Several types are available including pellets, resorbable microparticles, polymer implants, in situ–forming gel/solid implants, metal/plastic implants, and drug-eluting stents.

Pellet implants are small, sterile, solid masses of the active drug with or without excipients and are usually administered using a suitable special injector (e.g., trocar) or by surgical incision. The size and rate of erosion will influence the release rate, which is generally first-order kinetics.

Resorbable microparticles or microspheres generally range from 20 to 100 μm in diameter composed of the drug dispersed within a biocompatible, bioresorbable polymeric excipient (matrix). The microparticles are administered as an aqueous suspension subcutaneously or intramuscularly for systemic delivery, or they may be injected into a specific location in the body.

Polymer implants can be formed as a single mass, such as a cylinder. The polymer matrix must be biocompatible and can be either biodegradable or nonbiodegradable. Shaped implants are administered by means of a suitable injector; release rates are not zero order but can approach zero-order kinetics. They are used to deliver potent small molecules, including steroids, and large molecules, including peptides. An advantage to the biodegradable implants is that they do not require removal after release of all the drug.

Liquid–gel/solid implants are initially liquid formulations comprising a polymer, active drug, and solvent (either aqueous or organic). After administration, a gel or a solid polymeric matrix is formed trapping the drug and extending the release of the drug for days or months.

Metal/plastic implants may be formulated from titanium or other suitable materials and are administered by an injector or surgical installation. A solution of the drug, located inside the implant, is released via an osmotically driven pump inside the implant and may last as long as 1 year or more; release follows zero order.

Drug-eluting stents combine the mechanical effect of the stent with a prolonged pharmacologic effect of the incorporated drug. The metal stent can be coated with a nonbiodegradable or biodegradable polymer–containing drug.

Historically, pellets or implants were sterile, small, usually cylindrical solid objects about 3.2 mm in diameter and 8 mm long, prepared by compression and intended to be implanted subcutaneously to provide continuous release of medication over time. The pellets that are implanted under the skin (usually of the thigh or abdomen) with a special injector or by surgical incision are used for potent hormones. Implantation provides the patient with an economical means of obtaining long-lasting effects (up to many months after a single implantation) and obviates frequent parenteral or oral hormone therapy. The implanted pellets, which may contain 100 times the amount of drug (e.g., desoxycorticosterone, estradiol, testosterone) given by other routes of administration, release the drug slowly into the general circulation.

Pellets were formulated with no binders, diluents, or excipients, to permit total dissolution and absorption of the pellet from the site of implantation. Recently, a levonorgestrel implant contraceptive system was developed. Rather than dissolve entirely, the surgically implanted capsules are intended to be removed by surgery after an appropriate amount of time (up to 5 years).

Levonorgestrel Implants

Levonorgestrel implants are a set of six flexible closed capsules of a dimethylsiloxane–methyl vinyl siloxane copolymer, each containing 36 mg of the progestin (18). They are found in an insertion kit to facilitate subdermal implantation through a 2-mm incision in the mid–upper arm about 8 to 10 cm above the elbow crease. They are implanted in a fanlike pattern about 15 degrees apart for a total of 75 degrees. Appropriate insertion facilitates removal by the end of the 5th year. This system provides long-term (up to 5 years) reversible contraception.

Diffusion of the levonorgestrel through the wall of each capsule provides a continuous low dose of progestin. Initially, the dose of levonorgestrel is about 85 μg/d, declining to about 50 μg/d by 9 months, about 35 μg/d by 18 months, and thereafter to about 30 μg/d. The resulting blood levels are substantially below those generally observed among users of combination oral contraceptives containing the progestins norgestrel and levonorgestrel. Because of the range of blood levels and variation in individual response, blood levels alone are not predictive of the risk of pregnancy in an individual woman (19).

Gliadel Wafer Implant

Polifeprosan 20 with carmustine implant (Gliadel Wafer), shown in Figures 20.10 to 20.12, is a sterile off-white to pale yellow wafer approximately 1.45 cm in diameter and 1 mm thick. Each wafer contains 192.3 mg of a biodegradable polyanhydride copolymer and 7.7 mg of carmustine. Polifeprosan 20 consists of poly[bis(p-carboxyphenoxy) propane–sebacic acid] in a 20:80 molar ratio and is used to control the local delivery of carmustine, which is distributed uniformly throughout the copolymer matrix.

FIGURE 20.10. Gliadel wafer (polifeprosan 20 with carmustine implant) and packaging components. (Courtesy of Drugs.com.)

Gliadel is designed to deliver the carmustine directly into the surgical cavity created when a brain tumor is resected, with numerous wafers being used depending upon the desired dose. When exposed to the aqueous environment in the resection cavity, the anhydride bonds in the copolymer are hydrolyzed, releasing the carmustine, carboxyphenoxypropane, and sebacic acid. The active drug, carmustine, is released from the wafer and diffuses into the surrounding brain tissue, producing an antineoplastic effect by alkylating DNA and RNA.

In 3 weeks, more than 70% of the copolymer degrades, with carboxyphenoxypropane being eliminated by the kidney and sebacic acid being metabolized by the liver and expired as carbon dioxide.

Each wafer contains 7.7 mg of carmustine, and when eight wafers (the recommended dose) are used, a dose of 61.6 mg is delivered. The wafers are supplied in a single-dose treatment box containing eight individually pouched wafers. Each wafer is double-pouched in foil. The inner pouch is sterile; upon removing the outer foil pouch in an aseptic working environment, the inner pouch is treated as a sterile item. Gliadel wafers must be stored at or below −20°C (20).

FIGURE 20.11. Gliadel wafer removed from sterile foil pouch in preparation for implantation. (Courtesy of Drugs.com.)

Goserelin Implant (Zoladex)

Goserelin acetate implant (Zoladex, AstraZeneca) is a sterile, biodegradable product containing goserelin acetate, equivalent to 3.6 mg of drug, designed for subcutaneous injection with continuous release over 28 days. Goserelin acetate is dispersed in a matrix consisting of D,L-lactic and glycolic acid copolymer (13.3 to 14.3 mg/dose) containing less than 2.5% acetic acid and up to 12% goserelin-related substances. It is a sterile white to cream-colored cylinder 1

FIGURE 20.12. Gliadel wafer implanted in the brain. (Reprinted with permission from Cuartero-Martinez E, Asenjo B, et al. Use of Gliadel wafer in the surgical treatment of malignant glioma: Common and uncommon complications. ECR 2010:Poster C-2643. doi: 10.1594/ecr2010/C-2643. © European Society of Radiology.)

mm in diameter, preloaded in a special single-use syringe with a 16-gauge needle. The unit is packaged in a sealed light- and moisture-proof aluminum foil laminate pouch containing a desiccant capsule.

Zoladex is indicated for a number of disorders, including the palliative treatment of advanced carcinoma of the prostate, offering an alternative to orchiectomy and/or estrogen administration when the standard treatments are not indicated or are unacceptable to the patient. It is also used in the treatment of endometriosis and advanced breast cancer.

Zoladex is also available as Zoladex 3-Month, containing the equivalent of 10.8 mg of goserelin. The base consists of a matrix of D,L-lactic and glycolic acid copolymer (12.82 to 14.76 mg/dose) containing less than 2% acetic acid and up to 10% goserelin-related substances and presented as a sterile white to cream-colored cylinder 1.5 mm in diameter, preloaded in a special single-use syringe with a 14-gauge needle and overwrap, as previously described. This preparation is designed for administration every 3 months (21).

In 1998, the FDA approved the combination of Zoladex (3.6- and 10.8-mg goserelin acetate depots) and Eulexin (flutamide) for the management of locally confined stage B2 to C prostate carcinoma. The treatment is initiated 8 weeks prior to radiation therapy and continued during radiation therapy. The treatment regimen for prostate cancer uses one 3.6-mg implant subcutaneously into the upper abdomen every 28 days or a 10.8-mg implant subcutaneously into the abdominal wall every 12 weeks.

Goserelin is administered as a subcutaneous implant. Along with leuprolide acetate (Lupron Depot), it was one of the first polymer systems to have received FDA approval for controlled release of a peptide. This drug is available in a 3.6-mg biodegradable and biocompatible sterile white to cream-colored 1-mm by 1.5-mm cylinder about the size of a grain of rice preloaded into a special single-use syringe. The drug is dispersed in a matrix of D,L-lactic acid and glycolic acid copolymer.

Histrelin (Vantas) Implant

The Vantas (histrelin) implant is a sterile nonbiodegradable, diffusion-controlled reservoir drug delivery system designed to deliver histrelin continuously for 12 months upon subcutaneous implantation. It contains 50 mg of histrelin acetate, a synthetic nonapeptide analog of the naturally occurring gonadotropin-releasing hormone (GnRH) or luteinizing hormone–releasing hormone (LH-RH). The device must be removed after 12 months, and another implant may be inserted to continue therapy.

The sterile implant contains a 50-mg histrelin acetate drug core inside a nonbiodegradable, 3.5-cm by 3-mm cylindrically shaped hydrogel reservoir that also contains stearic acid. The hydrogel reservoir consists of a hydrophilic polymer cartridge composed of 2-hydroxyethyl methacrylate, 2-hydroxypropyl methacrylate, trimethylolpropane trimethacrylate, benzoin methyl ether, Perkadox-16, and Triton X-100. It is packaged in a glass vial containing 2 mL of 1.8% sodium chloride solution and is primed for release upon insertion (22).

Leuprolide Acetate (Lupron, Lupron Depot-Ped, Lupron Depot-3 Month)

Leuprolide is a synthetic GnRH analog. Like the naturally occurring LH-RH, initial and intermittent administration of this drug stimulates the release of LH and FSH from the anterior pituitary. As with goserelin, continuous administration of leuprolide suppresses the secretion of LH and FSH, with a concomitant drop in testosterone concentrations and subsequent medical castration.

The usual adult dose for prostatic carcinoma is a subcutaneous injection of 1 mg/d. There is also a monthly (every 28 to 33 days) depot intramuscular injection. The 7.5-mg strength is used for prostatic carcinoma. The powder for intramuscular injection is reconstituted with a special diluent composed of D-mannitol, purified gelatin, D,L-lactic and glycolic acid copolymer, polysorbate 80, and acetic acid.

Lupron should be refrigerated until dispensed, but patients may store the product at room temperature (no more than 30°C, or 86°F). The product should be protected from light and the vial stored in the carton until use. Following reconstitution, the suspension is stable for 1 day. However, because the product has no preservative, it should be discarded if not used immediately.

Viadur Implant

The Viadur (leuprolide acetate) implant is a sterile, non-biodegradable, osmotically driven miniaturized implant designed to deliver leuprolide acetate for 12 months at a controlled rate. It contains 65 mg of leuprolide (as 72 mg of the acetate), which is a synthetic nonapeptide analog of naturally occurring GnRH or LH-RH. After 12 months, the implant must be removed, and another may be inserted if indicated. Viadur is indicated in the palliative treatment of advanced prostate cancer. The drug is dissolved in 104 mg of dimethyl sulfoxide. The reservoir houses a polyurethane rate-controlling membrane, an elastomeric piston, and a polyethylene diffusion moderator. The contained osmotic tablets are composed of sodium chloride, sodium carboxymethylcellulose, povidone, magnesium stearate, and sterile water for injection. PEG fills the space between the osmotic tablets and the reservoir. The implant weighs about 1.1 g. As aqueous fluid diffuses through the membrane and is slowly taken up by the osmotic tablets, the piston will move and force out a controlled amount of the drug through the diffusion moderator orifice (23).

Vitrasert Implants

Vitrasert implants contain 4.5 mg of the antiviral drug ganciclovir and are used to treat AIDS-related cytomegalovirus (CMV) retinitis. Ganciclovir does not cure the CMV retinitis, but helps to decrease its progression. The dosage form is surgically implanted into the vitreous cavity of the eye in an outpatient intraocular procedure.

Each implant contains 4.5 mg of ganciclovir, contains magnesium stearate (0.25%) as an inactive ingredient, and is embedded into a polymer-based system that slowly releases the drug over a 5- to 8-month period. Follow-up ophthalmological examinations are required, and the Vitrasert is removed and replaced with a new implant once the contents of the original implant have been depleted. The Vitrasert implant only treats the eye in which it has been implanted and does not demonstrate any systemic effect. Clinical trials reported adverse effects, for example, loss of visual acuity, vitreal hemorrhage, and retinal detachment, which were observed in 10% to 20% of patients. Most patients experienced a loss in visual acuity from 2 to 4 weeks after implantation. Currently, Vitrasert is pregnancy category C, and its use in pediatric patients less than 9 years of age has not been established. Vitrasert is associated with carcinogenicity and mutagenicity and should be handled and disposed of properly according to antineoplastic guidelines.

OTHER NOVEL DELIVERY SYSTEMS

Definity is a vial of perflutren lipid microspheres for preparing an injectable suspension. The vial contains components that upon activation yield perflutren lipid microspheres that are used as a diagnostic agent for contrast enhancement during echocardiographic procedures; it is administered intravenously. Prior to activation, the Definity vial contains 6.52 mg/mL octafluoropropane in the head space; each milliliter of the clear liquid contains 0.75 mg of a specific lipid blend, 103.5 mg of propylene glycol, 126.2 mg of glycerin, and 6.8 mg of sodium chloride in water for injection. The pH may be adjusted to 5.8 to 7.0 with either sodium hydroxide or hydrochloric acid. The perflutren vial must be activated prior to use with a mechanical shaking device (Vialmix). Upon activation, each milliliter of the milky white suspension contains a maximum of 1.2×10^{10} perflutren lipid microspheres and about 150 µL/mL of octafluoropropane. The microsphere particles have an average diameter of 1.2 to 3.3 mm (24).

Minocycline hydrochloride (Arestin) microspheres are subgingival sustained-release products containing minocycline hydrochloride in a bioresorbable polymer, poly(glycolide-co-D,L-lactide), or PGLA; it is for professional administration into periodontal pockets. Each unit dose cartridge delivers minocycline hydrochloride equivalent to 1 mg of minocycline free base (25).

Doxycycline hyclate (Atridox) 10% in the Atrigel delivery system is for controlled release in subgingival applications. It is composed of a two-syringe mixing system. Syringe A contains 450 mg of the Atrigel delivery system, which is a bioabsorbable, flowable polymeric formulation composed of 36.7% poly(D,L-lactide) dissolved in 63.3% N-methyl-2-pyrrolidone.

Syringe B contains doxycycline hyclate that is equivalent to 42.5 mg doxycycline. Once prepared, the product is a pale yellow to yellow viscous liquid with a concentration of 10% doxycycline hyclate in the gel. After professional application and upon contact with the crevicular fluid, the liquid product solidifies and allows for controlled release of drug over 7 days. Doxycycline is a broad-spectrum semisynthetic bacteriostatic tetracycline (26).

Autoinjection Systems

The EpiPen and EpiPen Jr. automatic injectors contain 2 mL of epinephrine injection for emergency intramuscular use. Each latex-free injector delivers 0.3 mg of Epinephrine Injection, USP, 1:1,000 in a 0.3-mL volume. The remaining 1.7 mL (2.0 to 0.3 mL) remains in the injector after use and is not to be used. Each 0.3 mL of the solution contains 0.3 mg epinephrine, 1.8 mg sodium chloride, 0.5 mg sodium metabisulfite, hydrochloric acid to adjust the pH of the solution to 2.2 to 5.0, and water for injection (27).

Both EpiPen autoinjectors are designed as emergency supportive therapy of allergic reactions (anaphylaxis) and are not a replacement or substitute for immediate medical or hospital care. Epinephrine is a sympathomimetic amine that deteriorates rapidly on exposure to air or light, turning pink from oxidation to adrenochrome and brown from the formation of melanin. The EpiPen injectors should be checked immediately prior to use, and if there is any evidence of discoloration, they should be replaced. The activation cap on the units should not be removed until ready for use. The EpiPen injector should be stored in the provided tubes, because it is light sensitive, at room temperature; the units are not to be refrigerated. Figures 20.13 and 20.14 show prefilled pen injection systems.

Humulin N Pen contains NPH human insulin (rDNA origin) isophane suspension in a disposable insulin delivery device. It is packaged containing five 3-mL disposable insulin delivery devices containing NPH insulin 100 U/mL.

Safe Needle Systems

With the implementation of the Needlestick Safety and Prevention Act, which requires the evaluation and implementation of "safer medical devices" as well as Occupational Safety and Health Administration (OSHA) requirements, new devices will be entering the market to enhance the safety of personnel responsible for injecting medications in patients.

Enoxaparin sodium injection (Lovenox) is available in a prefilled syringe with an automatic safety device (28). The device allows the use of normal injection technique; the needle shield is removed; the injection proceeds as usual; and the syringe/needle is removed from the injection site with the finger still on the plunger rod. Next, the syringe/needle is pointed away from the administrator of the injection and others, and the safety device is activated by firmly pushing on the plunger rod. The protective sleeve automatically covers the needle, and an audible click is heard

FIGURE 20.13. EpiPen 2-Pak commercial epinephrine autoinjectors, each containing 0.3 mg of epinephrine. (Courtesy of Amy Kerkemeyer/Shutterstock.)

to confirm that the shield has been activated and covers the needle. The syringe/needle is then safely disposed of in the nearest sharps container.

Microneedle Arrays

Microneedle arrays are promising devices for the delivery of drugs and vaccines into or the skin. Unique microneedle arrays can be prepared from various materials and can be either solid or hollow. They rapidly take up skin interstitial fluid upon skin insertion to form continuous, unblockable, conduits from attached patch-type drug reservoirs to the dermal microcirculation. Microneedles that can be fabricated in a wide range of patch sizes and microneedle geometries can be easily sterilized, resist hole closure while in place, and are removed completely intact from the skin. Delivery of macromolecules is no longer limited to what can be loaded into the microneedles themselves, and transdermal drug delivery can now be controlled by the cross-link density of the hydrogel system rather than the stratum corneum. This technology has the potential to overcome the limitations of conventional microneedle designs and to greatly increase the range of the type of drug

FIGURE 20.14. Exenatide 250 μg/mL; 1.2-mL prefilled pen injection. Each prefilled pen will deliver 60 subcutaneous doses at 5 μg/dose.

that is deliverable transdermally, with ensuing benefits for industry, health care providers, and, ultimately, patients.

However, little is known about the safety of the microneedles. One study reported on the ability of microneedles to disrupt the skin barrier, which was evaluated by transepidermal water loss (TEWL). The study also determined the safety in terms of skin irritation (skin redness and blood flow) and pain sensation. The microneedle arrays used in the study are able to overcome the barrier function of the skin in human volunteers, are painless, and cause only minimal irritation. This opens the opportunity for dermal and transdermal delivery of drugs and vaccines.

Needle-free delivery has the potential to enhance parenteral administration efficacy and safety, as well as facilitate cost-effective global vaccine distribution and storage, especially for vaccines. To this end, microneedle arrays provide the ability for pain-free, safe, and convenient materials delivery through disruption of the outer layers of the skin to access potent immunocompetent cell populations residing within the epidermal/dermal tissues. These systems also have the capability of two-way activities: drug delivery and sensing capabilities potentially to monitor and adjust drug delivery (29).

3D PRINTING

3D Printing is already used for one commercial product, SPRITAM (levetiracetam) and this preparation method is ideal for individualized medications, based on a patient's medical, biological, and pharmaceutical profile; this may be utilized in the future utilizing three-dimensional (3D) printing. New products, based on a patient's weight, race, kidney, and liver functions, may be possible utilizing 3D printing to increase medication effectiveness and reduce side effects. When realized, one should be able to input the patient's information for a specific drug, and the software will calculate the dosage required and then generate the 3D printed medication. Tablets with wide dosage ranges, high reproducibility, and tight standard deviations have been prepared. These tablets can be varied each time the patient refills his or her medication, and this adds a new dimension to pharmaceutical compounding.

3D printing is a layer-by-layer production of three-dimensional objects from digital designs. The technology has developed as a combination of chemistry, optics, and robotics over about 30 years. 3D Printing quickly became a standard tool in the automotive, aerospace, and consumer goods in industry and, recently, 3D printing is gaining traction in pharmaceutical manufacturing. 3D Printing has been steadily growing and has received a boost with U.S. Food and Drug Administration (FDA) approval of the 3D-printed orodispersible tablet, SPRITAM (levetiracetam). This new product supports the application of 3D printing to manufacturing complex and customized dosage forms. 3D Printing supports a move from the "centralization" of manufacturing to "decentralization" and closer to the patient (30,31).

Briefly, underlying all current techniques is the construction of a CAD model, which describes the geometry and size of the dosage form(s); it contains the coordinates of the design that together make up the surface of the design 3D structure. The 3D printer processes the file by creating sliced layers of the model. Three dimensions are built by subsequent overprinting and, when the first layer is deposited, the model is reduced by the thickness of the next layer. The process is repeated until completion of the desired structure.

Personalization

Personalized dosing allows for individualizing the amount of drug delivered based on a patient's mass and metabolism. Also, another personalized dosing concept is preparing multidrug poly pills to combine all of the patient's medications into a single daily dose. Personalized implants allow for printing implants that match patients' anatomical features; this technique is gaining traction for medical devices such as tracheal splints and bone grafts.

On-Demand Manufacturing/Compounding

A 3D printer can make a variety of quality products within minutes. Three situations where this on-demand capability may be applicable include the following:

- Printing directly on the patients, that is, 3D printer as a drug administration device
- Printing "in-time" or in other resource-constrained settings
- Printing low-stability drugs for immediate consumption

Extrusion and ink-jet techniques have been used to create wound-healing gels on demand.

3D printing also can be used to

- Avoid incompatibilities between drugs
- Design multiple-release dosage forms
- Increase the solubility of poorly soluble drugs by producing an amorphous form
- Produce very porous material with the rapid onset of action
- Limit degradation of biological molecules

Additional novel characteristics that can be developed include the following:

- Creating radial gradients of diffusion controlling excipients, such as ethylcellulose, to achieve near-zero order release
- Joining osmotic pumps (composed of cellulose acetate, D-mannitol, and PEG) and hypromellose-based structures to create a single product with multiple-release modalities
- Altering the in-fill of polyvinyl alcohol products as a means of accelerating or decelerating drug release
- Implementing structured breakaway components to deposit different parts of a solid, oral dosage form in different parts of the lumen

- Printing solid, oral dosage forms with all but one side covered by an impermeable membrane so that the dissolvable portion maintains a constant surface area during drug release
- Stacking six or more distinct layers in a single product for multiphasic release
- Printing toroidal solid, oral dosage forms that achieve near-zero order release

The high degree of flexibility and control with 3D printing enables the preparation of dosage forms with multiple APIs with complex and tailored release profiles. This technique has been used to prepare PEG droplets of ibuprofen that could be imbibed into a porous substrate made of hydroxypropyl methylcellulose.

Available methods/techniques used in 3D printing are shown in Table 20.8; additional presentations on 3D Printing have been published (30–32) and examples of commercial products listed in Table 20.9.

An advantage of FDM 3DP is that the printer can be used to prepare tablets of almost any geometry.

TABLE 20.8. 3D Printing Technologies

Inkjet

Continuous Inkjet Printing (CIJ)

Drop on Demand (DOD)

  Drop on Drop (DOD)

  Drop on Solid (DOS)

    Drop on Powder (DOP)

    Drop on Bed (DOB)

Extrusion

Global

Hot-Melt Extrusion (HME)

Fused Filament Fabrication (FFF, FDM)

Pen-Based

Pressure-Assisted Microsyringes (PAM)

Powder Bed Fusion

Selective Laser Sintering

Polymerization (Laser or UV-Based, Stereolithography)

TABLE 20.9. Examples of 3D Printed Drug Dosage Forms

Drug	Carrier	Dosage Form	Technology
Acetaminophen	PVA	Devices	FDM
Acetaminophen	Ethylcellulose, HPMC E50, PVP K30	Tablets	DOP
Acetaminophen	Ethylcellulose	Devices	DOP
Acetaminophen	Lactose, PVP K30/mannitol	Devices	DOP
4-ASA	PVA	Tablets	FDM
5-ASA	PVA	Tablets	FDM
Aspirin	—		
Aspirin, hydrochlorothiazide, pravastatin, atenolol, ramipril	HPMC	Polypill	PAM
Captopril	HPMC/Cellulose acetate	Tablets	PAM
Captopril	Mannitol/PVP K25, maltitol, maltodextrin	Theriflash RDT	—
Chlorpheniramine maleate	Eudragit E1000 and Eudragit RLPO	Tablets	DOP
Dexamethasone sodium phosphate	PVA/PLGA	Implants	Inkjet
Diclofenac	Eudragit L100	Tablets	DOP
Ethinyl estradiol	PCL	Implants	DOP
Fenofibrate	—	Coated stent	Inkjet
Gentamicin sulfate and methotrexate	PLA	Device	Inkjet
Glipizide	HPMC/Cellulose Acetate	Tablets	PAM
Guaifenesin	HPMC/Polyacrylic acid	Tablets	PAM, Nozzle Deposition
Isoniazid	PLLA	Implants	DOP
Levofloxacin	PLLA	Implants	DOP
Nifedipine	HPMC/Cellulose Acetate	Tablets	PAM
Paclitaxel	PLGA	Microparticles	DOP
Prednisolone	PVA	Tablets	FDM
Pseudoephedrine hydrochloride	Kollidon SR/HPMC	Devices	DOP
Theophylline	Methacrylic polymers	Tablets	FDM

HPMC, hydroxypropyl methylcellulose; DOP, Drop on Powder; FDM, Fused Deposition Modeling; PAM, pressure-assisted microsyringes; PCL, polycaprolactone; PLGA, poly lactic-co-glycolic acid; PLLA, poly-L-lactide acid; PVA, polyvinyl alcohol; PVP, polyvinylpyrrolidone; RDT, rapid-dissolving tablet.

Even doughnut-shaped polymer matrices that show zero order release under certain conditions have been developed. Also, it has been shown that changing a tablet shape can modify drug release. The optimum shape to obtain a specific release profile could possibly be determined if select data are available. 3DP may be the only suitable and available method to design and develop elaborate shapes that would be impossible to do using typical tableting methods of compressing powers. A published study summarized the following:

- Geometry affects not only the dissolution release in vitro but also the transit time in vivo.
- Drug release kinetics from these tablets showed no dependence on surface area but dependence on surface area/volume ratio. This indicates the influence of geometrical shape on drug release profile.
- Objects with a larger surface area/volume values have a faster drug release (33).

In one 3DP study, the extrusion method was used to prepare a multi-active solid dosage form containing two instant-release and three sustained-release drugs (34). This was designed for a cardiovascular patient and consisted of aspirin and hydrochlorothiazide in the immediate release layer setting on top of the tablet and pravastatin, atenolol, and ramipril in three separate pie-shaped layers of segregated compartments immediately below; the tablet was 12 mm in diameter and 5.85 mm in height.

Commercial 3D Printing Product

SPRITAM (levetiracetam), the first drug using 3D technology, has been approved by the FDA. SPRITAM uses ZipDose technology, which combines formulation science with the unique manufacturing capabilities of 3-dimensional printing (3DP). Using 3DP technology, Aprecia is developing formulations of medicines that rapidly disintegrate with a sip of liquid, even at high-dose loads.

The 3D printing technology involves the following steps:

- A powder blend is deposited as a single layer.
- The binding fluid is applied to bind the particles.
- This process is repeated several times to manufacture orodispersible dosage forms.

This produces a porous formulation that rapidly disintegrates with a sip of liquid.

SPRITAM (levetiracetam) is for oral use as a prescription adjunctive therapy in the treatment of partial-onset seizures, myoclonic seizures, and primary generalized tonic–clonic seizures in adults and children with epilepsy and marks the first time a drug product manufactured with this technology has been approved by the FDA. SPRITAM is an antiepileptic drug available as 250-, 500-, 750-, and 1,000-mg round, white to off-white, spearmint-flavored tablets for oral suspension. Levetiracetam is a white to off-white crystalline powder with a faint odor and a bitter taste and is very soluble in water.

SPRITAM tablets for oral suspension contain 250, 500, 750, or 1,000 mg levetiracetam and the following inactive ingredients: colloidal silicon dioxide, glycerin, mannitol, microcrystalline cellulose, polysorbate 20, povidone, sucralose, butylated hydroxyanisole, and natural and artificial spearmint flavor. The tablets for oral suspension are unitary porous structures produced by a three-dimensional printing process that binds the powders without compression; they disintegrate in a mean time of 11 seconds (ranging from 2 to 27 seconds) in the mouth, when taken with a sip of liquid, to produce small particles that may be swallowed (35).

PATIENT COUNSELING

INSERTING VAGINAL RING INSERTS

1. Wash and dry hands and the vaginal area.
2. Stand or lie on the back to place the insert.
3. Remove the vaginal ring from its pouch.
4. Hold the vaginal ring between the thumb and index finger and press the opposite sides of the ring together.
5. Gently push the compressed ring into the vagina as far as possible into the upper third of the vagina.
6. When the ring is in place, nothing should be felt.
7. Wash and dry hands again.
8. One can continue to participate in regular activities while using the ring.
9. Replace the ring as often as prescribed.

REMOVING VAGINAL RING INSERTS

1. Wash and dry hands thoroughly.

2. Assume a comfortable position, either standing with one leg up or lying down.
3. Loop a finger through the ring and gently pull it out. Discard the used ring in a waste receptacle in an area where children or pets cannot get it; do NOT flush it.
4. Replace with a new ring as instructed.
5. Wash and dry hands.

GUMS

1. Chew the dosage form, but do not swallow it.
2. The saliva being produced can be swallowed.
3. If a nicotine gum is used and tingling occurs, move the dosage form to between the cheek and the gum; when the tingling disappears, begin chewing again; repeat as necessary.
4. Do not eat or drink for 15 minutes before chewing nicotine gum or while chewing a piece of the gum.

APPLYING THE PRINCIPLES AND CONCEPTS

GROUP ACTIVITIES

1. In groups of three, create a brief patient handout describing the appropriate use and varying administration techniques for Lamictal chewable dispersible tablets. Be specific in your recommendations and suggestions.

2. Select two ophthalmic and one oral inhalation products. In groups of three, one student serves as the pharmacist, the second the patient, and the third the observer. The pharmacist–student role-player will counsel (and demonstrate) the patient on the specific product. After the session, the observer and patient provide constructive feedback on the session. The roles then are rotated utilizing a different product until each of the three students has participated in each of the three roles.

3. To realize the need for novel dosage forms of vaginal administration, access http://www.livestrong.com/video/1945-menopause-health-byte/. View the menstrual cycle health video (1:18 minutes) and the menopause health video (2:09 minutes). Brainstorm possible delivery systems that might be used for intravaginal administration.

4. Interview a classmate who acknowledges using an oral inhalation product, for example, Advair Diskus. Discuss with the classmate his or her ability to use the product appropriately, the product's effectiveness, and any concerns he or she might have had when it was prescribed and/or might have presently.

5. In groups of two (one student serves as the pharmacist, the second the patient), have the pharmacist explain to the patient the reason for dispensing a pilocarpine (Ocusert) versus his/her traditional pilocarpine eye drop solution. This is intended to be an interactive exercise; the patient is expected to ask a series of pertinent follow-up questions.

INDIVIDUAL ACTIVITIES

1. Conduct a literature search to discover five different drugs that utilize liposomal injection technology.

2. Create a pharmacokinetic figure that demonstrates general pharmacokinetic properties (i.e., absorption, distribution, metabolism, excretion) of the Striant mucoadhesive testosterone buccal system against an orally administered testosterone medication.

3. Provide examples of drugs administered parenterally for a long-acting effect utilizing techniques shared in this chapter, for example, slowly dissolving chemical complexes of the drug entity, solutions or suspensions of drugs in slowly absorbed carriers or vehicles, and large drug particles in suspension.

4. Compare and contrast the administration techniques utilized for the EpiPen, Humulin N Pen, Byetta Pen, and a Glucagon Emergency Rescue Kit.

REFERENCES

1. Dutet J, Delgado-Charro M. Assessment of iontophoretic and passive ungula penetration by laser scanning confocal microscopy. Pharm Res 2012;29:3464–3474.

2. Product Information. Available at: https://www.drugs.com/pro/striant.html. (Accessed July 21, 2020)

3. Physicians' Desk Reference. 67th Ed. Montvale, NJ: Thomson PDR, 2013:658–664.

4. Product Information. Available at: http://www.drugs.com/mmx/progestasert.html. (Accessed July 21, 2020)

5. Product Information. Available at: http://www.cervidel.com. (Accessed July 21, 2020)

6. Madan PL. Sustained-release drug delivery systems, part VI: Special devices. Pharm Manufact 1985;2:33–40.

7. Madan PL. Sustained-release drug delivery systems, part V: Parenteral products. Pharm Manufact 1985;2:51.

8. Product Information. Available at: http://www.rxlist.com/abelcet-drug.htm. (Accessed July 21, 2020)

9. Product Information. Available at: http://www.drugs.com/cdi/amphotec.html. (Accessed July 21, 2020)

10. Product Information. Available at: http://www.daunoxome.com. (Accessed July 21, 2020)

11. Physicians' Desk Reference. 67th Ed. Montvale, NJ: Thomson PDR, 2013:1284–1291.

12. Allen Jr LV. Compounding self-emulsifying drug delivery systems and other self-emulsifying lipid formulations, part 1. Int J Pharm Compd May-June 2018;22(3):220–228.

13. Allen Jr LV. Compounding self-emulsifying drug delivery systems and other self-emulsifying lipid formulations, part 2. Int J Pharm Compd July-Aug 2018;22(4):294–300.

14. DePasquale S. Hot melt extrusion. Int J Pharm Compd Nov/Dec 2017;21(6):471–479.

15. Product Information. Available at: http://www.pegasys.com. (Accessed July 21, 2020)

16. Product Information. Available at: http://www.pegIntron.com. (Accessed July 21, 2020)

17. Product Information. Available at: http://www.Ontak.com. (Accessed July 21, 2020)

18. Fung S, Ferrill M. Contraceptive update: Subdermal implants. Calif Pharmacist 1992;40:35–41.

19. Munzenberger PJ, Levin S. Home parenteral antibiotic therapy for patients with cystic fibrosis. Hosp Pharm 1993;28:20–28.

20. Product Information. Available at: http://www.gliadel.com. (Accessed July 21, 2020)

21. Product Information. Available at: http://www.zoladex.com. (Accessed July 21, 2020)

22. Product Information. Available at: http://www.vantasimplant.com. (Accessed July 21, 2020)

23. Product Information. Available at: http://www.Rxlist.com/viadur-drug.htm. (Accessed July 21, 2020)

24. Product Information. Available at: http://www.definityimaging.com. (Accessed July 21, 2020)

25. Product Information. Warminster, PA: OraPharma, 2004.

26. Product Information. Newtown, PA: CollaGenex Pharmaceuticals, 2005.

27. Physicians' Desk Reference. 67th Ed. Montvale, NJ: Thomson PDR, 2013:1859–1861.

28. Product Information. Available at: http://www.lovenox.com. (Accessed July 21, 2020)

29. Bal SM, Caussin J, Pavel S, et al. In vivo assessment of safety of microneedle arrays in human skin. Eur J Pharm Sci 2008; 35(3):193–202.

30. Allen Jr LV. 3D printing: Pharmacy applications, part 1. Int J Pharm Compd Mar/April 2017;21(2):127–130.

31. Allen Jr LV. 3D printing: Pharmacy applications, part 2. Int J Pharm Compd May/June 2017;21(3) 215–220.

32. Allen Jr LV. 3D printing: Pharmacy applications, part 3: Compounding, formulation considerations, and the future. Int J Pharm Compd July/August 2017;21(4):293–298.

33. Goyanes A, et al. Effect of geometry on drug release from 3D printed tablets. Int J Pharm 2015;494:657–663.

34. Khaled SA, et al. 3D printing of five-in-one dose combination polypill with defined immediate and sustained release profiles. J Control Release 2015;217:308–314.

35. Product Information. Available at: http://www.spritam.com. (Accessed April 18, 2016)

Clinical Pharmaceutics

OBJECTIVES

After reading this chapter, the student will be able to:

1. Discuss the importance of clinical pharmaceutics in therapeutics
2. Describe the chemical phenomena responsible for some clinical pharmaceutic issues
3. Differentiate between chemical and physical phenomena involved in clinical pharmaceutics
4. Explain the rationale behind selected drug interactions and their correction
5. Discuss the different areas of clinical pharmaceutics as they relate to specific dosage forms

▌ INTRODUCTION

Pharmaceutics is relevant far beyond the pharmaceutical industry, compounding, and the laboratory. Pharmaceutics can be used to solve many problems in medication therapy. A pharmacist's knowledge of the physicochemical aspects of drugs and drug products should help the patient, physician, and health care personnel resolve issues in the increasingly complex world of modern medicine. Pharmacy is unique as it contains a knowledge base significantly different from that of physicians, nurses, and other health-related practitioners. The separation of the science and the practice of pharmacy have prevented the complete utilization of pharmaceutical sciences in the clinical environment far too long.

Some may wonder how surface tension, crystallinity, precipitation, viscosity, adsorption, and solubility are relevant in clinical situations. Also, how does the nature of the dosage form and its properties influence outcomes or even cause adverse events? Why do drugs precipitate before, during, or after administration? One of the most important relationships is that of pH, pK_a, and the solubility of acids and bases. Why do infusion pumps become blocked when proteins aggregate? Why do some oral dosage forms adhere to the esophagus and irritate/ulcerate? Last, how does knowing the nature and properties of the drug substances and excipients influence the clinical situation?

The emerging combination of the sciences and clinical aspects result in the discipline of clinical pharmaceutics, that is, the application of the unique knowledge base in pharmaceutical sciences to clinical situations. Clinical pharmaceutics involves applying basic scientific facts to solving problems in medication therapy. Where pharmaceutics has been looked at as being important primarily to those going into the pharmaceutical industry, teaching, and compounding, it is now becoming more apparent that therapeutic regimens can be effective or ineffective based upon pharmaceutics and the relationship with the patient. Chemistry and pharmaceutics are inseparable. Many topics that are applicable in clinical pharmaceutics include those shown in Table 21.1.

Examples are presented, both positive and negative, of how the above considerations have resulted in change(s) in patient responses from the formulation. Also, we will look at the effect of a change in diluent in phenytoin capsules and the resulting phenytoin intoxication in patients. Throughout this chapter, the scientific pharmaceutic principles associated with the case studies in this chapter will be discussed. First, let's look at some example general definitions of related terms to clinical pharmaceutics.

- Pharmacy: The science or practice of the preparation and dispensing of medicinal drugs
- Clinical pharmacy: A discipline in which pharmacists provide patient care that optimizes medication therapy and promotes health, wellness, and disease prevention

TABLE 21.1. Factors and Characteristics That Can Be Involved in Clinical Pharmaceutics

Adsorption/adhesion

Buffer capacity

Colligative properties

Complex organic molecules

Crystallinity

Dosage form selection and properties

Endotoxin calculations/levels

Hydrates and solvates

Melting point

Organic salts and esters

Particle size and surface area

Partition coefficient

pH

pK_a/dissociation constant

Potency designations

Precipitation

Preservation

Rate reactions

Rheology/viscosity

Sedimentation

Solubility

Surface tension/wetting

Transporter interactions

- Pharmaceutics: The study of drug formulations and their design, manufacture, and delivery to the body
- Clinical pharmaceutics: The application of the unique knowledge base in pharmaceutics to patients and to clinical situations
- Biopharmaceutics: The study of the factors influencing the bioavailability of a drug in man and animals

Pharmaceutics is a science involving the application of drug chemistry, drug biology, and formulation principles for the purpose of delivering drugs to target tissues in a biological system. During preformulation, important chemical and physical properties of the drug are important to rationally design a drug delivery system and predict the fate of the drug after administration. Some of these properties include water solubility, Log P, stability, enzymatic degradation, receptor location, and transporter interaction.

The quality and quantity of a drug effect is dependent upon pharmaceutic principles. Pharmaceutics is involved with taking a drug substance and knowledge of its characteristics and incorporating it into a suitable, safe, stable, and effective formulation or dosage form. Clinical pharmaceutics goes one step further with more of an emphasis on patient aspects while retaining the necessary product aspects of the drug. In this chapter, we will utilize pharmaceutic case examples to illustrate the scientific principles and clinical effects involved. We will also cover many of the scientific principles in typical pharmaceutics courses and their application to patient care. The onset of action of a drug can be very important; Table 21.2 provides an average onset of action depending upon the route of administration and dosage forms involved. These can be affected by the formulation. One of the first areas we will discuss is that of incompatibilities, which can directly affect a clinical outcome.

INCOMPATIBILITIES

Incompatibilities have generally been discussed in the past as being therapeutic, physical, or chemical. Therapeutic incompatibilities are now often referred to as drug interactions. Physical incompatibilities are those in which the physical properties of the ingredients produce a mixture or preparation that is unacceptable in appearance or in accuracy of dosage; chemical incompatibilities are

TABLE 21.2. Routes, Dosage Forms, and Average Onsets of Action

Route	Dosage Form	Onset of Action
Intravenous	Aqueous solutions, emulsions	Within 60 s
Intramuscular	Aqueous solutions, oily solutions, suspensions	15–30 min for aqueous solutions
Subcutaneous	Aqueous solutions, suspensions, implants	15–60 min for aqueous solutions
Sublingual	Tablets, solutions, aerosols	1–3 min
Buccal	Tablets, lozenges, chewing gum	2–3 min
Oral	Tablets, solutions, suspensions	30–60 min for immediate-release dosage forms
Rectal	Suppositories, ointments, creams, solutions, suspensions, foams	30–60 min
Vaginal	Inserts, creams, gels, tablets, rings	Slow for systemic effects
Skin (transdermal)	Patches, ointments, gels	1–4 h
Nose	Aerosolized solutions or suspensions	Within min
Lung	Aerosolized solutions, suspensions or powders	Within 5 min

Adapted from Remington Education: Pharmaceutics, by Shelley Chambers Fox.

those in which the ingredients interact or decompose to give new compounds; these may or may not produce visible changes.

Physical Incompatibilities

Pharmacists usually encounter physical incompatibilities when they mix two products together, as in parenteral admixtures, or when they use a manufactured drug product in a compounded formulation. Physical incompatibilities usually involve properties such as solubility, melting point, polymorphic forms, freezing point, dielectric constant, etc. Physical incompatibilities usually cause nonuniform, unsightly, or unpalatable mixtures, which pose the potential danger of nonuniform dosage. Examples are listed in Table 21.3. Incomplete solution can occur when two or more substances are combined and may not give a homogeneous product because of immiscibility or insolubility. Sometimes a change in pH or addition of a cosolvent may correct it. Precipitation can occur when a vehicle is added to a substance that is soluble in one solvent and is not soluble in this second vehicle or solvent. An example would be precipitation of phenytoin when the cosolvent-based injection is diluted with water. Immiscibility occurs when a vehicle is added to a solution of something like an oil, but the oil is not soluble in the second vehicle. A simple example would be the addition of water to peppermint spirit where the peppermint oil may come out of solution. Liquefaction of solid ingredients may occur with drug substances that form eutectics or crystalline hydrates that liberate their water of crystallization. It should be noted that some incompatibilities are intentional, as in the preparation of a product called White Lotion, and others are not intentional, as in the lowering of the pH of a dissolved sodium or potassium salt of the drug with the precipitation of the free form of the drug.

Chemical Incompatibilities

Pharmacists are usually concerned with chemical compatibilities in terms of the beyond-use date for the prescriptions they compound and dispense. Chemical incompatibilities generally can occur immediately upon mixing, whereas others may occur over time. Some of these incompatibilities are also instabilities. Instability describes degradation, including hydrolysis, oxidation, and covalent chemical reactions. These incompatibilities may be instantaneous (precipitate, color change, effervescence) or delayed (drug stability, precipitate) and occur at such a slow rate that no visible change occurs for a time. These incompatibilities should not be dispensed without correction, as they directly impact the potency and therapeutic efficacy of the product. A more complete list is detailed in Table 21.3.

Correction of Incompatibilities

Incompatibilities are easier to prevent than to correct. Pharmacists should exercise caution any time they modify or repackage a drug commercial drug product or mix two products together. If one can recognize a potential incompatibility and correct it, then it can save time, materials, and money. One must be cautious to not "imagine" incompatibilities where they may not exist. If one cannot be certain, it may be beneficial to prepare a small quantity of a preparation for observation. Assigning a conservative beyond-use date to products further protects patients from the effects of possible incompatibilities.

It has been generally accepted that it is unnecessary to consult the prescriber if adding official emulsifying or suspending agents or adding inert ingredients, that is, diluents, stabilizers, solvents, buffers, stiffening agents, and preservatives to a formulation. However, one should notify the prescriber if adding materials to change the dose and adding nonofficial suspending agents, emulsifying agents, chelating agents, or other materials that may interfere with the therapeutic effectiveness of a product. Also changes that may adversely affect the stability, omission of troublesome ingredients, dispensing ingredients separately, and changing the dosage form are situations where the physician should be notified. General methods and techniques used to correct incompatibilities are shown in Table 21.4.

DRUG FORM

The following are examples of the application and importance of clinical pharmaceutics covering different characteristics.

TABLE 21.3. Examples of Physical and Chemical Incompatibilities

Physical Incompatibilities
  Incomplete solution
  Precipitation
  Separation of immiscible liquids
  Liquefaction of solid ingredients
  Incorrect form prescribed

Chemical Incompatibilities
  Oxidation
  Reduction
  Racemization
  Precipitation
  Evolution of a gas
  Color changes
  Explosive combinations
  Cementation
  Separation of immiscible liquids
  Gelatinization
  Development of heat or cold
  Hydrolytic changes
  Invisible changes
  Development of poisonous substances
  Implosion
  Polymerization
  Double decomposition
  Substitution reactions
  Addition reactions
  Miscellaneous

TABLE 21.4. Methods and Techniques Used to Correct Incompatibilities

Modify the mixing order

Dispense with a "Shake Well" label

Dispense with a "Store in Refrigerator" label

Complete the reaction before packaging

Protect from air, light, heat, moisture

Addition of an ingredient
  Suspending agent
  Emulsifying agent
  Solubilizing agent
  Diluent
  Stiffening or softening agent

Removal of an ingredient
  Discard inactive sediment
  Separate into 2 prescriptions

Change the vehicle
  Increase the volume → increase dose
  Decrease volume → decrease dose
  Change vehicle → same dose
  Change an ingredient
  Change the dosage form

Example: Griseofulvin Solubility, Particle, Matrix, and Dose

Griseofulvin is very slightly soluble in water. "Very slightly soluble" is defined as 1 part in 1,000 to 10,000 parts (1 g in 1,000 to 10,000 mL of water). Commercial forms of the powder and their relative doses include the following:

Form	Particle Size	Comparative Dose
Microsize	Mostly <4 μm	500 mg to 1 g/d
Ultramicrosize	Mostly <1 μm	375–750 mg/d

Note: The ultramicrosize griseofulvin is composed of ultramicrosize crystals of griseofulvin dispersed in polyethylene glycol 6,000 or dispersed by other suitable means.

As is evident, there is a decrease in dose with a decrease in particle size. Decreasing particle size to increase the surface area available for dissolution is a common strategy to improve the bioavailability of poorly soluble drugs. When the particle size of a very poorly soluble drug is decreased, however, there is a tendency for the particles to agglomerate. By incorporating the ultramicrosize particles into polyethylene glycol, which tends to surround/coat the particles of griseofulvin, the particles are separated, and when they are placed in a fluid environment, they are wetted better and dissolve much faster for absorption. A decrease in particle size may or may not enhance bioavailability; it depends upon other factors such as wettability, agglomeration, etc. (1).

Example: Nitrofurantoin: Bigger Particle Size, Less GI Intolerance

Nitrofurantoin (Furadantin) has been available for the treatment of urinary tract infections (UTIs) since 1953. Its current uses include the treatment of uncomplicated UTIs and prophylaxis against UTIs in people prone to recurrent UTIs. Nausea, vomiting, and diarrhea occurred in an appreciable number of patients, related to the rapid absorption of the drug. A reduction in dosage or administration with food or milk lessened the incidence.

To address the issue, the manufacturer developed a macrocrystalline particle form (Macrodantin) that is more slowly absorbed than the microcrystalline form and is useful for patients who cannot tolerate the microcrystalline form. The absorption is slower and the excretion of Macrodantin is somewhat less, when the two are compared, leading to reduced incidence of GI intolerance with Macrodantin; this did not significantly reduce the clinical effectiveness. Generally, the trend is to reduce particle size to enhance bioavailability in product development; however, this is a situation where increased particle size is better for patients (2,3).

Example: Nitrofurantoin—Two Particle Sizes and a Gel

Another approach decrease nausea associated with nitrofurantoin was to develop a dual-release capsule that contained 25 mg of nitrofurantoin macrocrystals and 75 mg of nitrofurantoin monohydrate. In this formulation, there are two different approaches to slow down the absorption rate of the drug:

1. A large particle size for 25 mg of nitrofurantoin to retard the dissolution rate, and
2. 75 mg of regular size nitrofurantoin monohydrate in combination with an excipient to form a viscous gel and slow the diffusion of the nitrofurantoin to the mucosal surface after it dissolves

As a result, the drug slowly releases over time, slowing the rate of absorption. This product also has the advantage of requiring only two doses per day, while the capsule containing all macrocrystalline nitrofurantoin is typically taken four times per day. This is an example where dissolution and absorption can be affected by the use of a larger particle size and a smaller particle size inside a gel matrix (2,3).

Example: Solids to Liquids—Taking Advantage of a Physical Phenomenon

The melting point of lidocaine is 68°C and that of prilocaine is 38°C. When the dry solids are mixed together, they form eutectic mixtures and turn into a liquid. A eutectic mixture consists of two often similar materials whose melting point is below that of either individual component and is generally close to room temperature. In this case, the mixture of lidocaine and prilocaine forms a eutectic with a melting point reduction to 16°C. The resulting "oil" is then used as the internal or dispersed phase of an oil-in-water emulsion, forming EMLA (Eutectic Mixture of Local Anesthetics). A 5% EMLA cream consists of 2.5% lidocaine and 2.5% prilocaine (4). The eutectic mixture allows for a smooth cream with high thermodynamic activity of the active ingredients. Furthermore, as an oily liquid, the eutectic mixture does not require organic solvents to solubilize the drugs.

DRUG DOSAGE FORM

Posaconazole oral formulations cannot be substituted one to one. The two oral formulations are dosed differently as the delayed-release tablet has a higher bioavailability than does its oral suspension counterpart; the oral suspension has a lower bioavailability. If a milligram to milligram substitution is used, it can result in under- or overdosing the patient. The labels of the two formulations have been revised to reflect this problem (5,6). Similarly, compounded valsartan suspension has 60% higher bioavailability than valsartan tablets, necessitating a dose adjustment when switching between the two dosage forms.

EXCIPIENTS

Excipients are rarely inert! They may be incompatible or affect drug product quality. Also, patients may react to them. Excipients play a wide variety of roles in dosage forms that include (*a*) modulating solubility and bioavailability of APIs; (*b*) increasing the stability of active ingredients in the dosage forms; (*c*) helping APIs to maintain preferred polymorphic forms; (*d*) maintaining the pH and/or osmolarity of liquid formulations; (*e*) acting as antioxidants, emulsifying agents, aerosol propellants, tablet binders, and disintegrants; (*f*) preventing aggregation of dissociation; and (*g*) modulating immunogenic responses of APIs. An excipient is selected and used because it contributes one or more functional attributes to a product's characteristics.

Example: Phenytoin Intoxication

A change in an excipient in the late 1960s led to an outbreak of phenytoin intoxication in Australia, related to drug solubility. Upon investigation, the contents of the phenytoin capsules in question were analyzed and were not overfilled with the drug; therefore, there must have been some other reason for the toxicity. The affected patients all received one brand of 100 mg phenytoin sodium capsules. It was discovered that the manufacturer had changed the diluent from calcium sulfate to lactose along with a slight increase in the contents of both magnesium silicate and magnesium stearate in the capsules.

Calcium sulfate is only "slightly soluble in water," whereas lactose is "freely soluble in water." This increased solubility of the diluent can serve to more rapidly "wet" the phenytoin sodium (freely soluble in water) powder particles, and "wetting" is the first step in the dissolution process. Like griseofulvin, the absorption of phenytoin is strongly affected by the dissolution rate. The enhanced wetting with lactose led to more

rapid dissolution of the phenytoin sodium as compared to when calcium sulfate was used. Both substances are listed as "diluents," but their solubility properties are different. Upon changing back to the previous formula using calcium sulfate, the blood levels of the patients returned to previous values.

From this experience, it became apparent to manufacturers back in the 1960s that excipients are not "inert" substances and must be carefully evaluated for their effect on the drug dosage form (7).

ADVERSE EVENTS

Adverse effects could be the result of the following:

- Unusual bioavailability caused by a product or manufacturing defect
- Sensitivity to ingredients
- Reactions to impurities and/or breakdown products
- Aggregation of protein drugs in devices
- Device failure, as with medicated stents or infusion pumps
- Nature of the formulation as in adhesive tablets lodging in the esophagus or drug precipitation from injections

Some example adverse events related to different formulations include intestinal perforation (indomethacin osmotic minipump tablets), tissue necrosis at site of injection (fluspirilene IM injection), mild paralysis (epidural injection of prednisolone injection containing benzyl alcohol), bronchoconstriction (inhalation of nebulized ipratropium bromide containing benzalkonium chloride), anaphylactoid reaction (vaginal application of povidone iodine solution), and respiration depression and death (fentanyl transdermal patch).

Reactions to impurities and breakdown products may be initiated by interactions with moisture or acidity or with excipients or materials from containers and packaging. The manufacturing process may contribute some impurities.

Adverse reactions to preservatives, gluten, and other common ingredients must be checked with each patient and, if necessary, an alternate drug used or compounded.

SOLID ORAL

Example: Tetracyclines and Calcium

The patient has been prescribed tetracycline 500 mg three times daily for an infection and is also taking a calcium supplement (see Fig. 21.1). The complexation of tetracyclines with calcium poses a problem as it can reduce the actual amount of tetracycline absorbed systemically. If there is no alternative drug for the patient, the recommendation should be to separate the administration of the calcium supplement by at least 2 hours from the tetracycline administration (8).

FIGURE 21.1. Example products of tetracycline hydrochloride capsules and calcium supplement table.

Example: Drug-Induced Esophageal Injury

If a tablet or capsule adheres to the esophageal wall during swallowing, drug particles may be released onto the esophageal mucosa. As the drug particles dissolve, they create high local drug concentrations that can lead to erosion or ulceration of the mucosa. The esophageal injury can cause pain when swallowing and may potentially lead to more serious injury. Drug-induced esophageal injury usually occurs when a patient takes a tablet or capsule without a sufficient volume of water to ensure transit to the stomach or when the patient lies down soon after taking it. Drugs that are particularly associated with esophageal injury include doxycycline, alendronate, nonsteroidal anti-inflammatory drugs, and potassium chloride. Patients should be counseled to take tablets and capsules with at least 4 ounces of water and to not lie down for at least 15 to 30 minutes (9).

▌LIQUID ORAL

Example: Dosing Issues Using Hot Drink Dosage Forms

The same dose of a drug can be administered but can vary significantly in its rate of absorption, distribution, etc. A recent study demonstrated that an acetaminophen (APAP) hot drink product was much more rapid acting than an APAP tablet.

The study compared a hot drink product (Beechams Flu Plus Hot Lemon sachets) with standard APAP tablets (Panadol Original Tablets) (see Fig. 21.2).

The APAP dose was the same (1,000 mg) in both products, but the sachets also contained phenylephrine and ascorbic acid. The study involved 25 healthy male volunteers with no GI disorders that may impact the "normal" behavior of the formulations following administration. The sachets were administered with 150 mL of hot water and the tablets with 150 mL of room temperature water.

FIGURE 21.2. An acetaminophen (APAP) hot drink product (Theraflu) acts more rapidly than does an APAP tablet (Tylenol).

Samples were collected at predosing and then at 3, 5, 7, 9, 11, 15, 20, 30, 45, 90, 120, and 180 minutes postdosing and analyzed.

The results following the hot drink showed APAP absorption was both significantly faster and greater over the first 60 minutes postdose compared with the tablet; this is evidenced by the median time to reach a plasma APAP concentration of 0.25 µg/mL, which was 4.6 and 23.1 minutes for the hot drink and tablet, respectively, with AUC_{0-60} of 4,668 and 1,331 h*ng/mL, respectively. Using pharmacoscintigraphy, the onset of gastric emptying after the hot drink was significantly faster than after the standard tablet (7.9 vs. 54.2 minutes, respectively).

This study shows that a hot drink formulation provides faster absorption of APAP potentially because more rapid gastric emptying along with enhanced dissolution in the hot liquid. This may provide a counseling opportunity for pharmacists when discussing how to take selected medications where a rapid onset may or may not be desired; more study needs to be done to determine the significance with different medications (10).

Example: Isoniazid Bioavailability Reduced with Applesauce

An 8-month-old infant with tuberculous meningitis treated with isoniazid was unsuccessful and exhibited lower than expected plasma concentration (0.1 µg/mL). The isoniazid tablet was crushed and mixed with applesauce (see Fig. 21.3). When an injectable isoniazid solution was mixed with apple juice, a higher concentration (2.9 µg/mL) was achieved and the child improved. A study was then conducted using the aforementioned preparations along with a commercially available syrup

FIGURE 21.3. Isoniazid tablets and applesauce.

containing isoniazid and pyridoxine; the latter produced the highest concentrations of 8.3 and 6.9 μg/mL. Research suggests that isoniazid is absorbed from the small intestine with the assistance of an active transporter. One or more components of applesauce may inhibit the transporter, decreasing the rate of isoniazid absorption (11). In summary, before mixing with a food, one must be aware that there may be a decrease in the absorption of the drug, depending of course on the drug, drug formulation, and the food (12).

Example: Changing Salt–Ester Form for Compliance (Taste)

A pharmacist is asked to prepare an oral erythromycin dosage form for a child, and the following information is found.

Erythromycin occurs as a white or slightly yellow, odorless or practically odorless, bitter, crystalline powder. The drug has a solubility of approximately 1 mg/mL in water and is soluble in alcohol.

The bitter taste is going to cause an issue with the child, so they look for other options and find the following:

Erythromycin estolate, the sodium lauryl sulfate salt of the propionate ester of erythromycin, occurs as a white, odorless or practically odorless, practically tasteless, crystalline powder. The drug is practically insoluble in water and has a solubility of approximately 50 mg/mL in alcohol.

It becomes apparent that the estolate form of erythromycin would be a good choice because it is practically tasteless and is insoluble in water. It is well known that keeping a drug in suspension rather than in solution will also decrease its taste.

Upon further investigation, the following is also found.

Erythromycin ethylsuccinate occurs as a white or slightly yellow, odorless or practically odorless, practically

tasteless, crystalline powder that is very slightly soluble in water and freely soluble in alcohol and soluble in polyethylene glycol.

With this information at hand, one has the decision to select the erythromycin estolate or the erythromycin ethylsuccinate as the form of erythromycin to use. Either one can be used to effectively produce an acceptable-tasting suspension of the drug. The molecular weights of the different forms (Erythromycin 733.93, erythromycin estolate 1,056.39) will need to be considered to deliver the required dose of erythromycin. Because of the different absorption characteristics of erythromycin ethylsuccinate, the equivalent of erythromycin 250 mg is erythromycin ethylsuccinate 400 mg. The next step is to formulate a good-tasting and stable suspension of the drug for the patient.

Example: Diazepam Liquid

A physician has prescribed diazepam 1 mg/mL oral liquid for a patient. The hospital formulary had the following standard formula:

Diazepam amp (10 mg/2 mL)		20 mL
Ethanol 95%		5 mL
Propylene glycol		30 mL
Methylcellulose 0.5% solution	qs	100 mL

Because of the taste, the pharmacist diluted the methylcellulose 0.5% solution 1:1 with simple syrup. The pharmacist mixed the diazepam injection with the propylene glycol and methylcellulose:simple syrup solution, but it turned cloudy. The issue here is that diazepam is not water soluble and requires a high concentration of cosolvents (ethanol and propylene glycol) to be maintained during preparation. Mixing the diazepam injection with the ethanol 95% and the propylene glycol first followed by the addition of the methylcellulose 0.5% solution corrects the problem.

Example: Captopril Solution Stability

There are numerous publications involving captopril for pediatric use reporting stability issues related to different formulations. Captopril is degraded by oxidation that is catalyzed by metal ions. The addition of EDTA helps to prevent this degradation and provides a stable captopril oral liquid with stability reported up to 2 years at refrigerated temperature (13).

Example: Drugs in Triglyceride Oils

When poorly water-soluble drugs are to be administered orally, one option is to mix the drug with triglyceride oils, such as soybean oil, and administer as soft gelatin capsules. After administration and dissolution of the gelatin capsule, the drug–oil contents are acted upon by pancreatic lipase in the intestine to form monoglycerides and fatty acids that interact with bile salts to form small droplets or vesicles in which the drug is solubilized. These vesicles continue to be broken down to form mixed micelles of about 3 to 10 nm. These mixed micelles can solubilize the drug in the small intestine and promote much faster absorption than when the drug is given in an oil-free formulation.

Example: SEDDS–Microemulsion Preconcentrates

Self-emulsifying drug-delivery systems (SEDDS) can be prepared as a "preconcentrate" containing the drug in a mixture of surfactants and nonaqueous solvents that, upon dilution, forms a microemulsion. A microemulsion is characterized by internal phase droplets with diameter of 10 to 100 nm. (14) Sandimmune was an emulsion preconcentrate consisting of cyclosporine in a vegetable oil (olive or corn) and ethanol; it also contained a polyglycolyzed glyceride (Labrafil M-1944CS) as a surfactant. It was prepared for oral administration by mixing with several milliliters of a noncarbonated liquid, generally water, milk, or orange juice. This formed a coarse oil-in-water dispersion prior to drinking the dose. The product was also available as a soft gelatin capsule containing a preconcentrate (surfactants Cremophor RH40 and Labrafil M-2125CS and a cosolvent of propylene glycol) that formed a microemulsion upon mixing with the aqueous environment of the stomach to provide fast absorption (15). This topic is covered in more detail in Chapter 20 Novel Dosage Forms and Drug Delivery Technologies.

TOPICAL TRANSDERMAL

Example: Alternate Dosage Form to Minimize GI Distress

A physician has called and described a patient with musculoskeletal pain affecting the elbow and forearm area and wants to prescribe a nonsteroidal anti-inflammatory drug (NSAID). The patient has a history of GI ulcers, so the physician would like an alternative route of administration other than oral.

Options include the parenteral, rectal, and transdermal routes of administration, and you recommend the transdermal route. The physician may prescribe one of the commercially available diclofenac sodium topical products or opt for a compounded preparation. You explain good success has been obtained using a transdermal gel formulation of ketoprofen 10% or a combination of ibuprofen 20% with piroxicam 1%. You explain that the transdermal gel vehicle consisting of a blend of a poloxamer, lecithin, and isopropyl palmitate has the ability to deliver the NSAIDs across the epidermal skin barrier for a prolonged effect. Also, with the flexibility of compounding, the prescriber has many options for different combinations or drugs and different strengths, to accommodate different patients. Compounded transdermal NSAIDs offer the practitioner a viable treatment option and alternative dosage form for NSAID therapy with decreased systemic side effects (16).

Androgel-Enhanced Penetration by Topical Miconazole

A 30-year-old adult was using topical miconazole cream for a fungal infection on the skin. A recent visit to the doctor resulted in a prescription for Androgel for possible testosterone deficiency. After a couple of weeks, he complains of acne, breast swelling, headache, blurred vision, and intermittent weakness in the left arm and leg. When asked, the patient said he applied both medications to the same area. What is occurring is that the miconazole cream contains excipients that can serve as penetration enhancers and can result in enhanced absorption of the testosterone when applied to the same area. Options include administering the drugs to separate parts of the body or decreasing the dose of the Androgel; the first option seems to be more appropriate (17).

Example: "To occlude or not to occlude, ..."

It is well known that occlusive dressings applied to the site of application of a transdermal formulation increases drug delivery from most formulations. In fact, there have been deaths reported from excessive application of lidocaine creams with occlusion to prepare the skin for various procedures in clinics.

Occlusion serves to hydrate the skin by preventing moisture from evaporating into the atmosphere; thus, it remains on or in the skin and the water content of the stratum corneum can increase up to 4-fold of the tissue dry weight and drug (steroid) delivery can improve up to 100-fold when the skin tissue is covered. Other examples show lesser improvements in skin penetration, but even a 10 to 100 percent improvement may be significant. Occlusion does not always involve a plastic film or an occlusive ointment vehicle. In some cases, an infant's tightly fitting waterproof pants may occlude the area and increase drug delivery. Patch-delivery systems also take advantage of skin occlusion to enhance drug delivery.

However, the continued hydration of the skin may be problematic with microbial growth and irritation; these effects are usually reversible. An alternative is to use a volatile delivery vehicle. As the volatile delivery vehicle evaporates, it serves to increase the concentration of the drug to supersaturation so that increased amounts can penetrate into the stratum corneum.

To summarize, occlusion may be of benefit when enhanced drug penetration is needed over a prolonged period of time; it must be used cautiously to address specific problems in drug absorption rather than as a routine practice.

Example: "Equivalence" of Topicals

With cost considerations and pricing variations between products, it is often assumed by many that the formulations containing the same drug concentrations are generally equivalent. However, there is a great deal of clinical and scientific evidence showing that formulation changes or different manufacturing processes can alter the clinical efficacy of a drug. Showing bioequivalence between topical formulations, however, is more difficult and complex than the use of bioavailability AUC numbers like those used from oral and parenteral administration. It seems that vasoactive assays provide some benefit in comparing formulations; however, not all topically applied drugs are vasoactive.

The bioavailability from topically applied formulations is in the order of 1% to 3% of the dose applied. It is possible to reduce the concentration of a product like hydrocortisone in a cream vehicle to 0.1% and still be able to deliver the same amount of the steroid as from a 1% formulation. To add more confusion to the issue, there are preparations using different forms of the same drug with different salts or esters. As examples, hydrocortisone is formulated as the free base (1%, mild or low potency), as the acetate (1%, mild potency), and as the butyrate (0.1%, i.e., at one-tenth the free base concentration, but classified as potent or high potency). To this, add the variability in skin permeability between different body sites and between different individuals that may be in the order of 30% to 40%.

Some in vitro testing methods are applicable for confirming batch-to-batch uniformity during production/preparation but not applicable for bioequivalence testing for those topicals. For drugs that penetrate through the skin and enter the systemic circulation, plasma levels and C_{max} can be determined; but for drugs acting on or within the skin, biopsies need to be taken to determine drug levels: punch biopsies for drugs within the stratum corneum and shave biopsy for upper stratum corneum, viable epidermis, and some dermal tissue. This type of testing is impractical for clinical situations.

In summary, it is apparent that ensuring equivalence between different formulations of the same drug is not a simple task. A reasonable approach would be that if a specific formulation is working well, maybe it should not be changed.

Example: "Delivery Through a Repairing Barrier"

The delivery of a drug through compromised skin is different than through intact skin and may present a problem for drug delivery. Skin conditions range from psoriasis and eczema to ulcers, herpes infections (warts and cold sores), and dermatophytoses (fungal infections), and the affected stratum corneum may allow for greater uptake of the active drug than when intact. As an example, the uptake of 8-methoxypsoralen into psoriatic plaques is greater than in intact stratum corneum as plaques are largely devoid of the intracellular lipoidal content. Also, salicylic acid has been shown to be concentrated in the core of a wart and has been shown to be bound to the affected tissue. But it is also possible that drug delivery can be reduced compared to normal tissue, for example, when the skin is thickened but intact (callus tissue).

As the skin barrier changes during therapy, the amount of drug delivery into the tissue also changes, and the dynamics of this process are complex. One has several options available to address this situation:

- Alter the concentration of the API in the formula.
- Leave the formula on the affected area either longer or for a shorter period of time.
- Apply the product over a larger or smaller area.

These approaches can simply compensate for the altered/reduced efficiency of drug permeation as the barrier changes and the stratum corneum restores its integrity.

Example: "Supersaturation and Thermodynamic Effects"

The driving force for permeation is the thermodynamic activity of the active pharmaceutical ingredient (API) in the vehicle. Optimal transdermal drug delivery may be achieved from a saturated solution of the drug. However, a drug solution that is saturated at room temperature may no longer be saturated upon application to the skin with a surface temperature of about 32°C.

It may be possible to further increase the thermodynamic activity in a formulation beyond unity by using supersaturated systems. A supersaturated system contains a solute at a higher concentration than the equilibrium solubility (where the dissolved molecules are in equilibrium with solid). These systems are thermodynamically unstable, but supersaturation may be maintained over short periods of time by appropriate formulation and product application.

Supersaturation can be accomplished in a topical dosage form by evaporation of a solvent from the system after application to the skin, driving the drug activity on the skin higher than it was before product application. The degree of supersaturation decreases as the drug penetrates into the skin, decreasing the probability of drug crystallizing out of the system. Even though it may be uncontrolled and unpredictable, supersaturation of the API in the donor phase as the vehicle evaporates from the skin surface is a mechanism that is probably operating in many topically applied formulations.

For permeation, thermodynamic activity is the driving force, not concentration. Depletion of the drug in some cases may be problematic but can be overcome by the use of microcrystalline suspensions (18).

Clinical Pharmaceutics Example: "An Order of Magnitude"

Selection of an appropriate candidate in the appropriate form is a first step in this process. Keeping in mind that in vitro data only provide an estimate for in vivo delivery; it is a good place to start if the data are available. Some of the factors we have previously discussed can each contribute somewhat to enhanced delivery transdermally, including

- Solvent selection
- Penetration enhancers
- Surfactants
- Fragrance with penetration-enhancing capabilities
- Volatile substances that evaporate upon application to skin leading to supersaturation
- Hydration of the skin (occlusion from vehicle, plastic, etc.)

All these various factors considered, drug flux can be promoted often by about an order of magnitude using formulation manipulation.

Example: Why Was the Duragesic (Fentanyl Transdermal System) Changed?

The following is an interesting example of clinical pharmaceutics involving transdermal drug delivery and dosage form design, after reported deaths.

Read the following two descriptions (see Fig. 21.4).

PDR 1997—Proceeding from the outer surface toward the surface adhering to skin, these layers are

1. A backing layer of polyester film.
2. A *drug reservoir of fentanyl* and alcohol USP gelled with hydroxyethyl cellulose.
3. An ethylene-vinyl acetate copolymer membrane that controls the rate of fentanyl delivery to the skin surface.
4. A *fentanyl containing silicone adhesive.*
5. Before use, a protective liner covering the adhesive layer is removed and discarded (19).

PDR 2010–Proceeding from the outer surface toward the surface adhering to skin, these layers are as follows:

1. A backing layer of polyester/ethyl vinyl acetate film.
2. A *drug-in-adhesive layer*.
3. Before use, a protective liner covering the adhesive layer is removed and discarded (20).

A

B

FIGURE 21.4. Diagrams of the former Duragesic **(A)** and revised Duragesic **(B)** transdermal delivery systems.

Why the change? In the original version, the drug in the silicone adhesive served to assist in rapidly producing a depot of fentanyl in the skin; in other words, it worked like a "loading dose." There were some deaths associated with obese patients who had difficulty getting the "system" to stick to the skin, and, in some cases, after a few hours, the patch would loosen and the patient could not get it to stay on. So, they applied another patch, and then another, etc. This continually increased the quantity of drug being administered because each patch had a "loading dose" that kept building up in the skin and accumulating to a toxic level. The newer system provides a more evenly released dose and reaches a leveling off in the serum concentrations after 12 to 24 hours, the same as before. The advantage to the new system is less likelihood of accidental overdosing.

PARENTERAL

Example: Avastin Repackaging

Some publications have directed criticism at compounding pharmacists for "contaminating" Avastin˙ (bevacizumab) with silicone oil during the process of repackaging intravitreal injections. Most syringes contain silicone oil as a lubricant to reduce friction between the plunger and the barrel. Studies show that the silicone oil within the syringe is "immediately" mixed with solutions such as Avastin and is injected into the eye.

A study utilizing multiple sophisticated analytic methods found that "the commercial solution of bevacizumab can be safely repackaged in polypropylene syringes and stored for up to 3 months at 4°C without alteration of its primary, secondary and tertiary structure. The only difference observed is the contamination of the syringe content by silicone oil microdroplets, which is quite immediate and does not change significantly during the storage in terms of number and size."

The amount of silicone droplets in the injection does not appear to change significantly during storage. However, it is stated in this article that the "contamination" of the Avastin with silicone oil is immediate and results from the action of withdrawing into a syringe containing silicone oil. Injecting silicone droplets into the eye is of concern whether drawing up a solution directly from the manufacturer's vial or repackaging doses. The only way to avoid the problem is to use silicone-free syringes for intravitreal injections. It should be noted that there is no warning concerning this in the package label of Avastin (21).

Example: Paclitaxel Infusion and Special Tubing

A nurse calls the infusion pharmacy asking why the paclitaxel dose that was sent from the pharmacy also had a special infusion tubing set. Paclitaxel is poorly water soluble and requires a specific vehicle to dissolve it; the vehicle is Cremophor EL, or polyoxyl 35 castor oil, and ethanol. The vehicle can leach or extract the plasticizer DEHP (diethylhexyl phthalate) from standard infusion sets into the drug solution, which can cause hepatotoxicity. Therefore, paclitaxel is prepared in a non-PVC container and is administered via a non-PVC infusion set to avoid the risk of exposing the patient to DEHP (22).

Example: Insulin Adsorption

The adsorption of insulin onto the surface of glass containers and plastic IV tubing has been well documented. The adsorption occurs very rapidly, and the adsorbed insulin is unavailable to the patient. A common practice to prevent insulin adsorption is to add albumin to the insulin solution. The albumin preferentially adsorbs to the glass or plastic surface and significantly reduces the amount of insulin adsorbed to the surface (23).

SUPPOSITORIES AND INSERTS

Example: Wrong Suppository Vehicle Results in Seizures

The water solubility of a suppository base can strongly influence the absorption of lipophilic drugs. For example, a teenager with epilepsy was prescribed diazepam 10 mg suppositories. It was compounded using diazepam powder and cocoa butter as the vehicle. However, the teen has been to the emergency room twice with uncontrolled seizures, even after using the suppositories in an effort to try to bring the seizures under control.

Cocoa butter is a fatty acid (lipid) base and diazepam is a lipophilic drug with lipid–water partition coefficient of approximately 630:1. When diazepam is placed in a cocoa butter base and administered rectally, the cocoa butter base melts quickly at body temperature. Diazepam has a much greater tendency to remain within the melted cocoa butter than to partition into the aqueous mucosal fluids of the rectal mucosa. Diazepam absorption from the cocoa butter suppository is therefore very slow in this situation. The suppository should be reformulated using a water-soluble base, such as polyethylene glycol. When the lipid-free polyethylene glycol base dissolves in the aqueous mucosal fluids, the diazepam will disperse and come into greater contact with the membrane wall and be available for absorption.

Diastat is a rectal gel composed of 5 mg/mL diazepam, propylene glycol, ethyl alcohol (10%), hydroxypropyl methylcellulose, sodium benzoate, benzyl alcohol (1.5%), benzoic acid, and water (see Fig. 21.5). This product should function in a similar manner by spreading out over the mucosal fluids and mixing with them providing good contact with the membrane for absorption (24).

CLINICAL PHARMACEUTICS AND COMPOUNDING

A pharmacist must be well aware of the fact that almost anything placed into a "dosage form" can alter the clinical result when administered to a patient. Inherent in

FIGURE 21.5. Diastat rectal gel product.

compounding a drug dosage form are the following considerations of both APIs and excipients in dosage forms that should be addressed as they can affect both the clinical response and cause adverse events.

Example: Problems, PBMs, and Clinical Pharmaceutics

An unfortunate encounter a pharmacy experienced with a pharmacy benefit manager (PBM) occurred. The PBM denied coverage of most compounds by means of National Drug Code (NDC) rejection on over-the-counter (OTC) vehicles that are Generally Recognized as Safe (GRAS) by the FDA.

The pharmacy had a newborn baby patient with a life-threatening arrhythmia in the NICU who needed the antiarrhythmic propafenone. It was a very tense situation for a while until the patient was stabilized on the compounded medication in the hospital. Upon discharge, the insurance rejected the compounded formulation and would only pay for the tablets. The PBM did not give the pharmacy or the physician any type of prior authorization option other than the parents seeking some sort of formalized appeal process "down the road." The cash cost for the compounded medication was too much out of pocket for the family. So, unfortunately, the pharmacy had to send them home with tablets where they were to dissolve a tablet in 10 mL of water and then give a partial amount to try to best approximate the desired dose. As one can imagine, this is not an ideal situation, especially for a neonatal patient with an arrhythmia. This action is deplorable and the PBM is determining drug therapy and should be held accountable for what happens to the child.

Note: Propafenone is listed as "slightly soluble" in water; this encompasses from 10 to 1 mg/mL water. Tablets contain either 150 or 225 mg of drug. Using the 150 mg tablet, it would take between 15 and 150 mL of water to dissolve the drug to obtain a "uniform dose." It is quite evident that all the drug will not dissolve in 10 mL, and the patient may not be aware they must obtain a uniform suspension in order to accurately measure the required dose for the infant.

Example: Improper Dissolution/Mixing of Cremophor EL Leads to Anaphylactoid Reactions

A number of anaphylactoid reactions were observed during a phase I/II trial of high-dose intravenous cyclosporine (CsA) therapy to attenuate tumor multidrug resistance (25). Five of twenty-one children experienced the reactions shortly after initiation of either the first or second CsA infusion. Interviews of the health care professionals administering the drug regarding their technique of preparing the infusion and the occurrence of the anaphylactoid reactions were conducted. An evaluation of the effect of various mixing techniques on the distribution of Cremophor EL in the infusion showed a significant correlation between suboptimal mixing and the occurrence of the anaphylactoid reactions. CsA solutions that were mixed completely did not result in the anaphylactoid reactions. The study authors concluded that "improper mixing of high-dose CsA infusions causes nonsolubilized Cremophor EL to sink to the outflow area of the bottle. An initial bolus infusion of highly concentrated Cremophor EL may produce an anaphylactoid-like response."

Cremophor EL, or polyoxyl 35 castor oil, is soluble in water and has a density of 1.05 to 1.06. It is used as an emulsifying agent, nonionic surfactant, and a solubilizing agent. It is a complex mixture of various hydrophobic and hydrophilic components. The relatively hydrophobic constituents constitute about 83% of the total mixture (the main component is glycerol polyethylene glycol ricinoleate). The hydrophilic part (17%) consists of free polyethylene glycols and glycerol ethoxylates. It occurs as a pale yellow, oily liquid that is clear at temperatures above 26°C and it has a faint, but characteristic odor and can be completely liquefied by heating to 26°C. On heating aqueous solutions to higher temperatures, the solubility is reduced and the solution becomes turbid (22). Complex formulations such as the solubilized high-dose CsA solution require special attention to ensure that patients consistently receive the proper dose in a homogenous distribution.

GENERIC DRUGS

Example: Generic ADHD Drugs Not Bioequivalent?

In November 2014, the FDA changed the ratings for two generic versions of Concerta to BX, meaning "the data are insufficient to determine therapeutic equivalence" (26). The generics can no longer be substituted for the brand-name drug. These products are among the few approved generics that are not rated as therapeutic equivalents. The products had previously been approved as therapeutic equivalents to Concerta under abbreviated new drug applications. After the products were marketed, side effect reports indicated some patients were not getting

the expected drug effect. The FDA analyzed the generics and found they were not bioequivalent to Concerta. The generic companies questioned the FDA's action. The question they raise is "To what extent should the FDA be allowed to reclassify a generic drug when the agency believes it is no longer equivalent to the brand-name version?"

The issue involves an unusual lawsuit claiming the agency overstepped its bounds by deciding two generic drugs used to treat ADHD should no longer be substituted for the widely used Concerta treatment. And the outcome of the case may have implications for generic drug makers and the FDA.

The FDA gave the generic companies 6 months to provide data showing bioequivalency to Concerta or their drugs should be withdrawn from the market. The deadline passed, but the generics remain available, and it is unclear how the FDA will proceed. An agency spokeswoman would not comment.

One generic company spokesperson explains it is working with the FDA to meet its requirement. The other generic company, however, is not showing any signs of complying with the agency mandate and has challenged the authority of the agency to reclassify its generic by arguing that the FDA failed to provide sufficient notice of its decision and violated its constitutional rights. In addition, they state that the FDA has acknowledged there are no safety issues and patients should continue taking the generics if they are not experiencing problems.

The FDA has reclassified generic drugs over equivalency before this case; in 2012, the agency changed ratings for some generic antidepressants. These events pose an interesting situation because we now have two "categories" of generic Concerta available that are not bioequivalent; "Clinical Pharmaceutics" is the basis for this unique regulatory situation.

The FDA did state that it considered the drugs to be safe; data show that their effectiveness began to wear off much more quickly—after about 7 hours. Concerta's mechanism of drug release is that it absorbs fluid and pumps the active drug out of a laser-cut hole. Under FDA rules, generic companies do not need to use the same mechanisms to produce copies of long-acting drugs. The generic product must simply release the drug into the body at the same rate as the brand-name drug. The two generic company products use different techniques, which may account for the shorter effectiveness (27–30).

Example: Changing Excipients for Special Needs Patients

Some patients cannot take various drug products (Rx and OTC) because they have allergies or are intolerant to various substances, including dyes, flavorings, sweeteners, preservatives, gelatins, milk products, gluten, corn, soy, nuts, alcohol, chocolate, and animal-derived ingredients. Sometimes the specific allergy or intolerance is difficult to determine. Once known, the compounding pharmacist can work with the patient to circumvent the offending agent and resolve the problem.

Oftentimes, the offending agent is an excipient in a commercial drug product. The source that can be used for compounding of the active drug may be a raw material or possibly an injection or dosage form with minimal excipients and not containing the offending agent. Next, there are numerous excipients in each group that may be substituted for different patients with a little bit of literature research. In some cases, the issue can be resolved by changing brands or even generics manufacturers, as many different generics of the same drug product contain different excipients. The package insert should list the excipients contained in their products. Manufacturers of generics are not required to have identical excipients in their products; this can sometimes be an issue (31–34).

PACKAGING

Example: Packaging and Storage Issues with Misoprostol Tablets

Misoprostol tablets must be stored in tight containers in a dry place at controlled room temperature; they should not be removed from original packaging. However, they are sometimes packaged as multiple tablets within an aluminum strip, each cavity holding multiple tablets. When this cavity is opened, tablets are exposed to atmospheric conditions.

A study reports on an investigation to compare the pharmaceutical characteristics (weight, friability), water content, misoprostol content, and decomposition of misoprostol tablets (Cytotec, Pfizer) exposed to air (2°C/60% relative humidity) for periods of 1 to 720 hours (30 days) to those of identical nonexposed tablets. By 48 hours, exposed tablets had increased in weight (+4.5%), friability, and water content (+80%) as compared to controls. There was a decrease in misoprostol content by 5.1% after 48 hours.

Misoprostol occurs as a light yellow viscous oil with a musty odor that is stated to be soluble in water. Misoprostol is known to be unstable and is stabilized in the form of a solid dispersion with HPMC to protect the misoprostol and decrease water penetration. The 48-hour increase in weight corresponds to the maximum penetration of water into the tablets; this initiates the degradation of misoprostol. This degradation reaches 5% loss at 48 hours and more than 10% loss after 7 days. Studies have shown that the first-order rate constants increased as the water content of misoprostol increased. Misoprostol tablets should be stored in original containers or in small tight containers if repackaged.

Regarding compounding with misoprostol, studies of misoprostol suppositories in Suppocire base remained stable with loss of 7% in 180 days refrigerated and about 9% in 120 days at room temperature. In Polybase, the suppositories were stable for up to 12 months refrigerated but only 1 week at room temperature (35).

Example: It's All in the Package!

The USP states:

Packaging must not interact physically or chemically with official articles in any way that causes their safety, identity, strength, quality, or purity to fail to conform to requirements.

The packaging system (also referred to as a container-closure system) is the sum of packaging components that together contain and protect the article.

Syringe companies have announced that their syringes were not developed for long-term storage of medications. The FDA released a notice entitled "Compounded or Repackaged Drugs Stored in Becton-Dickinson (BD) 3 mL and 5 mL Syringes: FDA Alert-Do Not Use Unless There Is No Suitable Alternative" (36). The notice states, "Hospital and pharmacy staff should check supply stocks and remove drug products that were filled by pharmacies or outsourcing facilities and stored in general purpose BD 3 mL and 5 mL syringes."

It has been well known for years that some drugs will sorb (adsorb, absorb) to plastic containers, especially soft plastic IV bags, etc. It has also been known that some will "sorb" to syringes/plunger tips. This is especially critical in high-potency, low-concentration drugs but not as critical in drugs in high concentration. There are many published studies that address this clinical pharmaceutic situation.

PRACTICE CONSIDERATIONS IN CLINICAL PHARMACEUTICS

As has been stated, clinical pharmaceutics impacts drug therapy and involves applying basic scientific facts to solving problems in medication therapy. However, other aspects of practice impact clinical pharmaceutics and involve dispensing and reimbursement and the requirements of the PBMs (previously mentioned) and their requirements. In other words, reimbursement often dictates therapy and there are requirements by PBMs that are not in the patient's best interests, as below.

1. Sometimes, medications are not manufactured in the appropriate dosage form or strength needed by many patients.
2. PBMs often require a drug to be "FDA approved" for reimbursement. However, there are thousands of drug products that are not FDA approved. For example, pre-1938 drugs have never been FDA approved. Compounded medications are not FDA approved. Intravenous admixtures are not FDA approved. Total parenteral nutrition solutions (TPNs) are not FDA approved. Even though an admixture has been compounded using FDA-approved drugs, the final preparation is not FDA approved.

3. Most compounded oral preparations are made using FDA-approved dosage forms or powder and liquid medicines in their bulk chemical form that are in FDA-approved dosage forms. It is generally best to use bulk chemicals (USP/NF) in compounding as they are simpler to use. Manufactured drug products contain excipients that can be problematic and cause incompatibility and patient compliance issues.

4. Because of the number of tablets or capsules or the volume of injections required, it is not always possible to use commercial dosage forms of many drugs to compound many prescriptions ordered by physicians.

5. Without individualized medications, patients may not recover and lead useful lives but may continue with their disease/disorder that will lead to long-term costs to the PBMs that they will pass onto employers and patients who are the ultimate payors.

6. A patient having undergone a stem cell transplant costing hundreds of thousands of dollars may not be able to receive the compounded oral preparations necessary to sustain this costly procedure after discharge because they are "compounded preparations"; the additional cost of the patient not doing well because of a lack of medication they were stabilized on in the hospital may lead to additional costs passed from the PBM to employers and their employees (the patient or patient's family).

7. Without individualized medications, patients may die as a result of the PBM decisions controlling drug therapy!

In summary, clinical pharmaceutics goes far beyond the science and therapeutic aspects of patient care as it is also deeply involved in economic, compliance, and practical issues.

APPLYING THE PRINCIPLES AND CONCEPTS

GROUP ACTIVITIES

1. Link some therapeutic failures caused by situations related to clinical pharmaceutics.
2. Relate some clinical pharmaceutics phenomena to certain classes/categories of drugs.
3. List some current examples of potential drug incompatibilities.
4. Describe some counseling points related to clinical pharmaceutics for patients.
5. Select a reported drug incompatibility and prepare a report on its chemical or physical causation.
6. Discuss how you would explain therapeutic inequivalent generics to a physician and to a patient. Describe the practical impact of the likely therapeutic differences on patient care.

INDIVIDUAL ACTIVITIES

1. Distinguish between a physical and chemical drug incompatibility and provide three examples of each.

2. Discuss the importance of pH as it relates to solubility.
3. From the literature, find a clinical situation where dosing was compromised because of a clinical pharmaceutics situation and discuss how it could have been corrected.
4. Prepare a list of situations where packaging can adversely affect a drug product and how it is handled by the pharmaceutical industry.
5. Discuss an example of how pharmaceutical compounding can be used to eliminate an example situation involving clinical pharmaceutics.
6. Find the list of excipients in the "Description" section of drug package insert. Identify the function of each excipient and determine which ones could be eliminated (e.g., colorants) without affecting the product quality.
7. List examples of excipients with known intolerance issues for many patients, and list potential substitutes that could be used in their place.

REFERENCES

1. Lin C, Lim J, DiGiore C, et al. Comparative bioavailability of a microsize and ultramicrosize griseofulvin formulation in man. J Int Med Res 1982;10(4):274–277.
2. Gaginella TS. GI intolerance and nitrofurantoin. J Pharm Sci 1977;66(10):IV.
3. Anonymous. Physician's Desk Reference. 58th Ed. Montvale, NJ: Thomson PDR, 2004:2835–2837.
4. Kaplun-Firschoff Y, Touitou E. Testosterone skin permeation enhancement by menthol through formation of eutectic with drug and interaction with skin lipids. J Pharm Sci 1997;86(12): 1394–1399.
5. Durani U, Tosh PK, Barreto JN, et al. Retrospective comparison of posaconazole levels in patients taking the delayed-release tablet versus the oral suspension. Antimicrob Agents Chemother 2015;59(8):4914–4918.
6. www.medscape.com/viewarticle/856724. (Accessed March 2, 2016)
7. Tyrer JH, Eadie MJ, Sutherland JM, et al. Outbreak of anticonvulsant intoxication in an Australian city. Br Med J 1970;4(5730):271–273.
8. Burgess DS. Antimicrobial regimen selection. In: Pharmacotherapy: A Pathophysiologic Approach. 7th Ed. New York, NY: McGraw Hill, 2008:1735.
9. O'Neill JL, Remington TL. Drug-induced esophageal injuries and dysphagia. Ann Pharmacother 2003;37(Nov):1675–1684.
10. Hodges LA, Hughes A, Targett D, et al. Does a hot drink provide faster absorption of paracetamol than a tablet? A pharmacoscintigraphic study in healthy male volunteers. Pharm Res 2014;31(8):2078–2085.
11. Parvez MM, Kaisar N, Shin HJ, Yoon JL, Shin J-G. Comprehensive substrate characterization of 22 antituberculosis drugs for multiple

solute carrier (SLC) uptake transporters in vitro. Antimicrob Agent Chemother 2018;62(9):e00512-18.

12. Notterman DA, Nardi M, Saslow JG. Effect of dose formulation on isoniazid absorption in two young children. Pediatrics 1986;77(6):850–852.

13. Kristensen S, Lao YE, Brustugun J, et al. Influence of formulation properties on chemical stability of captopril in aqueous preparations. Pharmazie 2008;63(12):872–877.

14. Callender SP, Mathews JA, Kobernyk K, et al. Microemulsion utility in pharmaceuticals: Implications for multi-drug delivery. Int J Pharm 2017;526:425–442.

15. http://www.rxlist.com/sandimmune-drug.htm. (Accessed March 2, 2016)

16. Bassani AS, Banov D, Phan H. Characterization of the percutaneous absorption of ketoprofen using the Franz skin finite dose model. Postgrad Med 2016;7:1–6.

17. Baert B, Roche N, Burvenich C, et al. Increase of the transdermal penetration of testosterone by miconazole nitrate. Arch Pharm Res 2012;35(12):2163–2168.

18. Santos P, Watkinson AC, Hadgraft J, et al. Enhanced permeation of fentanyl from supersaturated solutions in a model membrane. Int J Pharm 2011;407(1–2):72–77.

19. Anonymous. Physician's Desk Reference. 51st Ed. Montvale, NJ: Medical Economics Company, Inc., 1997:1336–1340.

20. Anonymous. Physician's Desk Reference. 64th Ed. Montvale, NJ: PDR Network, LLC, 2010:2604–2611.

21. Paul M, Vieillard V, Roumi E, et al. Long-term stability of bevacizumab repackaged in 1 mL polypropylene syringes for intravitreal administration. Ann Pharm Fr 2012;70(3):139–154. doi: .1016/j. pharma.2012.03.006.

22. Waugh WN, Trissel LA, Stella VJ. Stability, compatibility, and plasticizer extraction of taxol (NSC-125973) injection diluted in infusion solutions and stored in various containers. Am J Hosp Pharm 1991;48(7):1520–1524.

23. McEvoy GK, ed. Handbook of Injectable Drugs. 18th Ed. Bethesda, MD: American Society of Health-Systems Pharmacists, 2015:675–681.

24. Allen Jr LV. Suppositories. London: Pharmaceutical Press, 2008:3, 63, 65, 83, 88, 185.

25. Theis JG, Liau-Chu M, Chan HS, et al. Anaphylactoid reactions in children receiving high-dose intravenous cyclosporine for reversal of tumor resistance: The causative role of improper dissolution of Cremophor EL. J Clin Oncol 1995;13():2508–2516.

26. Anonymous. Approved Drug Products with Therapeutic Equivalence Evaluations. 40th Ed. Washington, DC. U.S. Department of Health and Human Services, 2020.

27. http://www.nytimes.com/2015/06/17/business/generic-ritalin-drug-not-equivalent-to-the-brand-is-in-use-anyway.html?_r=0. (Accessed March 3, 2016)

28. Lally MD, Kral MC, Boan AD. Not all generic Concerta is created equal: Comparison of OROS versus non-OROS for the treatment of ADHD. Clin Pediatr (Phila) 2016;55(13):1197–1201. Pii: 0009922815611647.

29. http://www.webmd.com/add-adhd/news/20141114/two-generic-versions-of-adhd-drug-not-as-effective-fda. (Accessed March 3, 2016)

30. http://www.fdalawblog.net/fda_law_blog_hyman_phelps/2014/11/mallinckrodt-sues-fda-after-agency-downgrades-therapeutic-equivalence-rating-for-generic-concerta.html. (Accessed March 3, 2016)

31. Nagel-Edwards KM, Ko JY. Excipient choices for special populations. Int J Pharm Compd 2008;12(5):426–430.

32. Cacace JL. Formulating for the gluten-sensitive individual. Int J Pharm Compd 2005;9(5):357–358.

33. Lcaycomb J. Pharmacists Must Guard Vulnerable Patients Against Inactive Ingredients in Medications. http://drugtopics.modernmedicine.com/drug-topics/news/pharmacists-must-guard-vulnerable-patients-against-inactive-ingredients-medications. (Accessed March 3, 2016)

34. www.Glutenfreedrugs.com. (Accessed March 3, 2016)

35. Berard V, Fiala C, Cameron S, et al. Instability of misoprostol tablets stored outside the blister: A potential serious concern for clinical outcome in medical abortion. PLoS One 2014;9(12). http://journals.plos.org/plosone/article?id=.1371/journal.pone.0112401. (Accessed March 3, 2016)

36. Compounded or Repackaged Drugs Stored in Becton-Dickinson (BD) 3 mL and 5 mL Syringes: FDA Alert-Do Not Use Unless There Is No Suitable Alternative. Available at: http://www.fda.gov/Safety/MedWatch/SafetyInformation/SafetyAlertsforHumanMedicalProducts/ucm458955.htm. (Accessed March 3, 2016)

Definitions of Selected Drug Categories (Including Those Recognized by USP)

A

Abortifacient an agent that will induce an abortion.

Abradant an agent that removes an external layer, such as dental plaque (pumice).

Absorbent a drug that takes up other chemicals into its substance; it is used to reduce the free availability of toxic chemicals (polycarbophil, gastrointestinal absorbent).

ACE Inhibitor see Angiotensin-Converting Enzyme Inhibitor.

Acidifier, Systemic a drug that lowers the internal body pH; it is useful in restoring normal pH in patients with systemic alkalosis (ammonium chloride).

Acidifier, Urinary a drug that lowers the pH of the renal filtrate and urine (sodium dihydrogen phosphate).

Adrenergic a drug that activates organs innervated by the sympathetic nervous system; a sympathomimetic drug (epinephrine, norepinephrine).

Adrenocorticosteroid, Anti-inflammatory an adrenal cortex hormone that regulates organic metabolism and inhibits inflammatory response; a glucocorticoid (prednisolone, prednisone).

Adrenocorticosteroid, Salt-Regulating an adrenal cortex hormone that regulates sodium/potassium balance in the body; a mineralocorticoid (desoxycorticosterone acetate).

Adrenocorticotropic Hormone a hormone that stimulates the adrenal cortex to produce glucocorticoids (corticotropin).

Adsorbent a drug that binds other chemicals onto its surface; it is used to reduce the free availability of toxic chemicals (kaolin, gastrointestinal adsorbent).

Agonist a drug that reacts with and activates physiological receptors and induces the associated biologic response (morphine, opioid receptor agonist; isoproterenol, beta-adrenergic receptor agonist).

Alcohol-Abuse Deterrent a drug that alters physiology so that unpleasant symptoms follow ingestion of ethanol-containing products (disulfiram).

Aldehyde Dehydrogenase Inhibitor a drug that blocks the conversion of acetaldehyde to acetic acid by aldehyde dehydrogenase (disulfiram).

Alkalinizer, Systemic a drug that raises the internal body pH; it is useful in restoring normal pH in patients with systemic acidosis (sodium bicarbonate).

Alkylating Agent an antineoplastic drug that attacks malignant cells by reacting covalently with their DNA (chlorambucil).

Alpha Glucosidase Inhibitor a drug that blocks the digestion of carbohydrates into simple sugars that will increase blood sugar levels (oral diabetic drugs).

Alpha Receptor Agonist a drug that activates sympathetic nervous system alpha receptors, for example, to induce vasoconstriction (norepinephrine).

Alpha Receptor Antagonist a drug that reacts asymptomatically with sympathetic nervous system alpha receptors and prevents their endogenous activation, for example, to induce vasodilation (phentolamine).

Alpha Reductase Inhibitor a drug that decreases the levels of available 5α-reductase prior to testosterone's binding with the enzyme, reducing levels of dihydrotestosterone.

Amebicide an agent used to treat amoebozoa infections (metronidazole).

Anabolic Steroid an androgen analogue with relatively greater anabolic activity; it is used to treat catabolic disorders (methandrostenolone).

Analeptic a central nervous system stimulant, sometimes used to stimulate respiration during severe central nervous system depression (doxapram, modafinil).

Analgesic a drug that suppresses pain perception (nociception) without inducing unconsciousness (morphine sulfate, opioid analgesic; aspirin, nonopioid analgesic).

Androgen a hormone that stimulates and maintains male reproductive function and sex characteristics (testosterone).

Anesthetic, General a drug that eliminates pain perception by inducing unconsciousness (ether, inhalation anesthetic; thiopental sodium, intravenous anesthetic; midazolam).

Anesthetic, Local a drug that eliminates pain perception in a limited body area by local action on sensory nerves (procaine, lidocaine).

Anesthetic, Topical a local anesthetic that is effective upon application to mucous membranes (tetracaine).

Angiotensin-Converting Enzyme Inhibitor a drug that inhibits biotransformation of angiotensin I into vasoconstricting angiotensin II; it is used to treat hypertension (captopril, ramipril).

Anorexiant a drug that acts on the brain to reduce the appetite.

Anorexic a drug that suppresses appetite, usually by elevating mood (phentermine, sibutramine).

Antacid a drug that neutralizes excess gastric acid (calcium carbonate).

Antagonist a drug that reacts asymptomatically with physiological receptors and prevents their endogenous activation (naloxone, opioid receptor antagonist; propranolol and metoprolol, beta-adrenergic receptor antagonists).

Anthelmintic a drug that eradicates intestinal worm infestations (mebendazole).

Antiacne Agent a drug that combats the lesions of acne vulgaris (isotretinoin).

Antiadrenergic a drug that inhibits response to sympathetic nerve impulses and adrenergic drugs; a sympatholytic drug (phentolamine, alpha adrenergic antagonist; metoprolol, beta-adrenergic antagonist).

Antiamebic a drug that kills or inhibits protozoan parasites such as *Entamoeba histolytica*, causative agent of amebiasis (metronidazole, intestinal antiamebic; chloroquine, extraintestinal antiamebic).

Antiandrogen a drug that inhibits response to androgenic hormones.

Antianemic a drug used to treat anemia; see Hematopoietic, Hematinic (ferrous sulfate).

Antianginal a coronary vasodilator useful in preventing or treating attacks of angina pectoris (nitroglycerin).

Antiarrhythmic a cardiac depressant useful in suppressing rhythm irregularities of the heart (amiodarone HCl; procainamide).

Antiarthritic a drug that reduces the joint inflammation of arthritis (anakinra, celecoxib, ibuprofen).

Antibacterial a drug that kills or inhibits pathogenic bacteria (penicillin G, systemic antibacterial; nitrofurantoin, urinary antibacterial; bacitracin, topical antibacterial).

Antibiotic a drug originally of microbial origin used to kill or inhibit bacterial and other infections (clarithromycin, penicillin, levofloxacin).

Anticholesterol Agent a drug that lowers plasma cholesterol level (cholestyramine resin; atorvastatin, rosuvastatin calcium; simvastatin; ezetimibe).

Anticholinergic a drug that inhibits response to parasympathetic nerve impulses and cholinergic drugs; a parasympatholytic drug (ipratropium bromide).

Anticholinesterase Antidote a drug that reactivates cholinesterase enzyme after its inactivation by organophosphate poisons (pralidoxime).

Anticoagulant Antagonist a drug that opposes overdosage of anticoagulant drugs (phytonadione, supplies vitamin K to oppose vitamin K–antagonist anticoagulants).

Anticoagulant, for Storage of Whole Blood a nontoxic agent added to collected blood to prevent clotting (anticoagulant citrate dextrose solution).

Anticoagulant, Systemic a drug administered to slow the clotting of circulating blood (warfarin sodium).

Anticonvulsant an antiepileptic drug administered prophylactically to prevent seizures, or a drug that arrests convulsions by inducing general central nervous system depression (phenytoin, antiepileptic prophylactic; diazepam, central nervous system depressant anticonvulsant).

Antidementia Agent a drug used to treat declining mental abilities in the elderly.

Antidepressant a centrally acting drug that induces mood elevation, useful in treating mental depression (amitriptyline).

Antidiabetic a drug that supplies insulin or stimulates the secretion of insulin; it is useful in treating diabetes mellitus (insulin injection, supplies insulin; glipizide, stimulates insulin secretion; pioglitazone HCl, exenatide).

Antidiarrheal a drug that inhibits intestinal peristalsis; it is used to treat diarrhea (diphenoxylate; bismuth subsalicylate; loperamide HCl).

Antidiuretic a drug that promotes renal water reabsorption, thus reducing urine volume; it is used to treat neurogenic diabetes insipidus (desmopressin).

Antidote, General Purpose a drug that reduces the effects of ingested poisons (or drug overdoses) by adsorbing toxic material (activated charcoal).

Antidote, Specific a drug that reduces the effects of a systemic poison (or drug overdose) by a mechanism that relates to the particular poison (dimercaprol, specific antidote for arsenic, mercury, and gold poisoning; flumazenil, complete or partial reversal of the sedative effects of benzodiazepines).

Antieczematic a topical drug that aids in control of chronic exudative skin lesions (coal tar).

Antiemetic a drug that suppresses nausea and vomiting (ondansetron hydrochloride).

Antienuritic a drug that aids in control of bed-wetting (enuresis) (imipramine).

Antiepileptic a drug that prevents epileptic seizures upon prophylactic administration (valproic acid; topiramate).

Antiestrogen a drug that inhibits the action of estrogenic hormones (tamoxifen).

Antifibrinolytic a drug that promotes hemostasis by inhibiting clot dissolution (fibrinolysis) (aminocaproic acid).

Antifilarial a drug that kills or inhibits pathogenic filarial worms (diethylcarbamazine).

Antiflatulent a drug that reduces gastrointestinal gas (simethicone).

Antifungal, Systemic a drug that kills or inhibits pathogenic fungi (fluconazole).

Antifungal, Topical a drug applied externally to kill or inhibit pathogenic fungi (tolnaftate).

Antiglaucoma Agent a drug that lowers intraocular fluid pressure; it is used to treat glaucoma (methazolamide and acetazolamide reduce fluid formation; isofluorophate promotes fluid drainage).

Antigonadotropin a drug that inhibits anterior pituitary secretion of gonadotropins; it is used to suppress ovarian malfunction (danazol).

Antigout Agent a drug that reduces tissue deposits of uric acid in chronic gout or suppresses the intense inflammatory reaction of acute gout (allopurinol for chronic gout; indomethacin for acute gout).

Antihemophilic a drug that replaces blood clotting factors absent in the hereditary disease hemophilia (antihemophilic factor).

Antiherpes Agent a drug that inhibits replication of herpes simplex virus; it is used to treat genital herpes (acyclovir).

Antihistaminic a drug that antagonizes histamine action at H_1 histamine receptors; it is useful in suppressing the histamine-induced symptoms of allergy (chlorpheniramine maleate; cetirizine, fexofenadine HCl).

Antihyperlipidemic a drug that lowers plasma cholesterol and lipid levels (atorvastatin).

Antihypertensive a drug that lowers arterial blood pressure, especially the elevated diastolic pressure of hypertension (metoprolol; atenolol).

Antihypocalcemic a drug that elevates plasma calcium level; it is useful in treating hypocalcemia (parathyroid injection).

Antihypoglycemic a drug that elevates plasma glucose level; it is useful in treating hypoglycemia (glucagon).

Anti-infective, Topical (or Local) a drug that kills or inhibits pathogenic microorganisms and is suitable for sterilizing skin and wounds (povidone iodine liquid soap).

Anti-inflammatory a drug that inhibits physiological response to cell damage (inflammation) (prednisolone, adrenocorticosteroid; ibuprofen, nonsteroid).

Antileishmanial a drug that kills or inhibits pathogenic protozoa of the genus *Leishmania* (hydroxystilbamidine isethionate).

Antileprotic a drug that kills or inhibits *Mycobacterium leprae*, the causative agent of leprosy (dapsone).

Antilipemic an agent that reduces lipid levels in the blood (atorvastatin).

Antimalarial a drug that kills or inhibits protozoa of the genus *Plasmodium*, the causative agents of malaria (chloroquine).

Antimanic a drug that suppresses the excitement phase (mania) of bipolar disorder (lithium carbonate).

Antimetabolite a drug that attacks malignant cells or pathogenic cells by serving as a nonfunctional substitute for an essential metabolite (fluorouracil, antineoplastic antimetabolite).

Antimigraine Agent a drug that reduces incidence or severity of migraine vascular headaches (sumatriptan).

Anti–Motion Sickness Agent a drug that suppresses motion-induced nausea, vomiting, and vertigo (dimenhydrinate hydrochloride).

Antimuscarinic an anticholinergic drug that inhibits symptoms mediated by acetylcholine receptors of visceral organs (muscarinic receptors) (atropine sulfate).

Antimyasthenic Agent a drug used to correct or treat the symptoms of myasthenia gravis.

Antimycobacterial a drug used to treat fungal infections.

Antinauseant a drug that suppresses nausea and vomiting; an antiemetic (ondansetron).

Antineoplastic a drug that attacks malignant (neoplastic) cells in the body (chlorambucil, alkylating agent).

Antiparasitic a drug that eradicates parasitic arthropods, helminths, protozoa, etc. (permethrin for scabies, mebendazole for intestinal worms, metronidazole for amebic dysentery, malathion for head lice).

Antiparkinsonian (Antidyskinetic) a drug that suppresses the neurologic disturbances and symptoms of parkinsonism (levodopa).

Antiperistaltic a drug that inhibits intestinal motility; an antidiarrheal drug (diphenoxylate hydrochloride).

Antiplatelet Agent a drug that inhibits aggregation of blood platelets; it is used to prevent heart attack (aspirin; clopidogrel bisulfate).

Antiprogestin a type of hormone antagonist that antagonizes or suppresses the actions of progesterone (mifepristone).

Antiprotozoal a drug that kills or inhibits pathogenic protozoa (metronidazole).

Antipruritic a drug that reduces itching (pruritus) (trimeprazine, systemic antipruritic; menthol, topical antipruritic).

Antipsoriatic a drug that suppresses the lesions and symptoms of psoriasis (methotrexate, systemic antipsoriatic; anthralin, topical antipsoriatic).

Antipsychotic a drug that suppresses the symptoms of psychoses of various diagnostic types (haloperidol).

Antipyretic a drug that restores normal body temperature in the presence of fever (acetaminophen).

Antirachitic a drug with vitamin D activity; it is useful in treating vitamin D deficiency and rickets (cholecalciferol).

Antiretroviral a group of drugs used to treat infections caused by retroviruses, especially HIV.

Antirheumatic an anti-inflammatory drug used to treat arthritis and rheumatoid disorders (indomethacin).

Antirickettsial a drug that kills or inhibits pathogenic microorganisms of the genus *Rickettsia* (chloramphenicol).

Antischistosomal a drug that kills or inhibits pathogenic flukes of the genus *Schistosoma* (oxamniquine).

Antiscorbutic a drug with vitamin C activity; it is useful in treating vitamin C deficiency and scurvy (ascorbic acid).

Antiseborrheic a drug that aids in the control of seborrheic dermatitis (dandruff) (selenium sulfide).

Antisecretory an agent that acts to reduce or inhibit gastric secretions (omeprazole).

Antispasmodic a drug that inhibits the motility of visceral smooth muscles (atropine).

Antithyroid Agent a drug that reduces thyroid hormone action, usually by inhibiting hormone synthesis (methimazole).

Antitoxins antibodies formed in response to antigenic poisonous substances of biologic origin.

Antitreponemal a drug that kills or inhibits *Treponema pallidum*, the causative agent of syphilis (penicillin).

Antitrichomonal a drug that kills or inhibits pathogenic protozoa of the genus *Trichomonas* (metronidazole).

Antitubercular a drug that kills or inhibits *Mycobacterium tuberculosis*, the causative agent of tuberculosis (isoniazid).

Antitussive a drug that suppresses coughing (dextromethorphan hydrobromide).

Antiviral a drug that kills or inhibits viral infections (idoxuridine, ophthalmic antiviral).

Antiviral, Prophylactic a drug useful in preventing (rather than treating) viral infections (amantadine, prophylactic for influenza).

Antixerophthalmic a drug with vitamin A activity; it is useful in treating vitamin A deficiency and xerophthalmia (vitamin A).

Anxiolytic a drug that suppresses symptoms of anxiety (diazepam; alprazolam).

Astringent a drug used topically to toughen and shrink tissues (aluminum acetate solution).

Astringent, Ophthalmic a mild astringent suitable for use in the eye (zinc sulfate).

B

Barbiturate a sedative–hypnotic drug that contains the barbituric acid moiety in its chemical structure (phenobarbital).

Belladonna Alkaloid a plant principle derived from *Atropa belladonna* and related species, with anticholinergic action (atropine).

Benzodiazepine a sedative–anxiolytic–muscle relaxant drug that contains the benzodiazepine moiety in its chemical structure (diazepam).

Beta Receptor Agonist a drug that activates sympathetic nervous system beta receptors, for example, to induce bronchodilation (isoproterenol).

Beta Receptor Antagonist a drug that reacts asymptomatically with sympathetic nervous system beta receptors and prevents their endogenous activation, for example, to oppose sympathetic stimulation of the heart (atenolol, metoprolol, propranolol).

Bipolar Agents drugs used to treat a mental disorder characterized by periods of depression and abnormally elevated moods.

Bisphosphonate also called diphosphonates, are a class of drugs that are used to prevent the loss of bone mass.

Blood Glucose Regulators drugs used to maintain the levels of blood glucose within a narrow range, referred to as glucose homeostasis.

Blood Products this includes human serum, recovered plasma, source plasma, whole blood, red blood cells, leukocytes, platelet rich plasma, platelet concentrates, and possibly other specialized products.

Bone Metabolism Regulator a drug that slows calcium turnover in bone; it is used to treat Paget disease (etidronate).

Bronchodilator a drug that expands bronchiolar airways; it is useful in treating asthma (albuterol and isoproterenol, adrenergic bronchodilators; oxtriphylline, smooth muscle relaxant bronchodilator).

C

Calcium Channel Blocker an antianginal drug that acts by impairing the function of transmembrane calcium channels of vascular smooth muscle cells (verapamil).

Carbonic Anhydrase Inhibitor a drug that inhibits the enzyme carbonic anhydrase, the therapeutic effects of which are diuresis and reduced formation of intraocular fluid (acetazolamide).

Cardiac Depressant, Antiarrhythmic a drug that depresses myocardial function; it is useful in treating cardiac arrhythmias (procainamide).

Cardiac Glycoside a plant principle derived from *Digitalis purpurea* and related species, with cardiotonic action (digoxin).

Cardiotonic a drug that increases myocardial contractile force; it is useful in treating congestive heart failure (digoxin).

Cardiovascular Agents drugs used to treat conditions related to the heart and blood vessels or the circulation.

Catecholamine Synthesis Inhibitor a drug that inhibits the biosynthesis of catecholamine neurotransmitters such as norepinephrine (metyrosine).

Cathartic a drug that promotes defecation, usually considered stronger in action than a laxative (bisacodyl).

Caustic a topical drug that destroys tissue on contact; it is useful in removing skin lesions (toughened silver nitrate).

Cauterizing Agent an agent that "burns" off a part of the body to remove or close it off (silver nitrate).

Central Nervous System Agent see Centrally Acting Drug

Centrally Acting Drug a drug that produces its therapeutic effect by action on the central nervous system, usually designated by the type of therapeutic action (sedative, hypnotic, anticonvulsant, etc.).

Cephalosporin an antimicrobial drug that contains the cephalosporin moiety in its chemical structure (cefotaxime; cefdinir).

Chelating Agent a complexing agent that binds metal ions into stable ring structures (chelates); it is useful in treating poisoning (edetate calcium disodium, chelating agent for lead).

Cholelitholytic a drug that promotes dissolution of gallstones (ursodeoxycholic acid).

Choleretic a drug that increases bile secretion by the liver (dehydrocholic acid).

Cholinergic a drug that activates organs innervated by the parasympathetic nervous system; a parasympathomimetic drug (neostigmine, systemic cholinergic; pilocarpine, ophthalmic cholinergic).

Chrysotherapeutic a drug containing gold; it is used to treat rheumatoid arthritis (auranofin).

Coagulant see Hemostatic, Systemic.

Contraceptive, Oral an orally administered drug that prevents conception. Currently available oral contraceptives are for use by females (norethindrone acetate and ethinyl estradiol tablets).

Contraceptive, Topical a spermicidal agent used topically in the vagina to prevent conception (nonoxynol-9).

Contraceptive, Transdermal topically administered drugs that prevent conception (norelgestromin/ethinyl estradiol).

Contraceptive, Vaginal intravaginal ring inserted releasing drugs that prevent conception (etonogestrel/ethinyl estradiol).

Corticosteroid an agent that includes the steroid hormones naturally produced in the adrenal cortex; it includes cortisol (hydrocortisone) and others.

Cycloplegic an anticholinergic drug used topically in the eye to induce paralysis of accommodation (cycloplegia) and dilation of the pupil (cyclopentolate).

D

Decongestant, Nasal an adrenergic drug used orally or topically to induce vasoconstriction in nasal passages (phenylephrine HCl; pseudoephedrine HCl).

Demulcent a bland viscous liquid, usually water based, used to coat and soothe damaged or inflamed skin or mucous membranes (methylcellulose).

Dental and Oral Agents drugs used to treat conditions of the teeth and the oral cavity.

Dental Caries Prophylactic a drug applied to the teeth to reduce the incidence of cavities (sodium fluoride).

Dentin Desensitizer a drug applied to the teeth to reduce the sensitivity of exposed subenamel dentin (potassium nitrate).

Depigmenting Agent a drug that inhibits melanin production in the skin; it is used to induce general depigmentation in certain splotchy depigmented conditions (e.g., vitiligo) (hydroquinone).

Dermatological (Skin) Agents drugs used to treat various conditions of the skin.

Detergent an emulsifying agent used as a cleanser (hexachlorophene liquid soap, anti-infective detergent).

Diagnostic Aid a drug used to determine the functional state of a body organ or to determine the presence of a disease (Peptavlon, gastric secretion indicator; fluorescein sodium, corneal trauma indicator).

Digestive Aid a drug that promotes digestion, usually by supplementing a gastrointestinal enzyme (pancreatin).

Disinfectant an agent that destroys microorganisms on contact and is suitable for sterilizing inanimate objects (formaldehyde solution).

Diuretic a drug that promotes renal excretion of electrolytes and water; it is useful in treating generalized edema (furosemide, loop diuretic; hydrochlorothiazide, thiazide diuretic; triamterene, potassium-sparing diuretic).

Dopamine Receptor Agonist a drug that activates dopamine receptors, for example, to inhibit anterior pituitary secretion of prolactin (bromocriptine; pramipexole dihydrochloride; ropinirole HCl).

E

Emetic a drug that induces vomiting; it is useful in expelling ingested but unabsorbed poisons (ipecac syrup).

Emollient a topical drug, especially an oil or fat, used to soften the skin and make it more pliable (cold cream).

Endothelin Receptor Antagonist a drug that blocks endothelin receptors for treatment of a number of diseases, including pulmonary arterial hypertension.

Enzyme a molecule that catalyzes a chemical reaction.

Enzyme Replacement Agent an enzyme or related agent used to replace, enhance production of or act in lieu of an enzyme in the body.

Epidermal Growth Factor a growth factor that stimulates cell growth, proliferation, and differentiation by binding to its receptor EGFR.

Ergot Alkaloid a plant principle derived from the fungus *Claviceps purpurea* grown on rye or other grains (ergonovine, uterine contractant; ergotamine, migraine therapy).

Estrogen a hormone that stimulates and maintains female reproductive organs and sex characteristics and functions in the uterine cycle (ethinyl estradiol).

Expectorant a drug that increases respiratory tract secretions, lowers their viscosity, and promotes removal (guaifenesin).

F

Fecal Softener a drug that promotes defecation by softening the feces (docusate sodium).

Fertility Agent a drug that promotes ovulation in women of low fertility or spermatogenesis in men of low fertility (clomiphene).

Fibrinolytic Proteolytic an enzyme drug used topically to hydrolyze the exudates of infected and inflammatory lesions (fibrinolysin and desoxyribonuclease, bovine).

G

GABA Agonist a drug that acts to stimulate or increase the action at the GABA receptor, producing typically sedative effects, and may cause other effects such as anxiolytic and muscle relaxant effects.

Galactokinetic a drug used to initiate lactation after childbirth (oxytocin nasal spray).

Gastric Acid Secretion Inhibitor a drug that inhibits the secretion of gastric acid, as shown by the proton pump inhibitors.

Gastrointestinal Agents drugs related to therapy involving the stomach and intestines, for example, H2 blockers, proton pump inhibitors, etc.

Gastroprokinetic a drug that increases gastrointestinal motility by increasing the frequency of contractions in the small intestine or making them stronger, without disrupting their rhythm.

Genitourinary Agents (Genital and Urinary Tract Agents) drugs related to therapy involving the genital and urinary tract.

Glucocorticoid an adrenocortical hormone that regulates organic metabolism and inhibits inflammatory response (betamethasone; prednisone).

Glutamate Inhibitor a drug that will block the action of glutamic acid/glutamate.

Gonadotropin a drug that supplies the gonad-stimulating actions of follicle-stimulating hormone (FSH) and/or luteinizing hormone (LH); it is used to promote fertility (menotropins contain FSH and LH; human chorionic gonadotropin has LH-like activity).

Growth Hormone, Human a drug that duplicates endogenous growth hormone; it is used in children to treat growth failure due to the lack of growth hormone (somatrem).

H

Heavy Metal Antagonist a drug used as an antidote to poisoning with toxic metals such as arsenic and mercury (dimercaprol).

Hematinic a drug that promotes hemoglobin formation by supplying iron (ferrous sulfate).

Hematopoietic a vitamin that stimulates the formation of blood cells; it is useful in treating vitamin deficiency anemia (cyanocobalamin).

Hemorheologic Agent a drug that improves the flow properties of blood by reducing viscosity (pentoxifylline).

Hemostatic, Local a drug applied to a bleeding surface to promote clotting or to serve as a clot matrix (thrombin, clot promoter; oxidized cellulose, clot matrix).

Hemostatic, Systemic a drug that stops bleeding by inhibiting systemic fibrinolysis (aminocaproic acid).

Histamine H_1 Receptor Antagonist a drug used to combat the histamine-induced symptoms of allergy; an antihistamine (diphenhydramine hydrochloride).

Histamine H_2 Receptor Antagonist a drug that inhibits histamine-mediated gastric acid secretion; it is used to treat peptic and duodenal ulcers (famotidine).

HMG-CoA Reductase Inhibitor a drug that inhibits the rate-controlling enzyme of the mevalonate pathway, the metabolic pathway that produces cholesterol and other isoprenoids (statins, atorvastatin).

Hormonal Agents drugs related to therapy involving replacement or stimulation of production of hormones of the adrenal and pituitary glands as well as prostaglandins, sex hormones, and thyroid.

Hormonal Suppressants (Adrenal, Parathyroid, Pituitary, Sex Hormones, Thyroid) drugs related to therapy involving suppression of excess production of hormones of the adrenal and pituitary glands as well as prostaglandins, sex hormones, and thyroid.

Hormone a drug that duplicates the action of a physiological cell regulator (hormone) (insulin, estradiol, thyroxine).

Hydantoin an antiepileptic drug that contains the hydantoin moiety in its chemical structure (phenytoin sodium).

Hydrolytic, Injectable an enzyme drug that promotes the diffusion of other injected drugs through connective tissues (hyaluronidase).

Hyperglycemic a drug that elevates blood glucose level (glucagon).

Hypnotic a central nervous system depressant used to induce sleep (eszopiclone, flurazepam, zolpidem tartrate).

Hypoglycemic a condition of low blood sugar.

Hypotensive see Antihypertensive.

I

Immunizing Agent, Active an antigen that induces antibody production against a pathogenic microorganism; it is used to provide permanent but delayed protection against infection (tetanus toxoid).

Immunizing Agent, Passive a drug containing antibodies against a pathogenic microorganism; it is used to provide immediate but temporary protection against infection (tetanus immune globulin, rabies immune globulin).

Immunoglobulin antibody protein derived from blood serum; it is used to confer passive immunity to infectious diseases (see Immunizing Agent, Passive).

Immunological Agents drugs related to therapy involving various phenomena of immunity, induced sensitivity and allergy; including vaccines and disease-modifying antirheumatic drugs.

Immunosuppressant a drug that inhibits immune response to foreign materials; it is used to suppress rejection of tissue grafts (azathioprine).

Inflammatory Bowel Disease Agents drugs used for therapy involving the inflammation of the bowel.

Inotropic Agent a drug that increases the contractile strength of heart muscle; a cardiotonic (digoxin, digitoxin, dopamine).

Ion Exchange Resin a drug in the gastrointestinal tract that takes up ions present in a toxic amount with an equivalent release of nontoxic ions (sodium polystyrene sulfonate, takes up potassium ions with the release of sodium ions).

Irritant, Local a drug that reacts weakly and nonspecifically with biologic tissue; it is used topically to induce a mild inflammatory response (camphor).

K

Keratolytic a topical drug that toughens and protects skin (compound benzoin tincture, salicylic acid).

L

Laxative a drug that promotes defecation, usually considered milder in action than a cathartic (psyllium mucilloid, bulk laxative; mineral oil, lubricant laxative; sodium phosphates oral solution, saline laxative; bisacodyl, irritant laxative).

Leprostatic see Antileprotic.

Leukotriene Receptor Antagonist a drug that inhibits its leukotrienes or fatty compounds produced by the immune system that cause inflammation in asthma and bronchitis and constrict airways (montelukast).

Lipase Inhibitor a drug used to reduce the activity of lipases found in the intestine secreted by the pancreas when fat is present (orlistat).

Loop Diuretic a diuretic with renal site of action in the thick ascending loop of Henle (furosemide).

Lung Surfactant a surface-active lipoprotein complex (phospholipoprotein) formed by type II alveolar cells.

M

MAO Inhibitor see Monoamine Oxidase Inhibitor.

Metabolic Bone Disease Agent a drug related to therapy involving a metabolic function of bone disease.

Metal Complexing Agent a drug that binds metal ions; it is useful in treating metal poisoning (dimercaprol, complexing agent for arsenic, mercury, and gold).

Mineralocorticoid an adrenocortical hormone that regulates sodium/potassium balance in the body (desoxycorticosterone acetate).

Miotic a cholinergic drug used topically in the eye to induce constriction of the pupil (miosis) (pilocarpine).

Monoamine Oxidase Inhibitor an antidepressant drug that inhibits the enzyme monoamine oxidase, thereby increasing catecholamine levels of neurons (isocarboxazid).

Monoclonal Antibody a highly specific immunoglobulin produced by cell culture cloning (muromonab CD3, inactivates T lymphocytes that reject tissue grafts).

Mucolytic a drug that hydrolyzes mucoproteins; it is useful in reducing the viscosity of pulmonary mucus (acetylcysteine).

Muscle Relaxant, Skeletal a drug that inhibits the contraction of voluntary muscles (cyclobenzaprine HCl, dantrolene, succinylcholine).

Muscle Relaxant, Smooth a drug that inhibits the contraction of visceral smooth muscles (aminophylline).

Mydriatic an adrenergic drug used topically in the eye to induce dilation of the pupil (mydriasis) (phenylephrine).

N

Narcotic a drug that induces action by reacting with opioid receptors of the central nervous system or a drug that is legally classified as a narcotic with regard to prescribing regulations.

Narcotic Antagonist a drug that reacts with opioid receptors asymptomatically; it is used to terminate the action of narcotic drugs (naloxone).

Neuraminidase Inhibitor a drug in a class of antiviral drugs targeted at the influenza virus, which works by blocking the function of the viral neuraminidase protein, preventing the virus from reproducing by budding from the host cell (oseltamivir).

Neuromuscular Blocking Agent a drug that paralyzes skeletal muscles by preventing transmission of neural impulses to them (succinylcholine).

Nonsteroidal Anti-inflammatory Drug an analgesic, anti-inflammatory drug that inhibits prostaglandin synthesis (ketoprofen).

NSAID see Nonsteroidal Anti-inflammatory Drug.

O

Ophthalmic Agent a drug used for a condition involving the eye.

Opioid see Narcotic.

Opioid Antagonist see Narcotic Antagonist.

Otic Agent a drug used for a condition involving the ear.

Ovulation Stimulator a drug that is similar to estrogen and binds to the estrogen receptor causing a negative feedback that stimulates the release of gonadotropin releasing hormone that activates the pituitary gland to release follicle-stimulating hormone and luteinizing hormone with resultant release of an egg (clomifene).

Oxytocic a drug that stimulates uterine motility; it is used in obstetrics to initiate labor or to control postpartum hemorrhage (oxytocin).

P

Parasympatholytic a drug that inhibits response to parasympathetic nerve impulses and to parasympathomimetic drugs; an anticholinergic drug (atropine).

Parasympathomimetic a drug that activates organs innervated by the parasympathetic nervous system; a cholinergic drug (metoclopramide HCl; neostigmine).

Pediculicide an insecticide suitable for eradicating louse infestations (pediculosis) (malathion; permethrin).

Penicillin Adjuvant a drug that extends the systemic duration of penicillin by inhibiting its renal excretion (probenecid).

Phenothiazine an antipsychotic or antidepressant drug that contains the phenothiazine nucleus in its chemical structure (chlorpromazine, antipsychotic; imipramine, antidepressant).

Phosphate Binder an agent that reduces the absorption of phosphate when taken with meals and snacks.

Photosensitizer a drug that increases cutaneous response to ultraviolet light; it is used with ultraviolet light to treat certain skin diseases (e.g., psoriasis) (methoxsalen).

Pigmenting Agent a drug that promotes melanin synthesis in the skin (trioxsalen, oral pigmenting agent; methoxsalen, topical pigmenting agent).

Plasma Volume Expander a substance that can be transfused to maintain fluid volume of the blood.

Platelet Growth Factor contained in platelet-rich plasma that is a blood plasma that has been enriched with platelets, different growth factors, and cytokines.

Platelet-Reducing Agent a drug that slows down platelet production in the body (anagrelide).

Posterior Pituitary Hormone, Antidiuretic a hormone that promotes renal reabsorption of water; it is useful in treating diabetes insipidus (vasopressin injection).

Potassium-Sparing Diuretic a diuretic that does not induce systemic potassium depletion as a side effect (triamterene).

Potentiator an adjunctive drug that enhances the action of a primary drug, the total response being greater than the sum of the individual actions (hexafluorenium, potentiator for succinylcholine).

Progestin a progesterone-like hormone that stimulates the secretory phase of the uterine cycle (norethindrone).

Prostaglandin Synthetase Inhibitor a drug that inhibits prostaglandin synthesis and prostaglandin-induced symptoms such as inflammation; a nonsteroidal anti-inflammatory drug (ibuprofen).

Prostaglandin a drug from the classes of cell-regulating hormones cyclized from arachidonic acid (alprostadil, maintains ductus arteriosus patency in newborn infants pending corrective surgery for congenital heart defects).

Protease Inhibitor is a drug used to treat or prevent infection by viruses, including HIV and hepatitis C (saquinavir).

Proteasome Inhibitor a drug that blocks the action of proteasomes, cellular complexes that break down proteins (bortezomib).

Protectant a topical drug that provides a physical barrier to the environment (zinc gelatin, skin protectant; methylcellulose, ophthalmic protectant).

Proteolytic, Injectable an enzyme drug for injection into herniated lumbar intervertebral discs to reduce interdiscal pressure (chymopapain).

Prothrombogenic a drug with vitamin K activity; it is useful in treating the hypoprothrombinemia of vitamin K deficiency or overdosage with a vitamin K antagonist (phytonadione).

Proton Pump Inhibitor a drug that inhibits gastric acid production (omeprazole).

Psychedelic a drug (especially a street drug) that induces vivid sensory phenomena and hallucinations (mescaline).

Psychotherapeutic a drug used to treat abnormal mental or emotional processes (chlorpromazine, haloperidol).

R

Radiographic Agent see X-Ray Contrast Medium.

Radiopaque Agent a drug used to help diagnose certain medical diseases by absorbing X-rays.

Radiopharmaceutical a drug containing a radioactive isotope; it is used for diagnostic or therapeutic purposes (iodinated albumin with ^{125}I or ^{131}I).

Rauwolfia Alkaloid a plant principle derived from *Rauwolfia serpentina* and related species, with antihypertensive and antipsychotic actions (reserpine).

Resin, Electrolyte Removing see Ion Exchange Resin.

Respiratory Stimulant a drug that serves to increase the action of the respiratory system; it increases breathing.

Respiratory Tract Agents (Including Antihistamines and Bronchodilators) drugs used for various conditions involving the respiratory tract, including antihistamines and bronchodilators.

Retinoic Acid Derivative a derivative of vitamin A (retinol).

Reverse COMT Inhibitor a drug that inhibits the action of catechol-*O*-methyltransferase.

Rubefacient a topical drug that induces mild skin irritation with erythema; it is used as a toughening agent (rubbing alcohol).

S

Salt Substitute a sodium-free alternative to sodium chloride used for flavoring foods (potassium chloride).

Scabicide an insecticide suitable for the eradication of the itch mite *Sarcoptes scabiei* (scabies) (crotamiton).

Sclerosing Agent an irritant drug suitable for injection into varicose veins to induce their fibrosis and obliteration (morrhuate sodium injection).

Sedative a central nervous system depressant used to induce mild relaxation (phenobarbital).

Selective Estrogen Receptor Modulator (SERM) a compound that acts on the estrogen receptor to selectively inhibit or stimulate estrogen-like action in various tissues (clomifene).

Serotonin Agonist a compound that activates serotonin receptors, mimicking the effect of the neurotransmitter serotonin.

Serotonin Antagonist a drug used to inhibit the action at serotonin receptors.

Skeletal Muscle Relaxants drugs used to treat conditions related to the skeletal muscles, including cramping, spasms, etc.

Smoking Deterrent a drug that serves to minimize the desire to smoke.

Somatostatin Analog a hormone chemically and functionally similar to somatostatin.

Specific a drug specially adapted in its indicated use, usually because of a functional relationship between drug mechanism and disease pathophysiology.

Stimulant, Central a drug that increases the functional state of the central nervous system, sometimes used in convulsive therapy of mental disorders (flurothyl, modafinil).

Stimulant, Respiratory a drug that selectively stimulates respiration, either by peripheral initiation of respiratory reflexes or by selective central nervous system stimulation (carbon dioxide, reflex respiratory stimulant; ethamivan, central respiratory stimulant).

Stool Softener a drug used to soften the stool by enhancing the incorporation of water to ease evacuation.

Sulfonylurea an oral antidiabetic drug that contains the sulfonylurea moiety in its chemical structure (glimepiride, glipizide).

Sunscreening Agent a skin protectant that absorbs light energy at wavelengths that cause sunburn (paraaminobenzoic acid, PABA).

Suppressant a drug that inhibits the progress of a disease but does not cure it.

Sympatholytic a drug that inhibits response to sympathetic nerve impulses and to sympathomimetic drugs; an antiadrenergic drug (phentolamine, *alpha* sympatholytic; propranolol, *beta* sympatholytic; clonidine, $alpha_2$ sympatholytic; doxazosin mesylate, *alpha* sympatholytic).

Sympathomimetic a drug that activates organs innervated by the sympathetic nervous system; an adrenergic drug (epinephrine).

Systemically Acting Drug a drug administered so as to reach systemic circulation, from which the drug diffuses into all tissues, including the site of the therapeutic action.

T

Therapeutic Nutrients, Minerals, and Electrolytes nutrients, minerals, and electrolytes used for replacement and enhancement in malnourished or nutritionally problematic patients.

Thiazide Diuretic a diuretic that contains the benzothiadiazide (thiazide) moiety in its chemical structure (hydrochlorothiazide).

Thrombolytic an enzyme drug administered parenterally to solubilize blood clots (enoxaparin sodium, urokinase, warfarin sodium).

Thyroid Hormone a hormone that maintains metabolic function and normal metabolic rate of tissues (levothyroxine).

Topically Acting Drug a drug applied to the body surface for local therapeutic action.

Toxoid a modified antigen from an infectious organism used as a vaccine (tetanus toxoid).

Trace Element a chemical element required by living organisms in minute amounts (chromium).

Tranquilizer a drug (such as antipsychotic) used to suppress an acutely disturbed emotional state (trifluoperazine, antipsychotic).

Tranquilizer, Minor an old term for an anxiolytic drug.

Tricyclic Antidepressant an antidepressant that contains the tricyclic phenothiazine nucleus in its chemical structure (amitriptyline, imipramine).

Tuberculostatic see Antitubercular.

U

Urea Cyclic Disorder Agent a drug used to treat a severe disease of newborns in which ammonia is not correctly metabolized in the liver.

Uricosuric a drug that promotes renal excretion of uric acid; it is useful in treating chronic gout (probenecid).

Urinary Acidifier an agent used to adjust the pH of the urine to be more acidic (ammonium chloride).

Uterine Contractant an obstetric drug used after placenta delivery to induce sustained uterine contraction to reduce bleeding (methylergonovine).

Uterine Contraction Inhibitor a drug that inhibits uterine muscle contraction; it is used in preterm labor to prolong gestation (ritodrine).

V

Vaccine an antigen-containing drug used to induce active immunity against an infectious disease (hepatitis B vaccine, rabies vaccine).

Vasoconstrictor a drug that narrows arterioles, usually to elevate blood pressure. See Vasopressor.

Vasodilator, Coronary a drug that expands blood vessels in the heart and improves coronary blood flow; it is useful in treating angina pectoris; an antianginal drug (nitroglycerin).

Vasodilator, Peripheral a drug that expands peripheral blood vessels and improves blood flow to the extremities of the body (minoxidil).

Vasopressor an adrenergic drug administered to constrict arterioles and elevate arterial blood pressure (norepinephrine).

Vesicant a blistering agent or blister-producing agent (cantharidin).

Vinca Alkaloid a plant principle derived from *Vinca rosea* and related species, with antineoplastic action (vincristine).

Vitamin an organic chemical essential in small amounts for normal metabolism; it is used therapeutically to supplement the vitamin content of foods (ascorbic acid, thiamine HCl, pyridoxine HCl).

X

Xanthine Alkaloid a plant principle chemically related to xanthine, with central nervous system stimulant, smooth muscle relaxant, and diuretic actions (caffeine).

Xanthine Oxidase Inhibitor a substance that inhibits the activity of xanthine oxidase, an enzyme involved in purine metabolism (allopurinol).

X-Ray Contrast Medium a drug opaque to x-rays that assists visualization of an internal organ during radiographic examination (barium sulfate, iopanoic acid).

Glossary of Pharmaceutical Terms and Dosage Forms

A

Active Ingredient the ingredient or ingredients of a pharmaceutical product responsible for its pharmacologic activity (also medicament, drug substance, active pharmaceutical ingredient [API]).

Aerosol a dosage form that is packaged under pressure and contains therapeutically active ingredients that are released upon activation of an appropriate valve system. A dosage form consisting of a liquid or solid preparation packaged under pressure and intended for administration as a fine mist. The descriptive term aerosol also refers to the fine mist of small droplets or solid particles that are emitted from the product.

Aerosol Foam a dosage form containing one or more active ingredients, surfactants, aqueous or nonaqueous liquids, and the propellant; if the propellant is in the internal (discontinuous) phase (i.e., of the oil-in-water type), a stable foam is discharged, and if the propellant is in the external (continuous) phase (i.e., of the water-in-oil type), a spray or a quick-breaking foam is discharged.

Aerosol, Metered a pressurized dosage foam consisting of metered-dose valves, which allow for the delivery of a uniform quantity of spray upon each activation.

Ampul a final container that is all glass in which the open end, after filling with product, is sealed by heat (also ampoule, ampule, [French] carpule).

Aromatic Water a clear, saturated, aqueous solution of volatile oils or other aromatic or volatile substances.

Aseptic lacking disease-producing microorganisms; not the same as sterile.

Aseptic Processing manufacturing dosage forms without terminal sterilization. The dosage form is sterile filtered, aseptically filled into the final package, and then aseptically sealed.

Aural (Auricular) for administration into, or by way of, the ear.

B

Bead a solid dosage form in the shape of a small sphere. The dosage form generally contains multiple beads (also pellet).

Blocks large veterinary products intended to be licked by animals and containing API(s) and nutrients such as salts, vitamins, and minerals.

Bolus a large, long tablet intended for administration to animals.

C

Caplet tablet dosage form in the shape of a capsule.

Capsule a solid dosage form in which the drug is enclosed within a hard or soft soluble container or shell.

Capsule, Delayed-Release a coated capsule or more commonly encapsulated granules that may be coated to resist releasing the drug in the stomach because the drug will irritate gastric mucosa or gastric fluid will inactivate the drug.

Capsule, Extended-Release a capsule that is formulated in such a manner as to make the contained medication available over an extended period following ingestion.

Capsule, Film-Coated Extended-Release a solid dosage form in which the drug is enclosed within either a hard or soft soluble container or "shell" made from a suitable form of gelatin; additionally, the capsule is covered in a designated film coating, which releases a drug (or drugs) in such a manner to allow at least a reduction in dosing frequency as compared to that drug (or drugs) presented as a conventional dosage form.

Capsule, Gelatin-Coated a solid dosage form in which the drug is enclosed within either a hard or soft soluble container made from a suitable form of gelatin; through a banding process, the capsule is coated with additional layers of gelatin so as to form a complete seal.

Capsule, Liquid-Filled a solid dosage form in which the drug is enclosed within a soluble, gelatin shell, which is plasticized by the addition of a polyol, such as sorbitol or glycerin, and is therefore of a somewhat thicker consistency than that of a hard-shell capsule; typically, the active ingredients are dissolved or suspended in a liquid vehicle.

Chewable attribute of a solid dosage form that is intended to be chewed or crushed before swallowing.

Coated attribute of a solid dosage form that is covered by deposition of an outer solid that is different in composition from the core material.

Collodion a liquid preparation composed of pyroxylin dissolved in a solvent mixture of alcohol and ether and applied externally.

Colloidal Dispersion an attribute of a preparation or formulation in which particles of colloidal dimension (i.e., typically between 1 nm and 1 μm) are distributed uniformly throughout a liquid.

Concentrate a liquid preparation of increased strength and reduced volume, which is usually diluted prior to administration or use.

Concentrate for Dip a preparation containing one or more active ingredients usually in the form of a paste or solution; it is used to prepare a diluted suspension, emulsion, or solution of the active ingredient(s) for the prevention and treatment of ectoparasitic infestations of animals.

Conventional-Release descriptive term for a dosage form in which no deliberate effort has been made to modify the release rate of the API. In the case of capsules and tablets, the inclusion or exclusion of a disintegrating agent is not interpreted as a modification.

Cream a semisolid dosage form containing one or more drug substances dissolved or dispersed in a suitable base. An emulsion dosage form often containing more than 20% water and volatiles and/or containing less than 50% hydrocarbons, waxes, or polyols, as the vehicle for the API. Creams are generally intended for external application to the skin or mucous membranes.

D

Delayed-Release a type of modified-release dosage form. A descriptive term for a dosage form deliberately modified to delay release of the API for some period of time after initial administration. For example, release of the API is prevented in the gastric environment but promoted in the intestinal environment; this term is synonymous with enteric-coated or gastro-resistant.

Dental descriptive term for a preparation that is applied to the teeth or gums for local action.

Dermal a topical route of administration where the article is intended to reach or be applied to the dermis.

Dosage Form a formulation that typically contains the API(s) and excipients in quantities and physical form designed to facilitate the accurate and efficient administration of the API to the human or animal patient.

Douche a liquid preparation intended for the irrigative cleansing of the vagina; prepared from powders, liquid solutions, or liquid concentrates.

Dressing the application of various materials for protecting a wound.

Drops, Oral a solution, emulsion, or suspension that is administered in small volumes, such as drops, by means of a suitable device.

Drug Delivery System modern technology, distributed with or as a part of a drug product that allows for the uniform release or targeting of drugs to the body.

Dry Powder Inhaler a device used to administer an inhalation powder in a finely divided state suitable for oral inhalation by the patient.

E

Effervescent a dosage form containing ingredients that rapidly release carbon dioxide when in contact with water.

Elixir a clear, pleasantly flavored, sweetened hydroalcoholic liquid containing dissolved active ingredients intended for oral use.

Emollient attribute of a cream of ointment indicating an increase in the moisture content of the skin following application of bland, fatty, or oleaginous substances.

Emulsion a two-phase system in which one liquid is dispersed throughout another liquid in the form of small droplets. A dosage form consisting of a two-phase system composed of at least two immiscible liquids, one of which is dispersed as droplets (internal or dispersed phase) within the other liquid (external or continuous phase), generally stabilized with one or more emulsifying agents.

Enema a rectal preparation for therapeutic, diagnostic, or nutritive purposes.

Enteric-Coated descriptive term for a solid dosage form in which a polymer coating has been applied to prevent the release of the API in the gastric environment.

Excipient an ingredient of a dosage form other than an API.

Extended-Release descriptive term for a dosage form that is deliberately modified to protract the release of the API compared to that observed for an immediate-release dosage form. The term is synonymous with prolonged or sustained release. Many extended-release dosage forms have a pattern of release that begins with a "burst effect" that mimics an immediate release followed by a slower release of the remaining API in the dosage form.

Extract a concentrated preparation of vegetable or animal drug obtained by removal of the active constituents with suitable menstrua, by evaporation of all or nearly all of the solvent, and by adjustment of the residual mass or powder to the prescribed standards.

F

Film a thin layer or coating. A term used to describe a thin, flexible sheet of material, usually composed of a polymer. Films are used in various routes of administration including as a means of oral administration of material in a rapidly dissolving form. The term may also be used as an attribute when applied to solid oral dosage forms for taste masking, product identification, and aesthetic purposes.

Fluidextract a liquid preparation of a vegetable drug containing alcohol as a solvent, preservative, or both and so made that unless otherwise specified in an individual monograph, each milliliter contains the therapeutic constituents of 1 g of the standard drug.

Foam an emulsion packaged in a pressurized aerosol container that has a fluffy, semisolid consistency when dispensed. An emulsion dosage form containing dispersed gas bubbles.

For Solution a product, usually a solid, intended for solution prior to administration.

For Suspension a product, usually a solid, intended for suspension prior to administration.

G

Gas one of the states of matter having no definite shape or volume and occupying the entire container when confined.

Gastro-Resistant descriptive term for a solid dosage form in which a polymer coating has been applied to prevent the release in the gastric environment.

Gel a semisolid system consisting of either a suspension of small inorganic particles or large organic molecules interpenetrated by a liquid. It may contain suspended particles. It may contain a gelling agent to promote stiffness.

Gel, Dentifrice a combination of a dentifrice (formulation intended to clean and/or polish the teeth and which may contain certain additional agents) and a gel. It is used with a toothbrush for the purpose of cleaning and polishing the teeth.

Gel, Metered a gel preparation, with metered-dose valves, which allow for the delivery of a uniform quantity of gel upon each activation.

Globule also called pellets or pilules, are made of pure sucrose, lactose, or other polysaccharides. They are formed into small globular masses of various sizes and are medicated by placing them in a vial and adding the liquid drug attenuation in the proportion not less than 1% (w/v). After shaking, the medicated globules are dried at temperatures not to exceed 40°C.

Granules a preparation of dry aggregates of powder particles that may contain one or more active ingredients with or without other ingredients. They may be swallowed as such, dispersed in food, or dissolved in water. Granules are frequently compacted into tablets or filled into capsules, with or without additional ingredients.

Gum a mucilaginous excretion from various plants. A dosage form in which the base consists of a pliable material that, when chewed, releases the API into the oral cavity.

Gum, Chewing a sweetened and flavored insoluble plastic material that, when chewed, releases a drug substance into the oral cavity.

Gum, Resin natural mixture of gum and resin, usually obtained as exudations from plants.

H

Hard-Shell Capsule a type of capsule in which one or more APIs, with or without other ingredients, are filled into a two-piece shell.

I

Immediate-Release descriptive term for a dosage form in which no deliberate effort has been made to modify the API release rate. In the case of capsules and tablets, the inclusion or exclusion of a disintegrating agent is not interpreted as a modification.

Implant see Pellet. A small sterile solid mass consisting of a highly purified drug with or without excipients made by compression or molding and put in place by injection or incision.

Infusion, Intramammary a suspension of a drug in a suitable oil vehicle; intended for veterinary use only.

Inhalant a special class of inhalations consisting of a drug or combination of drugs that by virtue of their high vapor pressure can be carried by an air current into the nasal passage where they exert their effect; the container from which the inhalant generally is administered is known as an inhaler.

Inhalation a route of administration for aerosols characterized by dispersion of the API into the airways during inspiration.

Injection, Liposomal an injection, which either consists of or forms liposomes (a lipid bilayer vesicle usually composed of phospholipids, which is used to encapsulate an active drug substance).

Injection a preparation intended for parenteral administration or for constituting or diluting a parenteral product prior to administration. A route of administration of a liquid or semisolid deposited into a body cavity, fluid, or tissue by use of a needle.

Insert a specially formulated and shaped nonencapsulated solid preparation intended to be placed into a nonrectal orifice of the body, where drug is released, generally for localized effects.

Intraocular a route of administration to deliver a sterile preparation within the eye.

Intrauterine Device a device inserted and left in the uterus to prevent effective conception.

Irrigation a sterile solution intended to bathe or flush open wounds or body cavities.

J

Jelly see Gel.

L

Liniment an alcoholic or oleaginous solution or emulsion applied by rubbing on the skin for treating pain and stiffness of underlying musculature.

Liposomes microvesicles composed of a bilayer and/or concentric series of multiple bilayers separated by aqueous compartments formed by amphipathic molecules such as phospholipids, which enclose a central aqueous compartment.

Lipstick a waxy solid, usually colored cosmetic, in stick form for the lips.

Liquid a dosage form consisting of a pure chemical in its liquid state. This dosage form term should not be applied to solutions.

Lotion a fluid emulsion applied to the surface of the skin. See Solution or Suspension. The term has also been applied to suspensions and solutions.

Lozenge a solid preparation that is intended to dissolve or disintegrate slowly in the mouth (also called a troche).

Lyophilization removal of water or other solvent from a frozen solution by sublimation caused by a combination of temperature and pressure differentials (also called freeze drying).

M

Modified-Release a release pattern of the active ingredient from the dosage form that has been deliberately changed from that of the conventional form. It includes accelerated release, delayed release, extended release, pulsatile release, and targeted release.

Molded Tablet a tablet that has been formed by dampening the ingredients and pressing them into a mold, then removing and drying the resulting solid mass.

Mouthwash an aqueous solution used to rinse the oral cavity.

N

Nasal route of administration (mucosal) characterized by deposition in the nasal cavity for local or systemic effect.

O

Ocular route of administration indicating deposition of the API within the eye.

Oil an unctuous, combustible substance that is liquid, or easily liquefiable, on warming and is soluble in ether but insoluble in water. Such substances, depending on their origin, are classified as animal, mineral, or vegetable oils.

Ointment a semisolid preparation intended for external application to the skin or mucous membrane. A semisolid dosage form, usually containing less than 20% water and volatiles and more than 50% hydrocarbons, waxes, or polyols as the vehicle. This dosage form generally is for external application to the skin or mucous membranes.

Ophthalmic a route of administration characterized by application of a sterile preparation to the external parts of the eye.

Ophthalmic Ointment a sterile ointment intended for application to the eye.

Ophthalmic Preparation drug in a dosage form intended to be applied to the eye.

Ophthalmic Solution a sterile solution, essentially free from foreign particles, suitably prepared and packaged for application to the eye.

Ophthalmic Strip a sterile single-use container or sterile impregnated paper strip containing the drug to be applied to the eye.

Ophthalmic Suspension a sterile liquid preparation containing solid particles dispersed in a liquid vehicle intended for application to the eye.

Orally Disintegrating a descriptive term for a solid oral dosage form that disintegrates rapidly in the mouth prior to swallowing. The API is generally intended for gastrointestinal delivery and/or absorption.

Oropharyngeal a route of administration characterized by deposition of a preparation into the oral cavity and/or pharyngeal region to exert a local or systemic effect.

Otic a route of administration characterized by deposition of a preparation into, or by way of, the ear. Also referred to as aural.

Otic Solution a solution intended for instillation in the outer ear.

Otic Suspension a liquid preparation containing micronized particles intended for instillation in the outer ear.

P

Paste a semisolid dosage form that contains one or more drug substances intended for topical application. It generally contains a high concentration of solids (20% to 50%) and has a stiff consistency. It is intended for application to the skin, oral cavity, or mucous membranes.

Pastille an aromatic preparation, often with a pleasing flavor, usually intended to dissolve in the mouth.

Patch a drug delivery system that often contains an adhesive backing usually applied to an external site on the body. Its ingredients either passively diffuse from or are actively transported from some portion of the patch.

Pellet see Bead. A small solid dosage form of uniform, often spherical, shape. Spherical pellets are sometimes referred to as beads. Pellets intended as implants must be sterile. (Also a solid granule or regular shape prepared by compaction, molding, or granulation.)

Periodontal descriptive term for a preparation that is applied around a tooth for localized action.

Pill a solid spherical dosage form usually prepared by a wet massing technique.

Plaster a solid or semisolid mass supplied on a backing material and intended to provide prolonged contact with the skin.

Pledget a small compress or tuft, usually of cotton or cotton wool, used to apply disinfectant or medicament to the skin.

Poultice a soft, moist mass of meal, herbs, seed, etc., usually applied hot on a cloth that consists of gruel-like consistency.

Powder an intimate mixture of dry, finely divided drug and/or chemicals that may be intended for internal (oral) or external (topical) use.

Powder, Inhalation a powder containing an API for oral inhalation. The powder is used with a device that aerosolizes and delivers an accurately metered amount.

Premix a mixture of one or more drug substances with a suitable vehicle.

Prolonged-Release see Extended-Release.

Pulsatile Release a release pattern of the active ingredient from the dosage form modified to release aliquots of the total dose at two or more time intervals.

R

Radiopharmaceuticals "radioactive pharmaceuticals," or substances labeled with radioisotope and used for diagnostic imaging or therapy. Each name specifies the substance, the isotope, and the dosage form.

Rectal a route of administration (mucosal) characterized by deposition into the rectum to provide local or systemic effect.

Rinse a solution used to cleanse by flushing.

S

Salve a thick ointment or cerate (a fat- or wax-based preparation with a consistency between an ointment and a plaster).

Semisolid attribute of a material characterized by a reduced ability to flow or conform to its container at room temperature. A semisolid does not flow at low shear stress and generally exhibits plastic flow behavior.

Shampoo a solution, emulsion, or suspension used to clean the hair and scalp.

Soap the alkali salt(s) of one or more fatty acids.

Soft Gel Capsule a specific capsule type characterized by increased levels of plasticizers producing a more pliable and thicker-walled material than hard gelatin capsules. Soft gel capsules are further distinguished because they are single-piece sealed dosages. Frequently used for delivering liquid compositions.

Solution a liquid preparation that contains one or more dissolved (molecularly dispersed) chemical substances in a suitable solvent or mixture of miscible solvents; it may be oral, topical, otic, or ophthalmic. A clear, homogenous liquid dosage form that contains one or more chemical substances dissolved in a solvent or mixture of mutually miscible solvents.

Solution, Concentrate a liquid preparation (i.e., a substance that flows readily in its natural state) that contains a drug dissolved in a suitable solvent or mixture of mutually miscible solvents; the drug has been strengthened by the evaporation of its nonactive parts.

Spirit an alcoholic or hydroalcoholic solution of volatile substances prepared usually by simple solution or by admixture of the ingredients.

Sponge a porous, interlacing, absorbent material that contains a drug. It is typically used for applying or introducing medication or for cleansing. A sponge usually retains its shape.

Spray a liquid minutely divided as by a jet of air or steam; used to facilitate application to the intended area

Stent, Drug-Eluting a specialized form of implant used for extended local delivery of the API to the immediate location of stent placement.

Sterile completely lacking living (viable) microbial life.

Sterility an acceptably high level of probability that a product processed in an aseptic system does not contain viable microorganisms.

Stick a slender, cylindrical dosage form of rigid consistency.

Strip see Tape, Medicated.

Sublingual a route of administration (mucosal) characterized by placement underneath the tongue and for release of the API for absorption in that region.

Suppository a solid dosage form in which one or more APIs are dispersed in a suitable base and molded or otherwise formed into a suitable shape for insertion into the rectum to provide local or systemic effect.

Suspension a liquid preparation that consists of solid particles dispersed throughout a liquid phase in which the particles are not soluble; it may be oral, topical, otic, or ophthalmic.

Swab a small piece of relatively flat absorbent material that contains a drug. A swab may also be attached to one end of a small stick. A swab is typically used for applying medication or for cleansing.

Syrup a solution containing a high concentration of sucrose or other sugars. See Solution.

System a dosage form developed to allow for uniform release or targeting of drugs to the body.

System, Intrauterine a system that is intended for release of drug to the uterus over a long period, such as a year.

System, Ocular a dosage form intended for placement in the lower conjunctival fornix, from which the drug diffuses through a membrane at a constant rate.

System, Transdermal a self-contained, discrete dosage form that is designed to deliver drug(s) through the intact skin to the systemic circulation.

T

Tablet a solid dosage form containing medicinal substance(s) with or without diluents.

Tablet, Chewable a tablet formulated so that it may be chewed, producing a pleasant-tasting residue that is easily swallowed and does not leave a bitter or unpleasant aftertaste.

Tablet, Delayed-Release a tablet with a coating that is intended to postpone the release of the medication until the tablet has passed through the stomach.

Tablet, Effervescent a solid dosage form containing mixtures of acids and sodium bicarbonate, which release carbon dioxide when dissolved in water; it is intended to be dissolved or dispersed in water before administration.

Tablet, Extended-Release a tablet that is formulated so as to make the contained medication available over an extended period following ingestion.

Tablet, Orally Disintegrating a solid dosage form containing medicinal substances, which disintegrates rapidly, usually within a matter of seconds, when placed upon the tongue.

Tape, Medicated a dosage form or device composed of a woven fabric or synthetic material onto which an API is placed, usually with an adhesive on one or both sides to facilitate topical application.

Targeted Release release of the active ingredient from a dosage form modified to preferentially deliver most of the drug to a specific region, organ, or tissue.

Terminal Sterilization a process used to produce sterility in the final product contained in its final packaging system.

Tincture an alcoholic or hydroalcoholic solution prepared from vegetable materials or from chemical substances.

Topical a route of administration characterized by application to the outer surface of the body.

Transdermal Delivery System, Electroporation a transdermal delivery system enhanced by the application of short, high-voltage electric pulses to create aqueous pores in the lipid bilayer of the skin and thereby facilitate drug diffusion.

Transdermal Delivery System, High-Velocity Powder Particles a transdermal drug delivery system using supersonic shock waves of helium gas to enhance drug diffusion through the skin.

Transdermal Delivery System, Iontophoresis a transdermal drug delivery system enhanced by the use of applied electric current to facilitate drug diffusion through the skin.

Transdermal Delivery System, Phonophoresis a transdermal drug delivery system enhanced by the application of low-frequency ultrasound to facilitate drug diffusion through the skin (also ultrasound, sonophoresis, ultrasonophoresis, ultraphonophoresis).

Transdermal Matrix Patch a transdermal system using a polymeric matrix containing drug intended for systemic delivery through the skin; generally, the skin is the rate-controlling membrane for drug diffusion.

Transdermal Membrane Patch a transdermal system containing a drug reservoir entrapped between backing and adhesive layers and a drug diffusion-controlling membrane; the reservoir is usually a semisolid dispersion or solution of the drug.

Troche see Lozenge.

U

Urethral a dosage form intended for insertion into the urethra to provide a local effect of the active ingredient.

V

Vaginal a route of administration (mucosal) characterized by deposition into the vagina.

Vaginal Tablet or Insert a vaginal insert prepared by compression of powdered materials into a suitable shape; it can also be prepared by encapsulation in soft gelatin.

Validation scientific study to prove that a process is doing what it is supposed to do and is under control.

Vehicle a term commonly encountered that refers to a component for internal or external use that is used as a carrier or diluent in which liquids, semisolids, or solids are dissolved or suspended. Examples include water, syrups, elixirs, oleaginous liquids, solid and semisolid carriers, and proprietary products.

Veterinary descriptive term for dosage forms intended for nonhuman use.

W

Wafer a thin slice of a material containing a medicinal agent.

Water, Aromatic a clear, saturated aqueous solution (unless otherwise specified) of one or more volatile oils or other aromatic or volatile substances.

C Systems and Techniques of Pharmaceutical Measurement

INTRODUCTION

Knowledge and application of the systems of pharmaceutical measurement are essential to the practice of pharmacy. Whether applied to the compounding and dispensing of prescriptions in the community pharmacy, the filling of medication orders in the institutional pharmacy, or the large-scale industrial manufacture of pharmaceuticals, quantitative accuracy is essential in the preparation of safe and effective medications.

Pharmaceuticals prepared industrially undergo rigid in-process controls and final product assays to ensure conformance with the applicable standards for drug content. Prescriptions and medication orders filled extemporaneously in the community and institutional pharmacy often lack the advantage of control by assay, and thus, the pharmacist must be absolutely certain of the accuracy of all calculations and measurements employed. Calculations should be double-checked by the pharmacist and, whenever possible, by a colleague. The importance of accurate calculations and measurements cannot be overstated. For example, an error in the placement of a decimal point represents a *minimum* error of a factor of 10, and if it is applicable to the active ingredient, a critical drug underdosage or overdosage results.

The pharmacy student must have a working knowledge of the systems of pharmaceutical measurement, their application in pharmaceutical calculations, the factors used for conversion between the systems, and the proper techniques of weighing and measuring.

SYSTEMS OF PHARMACEUTICAL MEASUREMENT

Although pharmacy has moved toward the exclusive use of the metric system, two other systems of measurement, namely, the *apothecary system* and the *avoirdupois system*, occasionally may be encountered. The metric system includes units of weight, volume, and linear measure; the apothecary system includes units of weight and volume; and the avoirdupois system includes only units of weight. The metric system has replaced the apothecary system in virtually all pharmaceutical measurements and calculations, although some use

remains, such as common reference to the dose of thyroid in *grains*, an apothecary system unit. The avoirdupois system is the *common* commercial system of weight used in the United States. It too is being replaced by the metric system, but at a much slower pace. The avoirdupois system is encountered by the pharmacist in the purchase of bulk chemicals and other items packaged and sold by the ounce or pound.

The Metric System

The metric system is the most widely used system in pharmacy. It is the system used in the *United States Pharmacopeia* (USP) and *National Formulary* (NF), by the federal Food and Drug Administration, in manufacturers' labeling of pharmaceutical products, and in most physicians' writing of prescriptions and medication orders.

In the metric system, the *gram* is the main unit of weight, the *liter* the main unit of volume, and the *meter* the main unit of length. Subunits and multiples of these basic units are indicated by the prefix notations and symbols shown in Table C.1.

In pharmacy, these are the most commonly used metric units:

Weight is expressed in terms of the kilogram (kg), gram (g), milligram (mg), or microgram (μg).

Liquid measure is expressed in terms of the liter (L) or milliliter (mL).

Linear measure is expressed in terms of the meter (m), centimeter (cm), or millimeter (mm).

Area measure is expressed in terms of the square meter (m²) or square centimeter (cm²).

The metric weight scale in Figure C.1 is intended to depict the relationship between the units of weight in the metric system and to demonstrate an easy method of converting from one unit to another (1). In the example, 1.23 kg is to be converted to grams. On the scale, the gram position is three decimal places from the kilogram position. Thus, the decimal point is moved three places toward the right. In the other example, the conversion from milligrams to grams also requires movement of the decimal point three places, but this time to the left. The same method may be used to convert metric units of volume or length.

TABLE C.1. Metric System Unit Prefixes

Multiplication Factor	Prefix	Symbol	Term (USA)
1 000 000 000 000 000 000 = 10^{18}	exa	E	one quintillion
1 000 000 000 000 000 = 10^{15}	tera	T	one quadrillion
1 000 000 000 000 = 10^{12}	giga	G	one trillion
1 000 000 000 = 10^{9}	mega	M	one billion
1 000 000 = 10^{6}	kilo	k	one million
1 000 = 10^{3}	hecto	h	one thousand
100 = 10^{2}	deka	da	one hundred
10 = 10	peta	P	ten
0.1 = 10^{-1}	deci	d	one-tenth
0.01 = 10^{-2}	centi	c	one-hundredth
0.001 = 10^{-3}	milli	m	one-thousandth
0.000 001 = 10^{-6}	micro	μ	one-millionth
0.000 000 001 = 10^{-9}	nano	n	one-billionth
0.000 000 000 001 = 10^{-12}	pico	p	one-trillionth
0.000 000 000 000 001 = 10^{-15}	femto	f	one-quadrillionth
0.000 000 000 000 000 001 = 10^{-18}	atto	a	one-quintillionth

The table is based on the International System of Units (SI, from the French, Le Système International d'Unites), as modified for use in the United States by the Secretary of Commerce.

Table of Metric Weight

1 kg = 1,000.000 g
1 hg = 100.000 g
1 Dg = 10.000 g
1 g   = 1.000 g
1 dg = 0.100 g
1 cg = 0.010 g
1 mg = 0.001 g
1 μg = 0.000001 g
1 ng = 0.0000000001 g
1 pg = 0.000000000001 g

hg, hectogram; Dg, dekagram; dg, decigram; cg, centigram; ng, nanogram; pg, picogram.

or

1 g = 0.001 kg
    = 0.010 hg
    = 0.100 Dg
    = 10 dg
    = 100 cg
    = 1,000 mg
    = 1,000,000 μg
    = 1,000,000,000 ng
    = 1,000,000,000,000 pg

DECIMAL MOVEMENT
⊙➝ TO CONVERT FROM LARGER TO SMALLER UNITS
◀⊙ TO CONVERT FROM SMALLER TO LARGER UNITS

FIGURE C.1. Metric weight scale.

Table of Metric Volume

1 kL = 1,000.000 L
1 hL = 100.000 L
1 DL = 10.000 L
1 L = 1.000 L
1 dL = 0.100 L
1 cL = 0.010 L
1 mL = 0.001 L
1 μL = 0.000001 L

kL, kiloliter; hL, hectoliter; DL, dekaliter; L, liter; dL, deciliter; cL, centiliter; mL, milliliter; μL, microliter.

or

1 L = 0.0001 kL
  = 0.010 hL
  = 0.100 DL
  = 10 dL
  = 100 cL
  = 1,000 mL
  = 1,000,000 μL

Table of Metric Length

1 km = 1,000.000 m
1 hm = 100.000 m
1 Dm = 10.000 m
1 m = 1.000 m
1 dm = 0.100 m
1 cm = 0.010 m
1 mm = 0.001 m
1 μm = 0.000001 m
1 nm = 0.000000001 m

km, kilometer; hm, hectometer; Dm, dekameter; m, meter; dm, decimeter; cm, centimeter; mm, millimeter; μm, micrometer; nm, nanometer.

or

1 m = 0.001 km
  = 0.010 hm
  = 0.100 Dm
  = 10 dm
  = 100 cm
  = 1,000 mm
  = 1,000,000 μm
  = 10,000,000,000 nm

The Apothecary System

The apothecary system provides for the measurement of both weight and volume. The tables of the system are presented below.

Table of Apothecaries' Fluid Measure

60 ♏ = 1 f♌^{a}
8 f♌ (480 ♏) = 1 f♌^{a}
16 f♌ = 1 pt
2 pt (32 f♌) = 1 qt
4 qt (8 pt) = 1 gal

^{a}When there is no doubt that the material referred to is a liquid, Э the *f* is usually omitted from this symbol. *Drachm* is also spelled *dram*.
♏, minim; f♌, fluidrachm; f♌, fluidounce; pt, pint; qt, quart; gal, gallon.

Table of Apothecaries' Measure of Weight

20 gr = 1 Э
3 Э (60 gr) = 1
8 ♌ (480 gr) = 1
12 (5,760 gr) = 1 lb

gr, grain; Э, scruple; lb, pound.

The Avoirdupois System

The avoirdupois system is used in commerce to supply bulk chemicals and other items by weight, in ounces or pounds (e.g., Epsom salts).

The grain is the same weight in the apothecary and avoirdupois systems. However, the ounce and the pound in the two systems differ in the number of grains per unit. The apothecary ounce contains 480 grains, whereas the avoirdupois ounce contains 437.5 grains. The apothecary pound contains 5,760 grains, whereas the avoirdupois pound contains 7,000 grains. Also, the symbols for the ounce and pound are different in the two systems.

Table of Avoirdupois Measure of Weight

437.5 gr = 1 oz

16 oz (7,000 gr) = 1 lb

oz, avoirdupois ounce.

Intersystem Conversion

A pharmacist may convert the weight, volume, or dimensions of length from one system to another with conversion factors. Depending on the circumstances and requirements for accuracy, conversion factors of different exactness may be used. The following is a table of the factors commonly used in prescription practice. They are exact equivalents rounded off for practical application. Exact equivalents, used in the conversion of specific quantities in pharmaceutical formulas, may be found in the USP.

Useful Conversion Equivalents of Weight

1 g = 15.432 gr
1 kg = 2.2 lb (avoir)
1 gr = 0.0648 g or 64.8 or 65 mg
1 ♌ = 31.1 g
1 oz (avoir) = 28.35 g
1 lb (apoth) = 373.2 g
1 lb (avoir) = 453.6 or 454 g

Useful Conversion Equivalents of Volume

1 mL = 16.23 ♏
1 ♏ = 0.06 mL
1 ♌ = 3.69 mL
1 ♌ = 29.57 mL
1 pt = 473 mL
1 gal (US) = 3,785 mL
1 gal (British Imperial) = 4,546 mL

Useful Conversion Equivalents of Length

1 in = 2.54 cm
1 m = 39.37 in

Today, there are very few occasions on which intersystem conversion is needed, owing to the almost exclusive use of the metric system in both product formulation and prescription compounding. However, when conversion is necessary or desired, it is a simple matter of selecting and applying the appropriate intersystem conversion factor.

For example, if one wishes to determine the number of milliliters in 8 fℨ, the conversion factor that most directly relates milliliters and fluidounces is selected. That factor is 1 fℨ = 29.57 mL; thus, 8 fℨ = 8 × 29.57 mL, or 236.56 mL.

Another example: How many 30-mL containers may be filled from 10 gal of a formulation? 1 gal = 3,785 mL. Thus, 10 gal = 10 × 3,785 mL, or 37,850 mL. By dividing this total number of milliliters by 30, the number of containers that may be filled is found to be 1,261.

Another example: How many 0.5-gr tablets may be prepared from 1 kg of a drug substance? Because 1 gr = 64.8 mg, 0.5 gr = 32.4 mg. Also, 1 kg = 1,000 g, or 1,000,000 mg. Because 32.4 mg is required for one tablet, 1,000,000 mg divided by 32.4 mg = 30,864 tablets. Hence, 30,864 tablets may be prepared from 1 kg of the drug substance.

A final example: If a transdermal patch measures 30 mm^2, what is this dimension in inches? The conversion factor, 1 inch = 2.54 cm, may be expressed as 1 inch = 25.4 mm, so 1 inch^2 = $(25.4)^2$ mm^2 or 645.16 mm^2. Thus, by dividing 30 mm by 645.16 mm^2/inch^2, one finds the patch is 0.0465 inch^2.

Quantitative Product Strength

The quantitative composition of certain pharmaceuticals, particularly liquids and semisolid dosage forms, often is expressed in terms of the *percentage strength* of the active and sometimes inactive ingredients. For some dilute solutions, the strength may be expressed in terms of their *ratio strength*. For most injections, many oral liquids, and some semisolid dosage forms, the quantity of active ingredient commonly is expressed as weight of drug per unit volume basis, such as milligrams of drug per milliliter of injection or oral liquid, or as weight of drug per unit weight of preparation, such as milligrams of drug per gram of ointment. The strength of solid dosage forms is given as the drug content (e.g., 5 mg) per dosage unit (e.g., tablets and capsules).

Percent, by definition, means parts per hundred. In pharmacy, percentage concentrations have specific meanings based on the physical character of the particular product or formulation, that is,

Percent weight in volume: Expressed % w/v, this defines grams of a constituent in 100 mL of a preparation (generally a liquid).

Percent volume in volume: Expressed % v/v, this defines milliliters of a constituent in 100 mL of a preparation (generally a liquid).

Percent weight in weight: Expressed % w/w, this defines grams of a constituent in 100 g of a preparation (generally a solid or semisolid, but also for liquid preparations prepared by weight).

Thus, a 5% w/v solution or suspension of a drug contains 5 g of the substance in each 100 mL of the product, a 5% v/v preparation contains 5 mL of the substance in each 100 mL of the product, and a 5% w/w preparation contains 5 g of the substance in each 100 g of the product.

In the manufacture or compounding of pharmaceutical preparations, the pharmacist may calculate (*a*) the strength of an individual component in a product or (*b*) the amount of a component needed to achieve a desired percentage strength.

For example, what is the percentage strength, w/v, of a solution containing 15 g of drug in 500 mL? Because by definition percentage strength is in parts per hundred, just determine how many grams of the drug are present in each 100 mL solution. Solving by proportion: 15 g/500 mL = (×) g/100 mL. The answer is 3 g, and thus, the solution is 3% w/v in strength.

Other examples: 3 mL of a liquid in 1 L of solution = 0.3% v/v, 4 g of drug in 250 mL = 1.6% w/v, and 8 g of drug in 40 g of product = 20% w/w.

How many grams of drug are needed to prepare 400 mL of a 5% w/v preparation? In w/v problems, the specific gravity *of the preparation* is assumed to be the same as that of water (sp. gr. 1.0), so 1 mL is assumed to weigh 1 g. Therefore, in the problem example, the 400 mL is assumed to weigh 400 g, and 5% of 400 g = 20 g, the amount of drug needed.

A v/v problem example: How many mL of a liquid is needed to make 1 pt of a 0.1% v/v solution? 1 pt = 473 mL, and 0.1% of that is 0.473 mL, the answer.

A w/w problem example: How many grams of zinc oxide powder should be used in preparing 120 g of a 20% w/w ointment? The answer is 20% of 120 g = 24 g.

Ratio strength is sometimes used to express the strength of or to calculate the amount of a component needed to make a relatively dilute preparation. Compared to percentage strength designations, for example, a 0.1% w/v preparation (0.1 g/100 mL) is equivalent to 1 g/1,000 mL and may be expressed as a ratio strength of 1:1,000 w/v. Ratio strength expressions use the w/v, v/v, and w/w designations in the same manner as percentage strength expressions. For example:

A 1:1,000 w/v preparation of a solid constituent in a liquid preparation = 1 g of the solid constituent in 1,000 mL of preparation

A 1:1,000 v/v preparation of a liquid constituent in a liquid preparation = 1 mL of the constituent in 1,000 mL of preparation

A 1:1,000 w/w preparation of a solid constituent in a solid or semisolid preparation = 1 g of the constituent in 1,000 g of preparation

A ratio strength calculation: What is the ratio strength of 6,000 mL of solution containing 3 g of drug? Whenever possible, it is preferable for ratio strengths to be expressed as 1. In this example, if 3 g of drug is in 6,000 mL of solution, 1 g of drug is contained in 2,000 mL, and thus, the ratio strength is 1:2,000 w/v. Sometimes, the answers do not come out as evenly, for example, what is the ratio strength of 0.3 mL of a liquid in 1 L of solution? In this instance, there is 0.3 mL in 1,000 mL, equivalent to 3 mL in 10,000 mL, or a ratio strength of 3:10,000 v/v, or 1:3,333.3 v/v.

Another ratio strength calculation: In grams, how much drug is needed to make 5 L of a 1:400 w/v solution? By definition (of 1:400 w/v), 1 g of drug is needed for each 400 mL of the solution. Because 5 L, or 5,000 mL, of solution is to be prepared, the amount of drug required is found by solving 1 g/400 mL = (×) g/5,000 mL, or 12.5 g.

Rather than being expressed in terms of percentage strength or ratio strength, the strength of some pharmaceutical preparations, particularly injections and sometimes oral liquids, is based on drug content per unit of volume, as milligrams per milliliter. Thus, flexibility in dosing can be achieved by administering the volume of preparation that contains the desired dose.

Reducing and Enlarging Formulas

In the course of pharmaceutical manufacturing and in professional practice activities, it is often necessary to reduce or enlarge a pharmaceutical formulation to prepare the desired amount of product. A standard manufacturing formulation, or *master formula*, contains the quantitative amounts of each ingredient needed to prepare a specified quantity of product. When preparing other quantities, larger or smaller, the *quantitative relationship* of each component to the other in the formula must be maintained. For example, if there is 2 g of ingredient A and 10 mL of ingredient B (among other ingredients) in a formula for 1,000 mL, one must use 0.2 g of ingredient A and 1 mL of ingredient B to make 100 mL, or one-tenth of the formula. If, on the other hand, a formula is to be enlarged— for example, from 1 L (1,000 mL) of product to a gallon (3,785 mL)—the amount of each ingredient required is 3.785 times that needed to prepare 1 L of product.

In these examples, the quantity of product prepared is reduced or enlarged, but the quantitative relationship between each ingredient and the product strength remains unchanged.

Dosage Units

Drug dosage is selected by the prescriber based upon clinical considerations and the characteristics of the pharmacologic agent. Dosage forms (e.g., tablets, injections, transdermal patches) are used to administer the drug to the patient. Solid dosage forms, such as tablets and capsules, are generally prepared in various strengths to allow flexibility in dosing. The desired dose for a drug prepared in a liquid form may be provided by the volume administered. For example, if a liquid dosage form contains 5 mg of drug per milliliter and if a dose of 25 mg of drug is desired, 5 mL of the liquid may be administered. Commercially manufactured products are formulated to provide the drug in dosage forms and amounts convenient for administration. When the desired dosage or dosage form is commercially unavailable, the pharmacist may be called upon to compound the desired preparation.

Common Household Measure

Liquid and powder medications not packaged in unit-dose systems are usually measured at home by the patient with

FIGURE C.2. Oral measuring devices of different styles, shapes, and capacities. (Courtesy of wk1003mike/Shutterstock.)

common household measuring devices, such as the teaspoon or tablespoon. Although the household teaspoon may vary in volume capacity from approximately 3 to 8 mL, the American Standard Teaspoon has been established as having a volume of 4.93 ± 0.24 mL by the American National Standards Institute. For practical purposes, most pharmacy practitioners and pharmacy references use 5 mL as the capacity of the teaspoon. This is approximately equivalent to 1.33 ʒ, although physicians commonly use the drachm symbol to indicate a teaspoonful in their prescription directions to be transcribed by the pharmacist to the patient. The tablespoon is considered to have a capacity of 15 mL, equivalent to three teaspoonfuls or approximately 0.5 fʒ.

Occasionally, the pharmacist will provide a special medicinal spoon for the patient to use in measuring this medication. These spoons are available in half-teaspoon, teaspoon, and tablespoon capacities. Some manufacturers provide specially designed devices to be used by the patient in measuring medication. These include specially calibrated droppers, oral syringes, measuring wells or tubes, and calibrated bottle caps. In health care institutions, disposable measuring cups and unit-dose containers are commonly employed in administering liquid medication. Examples of measuring devices are shown in Figure C.2.

TECHNIQUES OF PHARMACEUTICAL MEASUREMENT

Weighing and the Prescription Balance

In weighing materials, the selection of the instrument is based on the amount of material and the accuracy desired. In the large-scale manufacture of pharmaceuticals, large industrial *scales* of varying capacity and sensitivity are employed, and, later, highly sensitive analytical balances are used in the quality control and analytical work.

In the hospital and community pharmacy, most weighing is done on either a *prescription balance* or an *electronic balance* (Fig. C.3). Prescription balances are termed *class III* (formerly class A) balances, which meet the prescribed standards of the National Institute of Standards and Technology. Every prescription department is required by law to have a prescription or electronic balance.

FIGURE C.3. Prescription balances: **(A)** torsion balance (courtesy of Torbal, a division of Scientific Industries, Inc.) and **(B)** electronic balance (courtesy of OHAUS Corp.).

The sensitivity of a balance is usually represented by the term *sensitivity requirement* (SR), the maximum change in load that will cause a specified change, one subdivision on the index plate, in the position of rest of the indicating element of the balance. The SR is determined in the following manner: (*a*) level the balance, (*b*) determine the rest point, (*c*) place a 6-mg weight on one of the empty pans, and (*d*) look at the readout. The rest point should shift *not less than* one division on the index plate. The entire operation is repeated with a 10-g weight placed in the center of each balance pan. A class III balance has an SR of 6 mg with no load as well as with 10 g on each pan. This means that under these conditions, the addition of 6 mg of weight to one pan of the balance will disturb the equilibrium and move the balance pointer one division marking on the scale.

The USP directs that to avoid weighing errors of 5% or greater, which may be due to the limits of accuracy of the prescription balance, one must weigh a minimum of 120 mg of any material in each weighing (5% of 120 mg being the 6 mg SR, or error inherent with the balance). If a smaller weight of the material is desired, it is directed that the pharmacist mix a larger calculated weight of the ingredient (120 mg or more), dilute it with a known weight of an inert dry diluent (as lactose), mix the two uniformly, and weigh an aliquot portion of the mixture (again 120 mg or more) calculated to contain the desired amount of agent. The class III balance with a capacity of 120 g should be used for all weighing required in prescription compounding.

The electronic balance is available in various sensitivities. The one most commonly used in prescription compounding has a readability of 0.001 g; consequently, the least amount that can be weighed is 20 times that, or 20 mg. The electronic balance is much faster and easier to use than the prescription balance. The digital readout is easy to read and the balance is quite versatile and easy to clean, and it has a relatively small footprint.

Weights

Today, most pharmacies have a set of metric weights. Some commercial weight sets contain both the metric

and apothecary systems. Prescription weights meet the National Bureau of Standards' specifications for analytical weights. Metric weights of 1 g and more and apothecaries' weights of 1 scruple and more are generally conical, with a narrow neck and head that allow them to be easily picked up with small forceps. Most of these weights are made of polished brass, and some are coated with nickel, chromium, or another material to resist corrosion. Fractional gram weights are made of aluminum and are generally square and flat with one raised end or corner for picking up with the forceps (Fig. C.4). Apothecaries' weights of 0.5 scruple are frequently coin-shaped brass, and those of 5 gr and less are usually bent aluminum wires, with each straight side representing 1 gr of weight. The half-grain weight is usually a smaller gauge wire bent in half.

FIGURE C.4. Prescription weights: combination set of metric and apothecary. (Courtesy of Torbal, a division of Scientific Industries, Inc.)

To prevent moisture and oils from the fingertips being deposited on the weights, all weights should be transferred with the forceps provided in each weight set.

Care and Use of a Balance

First and foremost, the balance should be kept in a well-lighted location, placed on a firm level counter approximately waist high to the operator. The area should be as free from dust as possible and in an area that is draft-free. There should be no corrosive vapors, high humidity, or vibration. When not in use, the balance should be clean and covered with the balance cover. Any agent spilled on the balance during use should be wiped off immediately with a soft brush or cloth. When not in use, the balance should always be kept with the weights off and the beam in the fixed or locked (arrested) position.

Before weighing an article, the balance must be made level. This is accomplished with the leveling screws on the bottom of the balance, according to the instructions accompanying the balance. The balance should be level both front to back and side to side, as indicated by the leveling bubble.

In using a prescription balance, neither the weights nor the substance to be weighed should be placed on the balance while the beam is free to oscillate. Before weighing, powder papers or weigh boats of equal size should be placed on both pans of the balance and the equilibrium of the balance tested by releasing the arresting knob. If the balance is off because of differences in the weight, additional weight may be added to the light pan by adding small tearings of powder papers. When balanced, the balance is placed in the arrested position, and the desired weight added to the right-hand pan. Then, an amount of substance considered to be approximately the desired weight is carefully placed on the left-hand pan with a spatula. The beam should then be slowly released by means of the locking device in the front of the balance. If the substance is in excess, the beam is fixed again, and a small portion of the substance removed with the spatula. The process is continued until the two pans balance, as indicated by the central position of the balance pointer. If the amount of weight on the balance is initially too little, the reverse process is undertaken. The powder paper used on the left-hand pan, intended to hold the substance to be weighed, is usually folded diagonally, or its edges are turned up to contain the material being weighed.

In transferring material by spatula, the material may be lightly tapped from the spatula when the correct amount to be measured is approached. Usually this is done by holding the spatula with a small amount of material on it in the right hand and tapping the spatula with the forefinger. As material comes off the spatula, the left hand is working the balance-arresting mechanism, and the status of the weight is observed alternately with the tapping of the spatula. Most balances have a damping mechanism that slows down the oscillations and permits more rapid determinations of the balance or imbalance positions of the pans.

Once the material has been weighed, the balance beam is again put in the fixed position, and the paper or weigh boat holding the weighed substance carefully removed. If more than a single weighing is to be performed, the paper or weigh boat is usually marked with the name of the substance it holds. After the final weighing, all weights are removed with the forceps and the balance is cleaned, closed, and covered.

Most prescription balances contain built-in mechanisms whereby external weights are not required for weighing less than 1 g. Some balances use a rider, which may be shifted from the zero position toward the right side of the balance to add increments of weight marked on the scale in 10-mg units, up to 1 g. Another type of balance uses a central dial, calibrated in 10-mg units, to add weight up to 1 g. Both types of devices add the weight to the right-hand pan internally. In each case, the pharmacist may use a combination of the internal and external weights. For instance, if 1.2 g is to be weighed, the pharmacist can place a 1-g weight on the right-hand pan and place the rider or adjust the dial to add 0.2 g. Care must always be exercised to bring the rider or dial to zero between weighings to maintain accuracy.

Most use of the prescription balance is weighing of powders or semisolid materials, such as ointments. However, liquids may also be weighed in tared (weighed) vessels of appropriate size. The pharmacist must always be certain to account for the weight of the vessel in calculating the amount of liquid weighed.

Materials should never be downweighed, that is, substances should never be placed on the pan with the balance in the unarrested position, forcing the pan to drop suddenly and forcefully. The sudden slamming down of the pan can do serious damage to the balance, affecting its sensitivity and accuracy.

The most common type of prescription balance is the torsion balance. It operates on the tension of taut wires, which, when twisted by addition of weight, tend to twist back to the original position (Fig. C.3).

In using an electronic balance, first make sure the balance is clean and level. The balance should be calibrated daily. Many of these balances have internal calibration, and some use an external 200- or 300-g weight. After calibration, a weighing boat or paper is placed on the balance pan, and the tare button is depressed to a reading of 0.000. Then, the required quantity of material is added to the weighing boat or paper; the dial constantly reads out the weight of material on the pan. Material can be easily removed or added to obtain the desired quantity.

Measuring Volume

The common instruments for pharmaceutical measurement are presented in Figure C.5. Two types of graduates, *conical* and *cylindrical*, are used in pharmacy. Cylindrical graduates are generally calibrated in metric units, whereas conical graduates may be graduated in both metric and apothecary units or with a single scale of either of the

FIGURE C.5. Typical equipment for the pharmaceutical measurement of volume. **Left:** Conical graduates. **Right:** Cylindrical graduates. **Front:** A pipet for measurement of small volumes. Behind the pipet is a pipet filler used instead of the mouth to draw acids and other dangerous liquids into the pipet.

systems. Graduates of both shapes are available in a wide variety of capacities, ranging from 5 to 1,000 mL or more. Most graduates are made of a good-quality heat-treated glass, although graduates of polypropylene are also available. In measuring small volumes of liquids, less than 1.5 mL, the pharmacist should use a pipet as the one shown in Figure C.5. The bulky-looking device shown with the pipet is a pipet filler, used for drawing acids or other toxic solutions into the pipet without the mouth. The device, without being removed from the pipet, also allows for accurate delivery of the liquid.

In measuring volumes of liquids, the pharmacist should select the measuring device most appropriate to the volume of liquid to be measured and the desired degree of accuracy. With liquids, the more narrow the column of the liquid, the more accurate is likely to be the measurement. Figure C.6 demonstrates this point. A reading error of the same dimension will produce a small-volume error with a

FIGURE C.6. The difference in the volume error occurring with the same reading error in measuring devices of different diameters.

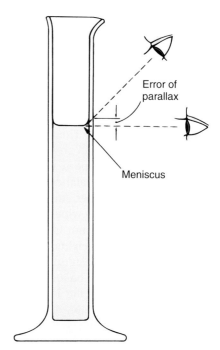

FIGURE C.7. Error in reading the meniscus of a liquid in a graduated cylinder when the reading is made from above the level of the liquid rather than at the same level.

pipet, a greater-volume error with a cylindrical graduate, and the largest error of volume with conical graduate. The greater the flare in the design of the conical graduate, the greater is the volume error.

In reading the level of liquid in a graduate, it is important to recognize the possibility of parallax error. Figure C.7 depicts this point. A liquid in a graduate tends to be drawn to the inner surface of the graduate and rises slightly against that surface and above its true meniscus. If one measures looking downward, it appears that the meniscus of the liquid is at this upper level, whereas it is slightly lower, at the actual level of the liquid, the center of the graduate. Thus, measurements of liquids in graduates should be taken with the eyesight level with the liquid in the graduate.

If a pharmacist misreads a graduate, the *percentage of error* is affected by the volume of liquid. According to the USP, an acceptable 10-mL graduate cylinder with an internal diameter of 1.18 cm contains 0.109 mL of liquid in each millimeter of column. A reading error of 1 mm causes a percentage error of only 1.09% when 10 mL is being measured, 2.18% when 5 mL is being measured, 4.36% when 2.5 mL is being measured, and 7.26% when 1.5 mL is being measured. It is apparent that the greatest percentage error occurs when the smallest amount is being measured. Thus, the rule of thumb for measuring liquids in graduates is that a graduate should be used having a capacity *equal to or just exceeding* the volume to be measured.

According to Goldstein and Mattocks (2), based on a deviation of 1 mm from the mark and an allowable error of 2.5%, the smallest amounts that should be measured in cylindrical graduates having the stated internal diameters are as follows:

Graduated Cylinder Size (mL)	Internal Diameter (cm)	Deviation in Actual Volume (mL)	Minimum Volume Measurable (mL)
5	0.98	0.075	3.00
10	1.18	0.109	4.36
25	1.95	0.296	11.84
50	2.24	0.394	15.76
100	2.58	0.522	20.88

For a 5% error, the minimum volumes measurable would be one-half of those stated. It is apparent that for accuracy, one should not use a graduate when the measurement would use only the bottom portion of the scale.

In using graduates, the pharmacist pours the liquid into the graduate slowly, observing the level. In measuring viscous liquids, adequate time must be allowed for the liquid to settle in the graduate, as some may run slowly down the inner sides of the graduate. It is best to attempt to pour such liquids toward the center of the graduate, avoiding contact with the sides. In emptying the graduate of its measured contents, adequate drain time should be allowed.

When pouring liquids from bottles, good pharmaceutical technique is to keep the label on the bottle facing up; this avoids the possibility of any errant liquid running down over the label as the bottle is righted after use. The bottle orifice should be wiped clean after each use.

REFERENCES

1. Ansel HC, Stockton SJ. Pharmaceutical Calculations. 15th Ed. Baltimore, MD: Wolters Kluwer, 2017.

2. Goldstein SW, Mattocks AM. How to measure accurately. J Am Pharm 1951;23:421.

INDEX